MASSACHUSETTS GENERAL HOSPITAL HANDBOOK OF GENERAL HOSPITAL PSYCHIATRY

John Pozokam

2004

MASSACHUSETTS GENERAL HOSPITAL HANDBOOK OF GENERAL HOSPITAL PSYCHIATRY

Fifth Edition

Theodore A. Stern, M.D.

Professor of Psychiatry, Harvard Medical School;
Psychiatrist and Chief, Psychiatric Consultation Service,
Massachusetts General Hospital, Boston, Massachusetts

Gregory L. Fricchione, M.D.

Associate Professor of Psychiatry, Harvard Medical School;
Associate Chief of Psychiatry and Director, Division of Psychiatry and Medicine,
Massachusetts General Hospital, Boston, Massachusetts

Ned H. Cassem, M.D., S.J.

Professor of Psychiatry, Harvard Medical School; Psychiatrist,
Massachusetts General Hospital, Boston, Massachusetts

Michael S. Jellinek, M.D.

Professor of Psychiatry and Pediatrics, Harvard Medical School; Chief,
Child Psychiatry Service, Massachusetts General Hospital, Boston, Massachusetts

Jerrold F. Rosenbaum, M.D.

Professor of Psychiatry, Harvard Medical School; Chief of Psychiatry,
Massachusetts General Hospital, Boston, Massachusetts

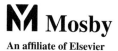 Mosby

An affiliate of Elsevier

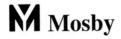 Mosby

Editor: Susan F. Pioli
Editorial Assistant: Joan Ryan
Publishing Services Manager: Joan Sinclair
Project Manager: Mary Stermel

Fifth Edition

Mosby is an affiliate of Elsevier.

Copyright © 2004, 1997, 1991, 1987, 1978 by Mosby, Inc.

Medicine is an ever-changing field. Standard safety precautions must be followed but as new research and clinical experience broaden our knowledge, changes in treatment and drug therapy may become necessary or appropriate. Readers are advised to check the most current product information provided by the manufacturer of each drug to be administered to verify the recommended dose, the method and duration of administration, and contraindications. It is the responsibility of the treating physician, relying on experience and knowledge of the patient, to determine dosages and the best treatment for each individual patient. Neither the Publisher nor the author assumes any liability for any injury and/or damage to persons or property arising from this publication.

Every effort has been made to ensure that the drug dosage schedules within this text are accurate and conform to standards accepted at time of publication. However, as treatment recommendations vary in the light of continuing research and clinical experience, the reader is advised to verify drug dosage schedules herein with information found on product information sheets. This is especially true in cases of new or infrequently used drugs.

Recognizing the importance of preserving what has been written, Elsevier Science prints its books on acid-free paper whenever possible.

Library of Congress Cataloging-in-Publication Data

Massachusetts General Hospital handbook of general hospital psychiatry/[edited by]
   Theodore A. Stern . . . [et al.] – 5th ed.
    p. ; cm.
   Includes bibliographical references and index.
   ISBN 0-323-02767-9
    1. Psychiatric consultation—Handbooks, manuals, etc. 2. Hospital patients—Mental health—Handbooks, manuals, etc. 3. Sick—Psychology—Handbooks, manuals, etc. I. Title: Handbook of general hospital psychiatry. II. Stern, Theodore A. III. Massachusetts General Hospital.
    [DNLM: 1. Mental Disorders. 2. Hospitalization. 3. Patients—psychology. 4. Psychology, Medical. 5. Referral and Consultation. WM 140 M414 2004]
   RC455.2.C65M365 2004
   616′.001′9—dc22

                            2003057853

The publisher offers special discounts on bulk orders of this book.
For information, please contact:

Manager of Special Sales
Elsevier
170 So. Independence Mall West 300 E
Philadelphia, PA 19106
Tel: 215-238-7800
Fax: 215-238-8483

10 9 8 7 6 5 4 3 2 1

Printed in the United States of America

To our patients, our students, our colleagues, and our mentors . . .

Contributing Authors

Annah N. Abrams, M.D.
Instructor in Psychiatry, Harvard Medical School; Clinical Assistant in Psychiatry, Massachusetts General Hospital, Boston, Massachusetts

Marilyn S. Albert, Ph.D.
Director, Division of Cognitive Neuroscience, Johns Hopkins University School of Medicine; Department of Neurology, Johns Hopkins Hospital, Baltimore, Maryland

Vincent P. Alessandrini
Director of Patient Accounts, Non-Acute Services, Department of Finance, Partners HealthCare System Psychiatry, Boston, Massachusetts

Menekse Alpay, M.D.
Instructor in Psychiatry, Harvard Medical School; Clinical Assistant in Psychiatry, Massachusetts General Hospital, Boston, Massachusetts

Jonathan E. Alpert, M.D., Ph.D.
Assistant Professor of Psychiatry, Harvard Medical School; Associate Director, Depression Clinic and Research Program, Massachusetts General Hospital, Boston, Massachusetts

Arthur J. Barsky, M.D.
Professor of Psychiatry, Harvard Medical School; Director of Psychiatric Research, Brigham and Women's Hospital, Boston, Massachusetts

B. J. Beck, M.S.N., M.D.
Clinical Instructor in Psychiatry, Harvard Medical School; Psychiatrist, Robert B. Andrews Unit, Massachusetts General Hospital; Medical Director of Mental Health/Social Services, East Boston Neighborhood Health Center, East Boston, Massachusetts

Anne E. Becker, M.D., Ph.D.
Assistant Professor of Medical Anthropology and Psychiatry, Departments of Social Medicine and Psychiatry, Harvard Medical School; Director, Adult Eating and Weight Disorders Program, Massachusetts General Hospital, Boston, Massachusetts

Jerrold G. Bernstein, M.D.*
Former Assistant Clinical Professor of Psychiatry, Harvard Medical School;
Visiting Scientist, Clinical Research Center, Harvard Medical School and
Massachusetts Institute of Technology; Assistant Psychiatrist, Massachusetts
General Hospital, Boston, Massachusetts

Joseph Biederman, M.D.
Professor of Psychiatry, Harvard Medical School; Chief, Clinical and Research
Programs in Pediatric Psychopharmacology and Adult ADHD, Massachusetts
General Hospital, Boston, Massachusetts

Mark A. Blais, Psy.D.
Associate Professor of Psychology in Psychiatry, Harvard Medical School;
Associate Chief of Psychology, Massachusetts General Hospital, Boston,
Massachusetts

Rebecca W. Brendel, M.D., J.D.
Clinical Fellow in Psychiatry, Harvard Medical School; Chief Resident in
Consultation-Liaison Psychiatry and Fourth Year Resident in Psychiatry,
Massachusetts General Hospital/McLean Hospital, Boston, Massachusetts

George Bush, M.D., M.M.Sc.
Assistant Professor of Psychiatry and Research Fellow in Radiology, Harvard
Medical School; Assistant in Psychiatry and Assistant Director of Psychiatric
Neuroimaging Research, Massachusetts General Hospital, Boston, Massachusetts

Ned H. Cassem, M.D.
Professor of Psychiatry, Harvard Medical School; Psychiatrist, Massachusetts
General Hospital, Boston, Massachusetts

Lee S. Cohen, M.D.
Associate Professor of Psychiatry, Harvard Medical School; Director, Perinatal
and Reproductive Psychiatry Clinical Research Program, Massachusetts General
Hospital, Boston, Massachusetts

M. Cornelia Cremens, M.D., M.P.H.
Instructor in Psychiatry and Medicine, Harvard Medical School; Geriatric
Psychiatrist, Massachusetts General Hospital Senior Health Practice, Geriatric
Psychopharmacology, Massachusetts General Hospital, Boston, Massachusetts

William E. Falk, M.D.
Assistant Professor of Psychiatry, Harvard Medical School; Director, Geriatric
Psychopharmacology, Massachusetts General Hospital, Boston, Massachusetts

Maurizio Fava, M.D.
Professor of Psychiatry, Harvard Medical School; Associate Chief of Psychiatry for
Clinical Research and Director of the Depression Clinical and Research Program,
Massachusetts General Hospital, Boston, Massachusetts

* Deceased

Christine T. Finn, M.D.
Clinical Fellow in Medicine, Department of Genetics, Harvard Medical School; Clinical Associate in Psychiatry, Massachusetts General Hospital, Boston, Massachusetts

Oliver Freudenreich, M.D.
Instructor in Psychiatry, Harvard Medical School; Director, First-Episode and Early Psychosis Program, Massachusetts General Hospital, Boston, Massachusetts

Gregory L. Fricchione, M.D.
Associate Professor of Psychiatry, Harvard Medical School; Associate Chief of Psychiatry and Director, Division of Psychiatry and Medicine, Massachusetts General Hospital, Boston, Massachusetts

David R. Gastfriend, M.D.
Associate Professor of Psychiatry, Harvard Medical School; Director, Addiction Research Program, Massachusetts General Hospital, Boston, Massachusetts

Donald C. Goff, M.D.
Associate Professor of Psychiatry, Harvard Medical School; Director, Schizophrenia Program, Massachusetts General Hospital, Boston, Massachusetts

Donna B. Greenberg, M.D.
Associate Professor of Psychiatry, Harvard Medical School; Director, Medical Student Education, Department of Psychiatry, Massachusetts General Hospital, Boston, Massachusetts

James E. Groves, M.D.
Associate Clinical Professor of Psychiatry, Harvard Medical School; Psychiatrist, Department of Psychiatry Service, Massachusetts General Hospital, Boston, Massachusetts

Thomas P. Hackett, M.D.*
Former Eben S. Draper Professor of Psychiatry, Harvard Medical School; Chief of Psychiatry, Massachusetts General Hospital (1976–1988), Boston, Massachusetts

Stephan Heckers, M.D.
Assistant Professor of Psychiatry, Harvard Medical School; Director, Schizophrenia and Bipolar Disorder Program, McLean Hospital, Belmont, Massachusetts

David C. Henderson, M.D.
Assistant Professor of Psychiatry, Harvard Medical School; Associate Director, Schizophrenia Program and Director, Schizophrenia Weight Reduction and Glucose Metabolism Research Program, Massachusetts General Hospital, Boston, Massachusetts

Jeff C. Huffman, M.D.
Clinical Fellow in Psychiatry, Harvard Medical School; Consultation Fellow, Department of Psychiatry, Massachusetts General Hospital, Boston, Massachusetts

* Deceased

Esther Jacobowitz Israel, M.D.
Assistant Professor of Pediatrics, Harvard Medical School; Associate Chief, Pediatric Gastroenterology and Nutrition, Massachusetts General Hospital, Boston, Massachusetts

James L. Januzzi, M.D.
Assistant Professor of Medicine, Cardiology Division, Harvard Medical School; Assistant Physician, Department of Internal Medicine/Cardiology, Massachusetts General Hospital, Boston, Massachusetts

Karsten Kueppenbender, M.D.
Clinical Fellow in Psychiatry, Harvard Medical School; Resident, Department of Psychiatry, Massachusetts General Hospital, Boston, Massachusetts

Jennifer M. Lafayette, M.D.
Instructor of Psychiatry, Harvard Medical School; Associate Director, Acute Psychiatry Service, Massachusetts General Hospital, Boston, Massachusetts

Isabel T. Lagomasino, M.D.
Assistant Professor of Psychiatry and Behavioral Sciences, University of Southern California Keck School of Medicine; Attending Psychiatrist, Adult Outpatient Psychiatry, LAC + USC Medical Center, Los Angeles, California

Bruce J. Masek, Ph.D.
Associate Professor of Psychology (Psychiatry), Harvard Medical School; Clinical Director, Child and Adolescent Psychiatry, Massachusetts General Hospital, Boston, Massachusetts

Anna C. Muriel, M.D., M.P.H.
Instructor in Psychiatry, Harvard Medical School; Clinical Assistant in Psychiatry, Massachusetts General Hospital, Boston, Massachusetts

George B. Murray, M.D.
Associate Professor of Psychiatry, Harvard Medical School; Senior Psychiatrist, Massachusetts General Hospital, Boston, Massachusetts

Dana Diem Nguyen, M.D.
Director of Neuropsychological Testing, Schizophrenia Weight Reduction and Glucose Metabolism Research Program, Massachusetts General Hospital, Boston, Massachusetts

Ruta Nonacs, M.D., Ph.D.
Clinical Instructor in Psychiatry, Harvard Medical School; Clinical Assistant, Perinatal and Reproductive Psychiatry Clinical Research Program, Massachusetts General Hospital, Boston, Massachusetts

Dennis K. Norman, Ed.D.
Associate Professor of Psychology, Harvard Medical School; Chief of Psychology, Massachusetts General Hospital, Boston, Massachusetts

Sheila M. O'Keefe, Ed.D.
Instructor in Psychology, Department of Psychiatry, Harvard Medical School;
Director of Psychology Training, Massachusetts General Hospital, Boston,
Massachusetts

Michael W. Otto, Ph.D.
Associate Professor of Psychology, Harvard Medical School; Director, Cognitive-
Behavior Therapy Program, Massachusetts General Hospital, Boston, Massachusetts

George I. Papakostas, M.D.
Instructor in Psychiatry, Harvard Medical School; Clinical Assistant, Department of
Psychiatry, Massachusetts General Hospital, Boston, Massachusetts

Roy H. Perlis, M.D.
Instructor in Psychiatry, Harvard Medical School; Director, Mood and Anxiety
Disorder Institute Outpatient Consultation Service, Massachusetts General
Hospital, Boston, Massachusetts

William F. Pirl, M.D.
Instructor in Psychiatry, Harvard Medical School; Clinical Assistant in Psychiatry,
Massachusetts General Hospital, Boston, Massachusetts

Mark H. Pollack, M.D.
Associate Professor of Psychiatry, Harvard Medical School; Director, Center for
Anxiety and Traumatic Stress Related Disorders, Massachusetts General Hospital,
Boston, Massachusetts

Laura M. Prager, M.D.
Clinical Instructor in Psychiatry (Child Psychiatry), Harvard Medical School;
Psychiatrist, Department of Child Psychiatry, Massachusetts General Hospital,
Boston, Massachusetts

Jefferson B. Prince, M.D.
Instructor in Psychiatry, Harvard Medical School; Staff, Child Psychiatry,
Massachusetts General Hospital, Boston; Director of Child Psychiatry, North Shore
Medical Center, Salem, Massachusetts

John Querques, M.D.
Instructor in Psychiatry, Harvard Medical School; Associate Director, Psychiatry
Consultation Service, Beth Israel Deaconess Medical Center, Boston, Massachusetts

Terry Rabinowitz, M.D., D.D.S.
Associate Professor of Psychiatry and Family Practice, University of Vermont
College of Medicine; Director, Psychiatric Consultation Service, Fletcher Allen
Health Care, Burlington, Vermont

Paula K. Rauch, M.D.
Assistant Professor of Psychiatry, Harvard Medical School; Chief, Child Psychiatry
Consultation Service to Pediatrics, Massachusetts General Hospital, Boston,
Massachusetts

Scott L. Rauch, M.D.
Associate Professor of Psychiatry, Harvard Medical School; Associate Chief of
Psychiatry (for Neuroscience Research), Massachusetts General Hospital, Boston,
Massachusetts

John A. Renner, Jr., M.D.
Associate Professor of Psychiatry, Boston University School of Medicine;
Associate Psychiatrist, Massachusetts General Hospital, Boston, Massachusetts

Joshua L. Roffman, M.D.
Clinical Fellow in Psychiatry, Harvard Medical School; Adult Psychiatry Resident,
Massachusetts General Hospital/McLean Hospital, Boston, Massachusetts

Jerrold F. Rosenbaum, M.D.
Professor of Psychiatry, Harvard Medical School; Chief of Psychiatry,
Massachusetts General Hospital, Boston, Massachusetts

Kathy M. Sanders, M.D.
Associate Professor of Psychiatry, Harvard Medical School; Director, Adult
Psychiatry Resident Training, Massachusetts General Hospital/McLean Hospital,
Boston, Massachusetts

Lisa Scharff, Ph.D.
Assistant Professor of Psychiatry, Harvard Medical School; Associate Director,
Pain Treatment Service, Children's Hospital, Boston, Massachusetts

Steven C. Schlozman, M.D.
Clinical Instructor in Psychiatry, Harvard Medical School; Lecturer in Education,
Human Development Program, Harvard Graduate School of Education; Staff
Psychiatrist, Child Psychiatrist, and Psychiatric Consultant to Pediatric
Transplantation Service, Massachusetts General Hospital, Boston, Massachusetts

Ronald Schouten, M.D., J.D.
Associate Professor of Psychiatry, Harvard Medical School; Director, Law and
Psychiatry Service, Massachusetts General Hospital, Boston, Massachusetts

Patrick Smallwood, M.D.
Assistant Professor of Psychiatry, University of Massachusetts Medical
School; Medical Director, Consultation-Liaison Psychiatry and Emergency
Mental Health, University of Massachusetts Medical Center, Worcester,
Massachusetts

Felicia A. Smith, M.D.
Clinical Fellow in Psychiatry, Harvard Medical School; Chief Resident, Acute
Psychiatry Service, Massachusetts General Hospital, Boston, Massachusetts

Jordan W. Smoller, M.D., Sc.D.
Assistant Professor of Psychiatry, Harvard Medical School; Director, Psychiatric
Genetics Program in Mood and Anxiety Disorders, Outpatient Division,
Massachusetts General Hospital, Boston, Massachusetts

Thomas J. Spenser, M.D.
Assistant Professor of Psychiatry, Harvard Medical School; Assistant Chief of the
Pediatric Psychopharmacology Research Program, Massachusetts General Hospital,
Boston, Massachusetts

Robert M. Stern, M.D.
Associate Director, Behavioral Health Services, Emerson Hospital, Concord,
Massachusetts

Theodore A. Stern, M.D.
Professor of Psychiatry, Harvard Medical School; Psychiatrist and Chief, Psychiatric
Consultation Service, Massachusetts General Hospital, Boston, Massachusetts

Thomas D. Stewart, M.D.
Associate Clinical Professor of Psychiatry, Yale University School of Medicine;
Consultant Psychiatrist, Yale New Haven Hospital, New Haven, Connecticut

Frederick J. Stoddard, Jr., M.D.
Associate Clinical Professor of Psychiatry, Harvard Medical School; Chief of
Psychiatry, Shriners Burns Hospital; Senior Attending Psychiatrist, Massachusetts
General Hospital Burn Unit, Boston, Massachusetts

Joan M. Stoler, M.D.
Assistant Professor of Pediatrics, Harvard Medical School; Assistant Pediatrician,
Medical Geneticist, Massachusetts General Hospital, Boston, Massachusetts

Paul Summergrad, M.D.
Associate Professor of Psychiatry, Harvard Medical School; Network Director,
Partners Psychiatry and Mental Health, Massachusetts General Hospital, Boston;
Psychiatrist-in-Chief, North Shore Medical Center, Salem, Massachusetts

Owen S. Surman, M.D.
Associate Professor of Psychiatry, Harvard Medical School; Psychiatrist,
Massachusetts General Hospital, Boston, Massachusetts

Adele C. Viguera, M.D., M.P.H.
Assistant Professor in Psychiatry, Harvard Medical School; Associate Director of
the Perinatal and Reproductive Psychiatric Program, Massachusetts General
Hospital, Boston, Massachusetts

Halyna Vitagliano, M.S., M.D.
Instructor in Psychiatry, Harvard Medical School; Clinical Assistant in Psychiatry,
Massachusetts General Hospital, Boston, Massachusetts

Avery D. Weisman, M.D.
Professor Emeritus of Psychiatry, Harvard Medical School; Senior Psychiatrist
(Retired), Massachusetts General Hospital, Boston, Massachusetts

Anthony P. Weiss, M.D.
Instructor in Psychiatry, Harvard Medical School; Psychiatric Neuroimaging
Group, Massachusetts General Hospital, Boston, Massachusetts

Charles A. Welch, M.D.
Instructor in Psychiatry, Harvard Medical School; Psychiatrist, Massachusetts General Hospital, Boston, Massachusetts

Timothy E. Wilens, M.D.
Associate Professor of Psychiatry, Harvard Medical School; Director of Substance Abuse Services, Pediatric Psychopharmacology Research Program, Massachusetts General Hospital, Boston, Massachusetts

Marketa M. Wills, M.D.
Clinical Fellow in Psychiatry, Harvard Medical School; Psychiatry Resident, Massachusetts General Hospital, Boston, Massachusetts

Jonathan L. Worth, M.D.
Instructor in Psychiatry, Harvard Medical School; Director, Psychiatry Outpatient Department, Massachusetts General Hospital, Boston, Massachusetts

Preface

This book, revised and substantially expanded, was put together by a stalwart group of general hospital psychiatrists. It was designed to help busy practitioners care for patients on medical and surgical wards and in outpatient practices filled by comorbid medical and psychiatric illness. Its chapters, which cover specific illnesses and care settings, were crafted for readability. Moreover, clinical vignettes strategically placed throughout the book were meant to act as a nidus upon which clinical pearls would grow.

Consultation psychiatry is a field whose time has come. In fact, it has recently been minted as a new subspecialty called *psychosomatic medicine*. Regardless of the appellation of the field, clinicians who practice this art are required to rapidly recognize and evaluate psychiatric problems in the medical setting; they must also deal effectively with psychiatric reactions to medical illness, with psychiatric complications of medical illness and its treatment, and with psychiatric illness in those who suffer from medical or surgical illness. Because problems related to the affective, behavioral, and cognitive realms of dementia, depression, anxiety, substance abuse, disruptive personalities, and critical illness are faced on a daily basis, emphasis has been placed in this book on successful strategies for their management by the consultant and by the physician of record.

More than twenty new chapters were added to this (fifth) edition, and previously written chapters were revised and updated; as a result, its length has nearly doubled. Additions include discussions of functional neuroanatomy and the neurological examination; diagnostic rating scales and laboratory tests; psychological and neuropsychological assessment; psychotherapy of the medically ill; care of ICU patients; end of life issues; principles of care and ethics; care of the geriatric patient; patients with neurological conditions; aggressive and impulsive patients; catatonia, NMS, and serotonin syndrome; patients with disordered sleep; patients with cancer; psychiatric management of patients with cardiac disease; patients with eating disorders; patients with chronic medical illness and rehabilitation; genetics and genetic disorders; the impact of culture; behavioral medicine; complementary medicine and natural medications; collaborative care; and billing documentation and cost effectiveness of consultation.

This book would not have been possible were it not for the steady hands of our editors at Mosby/Elsevier, Susan Pioli and Joan Ryan. At the Massachusetts General Hospital (MGH), Judi Greenberg of the MGH General Counsel's office once again steered us through legal currents, and Sara Nadelman, Judy Byford, and John Morton helped shepherd us through hundreds of emails, voice mails, FAXes, photocopies, and express mail packages associated with 46 chapters and 79 authors.

On behalf of the patients who suffer, we hope this edition improves the detection and treatment of psychiatric problems and brings much needed relief.

T.A.S.
G.L.F.
N.H.C.
M.S.J.
J.F.R.

Contents

Chapter 1

Beginnings: Psychosomatic Medicine and Consultation Psychiatry in the General Hospital

Thomas P. Hackett, M.D.
Ned H. Cassem, M.D., S.J.
Theodore A. Stern, M.D.
George B. Murray, M.D.
Gregory L. Fricchione, M.D.

Psychosomatic Medicine

A keen interest in the relationship between the psyche and the soma has been maintained in medicine since early times, and certain ancient physicians such as Hippocrates have been eloquent on the subject. A search for the precise origins of *psychosomatic medicine* is, however, a difficult undertaking unless one chooses to focus on the first use of the term itself. Johann Heinroth appears to have coined the term "psychosomatic" in reference to certain causes of insomnia in 1818.[1] The word *medicine* was apparently added to *psychosomatic* first by the psychoanalyst Felix Deutsch in the early 1920s.[2] Deutsch later emigrated to the United States with his wife Helene, and both worked at Massachusetts General Hospital (MGH) for a time in the 1930s and 1940s.

Three streams of thought flowed into the area of psychosomatic medicine, providing fertile ground for the growth of general hospital and consultation psychiatry.[3,4] The psychophysiologic school, perhaps best personified by the Harvard physiologist Walter B. Cannon, emphasized the effects of stress on the body.[5] The psychoanalytic school, best personified by the psychoanalyst Franz Alexander, focused on the effects that psychodynamic conflicts had on the body.[6] The organic synthesis point of view, ambitiously pursued by Helen Flanders Dunbar, tried with very limited success to unify the physiologic and psychoanalytic approaches.[7]

History

The history of general hospital psychiatry in the United States in general,[8] and consultation-liaison (C-L) psychiatry in particular,[9] has been extensively reviewed elsewhere. For those interested in a more detailed account of both historic trends and conceptual issues of C-L psychiatry, the writings of Lipowski[10–15] are highly recommended.

In years gone by, controversy surrounded the use of the term *liaison* in C-L psychiatry. We believed that using the term *liaison* was confusing and unnecessary. It was confusing because no other service in the practice of medicine employed the term for its consultation activities. In addition, the meaning it conveyed—to teach nonpsychiatrists psychiatric and interpersonal skills—is done as a matter of course during the routine consultation. The term *liaison*, although still used, has to some extent thankfully fallen out of fashion.

In March 2003, the American Board of Medical Specialties unanimously approved the American Board of Psychiatry and Neurology's (ABPN's) issuance of subspecialty certification in "Psychosomatic Medicine." The ABPN will now embark on a process for development of a certifying examination and for requirements and training in Psychosomatic Medicine. The term *psychosomatic medicine* encompasses the interactions between mind, brain, and body that have always formed the core knowledge base for the work of consultation psychiatrists. Much credit is owed to the members of the Academy of Psychosomatic Medicine (APM) for helping to organize the application that won approval from an assortment of governing bodies.

When the course of consultation psychiatry is examined, 1975 seems to be the watershed year. Before 1975, scant attention was given to the work of psychiatrists in medicine. Consultation topics were seldom presented at the national meetings of the American Psychiatric Association. Even the American Psychosomatic Society, which has many strong links to consultation work, rarely gave more than a nod of acknowledgment to presentations or panels discussing this aspect of psychiatry. Residency training programs on the whole were no better. In 1966 Mendel[16] surveyed training programs in the United States to determine the extent to which residents were exposed to a training experience in consultation psychiatry. He found that 75% of the 202 programs surveyed offered some training in consultation psychiatry, but most of it was informal and poorly organized. Ten years later, Schubert and McKegney[17] found only "a slight increase" in the amount of time devoted to C-L training in residency programs. Today, C-L training is mandated by the ABPN and a Consultation Psychiatry Fellowship will be a requirement for obtaining "added qualifications" in the subspecialty of Psychosomatic Medicine.

Several reasons account for the growth of C-L psychiatry. One was the leadership of Dr. James Eaton, former director of the Psychiatric Education Branch of the National Institute of Mental Health (NIMH). Eaton provided the support and encouragement that enabled the creation of C-L programs throughout the United States. Another reason for this growth was the burgeoning interest in the primary-care specialties, which required skills in psychiatric diagnosis and treatment. The growth of consultation psychiatry has also been stimulated by the attack on psychiatry from an army of self-appointed counselors and psychotherapists, all claiming to possess the same order of skill as the psychiatrist and all demanding recognition by third-party payers. The vigor of competition for patients has caused even those psychiatrists who most avidly sought a career in pure psychotherapy to start closing ranks with their fellow physicians to form a phalanx against the opposition. The medical model has become the guidon around which embattled psychiatrists are attempting to rally. Little in the training of the psychiatrist is more germane to the medical model than consultation psychiatry. For these reasons, as well as the natural growth of medicine in psychiatry and of neuropsychiatry, consultation work has enjoyed a renaissance.

The origins of organized interest in the mental life of patients at the MGH dates back to 1873, when James Jackson Putnam, a young Harvard neurologist, returned from his grand tour of German departments of medicine to practice his specialty. He was awarded a small office under the arch of one of the famous twin flying staircases of the Bulfinch Building. The office was the size of a cupboard and was designed to house electrical equipment. Putnam was given the title of "electrician." One of his duties was to ensure the proper functioning of various galvanic and faradic devices then used to treat nervous and muscular disorders. It is no coincidence that his office came to be called the "cloaca maxima" by Professor of Medicine George Shattuck. This designation stemmed from the fact that patients whose maladies defied diagnosis and treatment—in short, "the crocks"—were referred to young Putnam. With such a beginning, it is not difficult for today's consultation psychiatrist to affiliate with Putnam's experience and mission. Putnam eventually became a Professor of Neuropathology and practiced both neurology and psychiatry. He treated medical and surgical patients who developed mental disorders. Putnam's distinguished career, interwoven with the acceptance of Freudian psychology in the United States, is chronicled elsewhere.[18]

In the late 1920s Dr. Howard Means, chief of medicine, appointed Boston psychiatrist William Herman to study patients who developed mental disturbances in conjunction with endocrine disorders. Herman's studies are hardly remembered today, although he was honored by having a conference room at the MGH named after him.

In 1934 a department of psychiatry took shape when Stanley Cobb was given the Bullard Chair of Neuropathology and granted sufficient money by the Rockefeller Foundation to establish a ward for the study of psychosomatic conditions. Under Cobb's tutelage, the department expanded and became known for its eclecticism and for its interest in the mind-brain relationship. A number of European emigrants fled Nazi tyranny and were welcomed to the department by Cobb. Felix and Helene Deutsch, Edward and Grete Bibring, and Hans Sachs were early arrivals from the continent. Erich Lindemann came in the mid-1930s and worked with Cobb on a series of projects, the most notable being his study of grief. This came as a result of his work with victims of the 1942 Coconut Grove fire. Ironically, the most severely burned victims of the most recent horrific nightclub fire that occurred in February 2003 in Warwick, Rhode Island, were also cared for at the MGH.

When Lindemann became Chief of the Psychiatric Service in 1954, the consultation service had not yet been established. Customarily the resident assigned to night call in the emergency department saw all medical and surgical patients in need of psychiatric evaluation. This was regarded as an onerous task, and such calls were often set aside until after supper in the hope that the disturbance might quiet in the intervening hours. Notes in the chart were terse and often impractical. Seldom was there a follow-up. As a result, animosity toward psychiatry grew. To remedy this, Lindemann officially established the Psychiatric Consultation Service under the leadership of Avery Weisman in 1956. As Weisman's resident, Hackett divided his time between doing consultations and learning outpatient psychotherapy. During the first year of the consultation service, 130 consultations were performed. In 1958 the number of consultations increased to 370, and an active research program was organized that later became one of the cornerstones of the overall operation.

By 1960 a rotation through the consultation service had become a mandatory part of the MGH residency in psychiatry. Second-year residents were each assigned two wards. Each resident spent 20 to 30 hours a week in the consultation service for a 6-month period. Between 1956 and 1960, the service attracted the interest of fellowship students, who contributed postgraduate work on psychosomatic topics. Medical students also began to choose the consultation service as part of their elective in psychiatry during this period. From our work with these fellows and medical students, collaborative research studies were initiated with other services. Examples of these early studies are (1) the surgical treatment of intractable pain,[19,20] (2) the compliance of duodenal ulcer patients with their medical regimen,[21] (3) postamputation depression in the elderly patient,[15] (4) emotional maladaptation in the surgical patient,[22–26] and (5) the psychological aspect of acute myocardial infarction.[27,28]

By 1970 Hackett, then Chief of the Consultation Service, had one full-time (postgraduate year [PGY]-IV) chief resident and six half-time (PGY-III) residents to see consultations from the approximately 400 house beds. A private psychiatric consultation service was begun to systematize consultations for the 600 private beds of the hospital. A somatic therapies service began and offered electroconvulsive therapy (ECT) to treat refractory patients. Three fellows and a full-time faculty member were added to the roster in 1976. Cassem became Chief of the Consultation Service, and Murray was appointed Director of a new fellowship program in psychosomatic medicine/consultation psychiatry. Then in 1995 Stern was named Chief of the Avery Weisman Psychiatric Consultation Service. Now both fellows and residents take consultations in rotation from throughout the hospital. Our child psychiatry division composed of residents, fellows, and attendings provides full consultation to the 40 beds of the MGH Hospital for Children.

In July 2002 Fricchione was appointed Director of the new Division of Psychiatry and Medicine with a mission to integrate the various inpatient and outpatient medical-psychiatry services at the MGH and its affiliates while maintaining the diverse characters and strengths of each unit. The Division includes the Avery D. Weisman Psychiatry Consultation Service, the Cox Psychooncology Service, the Transplant Consultation Service, the Burn Psychiatry Service, the Women's Consultation Service, the Cardiovascular Health Center Service, and the Spaulding Rehabilitation Hospital's Behavioral and Mental Health Service.

Patient Care, Teaching, and Research

The three functions provided by any consultation service are patient care, teaching, and research. Each of these is considered separately here.

Patient Care

At the MGH, approximately 7% of all admissions are seen by a psychiatrist; roughly 3000 initial consultations are performed each year. The problems discovered run the gamut of conditions listed in the *Diagnostic and Statistical Manual of Mental Disorders*, fourth edition (DSM-IV)[29]; however, the most common reasons for consultation are related to depression, delirium, anxiety, substance abuse, character pathology, dementia, and the evaluation of capacity and pain.

Patients are seen in consultation only at the request of another physician, who must write a specific order for the consultation. Similar to consultations performed by other physicians, the psychiatrist called to see a patient is expected to provide diagnosis and treatment. This includes defining the reason for the consultation; reading the chart; gathering information from nurses and family members when indicated; interviewing the patient; performing the appropriate physical and neurologic examinations; writing a clear clinical impression and treatment plan; ordering or suggesting laboratory tests, procedures, and medications; speaking with the referring physician when indicated; and making follow-up visits until the patient's problems are resolved, the patient is discharged, or the patient dies.

Interviewing style is indelibly individual. In contrast to most psychotherapy sessions, consultation usually involves a patient who did not ask for a psychiatrist and may experience embarrassment at having a consultation because of a mental malfunction. The stigma of mental illness is universal; it is part of every psychiatrist's territory. Each psychiatrist learns to deal with it in a unique way. Because the consultation usually requires getting a great deal of personal information from a patient, the patient's cooperation is essential. Residents learn to do this more by trial and error, self-understanding, and observing role models than from any formulas. Interest in the patient's medical illness is indispensable and is often the most natural topic on which to focus the opening conversation. One helpful approach to reduce the stigma of being seen by a psychiatrist is to discuss early on the role of stress in exacerbating many medical illnesses. In any event, patients should rapidly understand from the consultant's manner, tone, and examination that they are seeing a specialist not unlike other physician specialists who have consulted on them.

The location of the consultation is most often the patient's hospital room. Interviews are conducted there unless the patient objects. Even if other patients are present, drawn curtains usually provide adequate privacy. A thorough examination requires the usual information: chief complaint; personal, family, and psychosocial histories; medical history; current medications; and (from the chart) relevant laboratory values. Seldom can a formal mental status be omitted; we recommend that the Mini-Mental State Examination of Folstein, Folstein, and McHugh[30] be performed routinely. Clock drawing is also often of benefit, as is the elicitation of frontal release signs.

Teaching

Many consultation psychiatrists believe that teaching psychiatry to medical and surgical house officers cannot be done on a formal basis. When teaching is formalized in weekly lectures or discussion groups, attendance invariably lags. More than 30 years ago, Lindemann, in an attempt to educate medical house officers about the emotional problems of their patients, enlisted the help of several psychiatric luminaries from the Boston area. A series of biweekly lectures was announced in which Edward and Grete Bibring, Felix and Helene Deutsch, Stanley Cobb, and Carl Binger, among others, shared their knowledge and skills. In the beginning, approximately one fifth of the medical house officers attended. Attendance steadily dwindled in subsequent sessions until finally the psychiatry residents had to be forced to attend to infuse the lecturers with enough spirit to continue. If Freud could have been resurrected and persuaded to hold luncheon meetings every other week for the medical staff, his reception would have been no more enthusiastic.

Teaching, to be most effective and reliable, is best done at the bedside on a case-by-case basis. With the residents, rounds held three times a week with Stern, the Chief of the Avery D. Weisman Psychiatry Consultation Service, and the chief resident accomplish this. In 90 to 120 minutes, follow-ups on all current cases are presented and discussed, and all new cases are presented by the consulting resident. New patients are interviewed by Stern and other C-L attendings at the bedside. Each resident is paired with an attending for bedside supervision of all cases seen. Residents teach as well. Medical students are supervised by PGY-III residents, the chief resident, and by Stern during each 4-week clerkship.

Fellows attend the rounds of the Fellows Consultation Service, with Murray and Fricchione presiding four times per week; they see patients at the bedside with Murray, Cassem, and Fricchione several times each week. Fellows have an additional 4 hours per week of didactic sessions with Murray on topics of consultation psychiatry, psychosomatic medicine, and neuropsychiatry, and individual supervision with Fricchione also takes place each week. The Fellowship Program in Consultation Psychiatry, under the leadership of Murray, celebrated its twenty-fifth anniversary in 2001; it has trained 79 fellows through June 2003. Many have gone on to direct C-L programs across the United States.

When each group of residents begins their 4-month half-time rotation in July, November, and March, they have had 25 introductory 45-minute lectures on practical topics in consultation (e.g., how to write the note, how to perform the neurologic examination, understanding the nature of psychotherapy in consultation, how to rule out organic causes of psychiatric symptoms, how to diagnose delirium and dementia, how to use intravenous haloperidol, how to use psychostimulants, how to use psychotropic medications in the medically ill, how to evaluate competency, how to perform hypnosis, and how to manage functional somatic symptoms). In concert with the orientation lecture series, we provide residents with relevant articles and with an annotated bibliography.[31] The overall curriculum we provide is quite similar to that recommended by the Academy of Psychosomatic Medicine's Task Force on Residency Training in C-L Psychiatry.[32]

Each resident makes two formal presentations (i.e., a 45-minute review of a topic chosen by the resident, which is elaborated on by a senior discussant for 45 minutes) during the 4-month rotation. These weekly Psychosomatic Conferences not only produce presentations of high quality, but also lead to improved speaking skills, occasional publications, and the beginning of specialized interests and expertise for the resident.[33–42]

Stern, who joins medical house staff for work rounds three times a week in the medical intensive care unit, has run "autognosis" rounds on a weekly basis since 1979.[43] At these rounds, the feelings of the medical house officers toward the patients are examined so that patients can be managed more effectively. Since their inception, only two house officers have refused to attend.

Research

Research activity by the consultation service, besides answering important questions, builds bridges between medical specialties. When physicians from other services are involved in research planning and when there is dual authorship of published accounts, friendships are firmly bonded, and differences fade. The general hospital population provides such a cornucopia of research material that a consultation service would be lax or unresponsive not to take advantage of it. Many examples are cited in the chapters that follow.[44–51]

Small research projects are the cornerstone of larger ones. Research need not be funded through federal or state agencies. Projects can be assigned as such to medical students during their month on the service. They can also be suggested to fellows for more extensive development over the course of the year. What begins as a project with results and conclusions to be presented at Psychiatric Grand Rounds can, over a period of a year, develop into full-fledged publication. This, in turn, might be the starting point for a larger investigation.

A filing system should be designed to keep potential research materials readily accessible.

Systems of computer-based records in consultation services have been described. Strain and associates have devised one of them, and it is now in use in a number of C-L services throughout the United States.[52,53]

Once the direction of the consultation team has been pointed toward research and publication, the results usually fall into line. One of the distressing roadblocks en route to publication is the poor writing skill of many physicians. One or two resource people who can serve as editors and teachers can be of great help. For more than two decades, we have held a biweekly writing seminar in which members submit manuscripts that are reviewed by the seminar group and two senior members of our department (Dr. Stern and Mrs. Eleanor Hackett). All efforts seem worthwhile once the printed page is in the author's hand. When a service begins to develop a shelf of publications authored by various members of the team, a pride of accomplishment exists, and this compounds the excitement of the research and stimulates renewed academic effort.

Summary

From early on in medical history, curious physicians have investigated the mysteries of the mind-body relationship, developing a field of study called Psychosomatic Medicine. The energy of this intellectual enterprise has led to the growth of general hospital psychiatry, initially helped along by Rockefeller Foundation funding in 1934, as well as the development of consultation psychiatry, supported through the funding of Eaton's NIMH Program in the 1970s and 1980s. A subspecialty of psychiatry called *Psychosomatic Medicine* has now been approved, a fact that recognizes the maturation of the field and the growth that lies ahead.

At each step of the way, MGH Consultation Psychiatry has played an important role. This book, which reviews the essentials of general hospital psychiatry, is a testimony to the caring, creativity, and diligence of those who have come before us.

References

1. Heinroth JC: *Lehrbuch der storungen des seelenlebens*, FCW Vogel, 1818, Leipzig, Germany.

2. Deutsch F: Der gesunde und der kranke korper in psychoanalytischer betrachtun. *Int Zeit Psa* 8:290, 1922.

3. Heldt TJ: Psychiatric services in general hospitals. *Am J Psychiatry* 95:865–871, 1939.

4. Henry GW: Some modern aspects of psychiatry in general hospital practice. *Am J Psychiatry* 86:481–499, 1929.

5. Cannon WB: *Bodily changes in pain, hunger, fear, and rage: an account of recent researchers into the function of emotional excitement*, New York, 1915 Appleton and Company.

6. Alexander F: *Psychosomatic medicine: its principles and applications*, New York, 1950, Norton, pp 68, 72, 196.

7. Powell RC: Helen Flanders Dunbar (1902–1959) and a holistic approach to psychosomatic problems: II. the role of Dunbar's nonmedical background. *Psychiatr Q* 50:144–157, 1978.

8. Summergrad P, Hackett TP: Alan Gregg and the rise of general hospital psychiatry, *Gen Hosp Psychiatry* 9:439–445, 1987.

9. Schwab JJ: Consultation-liaison psychiatry: a historical overview, *Psychosomatics* 3:245–254, 1989.

10. Lipowski ZJ: Review of consultation psychiatry and psychosomatic medicine: I. general principles, *Psychosom Med* 29:153–171, 1967.

11. Lipowski ZJ: Review of consultation psychiatry and psychosomatic medicine: II. clinical aspects, *Psychosom Med* 29:201–224, 1967.

12. Lipowski ZJ: Review of consultation psychiatry and psychosomatic medicine: III. theoretical issues, *Psychosom Med* 30:395–421, 1968.

13. Lipowski ZJ: Consultation-liaison psychiatry: an overview, *Am J Psychiatry* 131:623–630, 1974.

14. Lipowski ZJ: Psychiatric consultation: concepts and controversies, *Am J Psychiatry* 134:523–528, 1977.

15. Lipowski ZJ: Consultation-liaison psychiatry: the first half century, *Gen Hosp Psychiatry* 8:305–315, 1986.

16. Mendel WM: Psychiatric consultation education—1966, *Am J Psychiatry* 123:150–155, 1966.

17. Schubert DSP, McKegney FP: Psychiatric consultation education—1976, *Arch Gen Psychiatry* 33:1271–1273, 1976.

18. Hale NG: *Freud and the Americans*, New York, 1971, Oxford University Press.

19. White JC, Sweet WH, Hackett TP: Radiofrequency leukotomy for the relief of pain, *Arch Neurol* 2:317–330, 1960.

20. Mark VH, Hackett TP: Surgical aspects of thalamotomy in the human, *Trans Am Neurol Assoc* 84:92–94, 1959.

21. Hernandez M, Hackett TP: The problem of nonadherence to therapy in the management of duodenal ulcer recurrences, *Am J Dig Dis* 7:1047–1060, 1962.

22. Caplan LM, Hackett TP: Prelude to death: emotional effects of lower limb amputation in the aged, *N Engl J Med* 269:1166–1171, 1963.

23. Weisman AD, Hackett TP: Psychosis after eye surgery: establishment of a specific doctor-patient relation and the prevention and treatment of "black patch delirium," *N Engl J Med* 258:1284–1289, 1958.

24. Weisman AD, Hackett TP: Predilection to death: death and dying as a psychiatric problem, *Psychosom Med* 23:232–257, 1961.

25. Hackett TP, Weisman AD: Psychiatric management of operative syndromes: I. the therapeutic consultation and the effect of noninterpretive intervention, *Psychosom Med* 22:267–282, 1960.

26. Hackett TP, Weisman AD: Psychiatric management of operative syndromes: II. psychodynamic factors in formulation and management, *Psychosom Med* 22:356–372, 1960.

27. Olin HS, Hackett TP: The denial of chest pain in thirty-two patients with acute myocardial infarction, *JAMA* 190:977–981, 1964.

28. Cassem NH, Hackett TP: Psychiatric consultation in a coronary care unit, *Ann Intern Med* 75:9–14, 1971.

29. American Psychiatric Association: *Diagnostic and statistical manual of mental disorders*, ed 4 *(DSM-IV)*, Washington, DC, 1994, American Psychiatric Association.

30. Folstein MF, Folstein SE, McHugh PR: Mini-mental state: a practical method for grading the cognitive state of patients for the clinician, *J Psychiatr Res* 12:189–198, 1975.

31. Cremens MC, Calabrese LV, Shuster JL, et al: The Massachusetts General Hospital annotated bibliography for residents training in consultation-liaison psychiatry, *Psychosomatics* 36:217–235, 1995.

32. Gitlin DF, Schindler BA, Stern TA, et al: Recommended guidelines for consultation-liaison psychiatric training in psychiatry residency programs: a report from the Academy of Psychosomatic Medicine Task Force on psychiatric residency training in consultation-liaison psychiatry, *Psychosomatics* 37:3–11, 1996.

33. Stern TA: Munchausen's syndrome revisited, *Psychosomatics* 21:329–336, 1980.

34. Jenike MA: Obsessive-compulsive disorders, *Compr Psychiatry* 24:99–115, 1983.

35. Brotman AW, Stern TA: Cardiovascular abnormalities in anorexia nervosa, *Am J Psychiatry* 140:1227–1228, 1983.

36. Summergrad P: Depression in Binswanger's encephalopathy responsive to tranylcypromine, *J Clin Psychiatry* 46:69–70, 1985.

37. Pollack MH, Rosenbaum JF: The treatment of antidepressant induced side effects, *J Clin Psychiatry* 43:3–8, 1987.

38. Malone DA, Stern TA: Successful treatment of acquired Tourettism and major depression, *J Geriatr Psychiatry Neurol* 1:169–171, 1988.

39. Fava M, Copeland PM, Schweiger V, et al: Neurochemical abnormalities of anorexia nervosa and bulimia nervosa, *Am J Psychiatry* 146:963–971, 1989.

40. Peterson B, Summergrad P: Binswanger's disease: II. Pathogenesis of subcortical arteriosclerotic encephalopathy and its relation to other dementing processes, *J Geriatr Psychiatry Neurol* 2:171–181, 1989.

41. Cohen LS, Heller VL, Rosenbaum JF: Treatment guidelines for psychotropic use in pregnancy, *Psychosomatics* 30:25–33, 1989.

42. Frank C, Smith S: Stress and the heart: biobehavioral aspects of sudden cardiac death, *Psychosomatics* 31:255–264, 1990.

43. Stern TA, Prager LM, Cremens MC: Autognosis rounds for medical housestaff, *Psychosomatics* 34:1–7, 1993.

44. Dec GW, Stern TA, Welch C: The effects of electroconvulsive therapy on serial electrocardiograms and serum cardiac enzymes: a prospective study of depressed hospitalized inpatients, *JAMA* 253:2525–2529, 1985.

45. Stern TA, Mulley AG, Thibault GE: Life-threatening drug overdose: precipitants and prognosis, *JAMA* 251:1983–1985, 1984.

46. Stern TA, O'Gara PT, Mulley AG, et al: Complications after overdose with tricyclic antidepressants, *Crit Care Med* 13:672–674, 1985.

47. Mahoney J, Gross PL, Stern TA, et al: Quantitative serum toxic screening in the management of suspected drug overdose, *Am J Emerg Med* 8:16–22, 1990.

48. Wilens TE, Stern TA, O'Gara PT: Adverse cardiac effects of combined neuroleptic ingestion and tricyclic antidepressant overdose, *J Clin Psychopharmacol* 10:51–54, 1990.

49. Stern TA, Gross PL, Pollack MH, et al: Drug overdose seen in the emergency department: assessment, disposition, and follow-up, *Ann Clin Psychiatry* 3:223–231, 1991.

50. Sanders KM, Stern TA, O'Gara PT, et al: Delirium during intraaortic balloon pump therapy: incidence and management, *Psychosomatics* 33:35–44, 1992.

51. Sanders KM, Stern TA, O'Gara PT, et al: Medical and psychiatric complications associated with the use of the intraaortic balloon pump, *J Intensive Care Med* 7:154–160, 1992.

52. Hammer JS, Hammond D, Strain JJ, et al: Microcomputers and consultation psychiatry, *Gen Hosp Psychiatry* 7:119–124, 1985.

53. Popkin MK, Mackenzie JB, Callies AL: Data-based psychiatric consultation: applying mainframe computer capability to consultation, *Gen Hosp Psychiatry* 7:109–112, 1985.

Chapter 2

Approach to Consultation Psychiatry: Assessment Strategies

John Querques, M.D.
Theodore A. Stern, M.D.

My emphasis to the residents is: "Now that you've learned a lot about compassion and human dignity . . . you must learn to be competent," adding "or else." The goals for the trainee are specialty-competence, that is, some specific things about consultation: accountability, commitment, industry, discipline; these are the components that go into the make-up of a professional.

Ned H. Cassem, M.D.[1]

This chapter provides a practical approach to the assessment of affective, behavioral, and cognitive problems of patients in the general hospital. We first survey the landscape of consultation psychiatry and then identify six broad domains of psychiatric problems commonly encountered in the medical setting. Next, we describe the differences in clinical approach, environment, interactive style, and use of language that distinguish psychiatry in the general hospital from practice in other venues. Then we offer a step-by-step guide to the conduct of a psychiatric consultation. The chapter concludes with a review of treatment principles critical to caring for the medically ill. Throughout this chapter, we emphasize the hallmarks of competence identified by Cassem[1] almost two decades ago: accountability, commitment, industry, and discipline.

Categories of Psychiatric Differential Diagnosis in the General Hospital

The "borderland" between psychiatry and medicine in which consultation psychiatrists ply their trade can be visualized as the area shared by two intersecting circles in a Venn diagram (Figure 2-1). As depicted in the figure and consistent with the fundamental tenet of psychosomatic medicine (i.e., that mind and body are indivisible), the likelihood that either a psychiatric or a medical condition will have no impact on the other is incredibly slim. Within the broad region of bidirectional influence (the area of overlap in the Venn diagram), the problems most commonly encountered on a consultation-liaison (C-L) service can be grouped into six categories (modified from Lipowski[2]; see Figure 2-1). Examples of each classification follow; later in the chapter we provide clinical vignettes to illustrate the issues raised.

Psychiatric Presentations of Medical Conditions

An elderly man underwent neurosurgery for clipping of an aneurysm of the anterior communicating artery. A few days after surgery, he became diaphoretic, confused, and agitated (with tachycardia and hypertension). Because of a history of alcoholism (reportedly in remission but suspected

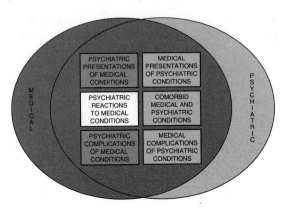

Figure 2-1. A representation of the overlap between medical and psychiatric care.

to be active), a diagnosis of alcohol withdrawal delirium was made. He remained confused despite aggressive benzodiazepine treatment. When he later became febrile, a lumbar puncture was done and the cerebrospinal fluid (CSF) analysis was consistent with herpes simplex virus (HSV) infection. His sensorium cleared after a course of acyclovir. *In this case, infection of the central nervous system (CNS) by HSV was heralded by delirium.*

Psychiatric Complications of Medical Conditions or Treatments

Newly diagnosed with human immunodeficiency virus (HIV) infection with a high viral load, a young man with no prior psychiatric history began treatment with efavirenz, a nonnucleoside reverse transcriptase inhibitor. Within a few days, he experienced vivid nightmares, a known side effect of efavirenz. Over the next several weeks, the nightmares resolved. He continued with antiretroviral treatment, but he became increasingly despondent with a full complement of neurovegetative symptoms of major depression. *A chronic, incurable viral illness—whose treatment caused a neuropsychiatric complication—precipitated a depressive episode.*

Psychological Reactions to Medical Conditions or Treatments

A woman with a history of preeclampsia during her first pregnancy was admitted with hyperten-

sion in the 38th week of her second pregnancy. Preeclampsia was diagnosed, and she delivered a healthy baby. As she prepared for discharge, and despite her obstetrician's reassurance, she fretted that a hypertensive catastrophe was going to befall her at home. *Pathologic anxiety resulted from an acute obstetric condition.*

Medical Presentations of Psychiatric Conditions

A young female graduate student from another country who for several years had habitually induced vomiting to relieve persistent abdominal pain presented with generalized weakness and was found to have a serum potassium of 2.2 mEq/L. She had long since been diagnosed with bulimia nervosa, but the psychiatric consultant found no evidence for this disorder and instead diagnosed conversion disorder, construing her chronic abdominal pain as a converted symptom of psychological distress over leaving her family to study abroad. *Conversion disorder presented as persistent abdominal pain.*

Medical Complications of Psychiatric Conditions or Treatments

An obese man with schizophrenia treated with olanzapine (20 mg daily) gained 30 pounds in 6 months. Repeated measurements of fasting serum glucose were more than 126 mg/dl. *Treatment with an atypical antipsychotic was complicated by an endocrine condition.*

Comorbid Medical and Psychiatric Conditions

A middle-aged man with long-standing obsessive-compulsive disorder (OCD) effectively treated with high-dose fluoxetine presented with cough, dyspnea, and fever. Chest radiography showed a left lower-lobe infiltrate, consistent with pneumonia. He defervesced after a few doses of intravenous (IV) antibiotics and was discharged to complete the antibiotic course at home. His OCD remained in remission. *Infectious and psychiatric conditions existed independently.*

The Art of Psychiatric Consultation in the General Hospital

Determining where on the vast border between psychiatry and medicine an individual's pathologic condition is located is the psychiatric consultant's fundamental task. As for any physician, his or her chief responsibility is diagnosis. The C-L psychiatrist is aided in this enterprise by appreciation of four key differences between general hospital psychiatry and practice in other venues: clinical approach, environment, style of interaction, and use of language.

Clinical Approach

A senior psychiatrist at the Massachusetts General Hospital (MGH) and director of its Psychosomatic/Consultation Psychiatry Fellowship Program for more than 25 years, Dr. George Murray advises his students to think in three ways when consulting on patients: physiologically, existentially, and "dirty." Each element of this tripartite conceptualization is no more or less important than the other, and the most accurate formulation of a patient's problem will prove elusive without attention to all three.

First and foremost, psychiatrists are physicians and, as such, subscribe to the medical model: altered bodily structures and functions lead to disease; their correction through physical means leads to restoration of health. Although allegiance to this model may be impolitic in this era of biopsychosocial holism, the degree of morbidity in general hospitals is ever more acute and the technology brought to bear against it is increasingly more sophisticated.[3] Consultation psychiatrists who fail to keep pace with their medical and surgical colleagues jeopardize their usefulness to physicians and patients alike.

Alongside the physiologic frame of mind, consultation psychiatrists must think existentially; that is, they must nurture a healthy curiosity about the circumstances in which their patients find themselves at particular moments in the course of an illness. What does it mean to a burn victim that he was brought by helicopter to a hospital in a neighboring state? What was he thinking during the airlift? Would he have thought differently if an ambulance had brought him to his local hospital? To be curious about such matters, the consulting psychiatrist must first *know* the details of the patient's situation, largely achieved by a careful reading of the chart. For example, ambulance (or helicopter) "run" sheets and emergency department notes often contain interesting and meaningful data about a patient's mental state in the aftermath of a tragic event. Armed with this information, the consultant can then *ask* the patient what the whole ordeal was like for him or her.

Consultation psychiatrists are wise to maintain a measured skepticism toward patients' and others' statements, motivations, and desires. In other words, they should consider the possibility that the patient (or another informant) is somehow distorting information to serve his or her own agenda. Providers of history can distort the truth in a myriad of ways, ranging from innocuous exaggeration of the truth to outright lies; their aims are equally legion: money, revenge, convenience, cover-up of peccadilloes, infidelities, or crimes. For example, the beleaguered mother of a young woman with borderline personality disorder embellished her daughter's suicidal comments in an effort to secure involuntary commitment for her daughter and respite for herself. By paying attention to his or her own countertransference—his or her personal read of the "limbic music"[4] emanating from the mother-daughter dyad—the psychiatric consultant called in to assess the patient's suicidality ably detected the mother's self-serving distortion and thus avoided unwittingly colluding with it. This special case of distortion to remove a relative to a mental or other hospital has been termed the *Gaslight phenomenon*.[5–7] Although thinking "dirty" is merely a realization that people refract reality through the lens of their own personal experience, other health professionals—even some psychiatrists—bristle at even a consideration, let alone a suggestion, that patients and their families harbor unseemly ulterior motives. Consequently, this perspective does not make the consultation psychiatrist many friends; his thinking "dirty" may even earn him an unsavory reputation. However, neither an ever-widening social circle nor victory in popularity contests is the C-L psychiatrist's raison d'être; competent doctoring is.

Environment

The successful psychiatric consultant must be prepared to work in an atmosphere less formal, rigid, and predictable than one typically found in an office or a clinic; flexibility and adaptability are crucial. Patients are often seen in two-bedded rooms with nothing but a thin curtain providing only a semblance of privacy; roommates—as well as nurses, aides, dietary personnel, and other physicians—are frequent interlocutors. Cramped quarters are the rule, with IV poles, tray tables, and one or two chairs leaving little room for much else. When family members and other visitors are present, the physician may ask them to leave the room; alternatively, he may invite them to stay to "biopsy" the interpersonal dynamics among the family and friends, as was done in the case of the borderline patient described previously. The various alarms and warning signals of medical equipment (e.g., IV pumps, cardiac monitors, and ventilators) and assorted catheters and tubes traveling into and out of the patient's body add to the unique ambiance of the bedside experience that distinguishes it from the quiet comfort afforded by a private office. Perhaps off-putting at first, for the psychiatrist who, as Lewis Glickman in his book on consultation put it (as cited in Cassem[1]), loves medicine and is fascinated with medical illness, the exigencies of life and work in a modern hospital quickly become exciting and ultimately captivating.

Style of Interaction

The adaptability required by these environmental circumstances permits—in fact, demands—that the psychiatric consultant to be more flexible in his or her relations with the patient. For example, psychiatric consultants should permit themselves to crouch at the bedside; lowering themselves to the recumbent patient's level may diminish apprehension. Shaking hands or otherwise laying on of hands may achieve the same end. Performance of a physical examination provides an excellent opportunity to allay anxiety and distinguishes dramatically consultation work from office-based psychiatry, where any touching of a patient—let alone physical examination—is considered taboo. An offer to make the person more comfortable by adjusting the bed or getting the patient a drink before beginning the interview goes a long way to building rapport. When the patient is unable to do even these simple things unaided, it is simply a kind, human gesture. When the patient tends toward the cantankerous and irascible, concern for his comfort may prevent his expelling the consultant from the room.

Use of Language

Allowance for flexibility also extends to the psychiatrists' use of language; they can feel freer than they might in other practice settings to use humor, slang expressions, and perhaps even foul language. All of these varieties of verbal expression create a temporarily jarring juxtaposition between the stereotypical image of the austere, reserved physician and the present one; defenses may be briefly disabled just long enough to connect with the truth and allow connection with the patient. For example, in a technique taught by Murray, the psychiatrist raises a clenched fist in front of an angry but anger-phobic patient and asks him, "If you had one shot, where would you put it?" In this case, the sight and sound of a "healer" in boxer's pose inquiring about placement of a "shot" creates a curious, or even humorous, incongruity that disarms the patient's defenses and allows an otherwise intolerable affect (anger) to emerge (if it is there in the first place). A variant of this maneuver, substitution of a verbal expression of anger for the physical one, is also possible. For example, a 30-year-old man with leukemia refractory to bone-marrow transplantation was admitted with graft-versus-host disease. His mother and sister kept a near-constant vigil at his bedside. When he refused to eat and to talk to his family and the nurses, the psychiatrist was summoned. Quickly sizing up the situation, the consultant said to the young man, "It must be a pain to have your mother constantly hovering over you." The patient grinned slightly and answered in the affirmative. Use of a foul expression of the same sentiment would predictably have achieved a more robust response. Lack of the formal arrangements of office-based psychiatric practice make such techniques permissible in the general hospital, often to the delight of residents who sometimes feel unnecessarily constrained in their interpersonal comportment and in whom even a little training unfortunately does much to limit their natural spontaneity.

The Process of Psychiatric Consultation in the General Hospital

With this general overview of the art of consultation, we next outline the step-by-step approach to the actual performance of a psychiatric consultation. Table 2-1 summarizes the key points elaborated in the following text.

Speak Directly With the Referring Clinician

The consultative process begins with the receipt of the referral. With experience, the sensitive consultant begins to formulate preliminary hypotheses even at this early stage. For example, he or she recognizes a particular unit within the hospital or an individual physician and recollects previous consultations that originated from these sources. In addition, he or she may discern a difference in the way this consult request was communicated compared with the form of previous requests. In a form of parallel process, this alteration in the usual routine—even if subtle and only in retrospect—often reflects something about the patient. Throughout the consultative process, these crude preliminary hypotheses thus formed are refined and ultimately either accepted or rejected.

Table 2-1. Procedural Approach to Psychiatric Consultation

- Speak directly with the referring clinician.
- Review the current and pertinent past records.
- Review the patient's medications.
- Gather collateral data.
- Interview and examine the patient.
- Formulate a diagnosis and management plan.
- Write a note.
- Speak directly with the referring clinician.
- Provide periodic follow-up.

The continual revision of previous theories as additional data become available is one of the pleasures of psychiatric consultation.

The reason for the consultation stated in the request may differ from the "real" reason for the consult. The team may accurately sense a problem with the patient but not capture it precisely. In some cases, they may be quite far afield, usually when the "real" reason for the consultation is difficulty in the management of a hateful patient.[8] It is up to the consultant to identify the core issue and ultimately address it in the consultation. Practically speaking, a special effort to contact the consultee is not usually required, because, in general, in the course of reading the chart or reviewing laboratory data, one encounters a member of the team and can inquire then about the consultation request.

Review the Current and Pertinent Past Records

A careful review of the current medical record is indispensable to a thorough and comprehensive evaluation of the patient. Perhaps no other element of the consultative process requires as much discipline as this one. The seasoned consultant is able to accomplish this task quite efficiently, knowing fruitful areas of the chart to mine. For example, nursing notes often contain behavioral data often lacking from other disciplines' notes; a well-written consultation provided by another service (at the MGH, infectious-disease consultations are particularly meticulous) can provide a general orientation to a case, although the consultant must take care not to propagate error by failing to check primary data himself or herself. Other bountiful areas of the chart include notes written by medical students (who tend to be the most thorough of all), physical and occupational therapists (for functional data), and speech pathologists (for cognitive data). In reading the chart, the focus of the psychiatric consultant's attention varies according to the nature of the case and the reason for the consultation. In cases in which sensorium is altered, for example, careful note of changes in level of awareness, behavior, and cognition should be made, especially as they relate to changes in the medical condition and treatment.

Review the Patient's Medications

Regardless of the particulars of a case, detailed evaluation of medications, paying special attention to those recently initiated or discontinued, is always in order. For example, in the vignette presented previously, knowledge that the young HIV-positive man had recently initiated treatment with efavirenz was key to diagnosing accurately the cause of his nightmares. Important medications the patient may have taken before admission, including those on which he may be physiologically dependent (e.g., benzodiazepines and narcotic analgesics), may inadvertently have been excluded from his current regimen. Patients who have been transferred among various units in the hospital may be at particular risk of such inadvertent omissions. In cases in which status changes resulting from withdrawal phenomena top the list of differential diagnoses, careful construction of a timeline of the patient's receipt of psychoactive agents is often the only way to identify the problem. In much the same way as infectious-disease specialists chart the administration of antibiotics in relation to culture results and dermatologists plot newly prescribed medications against appearance of rashes, the psychiatric consultant tabulates mental status changes, vital signs, and dosages of psychoactive medications to clarify the diagnostic picture. Such a procedure exemplifies the industry and discipline required of the competent consultant.

Gather Collateral Data

The gathering of collateral information from family, friends, and outpatient treaters is no less important in consultation work than in other psychiatric settings. For several reasons (e.g., altered mental status, denial, memory impairment, and malingering), patients' accounts of their history and current symptoms are often vague, spotty, and unreliable. Although data from other sources is therefore vital, the astute psychiatrist recognizes that their information, too, may be distorted by the same factors and by selfish interests, as already described. Consultation psychiatrists must guard against accepting any one party's version of events as gospel and maintain an open mind in collecting a history informed from many angles.

Interview and Examine the Patient

Next follows the interview of the patient and performance of a mental status examination, in addition to relevant portions of the physical and neurologic examinations. We discussed earlier the differences between patient encounters in the general hospital and those in other venues.

A detailed assessment of cognitive function is not necessary in all patients. If there is no evidence that a patient has a cognitive problem, a simple statement to the effect that no gross cognitive problem is apparent is sufficient. However, even a slight hint that a cognitive disturbance is present should trigger performance of a more formal screen. We recommend the Folstein Mini-Mental State Examination (MMSE)[9] for this purpose and supplement this test with others that specifically target frontal executive functions (e.g., clock drawing, Luria maneuvers, and cognitive estimations). Any abnormalities that turn up on these bedside tests should be comprehensively evaluated by formal neuropsychological testing. It is convenient if a psychologist—especially one trained specifically in neuropsychology—is affiliated with the consultation service. Conversely, if a patient is obviously inattentive, we would argue that performance of the MMSE (or similar tests) is not indicated, because one can predict *a priori* poor performance resulting from the subject's general inattention to the required tasks.

The consultant should at the very least review the physical examinations performed by other physicians. This does not, however, preclude doing his or her own examination of relevant systems, including the CNS, which, unless the patient is on the neurologic service or is known to have a motor or a sensory problem, has likely been left unexamined. A number of physical findings can be discerned simply by observation: pupillary size (which is noteworthy with opioid withdrawal or intoxication); diaphoresis, either present (from fever, alcohol, or benzodiazepine withdrawal) or absent (associated with anticholinergic intoxication); and adventitious motor activity (e.g., tremors, tremulousness, or agitation). Vital signs are especially relevant in cases of substance withdrawal, delirium, and other causes of agitation. Primitive reflexes (e.g., snout, glabellar, and grasp), deep-tendon reflexes, extraocular movements, pupillary reaction to light, and muscle tone are among the key elements of the neurologic examination that the psychiatrist frequently checks.

Formulate a Diagnosis and Management Plan

Any physician's tasks are two-fold: diagnosis and treatment; this dictum is no different for the psychiatrist—whether in the general hospital or elsewhere. In arriving at a diagnosis, after history and examination comes laboratory testing. By the time a psychiatric consultation is requested, most hospitalized patients have already undergone extensive laboratory testing, including comprehensive metabolic panels and complete blood cell counts; these should be reviewed. In constructing the initial parts of a management plan, the psychiatric consultant should attend to diagnostics and specifically consider each of the tests listed in Table 2-2, which we review presently. Therapeutic strategies are discussed in a later section.

Toxicologic screens of both serum and urine are required any time a substance-use disorder is suspected and in cases of altered sensorium, intoxication, or withdrawal.

Well-known by every student of psychiatry, syphilis, thyroid dysfunction, and deficiencies of

Table 2-2. Laboratory Tests in Psychiatric Consultation

- Toxicology
  - Serum
  - Urine
- Serology
  - RPR test
  - VDRL test
- TSH, thyrotropin
- Vitamin B_{12} (cyanocobalamin)
- Folic acid (folate)
- Neuroimaging
  - CT
  - MRI
- EEG
- CSF analysis

CSF, Cerebrospinal fluid; *CT*, computed tomography; *EEG*, electroencephalography; *MRI*, magnetic resonance imaging; *RPR*, rapid plasma reagin; *TSH*, thyroid stimulating hormone; *VDRL*, Venereal Disease Research Laboratory.

vitamin B_{12} and folic acid are always included in exhaustive lists of the differential diagnoses of virtually every neuropsychiatric disturbance. Although it is certainly possible that these conditions can *cause* any manner of psychiatric perturbation (e.g., dementia, depression, or mania), more commonly these ailments coexist with other conditions, which together *contribute* to psychiatric disturbances. Because blood tests and treatments for these diseases are relatively easily accomplished, we routinely recommend that these tests be completed in hospitalized patients with an abnormal mental status.

For purposes other than evaluation of acute intracranial hemorrhage, cerebral magnetic resonance imaging (MRI) is preferred to computed tomography. MRI provides higher resolution and greater detail, particularly of subcortical structures of interest to the psychiatrist. A thorough consultation is incomplete without a reading of the actual radiologic report of the study; merely reviewing the telegraphic summary in a house officer's progress note is insufficient, because important findings are often omitted. For example, an MRI scan that shows no abnormalities other than periventricular white matter changes is invariably recorded as "normal" or as showing "no acute change." Although periventricular white matter changes are not acute and their significance is arguable, they are certainly not normal and they should be documented in a careful psychiatric consultation note. They may be evidence of an "insulted" brain that forms a substrate for depression or dementia and may be a predictive sign of sensitivity to usual dosages of psychotropic medications.

Electroencephalograph (EEG) can be particularly helpful to document the presence of generalized slowing in patients thought by their primary physicians to have a so-called "functional" problem. Such indisputable evidence of electric dysrhythmia often puts a sudden end to the primary team's skepticism. In cases of suspected complex partial seizures, depriving the patient of sleep the night before the EEG increases the likelihood that he will sleep during the test; against a background of slow activity in the sleeping state, any spikes or sharp waves indicative of seizure activity are more easily detected. Continuous EEG and video monitoring or ambulatory EEG monitoring may be necessary to "catch" aberrant electric activity. As with neuroimaging reports, the consultant psychiatrist must read the EEG report him or herself; nonpsychiatrists commonly equate absence of "organized electrographic seizure activity" with normality, even though focal slowing may be evidence of seizure activity.

CSF analysis is frequently overlooked by psychiatrists and other physicians alike. However, it should be considered in cases of altered mental status with fever, leukocytosis, or meningismus and when causes of beclouded consciousness are not obvious. In some cases (e.g., in the vignette of the man with HSV presented previously), some conditions initially considered causative are not and the true culprit is identified only after lumbar puncture.

Any suspicion of a somatoform disorder (especially conversion disorder) should trigger referral for psychological testing with the Minnesota Multiphasic Personality Inventory (MMPI) or the shorter Personality Assessment Inventory. For example, MMPI results of the young female graduate student described previously may demonstrate the so-called "conversion (or psychosomatic) V" pattern of marked elevations on the hypochondriasis and hysteria scales and a normal or slightly elevated result on the depression scale. These pencil-and-paper tests can also be useful in assessments of psychological contributions to pain. Projective testing (e.g., Rorschach inkblots) is more common in outpatient venues.

Write a Note

The psychiatric consultation note should be a model of clear, concise writing with careful attention to specific, practical diagnostic and therapeutic recommendations. Several reviews of this topic are available.[10,11] If the stated reason for the consultation differs from the consultee's more fundamental concern, both should be addressed in the note. If the referring physician adopts the consultant's recommendations, he or she should be able to transcribe them directly onto the order sheet or (increasingly frequently) into computerized order-entry systems. "Note wars," criticism of the consultee, accusations of shoddy work, pejorative labels, and jargon should all be avoided. If the consultee chooses a diagnostic

or therapeutic course equally appropriate to the consultant's suggested choice, an indication of agreement is more prudent than rigid insistence on the psychiatrist's preference. The consultant should avoid prognostication (e.g., "This patient will probably have decision-making capacity after his infection has resolved" or "This patient will likely need psychiatric hospitalization after he recovers from tricyclic antidepressant toxicity"). Such forecasts do not evince confidence in the consultant's skill if they prove inaccurate, may be invoked by the consultee even when they no longer apply, and are unnecessary if routine follow-up is provided (see later text).

Speak Directly With the Referring Clinician

The consultative process is not complete without contact, either by phone or in person, with the referring physician or other member of the patient's team, especially if the diagnosis or recommended intervention warrants immediate attention.

Provide Periodic Follow-Up

The committed consultant sees the patient as often as is necessary to treat him or her competently, and the consultant holds himself or herself accountable for tracking the patient's clinical progress, following up on laboratory tests, refining earlier diagnostic impressions, and modifying diagnostic and treatment recommendations. The consultation comes to an end only when the problem for which the consultant was called resolves, any other concerns identified by the consultant are fully addressed, or the patient is discharged or dies. Rarely do any of these outcomes occur after a single visit, making repeated visits the rule and availability, even at inopportune times, crucial. However, the consultant is not obligated to continue consulting on a case when his or her recommendations are clearly being ignored.[12] In these cases, it is appropriate to sign off. Although so-called "physician extenders" (e.g., clinical nurse specialists, nurse practitioners, physician assistants, and case managers) may be available to locate psychiatric beds and secure insurance coverage for inpatient psychiatric stays for patients who require them, the psychiatric consultant should be ready and able to perform these duties.

Principles of Psychiatric Treatment in the General Hospital

As in other practice settings, in the general hospital, psychiatric treatment proceeds along three fronts: biologic, psychological, and social.

Biologic Management

When prescribing psychopharmaceuticals for medically ill patients taking other medications, the consultant must be aware of pharmacokinetic profiles, drug-drug interactions, and adverse effects. These topics are considered in depth in Chapter 18.

Pharmacokinetic Profiles

Pharmacokinetics refers to a drug's absorption, distribution, metabolism, and excretion. Because an acutely medically ill patient may not be able to take medications orally, absorption is a primary concern in the general hospital setting. Often in such situations (e.g., in an intubated patient), a nasogastric (NG) tube is in place and medications can be crushed and administered through the NG tube. However, if one is not in place, the psychiatric consultant is obliged to consider medications that can be given intramuscularly, intravenously, or in suppository form. In addition, mirtazapine and olanzapine are now available in orally disintegrating formulations.

Many psychotropic medications are metabolized in the liver and excreted through the kidneys. Thus impaired hepatic and renal function can lead to increased concentrations of parent compounds and pharmacologically active metabolites. This problem is readily overcome by use of lower initial doses and by slower titration. However, concern for metabolic alterations in medically ill patients should not justify use of homeopathic doses for indeterminate durations, because most patients ultimately tolerate and require standard regimens.

Drug-Drug Interactions

Many psychopharmaceuticals are metabolized by the cytochrome P-450 isoenzyme system; many also inhibit various isoforms in this extensive family of hepatic enzymes and the metabolism of many is, in turn, inhibited by other classes of medication, thus creating fertile ground for drug-drug interactions in patients taking several medications. This topic is reviewed extensively in Chapter 18. Psychiatric consultants should also be aware that cigarette smoking induces the metabolism of many drugs. When patients are hospitalized and thus stop or curtail smoking, serum concentrations of these drugs (e.g., clozapine) increase and propensity for adverse effects thus also increases.

Adverse Effects

Depending on the practice venue, the profile of adverse effects of concern to the psychiatrist vary. For example, the likelihood that tricyclic antidepressants will cause dry mouth and sedation may be of more concern in the outpatient setting than in the general hospital, where concern about the cardiac-conduction and gut-slowing effects will likely be of greater importance in patients recovering from myocardial infarction (MI) or bowel surgery. Traditional neuroleptics—relegated to the second line in otherwise healthy patients with psychosis—may be preferable to the atypical agents in general medical settings, where patients with obesity, diabetes mellitus, and dyslipidemia may be seen for the complications of these conditions (e.g., MI, stroke, and diabetic ketoacidosis).

Psychological Management

Psychological management of the hospitalized, medically ill patient begins—as does all competent treatment—with diagnosis, in this case, personality diagnosis. That is, the psychiatric consultant first appraises the patient's psychological strengths and vulnerabilities. Armed with this psychological balance sheet, the psychiatrist then uses this information therapeutically in how he or she phrases questions and comments to the patient and describes the patient to the medical and nursing staff. Several

Table 2-3. Personality Assessment and Management in the General Hospital

Personality Type	Major Traits	Reaction to Illness	Recommended Strategies
Dependent	Craves special attention. Expects services on demand. Requires constant reassurance.	Perceived abandonment generates feeling of helplessness. Increased anxiety prompts more demands.	Express desire to provide comprehensive care. Make minor concessions if possible.
Obsessive	Values detail and order. Becomes anxious with uncertain outcomes. Well defended against fear and pain.	Illness represents threat to self-control. Need for certainty and control prevents questioning of staff, thus increasing anxiety.	Provide ample information, using and defining medical terms. Ally with patient's desire for mastery. Allow patient to participate in medical decisions.
Histrionic	Prematurely trusts others. Uses repression, denial, and avoidance. Dramatizes feelings.	Illness represents threat to masculinity or femininity.	Recognize patient's grace under pressure. Omit details in reassuring patient.
Masochistic	Plays the martyr role. Seems to enjoy suffering. Feels unappreciated.	Illness represents deserved punishment. Illness is welcomed as form of suffering. Lack of recognition of martyr status risks noncompliance.	Appreciate patient's suffering. Recommend treatment as an additional burden that will aid others.
Paranoid	Is suspicious, wary, and guarded. Readily feels slighted. Bickers when feels persecuted.	Illness represents an external assault. Medical interventions generate suspicions and fear of harm.	Inform patient completely about tests and treatments. Acknowledge difficulty of illness.
Narcissistic	Requests and receives help with difficulty. Strives to appear smart, strong, and superior. Fears dependence.	Illness challenges self-esteem and superior stance. Efforts to appear effectual and strong are redoubled.	Recognize patient's strengths and knowledge. Allow patient to participate in medical decisions. Expect gaps in history, because more illness connotes weakness.
Schizoid	Is aloof, uninvolved, and detached. Prefers solitary occupations.	Illness requires contact with caregivers. Rejection risk spurs greater withdrawal.	Recognize preference for isolation. Minimize intrusions. Assure patient of interest and concern.

Adapted from Shuster JL, Stern TA: Intensive care units. In Wise MG, Rundell JR, editors: *The American Psychiatric Publishing textbook of consultation-liaison psychiatry: psychiatry in the medically ill*, ed 2, Washington, 2002, American Psychiatric Publishing, pp 753–770; Kahana RJ, Bibring GL: Personality types in medical management. In Zinberg NE, editor: *Psychiatry and medical practice in a general hospital*, New York, 1965, International Universities Press, pp 108–123; and Wool C, Geringer ES, Stern TA: The management of behavioral problems in the ICU. In Rippe JM, Irwin RS, Alpert JS, et al, editors: *Intensive care medicine*, ed 2, Boston, 1991, Little, Brown, pp 1906–1916. Copyright 1991, Little, Brown and Company. Used with permission.

schemas have been developed to aid in such a personality assessment.[8,13,14] Groves' formulation is reviewed in Chapter 20; Table 2-3 in this chapter summarizes Kahana and Bibring's approach.

The consultant must realize that the patient may find the psychiatrist the only outlet available to vent his or her feelings about treatment in the hospital. This is an appropriate function of the consultant—and, in fact, may be the tacit reason for the consultation. Relieved of his or her feelings, often hostile and at odds with the team's treatment efforts, the patient is thus better able to work with the team.

Social Management

Psychiatric consultants may be called on to help make decisions about end-of-life care (e.g., do-not-resuscitate and do-not-intubate orders), disposition to an appropriate living situation (e.g., home with services, assisted living residence, skilled nursing facility, or nursing home), short-term disability, probate guardianship for a patient deemed clinically unable to make medical decisions for himself or herself, and involuntary psychiatric commitment. For patients who are agitated and thereby place themselves and others in harm's way, the consultant may recommend the use of various restraints (e.g., Posey vests, mitts [to prevent removing IV and other catheters], soft wrist restraints, and leather wrist and ankle restraints) and constant observation.

Summary

Regardless of the practice setting, the basics of competent psychiatric care remain the diagnosis of affective, behavioral, and cognitive disturbances and their treatment by pharmacologic, psychological, and social interventions. The psychiatrist in the general hospital applies these fundamentals while remaining *accessible* to the consultee and to the patient; *adaptable* to the exigencies of the hospital environment; and *flexible* in clinical approach and interpersonal style. The consultation psychiatrist adheres to the tenets of competent doctoring: accountability, commitment, industry, and discipline.

References

1. Cassem NH: *The consultation service.* In Hackett TP, Weisman AD, Kucharski A, editors: *Psychiatry in a general hospital: the first fifty years.* Littleton, MA, 1987, PSG Publishing Company, p 34.
2. Lipowski ZJ: Review of consultation psychiatry and psychosomatic medicine: II. Clinical aspects. *Psychosom Med* 29:201–224, 1967.
3. Murray GB: The liaison psychiatrist as busybody. *Ann Clin Psychiatry* 1:265–268, 1989.
4. Murray GB: *Limbic music.* In Cassem NH, Stern TA, Rosenbaum JF, et al, editors: *Massachusetts General Hospital handbook of general hospital psychiatry*, ed 4, St Louis, 1997, Mosby, pp 11–23.
5. Lund CA, Gardiner AQ: The Gaslight phenomenon: an institutional variant. *Br J Psychiatry* 131:533–534, 1977.
6. Smith CG, Sinanan K: The "Gaslight phenomenon" reappears: a modification of the Ganser syndrome. *Br J Psychiatry* 120:685–686, 1972.
7. Barton R, Whitehead TA: The Gaslight phenomenon. *Lancet* 1:1258–1260, 1969.
8. Groves JE: Taking care of the hateful patient. *N Engl J Med* 298:883–887, 1978.
9. Folstein MF, Folstein SE, McHugh PR: "Mini-Mental State": a practical method for grading the cognitive state of patients for the clinician. *J Psychiatr Res* 12:189–198, 1975.
10. Alexander T, Bloch S: The written report in consultation-liaison psychiatry: a proposed schema. *Austr New Zealand J Psychiatry* 36:251–258, 2002.
11. Garrick TR, Stotland NL: How to write a psychiatric consultation. *Am J Psychiatry* 139:849–855, 1982.
12. Kontos N, Freudenreich O, Querques J, et al: The consultation psychiatrist as effective physician. *Gen Hosp Psychiatry* 25:20–23, 2003.
13. Kahana RJ, Bibring GL: *Personality types in medical management.* In Zinberg NE, editor: *Psychiatry and medical practice in a general hospital.* New York, 1965, International Universities Press, pp 108–123.
14. Bibring GL: Psychiatry and medical practice in a general hospital. *N Engl J Med* 254:366–372, 1956.

Chapter 3
Limbic Music

George B. Murray, M.D.

"Limbic Music" is a strange title for a chapter in a handbook of psychiatry in the general hospital. It is meant to be clinically relevant, however. It must be stressed that this chapter is primarily heuristic. Some license is taken with philosophic assumptions not adequately substantiated, there are arguable statements, and the anatomy and physiology on which this structure is based may change, although probably not in a major way, in coming years. Mesulam[1] mentions that the concept of the limbic system has ebbed and welled to fit the preference of individual authors. This is another case of it. It is hoped that the use of *limbic music* will aid the clinician in assessing the affective component in the patient.

When discussing delirium and dementia and reading the literature, attention is paid to the cerebral hemispheres and to the arousal systems. It is rare to find any mention of the limbic system. Several reasons may account for this. First, the limbic system is difficult to reach within the brain; one has to traverse much cortex to get to it. Second, the limbic system is not a neatly discrete structure, and some, such as Brodal,[2] would say that it does not exist as a system at all. A third reason, not usually stated, but detectable in casual discussion, is that the limbic system does not subserve "higher function" and as a result has the bias associated with it as mediating man's "lower functions." Academicians usually pride themselves not on pro-football muscles but on their higher functions, and they therefore do not usually feel that the study of the "lower functions" (the four Fs) in human beings is an especially worthy, clean, intellectual, and liberalizing endeavor.

Mind-Brain

First, let us briefly review some aspects of the mind-body arena. *Psychobiology* was a word coined by Adolph Meyer to compress and unite the concept of mind-brain. Those of us who had an interest in the mind-brain connection thought that this concept of psychobiology would contain the kernel that would dispel the problems involved with mind-brain. Unfortunately, after carefully reading Meyer's works, we find that kernel is still difficult to attain. In the relatively recent tradition of psychosomatic medicine, a word again tries to compress the two ideas of mind-brain into one word, implying a unity therein. As one reads the literature in this area and discusses the term with experts in the field, one finds much left to be desired for an understanding of the relationship of mind to brain and vice versa.

An important feature with regard to psychosomatic medicine is that there are no residency training programs in the subject. This fact of no residencies tells us something about psychosomatic medicine in the pragmatic world. It tells us, in William James's words, that "it bakes no bread." It may be quite interesting in itself, but as a collected fund of knowledge, it does not allow the physician to do much with psychosomatic medical knowledge.

On the other hand, there is a certain animosity among psychosomaticists directed toward those who would split man into mind and brain. In traditional philosophic thinking, there are two core poles: realism and idealism. Those with a more idealistic bent strive for global unity; tend to dislike fractionation and atomization; tend to charge the so-called realists as being those who would disunite and reduce everything to its smallest biologic parts, that is, realists are practitioners of reductionism. The charge goes on to say that in reductionism what one reduces and gets rid of is, in fact, mind. The idealist smiles when the charge is made that the realist has a mindless brain only; however, when the idealist is charged with having a brainless mind as a subject of study, the smile turns to a frown.

The culprit for this great supposed split between brain and mind is usually thought to be Descartes. His most famous treatise, Discourse on Method of Rightly Conducting the Reason and Seeking for Truth in the Sciences,[3] outlined his philosophic approach to using methodic doubt in obtaining philosophic proof by the use of reason alone.

One often hears the phrase *Cartesian dualism*, and it is presupposed that Descartes, in isolating the mind from the body to study it more specifically, has in fact initiated the great nonunion of mind and brain.[4] I submit that it was primarily Descartes' followers who pragmatically operated on the premises of a split between brain and mind. Because Descartes is often quoted and rarely read, it is not difficult to see why he has been blamed for dualism. Descartes operated in no way differently than, for example, a cardiac surgeon does today. The cardiac surgeon isolates his interests and bears his intensity on how he may best make an intervention on the physiologic function of a failing heart, and he does not pay much attention to the gastrointestinal system, endocrine system, and so forth. Similarly, Descartes set his intensity on the mind and did not, in fact, negate the importance of the body, just as the cardiac surgeon would not negate the importance of the endocrine system and the fact that man lives by all of his physiologic systems as well as mind. Although Descartes' criteria of clarity and distinctness of ideas led him to emphasize a real distinction between mind and body—soul and body to him— he still did not accept the idea that the soul (mind) is just lodged in the body. What he does say in his *Objections and Replies to Objections* is "Mind and body are incomplete substances, viewed in relation to the man who is the unity which they form together."[5]

Most psychiatrists in using the term *Cartesian dualism* use it in a pejorative sense, as if to castigate someone for not being an idealistic upholder of "holism." Most persons interested in psychosomatic medicine have an interest in how the body may influence the mind and how the mind may influence the body, and there have been no clear, distinct theories that settle this question to everybody's satisfaction.

I submit here that a partial key to the understanding of the mind-brain or mind-body meld is the limbic system. The limbic system can be considered in the Cartesian manner as part mind and part body. Mind consists of many things—intellect, imagination, affect, cognition, and motivation among others. There is no one definition of *mind* that satisfies everybody. If the neocortex is more "intellectual," certainly the limbic system is more effectual. In fact, it is often stated that the limbic system is the substratum of emotion in man and animals.

History of the Limbic System

The history of the development of the concept of the limbic system is important in psychiatry. Of the many names in the history of its development, four stand out: Broca, Papez, MacLean, and Nauta. Broca (1824–1880), a French surgeon, founded the Societé d'Anthropologie in Paris in 1859 (the year of Darwin's *On the Origin of Species by Means of Natural Selection*). In 1861, a patient named Laborgne came under Broca's care. Laborgne had had aphasia for 21 years; all he could say was "tan-tan-tan." After his death, a postmortem examination was carried out, and Broca found a softened area in the left frontal cortex, now described as *Brodmann's area 44* and more popularly known as *Broca's area*.[6] In the medical sciences, Broca is best known for his work in aphasia. (Laborgne's brain is still extant, housed in L'École de Medicine in Paris, as is, interestingly enough, Broca's brain.)

Broca is less well known as an author of a remarkable 113-page monograph on the comparative neuroanatomy of mammals.[7] The title of this monograph is *Des Circonvolutions Cérébrals*. This work was published in Revue d'Anthropologie in 1878, 2 years before Broca's death. The monograph is a fascinating, comparative neuro-anatomic study of mammals and contains drawings of what the author called the *great limbic lobe* (*limbic* meaning *border*). What Broca called the *great limbic lobe* includes today the cingulate gyrus, retrosplenial cortex, and parahippocampal gyrus (gyrus fornicatus).

Neuroanatomic knowledge progressed with its characterizations of nuclei and connections, but there was no stimulating discussion of the limbic lobe until 1937, when Papez published his classic paper, "A Proposed Mechanism of Emotion."[8] Papez (1883–1958) was a 1911 graduate of the University of Minnesota Medical School; at the time of writing the paper cited, he was a neuroanatomist at Cornell University Medical School when it was still in Ithaca, New York. When he published the paper, it did not create much stir. According to MacLean,[9] Papez wrote this paper because of some ongoing discussion in England on the subject; Papez thought that the discussion did not reflect the tradition of emotion and neuroanatomic structures already known, and thus he elaborated the idea of the limbic structures subserving the emotions.

From this paper came the popular name of the *Papez circuit* (Figure 3-1). This circuit was so called because Papez himself hypothesized that a neuroimpulse could leave the hippocampus via the fornix, travel on up the fornix under the corpus callosum, and traverse the septal area into the mamillary bodies. At the mamillary bodies, a synaptic connection would be made to the anterior nucleus of the thalamus and then radiate up onto more primitive cortex, the cingulate gyrus. This impulse would then be captured at the level of the cingulate gyrus, be returned in a neurobundle, the cingulum, and brought down and again entered into the hippocampus.[10] Notice he did not include the amygdala.

Papez postulated that this circuit was the basis for the feeling of emotions in humans. The cingulate gyrus in particular, not a neocortical structure but composed of archicortex and mesocortex, allows a human to "know" that he is having his present feelings.

There was not much stir until 1947 when MacLean ran across Papez's paper in the library at Massachusetts General Hospital. At this time, MacLean was a U.S. Public Health Service Fellow.

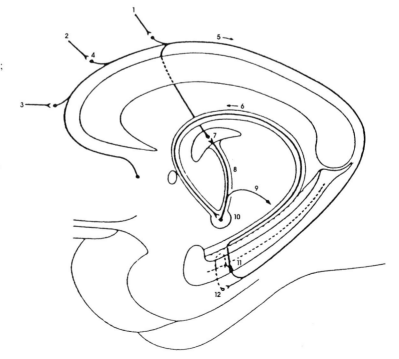

Figure 3-1. The Papez circuit.
1, Brodmann areas 6 and 8;
2, area 9; **3**, areas 10 and 11;
4, area 24; **5**, cingulum; **6**, fornix;
7, anterior nucleus of the thalamus;
8, mamillothalamic tract;
9, mamillotegmental tract;
10, mamillary body;
11, subiculum; **12**, area 28.
(From Nieuwenhuys SR, Voogd J, Van Huijzen CHR: *The human central nervous system.* New York, 1979, Springer-Verlag.)

MacLean, with Cobb as his mentor, was making electroencephalographic recordings of the meso-basal structures of the brain in patients with temporal lobe epilepsy. Discussion with Cobb about the significance of the Papez circuit resulted in MacLean's visiting Papez with Cobb's help.

After his discussion with Papez, MacLean wrote a paper entitled "Psychosomatic Disease and the 'Visceral Brain': Recent Developments Bearing on the Papez Theory of Emotion."[11] MacLean used the term *visceral brain* because he wanted to communicate the notion of "gut feeling." In those years, for the most part, this area of the brain was called the *rhinencephalon*, or the *nose brain*. It turned out that *visceral brain* did not catch the wind and soar effectively either.

In 1952, after further research, MacLean published another paper entitled "Some Psychiatric Implications of Physiological Studies on the Frontotemporal Portion of the Limbic System (Visceral Brain)."[12] This was the first coining of the words *limbic system*. This concept did catch the wind, and soars today as a concept for those structures that subserve emotion in man.

Nauta, neuroanatomist at Massachusetts Institute of Technology, was instrumental both in his own meticulous work and in influencing his students in careful delineation and expansion of the limbic system. In tracking down frontal lobe connections to the limbic system, he effectively expanded it forward. Connections to the midbrain indicate an expansion of the limbic concept backward or "downstream."[13,14]

More important, the limbic system can serve as an integrating concept for the clinical side of psychiatry and neurology. Various approaches to the study of the limbic system can be taken: morphologic,[15] evolutionary,[16] polymodal,[1] or an overview.[17] Perhaps Nauta gave us the most contemporary view—a look at emotions and their anatomy.[18]

Psychologists' Views

There has been disagreement in the field of cognitive psychology. Some say emotion is partially independent of cognition; others say that emotions are the products of cognition. It is my position that although emotions (mediated by the limbic system) are usually conjoined with cognition, they may stand on their own without prior cognitive process. Psychologist Lazarus, maintaining that emotions are the products of cognitions, says:

> Recent years have seen a major change in the way psychologists view emotion—the rediscovery that emotions are products of cognitive processes. The emotional response is elicited by an evaluative perception in lower animals, and in humans by a complex cognitive appraisal of the significance of events for one's well-being.[19]

Psychologist Zajonc elaborates a position seemingly more in accord with how the limbic system functions:

> Only a few years ago, I published a rather speculative paper entitled "Feeling and thinking" (Zajonc, 1980).[20]. . .In this paper I tried to make an appeal for more concentrated study of affective phenomena which have been ignored for decades, and at the same time to ease the heavy reliance on cognitive functions for the explanation of affect. The argument began with the general hypothesis that affect and cognition are partially independent systems and although they ordinarily function conjointly, affect could be generated without a prior cognitive process. It could, therefore, at times precede cognition in a behavioral chain.[21]

Zajonc also believes that there exists presently a form of cognitive imperialism, wherein there is a disdain for affect and only the cognitive is of priority in higher animals.

Sperry has shown movies of "split brain" subjects that had had corpus callosotomies for intractable epilepsy. In one film, the contents of a slide were flashed into the right cortex of a woman's brain, and, of course, she could not speak about it because there is no Broca's area in the right cortex. Every slide flashed into her left cortex only was described adequately in words; in those pictures flashed to her right cortex only, the left brain chattered on in a manner not relevant to the slide shown to the right mute brain. At one point, a risqué slide was shown to the right brain and the woman flushed and showed other aspects of autonomic arousal, for example, rapid respirations, increased systolic blood pressure, increased pulse rate. Not surprisingly, her left brain did not know why. All the left brain said was "Oh my! That's something isn't it!" Even though the left brain did not know what was occurring and the right brain did, the limbic system also "knew" what was occurring to have the affectual engagement of the autonomic system. It became clear that many things can happen affectually without all of the neocortex being aware of what is going on.

Emotional Valence

Humans' intellects are often not formally conscious of much that goes on within them. This is no great insight to psychotherapists who emphasize the unconscious. Kihlstrom[22] states, "People may reach conclusions about events—for example, their emotional valence—and act on these judgments without being able to articulate the reasoning by which they were reached." Behavioral activity can tell us often about the inner state of another or ourselves. For example, dogs have a visible "limbicometer," their tails. Whether a dog's tail wags or not, with what frequency, and with what vigor all tell us about the dog's feelings.

Probably the closest thing to a limbicometer in humans is the smile. In this context, a smile is the limbic recognition of reality before fully understood by intellect (neocortex). If someone smiles and is asked why he or she smiled or what made him or her smile, that person often cannot specify or will give an intellectual response not derived from the present smile-reality.

The traditional view of affective coloring on incoming sensory material has been that the incoming sensory signals went to thalamic relay nuclei and therein radiated to sensory receiving areas as, for example, occipital visual Brodmann area 18. From there, over many synapses, the now modified signal went to subcortical (limbic) regions, which attached an emotional tone to the signal (schematized in Figure 3-1). It is now clear, mainly through the work of LeDoux,[23] that pathways exist from sensory receptors that bypass the neocortex and wend straightway to the limbic system, specifically, the amygdala (Figure 3-2). If this bypass exists in humans, it could reshape current thinking about how the affective processing of incoming sensory material can be an unconscious function of the brain.

Hippocampus

The hippocampus has been termed a cognitive map by O'Keefe and Nadel.[24] The importance of the hippocampus in memory is well known since the hippocampectomies in the patient H.M., who ever since this surgery has been unable to lay down new memories.[25] Knowing one's place in the world, both internally and externally, appears to be another function of the hippocampus.

Because humans are an altricial species, that is, the infant undergoes much maturation after birth,

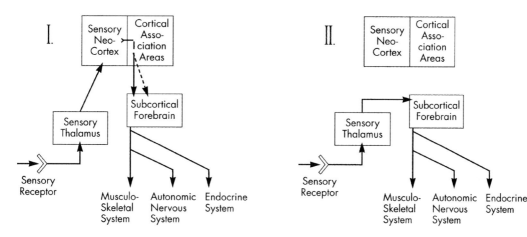

Figure 3-2. Diagrams of (I) the traditional perceptual process and (II) a recently found variant of the perceptual process. (Modified from LeDoux JE: Sensory systems and emotion: a model of affective processing, *Integr Psychiatry*, 4:237–248, 1986.)

there is a relatively enormous openness to environmental influence compared to the nonaltricial species. Some fibers to the hippocampus do not mature for years after birth. Although "the wires and the juices" have much to do in setting the individual's emotional life, it is this long maturation process that allows culture, teaching, and so forth to shape that emotional life.

The limbic system is involved with motivation, attention, emotion, and memory. It can also be looked at in an animal way or a human way. In a cavalier fashion, it is often said that the limbic system mediates the four Fs—fear, food, fight, and fornication. This is a view from the Olympian hill of the cerebral cortex. A more noble formulation is that the limbic system mediates gender role, territoriality, and bonding.[26] For example, as far as territoriality is concerned, the limbic system mediates how one feels about family, rights, "keep off the grass," and other areas that have a spatial or relational component. In bonding, the limbic system mediates strongly how one bonds to one's spouse, family, father, country, flag, religion—in sum, loyalty. If this is true, most of the actions performed daily are already set limbically before humans neocortically intellectualize, and these three elements constitute much of the work of the psychiatrist.

The neocortex, with Broca's area, is the substrate for the lyrics or the words of what one thinks and feels. The limbic system has no Broca's area, has no words, but is the locus of the music of one's affect. Psychiatric interviewers hear what people verbalize, but often much more important is what one sees, what one feels, and what one hears as the affective music or tune from the person interviewed.

Amygdala

Some general agreement exists that the amygdala is concerned with motivation in the organism. The classic view is that the amygdala attaches motivational significance to the information elaborated by the neocortex.[27] Kagan et al.[28] consider increased arousal in the amygdala to be a contributor to shyness in childhood and social avoidance in adults. A newer theory of how the amygdala functions in humans is proposed by Gloor of Montreal following his experience with implanted electrodes in the human limbic system:

I would like to propose that the site where this [the coalescence of experimental mechanisms] occurs is the limbic system, and in particular the amygdala. Visual and auditory perceptual data are first analyzed in the appropriate areas of the temporal neocortex. . . . Finally, the information is conveyed to the amygdala where affective tone is attached to it. I would like to suggest that this involvement of affect is necessary to make a perception or memory emerge into consciousness, thus enabling it to be experienced as an event "one is living or has lived through."[29]

Therefore, according to this proposal, it is primarily the amygdala and its role in affect that affects the brain's consciousness of the material. Thus the limbic system is responsible for what enters into consciousness—a long noble step from the Four Fs.

A crude analogy may be helpful in how the neocortex and limbic system may work in the human. If one views a slide of Death Valley, one perceives that slide neocortically in the primary visual area pretty much the same as all other humans. Limbically, however, one could have at least two different feeling states on seeing the slide. One could have a subtitle or label at the bottom of the slide reading "the sparse grandeur of the West," or at the other end of the spectrum one could label the Death Valley slide as "the devil's fiery hell." The limbic system supplies the personalized affective tone when information is perceived or recalled.

Clinical Aspect of the Limbic System

At the bedside, one can use the so-called Frank Jones story to test acute confusional states. The supposition here is that the neocortex is usually affected in confusional states earlier and more severely than the limbic system. Let us say that the psychiatrist has been called because there is suspicion of a postoperative acute confusional state. One of the things he can do is say to the patient, "Now, sir, how does this strike you? I have a friend, Frank Jones, whose feet are so big he has to put his pants on over his head." If the limbic system is grossly intact, the patient will smile or chuckle. There are usually three responses with patients at the bedside. With type 1—the normal response—the patient usually chuckles indicating that he "gits it" and when he's asked, "Can he do it?" he usually says, "No, it's goofy. . . . The crotch—he can't go up on both sides," meaning that he also "gets it," that is, he has intellectual insight. A type 2 answer usually indicates that the limbic system is intact, but the neocortex is impaired. When told the Frank Jones pants story, the patient usually smiles and laughs and gives the limbic music that there's something funny to it. When asked, however, "Can he do it?" he will usually say something like, "Well, whatever you say, doc," or "Well, if he tries hard enough." This type 2 patient "gits it" but does not "get it."

The type 3 response indicates that both the limbic system and the neocortex are impaired. When one tells the patient the story about putting the pants on over the head, the patient does not smile, shows no facial quizzicalness, gives no special limbic response at all, and then when one asks, "Can he do it?" the unsmiling answer usually is something like, "Well, doctor, he must have to have special shoes but sure he can do." He neither "gits it" nor "gets it." He has limbic and neocortical confusion. With a type 3 response, one has to suspect an underlying dementia.

Quietly confused hospital patients are frequently seen after surgery. They are often not recognized by the treating physician as having an impairment of higher cortical function. The impairment is usually missed because the patient is alert and gets along well with the physician. The patient smiles and says he's doing okay, but if he were pressed as to exactly where he is, or what year it is, he would not know. The point to emphasize here is that the limbic system, even without neocortical clarity, can take humans quite far in everyday life, and it is probably that which really gets us through the day. That is, the limbic system and not the higher intellectual activity of the neocortex, save for the primary motor and sensory areas, is where most of man's mental activity occurs. Much resistance to this notion exists, especially from intellectuals, theologians, humanists, and others who, perhaps unconsciously, have a bias against the limbic system because it mediates those raw, crude, baser elements of man, that is, the emotions.

Not long ago, I was asked to see a patient who was in the Massachusetts Eye and Ear Infirmary for presumed hysterical blindness. She had had an extensive workup, including visually evoked potentials, and no clinical findings were found to support an organic lesion. Unfortunately the diagnosis of a conversion disorder is often made without primary data for the diagnosis, but only on secondary, substantive corollary data from the psychosocial realm. This woman had quite a bit of psychosocial perturbation having to do with a violent husband and an appearance in court. In fact, the day she was seen, she was to have appeared in court against her husband, but "unfortunately" she was hospitalized.

As I stood before the patient and interviewed her I noticed that she looked away from me. Gradually I moved over in front of her again as I was talking and noticed that gradually her eyes moved off to the other side, looking away again. I continued to do this, moving in front of her gaze several times, and she always shifted her gaze. I performed the usual test of threatening her eyes with my hand. She did not blink. I then moved over in front of her gaze again and as I continued to speak I put both of my hands on the side of my head, contorted my face, and wiggled my fingers as children do. (The incongruity of finger wiggling and serious physician's voice should evoke some response in the normal patient.) There was a brief, slight smile on her lips, and her eyes shifted away again. I repeated this maneuver several times, and each time it was apparent that the patient revealed a slight smile, which immediately disappeared. Then it was clear: This woman sees. My interpretation of what happened is that the patient perceived in the occipital cortex my funny business with the hands and screwing-up of my face but heard in her auditory cortex a serious physician's voice. Before she could employ "neocortical squelch," her limbic system assigned a valence[29] to the incongruity of voice and pantomime, thus activating, presumably, the nucleus accumbens[30]— the limbic basal ganglion[31]—and evoking a slight smile that appeared just slightly out of her immediate neocortical control.

Conclusion

There are several points to emphasize:

1. The use of the term *limbic system* here is not hard, scientific usage; it partakes of metaphor.

2. The limbic system can be helpful in understanding the so-called rift between mind and body.
3. The stuff of clinical psychiatry is primarily mediated by the limbic system and not by the nonsensory structures of the neocortex.
4. *Limbic music* is a term that denotes the existential, clinical, "raw feel" emanating from the patient. It is a more true rendering of the patient's clinical state than articulate speech. Limbic music never lies.

References

1. Mesulam MM: *Patterns in behavioral neuroanatomy: association areas, the limbic system, and hemispheric specialization.* In Mesulam MM, editor: *Principles of behavioral neurology,* Philadelphia, 1985, FA Davis.
2. Brodal A: *Neurological anatomy,* ed 2, New York, 1969, Oxford University Press.
3. Descartes R: *Discourse on method of rightly conducting the reason and seeking for truth in the sciences, 1637.* In Adam C, Tannery P, translators-editors: *Works of Descartes,* 13 vols, Paris, 1897–1913.
4. Brown TM: *Descartes, dualism and psychosomatic medicine.* In Byrum WF, Porter R, Shepherd M, editors: *The anatomy of madness,* vol 1, New York, 1982, Tavistock.
5. Descartes R: *Objections and replies to objections.* In Adam C, Tannery P, translators-editors: *Works of Descartes,* vol 7, Paris, 1897–1913.
6. Broca PP: Perte de parole, ramolissement chronique et destruction du lobe anterieur gauche du cerveau, *Bull Soc Anthropol Paris* 2:235–238, 1861.
7. Broca P: Des circonvolutions cérébrales: le grand lobe limbique dans la serie des mammiferes, *Rev Anthropol* 1:385–498, 1878.
8. Papez JW: A proposed mechanism of emotion, *Arch Neural Psychiatry* 38:725–743, 1937.
9. MacLean PD: *Challenges of the Papez heritage.* In Livingston KE, Hornykievicz O, editors: *Limbic mechanisms,* New York, 1976, Plenum.
10. Nieuwenhuys SR, Voogd J, Van Huijzen CHR: *The human central nervous system,* New York, 1979, Springer-Verlag.
11. MacLean PD: Psychosomatic disease and the "visceral brain": recent developments bearing on the Papez theory of emotion, *Psychosom Med* 11:338–353, 1949.
12. MacLean PD: Some psychiatric implications of physiological studies on frontotemporal portion of limbic system (visceral brain) EEG, *Clin Neurophysiol* 4:407–418, 1952.
13. Nauta WJH: *Connections of the frontal lobe with the limbic system.* In Laitinen LV, Livingston KE, editors: *Surgical approaches in psychiatry,* Baltimore, 1973, University Park Press.
14. Nauta WJH, Domesick VB: *Neural associations of the limbic system.* In Beckman AL, editor: *The neural basis of behavior,* New York, 1982, Spectrum.
15. White LE: A morphologic concept of the limbic lobe, *Int Rev Neurobiol* 8:1–34, 1965.
16. MacLean PD: *A triune concept of the brain and behaviour,* Toronto, 1973, University of Toronto.
17. Swanson LW: *The hippocampus and the concept of the limbic system.* In Seifert W, editor: *Neurobiology of the hippocampus,* New York, 1983, Academic Press.
18. Nauta WJH, Feirtag M: *Affect and motivation: the limbic system.* In Nauta WJH, Feirtag M, editors: *Fundamental neuroanatomy,* New York, 1986, W.H. Freeman Co.
19. Lazarus RS: *Thoughts on the relations between emotion and cognitions.* In Scherer KR, Ekman P, editors: *Approaches to emotion,* Hillsdale, NJ, 1984, Lawrence Erlbaum Associates.
20. Zajonc RB: Feeling and thinking: preferences need no inferences, *Am Psychol* 35:151–175, 1980.
21. Zajonc RB: *On primary of affect.* In Scherer KR, Ehman P, editors: *Approaches to emotion,* Hillsdale, NJ, 1984, Lawrence Erlbaum Associates.
22. Kihlstrom JF: The cognitive unconscious, *Science* 237:1445–1452, 1987.
23. LeDoux JE: Sensory systems and emotion: a model of affective processing, *Integr Psychiatry,* 4:237–248, 1976.
24. O'Keefe J, Nadel L: *The hippocampus as a cognitive map,* New York, 1978, Oxford University Press.
25. Scoville WB, Milner B: Loss of recent memory after bilateral hippocampal lesion, *J Neural Neurosurg Psychiatry* 6:211–213, 1957.
26. Henry JP, Stephens PM: *Stress, health, and the social environment,* New York, 1977, Springer-Verlag.
27. Gloor P, Olivier A, Quesnay LF: *The role of the amygdala in the expression of psychic phenomena in temporal lobe seizures.* In Ben-Ari Y, editor: *The amygdaloid complex,* New York, 1981, Elsevier.
28. Kagan J, Reznick JS, Snidman N: Biological bases of childhood shyness, *Science* 240:167–171, 1988.
29. Gloor P: *Role of the human limbic system in perception, memory and affect: lessons from temporal lobe epilepsy.* In Doane BK, Livingston KF, editors: *The limbic system,* New York, 1986, Raven Press.
30. Graybiel AM: Input-output anatomy of the basal ganglia, in Basal Ganglia. In Barbeau A, editor: Health and disease, Soc Neurosci, Toronto, 1976.
31. Mogenson GJ, Jones DL, Yim CY: From motivation to action: functional interface between the limbic system and the motor system, *Prog Neurobiol* 14:69–97, 1980.

Chapter 4

Functional Neuroanatomy and the Neurologic Examination

Anthony P. Weiss, M.D.
Stephan Heckers, M.D.

The brain is a complex and mysterious organ. Sealed away in its cranial vault, it is immune from the poking, prodding, visualizing, and auscultating that are central to the examination of other organs. The assessment of the brain and its peripheral extensions requires an indirect approach, one that evaluates the integrity of its functional capacity. Because there are many faculties associated with the brain, this functional assessment is lengthy and complex. One component of this evaluation is the neurologic examination, which can intimidate both medical students and seasoned physicians alike. As a result, the neurologic examination is all too often omitted by the busy clinician, with the entire examination summarized as "grossly intact."

For the psychiatric consultant, the neurologic examination is an important component of every patient evaluation for several reasons. First, psychiatric symptoms (affective, behavioral, or cognitive) may result directly from underlying neurologic damage (e.g., stroke causing mood lability). It is the associated sensory-motor findings on examination that will uncover the root cause of these symptoms. Second, psychiatric symptoms are commonly seen in the context of neurologic disorders (e.g., depression in Parkinson's disease). In some cases, the psychiatric symptoms predate or predominate over the other features of the illness; a thorough examination by the psychiatrist may

therefore lead to early recognition and treatment. Third, knowledge of the neurologic examination is crucial in distinguishing "real" neurologic deficits from simulated deficits associated with conversion disorders or malingering. The consultation psychiatrist is often called on to clarify this diagnostic dilemma. Finally, the psychiatrist must be aware of the numerous ways in which psychotropic medications can affect the sensory and motor systems of the brain (e.g., dystonias and other movement disorders), and be capable of assessing the severity of these adverse effects.

In this chapter we hope to provide the consulting psychiatrist with both a theoretic and pragmatic framework for the neurologic examination. First, we introduce a systematic overview of functional neuroanatomy, examining at a basic level the actual role of the nervous system in the human, and providing a simplified approach to the otherwise unimaginable complexity of billions of interconnected neurons. Then we provide an outline for the neurologic examination itself, discussing the rationale for each component, and providing a few clinically relevant pointers. By enumerating the main components of the standard examination and attempting to relate them to the anatomic constructs developed herein, we hope to provide an organization to help in both the understanding and the recollection of each aspect of the examination.

Functional Neuroanatomy

Why do we have a nervous system? What is the reason for its complexity in humans? By addressing these questions we gain a greater understanding, not only of the nervous system as a whole, but also the component parts of this system.

At its most basic level, the nervous system allows us to interact with the external world, serving as a bridge between the environment and our internal mental and physical worlds. Put another way, the nervous system allows us to respond in some fashion to environmental stimuli. In simpler organisms, there is little or no gap between stimulus and response, allowing little or no variability of response to a specific stimulus. In humans, however, there is a large evaluation step, which allows for a carefully chosen response to a stimulus, one that may be influenced by the situational context.

Using an information-processing model, we can map these concepts onto three distinct steps: *input* of sensory information through perceptual modules, the internal integration and *evaluation* of this information, and the production of a *response*. These steps are carried out by four main anatomic systems within the brain: the *thalamus*, the *cortex*, the *medial temporal lobe*, and the *basal ganglia* (Figure 4-1).

Sensory organs provide information about physical attributes of incoming information. Details of physical attributes (e.g., temperature, sound frequency, or color) are conveyed through multiple segregated channels within each perceptual module. Information then passes through the thalamus, which serves as the gateway to cortical processing for all sensory data. Specifically, it is the relay nuclei (ventral posterior lateral, medial geniculate, and lateral geniculate) that convey sensory information from the sensory organs to the appropriate areas of primary sensory cortex (i.e., S1, A1, or V1) (Figure 4-2).

The first step in the integration and evaluation of incoming stimuli occurs in unimodal association areas of the cortex, where physical attributes of one sensory domain are linked together. A second level of integration is reached in multimodal association areas, including regions within the parietal lobe and prefrontal cortex, which link together the physical attributes from different sensory domains. A third level of integration is provided by input from limbic and paralimbic regions of the brain, including the cingulate cortex and regions of the medial temporal lobe (hippocampus and amygdala). It is at this third level of integration that the brain creates a representation of experience that has the spatio-temporal resolution and full complexity of the outside world, imbued with emotion and viewed in the context of prior experience. Evaluation and interpretation involves the comparison of new information with previously stored information and current expectations or desires. This allows the brain to classify information as new or old, threatening or non-threatening.

Based on the result of evaluation and interpretation, the brain then creates a response, most often through motor action. The regions involved in generating this response include motor cortex, motor nuclei of the thalamus, the basal ganglia, and the cerebellum. The basal ganglia, which includes the striatum (caudate + putamen) and the globus pallidus, is charged with a role of integrating and coordinating this motor output. The striatum receives input from the motor cortex and it projects to the globus pallidus. The globus pallidus in turn relays the neostriatal input to the thalamus. The thalamus then projects back to the cortical areas that gave rise to the cortico-striatal projections, thereby

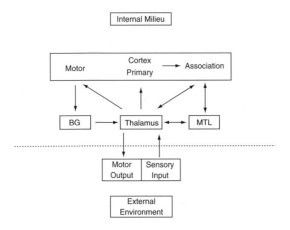

Figure 4-1. Basic circuitry of information processing. *BG*, Basal ganglia; *MTL*, medial temporal Idx.

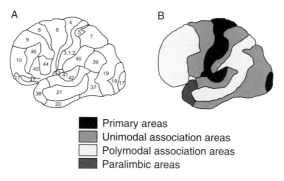

Primary areas
Unimodal association areas
Polymodal association areas
Paralimbic areas

Figure 4-2. Functional role of areas in the human cerebral cortex. (*A*) Map of cytoarchitectonic areas according to Brodmann. The parcellation of the cortical mantle into distinct areas is based on the microscopic analysis of neurons in the six layers of the cortex.(*B*) Map of functional areas according to Mesulam. The primary sensory areas (visual = area 17; auditory = areas 41–42; somatosensory = areas 3, 1, 2) and the primary motor area 4 are indicated in black. The association areas, dedicated to one stream of information processing (visual – areas 18–19, 20, 37; auditory – area 22; somatosensory = areas 5, 7, 40; motor = areas 6, 44), are indicated in dark gray. The polymodal association areas, where all sensory modalities converge, are indicated in light gray. The temporal pole is part of the paralimbic areas, which occupy large regions on the medial surface of the brain (i.e., cingulate cortex and parahippocampal cortex). (*A*) from Brodmann K: *Vergleichende lokalisationslehre der grosshirnrinde in ihren prinzipien dargestellt auf grund des zellenbaues*, Leipzig, Germany 1909, JA Barth; (*B*) from Mesulam M-M: *Principles of behavioral neurology*, Philadelphia, 1985, FA Davis.

closing the cortico-striato-pallido-thalamo-cortical loop. This loop is thought to be the means by which motor control is enacted; damage to regions within this loop lead to such disorders as Parkinson's disease and Huntington's disease.

The Neurologic Examination

The neurologic examination is a set of steps designed to probe the input, integration/evaluation, and output domains of information processing. In this section we provide an overview of the examination, using this framework. Our aim is to demystify the examination by presenting the rationale for its component parts. The examination presented here is not all encompassing; the reader is referred to standard texts of neurology for complete details.

Input

Sensory information enters the central nervous system (CNS) through two routes: spinal nerves and cranial nerves. The former handle tactile information presented to the body, and the latter handle tactile information presented to the face and each of the remaining special senses (vision, hearing, smell, and taste).

Peripheral Sensory Examination

Peripheral sensation allows tactile exploration of our environment. Even the most thorough examiner could not test every square inch of the body for intact sensation, nor would this be necessary. Knowledge of the full sensory examination is important for the patient with a focal sensory complaint, and the reader is referred to other texts for detailed information on this peripheral nerve examination.[1–9] The main sensory modalities include the following:

1. **Pain:** Tested by pinprick (using disposable sterile pins).
2. **Temperature:** Tested by touching the skin with a cold metal object (tuning fork).
3. **Light touch:** Tested by simply brushing the patient's skin with your hand or a moving wisp of cotton.
4. **Vibration sense:** Tested by applying a "buzzing" tuning fork to the distal lower extremities.

5. **Proprioception:** Best tested by the Romberg's maneuver (can be assessed during gait observation). Ask the patient to stand with his or her feet as close together as possible, while still maintaining stability. Ask the patient to close his or her eyes while assuring the patient that you will not let him or her fall. The patient with poor proprioception will begin to sway and lose balance after closing his or her eyes.

Sensory Cranial Nerves (I, II, V, VII, VIII)

Olfactory Nerve (Cranial Nerve I)

Testing of the first cranial nerve is almost uniformly neglected, with the entire cranial nerve examination often described as "II-XII within normal limits." This notation not only indicates little regard for the first cranial nerve, but also communicates little about the individual features of the examination.

The first cranial nerve runs along the orbital surface of the frontal lobe, an area that is otherwise clinically silent. Lesions in this area (e.g., frontal lobe meningioma) may produce unilateral anosmia, occasionally as a unitary symptom. Routine testing of smell is therefore quite important. Carrying a small vial of coffee is a simple and convenient method for testing smell. Each nostril should be tested separately.

Optic Nerve (Cranial Nerve II)

The optic nerve and its posterior radiations run the entire length of the brain and produce different patterns of symptoms and signs depending on where they are compromised. A thorough visual examination can therefore be quite informative; it involves five components:

1. **Funduscopic examination:** The optic nerve is the only nerve that can be visualized directly. The physician should take advantage of this fact in assessing its integrity. A good funduscopic examination also reveals much about the systemic vascular system, and it is a critical guide to the presence of increased intracranial pressure.

2. **Visual acuity:** Testing of visual acuity (i.e., the actual strength of vision) is frequently ignored in the adult patient. This is unfortunate because poor vision can profoundly impair a patient's functioning and is often reversible with corrective lenses or surgery. Acuity should be assessed in each eye separately while wearing current corrective lenses.

3. **Pupillary measurement:** Pupillary size represents the delicate balance between sympathetic and parasympathetic input to the cilliary muscles of the eye. The presence of abnormally large or small pupils reflects an imbalance, and may be an important sign of disease. Similarly, an inequality in pupillary size (anisocoria) can be an important hallmark of a severe intracranial pathologic condition. Each pupil should be measured in millimeters, with measurements clearly documented for future reference.

4. **Pupillary reaction:** The direct and consensual pupillary reaction to light, and the near reaction (accommodation), should be tested routinely. This assesses any damage in either the afferent or efferent pathways that compose the pupillary response. A penlight and close observation are all that are necessary.

5. **Confrontational visual fields:** As noted previously, the visual system runs from the retina to the occipital cortex, involving a substantial area of the CNS. Lesions anywhere along this pathway lead to visual field cuts. Importantly, the patient is almost never aware of this abnormality of vision; careful testing is therefore required to elucidate it. Sit directly in front of the patient, and have him or her look in your eyes. Test each eye separately by bringing an object (pin or wiggling finger) into each visual quadrant. For the patient who is unable to cooperate in this fashion, simply having him or her count fingers displayed in each quadrant is another option.

Trigeminal Nerve (Cranial Nerve V)

The sensory component of the trigeminal nerve provides tactile sense to the face. As with sensory testing in general (see previous text), testing sensory integrity of the face can be a frustrating exercise if the examiner insists on precision.

Unless the patient has a specific sensory complaint (e.g., a numb chin or facial pain), thorough testing of all sensory modalities is probably unnecessary. Testing light touch (by stroking the face with your fingers) or temperature sensitivity (using a cold metal tuning fork) is usually adequate. Asking the patient to "quantify" the degree of difference (e.g., "If this side is a dollar, how much is this side?") is generally not a fruitful exercise. Simply asking, "Does this feel normal on both sides?" saves time and will generally detect any abnormalities worth further investigation.

The trigeminal nerve also provides the input for the corneal reflex, the direct and the consensual blink seen in response to corneal irritation. Although testing for the corneal reflex can be helpful in localization of brainstem dysfunction (usually in the comatose patient), it is unfortunately both nonspecific and insensitive. It is therefore not done routinely.

Facial Nerve (Cranial Nerve VII)

The sensory component of the facial nerve (chorda tympani) transmits taste from the anterior two thirds of the tongue, running from the taste buds to the nucleus of the tractus solitarius in the medulla. Testing this aspect of the facial nerve involves the application of a sweet, sour, or salty solution (via a cotton tipped swab) to the outstretched tongue. The yield of this component of the examination in the patient without specific gustatory complaints is minimal.

Acoustic Nerve (Cranial Nerve VIII)

In addition to its role in the maintenance of equilibrium (via the vestibular branch) the eighth cranial nerve is the primary input channel for auditory information. The acoustic nerve carries information from the hair cells in the organ of Corti, traveling through the internal auditory meatus to the pontomedullary junction of the brainstem. For the consulting psychiatrist, the examination of auditory function can be kept to a cursory check, but should be included, particularly in geriatric patients. Rubbing fingers together near the ear may bring out high-pitched hearing deficits, a finding typically associated with presbyacusis.

Integration and Evaluation

Even the simplest unicellular organisms have means by which they can sense and react to the environment. These responses are automatic and limited; the same stimulus results in the same response regardless of context. There are a number of these automatic or reflexive responses that can be tested in the human, some of which have already been discussed as part of the sensory evaluation (e.g., the pupillary light reflex and the corneal reflex). Three additional sets of reflexes are commonly probed in a standard neurologic examination:

1. **Proprioceptive reflexes:** Proprioceptive reflexes, also known as deep tendon reflexes (DTRs), are based on the simple reflex arcs that are activated by stretching (or tapping). Because they are influenced by the descending corticospinal tracts, DTRs can provide important information on the integrity of this pathway at several levels. The reader is likely familiar with the methods used to elicit the five major DTRs: biceps, triceps, brachioradialis, quadriceps (knee), and Achilles (ankle). The grading of each reflex is on a 4-point scale, with a score of 2 (2 +) designated as normal.
2. **Nociceptive reflexes:** Nociceptive reflexes are based on reflex arcs located in the skin (rather than muscle tendons) and are therefore elicited by scratching or stroking. These include the abdominal reflexes, cremasteric reflex, and anal wink, none of which is extensively used clinically. The major nociceptive reflex of clinical value is the plantar reflex. Stroking the sole of the foot should elicit plantar flexion of the toes. Babinski's sign, marked by an extensor response (i.e., dorsiflexion) of the toes, often with fanning of the toes and flexion of the ankle, is seen in pyramidal tract disease. It has become one of the most famous eponymic signs in all of medicine.
3. **Primitive reflexes (release reflexes):** Primitive reflexes are present at birth but disappear in early infancy. Their reappearance later in life is abnormal and is often reflective of frontal lobe disease. Amongst others, they include the grasp reflex (stroking the patient's palm will lead to an automatic clutching of your finger between

his thumb and index finger) and the snout reflex (gentle tapping over the patient's upper lip will cause a puckering of the lips. Note that this may also elicit a suck response, or a turning of the head toward the stroking stimulus (root reflex).

The Mental Status Examination

The brains of higher mammals, particularly in the human, have the added capacity to integrate sensory information across domains, evaluate this information, and react in a manner consistent with past experience, current context, or future expectations. The ability to use these higher-level faculties is often considered as part of the mental status examination. For routine purposes, the following four components compose an adequate examination. Unlike other features of the neurologic examination, it is important that these components be done in order, because basic functions must be intact to perform more complex tasks.

1. **Level of consciousness:** Consciousness lies on a continuum from full alertness to coma. Although the two extremes are generally obvious, the middle ground of attentional deficit can be subtle. Because inattention is a hallmark of delirium (an acute confusional state), a common and emergent medical condition, attention should be tested in all patients. Sustained attention is also a critical component for all other cognitive functioning. Some common tests of attention include serial 7s (ask the patient to subtract 7 from 100, and then continue to serially subtract 7 from the remainder) and digit span. (Have the patient repeat a randomly presented list of digits. A normal capacity is between five and seven digits. Alternatively, have the patient spell a five-letter word [e.g., *world*] backward.)

2. **Language:** Language is the means by which we present our thoughts to each other. Like other cognitive functions, language can be extraordinarily complex, with entire texts of aphasiology dedicated to its study. In general, the following three simple questions allow the examiner to draw valid conclusions about language in the individual patient (Figure 4-3):

Type	Repetition	Comprehension	Speech
Global	Impaired	Impaired	Nonfluent
Wernicke's	Impaired	Impaired	Fluent
Broca's	Impaired	Intact	Nonfluent
Conduction	Impaired	Intact	Fluent
Transcortical			
Motor	Intact	Intact	Nonfluent
Sensory	Intact	Impaired	Fluent

Figure 4-3. Differential diagnosis of the main types of aphasias.

a. **Is the language *fluent* or *nonfluent*?** Independent of the actual words, does the speech sound like a language? Loss of the normal inflection and spacing of normal speech leads to nonfluent language production.

b. **Is *comprehension* normal or abnormal?** Does the patient seem to understand what you are saying? A request to complete a one to three-step command (although complex commands may test more than just receptive language function) best assesses this. Asking simple "yes/no" questions (e.g., "Were you born in Mexico?" or "Are we in the kitchen?") is another common method.

c. **Is *repetition* normal or abnormal?** Have the patient repeat a phrase such as "no ifs, ands, or buts." This particular phrase is quite sensitive, given the difficulty of repeating conjunctions.

3. **Memory:** Memory function is generally divided into the following three components:

a. **Immediate recall:** Immediate recall is the ability to hold information long enough to use it (e.g., remembering a phone number given by the operator long enough to dial it). Immediate recall is heavily dependent on attention and is tested by both digit span and phrase repetition (see previous text). Asking the patient to repeat three named items (e.g., piano, monkey, and blue) is another commonly used method.

b. **Short-term memory:** Short-term memory involves the ability to store information for later use. Asking the patient to reproduce the three previously named items after a span of 2 to 5 minutes is a common test.

   c. **Long-term memory:** Long-term memory involves the recall of past events. This is nearly impossible to test accurately at the bedside, because the examiner is rarely privy to details of remote events from the patient's life. Asking about well-known national events or people (e.g., How did JFK die?) depends on the age and educational background of the patient. Accurate assessment often requires a standardized battery of questions available in full neuropsychological testing.

4. Visual-spatial skills:

   a. **Writing:** Have the patient write his or her name, address, and a sentence about the weather. Look for grammatical errors, as well as errors in spacing and overall presentation.

   b. **Clock drawing:** Have the patient fill in a circle with numbers in the form of a clock. Then ask her or him to set the hands at 10 minutes to 2. Abnormalities can occur in planning (poor spacing of numbers) or in positioning of the hands, which may belie a frontal lobe lesion. Complete absence of detail on one side of the clock (usually left) may represent a hemineglect syndrome associated with a (right) parietal lobe lesion.

Output

Although there are many potential responses to environmental stimuli, including subtle changes in the internal hormonal or neurochemical milieu, most often the response requires some type of motor output. The examination of this output can be divided into a motor (or muscular) component and a coordination component.

Motor Examination

There are three aspects evaluated in the motor examination: muscle tone, muscle bulk, and muscle strength. The three aspects may be affected separately. *Motor tone* refers to the resistance of a limb to passive movement through its normal range of motion. To examine for tone, have the

patient fully relax his or her arms and legs to allow you to determine the degree of stiffness during passive motion. An increased level of tone, noted by rigidity or spasticity, is an important finding that may belie an upper motor neuron or extrapyramidal lesion (parkinsonism).

Muscle atrophy is an important sign of lower motor neuron disease. Assessment of muscle bulk can be extraordinarily difficult, even for the seasoned clinician, because of natural variations in body habitus and the role of weightlifting or exercise (i.e., "bulking up"). Muscles that are unaffected by weightlifting or exercise (e.g., the facial muscles or the intrinsic muscles of the hand) may therefore provide the best estimate of overall muscle bulk.

In testing muscle strength, it is impractical (and unnecessary) to test each of the several hundred muscles in the human body. Should the patient have a focal motor complaint, knowledge of major muscle groups in the proximal and distal limbs becomes important. Muscle strength is graded from 0 (no motion) to 5 (normal strength).

Observation of gait is an excellent screening test for the patient without focal weakness. If the patient is able to rise briskly and independently from a seated position and walk independently, gross motor deficits can be confidently ruled out. The ability to walk on heels and toes further ensures distal lower-extremity strength. Gait must be tested in all patients, particularly in older adults, for whom falls are a life-threatening event.

Coordination

Coordination reflects the ability to orchestrate and control movement, and is crucial in the translation of movement into productive activity. Although the cerebellum probably plays the lead role in motor coordination, several other structures (e.g., basal ganglia and red nucleus) are also clearly involved.

Walking is an extraordinarily complex motor skill that requires significant coordination of the trunk and limbs. Its actual complexity makes it an ideal screening test for coordination ability. The human has a particularly narrow base when standing upright; with any degree of incoordination (ataxia), the patient needs to widen the base to remain upright. Balance becomes even more difficult when other sensory information is removed, forming the basis for Romberg's maneuver. The sensitivity of screening is further increased by having the patient walk heel-to-toe (as on a tight rope). The ability to do this smoothly and quickly rules out any major impairment in coordination.

Diadochokinesia refers to the alternating movements made possible by the paired nature of agonist and antagonist muscle activity in coordinated limb movement. Abnormalities of this function are given the lengthy label *dysdiadochokinesia*, and are detected by several simple maneuvers, including finger-to-nose, heel-to-shin, and rapid alternating movements (rapid pronation/supination of the forearm [e.g., screwing in a light bulb], finger tapping, or toe tapping). Having the patient tap out a rhythm is an excellent way to assess coordination ability. With cerebellar damage, the rhythm is poorly timed, with emphases in the wrong places.

Conclusions

The brain is an organ that is unmatched in its eloquence. Unlike the anginal grip of cardiac disease or the choking dyspnea of respiratory dysfunction, illness of the brain can send many different messages. Deciphering these messages, using the neurologic examination, can be complex, and at times bewildering. This should not discourage the practicing psychiatrist from using the examination described in this chapter as a routine part of every patient evaluation.

References

1. DeGowin RL, Brown DD: *DeGowin's diagnostic examination*, ed 7, New York, 1999, McGraw-Hill.
2. Glick TH: *Neurologic skills*, Boston, 1993, Blackwell Science.
3. Haerer AF: *DeJong's the neurologic exam*, ed 5, Philadelphia, 1992, Lippincott Williams & Wilkins.
4. Heimer L: *The human brain and spinal cord: functional neuroanatomy and dissection guide*, ed 2, New York, 1995, Springer-Verlag.
5. Lishman WA: *Organic psychiatry*, ed 3, Oxford, England, 1998, Blackwell Science.
6. Mesulam MM: *Principles of behavioral and cognitive neurology*, ed 2, Oxford, England, 2000, Oxford University Press.
7. Samuels MA: *Video textbook of neurology for the practicing physician, vol 2: the neurologic exam.* Boston, 1996, Butterworth-Heinemann.
8. Samuels MA: *The manual of neurologic therapeutics*, ed 6, Philadelphia, 1999, Lippincott Williams & Wilkins.
9. Samuels MA, Feske S, Livingstone C: *Office practice of neurology.* Philadelphia, 2003, Saunders.

Chapter 5

Diagnostic Rating Scales and Laboratory Tests

Joshua L. Roffman, M.D.
Theodore A. Stern, M.D.

Although the interview and the mental status examination compose the primary diagnostic tools in psychiatry, the use of standardized rating scales and laboratory tests provide important adjunctive data. In addition to ruling out medical and neurologic explanations for new psychiatric symptoms, the quantitative instruments described in this chapter play important roles in clarifying disease severity, identifying patients who meet subsyndromal criteria within a particular diagnosis, assessing response to treatment, and monitoring for treatment-related side effects. Neuroimaging studies, which are emerging as increasingly versatile tools for analogous reasons, also are discussed.

Diagnostic Rating Scales

Useful in a variety of settings, diagnostic rating scales translate clinical observations or patient self-assessments into objective measures. Clinically, they can screen for individuals who need treatment, evaluate the accuracy of a diagnosis, determine the severity of symptoms, or gauge the effectiveness of a given intervention. These scales are employed ubiquitously in clinical research for similar reasons (e.g., to ensure diagnostic homogeneity of subject populations). Rating instruments should demonstrate good reliability (i.e., the ability to relate consistent and reproducible information) and validity (i.e., the ability to measure what they intend to measure). Although clinician-rated instruments are generally more valid and reliable, patient-rated instruments are often more readily administered and less time-consuming. In either case, consideration should be given to the clinical consequences of their results, as well as to cultural factors that could affect performance. The following sections summarize commonly used rating scales for general psychiatric diagnosis as well as specific disorders and treatment-related conditions.

General Psychiatric Diagnostic Instruments

The Structured Clinical Interview for the *Diagnostic and Statistical Manual for Mental Disorders*, fourth edition, (SCID)[1,2] is the most commonly used diagnostic instrument in psychiatry. An introductory segment relies on open-ended questions to elucidate demographic, medical, and psychiatric histories, as well as medication use. The remainder employs standardized questions in nine modules that reflect *Diagnostic and Statistical Manual for Mental Disorders*, fourth edition (DSM-IV), criteria for most major Axis I disorders: mood episodes, psychotic symptoms, psychotic disorders, mood disorders, substance use, anxiety, somatoform disorders, eating disorders, and adjustment disorders. Based on patient responses, the rater determines the likelihood that a DSM-IV diagnosis will be met. The SCID is reliable but time-consuming; for this reason it is used primarily in research. The derivative SCID-clinical version (SCID-CV) provides a modestly simplified format that is more appropriate for clinical use. A similar, but more compact structured diagnostic interview, perhaps better suited to clinical use, is the Mini-International Neuropsychiatric Interview (MINI).[3] Also administered by the clinician, the MINI utilizes "yes/no" questions that cover the major Axis I disorders as well as antisocial personality disorder. Particular attention is also given to the risk of suicide. Following administration of a diagnostic instrument, the seven-point Clinical Global Improvement (CGI) scale may be used to determine both severity of illness (CGI-severity [S]) and degree of improvement following treatment (CGI-improvement [I]).[4] On the CGI-S, a score of 1 indicates normal, whereas a score of 7 indicates severe illness; a 1 on the CGI-I corresponds to a high degree of improvement, whereas a 7 means the patient is doing much worse.

Mood Disorders

Considered the gold standard for evaluating the severity of depression in clinical studies, the Hamilton Rating Scale for Depression (HAM-D)[5] may be used to monitor the patient's progress during treatment, after the diagnosis of major depression has been established. This clinician-administered scale exists in several versions, ranging from 6 to 31 items; answers by patients are scored from 0 to 2 or 0 to 4 and tallied to obtain an overall score. Standard scoring for the 17-item HAM-D-17 instrument, frequently used in research studies, is listed in Table 5-1. A decrease of 50% or more in the HAM-D score is often considered to indicate a positive treatment response, whereas a score of 7 or less is considered equivalent to a remission. The HAM-D was developed prior to publication of the DSM-III and does not evaluate more recent criteria for depression (e.g., anhedonia); it also favors somatic signs and symptoms and can miss atypical symptoms, such as overeating and oversleeping.

The Beck Depression Inventory (BDI)[6] is a widely used 21-item self-rating scale that can be completed in a few minutes. Scores on the BDI can be used both as a diagnostic screen and as a measure of improvement over time. For each item, patients choose from among four answers, each corresponding to a severity rating from 0 to 3. The correlation between total scores and the severity of depression is provided in Table 5-2. Although easy to administer and to score, the BDI also excludes atypical neurovegetative symptoms.

Fewer rating scales have been designed to assess mania. Two instruments for assessing manic symptoms, the Manic State Rating Scale (MSRS)[7] and Young Mania Rating Scale (Y-MRS)[8] have been designed for use on inpatient units; they demonstrate high reliability and validity. Whereas the 26-item MSRS gives extra weight to grandiosity and to paranoid-destructive symptoms, the Y-MRS examines primarily symptoms related to irritability, speech, thought content, and aggressive behavior. Neither scale has been as extensively evaluated for reliability and validity as have its counterparts geared toward depression.

Psychotic Disorders and Related Symptoms

Instruments for assessing psychotic symptoms are nearly always administered by clinicians. Two of the broader and more frequently used instruments are the Brief Psychiatric Rating Scale (BPRS)[9] and Positive and Negative Symptoms Scale (PANSS).[10] The BPRS was designed to address symptoms common to schizophrenia and other psychotic

Table 5-1. Scoring the HAM-D

Score	Interpretation
0–7	Not depressed
7–15	Mildly depressed
15–25	Moderately depressed
>25	Severely depressed

HAM-D, Hamilton Rating Scale for Depression.

Table 5-2. Scoring the BDI

Score	Interpretation
0–7	Normal
7–15	Mild depression
15–25	Moderate depression
>25	Severe depression

BDI, Beck Depression Inventory.

disorders, as well as severe mood disorders with psychotic features. Therefore items assessed include hallucinations, delusions, and disorganization, as well as hostility, anxiety, and depression. The test is relatively easy to administer and it takes about 20 to 30 minutes. The total score, which is often used to gauge the efficacy of treatment, provides a global assessment and therefore lacks the ability to track subsyndromal items (e.g., positive versus negative symptoms). Alternatively, the PANSS includes separate scales for positive and negative symptoms, as well as a scale for general psychopathology. The PANSS requires more time to administer (30 to 40 minutes); related versions for children and adolescents are also available.

More focused attention to positive and negative symptoms characterize the Scale for the Assessment of Positive Symptoms (SAPS)[11] and the Scale for the Assessment of Negative Symptoms (SANS),[12] respectively. The 30-item SAPS is organized into domains that include hallucinations, delusions, bizarre behavior, and formal thought disorder; the SANS, which includes 20 items, covers affective flattening and blunting, alogia, avolition-apathy, anhedonia-antisociality, and attentional impairment. The scales are particularly useful to document specific target symptoms and measure their response to treatment, but their proper administration requires more training than do the global scales.

The proclivity of neuroleptics to induce motoric side effects has driven the creation of standardized rating scales to assess these treatment-related conditions. The Abnormal Involuntary Movement Scale[4] is the most widely used scale to rate tardive dyskinesia. Ten items evaluate orofacial movements, limb-truncal dyskinesias, and global severity on a 5-point scale; the remaining two items rule out contributions of dental problems or dentures. The Barnes Akathisia Rating Scale[13] evaluates both objective measures of akathisia as well as subjective distress related to restlessness. Both scales are administered easily and rapidly, and may be used serially to document the effects of chronic neuroleptic use or changes in treatment.

Anxiety Disorders

A variety of rating scales are available to assess anxiety symptoms as well as specific anxiety disorders

(e.g., panic disorder, social phobia, obsessive-compulsive disorder [OCD], posttraumatic stress disorder, and generalized anxiety disorder [GAD]). Two of the more frequently used scales, both clinically and for research purposes, are described here: the Hamilton Anxiety Rating Scale (HAM-A)[14] and Yale-Brown Obsessive-Compulsive Scale (Y-BOCS).[15,16] The HAM-A provides an overall measure of anxiety with particular focus on somatic and cognitive symptoms; worry, which is hallmark of GAD, receives less attention. The clinician-administered scale consists of 14 items, and when scored does not distinguish specific symptoms of a specific anxiety disorder. A briefer six-item version, the Clinical Anxiety Scale, is also available. The most widely used scale for assessing severity of OCD symptoms, the Y-BOCS is also clinician-administered and it yields global as well as obsessive and compulsive subscale scores. Newer self-report and computer-administered versions have compared favorably to the clinician-based gold standard. Again, the Y-BOCS has proven useful both in initial assessments and as a longitudinal measure.

Substance Abuse Disorders

The CAGE Questionnaire (Table 5-3)[17] is a brief, clinician-administered tool used to screen for alcohol problems in many clinical settings. CAGE is an acronym for the four "yes-no" items in the test, which requires less than 1 minute to administer. "Yes" answers to two or more questions indicate a clinically significant alcohol problem (sensitivity has been measured at 0.78 to 0.81, specificity at 0.76 to 0.96), and positive screening suggests the need for further evaluation. A widely used scale to assess past or present clinically significant drug-related diagnoses, the Drug Abuse Screening Test[18] is a 28- or 20-item self-administered

Table 5-3. The CAGE Questionnaire

C Have you ever felt you should **C**ut down on your drinking?
A Have people **A**nnoyed you by criticizing your drinking?
G Have you ever felt bad or **G**uilty about your drinking?
E Have you ever had a drink first thing in the morning to steady your nerves or get rid of a hangover (**E**ye opener)?

instrument that takes several minutes to complete. If the subject answers "yes" to five or more questions, a drug abuse disorder is likely. The instrument includes consequences related to drug abuse (without being specific about the drug); it is most useful in settings where drug-related problems are not the patient's chief complaint.

Cognitive Disorders

Cognitive scales are useful for screening out organic causes for psychopathologic conditions, and can help the clinician determine whether more formal neuropsychological, laboratory, or neuroimaging work-ups are warranted. It is important to consider the patient's intelligence, level of education, and literacy before interpreting results. The Folstein Mini-Mental State Exam (MMSE) (Table 5-4)[19] is used ubiquitously in diagnostic interviews as well as to follow cognitive decline over time in neurodegenerative disorders. The MMSE is administered by the clinician. It includes items that test orientation to place (state, county, town, hospital, and floor) and time (year, season, month, day, and date), registration and recall of three words, attention and concentration (serial 7s or spelling the word *world* backward), language (naming two items, repeating a phrase, understanding a sentence, following a three-step command), and visual construction (copying a design). The total score ranges from 0 to

Table 5-4. Scoring the MMSE

5 points	Orientation to state, country, town, hospital, floor
5 points	Orientation to year, season, month, day, date
3 points	Registration of three words
3 points	Recall of three words after 5 minutes
5 points	Serial 7s or spelling *world* backward
2 points	Naming two items
1 points	Understanding a sentence
1 points	Writing a sentence
1 points	Repeating "No if's, and's, or but's"
3 points	Following a three-step command
1 points	Copying a design
30 points	Total

Adapted from Folstein MF, Folstein SE, McHugh PR: "Mini-mental state": A practical method for grading the cognitive state of patients for the clinician, *J Psychiatr Res* 12:189–198, 1975.

30, with a score of 24 or lower indicating possible dementia. Although highly reliable and valid, the MMSE also demonstrates less sensitivity early in the course of Alzheimer's disease and other dementing disorders.

Earlier detection of neurodegenerative disorders can be achieved with the Mattis Dementia Rating Scale (DRS).[20] Administered by a trained clinician, the DRS consists of questions in five domains: attention, initiation and perseveration, construction, conceptualization, and memory. Subscale items are presented in hierarchical fashion, with the most difficult items presented first; if the subject can perform these correctly, many of the remaining items in the section are skipped and scored as correct. The total score ranges from 0 to 144 points. In addition to early detection, the DRS can be used in some cases to differentiate dementia resulting from different neuropathologic conditions, including Alzheimer's disease, Huntington's disease, Parkinson's disease, and progressive supranuclear palsy.

A simpler, bedside assessment of general cognitive dysfunction is the Clock Drawing Test.[21] When asked to draw a clock face with the hands set to a specified time, the patient must demonstrate several cognitive processes, including auditory comprehension of the instructions, access to the semantic representation of a clock, planning ability, and visuospatial/visuomotor skills, to successfully complete the task. Although performance can be assessed informally, several structured scoring measures have been described in the literature.[21–23]

Laboratory Tests

Although primary diagnoses in psychiatry are based on clinical phenomenology, physical examination and laboratory studies are often essential to rule out organic causes in the differential diagnosis for psychiatric symptoms.[24,25] Consideration should be given to dysfunction in multiple organ systems, toxins, malnutrition, infections, vascular abnormalities, neoplasm, and other intracranial problems (Table 5-5 organizes many of these using the mnemonic VICTIMS DIE). Certain presentations are especially suggestive of an organic cause, including the onset after the age of

Table 5-5. Organic Causes for Psychiatric Symptoms, Recalled by the Mnemonic VICTIMS DIE

Vascular	Multiinfarct dementia
	Other stroke syndromes
	Hypertensive encephalopathy
	Vasculitis
Infectious	Urinary tract infection and urosepsis
	Acquired immunodeficiency syndrome
	Brain abscess
	Meningitis
	Encephalitis
	Neurosyphilis
	Tuberculosis
	Prion disease
Cancer	Central nervous system tumors (primary or metastatic)
	Endocrine tumors
	Pancreatic cancer
	Paraneoplastic syndromes
Trauma	Intracranial hemorrhage
	Traumatic brain injury
Intoxication/ withdrawal	Alcohol or other drugs
	Environmental toxins
	Psychiatric or other medications (side effects or toxic levels)
Metabolic/ nutritional	Hypoxemia
	Hyper/hyponatremia
	Hypoglycemia
	Ketoacidosis
	Uremic encephalopathy
	Hyper/hypothyroidism
	Parathyroid dysfunction
	Adrenal hypoplasia (Cushing's syndrome)
	Hepatic failure
	Wilson's disease
	Acute intermittent porphyria
	Pheochromocytoma
	Vitamin B_{12} deficiency
	Thiamine deficiency (Wernicke-Korsakoff syndrome)
	Niacin deficiency (pellagra)
Structural Degenerative	Normal pressure hydrocephalus
	Alzheimer's disease
	Parkinson's disease
	Huntington's disease
	Pick's disease
Immune (autoimmune)	Systemic lupus erythematosus
	Rheumatoid arthritis
	Sjögren's syndrome
Epilepsy	Partial complex seizures/temporal lobe epilepsy
	Postictal or intraictal states

40 years, history of chronic medical illness, or a precipitous course. Laboratory tests are also important for following levels of certain psychiatric medications and for surveillance for treatment-related side effects. The following sections describe routine screening tests as well as specific serum, urine, cerebrospinal fluid (CSF), and other studies that are considered in the determination of the differential diagnosis and in treatment monitoring. The use of electroencephalography and neuroimaging studies is also described later in this chapter vis-à-vis diagnosis of neuropsychiatric conditions.

Routine Screening

The decision to order a screening test should take into account its ease of administration, the likelihood of an abnormal result, and the clinical implications of abnormal results (including management). Although no clear consensus exists about which tests to order in a routine screening battery for new-onset psychiatric symptoms, in practice routine screening tests include the complete blood cell (CBC) count; serum chemistries; erythrocyte sedimentation rate; and levels of vitamin B_{12}, folate, thyroid-stimulating hormone, and rapid plasma reagen (RPR). Often urine and serum toxicology screens, liver function tests (LFTs), and urinalysis are added as well.

Psychosis and Delirium

Evaluation of new-onset psychosis or delirium must include a full medical and neurologic workup; potential causes for mental status changes include central nervous system lesions, infections, intoxication, medication effects, metabolic abnormalities, and alcohol or benzodiazepine withdrawal. If an organic causal agent is not clearly established by virtue of the history, physical examination, and the screening studies listed previously, additional testing should include an electroencephalogram (EEG) and neuroimaging. Blood or urine cultures should be sent if there is suspicion for a systemic infectious process. Lumbar puncture is indicated (once an intracranial lesion has been ruled out) if patients present with fever, headache, photophobia, or meningeal symptoms; in addition to sending routine CSF studies (e.g., opening pressure, appearance, Gram's stain, culture, cell counts, and levels of protein and glucose), depending on the clinical circumstances, consideration should also be given to specialized markers (e.g., antigens for cryptococcus, herpes simplex virus, Lyme disease; acid-fast staining; and cytologic examination for leptomeningeal metastases). With appropriate clinical suspicion, other tests to consider include serum heavy metals (e.g., lead, mercury, aluminum, arsenic, and copper), ceruloplasmin (which is decreased in Wilson's disease), and bromides.

Patients receiving certain antipsychotic medications (e.g., thioridazine, droperidol, pimozide, and ziprasidone [as well as haloperidol when high-dose intravenous administration is required for the treatment of agitated delirious patients]) should have a baseline electrocardiogram (ECG) as well as periodic follow-ups to monitor for QTc prolongation. Serum levels of antipsychotics can be useful both as a measure of compliance and to monitor for drug interactions (e.g., carbamazepine can decrease haloperidol levels).[26] The atypical antipsychotic clozapine causes agranulocytosis in 1% to 2% of patients taking the medication, necessitating weekly CBC testing for the first 6 months, and biweekly testing after this for the duration of treatment. If the white blood cell (WBC) count drops significantly (by more than 3000), or in the case of mild leukopenia (3000 to 5000), the patient should be monitored closely and biweekly CBCs checked; if the WBC count drops below 2000 or the granulocyte count drops below 1500 cells, the medication should be stopped, and the patient should be admitted to the hospital, where daily CBC counts should be obtained. Clozapine is permanently discontinued if the WBC count falls below 2000 or the granulocyte count drops below 1000.

Other adverse neuropsychiatric side effects include the risk of seizure, changes in prolactin levels, and the onset of neuroleptic malignant syndrome (NMS). A baseline EEG can be helpful in patients taking more than 600 mg/day of clozapine because of an increased incidence of seizures at higher doses.

Patients taking typical antipsychotics and risperidone should have prolactin levels checked if they manifest galactorrhea. NMS should be suspected in patients who develop high fever, delirium, muscle rigidity and elevated serum creatine phosphokinase levels while taking antipsychotic medications.

Mood Disorders and Affective Symptoms

Although depressive symptoms often reflect a primary mood disorder, they may also be associated with a number of medical conditions, including thyroid dysfunction, folate deficiency, Addison's disease, rheumatoid arthritis, systemic lupus erythematosus, pancreatic cancer, Parkinson's disease and other neurodegenerative disorders. Clinical suspicion for any of these disorders should drive further laboratory testing, in addition to the routine screening battery listed previously. First-break manic symptoms warrant especially careful medical and neurologic evaluation, and patients who present with these symptoms often receive a laboratory work-up analogous to that described for a new-onset psychosis.

Patients who receive pharmacotherapy for mood disorders often require serum levels of the drug being prescribed (and its metabolite) to be checked periodically, as well baseline and follow-up screening for treatment-induced organ damage. Tricyclic antidepressants (TCAs) can cause cardiac conduction abnormalities, including prolongation of the PR, QRS, or QT intervals; patients taking TCAs should have a baseline ECG, especially if they have a history of cardiac pathologic conditions. TCA levels are useful in several clinical situations, including when the patient reports side effects at low doses, or in geriatric or medically ill patients, or when there is a question of compliance, or an urgent clinical situation that requires rapid achievement of therapeutic levels (e.g., in a severely suicidal patient). Steady-state levels are usually not achieved for 5 days after starting the medication or changing the dose; TCA trough levels should be obtained 9 to 12 hours after the last dose.

Lithium, a remarkably effective drug for bipolar disorder has a bevy of adverse effects spanning numerous organ systems. Lithium can induce adverse effects on the thyroid gland, the kidney, and the heart, as well as cause a benign elevation of the WBC count; accordingly, baseline and follow-up measures of the CBC count with a differential, serum electrolytes, blood urea nitrogen (BUN), creatinine, thyroid function tests (TFTs), urinalysis, and ECG should be obtained. Pregnancy tests should also be obtained in women of childbearing years given the risk of teratogenic effects (e.g., Ebstein's anomaly) that are associated with use in the first trimester. There is general consensus that therapeutic lithium levels range from 0.8 to 1.2 mEq/L, although certain patients may have idiosyncratic responses outside of this range. Steady-state levels can be checked after 4 to 5 days. Lithium levels can change dramatically during or immediately after pregnancy or if patients are taking thiazide diuretics, nonsteroidal antiinflammatory drugs, or angiotensin-converting enzyme inhibitors or in those who have deteriorating renal function or are dehydrated.

Patients taking carbamazepine or valproic acid for bipolar disorder should have baseline and follow-up CBC, electrolytes, and LFTs in addition to routine level monitoring. In the case of carbamazepine, which can cause agranulocytosis, CBC should be checked every 2 weeks for the first 2 months of treatment, and then once every 3 months thereafter. Again, pregnancy tests should be considered for women of childbearing age.

Anxiety

The medical differential for new-onset anxiety is broad; it includes drug effects, thyroid or parathyroid dysfunction, hypoglycemia, cardiac disease (including myocardial infarction and mitral valve prolapse), respiratory compromise (including asthma, chronic obstructive pulmonary disease, and pulmonary embolism), and alcohol or benzodiazepine withdrawal. Rare causes, such as pheochromocytoma, porphyria, and seizure disorder, should be investigated if suggested by other associated clinical features. Laboratory work-up may therefore include TFTs, serum glucose or glucose tolerance testing, chest x-ray examination, pulmonary function tests, cardiac work-up, urine vanillylmandelic acid or porphyrins, and an EEG.

Care of the Geriatric Population

Given the increased likelihood of medical conditions that cause psychiatric symptoms in older adults, special attention should be given to organic causal agents. Especially common are mental status changes resulting from urinary tract infections, anemia, thyroid disease, and dementia. Kolman[27] described five particularly useful tests for older adults: clean-catch urinalysis and culture, a chest x-ray examination, a serum B_{12} level, an ECG, and a BUN. Although the National Institutes of Health Consensus Development Conference identified the history and physical examination as the most important diagnostic tests in older adult psychiatric patients, they also specifically recommended a CBC count, serum chemistries, TFTs, a RPR, a B_{12} level, and a folate level. If clinically indicated, additional testing should include neuroimaging, an EEG, and a lumbar puncture. With suspected early dementia, in addition to the DRS (see "Diagnostic Rating Scales" section of this chapter), positron emission tomography (PET) may be useful diagnostically.[28]

Substance Abuse

Substance abuse and withdrawal should always be considered in patients with mental status changes. Substances available for testing in serum and urine are summarized in Table 5-6. Alcohol levels can be quickly assessed using breath analysis (breathalyzer). It is important to remember that serum

Table 5-6. Serum and Urine Toxicology Screens

Substance	Serum Detection	Urine Detection
Alcohol	1–2 days	1 day
Amphetamine	Variable	1–2 days
Barbiturates	Variable	3 days to 3 weeks
Benzodiazepines	Variable	2–3 days
Cocaine	Hours to 1 day	2–3 days
Codeine, morphine, heroin	Variable	1–2 days
Delta-9-THC	N/A	~30 days, longer if chronic use
Methadone	15–29 hours	2–3 days
Phencyclidine	N/A	8 days
Propoxyphene	8–34 hours	1–2 days

N/A, Not applicable.

levels of alcohol do not necessarily correlate with the timing of withdrawal symptoms. Patients who present with a history of alcohol abuse should have LFTs as well as a CBC count checked; if macrocytic anemia is present, B_{12} and folate levels should also be assessed. Chronic liver damage can lead to coagulopathy (as manifest by an elevated partial thromboplastin time) and other manifestations of synthetic failure (e.g., low albumin). In the case of cocaine abuse, there should be a low threshold for obtaining an ECG with any cardiac symptom.

Eating Disorders

As part of their medical evaluation, patients who present with severe eating disorders should have routine laboratory studies to evaluate electrolyte status and nutritional measures (e.g., albumin). Patients who are actively purging can present with metabolic alkalosis (manifested by an elevated bicarbonate), hypochloremia, and hypokalemia. Serum aldolase levels can be increased in those who abuse ipecac; chronic emesis can also lead to elevated levels of amylase. Cholecystokinin levels can be blunted in bulimic patients, relative to controls, following ingestion of a meal. Finally, patients who abuse laxatives chronically may present with hypocalcemia.

The Electroencephalogram

The EEG employs surface (and sometimes nasopharyngeal) electrodes to measure the low-voltage electric activity of the brain. Used primarily in the evaluation of epilepsy and other neurologic disorders, the EEG is often useful in evaluating organic causes of psychiatric symptoms.

EEG signals are presumed to reflect primarily cortical activity, especially from neurons in the most superficial cortical cell layers. The frequencies of electric activity have been divided into four bands: delta (0 to 4 Hz), theta (4 to 8 Hz), alpha (8 to 12 Hz), and beta (greater than 12 Hz). The awake state is characterized by an alpha predominance. Beta waves emerge during stage 1 sleep (drowsiness); during stage 2, vertex sharp theta and delta waves are observed. Delta waves are seen in stages 3 and 4 sleep. During rapid eye movement sleep, the EEG will record low-voltage fast waves with ocular movement artifacts. Sleep deprivation, hyperventilation, and photic stimulation can sometimes activate seizure foci. For patients with nonepileptiform EEGs but a residual high suspicion for seizure activity, serial studies, sleep-deprived studies, or long-term monitoring can produce a higher yield.

EEG patterns associated with neuropsychiatric conditions are summarized in Table 5-7. EEG

Table 5-7. EEG Findings Associated with Neuropsychiatric Conditions

Seizure	
– Generalized	– Bilateral, symmetric, synchronous, paroxysmal spike; sharp waves followed by slow waves
– Absence	– 3-Hz spike-wave complexes
– Complex partial	– Temporal lobe spikes, polyspikes, and waves
Pseudoseizure	Normal EEG
Delirium	Generalized theta and delta activity
– Hepatic or uremic encephalopathy	– Triphasic waves
Dementia	
– Alzheimer's and vascular	– Alpha slowing of the background
– Subacute sclerosing panencephalitis and Creutzfeldt-Jakob disease	– Periodic complexes accompanying myoclonic jerks
Locked-In Syndrome	Normal EEG
Persistent Vegetative State	Slow and disorganized EEG
Death	Electrocerebral silence
Medications	
– Benzodiazepines and barbiturates	– Beta activity
– Neuroleptics and antidepressants	– Nonspecific changes
Focal Lesion	Focal delta slowing
Increased Intracranial Pressure	FIRDA

EEG, Electroencephalogram; *FIRDA*, frontal, intermittent, rhythmic delta activity.

findings in generalized, absence, and partial complex seizures disorders are well characterized and are diagnostic. When interpreted within the context of the clinical presentation, abnormal EEG data can help support several other broad diagnostic categories, including delirium, dementia, medication-induced mental status changes, and focal lesions; normal data can provide support for diagnoses of pseudoseizures and locked-in syndrome but are not able to rule out a variety of ictal states. Although an increased number of EEG abnormalities have been described in a variety of primary psychiatric disorders, at present the EEG is not clinically useful to definitively rule in any primary psychiatric diagnosis.

Neuroimaging

Neuroimaging has emerged as a powerful tool in both neuropsychiatric research and in the clinical investigation of organic causal agents for psychiatric presentations; however, rarely do neuroimaging studies establish a primary psychiatric diagnosis. Although less invasive than other diagnostic tests, imaging studies come with their own risks to the patient, and they remain costly. Following a thorough initial evaluation, the decision to use neuroimaging needs to be made on a case-by-case basis; at present, the major objective of neuroimaging studies in patients with psychiatric symptoms is to prevent missing a treatable brain lesion. A suggested list of indications for brain imaging in psychiatric patients is given in Table 5-8. The following sections describe the major neuroimaging techniques currently available, as well as their clinical utility.

Table 5-8. Indications for Neuroimaging in Patients With Psychiatric Symptoms

New-onset psychosis*
New-onset delirium*
New-onset dementia
Onset of any psychiatric problem in a patient > 50 years old*
An abnormal neurologic examination
A history of head trauma
During an initial work-up for ECT

*When initial history, physical examination, and laboratory studies are not definitive.
ECT, Electroconvulsive therapy.

Computed Tomography

Computed tomography (CT) scans use multiple X rays to provide cross-sectional images of the brain. On CT films, areas of increased beam attenuation (e.g., of the skull) appear white, whereas those of low attenuation (e.g., gas) appear black, and those of intermediate attenuation (e.g., soft tissues) appear in shades of gray. Contrast material may be used to visualize areas where the blood-brain barrier has been compromised, for example, by tumors, bleeding, inflammation, and abscesses; however, up to 5% of patients can develop idiosyncratic reactions to contrast media manifest by hypotension, nausea, flushing, urticaria, and anaphylaxis. CT scans can be obtained rapidly and are the imaging modality of choice in identifying acute hemorrhage and trauma, as well as in situations in which magnetic resonance imaging (MRI) is contraindicated. CT scans are generally better tolerated by patients with anxiety or claustrophobia. Although useful in examining gross pathologic conditions, CT lacks the resolution to detect subtle white matter lesions or changes in smaller structures, such as the hippocampi and basal ganglia. Because CT scans use ionizing radiation, they are contraindicated in pregnancy.

Although CT scans have a well-established role in the identification of structural abnormalities responsible for psychiatric symptoms in patients with organic lesions, they cannot be used to diagnose primary psychiatric illness. However, there are nonspecific structural changes identifiable on CT that have been consistently identified in the brains of psychiatric patients. Since Weinberger et al.[29] first described increased ventricular-to-brain ratios in patients with schizophrenia, several investigators have observed enlarged ventricles in those with eating disorders, alcoholism, bipolar disorder, dementia, and depression.

Magnetic Resonance Imaging

MRI, which provides detailed images of the brain in axial, sagittal, and coronal plains, takes advantage of the interaction between protons and an external magnetic field. In the magnetic field of the MRI scanner, hydrogen protons in the water molecules of the brain become aligned as dipoles with, or against, the field. A radiofrequency pulse is applied, shifting the spin on the protons to a higher energy level; when the signal is turned off, spin returns to the ground state and the proton releases energy. The frequency of energy release (or relaxation) depends on the chemical environment surrounding the proton. A coil that detects the energy emission generates signals that are processed by the scanner to create images. Adjusting the relaxation time parameters (known as T1 and T2) can result in images that are "weighted" differently; whereas T1-weighted images provide anatomic detail and gray-white matter differentiation, T2-weighted images highlight areas of pathologic conditions.

MRI is considered superior to CT for differentiation of white and gray matter, identification of white matter lesions (e.g., in multiple sclerosis, vasculitis, and leukoencephalitis), and visualization of the posterior fossa. As with CT, contrast medium may be used to identify lesions where the blood-brain barrier has been compromised. MRI is contraindicated in patients with metallic implants (including pacemakers) and is often less tolerable to patients because of the length of the study, the enclosed space, and the noise.

MRI may be used clinically to rule out structural brain lesions in patients with psychiatric symptoms, including acute psychosis or delirium, severe mood disorder, and abrupt personality changes. In addition to the structural changes that CT scans are capable of detecting, MRI appears to be more sensitive at detecting atrophic changes in dementia, inflammation-induced edema, and white matter lesions. Compared with CT, MRI is capable of detecting acute strokes earlier, using a method called diffusion-weighted imaging.

Functional MRI (fMRI), which is primarily a research tool at present, uses a process of acquisition sequences to approximate cerebral blood flow; accordingly, one can infer regions of brain activation and deactivation at rest, as well as during execution of sensory, motor, or cognitive tasks. Certain patterns of activation have emerged consistently in dementia, major depression, schizophrenia, and obsessive-compulsive disorder, but again, fMRI is not currently considered a diagnostic tool.

A related imaging modality, magnetic resonance spectroscopy (MRS), permits in vivo measurements of certain markers of brain tissue metabolism and biochemistry. For example, using proton-based MRS, one can measure local concentrations of n-acetylaspartate (a putative marker of neuronal integrity), choline (a marker of membrane turnover), creatine (a marker of intracellular energy metabolism), glutamine, glutamate, and gamma aminobutyric acid. Localized reductions in n-acetylaspartate have been implicated in multiple neuropsychiatric disorders, including schizophrenia, temporal lobe epilepsy, Alzheimer's disease, acquired immune deficiency syndrome dementia, and Huntington's disease. In the near future, the combined use of fMRI and MRS holds great promise for delineating abnormal structure-function relationships underlying psychopathologic conditions.[30]

PET and SPECT

Positron emission tomography (PET) employs radioactive markers to visualize directly cortical and subcortical brain functioning. Some examples of these markers include[18] fluorodeoxyglucose (which provides a picture of brain glucose metabolism),[15]-oxygen (a surrogate for regional cerebral blood flow), and receptor-specific radioligands (which indicate activity at neurotransmitter receptors). Studies can be performed only where an on-site cyclotron is present to prepare the emitter tracers. Single photon emission computed tomography (SPECT) uses photon-emitting nucleotides measured by gamma detectors to localize brain activation or pharmacologic activity; commonly used tracers include 133-Xe and 99m-technetium hexamethylpropyleneamine (which measure cerebral blood flow) and, as in PET, radioligands with specific receptor activity. Although PET scans provide greater spatial and temporal resolution, signal-to-noise ratio, and variety of ligands, SPECT is more readily available, better tolerated, and less expensive.

Although both PET and SPECT are primarily used as research tools in delineating pathophysiology and rational drug designs, clinical use of these techniques is becoming increasingly common. PET and SPECT may be used in concert with the EEG to determine seizure foci, especially in patients with partial complex seizures; during a seizure, scans can demonstrate areas of increased metabolism, while interictally the focus will be hypometabolic and hypoperfused. Moreover, in both Alzheimer's disease and multiinfarct dementia, abnormal patterns of cortical metabolism and receptor function as evidenced on PET and SPECT appear to predate structural changes visible on MRI.[31,32] With the continued development of receptor-specific ligands and other functional markers, these imaging modalities may continue to find a more prominent role in clinical diagnosis and management.

Conclusion

Although diagnosis in psychiatry continues to rely primarily on the interview and other clinical phenomenology, laboratory testing and use of diagnostic rating scales serve important roles in eliminating organic causal agents from the differential diagnoses, monitoring the effects of treatment, and guiding further management decisions. Neuroimaging has provided a noninvasive means to detect subtle neurophysiologic dysfunction in psychiatric patients, and has begun to find meaningful clinical as well as research applications. It is clear that these quantitative measures will assume increasing prominence and importance in twenty-first century psychiatry.

References

1. Spitzer RL, Williams JB, Gibbon M, et al: The Structured Clinical Interview for DSM-III-R (SCID). I. History, rationale, and description, *Arch Gen Psychiatry* 49:624–629, 1992.
2. Williams JB, Gibbon M, First MB, et al: The Structured Clinical Interview for DSM-III-R (SCID): II. Multisite test-retest reliability, *Arch Gen Psychiatry* 49:630–636, 1992.
3. Sheehan DV, Lecrubier Y, Sheehan KH, et al: The Mini-International Neuropsychiatric Interview (M.I.N.I.): the development and validation of a structured diagnostic psychiatric interview for DSM-IV and ICD-10, *J Clin Psychiatry* 59(suppl 20):22–33, 1998.
4. Guy W: *ECDEU assessment manual for psychopharmacology—revised (DHEW Publ No ADM 76–338)*, Rockville, 1976, U.S. Department of Health, Education, and Welfare, Public Health Service, Alcohol, Drug Abuse, and Mental Health Administration, National Institutes of Mental Health Psychopharmacology Branch, Division of Extramural Research Programs.
5. Hamilton M: A rating scale for depression, *J Neurol Neurosurg Psychiatry* 23:56–62, 1960.
6. Beck AT, Ward CH, Mendelson M, et al: An inventory for measuring depression, *Arch Gen Psychiatry* 4:561, 1961.
7. Beigel A, Murphy D, Bunney W: The manic state rating scale: scale construction, reliability, and validity, *Arch Gen Psychiatry* 25:256, 1971.
8. Young RC, Biggs JT, Ziegler VE, et al: A rating scale for mania: reliability, validity and sensitivity, *Br J Psychiatry* 133:429–435, 1978.
9. Overall JE, Gorham DR: The brief psychiatric rating scale, *Psychol Rep* 10:799, 1962.
10. Kay SR, Fiszbein A, Opler LA: The Positive and Negative Syndrome Scale (PANSS) for schizophrenia, *Schizophr Bull* 13:261–276, 1987.
11. Andreasen NC: *Scale for the Assessment of Positive Symptoms (SAPS)*, Iowa City, 1984, University of Iowa.
12. Andreasen NC: *Scale for the Assessment of Negative Symptoms (SANS)*, Iowa City, 1983, University of Iowa.
13. Barnes TRE: A rating scale for drug-induced akathisia, *Br J Psychiatry* 154:672–676, 1989.
14. Hamilton M: The assessment of anxiety states by rating, *Br J Med Psychol* 32:50, 1959.
15. Goodman WK, Price LH, Rasmussen SA, et al: The Yale-Brown Obsessive Compulsive Scale: I. Development, use, and reliability, *Arch Gen Psychiatry* 46:1006–1011, 1989.
16. Goodman WK, Price LH, Rasmussen SA, et al: The Yale-Brown Obsessive Compulsive Scale: II. Validity, *Arch Gen Psychiatry* 46:1012–1016, 1989.
17. Mayfield D, McLeod G, Hall P: The CAGE Questionnaire: validation of a new alcoholism screening instrument, *Am J Psychiatry* 131:1121–1123, 1974.
18. Skinner HA: The Drug Abuse Screening Test, *Addict Behav* 7:363–371, 1982.
19. Folstein MF, Folstein SE, McHugh PR: "Mini-mental state:" A practical method for grading the cognitive state of patients for the clinician, *J Psychiatr Res* 12:189–198, 1975.
20. Mattis S: *Dementia rating scale: professional manual*, Odessa, Fla 1988, Psychological Assessment Resources.
21. Freedman M, Leach L, Kaplan E, et al: *Clock drawing: a neuropsychological analysis*, New York, 1994, Oxford University Press.
22. Tuokko H, Hadjistavropoulos T, Miller JA, et al: *The clock test: administration and scoring manual*, Toronto, 1995, Multi-Health Systems.
23. Wolf-Klein GP, Silverstone FA, Levy AP, et al: Screening for Alzheimer's disease by clock drawing, *J Am Geriatr Soc* 37:730–734, 1989.
24. Anfinson TJ, Kathol RG: Screening laboratory evaluation in psychiatric patients: a review, *Gen Hosp Psychiatry* 14:248–257, 1992.

25. Morihisa JM, Cross CD, Price S, et al: *Laboratory and other diagnostic tests in psychiatry*. In Hales RE, Yudofsky SC, editors: *The American psychiatric publishing textbook of clinical psychiatry*, ed 4, Washington, DC, 2003, American Psychiatric Publishing.

26. Arana GW, Goff DC, Friedman H, et al: Does carbamazepine-induced reduction of plasma haloperidol levels worsen psychotic symptoms? *Am J Psychiatry* 143:650–651, 1986.

27. Kolman PBR: The value of laboratory investigations of elderly psychiatric patients, *J Clin Psychiatry* 45:112–116, 1984.

28. Ishii K: Clinical application of positron emission tomography for diagnosis of dementia, *Ann Nucl Med* 16:515–525, 2002.

29. Weinberger DR, Torrey EF, Neophytides AN, et al: Lateral cerebral ventricular enlargement in chronic schizophrenia, *Arch Gen Psychiatry* 36:735–739, 1979.

30. Callicott JH: *Functional brain imaging in psychiatry: the next wave*. In Morihisa JM, editor: *Advances in brain imaging*, Washington, DC, 2001, American Psychiatric Publishing.

31. Fazekas F, Alavi A, Chawluk JB, et al: Comparison of CT, MR, and PET in Alzheimer's dementia and normal aging, *J Nucl Med* 30:1607–1615, 1989.

32. Kuhl DE, Metter EJ, Riege WH, et al: Determination of cerebral glucose utilization in dementia using positron emission tomography, *Dan Med Bull* 32(suppl 1):51–55, 1985.

Chapter 6

Psychological and Neuropsychological Assessment

Mark A. Blais, Psy.D.
Sheila M. O'Keefe, Ed.D.
Dennis K. Norman, Ed.D.

The intent of this chapter is to increase your knowledge of psychological and neuropsychological assessment. This will be accomplished by reviewing the scientific basis of psychological instruments, the major categories of psychological tests, and the application of these instruments in clinical assessment. The chapter also briefly touches on issues related to ordering psychological testing and understanding the final report of the assessment. The material contained in this chapter should allow you to better utilize psychological and neuropsychological assessments in your care of patients.

Psychological tests must be reliable and valid. Reliability represents the repeatability, stability, or consistency of a subject's test score. Reliability is usually represented as a correlation coefficient ranging form 0 to 1.0. Research instruments can have reliabilities in the low .70s, whereas clinical instruments should have reliabilities in the high .80s to low .90s. A number of reliability statistics are available for evaluating a test. For example, internal consistency measures the degree to which items in a test function in the same manner, and test-retest reliability shows the consistency of a test score over time. Inter-rater reliability measured by the Kappa statistic reflects the degree of agreement between raters, usually corrected for chance. Unreliability, or error, can be introduced into a test score by variability in the subject (changes in the subject over time), the examiner, or the test (given with different instructions).

Validity is a more complex concept and a hard property to demonstrate. The validity of a test reflects the degree to which the test actually measures the construct it was designed to measure. Measures of validity are usually represented as correlation coefficients ranging from 0 to 1.0. Multiple types of validity data are required before a test can be considered valid. Content validity assesses the degree that an instrument covers the full range of the target construct, and predictive validity indicates how well a test predicts future occurrences of the target variable. It is important to realize that no psychological test is universally valid. Tests are considered valid or not valid for a specific purpose.

Types of Psychological Tests

Test of Intelligence

Matarazzo states, "Intelligence . . . is the aggregate or global capacity of the individual to act purposefully, to think rationally, and to deal effectively with the environment."[1] This definition demonstrates what the modern intelligence quotient (IQ) tests try to measure (adaptive functioning) and why IQ tests can be important aids in clinical assessment particularly with regard to treatment planning. The Wechsler IQ tests are the most commonly used IQ tests; they cover almost the whole life span. The series starts with the Wechsler Preschool and Primary Scale of Intelligence (ages 4 to 6), progresses to the Wechsler Intelligence Scale for Children-III (5 to 16 years), and ends with the Wechsler Adult Intelligence Scale-III for ages 16 to 89.[2–4] A new abbreviated version of the Wechsler IQ test is now available (Wechsler Abbreviated Scale of Intelligence [WASI]).[5] All the Wechsler scales provide three major IQ tests scores: the full scale IQ, verbal IQ (VIQ), and performance IQ (PIQ). All three IQ scores have a mean of 100 and standard deviations (SDs) of 15. These statistical features mean that a 15-point difference between a subject's VIQ and PIQ is both statistically and clinically meaningful. Table 6-1 presents an overview of the IQ categories.

The Wechsler IQ tests are composed of 10 or 11 subtests that were developed to tap into two primarily intellectual domains, verbal intelligence (as measured by Vocabulary, Similarities, Arithmetic, Digit Span, Information, and Comprehension) and nonverbal visual spatial intelligence (as measured by Picture Completion, Digit Symbol, Block Design, Matrix Reasoning, and Picture Arrangement). Empirical studies have suggested that the Wechsler subscales can be reorganized into three cognitive domains: verbal ability, visual-spatial ability, and attention and concentration (which is assessed by the Arithmetic, Digit Span, and Digit Symbol subtests). All the Wechsler subtests have a mean score of 10 and SD of 3. Given this statistical feature, we know that if two subtests differ by 3 or more scaled score points, the difference is significant. All IQ scores and subtest scaled scores are adjusted for age. It is important to understand that IQ scores represent patients' ordinal position, their percentile ranking as it were, on the test relative to the normative sample. These scores do not represent a patient's innate intelligence, and there is no good evidence that they measure a genetically determined intelligence. They do to a considerable degree reflect the patient's current level of adaptive functioning.

Table 6-1. IQ Categories With Their Corresponding IQ Scores and Percentile Distribution

IQ Categories		
Full Scale IQ Score	Categories	Normal Distribution Percentile
≥130	Very superior	2.2
120–129	Superior	6.7
110–119	High average	16.1
90–109	Average	50.0
80–89	Low average	16.1
70–79	Borderline	6.7
≤69	Mentally retarded	2.2

IQ, Intelligence quotient.

At times it is difficult to sort out whether dysfunction in affect, behavior, or cognition can be primarily assessed with psychological instruments of psychiatric consultation or whether they require neuropsychological assessment. Requests for psychological assessment might be conveyed as follows:

A psychological assessment was requested on Ms. B, a 28-year-old, right-handed, single attorney. She was seen in the emergency department (ED) after she ingested extra pain medication for a painful back. When the ED physician found her to be mildly confused and disoriented, Ms. B was admitted to the medical service. By the next morning her mental status had improved; however, she continued to complain of extreme back pain and she made vague suicidal statements. A pain work-up and psychiatric consultation were both ordered.

Ms. B got into frequent struggles with the nursing staff over the hospital's smoking rules. A review of the medical chart revealed that she had graduated from a prestigious university and law school and was employed at a large legal firm. She had developed severe back pain secondary to multiple equestrian injuries that occurred while riding competitively in college. She had received various diagnoses for her pain and she had failed to respond to several medication trials, surgery, and one stay on an inpatient pain rehabilitation unit. Ms. B's current medications included: diazepam 5 mg bid, amitriptyline 100 mg qhs, and oxycodone/acetaminophen (Percocet) one tablet qhs. The pain service consultant was unsure about the diagnosis. The psychiatric consultant found her to be guarded (around her mood and the level of her suicidal ideation). She reported no history of depression or suicide attempts. Psychological testing was requested to help determine "if Ms. B was really depressed and suicidal or just character-disordered." Later that same day Ms. B completed a brief but fairly comprehensive psychological assessment.

The test battery for Ms. B consisted of several tests, including the WASI (which was given first); it was followed by the Rorschach inkblot test, four Thematic Apperception Test (TAT) cards, and the Personality Assessment Inventory (PAI). The WASI was selected for its brief administration time (20 to 30 minutes) and its ability to provide accurate IQ data (assessing cognitive functioning). The Rorschach was selected as the second test to be administered for two reasons: Given Ms. B's guardedness, projective test data seemed crucial for the personality assessment, and it was felt that the novelty of the Rorschach might help maintain Ms. B's involvement in the assessment. A self-report test of psychopathology was desired, but it seemed likely that Ms. B would neither complete one nor would she portray herself in an exceedingly favorable light. The PAI was selected for use due to its shorter length (344 items) and its ability to be scored with a short form of the test using only the first 199 items. Also, the PAI contains a number of treatment planning scales that can provide important information.

Ms. B's assessment was conducted in her semi-private room. Although this was not an ideal situation, it is commonly performed in this fashion. Surprisingly, Ms. B completed all of the testing without complaint or fuss. The WASI data provided a screen of Ms. B's cognitive functioning and assessed the quality and consistency of her functioning in highly structured situations. Her WASI scores were full scale IQ 102, VIQ 120, and PIQ 87. The WASI data can be thought of as providing an estimate of the patient's current best possible level of functioning. Her visual-spatial skills were weak relative to her verbal ability. In general, Ms. B's cognitive functioning was not as effective as one might have assumed, given her verbal abilities and her level of education. The VIQ > PIQ difference of an 18-point split could have represented either a long-standing learning

disability (somewhat less likely given her strong high school, college, and law school performance) or cognitive disruption secondary to depression and/or the effects of her current medications.

The Rorschach revealed Ms. B's deeper psychological functioning. The test was valid. The Rorschach depression index was positive, suggesting either current depression or a propensity to depressive experiences. The suicide constellation was negative (score = 4). Although her psychological resources were adequate, she had no established coping style, which detracted from the quality of her coping. Situational stress further reduced the quality of her functioning. Her affective experience was dominated by helplessness, painful internalized affect, and unmet dependency/nurturance needs. Together these findings suggested depression resulting from situational factors. Her thinking was marked by poor perceptual accuracy, mainly because of the overpersonalization of perceptions and the disruptive affect of anger on her thinking. However, she was not psychotic. She had an immature, self-centered personality style and a narcissistic character style. Excessive intellectualization, escape into fantasy, and the use of externalizing defenses dominated her defensive function.

The PAI (which the patient completed) could be considered to provide a more superficial picture of her psychological world. The PAI profile was valid. She reported minimal psychopathology. Her mean elevation on the 10 clinical scales was only 53 (T-score, well within the range of nonpatients), suggesting either that she was experiencing little overt distress or that she was reluctant to express emotional pain. Either way, she did not appear to others, including her caregivers, to be psychologically impaired. She reported mild clinical depression (T-score = 71) and excessive concern about her physical functioning (T-score = 85). Further, on clinical interview her excessive physical complaints and concerns overshadowed her depressive symptoms. A grandiose sense of self, consistent with the pronounced signs of a narcissistic character style on the Rorschach, was indicated by one of the PAI subscales. On the treatment consideration scales she indicated minimal interest in psychologically oriented treatments, a perception of high levels of social stress, and minimal suicidal ideation (T-score = 54). Impressions and recommendations:

Overall the assessment strongly suggested the presence of a clinical depression. Depression was likely masked to some extent by both the patient's focus on her physical functioning (the back pain) and her inability or unwillingness to express her emotional pain. As a result, her depression is likely more significant and disruptive to her functioning than she is reporting. In addition, character issues (Axis II pathology) in the form of an immature self-centered view of the world and narcissistic character traits (possibly a full-blown disorder) complicated Ms. B's treatment. Ms. B's functioning, at present, is greatly reduced because of both her depression and her situational stressors. These stressors affect both her emotional and intellectual function. Her ability to organize, plan, and initiate coping strategies is currently limited. As such, the advisability of her immediate return to full-time employment should be carefully reviewed. Her caregivers may have overestimated her level of functioning because of her strong verbal communication skills. On testing she does not appear to be actively suicidal (either on the self-report or projective tests). However, in her current state of being emotionally overwhelmed, depressed, and having reduced coping ability, Ms. B should be considered at an increased risk (over and above being depressed) for impulsive self-harm. Her safety should be monitored closely. Her psychotherapy, which will be challenging given her personality style, should first focus on practical efforts to improve her coping and functioning. Once her functioning stabilizes, the therapy focus might profitably expand to include her interpersonal style.

Tests of Personality, Psychopathology, and Psychological Functioning

Objective psychological tests, also called *self-report tests*, are designed to clarify and quantify a patient's personality functioning and psychopathology. Objective tests use a patient's response to a series of true/false or multiple-choice questions to broadly assess psychological functioning. These tests are called "objective" because their scoring involves little speculation. Objective tests provide excellent insight into how a patient sees him or herself and how the patient wants others to see and treat him or her.

The Minnesota Multiphasic Personality Inventory–2 (MMPI-2)[6] is a 567-item true/false, self-report test of psychological functioning. It was designed to provide an objective measure of abnormal behavior, basically to separate subjects into two groups (normal and abnormal) and then to further categorize the abnormal group into specific classes.[7] The MMPI-2 contains 10 clinical scales that assess major categories of psychopathology and 3 validity scales designed to assess test-taking attitudes. MMPI-2 validity scales are (L) lie, (F) infrequency, and (K) correction. The MMPI-2 clinical scales include (1) Hs—hypochondriasis, (2) D—depression, (3) Hy—conversion hysteria, (4) Pd—psychopathic deviate, (5) Mf—masculinity-femininity, (6) Pa—paranoia, (7) Pt—psychasthenia, (8) Sc—schizophrenia, (9) Ma—hypomania, and 10Si—social introversion. More than 300 "new" or experiential scales have also been developed for the MMPI-2. MMPI raw scores are transformed into T-scores; a T-score greater than or equal to 65 indicates clinical levels of psychopathology. The MMPI-2 is interpreted by determining the highest two or three scales, called a code type. For example, a 2–4–7 code type indicates the presence of depression (scale 2), impulsivity (scale 4), and anxiety (scale 7), along with the likelihood of a personality disorder (PD).[7]

The Millon Clinical Multiaxial Inventory–III (MCMI-III) is a 175-item true/false, self-report questionnaire designed to identify both symptom disorders (Axis I conditions) and PDs.[8] The MCMI-III is composed of 3 modifier indices (validity scales), 10 basic personality scales, 3 severe personality scales, 6 clinical syndrome scales, and 3 severe clinical syndrome scales. One of the unique features of the MCMI-III is that it attempts to assess both Axis I and Axis II psychopathology simultaneously. The Axis II scales resemble but are not identical to the Axis II disorders given in the *Diagnostic and Statistical Manual for Mental Disorders*, fourth edition. Given its relatively short length (175 items versus 567 for the MMPI-2), the MCMI-III has an advantage in the assessment of patients who are agitated, whose stamina is significantly impaired, or who are just suboptimally motivated.

The PAI[9] is one of the newest objective psychological tests available. The PAI uses 344 items and a 4-point response format (false, slightly true, mainly true, and very true) to make 22 nonoverlapping scales. These 22 scales include 4 validity scales, 11 clinical scales, 5 treatment scales, and 2 interpersonal scales. The PAI covers a wide range of Axis I and Axis II psychopathology and other variables related to interpersonal functioning and treatment planning, including suicidal ideation, resistance to treatment, and aggression. The PAI possesses outstanding psychometric features and is an ideal test for broadly assessing multiple domains of relevant psychological functioning.

A subject's response style can have an impact on the accuracy of his or her self-report. Validity scales are incorporated into all major objective tests to assess the degree to which a response style may have distorted the findings. The three main response styles are careless or random responding (which may indicate that someone is not reading or cannot understand the test), attempting to "look good" by denying pathology, and attempting to "look bad" by over reporting pathology (a cry for help or malingering).

Projective tests of psychological functioning differ from objective tests in that they are less structured and require more effort on the part of the patient to make sense of and to respond to the test stimuli. As a result, the patient has a greater degree of freedom to demonstrate his or her own unique personality characteristics. Projective tests are more like problem-solving tasks, and they provide us with insights into a patient's style of perceiving, organizing, and responding to external and internal stimuli. When data from objective and projective tests are combined, they can provide a fairly complete picture or description of a patient's range of functioning.

The Rorschach inkblot test[10] consists of 10 cards that contain inkblots (5 are black and white; 2 are black, red, and white; and 3 are various pastels) to which the patient is required to say what the inkblot might be. The test is administered in two phases. First, the patient is presented with the 10 inkblots one at a time and asked, "What might this be?" The patient's responses are recorded verbatim. In the second phase, the examiner reviews the patient's responses and inquires where on the card the response was seen (known as *location* in Rorschach language) and what about the blot made it look that way (known as the *determinants*). For example , a patient responds to Card V with "A flying bat." The practitioner asks, "Can you show me where you saw that?" The patient answers, "Here. I used the whole card." The practitioner asks, "What made it look like a bat?" The patient answers, "The color, the black made it look like a bat to me." This response would be coded as follows:

Wo FMa.FC'o A P 1.0.

The examining psychologist reviews these codes rather than the verbal responses to evaluate the patient's performance. Rorschach "scoring" has been criticized for being subjective. However, over the last 20 years Exner[11] has developed a Rorschach system (called the *Comprehensive System*) that has demonstrated acceptable levels of reliability. For example, inter-rater Kappas of .80 or better are required for all Rorschach variables reported in research studies. Rorschach data are particularly useful for quantifying a patient's reality contact and the quality of his or her thinking.

The TAT is useful in revealing a patient's dominant motivations, emotions, and core personality conflicts.[12] The TAT consists of a series of 20 cards depicting people in various interpersonal interactions. The cards were intentionally drawn to be ambiguous. The TAT is administered by presenting 8 to 10 of these cards, one at a time, with the instructions to "Make up a story around this picture. Like all good stories it should have a beginning, a middle, and an ending. Tell me how the people feel and what they are thinking." Although there is no standard scoring method for the TAT (making it more of a clinical technique than psychological test proper), when a sufficient number of cards are presented, reliable information can be obtained. Psychologists typically assess TAT stories for emotional themes, level of emotional and cognitive integration, interpersonal relational style, and view of the world (e.g., is it seen as a helpful or hurtful place). This type of data can be particularly useful in predicting a patient's response to psychotherapy.

Psychologists sometimes use projective drawings (free-hand drawings of human figures, families, houses, and trees) as a supplemental assessment procedure. These are clinical techniques rather than tests because there are no formal scoring methods. Despite their lack of psychometric grounding, projective drawings can sometimes be very revealing. For example, psychotic subjects may produce a human figure drawing that is transparent and shows internal organs. Still, it is important to remember that projective drawings are less reliable and less valid than the tests reviewed in this chapter.

Neuropsychological Assessment

The request for neuropsychological testing might be framed as follows:

Please perform a neuropsychological evaluation on Mr. A, a 20-year-old, white, single male, to assess his current cognitive function, to establish a baseline profile, to aid in diagnosis, and to guide treatment. Help figuring out whether his current problems are a result of psychiatric or neurologic conditions would be greatly appreciated.

Mr. A was recently discharged from a psychiatric unit where he was being treated for schizophrenic symptoms that included hallucinations (in multiple perceptual systems) and dysregulated behavior. Currently he is on the medical service for treatment of diabetic ketoacidosis. He is right-handed. Despite a long history of psychiatric and emotional problems (including a diagnosis of attention deficit hyperactivity disorder at the age of 9, and visual hallucinations that first developed at the age of 16), he has completed some college courses. During his mid- to late teens he was treated with a variety of antidepressants and antianxiety agents. Antipsychotics were started in the past year. Two years before this admission he sustained a closed head injury (CHI) in a motor vehicle accident. A question has arisen as to whether he has residual cognitive deficits from the CHI. Although he denies use of substances within the past 4 months, he had regularly smoked marijuana, taken mushrooms, and used inhalants.

Mr. A's evaluation included a review of his recent hospital discharge summary, an interview with Mr. A and his mother, and a discussion with his outpatient treaters. The following tests were also administered: WASI, Wechsler Memory Scale–III (WMS-III), Trials A & B, Boston Naming Test, Hooper Visual Organization Test, Rey-Ostterreith Complex Figure, Stroop Color Word Test, Digit Vigilance, and PAI. Mr. A cooperated fully with the evaluation. Overall, his performance appeared to be a valid reflection of his current behavior and level of functioning. All the psychological tests were valid

and interpretively useful. His WASI IQ scores were: Full Scale IQ 76 (borderline range fifth percentile); VIQ 83 (low average range, thirteenth percentile); and PIQ was 68 (second percentile). Age-adjusted scaled scores earned during this assessment were as follows:

Verbal	Scaled Score	Performance	Scaled Score
Vocabulary	8	Block design	5
Similarities	10	Matrix reasoning	6

Further analysis of Mr. A's WASI performance indicated a likely substantial decline from his premorbid level of functioning. Even if his estimated premorbid IQ had been just average (100), his current measured IQ has fallen 1.5 SDs. As such, the quality of his current functioning has also likely dropped substantially. Furthermore, his WASI profile reveals a significant 15-point difference between his VIQ and PIQ, favoring the former. A difference of this magnitude is unexpected and indicates that his nonverbal abilities have suffered more of a decline than his verbal/language-based abilities. Because nonverbal intellectual abilities are typically associated with right-hemisphere function, these findings point to a relative inefficiency in his right hemisphere.

Memory Functioning: His performance on the WMS-III was generally consistent with the WASI findings. His logical memory score (recalling a just-read paragraph) was at the fifty-seventh percentile on immediate recall (better than would be expected given his current VIQ), and it fell to the eighteenth percentile following a 30-minute delay (more consistent with his measured IQ). However, the quality of his memories was not as good as the percentile scores suggest. On this test, credit was given for any detail of a story recalled and no credit was lost if the details were recalled out of order or if errors were introduced into the stories. Mr. A's recall of these two stories was disjointed and some facts were misrepresented. His functional verbal memory was likely less adequate than his test scores suggest. His visual memory (ability to recall designs) fell at the twelfth percentile on immediate recall and at the eighteenth percentile following a 30-minute delay. Although weaker than his verbal memory scores, his recall of visual material was consistent with his current measured (nonverbal) PIQ. However, the quality of his visual memories was also quite poor. His strong immediate recall of verbal information compared with his generally weak recall of visual information again points to possible greater right-hemisphere dysfunction.

Language: On the Boston Naming Test he was able to correctly name 52 items (out of 60) spontaneously. This score was just slightly below the level expected for his age. However, when provided with a phonemic cue, he was able to improve his score to a 58 (out of 60). This degree of improvement suggests some mild word retrieval problems. He was able to comprehend complex instructions, suggesting that his receptive language skills were intact. His reading and writing abilities were not formally tested.

Visual-Spatial: Mr. A performed weakly, but inconsistently, on tests of visual spatial functioning. His performance on the WASI Block Design subtest was weak (scaled score of 5), and he frequently broke the "gestalt" of the design he was trying to copy. On the Hooper Visual Organization Test he obtained a score of 24, which was on the border of normal and impaired. However, his copy of the Rey Complex Figure was basically accurate. His inconsistent performance across these tests (all thought to tap basically the same function) suggested that fluctuations in his level of attention and motivation accounted for some of his poor performance.

Executive Functioning: On tests that tapped his ability to use abstract reasoning, and to plan and change his behavior based on external feedback, Mr. A again performed inconsistently. On the Trail Making Test Part B, a test that required him to draw a line that alternately connected numbers and letters in increasing order, he made three impulsive errors suggesting problems with inhibition of his behavior. Yet on the Stroop Color Word Test he scored at the expected level. Again, it is likely that alterations in his attention and motivation contributed to his inconsistent performance on these tasks that were thought to tap into frontal lobe functioning.

Emotional Functioning: The patient's PAI profile revealed elevations on the depression and schizophrenia scales. All three of the depression subscales (cognitive, affective, and physiologic) were elevated (indicating a strong likelihood of major depression), as were all three schizophrenia subscales (psychotic experiences, social isolation, and thought disorder).

Mr. A likely suffers from both a mood disorder and a psychotic condition. However, it is not clear whether or not these are independent conditions. Mr. A also reported having a stimulus-seeking personality style and little motivation for psychological treatment. Both of these features will complicate his treatment.

Impressions and Recommendations: The neuropsychological evaluation revealed three principle findings. (1) Mr. A's overall functional capacity (efficiency of his functioning) was greatly reduced from his premorbid level. (2) There were some consistent findings that point to a greater relative decline in right hemisphere function. (3) However, most of the areas tested revealed inconsistent findings that likely reflect minute-to-minute fluctuations in his attention, concentration, and level of motivation. The overall profile appears most consistent with the types of cognitive deficits usually associated with schizophrenia, and also point to a possible independent (but mild) problem that affects his right-hemisphere function. Perhaps this mild right-hemisphere impairment is a residual effect from his CHI. Still, the majority of difficulties seen on this testing (and likely in his daily functioning) appear related to his psychiatric condition (schizophrenia).

Mr. A will function best in a well-structured environment where expectations are clear and predictable. His medication regimen and treatment program should be simplified as much as possible to improve his adherence. His psychiatric conditions should be aggressively treated. His psychotherapy should be focused on concrete strategies to help him cope and deal with the problems of life.

Neuropsychological function assessment is a relatively recent development within applied psychology. In fact, it is only in the last 2 or 3 decades that neuropsychology has become established as a clinical specialty. Neuropsychologists assess brain-behavior relationships using standardized psychological instruments. The main goal of a neuropsychological evaluation is to relate a patient's test performance to both the status of his or her central nervous system and real-world functional capacity. In addition to assessing general intelligence, five major cognitive abilities are evaluated in a complete neuropsychological assessment: attention and concentration, language (expressive and receptive), memory (immediate and delayed), visual-spatial, and executive functioning and abstract thinking. This assessment is similar to the mental status examination used in neurology; it differs mainly in that it provides a deeper, more comprehensive, and better-quantified assessment. The application of a battery of tests covering these major cognitive areas allows for a broad assessment of the patient's strengths and deficits and provides some indication as to how these strengths and deficits will affect real world adaptation.

Types of Neuropsychological Assessment

The Halstead-Reitan (H-R) Battery is the oldest standardized neuropsychological assessment battery currently in use. The H-R Battery is an elaborate and time-intensive set of neuropsychological tests. Analysis of a H-R Battery is almost exclusively quantitative. The H-R profile is interpreted at four levels: an impairment index (a composite score reflecting the subject's overall performance), lateralizing signs, localizing signs, and a pattern analysis for inferences of causal factors.[13] The Boston process approach to neuropsychological assessment is a newer and more flexible style of neuropsychological assessment.[14] The Boston process approach starts with a small core test battery (usually containing one of the Wechsler IQ tests); subsequently, hypotheses regarding cognitive deficits are developed based on the patient's performance. Other instruments are administered to test and refine these hypotheses about the patient's cognitive deficits. The Boston approach focuses on both the quantitative and qualitative aspects of a patient's performance. By *qualitative*, we mean the manner or style of the patient's performance, not just the accuracy. In fact, reviewing how a patient failed an item can be more revealing than knowing which items were missed. In this way, the Boston approach reflects an integration of features from behavioral neurology and psychometric assessment.

Many neuropsychologists use a composite battery of tests in their day-to-day clinical work. A composite battery is usually composed of an IQ test (one of the Wechsler scales) and a number of selected tests matched to the patient and to the disorder being evaluated. Here we review some of the specific neuropsychological tests that might be used to compose a battery or to assess specific cognitive functions. For a description of these tests, see Spreen and Strauss.[15]

Attention and concentration are central to most complex cognitive processes; therefore it is important to adequately measure these functions in a neuropsychological test battery. In fact, some patients who complain of memory disorders turn out to have impaired attention and concentration, rather than pure memory dysfunction. Tests of attention and concentration include Trail Making Test Parts A & B and the mental control subtests of the WMS-III and the WAIS-III digit span, digit symbol, and arithmetic subtests. It is important to assess language from a number of perspectives, including simple word recognition, reading comprehension, verbal fluency, object naming ability, and writing. Frequently used measures of language functioning are the WAIS-III VIQ subtests, the Boston Naming Test, the Verbal Fluency Test, Reading (word recognition and reading comprehension), and Written Expression (a writing sample). The accurate measurement of reading ability (often using the North American Adult Reading Test) can provide an estimation of premorbid intelligence and allow the examiner to gauge the degree of overall cognitive decline. The assessment of memory is extremely important in a neuropsychological battery, because impaired memory is both a major reason for referral and a strong predictor of poor treatment outcome. An evaluation of memory should cover both visual and auditory memory systems, measure immediate and delayed recall, assess the pattern and rate of new learning, and explore for differences between recognition (memory with a retrieval cue) and unaided recall. The WMS-III[4] is one of the primary memory inventories. The WMS -III is composed of 11 subtests tapping into auditory and visual memory at both immediate and 30-minute delayed recall. It also provides indications of auditory and visual learning efficiency (new learning ability). Like the Wechsler IQ scales, this memory test is well standardized. The WMS-III produces three major memory scores that have a mean of 100 with an SD of 15. The memory subscales all have a mean of 10 and an SD of 3. These statistical properties allow for a detailed evaluation of memory function. In fact, the most recent revision of the Wechsler IQ and Memory Scales were jointly normed, allowing for more meaningful comparisons between IQ and memory. The Three Shapes and Three Words Memory Test[16] is a less demanding test of verbal (written) and nonverbal immediate and delayed memory. Unfortunately, it is not well normed. Visual-spatial tests (usually with a motor component—drawing) help evaluate right hemisphere functions in most (right-handed) adults. Because these deficits are nonverbal (sometimes called *silent*), they are often overlooked in briefer nonquantitative cognitive evaluations. Tests that tap visual-spatial functioning include the Rey-Ostterreith Complex Figure, the Hooper Visual Integration Tests, the Draw-a-Clock Test, and the PIQ subtests of the WAIS-III. Exccutive functioning refers to higher-order cognitive processes, such as judgement, planning, logical reasoning, and the modification of behavior bascd on external feedback. All of these functions are thought to be associated with the frontal and prefrontal lobes and are extremely important for effective real-world functioning. One of the most frequently used tests of executive functioning is the Wisconsin Card Sorting Test (WCST), which requires the patient to match 128 response cards to 1 of 4 stimulus cards using three possible dimensions (color, form, and number). While the patient matches these cards, the only feedback they receive is the response "right" or "wrong." After 10 consecutive correct matches the matching rule shifts to a new dimension (unannounced) and the patient must discover the "new" rule. One of the primary scores from the WCST is the number of perseverative errors committed (a perseverative error is scored when the patient continues to sort to a dimension despite clear feedback that the strategy is incorrect). Other tests of executive functioning include the Booklet Format Category Test, the Stroop Color Word Test, and the similarities and comprehension subtests of the WAIS-III (tapping abstract reasoning). Measures of tactile sensitivity and motor strength and speed are also important to measure in a neuropsycho-

logical examination. Typically, neuropsychologists are interested in both the absolute magnitude of the patients' performance (how well they performed in comparison with the test's norms) and any differences between the two body sides (the left-right discrepancies). Tests of motor functioning include the Finger Tapping Test (the average number of taps per 10 seconds with the index finger of each hand) and a test of grip strength (using the hand dynamometer). Sensory tests include Finger Localization Tests (naming and localizing fingers on the subject's and examiner's hand) and Two-Point Discrimination and Simultaneous Extinction Test (measuring two-point discrimination threshold and the extinction or suppression of sensory information by simultaneous bilateral activation).

Many psychiatric conditions, particularly anxiety and depression, can produce transient neuropsychological deficits. Therefore a complete neuropsychological assessment should also include a self-report test of psychopathology, such as the MMPI-2. Including such a test in the battery allows the neuropsychologist to assess the possible contribution of psychopathology to the cognitive profile. One of the main advantages of neuropsychological assessment is the ability to compare a patient's performance to that of a normative sample. This allows one to determine how well the patient performed relative to a comparison group. However, the usefulness of neuropsychological test data can be limited by the quality of such norms. Unfortunately, the quality of norms varies greatly from test to test. Tests like the Wechsler IQ and Memory Scales have excellent norms, whereas other frequently used tests (like the Boston Naming Test) have severely limited norms. When working with older adults, it is most helpful to have age- and education-adjusted norms, because both these variables have a substantial mediating effect on the normal (age-appropriate) decline of cognitive function. A number of brief neuropsychological assessment tools are used in clinical practice. Brief assessment tools are not a substitute for a comprehensive neuropsychological assessment, but they can be useful as screening instruments or when patients cannot tolerate a complete test battery. One such brief test is the Dementia Rating Scale–2 (DRS-2).[17] This test provides a brief but reasonable assessment of the major areas of cognitive functioning (attention, memory, language, reasoning, and construction). The test employs a screening methodology in evaluating these cognitive domains; the patient is first presented with a moderately difficult item, and, if that item is passed, the rest of the items in that domain are skipped (with the examiner moving on to the next domain). However, if the screening item is failed, then a series of easier items are given to more fully evaluate the specific cognitive ability.

The DRS-2 is a useful tool for assessing patients 55 and older who are suspected of having dementia of the Alzheimer's type (DAT). It takes between 10 and 20 minutes to administer, and it provides 6 scores. The total score and the scores from the Memory and Initiation/Perseveration subscales have been useful in the identification of patients with DAT. The DRS was designed to have a deep "floor." This means that the test contains many items that tap low levels of function and allow the test to track patients as their function declines. This quality makes the DRS a useful tool for monitoring patients with DAT along the course of their illness.

The differentiation of depression from dementia in older adults is the most common neuropsychological referral question. Depression in older adults is often accompanied by mild cognitive deficits, making the diagnostic picture somewhat confused with that of early dementia. By evaluating the profile of deficits obtained across a battery of tests, a neuropsychologist can help distinguish between these two illnesses. For example, depressed patients tend to have problems with attention, concentration, and memory (new learning and retrieval), whereas patients with early dementia have problems with delayed recall memory (encoding) and word-finding or naming problems. Both groups of patients can display problems with frontal lobe/executive function. However, the functioning of the depressed patient often improves with cues or suggestions about strategies; this typically does not help patients with dementia. Although this general pattern does not always hold true, it is this type of contrasting performance that allows neuropsychological assessment to aid differential diagnosis.

Whether or not a patient is capable of living independently is a complex and often emotionally charged question. Neuropsychological test data

can provide one piece of the information needed to make a reasonable medical decision in this area. In particular, neuropsychological test data regarding memory functioning (both new learning rate and delayed recall) and executive functioning (judgement and planning) have been shown to predict failure and success in independent living. However, any neuropsychological test data should be thoughtfully combined with information from an occupational therapy evaluation, assessment of the patient's psychiatric status, and input from the family (when available) before rendering any judgment about a patient's capacity for independent living.

Neuropsychological assessment has a role in the diagnosis and treatment of adults and children with attention deficit disorder (ADD). However, as in the question of independent living status, it provides just a piece of the data necessary for making this diagnosis. The evaluation of ADD should include a detailed review of academic performance, including report cards and school records. When possible, living parents should also be interviewed for their recollections of the patient's childhood behavior. The neuropsychological evaluation should focus on measuring intelligence, academic achievement (expecting to see normal or better IQ with reduced academic achievement), and multiple measures of attention and concentration (with tests of passive, active [shifting], and sustained attention). Although the neuropsychological testing profile might aid the diagnosis of ADD in adulthood, the diagnosis is usually based on historic data. The neuropsychological test data or profile is often more useful in helping the patient, the family, and the treater understand the impact of ADD on the patient's current cognitive abilities, as well as ruling out comorbid disorders (such as learning disabilities, which are very common in ADD).

Neuropsychological assessments can often aid in treatment planning for patients with moderate to severe psychiatric illness. Although this aspect of neuropsychological testing is somewhat underutilized at present, in the years to come this may prove to be the most beneficial use of these tests. Neuropsychological assessment benefits treatment planning by providing objective data (a test profile), regarding the patients cognitive skills (deficits and strengths). The availability of such data can help clinicians and family members develop more realistic expectations about the patient's functional capacity.[18] This can be particularly helpful for patients suffering from severe disorders, such as schizophrenia. The current literature indicates that neuropsychological deficits are more predictive of long-term outcome in schizophrenic patients than are either positive or negative symptoms.

Obtaining and Understanding Test Reports

Referring a patient for an assessment consultation should be like referring to any professional colleague. Psychological and neuropsychological testing cannot be done "blind." The psychologist will want to hear relevant information about the case and will explore with the practitioner asking for the referral what questions need to be answered (this is called the referral question). Based on this case discussion, the psychologist will select an appropriate battery of tests designed to obtain the desired information. It is helpful if the referrer prepares the patient for the testing by reviewing with him or her why the consultation is desired and telling him or her that it will likely take 3 or more hours to complete. The referrer should expect the psychologist to evaluate the patient in a timely manner and to provide verbal feedback, a "wet read" within hours after the testing. The written report should follow shortly thereafter (inpatient reports should be produced within 48 hours and outpatients reports should be available within 2 weeks).

The psychological assessment report is the written statement of the psychologist's findings. It should be understandable and it should plainly state and answer the referral question(s). The report should contain relevant background information, a list of the tests used in the consultation, a statement about the validity of the results and the confidence the psychologist has in the findings, a detailed integrated description of the patient, and clear recommendations. It should contain raw data (e.g., IQ scores) as appropriate to allow for meaningful follow-up testing. To a considerable degree, the quality of a report (and the assessment consultation) can be judged from the recommendations provided. A good assess-

ment report should contain a number of useful recommendations. The referrer should never read just the summary of a test report; this leads to the loss of important information, because the whole report is really a summary of a very complex consultation process.

In contrast to the written report from a personality assessment, the written neuropsychological testing report tends to be less integrated. The test findings are provided and reviewed for each major areas of cognitive functioning (intelligence, attention, memory, language, reasoning, and construction). These reports typically contain substantial amounts of raw data to allow for meaningful retesting comparison. However, the neuropsychological assessment report should provide a brief summary that reviews and integrates the major findings and also contains useful and meaningful recommendations. As with all professional consultations, the examining psychologist should be willing to meet with the referrer and/or the patient to review the findings.

References

1. Matarazzo J: *Wechsler's measurement and appraisal of adult intelligence*, New York, 1979, Oxford University Press.
2. Wechsler D: *Manual for the Wechsler intelligence scale for children-III*, New York, 1991, Psychological Corporation.
3. Wechsler D: *Manual for the Wechsler adult intelligence scale-III*, New York, 1997, Psychological Corporation.
4. Wechsler D: *Wechsler memory scale-III*, New York, 1997, Psychological Corporation.
5. Wechsler D: *Wechsler abbreviated scale of intelligence (WASI)*, New York, 1999, Psychological Corporation.
6. Butcher J, Dahlstrom W, Graham J, et al: *MMPI-2: manual for administration and scoring*, Minneapolis, 1989, University of Minnesota Press.
7. Greene R: *The MMPI-2/MMPI: an interpretive manual*, ed 2, Boston, 2000, Allyn and Bacon.
8. Millon T: *Millon clinical multiaxial inventory-III manual*, Minneapolis, 1994, National Computer Systems.
9. Morey L: *The personality assessment inventory: professional manual*, Odessa, FL, 1991, Psychological Assessment Resources.
10. Rorschach H: *Psychodiagnostics*, New York, 1942, Grune & Stratton.
11. Exner J: *The Rorschach: a comprehensive system, vol 1 basic foundations*, ed 3, New York, 1993, Wiley & Sons.

12. Murray H: *Explorations in personality*, New York, 1938, Oxford University Press.
13. Reitan R: *Theoretical and methodological bases of the Halstead-Reitan neuropsychological test battery.* In Grant I, Adams K, editors: *Neuropsychological assessment of neuropsychiatric disorders*, New York, 1986, Oxford University Press.
14. Milberg, W., Hebben, N., and Kaplan, E. (1986). *The Boston process neuropsychological approach to neuropsychological assessment.* In Grant I and Adams K, editors: *Neuropsychological Assessment of Neuropsychiatric Disorders*, New York: Oxford University Press.
15. Spreen O, Strauss E: *A compendium of neuropsychological tests*, ed 2, New York, 1998, Oxford University Press.
16. Weintraub S, Mesulam M-M: *Mental state assessments of young and elderly adults in behavioral neurology.* In Mesulam M-M, editor: *Principles of behavioral neurology.* Philadelphia, 1985, FA Davis.
17. Jurica P, Leitten C, Mattis S: *Dementia rating scale-2 (DRS-2): professional manual*, Odessa, Fla, 2001, Psychological Assessment Resources
18. Keefe R: The contribution of neuropsychology to psychiatry. *Am J Psychiatry*, 152:6–14, 1995.

Chapter 7

Coping With Illness and Psychotherapy of the Medically Ill

Steven C. Schlozman, M.D.
James E. Groves, M.D.
Avery D. Weisman, M.D.

Coping with illness can be a serious problem for both the patient and the physician. However, when addressing this phenomenon, it is important to recognize that few medical schools or residency programs train physicians to manage the interpersonal stress and discomfort in patients and in themselves that medical illness engenders. This absence stands in stark contrast to the way the art of medicine was conceptualized 100 years ago. Indeed, the irony of our increasing prowess in healing is our growing discomfort and our profound sense of impotence when a cure cannot be found, and when coping is the order of the day. This dilemma is both consciously realized and unconsciously experienced; patients and staff feel the ripple effect alike.

Fortunately, the consultation-liaison (C-L) psychiatrist is ideally suited to assist both patient and physician with the complexities of medical illness. From a psychological standpoint, the psychiatrist's scope directly involves an appreciation of the powerful emotions and defense mechanisms that swirl in and around the hospital bed. These observations are relevant in both the consultative setting and in the therapist's office. In fact, there is a growing body of literature that focuses on the specifics of psychotherapeutic techniques with the medically ill. This chapter addresses the fundamentals of coping, as well as the art of working psychotherapeutically with the medically ill.

What Exactly Is Coping?

For the patient and the physician, coping can be mutually beneficial and constructive, or depleting and deleterious. The coping strategies used by one can be complementary to the strategies used by the other or, unfortunately, be antagonistic.

Coping is best defined as problem-solving behavior that is intended to bring about relief, reward, quiescence, and equilibrium. Nothing in this definition promises permanent resolution of problems. It does imply a combination of knowing what the problems are and how to go about reaching a correct direction that will help resolution.

In ordinary language, the term *coping* is used to mean only the outcome of managing a problem, and it overlooks the intermediate process of appraisal, performance, and correction that most problem-solving entails. Coping is not a simple judgment about how some difficulty worked out. It is an extensive, recursive process of self-exploration, self-instruction, self-correction, self-rehearsal, and guidance gathered from outside sources.

Coping with illness and its ramifications cannot help but be an inescapable part of medical practice. Therefore the overall purpose of any intervention, physical or psychosocial, is to improve coping with potential problems beyond the limits of illness itself. Such interventions must take into account

61

both the problems to be solved and the individuals most closely affected by the difficulties.

How anyone copes depends on the nature of a problem as well as on the mental, emotional, physical, and social resources one has available for the coping process. The hospital psychiatrist is in an advantageous position to evaluate how physical illness interferes with the patient's conduct of life and to see how psychosocial issues impede the course of illness and recovery. This is accomplished largely by knowing which psychosocial problems are pertinent, which physical symptoms are most distressing, and what interpersonal relations support or undermine coping.

Assessment of how anyone copes, especially in a clinical setting, requires an emphasis on the here and now because that is the most practical. Long-range forays into past history are relevant only if they illuminate the present predicament. In fact, increasingly clinicians are adopting a focused and problem-solving approach to therapy with medically ill patients. For example, supportive therapies for medically ill children and adults in both group and individual settings have been found to not only reduce psychiatric morbidity, but also to have measurable effects on the course of nonpsychiatric illnesses.

Who Are Effective Copers?

There are few paragons who cope exceedingly well with every problem likely to occur. For virtually everyone, psychiatrists included, sickness imposes a personal and social burden, threat, and risk; these reactions are seldom precisely proportional to the actual dangers of the primary disease. Therefore effective copers may be regarded as individuals with a special skill or with personal traits that enable them to master many difficulties. What characterizes these individuals?

1. They are optimistic about mastering problems and, despite setbacks, generally maintain a high level of morale.
2. They tend to be practical and emphasize immediate problems, issues, and obstacles that must be conquered before even visualizing a remote or ideal resolution.
3. They select from a wide range of potential strategies and tactics, and their policy is not

to be at a loss for fallback methods. In this respect, they are resourceful.
4. They heed various possible outcomes and improve coping by being aware of consequences.
5. They are generally flexible and open to suggestions, but they do not give up the final say in decisions.
6. They are quite composed, although vigilant in avoiding emotional extremes that could impair judgment.

These are collective tendencies; they seldom typify any specific individual except the heroic or the idealized. No one copes superlatively at all times, especially with problems that impose a risk and might well be overwhelming. Notably, however, effective copers seem able to choose the kind of situation in which they are most likely to prosper. In addition, effective copers often maintain enough confidence to feel resourceful enough to survive intact. Finally, it is our impression that those individuals who cope effectively do not pretend to have knowledge that they do not have; therefore they feel comfortable turning to experts they trust. The clinical relevance of these characterizations is the extent to which we can assess how patients cope by more accurately pinpointing which traits they seem to lack.

Who Are Bad Copers?

Bad copers are not necessarily bad people, nor even incorrigibly ineffective people. In fact, it is too schematic merely to indicate that bad copers have the opposite characteristics of effective copers. Bad copers are those who have more problems in coping with unusual, intense, and unexpected difficulties because of the following traits:

1. They tend to be excessive in self-expectation, rigid in outlook, inflexible in standards, and reluctant to compromise or to ask for help.
2. Their opinion of how people should behave is narrow and absolute; they allow little room for tolerance.
3. Although prone to firm adherence to preconceptions, bad copers may show unexpected compliance or be suggestible on specious grounds, with little cause.

4. They are inclined to excessive denial and elaborate rationalization; in addition, they are unable to focus on salient problems.

5. Because they find it difficult to weigh feasible alternatives, bad copers tend to be more passive than usual and fail to initiate action on their own behalf.

6. Their rigidity occasionally lapses, and bad copers subject themselves to impulsive judgments or atypical behavior that fails to be effective.

Indeed, structured investigations into the psychiatric symptoms of the medically ill have often yielded many of the attributes of those who do not cope well. Problems such as demoralization, anhedonia, anxiety, pain, and overwhelming grief all have been documented in medical patients for whom psychiatric attention was indicated in a C-L setting.

The Role of Religion

The significance of religious or spiritual conviction in medically ill populations deserves special mention. Virtually every C-L psychiatrist works with patients as they wrestle with existential issues, such as mortality, fate, justice, and fairness. Such ruminations cannot help but invoke religious considerations in both patient and the physician; moreover, there is a growing appreciation in the medical literature for the important role that these considerations can play.

In some investigations,[1] being at peace with oneself and with one's sense of a higher power was predictive of both physical and psychiatric recovery. However, other studies[2] have suggested that resentment toward God, fears of God's abandonment, and a willingness to invoke Satanic motivation for medical illness were all predictive of worsening health and an increased risk of death.

In so much as the role of the therapist and the C-L psychiatrist is to identify and to strengthen those attributes that are most likely to aid a patient's physical and emotional well-being, effective therapy for the medically ill involves exploring the religious convictions of patients; fostering those elements is most likely to be helpful. It is *never* the role of the physician to encourage religious conviction de novo. At the same time, ignoring religious content risks omitting an important element of the psychotherapeutic armamentarium.

The Medical Predicament—Bringing It All Together

Coping refers to how a patient responds and deals with problems within a complex of factors that relates to disease, sickness, and vulnerability. Disease is the categoric reason for being sick and finding it difficult to cope. Sickness is the individual style of illness and patienthood. Vulnerability is the tendency to be distressed and to develop emotional extremes in the course of trying to cope.

A skilled psychiatrist, for example, focuses on the immediate illness and on surrounding circumstances (e.g., social and emotional). A key question to be answered is *why now?* What has preceded the request for consultation? Is the clinical situation too complicated? Is the clinician exasperated? How does the patient show his or her sense of futility and despair? How did the present trouble come about? Was there a time when such problems could have been thwarted?

If there is any doubt about the gap between how the staff and patents differ in cultural bias and social expectations, listen to the bedside conversation. Good communication may not only reduce potential problem areas, but also may actually help patients to cope better. Therefore coping well involves a kind of social compact of mutual respect that is formed by certain values and appropriate behavior. It also defines potential risks and pressure points. Because mutual values are concerned, how one copes is inevitably tied to how one is expected to cope, and therefore be judged. The psychiatrist, however, is by no means alone in professional concern about coping. Any specialist is expected to confer benefits through instruction and direction that will help coping with whatever interferes with recovery. There are, for instance, specialists in dialysis, nutrition, colostomy care, chaplaincy, social work, chemotherapy, pain control, and so on, to name only a few of the "coping experts" available in large modern hospitals. Long-term illness has its special psychosocial problems that merit assessment and intervention because coping is regularly impaired. As already mentioned, much of chronic disease evokes existential issues, such as death, permanent disability, low self-esteem, dependence, and alienation.

Given all of this, it is important to remember that psychiatry does not arbitrarily introduce psychosocial problems. If, for example, a patient is found to have an unspoken but vivid fear of death or to be suffering from an unrecognized and unresolved bereavement, fear and grief are already there, not superfluous artifacts of the evaluation procedure.

Being sick is, of course, much easier for some patients than for others, and for certain patients, it is preferred over trying to make it in the outside world. There is too much anxiety, fear of failure, inadequacy, pathologic shyness, expectation, frustration, and social hypochondriasis to make the struggle for holding one's own appealing. At key moments of life, sickness is a solution. Although healthy people are expected to tolerate defeat and to withstand disappointments, others legitimize their low self-esteem by a variety of excuses, denial, self-pity, and symptoms, long after other patients are back to work. Such patients thrive in a complaining atmosphere and even blame their physicians. These are perverse forms of coping.

These complexities substantially complicate the role of the hospital psychiatrist. The clinician must assess the motivation of staff and patient in asking for a psychiatric intervention. Additionally, clinicians need to be aware that the real question is not always the problem for which one is consulted. For example, the request for psychiatric consultation to treat depression and anxiety in a negativistic and passive-aggressive patient is inevitably more complicated than a simple recognition of certain key psychiatric symptoms. Such patients (through primitive defenses) can generate a profound sense of hopelessness and discomfort in their treaters. It is often an unspoken and unrecognized desire by physicians and ancillary staff that the psychiatrist shifts the focus of negativity and aggression onto him or herself and away from the remaining treatment team. If the consulting psychiatrist is not aware of these subtleties, the intent of the consultation will be misinterpreted and the psychiatrist's efforts will ultimately fall short.

Coping and Social Support

Every person needs or at least deserves a measure of support, sustenance, security, and self-esteem, even if they are not patients at all, but human beings encountered at a critical time.

No one gets far or feels well for long without drawing on someone significant or on something held valuable that sustains efforts to cope. Patients pointing themselves toward recovery simply need more support, sustenance, security, and self-esteem. Collectively, these factors constitute what can be called social support for the tasks of dealing with potential or actual problems.

In assessing problems and needs, the psychiatrist can help by identifying potential pressure points where trouble might arise. These include the following areas:

1. Health and well-being
2. Family responsibility
3. Marital and sexual roles
4. Job and money
5. Community expectations and approval
6. Religious and cultural demands
7. Self-image and sense of inadequacy
8. Existential issues

Social support is not a hodgepodge of interventions designed to cheer up or straighten out difficult patients. Self-image and self-esteem, for example, depend on the sense of confidence generated by various sources of social success and support. In a practical sense, social support reflects what society expects and therefore demands about health and conduct.

Social support is not a "sometime" thing, to be used only for the benefit of those too weak, needy, or troubled to get along by themselves. It requires a deliberate skill, which professionals can cultivate, in recognizing, refining, and implementing what any vulnerable individual needs to feel better and to cope better. In this light, it is not an amorphous exercise in reassurance but a combination of therapeutic gambits opportunistically activated to normalize a patient's attitude and behavior. Techniques of support range from concrete assistance to extended counseling.[3,4] Their aim is to help patients get along without professional support. Social support depends on an acceptable image of the patient, not one that invariably "pathologizes." If a counselor only corrects mistakes or points out what is wrong, bad, or inadequate, then insecurity increases and self-esteem inevitably suffers.

Courage to Cope

Most psychiatric assessments and interventions tend to pathologize, and to emphasize shortcomings, defects, and deviation from acceptable norms. Seldom does an examiner pay much attention to positive attributes such as confidence, loyalty, intelligence, hope, dedication, and generosity. One of the commonly neglected virtues in clinical situations is that of courage.

Courage in a clinical sense should not be confused with "bravery under fire." The derring-do of heroes is seldom found among ordinary people, who usually have more than their share of anxiety and apprehension when facing unfamiliar, unknown, and threatening events. Threats are manifest on many levels of experience, ranging from actual injury to situations that signify failure, disgrace, humiliation, embarrassment, and so forth. In a sense, threat is "negative support" because it may do or undo everything that positive support is supposed to strengthen. It pathologizes. The courage to cope is a real but seldom recognized element in the attributes that affect the coping process. Nevertheless, in coping well, the courage to cope means a wish to perform competently and to be valued as a significant person, even when threatened by risk and anonymity.

Hope, confidence, and morale go together and can be directly asked about because most patients know what these terms mean without translation. Naturally, few people readily admit their tendency to fail, shirk, or behave in unworthy ways. Nevertheless, a skillful interview gets behind denial, rationalization, posturing, and pretense without evoking another threat to security or self-esteem.

Courage requires an awareness of risk as well as a willingness to go it alone despite a substantial degree of anxiety, tension, and worry about being able to withstand pressure and pain. Courage is always accompanied by vulnerability, but it engages itself in the courage to cope.

Vulnerability is present in all humans, and it shows up at times of crisis, stress, calamity, and threat to well-being and identity.[5–11] Actually it has a double meaning: (1) the disposition or potential to undergo much distress and (2) the reality of distress itself, called *dysphoria.*

How does a patient visualize threat? What is most feared, say, in approaching a surgical procedure? The diagnosis? Anesthesia? Possible invalidism? Failure, pain, or abandonment by physician or family?

Coping and vulnerability have a loosely reciprocal relationship in that the better one copes, the less distress he or she experiences as a function of acknowledged vulnerability. In general, a good deal of distress often derives directly from a sense of uncertainty about how well one will cope when called on to do so. This does not mean that those who deny or disavow problems and concerns are superlative copers. The reverse may be true. Courage to cope requires anxiety confronted and dealt with, not phlegmatic indifference to outcome.

Table 7-1 shows 13 common types of distress. Table 7-2 describes how to find out about salient problems, the strategy used for coping, and the degree of the resolution attained.

Few coping strategies occur in an unamalgamated form, in pure culture. Most coping consists of a variety of specific tactics, but usually combines a number of more generic types, such as those listed in Table 7-2. Keeping their reciprocal relationship in mind, to find out about the specific dysphoria (e.g., anger, anxiety, depression, suspicion, futility, and hopelessness), the examiner must also find out how the patient tends to handle distress. Go over the potential pressure points for detectable problems, and see what misfortune the patient associates with not living up to what is expected and with not coping well enough. The psychiatrist cannot finesse questions of life and death, because no patient can be wholly exempt from such concerns.

Many interventions call on the consulting psychiatrist to ask patients to fill out forms indicating their degree of anxiety, level of self-esteem, perceived illness, and so on. Although such queries are often sources of valuable information, these standardized inquiries are no substitute for careful and compassionate interviews. There is a strong element of social desirability present in any attempt to assess how patients cope. How a patient deals with illness may not be the same as how he or she wishes to manage. Vulnerability, except in extreme forms (such as depression, anger, and anxiety), is difficult to characterize exactly, so the astute clinician must depend on a telling episode or metaphor that typifies a total reaction.

Table 7-1. Vulnerability

Hopelessness:	Patient believes that all is lost; effort is futile; there is no chance at all; a passive surrender to the inevitable
Turmoil/Perturbation:	Patient is tense, agitated, restless, hyperalert to potential risks, real and imagined
Frustration:	Patient is angry about an inability to progress, recover, or get satisfactory answers or relief
Despondency/Depression:	Patient is dejected, withdrawn, apathetic, tearful, and often unable to interact verbally
Helplessness/Powerlessness:	Patient complains of being too weak to struggle anymore; cannot initiate action or make decisions that stick
Anxiety/Fear:	Patient feels on the edge of dissolution, with dread and specific fears about impending doom and disaster
Exhaustion/Apathy:	Patient feels too worn out and depleted to care; there is more indifference than sadness
Worthlessness/Self-rebuke:	Patient feels persistent self-blame and no good; he or she finds numerous causes for weakness, failure, and incompetence
Painful Isolation/Abandonment:	Patient is lonely and feels ignored and alienated from significant others
Denial/Avoidance:	Patient speaks or acts as if threatening aspects of illness are minimal, almost showing a jolly interpretation of related events, or else a serious disinclination to examine potential problems
Truculence/Annoyance:	Patient is embittered and not openly angry; feels mistreated, victimized, and duped by forces or people
Repudiation of Significant Others:	Patient rejects or antagonizes significant others, including family, friends, and professional sources of support
Closed Time Perspective:	Patient may show any or all of the these symptoms, but in addition foresees an exceedingly limited future

Table 7-2. Coping (To Find Out How a Patient Copes)

Problem:	In your opinion, what has been the most difficult for you since your illness started? How has it troubled you?
Strategy:	What did you do (or are doing) about the problem?
	Get more information (rational/intellectual approach)
	Talk it over with others to relieve distress (share concern)
	Try to laugh it off; make light of it (reverse affect)
	Put it out of mind; try to forget (suppression/denial)
	Distract myself by doing other things (displacement/dissipation)
	Take a positive step based on a present understanding (confrontation)
	Accept, but change the meaning to something easier to deal with (redefinition)
	Submit, yield, and surrender to the inevitable (passivity/fatalism)
	Do something, anything, reckless or impractical (acting out)
	Look for feasible alternatives to negotiate (if *x*, then *y*)
	Drink, eat, take drugs, and so on, to reduce tension (tension reduction)
	Withdraw, get away, and seek isolation (stimulus reduction)
	Blame someone or something (projection/disowning/externalization)
	Go along with directives from authority figures (compliance)
	Blame self for faults; sacrifice or atone (undoing self-pity)
Resolution:	How has it worked out so far?
	Not at all
	Doubtful relief
	Limited relief, but better
	Much better; actual resolution

Adapted from Weisman AD: *The realization of death: a guide for the psychological autopsy*, New York, 1974, Jason Aronson Inc.

How to Find Out More About Coping

Thus far, we have discussed the following:

1. Salient characteristics of effective and less effective copers
2. Methods by which deficits in patients can be identified and how clinicians can intervene
3. Potential pressure points that alert clinicians to different psychosocial difficulties
4. Types of emotional vulnerabilities
5. A format for listing different coping strategies, along with questions about resolution

The assessment and identification of ways in which a patient copes or fails to cope with specific problems requires both a description by the patient and an interpretation by the psychiatrist. Even so, this may not be enough. Details of descriptive importance may not be explicit or forthcoming. In these situations, the clinician must take pains to elucidate the specifics of each situation. If not, the result is only a soft approximation that generalizes where it should be precise. Indeed, the clinician should ask again and again about a topic that is unclear and rephrase, without yielding to cliches and general impressions.

Psychiatrists have been imbued with the value of so-called empathy and intuition. Although immediate insights and inferences can be pleasing to the examiner, sometimes these conclusions can be misleading and totally wrong. It is far more empathic to respect each patient's individuality and unique slant on the world by making sure that the examiner accurately describes in detail how problems are confronted. To draw a quick inference without being sure about a highly private state of mind is distinctly unempathic. Like most individuals, patients give themselves the benefit of the doubt and claim to resolve problems in a socially desirable and potentially effective way. It takes little experience to realize that disavowal of any problem through pleasant distortions is itself a coping strategy, not necessarily an accurate description of how one coped.

Simple, straightforward problems are usually someone else's problems. It is difficult to translate complex events into understandable language without sounding pedantic or glossing over ambiguities. Good coping usually means less distress and little dysphoria, so it is hard to identify what patients do when coping is stressful. Consequently, relentless pursuit is guided by painful affect. Is the patient able to indicate any problem, or does he or she immediately set up a granitic denial? It is here that the examiner asks, "What if . . ." questions, such as "What if someone like you had a boss (or wife or husband) who was never satisfied and always picked you apart? How would that person handle it?"

Effective copers are not only flexible, resourceful, optimistic, and practical, but also good at indicating pressure points and problem areas and at instructing themselves what to do.

On the other hand, there are two groups of patients who are in general less effective in coping. One group adamantly denies any difficulty. The second group floods the interview with details of how badly the world and its occupants have treated them. In the first group, militant denial is the major strategy. In the second, the chief strategy is to put off the interviewer by appealing for pity and rescue. By seeking credit for having suffered so much, such patients reject any implication that they might have prevented, deflected, or corrected what has befallen them (see Table 7-2). Helping these patients does not necessarily require that they acknowledge their role in their particular predicament. Instead, the empathic listener identifies and provides comfort around the implicit fear that these patients harbor (i.e., that they somehow deserve their debilitation).

Suppression, isolation, and projection are common defenses. This makes it difficult to evaluate the scope of denial and to credit the reports that many patients give. To believe or not to believe is always an open question. Effective copers seem to pinpoint problems clearly, whereas bad copers, as well as those with strong defenses, seem only to seek relief from further questions without attempting anything suggesting reflective analysis.

In learning how anyone copes, a measure of authentic skepticism is always appropriate, especially when it is combined with a willingness to correction later on. The balance between denial and affirmation is always uncertain. The key is to focus on points of ambiguity, anxiety, and ambivalence while tactfully preserving a patient's self-esteem. A tactful examiner might say, for example, "I'm really not clear about what exactly bothered you, and what you really did . . ."

The purpose of focusing is to avoid premature formulations that gloss over points of ambiguity. An overly rigid format in approaching any evaluation risks overlooking individual tactics that deny, avoid, dissemble, and blame others for difficulties. Patients, too, can be rigid, discouraging alliance, rebuffing collaboration, and preventing an effective physician-patient relationship.

How To Be a Better Coper

Coping with illness is only one special area of human behavior. It is important to recognize that in evaluating how patients cope, examiners should learn their own coping styles and, in effect, learn from patients. Knowledge of medication, psychodynamic theory, and descriptive psychiatry has less to do with the outcome of psychotherapeutic intervention than the physician's integrity and informed compassion. Credentials, of course, are important, but it is uncertain which credentials are essential. Clearly, it is not enough to mean well, to have a warm heart, or to have a head filled with scientific information. Coping well requires open-ended communication and self-awareness. No technique for coping is applicable to one and all. In fact, the concept of technique may be antithetical to true understanding. A false objectivity obstructs appraisal; an exaggerated subjectivity only confuses what is being said about whom.

Psychiatrists and patients can become better copers by cultivating the characteristics of effective copers. Coping is, after all, a skill that is useful in a variety of situations, although many modifications of basic principles are called for.

Confidence in being able to cope can be enhanced only through repeated attempts at self-appraisal, self-instruction, and self-correction. Coping well with illness—with any problem—does not predict invariable success, but it does provide a foundation for becoming a better coper.

REFERENCES

1. Pargament KI, Koenig HG, Tarakeshwar N, et al: Religious struggle as a predictor of mortality among medically ill patients: a 2-year longitudinal study, *Arch Int Med* 161:1881–1885, 2001.
2. Clarke DM, Mackinnon AJ, Smith GC, et al: Dimensions of psychopathology in the medically ill: a latent trait analysis, *Psychosomatics* 41:418–425, 2000.
3. Stauffer MH: A long-term psychotherapy group for children with chronic medical illness, *Bull Menninger Clinic* 62:15–32, 1998.
4. Saravay SM: Psychiatric interventions in the medically ill: outcomes and effectiveness research, *Psych Clin North, Am* 19:467–480, 1996.
5. Bird B: *Talking with patients*, ed 2, Philadelphia, 1973, JB Lippincott.
6. Coelho G, Hamburg D, Adams J, editors: *Coping and adaptation*, New York, 1974, Basic Books Inc.
7. Jackson E: *Coping with crises in your life*, New York, 1974, Hawthorn Books Inc.
8. Kessler R, Price R, Wortman C: Social factors in psychopathology: stress, social support, and coping processes, *Annu Rev Psychol* 36:531–572, 1985.
9. Moos R, editor: *Human adaptation: coping with life crises*, Lexington, Mass, 1976, DC Heath & Co.
10. Murphy L, Moriarity A: *Vulnerability, coping and growth*, New Haven, Conn, 1976, Yale University Press.
11. Weisman A: *The coping capacity: on the nature of being mortal*, New York, 1984, Human Sciences.

Chapter 8
Mood-Disordered Patients

Ned H. Cassem, M.D., S.J.
George I. Papakostas, M.D.
Maurizio Fava, M.D.
Theodore A. Stern, M.D.

Most common among psychiatric disorders, depression sufficient to warrant professional care affects approximately 10% of the general population during their lifetime.[1] Both the Epidemiological Catchment Area Study and the National Comorbidity Survey Study have found that major depression is prevalent, with cross-sectional rates ranging from 2.3% to 4.9%, respectively.[2,3] Although this condition ranks first among reasons for psychiatric hospitalization (23.3% of total hospitalizations), it has been estimated that 80% of all persons suffering from it are either treated by nonpsychiatric personnel or are not treated at all.[4]

The presence of one or more chronic medical conditions raises the recent (6-month) and lifetime prevalence of mood disorder from 5.8% to 9.4% and from 8.9% to 12.9%. In general, the more severe the illness, the more likely depression is to complicate it.[5] At the Massachusetts General Hospital (MGH), the psychiatric consultant called to see a medical patient makes a diagnosis of major depression in approximately 20% of cases, making depression the most common problem that presents for diagnostic evaluation and treatment.

Failure to treat depression leaves the patient at even higher risk for further complications and death. Proceeding to cardiac surgery while in a state of major depression, for example, is known to increase the chances of a fatal outcome.[6] Depression in the first 24 hours after myocardial infarction (MI) was associated with significantly increased risk of early death, reinfarction, or cardiac arrest.[7] Even in depressed outpatients, the risk of mortality, chiefly as a result of cardiovascular disease, is more than doubled.[8] Some degree of depression in patients hospitalized for coronary artery disease (CAD) is associated with an increased risk of mortality and also with ongoing depression over the year following the admission.[9] The increased risk of cardiac mortality has also been confirmed in a large community cohort of individuals with cardiac disease who presented with either major or minor depression.[10] Those subjects without cardiac disease but with depression also had a higher risk (from 1.5- to 3.9-fold) of cardiac mortality.[10] Among type 1 or 2 diabetic patients, the occurrence of depression was associated with a significantly higher risk of diabetes-specific complications, such as diabetic retinopathy, nephropathy, neuropathy, macrovascular complications, and sexual dysfunction.[11] There remains a clinical sense, moreover, that any seriously ill person who has neurovegetative symptoms, and who has given up and wishes he or she were dead, is going to do worse than if he or she had hope and motivation. Major depression, even if the patient is healthy in every other way, requires treatment. When a seriously ill person becomes depressed, the failure to recognize and treat the disorder is even more unfortunate.

Making the Diagnosis of Depression

The criteria for major depression according to the *Diagnostic and Statistical Manual of Mental Disorders* (DSM-IV)[12] should be applied to the patient with medical illness in the same way as in a patient without medical illness. DSM-IV now has a category for mood disorders "due to" a general medical condition. A stroke in the left hemisphere, for example, is commonly followed by a syndrome clinically indistinguishable from major depression. It can now be referred to as a "major depression-like" condition when full criteria are met. Our recommendation is to diagnose a mood disorder using the DSM-IV criteria. Major depression can now be diagnosed as such, but there is still no term in DSM-IV to represent what the Research Diagnostic Criteria (RDC) referred to as minor depression—a distinction that is important in the medically ill.

Diagnosis is crucial to treatment. Three questions face the consultant at the outset: (1) On clinical examination, does the patient manifest depression? (2) If so, is it due to an organic cause, such as a medication, that can be eliminated, treated, or reversed? (3) Does it arise from the medical condition in such a way that treatment of that condition will alleviate it (e.g., Cushing's disease) or in such a way that it must be treated itself (e.g., poststroke depression)?

Major Depression

Depression is a term used by most to describe even minor and transient mood fluctuations. It is seen everywhere and is often thought to be normal; therefore it is likely to be dismissed even when it is serious. This applies all the more to a patient with serious medical illness: If a man has terminal cancer and meets full criteria for major depression, this mood state is regarded by some as "appropriate." Depression is used here to denote the disorder of major depression—a seriously disabling condition for the patient, capable of endangering the patient even to death, not just an emotional reaction of sadness or despondency. If while recovering from an acute stroke a patient has a severe exacerbation of psoriasis, no one says that the cutaneous eruption is appropriate, even though the stress associated with the stroke has almost

certainly caused it. Moreover, caregivers are swift to treat the exacerbation. When a patient with a prior history of depression lapses into severe depression 1 month after beginning radiation therapy for inoperable lung cancer, some may see a connection to the prior depressive illness and hasten to treat it. Far more common is the conclusion that "anyone with that condition" would be depressed. The majority of terminally ill cancer patients do not develop major depression no matter how despondent they feel at times. If a patient is hemorrhaging from a ruptured spleen, has lost a great deal of blood, becomes hypotensive, and goes into shock, no one says this is appropriate. Similar to shock, depression is a dread complication of medical illness that requires swift diagnosis and treatment. It is never appropriate.

Two assumptions are made here: (1) This depressive syndrome in medically ill patients shares the pathophysiology of (primary) major affective disorder, and (2) proper diagnosis is made by applying the same criteria. Because far less epidemiologic information is available on depression in the medically ill, the requirement that the dysphoria be present for 2 weeks should be regarded as only a rough approximation for medically ill patients. By DSM-IV,[12] at least five of the following nine symptoms should be present most of the day, nearly every day, and should include either depressed mood or loss of interest or pleasure:

1. Depressed mood, subjective or observed, most of the day, nearly every day
2. Markedly diminished interest or pleasure in all, or almost all, activities, nearly every day
3. Significant (more than 5% of body weight per month) weight loss or gain
4. Insomnia or hypersomnia, nearly every day
5. Psychomotor agitation or retardation, that is observable by others, nearly every day
6. Fatigue or loss of energy, nearly every day
7. Feelings of worthlessness or excessive or inappropriate guilt (which may be delusional), not merely about being sick, nearly every day
8. Diminished ability to think or concentrate, or indecisiveness, nearly every day
9. Recurrent thoughts of death (not just a fear of dying), recurrent suicidal ideation without a plan, or a suicide attempt or a specific plan for committing suicide.

These symptoms may seem invalid in medically ill patients. If the patient has advanced cancer, how can one attribute anorexia or fatigue to something other than the malignant disease itself? Four of the nine diagnostic symptoms could be viewed as impossible to ascribe exclusively to depression in a medically ill patient: sleep difficulty, anorexia, fatigue or energy loss, and difficulty concentrating. Endicott[13] has developed a list of symptoms that the clinician can substitute for and count in place of these four: fearful or depressed appearance; social withdrawal or decreased talkativeness; brooding, self-pity, or pessimism; and mood that is not reactive (i.e., cannot be cheered up, does not smile, or does not react to good news). Although this method is effective, Chochinov et al.[14] have compared diagnostic outcomes using both the regular (RDC) and the substituted criteria in a group of medically ill patients. If one holds the first two symptoms to the strict levels, that is, depressed mood must be present most of the day, nearly every day, and loss of interest applies to almost everything, the outcome for both diagnostic methods yielded exactly the same number of patients with the diagnosis of major depression.

The first help comes from discovery of symptoms that are more clearly the result of major depression, such as the presence of self-reproach ("I feel worthless"), the wish to be dead, or psychomotor retardation (few medical illnesses in and of themselves produce psychomotor retardation; hypothyroidism and Parkinson's disease are two of them). Insomnia or hypersomnia can also be helpful in the diagnosis, although the patient may have so much pain, dyspnea, or frequent clinical crises that sleep is impaired by these events. Although libidinous interests may not be high in an intensive care unit patient, some form of interest can usually be assessed, as when talk gets around to children or grandchildren, key interests, or people. Do they still find that their interest quickens or is it blunted? The ability to think or concentrate, similar to the other symptoms, needs to be specifically asked about in every case.

A second help for diagnosis is to free the search for specific neurovegetative symptoms from the patient's own misconceptions of depression. This label is often viewed as signifying that the patient's physician asked for psychiatric consultation because the symptoms were thought to be "in my head" or even the result of malingering. Depression is as much a somatic as a psychic disorder. Some patients who readily recognize a feeling like sadness mistakenly assume they should automatically "know" when they are depressed. This is no more logical than the assumption that one should know, in the presence of multiple symptoms, that one has systemic lupus erythematosus. (Moreover, some individuals lack awareness of even simple feelings, such as sadness.) The somatic manifestations of depression (e.g., insomnia, restlessness, and anhedonia) may even be construed as proof by patients that they have no "psychic" illness. "No, doctor, no way am I depressed; if I could just get rid of this pain, everything would be fine." Persistence and aggressive questioning are required to elicit the presence or absence of the nine symptoms.

If the history establishes six of nine symptoms, the consultant may not be certain that three of them have anything to do with depression but may just as likely stem from the medical illness itself. In this case, one must make a judgment whether there is anything in the treatment of the primary medical condition that can be improved. Of course, if the patient were found to be hypothyroid, the treatment of choice would not be antidepressants but judicious thyroid replacement. Usually, however, everything is being done for the patient to alleviate the symptoms of the primary illness. If this appears to be the case, our recommendation is to make the diagnosis of major depression and proceed with treatment.

States Commonly Mislabeled as Depression

Up to one third of patients referred for depression, on clinical examination, have neither major nor minor depression. By far the most common diagnosis found among these mislabeled referrals at the MGH has been an organic mental syndrome. A quietly confused patient often looks depressed. The patient with dementia or with a frontal lobe syndrome caused by brain injury can lack spontaneity and thus appear depressed. Only the complete physical and mental status examinations reveal the tell-tale abnormalities.

Although much less common, mental retardation may also be mistaken for depression, especially when failure to grasp or to comply with complex instructions makes no sense to those caring for the patient ("He seems not to care"). If suspected, mental retardation can be confirmed by history from family, by review of past records, or by formal intelligence testing.

Another unrecognized state, sometimes called depression by the consultee and easier for the psychiatrist to recognize, is anger. The patient's physician, realizing that the patient has been through a long and difficult illness, may perceive reduction in speech, smiling, and small talk on the patient's part as depression. The patient may thoroughly resent the illness, be irritated by therapeutic routines, and be fed up with the hospital environment but, despite interior fuming, remain reluctant to discharge overt wrath in the direction of the physician or nurses.

Excluding Organic Causes of Depression

When clinical findings confirm that the patient's symptoms are fully consistent with major depression, the consultant is still responsible for the differential diagnosis of this syndrome. Could the same constellation of symptoms be due to a medical illness or its treatment? The psychiatrist functions here as the last court of appeal. Should the patient's symptoms be due to an as yet undiagnosed illness, the last physician with the chance of detecting it is the consultant. Differential diagnosis in this situation is qualitatively the same as that described for excluding the organic causes of delirium (see Chapter 12). With depression, although the same process should be completed, certain conditions more commonly produce depressive syndromes and are worthy of comment.

A check on the medications that the patient is currently receiving generally tells the consultant whether or not the patient is receiving something that might cause a change in mood. Ordinarily, one would like to establish a relationship between the onset of depressive symptoms and either the start of, or a change in, the medication. If such a connection can be established, the simplest course is to stop the agent and monitor the patient for improvement. When the patient requires continued treatment, as for hypertension, the presumed offending agent can be changed, with the hope that

the change to another antihypertensive will be followed by resolution of depressive symptoms. When this fails or when clinical judgment warrants no change in medication, it may be necessary to start an antidepressant along with the antihypertensive drug. The literature linking drugs to depression is inconclusive at best. Clinicians have seen depression following use of reserpine and steroids, and with withdrawal from cocaine, amphetamine, and alcohol. The most common central nervous system (CNS) side effect of a drug is confusion or delirium, and this is commonly mislabeled as depression because a mental status examination has not been done.

Abnormal laboratory values should not be overlooked because they may provide the clues to an undiagnosed abnormality responsible for the depressive symptoms. Laboratory values necessary for the routine differential diagnosis in psychiatric consultation should be reviewed. A work-up is not complete if the evaluation of thyroid and parathyroid function is not included.

Many medical illnesses have been associated with depressive symptoms. The list is extensive and for all practical purposes can be included with the list of medical illnesses that can cause delirium (see Chapter 12).

Major depression is never "appropriate" (as in "This man has inoperable lung cancer metastatic to his brain and is depressed, which is appropriate"). Major depression is a common and dread complication of many medical illnesses as they become more severe. To call it anything else is to endanger the patient and neglect one of the worst forms of human suffering.

The disability associated with depressive illness is seldom recognized; yet it and mental illness in general show a stronger association with disability than with the severity of physical disease.[15] One of the most practical proofs of the capacity of major depression to undermine physical health is its association with decreases in trabecular bone in women (14% in the femoral neck),[16] a magnitude consistent with a 40% increase in hip fracture rates over a period of 10 years.

Major depression carries its own dangers and increases the risk of cardiovascular disease. Patients with coronary disease who are depressed show a significantly higher (24% versus 4%) prevalence of ventricular tachycardia[17] and a reduction in heart rate variability,[18] both of which increase the risk of sudden death. After acute MI, the presence of major depression is the strongest predictor of death at 6 months and depressive symptoms (defined as a Beck Depression Inventory score greater than 10) the strongest predictor of death at 18 months. Both of these predict lethality when combined with premature ventricular beats at a rate greater than 10 per hour.[19,20]

In general, the more serious the illness, the more likely the patient is to succumb to a depressive episode. Careful studies have found a high incidence of major depression in samples of hospitalized medical patients.[5] For more than 50 years, carcinoma of the pancreas has been associated with psychiatric symptoms, especially depression, which in some cases seems to be the first manifestation of the disease.[21] Two carefully controlled studies have shown these patients to have significantly more psychiatric symptoms and major depression than patients with other malignancies of gastrointestinal origin, leading some to suspect that depression in this case is a manifestation of a paraneoplastic syndrome.[22,23]

When medical illness is localized to the CNS, the incidence of depression is dramatically higher.[5] For example, patients with acquired immune deficiency syndrome (AIDS) and possibly even infection by the human immunodeficiency virus (HIV) can be expected to show higher than expected rates of depressive illness.[24,25]

Stroke

Direct injury to the brain can produce regular changes of affect that progress to a full syndrome of major depression. Robinson et al.[26–28] have intensively studied mood disorders resulting from strokes. Left-hemisphere lesions involving the prefrontal cortex or basal ganglia are the most likely to be associated with poststroke depression and to meet criteria for major depression or dysthymia.[28] Depressive symptoms appear in the immediate poststroke period in about two thirds of the patients, with the rest manifesting depression by the sixth month. Major and minor depression have different courses: major depression, left untreated, had a natural course of about 1 year, but minor depression had a more chronic (about a 2-year) course. Moreover, some untreated patients with minor depression went on to develop major depression. In depressed patients whose left-hemisphere strokes were in the posterior cerebral artery distribution, depression was not only less severe, but was also of shorter duration, with a natural history of about 6 months. Additional risk factors for developing major depression were a prior stroke, preexisting subcortical atrophy, and a family or personal history of affective disorder. Aphasia did not appear to cause depression, but nonfluent aphasia is associated with depression; both seem to result from lesions of the left frontal lobe. Although the severity of functional impairment at the time of acute injury did not correlate with the severity of depression, depression appeared to retard recovery. In patients with left-hemispheric damage, those who were depressed showed significantly worse cognitive performance, which was seen in tasks that assessed temporal orientation, frontal lobe function, and executive motor function. Successful treatment of poststroke depression has been demonstrated by double-blind studies with nortriptyline[29] and trazodone[30] and reported with electroconvulsive therapy (ECT)[31] and psychostimulants.[32] In fact, a recent study has shown nortriptyline to be more effective that fluoxetine in treating depressive symptoms in poststroke depression.[33] Early and aggressive treatment of poststroke depression is required to minimize the cognitive and performance deficits that this mood disorder inflicts on the patient in the recovery period.

Right-hemisphere lesions deserve special diagnostic attention. When the lesion was in the right anterior location, the mood disorder tended to be an apathetic, indifferent state associated with "inappropriate cheerfulness." The patient, however, seldom looks cheerful and may have complaints of loss of interest or even worrying. This disorder was found in 6 of 20 patients with solitary right-hemisphere strokes (and in none of 28 patients with single left-hemisphere lesions).

Prosody is also at risk with a right hemisphere injury. Ross and Rush[34] focused clinical attention on the presentation of aprosodia (lack of "prosody" or inflection, rhythm, and intensity of expression) when the right hemisphere is damaged. Such a patient could appear quite depressed and be so labeled by staff and family but simply lack the neuronal capacity to express or recognize emotion. If one stations oneself out of the patient's view, selects a neutral sentence (e.g., "The book is red"), asks the patient to identify the mood as mad, sad, frightened, or elated, and then declaims the sentence with the emotion to be tested, one should be able to identify those patients with a receptive aprosodia. Next the patient is presented with facial portrayals of the same emotions and asked to identify them (thereby separating visual from auditory clues). The patient then can be asked to portray facial or vocal expressions for the same emotions to test for the presence of an expressive aprosodia. There is no reason why a stroke patient cannot suffer from both aprosodia and depression, but separate diagnostic criteria and clinical examinations exist to recognize each one.

Dementia

Primary dementia, even of the Alzheimer's type, increases the vulnerability of the patient to suffer major depression, even though, as indicated subsequently, the incidence is not as high as it is in multiinfarct or vascular dementia. The careful postmortem studies of Zubenko et al.[35,36] fully support the hypothesis that the pathophysiology of secondary depression is fully consistent with theories of those for primary depression. Compared with demented patients without depression, demented patients with major depression showed a tenfold to twentyfold reduction in cortical norepinephrine levels.

Multiinfarct or vascular dementia so commonly includes depression as a symptom that Hachinski et al.[37] included it as part of the Ischemia Scale. Cummings et al.[38] compared 15 patients with multiinfarct dementia with 30 patients with Alzheimer's dementia and found that depressive symptoms (60% versus 17%) and episodes of major depression (4/15 versus 0/30) were more frequent in patients with the former.

Subcortical Dementias

Patients with Parkinson's disease and Huntington's disease commonly manifest major depres-sion. In fact, Huntington's disease may present as major depression before the onset of either chorea or dementia.[39] The diagnosis is made clinically, as described earlier. Some have noted that as depression in the Parkinson's patient is treated, the Parkinsonian symptoms also improve, even before the depressive symptoms have subsided. This is especially striking when ECT is used,[40,41] although the same improvement has been reported after use of tricyclic antidepressants (TCAs). Treatment of major depression in either disease may increase the comfort of the patient and is always worth a try. Because Huntington's patients may be sensitive to the anticholinergic side effects of TCAs (although not invariably), less anticholinergic drugs should be tried first.

Another subcortical dementia worth noting is Binswanger's encephalopathy, a state of white matter demyelination presumably based on arteriosclerosis; it is characterized by an insidious, slowly progressive state with abulia and a paucity of focal neurologic findings.[42] Whenever affective symptoms are discovered on clinical examination, a trial of an antidepressant medication may produce striking relief for the patient.

Because the HIV-1 is neurotropic, even asymptomatic HIV-seropositive individuals, when compared with seronegative controls, demonstrate a high incidence of electroencephalographic abnormalities (67% versus 10%) and more abnormalities on neuropsychological testing.[43] The unusually high lifetime and current rates of mood disorders in HIV-seronegative individuals at risk for AIDS[44] demand an exceedingly high vigilance for their appearance in HIV-positive persons. Depression, mania, or psychosis can appear with AIDS encephalopathy, but the early, subtler signs (e.g., impaired concentration, complaints of poor memory, blunting of interests, and lethargy) may respond dramatically to antidepressants, such as psychostimulants.[45,46] The selective serotonin reuptake inhibitors (SSRIs), such as sertraline, fluoxetine, and paroxetine have also been found to be effective in the treatment of depression in HIV-positive patients.[47–51] A small open trial also supports the use of bupropion in these patients.[52]

We recommend that pharmacologic treatment be considered seriously whenever a patient meets criteria for either minor or major depression.

Choice of an Appropriate Antidepressant Treatment

In Chapter 18, the properties, side effects, dosages, and drug interactions of antidepressant medications are discussed in detail. Whenever major depression is diagnosed, the effort to alleviate symptoms almost always includes somatic treatments. The consultant who understands the interactions of antidepressants and illnesses and with other drugs is best prepared to prescribe these agents effectively. ECT remains the single most effective somatic treatment of depression. A nationwide review has only sustained its merit. Indications for its use are discussed in Chapter 10.

Prescribing Antidepressants for the Medically Ill

Ever since sudden death in cardiac patients was first associated with amitriptyline,[53,54] physicians have tended to fear the use of TCAs when cardiac disease is present. However, depression itself is a life-threatening disease and it should be treated. Choice of an agent often begins with the knowledge of whether the patient is especially troubled by insomnia, but in patients with certain medical illnesses the decision must be made on a case-by-case basis, taking into consideration the side-effect profile (risk), the anticipated benefits, and potential drug-drug interactions. In diabetes, for instance, fluoxetine has been found in obese diabetic patients to ameliorate mean blood glucose levels, daily insulin requirements, and glycohemoglobin levels,[55–59] perhaps by improving insulin sensitivity.[60,61] In contrast, TCAs, such as nortriptyline, may actually worsen glycemic control.[62] However, TCAs have been found to be superior to fluoxetine in decreasing pain secondary to diabetic neuropathy.[63]

One could also make a similar argument in hypercholesterolemia, because the SSRI fluvoxamine has been found to decrease serum cholesterol,[64] whereas tricyclics appear to increase cholesterol levels.[65]

With respect to making a decision based on insomnia, the sedative potency of the available antidepressants can generally be predicted by their in vitro affinity for the histamine H_1-receptor. Table 8-1 includes these values.[66,67] The antihistaminic property of these drugs gives a reasonably good estimate of their sedative properties. Trazodone, which has low affinity for the H_1-receptor, is, however, sedating in clinical use.

This same property can also be used to predict how much weight gain may be associated with the antidepressant. Patients troubled by obesity may be at additional risk if treated with those agents higher on the list. For the most part, the SSRIs, bupropion, nefazodone, trazodone, and venlafaxine have negligible antihistaminic potency. The monoamine oxidase inhibitors (MAOIs) generally have low sedative potency, although phenelzine sulfate can produce patient complaints of drowsiness. Among the newer agents, mirtazapine,[68] a powerful antagonist of the H_1-receptor, is quite sedating and can be associated with significant weight gain.

All antidepressants in the cyclic, SSRI, and MAOI categories usually correct sleep disturbances (insomnia or hypersomnia) when these are symptoms of depression, a therapeutic effect not thought to be related to their effects on brain histamine. Therefore this discussion highlights a sedative effect of the drugs that occurs in addition to, and independent of, these agents' ability to correct the specific sleep disturbances of major depression (e.g., to lengthen rapid eye movement latency).

Occasionally the consultant may encounter a patient in whom antihistamines have been tried and have failed to achieve a therapeutic effect, such as in the treatment of an urticarial rash or the itching associated with uremia. Doxepin hydrochloride, the most potent antihistamine in clinical medicine, has demonstrated superiority with a 10-mg dose when compared to 25 mg of diphenhydramine hydrochloride.[69]

Threatening the successful use of antidepressants is the occurrence of unwanted side effects. Three groups of side effects are particularly relevant for the treatment of depression in the acute medical setting and are discussed individually. These three side-effect groups include (1) orthostatic hypotension (OH), (2) anticholinergic effects, and (3) cardiac conduction effects. The clinical ratings for these three side-effect groups in current antidepressants are presented in Table 8-2. Finally, we discuss side effects specific to each antidepressant class, and side effects associated with abrupt discontinuation of antidepressant treatment. Once these side effects are understood for each of

Table 8-1. Relationship of Antidepressants to Neurotransmitter Receptors

	Effect on Biogenic Amine Uptake: Potency*		Selectivity for Blocking Uptake of 5-HT over NE	Affinities† for Neurotransmitter Receptors							
	5-HT	NE		Histamine		Alpha		Serotonin		Muscarinic	Dopamine
				H1	H2	1	2	S_1	S_2	ACH	D-2
Doxepin	0.36	5.3	0.068	420.0	0.6	4.2	0.091	0.34	4.0	1.2	0.042
Amitriptyline	1.5	4.2	0.36	91.0	2.2	3.7	0.11	0.53	3.4	5.5	0.10
Imipramine	2.4	7.7	0.31	9.1	0.4	1.1	0.031	0.011	1.2	1.1	0.050
Clomipramine	18.0	3.6	5.2	3.2	—	2.6	0.031	0.014	3.7	2.7	0.53
Trimipramine	0.040	0.20	0.2	370	33.3	4.2	0.15	0.012	3.1	1.7	0.56
Protriptyline	0.36	100.0	0.0035	4.0	0.05	0.77	0.015	0.011	1.5	4.0	0.043
Nortriptyline	0.38	25.0	0.015	10.0	0.12	1.7	0.040	0.32	2.3	0.67	0.083
Desipramine	0.29	110.0	0.0026	0.91	0.08	0.77	0.014	0.010	0.36	0.50	0.030
Amoxapine	0.21	23.0	0.0094	4.0	—	2.0	0.038	0.46	170.0	0.10	0.62
Maprotiline	0.030	14.0	0.0022	50.0	—	1.1	0.011	0.0083	0.83	0.18	0.29
Trazodone	0.53	0.020	26.0	0.29	—	2.8	0.20	1.7	13.0	0.00031	0.026
Fluoxetine	8.3	0.36	23.0	0.016	—	0.017	0.008	0.0042	0.48	0.050	—
Bupropion	0.0064	0.043	0.15	0.015	—	0.022	0.0012	0.0059	0.0011	0.0021	0.00048
Sertraline	29.0	0.45	64.0	0.0041	—	0.27				0.16	0.0093
Paroxetine	136.0	3	45.0	0.0045	—	0.029				0.93	0.0031
Fluvoxamine	14.0	0.2	71.0								
Venlafaxine	2.6	0.48	5.4	0	—	0				0	0
Nefazodone	0.73	0.18	4.2								
Mirtazapine[44a]				200.00			0.2		5.0	0.2	0.040
(Dextromphetamine)‡	2.0										
(Diphenhydramine)‡				7.1							
(Phentolamine)‡						6.7					
(Yohimbine):)‡							62.0				
(Methysergide)‡									7.8		
(Atropine)‡										42	
(Haloperidol)‡											23

ACH Acetylcholine; *HT*, Serotonin; *NE*, Norepinephrine.
* $10^7 \times 1/K_i$, where K_i, = inhibitor constant in molarity.
† $10^7 \times 1/K_d$, where K_d = equilibrium dissociation constant in molarity.
‡ Not antidepressants.
Adapted from Richelson E: Pharmacology of antidepressants—characteristics of the ideal drug, *Mayo Clin Proc* 69:1069–1081, 1994.

the antidepressants, safe clinical prescription of the drugs is far more likely.

Orthostatic Hypotension

OH is not directly related to each drug's in vitro affinity for the α_1-noradrenergic receptor. Table 8-2 presents the drugs with a clinical rating of their respective likelihood of causing an orthostatic fall in blood pressure. In general, among the TCAs, tertiary amine agents are more likely to cause an orthostatic fall in blood pressure than are secondary amines. For reasons that are not clearly understood, imipramine, amitriptyline, and desipramine are the TCAs most commonly associated with

Table 8-2. Characteristics of Antidepressant Drugs

	Elimination Half-life (hr)*	Sedative Potency	Anticholinergic Potency	Orthostatic Hypotension	Cardiac Arrhythmia Potential	Target Dose (mg/day)	Dosage Range (mg/day)
Tricyclics							
Doxepine	17	High	Moderate	High	Yes	200	75–400
Amitriptyline	21	High	Highest	High	Yes	150	75–300
Imipramine	28	Moderate	Moderate	High	Yes	200	75–400
Trimipramine	13	High	Moderate	High	Yes	150	75–300
Clomipramine	23	High	High	High	Yes	150	75–300
Protriptyline	78	Low	High	Moderate	Yes	30	15–60
Nortriptyline	36	Moderate	Moderate	Moderate	Yes	100	40–150
Desipramine	21	Low	Moderate	Moderate	Yes	150	75–300
Others							
Citalopram	33	Low	Low	Low	Low	20	20–80
Maprotiline	43	High	Moderate	Moderate	Yes	150	75–300
Trazodone	3.5	High	Lowest	Moderate	Yes	150	50–600
Fluoxetine	87	Low	Low	Lowest	Low	20	40–80
Sertraline	26	Low	Low	Lowest	Low	50	50–200
Paroxetine	21	Low	Low-Moderate	Lowest	Low	20	20–60
Fluvoxamine	19	Low	Low	Low	Low	200	50–300
Bupropion	15	Low	Low	Lowest	Low	200	75–300
Venlafaxine	3.6	Low	Low	Low	Low	300	75–375
Nefazodone	3	Moderate	Low	Low	Low	300	300–600
Mirtazapine	30	High	Low	Low	Low	15	15–45
Monoamine oxidase inhibitors		Low	Low	High	Low		

clinical mishaps, such as falls and fractures of the head. The orthostatic effect appears earlier than the therapeutic effect for imipramine and is objectively verifiable at less than half the therapeutic plasma level. Hence, the drug may have to be discontinued long before a therapeutic plasma level is reached. Once postural symptoms develop, increasing the dose of the antidepressant may not make the symptoms worse.

Paradoxically, a pretreatment fall of more than 10 mm Hg in orthostatic blood pressure actually predicts a good response to antidepressant medication in older adult depressed patients.[70,71] Naturally, younger patients may tolerate a fall in pressure more easily than older patients, so an orthostatic fall in blood pressure may not produce symptoms serious enough to require discontinuation of the drug. The presence of cardiovascular disease increases the likelihood of OH. When patients with no cardiac disease take imipramine,

the incidence of significant OH is 7%. With conduction disease, such as a bundle-branch block (BBB), the incidence rises to 33%, and with congestive heart failure (CHF), it reaches 50%.[72] Of the traditional TCAs, nortriptyline has been shown to be the least likely to cause OH, an extremely valuable factor when depression in cardiac or older adult patients requires treatment.[73] MAOIs cause significant OH with about the same frequency as does imipramine (i.e., often). Moreover, the patient starting on an MAOI usually does not experience OH until the medication is having a significant therapeutic effect, roughly 2 to 4 weeks later.

Of the newer agents, trazodone is associated with OH moderately often. Mirtazapine has been associated with OH, although how clinically serious this is remains to be established. Fluoxetine, sertraline, paroxetine, citalopram, fluvoxamine, bupropion, venlafaxine, and psychostimulants are essentially free of this side effect. Bupropion, psychostimulants, and venlafaxine may raise systolic blood pressure slightly in some patients. Some have noted that even though the objective fall in standing pressure continues for several months, some patients with initial symptoms accommodate subjectively and no longer complain of the side effect.

Anticholinergic Effects

The anticholinergic effects of TCAs are a nuisance for many patients. Urinary retention, constipation, dry mouth, confusional states, and tachycardia are the most common. The increase in heart rate is usually manifest as a sinus tachycardia that results from muscarinic blockade of vagal tone on the heart. As many as 30% of normal individuals respond to amitriptyline with tachycardia.[74] This side effect correlates nicely with the in vitro affinity of each drug for the acetylcholine muscarinic receptor, presented in Table 8-1. As seen in the table, amitriptyline is the most anticholinergic of the antidepressants, with protriptyline a rather close second. These two agents regularly cause tachycardia in medically ill patients, and one should monitor the heart rate as the dosage is increased. If significant tachycardia results, another agent may have to be used. Many hospitalized patients, particularly those with ischemic heart disease, are already being treated with β-adrenergic blockers, such as propranolol. When this is the case, the β-blocker usually protects the patient from developing a significant tachycardia.

All of the cyclic agents except trazodone are significantly anticholinergic. If one switches from, for example, imipramine to desipramine because the patient developed urinary retention, the patient is quite likely to develop urinary retention again on desipramine. Amoxapine and maprotiline are not significantly less anticholinergic than desipramine. Trazodone is almost devoid of activity at the muscarinic receptor, and it is a reasonable choice when another agent has caused unwanted anticholinergic side effects.

Fluoxetine, bupropion, venlafaxine, and the MAOIs exert minimal activity at the acetylcholine muscarinic receptor; hence they can also be useful alternatives when these side effects impair access of a patient to an antidepressant. There is laboratory evidence (see Table 8-1) with anecdotal clinical support that paroxetine is more anticholinergic, close in in vitro potency to imipramine. Likewise, in Richelson's[67] laboratory, sertraline appears to have quite similar anticholinergic effects to maprotiline. For the latter, this effect is clinically noticeable (e.g., dry mouth) but usually mild. Similar mild effects seem to accompany the use of mirtazapine. Effects of fluvoxamine and nefazodone are generally mild, but the laboratory comparison values for muscarinic receptor affinity are not known.

Cardiac Conduction Effects

All TCAs appear to prolong ventricular depolarization. This tends to produce a lengthening of the P-R and QRS intervals as well as the Q-T interval corrected for heart rate (QTc) on the electrocardiogram (ECG). When the main effect of these agents is measured by His-bundle electrocardiography, the His-ventricular portion of the recording is preferentially prolonged. That is, these drugs, which are sodium-channel blockers, tend to slow the electric impulse as it passes through the specialized conduction tissue known as the His-Purkinje system. This makes them resemble in action the class IA arrhythmic drugs, such as quinidine and procainamide hydrochloride. In practical terms, this means that depressed cardiac patients with ventricular premature contractions, when started on an antidepressant, such as imipramine, are likely to experience improvement or resolution of their ventricular irritability, even if the abnormality is as serious as inducible ventricular tachycardia. Both imipramine and nortriptyline have proven efficacy as antiarrhythmics and share the advantage of a half-life long enough to permit twice-daily doses.[75–77]

Ordinarily, this property does not pose a problem for the cardiac patient who does not already have disease in the conduction system. The patient who already has conduction system disease is the focus of concern. First-degree heart block is the mildest pathologic form and probably should not pose a problem for antidepressant treatment. When the patient's abnormality exceeds this (e.g., right BBB, left BBB, bifascicular block, BBB with prolonged P-R, alternating BBB, or second-degree or third-degree atrioventricular [AV] block), extreme caution is necessary in treating the depression. Cardiology consultation is almost always already present for the patient. Electrolyte abnormalities, particularly hypokalemia or hypomagnesemia, increase the danger to these patients and they require careful monitoring.

Occasionally, the question arises clinically whether one of the cyclic agents is less likely than another to cause a quinidine-like prolongation in conduction, particularly when the patient already shows some intraventricular conduction delay. Maprotiline should be regarded as similar to the TCAs in its effects on cardiac conduction. Amoxapine has been touted to have fewer cardiac side effects, based on patients who had taken overdoses. Although these patients were noted to have suffered seizures, coma, and acute renal failure, the authors thought it worth noting that less cardiac toxicity resulted,[78,79] but atrial flutter and fibrillation have been reported in patients taking amoxapine.[80,81] Trazodone does not prolong conduction in the His-Purkinje system, but aggravation of the preexisting ventricular irritability has been reported.[82] Hence, clinical caution cannot be abandoned.

Bupropion, the SSRIs, venlafaxine, nefazodone, and mirtazapine are not known to cause cardiac arrhythmias, a definite advantage for cardiac patients with depression, although the newer agents have not been in use for a long time. There are also isolated reports of bradycardia associated with use of fluoxetine.

MAOIs are remarkably free of arrhythmogenic effects, although there are at least three case reports of atrial flutter or fibrillation, or both, with tranylcypromine. Consultees tend to dread them, fearing drug and food interactions.

How, then, should the consultant approach the depressed patient with conduction disease? Depression can itself be life-threatening and more damaging to cardiac function than a drug. Therefore it must be treated. In the case of a depressed patient with cardiac conduction problems, one can begin with an SSRI, bupropion, venlafaxine, nefazodone, or mirtazapine. Should the depression not remit completely, augmentation with a psychostimulant or switching to a psychostimulant are reasonable options. Should the patient improve, the stimulant can be continued as long as it is

helpful. By starting with a low dose (2.5 mg of either dextroamphetamine or methylphenidate), one is reasonably assured that toxicity will not result. The fragile patient can have his or her heart rate and blood pressure monitored hourly for 4 hours after receiving the drug. If no beneficial response is noted, the next day the dose should be raised to 5 mg (our usual starting dose), then to 10, 15, and 20 mg on successive days, if necessary. One should be able to see some response to the stimulant, even a negative one (e.g., feeling more tense, "wired," or agitated), so that a clear response is demonstrated. (It makes little sense to stop a stimulant trial without seeing any response unless the patient can report some subjective verification of a drug effect. Of course, an elevation of heart rate or blood pressure may be a reason to stop the trial. It can still be reasonable to add a TCA if the patient has failed a number of the previously listed antidepressants, which are considered safer, and if the patient has minimal history of cardiac conduction problems. The degree of clinical vigilance must match the clinical precariousness of the patient. Discussion of the type and intensity of monitoring takes place with the consultee.

The role of the psychiatric consultant is to recommend aggressive treatment for depression, with the consultee helping to decide what means are appropriate and to detect possible side effects. If the patient's depression failed to remit despite a number of adequate antidepressant trials, an MAOI is reasonable even with an unstable cardiac condition, provided that the patient can tolerate the OH that may result. The adage "start low, go slow," which is so appropriate in the treatment of older adult patients, is also a good rule for medically unstable patients.

If the depression has left the patient dangerously ill, suicidal, or catatonic, ECT is the treatment of choice. When an antidepressant can be used, monitoring must take into account both the development of a steady-state (which typically takes around five half-lives of the drug) and the rate at which the dose is being increased. When the patient requires a daily dose increase, a daily rhythm strip may be necessary as well as another one, five half-lives after reaching that level thought to represent the therapeutic dose. Plasma levels are especially useful when a 4- to 8-week drug trial is judged worthwhile. Reliable levels have been established only for nortriptyline hydrochloride (50 to 150 ng/ml), desipramine hydrochloride (greater than 125 ng/ml), and imipramine hydrochloride (greater than 200 ng/ml).

Myocardial Depression

Antidepressants have not been shown to impair left ventricular function significantly in depressed or nondepressed patients with either normal or impaired myocardial contractility.[83–86] Even with TCA overdose, impairment of left ventricular function is generally mild.[87] Hence, CHF is not an absolute contraindication to antidepressant therapy.[85,86,88] The patient with heart failure is far more vulnerable to OH; hence, the SSRIs, bupropion, venlafaxine, and nortriptyline, are the preferred agents.

A severely depressed patient could suffer an acute MI. Both conditions are a threat to survival, and the MI is no contraindication to antidepressant treatment. ECT or drugs may be mandatory. Using the previously mentioned principles, psychiatrists and cardiologists must combine their efforts to restore the patient's health.

Other Side Effects (Specific to Each Antidepressant Class)

Other common side effects of bupropion include anxiety and nervousness, agitation, insomnia, headache, nausea, constipation, and tremor. Bupropion is contraindicated in the treatment of patients with a seizure disorder or bulimia, because the incidence of seizures is approximately 0.4% at doses up to 450 mg/day, and increases almost tenfold at higher doses.

Common side effects of venlafaxine include nausea, lack of appetite, weight loss, excessive sweating, nervousness, insomnia, sexual dysfunction, sedation, fatigue, headache, and dizziness.

Mirtazapine's side effects include dry mouth, constipation, weight gain, and dizziness. The relative lack of significant drug-drug interactions with other antidepressants makes mirtazapine a good candidate for combination strategies (i.e., combining two antidepressants together at full doses).

Side effects of nefazodone include headache, fatigue, nausea, constipation, and sedation. There have also been some reports of severe hepatotoxicity associated with nefazodone. We recommend caution when nefazodone is prescribed with other drugs, especially those metabolized by CYP 450 3A4 isoenzyme system, or in patients with liver disease. Baseline and regular liver function tests should be obtained in all patients on nefazodone therapy for the first 6 months, and the drug should be discontinued if abnormalities are found.

Trazodone is an agent somewhat related to nefazodone, although it is much more sedating. The most common side effects of trazodone are drowsiness, dizziness, headache, and nausea, with priapism being an extremely rare but potentially serious side effect in men.

Antidepressant Discontinuation Syndrome

Recent reports describe discontinuation-emergent adverse events upon abrupt cessation of SSRIs and venlafaxine,[89,90] including dizziness, insomnia, nervousness, nausea, and agitation. The likelihood of developing these symptoms may be inversely related to the half-life of the SSRI employed, because these symptoms are more likely to develop after abrupt discontinuation of paroxetine and to a lesser degree with sertraline, with few symptoms seen with fluoxetine discontinuation.

Psychostimulant Use

Earlier MGH experience with the use of dextroamphetamine and methylphenidate, which showed them to be safe and effective in depressed mentally ill patients,[91] has been reconfirmed.[32] Their use as therapeutic agents was gradually discontinued a number of years ago,[92] but when patients with symptoms of major and minor depression continued to respond to stimulants, often achieving remission of their symptoms, these agents once again became independent antidepressants in our consultation practice. Their effects on heart rate and blood pressure have been trivial, even though any patient with hypertension or unstable cardiac rhythm requires monitoring of vital signs when started on these agents. The most common fear expressed about their use was that they would reduce appetite in patients who were already anorectic from their illness or their depression or both. Not a single case of interference with appetite was found associated with the use of these drugs. In several instances, increased appetite was reported by the patients—another striking and important benefit associated with their use.

Finally, in those patients who suffered both depressive symptoms and either dementia or an organic brain syndrome (e.g., from head injury), there was a fear that use of a stimulant would result in agitation, confusion, or psychosis. In 17 patients with an associated diagnosis of dementia, only 2 showed a worsening of confusion, which disappeared within 24 hours of discontinuation of the drug.[91] Hence, our practice is now to begin with a stimulant. If it helps (as it did to a moderate or marked degree in 48% of the patients), it does so within a short time: Approximately 93% of the patients who responded positively reached their maximum benefit by the second day. As long as it helps, the stimulant is maintained. Tolerance was not found in our patient sample. The same dosage of the stimulant was maintained until the depressive symptoms cleared or the patient was discharged. A small group of patients were discharged with instructions to continue taking the agent at home. The majority stopped the medication within 2 to 3 weeks. A few continued for 1 year or longer.

There is a strong bias against stimulants (dextroamphetamine more so than methylphenidate), because of associated street abuse. In the MGH review cited, neither tolerance nor abuse was found in the patients for whom these agents were prescribed.[92]

Hepatic Metabolism

Essentially all antidepressants are metabolized by the hepatic P450 microsomal enzyme system. The interactions produced by the competition of multiple drugs for these metabolic pathways is complex and covered in Chapter 18. For example, one of the newer agents, mirtazapine, is a substrate for, but not an inhibitor of, the 2D6, 1A2, and 3A4 isoenzymes.

How long antidepressants need to be maintained in major depression associated with medical illness is not known. Even though patients with primary affective disorder should be maintained on their antidepressant for more than 6 months, the same requirement is not clear for major depression in the medical setting. In poststroke depression and possibly in other instances in which primary brain disease or injury appears to cause depression, antidepressants should be continued for 6 months or longer.

Secondary Mania

Occasionally, a clinician is asked to see a patient with mania or hypomania of 1 (or more) week's duration, in whom no history of affective disorder can be obtained. Described by Krauthammer and Klerman,[93] this phenomenon results from an organic dysfunction. Table 8-3 lists some causes of secondary mania. The emergence of mania or hypomania usually signifies the presence of bipolar affective disease, but cases such as those in Table 8-3 continue to accumulate in the literature, indicating that alteration of brain states can lead to a clinical picture indistinguishable from primary mania.[94–103] Of clinical note was the report that in HIV-positive patients with mania, an abnormal magnetic resonance imaging (MRI) scan predicted poor response to lithium and neuroleptics. However, anticonvulsants were effective for these patients.[102]

Use of Lithium Carbonate in the Medically Ill

The treatment of secondary mania is the same as that for primary mania. Neuroleptics, lithium carbonate, or anticonvulsants are required in most cases, although lorazepam and clonazepam may prove to be helpful in the acute phase.

A word of caution is appropriate when lithium is used in older adults or in patients with cardiac disease. On the ECG of a patient taking lithium, a benign and reversible T-wave flattening is seen in approximately 50% of cases. Lithium appears to have some inhibitory effects on impulse generation and transmission within the atrium. Hence, the reports of adverse cardiac effects of lithium

Table 8-3. Reported Causes of Secondary Mania

Drugs	Alcohol intoxication, alprazolam, captopril, cimetidine, corticosteroids, cyclobenzaprine, cyproheptadine, disulfiram, felbamate, isoniazid, levodopa, L-glutamine, L-tryptophan, lysergic acid diethylamide, methylphenidate, metrizamide, metoclopramide, procainamide, procarbazine, propafenone, sympathomimetics, thyroxine, tolmetin, triazolam, yohimbine, zidovudine
Drug withdrawal	Clonidine, diltiazem, atenolol, isocarboxazid, propranolol
Metabolic	Hemodialysis, postoperative state, hyperthyroidism, vitamin B_{12} deficiency, Cushing's syndrome, cerebral hypoxia
Infection	Influenza, Q fever, post-St. Louis type A encephalitis, cryptococcosis, HIV, neurosyphilis
Neoplasm	Meningiomas, gliomas, thalamic metastases, brainstem tumor
Epilepsy	Complex partial seizures with right temporal focus
Surgery	Right hemispherectomy
Cerebrovascular accident	Thalamic stroke
Other	Cerebellar atrophy, head trauma, multiple sclerosis, Wilson's disease

HIV, Human immunodeficiency virus.

have been those of sinus node dysfunction and first-degree AV block.[104–106] Because older adults seem particularly prone to these effects, caution is essentially reserved for them and for patients who have preexisting disturbances of atrial conduction.[107]

Ordinarily, lithium's effects on the heart can be assumed to be benign, but as any serious illness becomes more complicated and as treatments increase, patients are at greater risk. Mania, similar to depression, can seldom be tolerated either by the patient or by caregivers. Whether the alternative treatments, such as use of calcium channel-blockers, or use of adjunctive measures, such as lorazepam, are useful in secondary mania remains to be established.

Thioridazine

A final caution about cardiovascular toxicity should include discussion of thioridazine. Notorious among neuroleptics for its potential cardiac side effects, this drug should not be used in combination with TCAs unless there is a special need. It, too, possesses quinidine-like properties, has been associated with reports of sudden death that antedate similar reports with TCAs,[108] and was more recently implicated in the causation of ventricular tachycardia alone[109] and in combination with desipramine.[110] Thioridazine's anticholinergic potency is high (roughly equivalent in vitro to that

of desipramine), which can be troublesome. This property, however, might make it particularly useful to treat the delirium of a patient with Parkinson's disease. As little as 5 to 10 mg can be helpful in such a patient. Again, it is important to avoid hypokalemia and hypomagnesemia, which predispose patients to cardiac rhythm disturbances.

Other DSM-IV Diagnoses of Depression

Dysthymia

For the diagnosis of dysthymia (300.40), DSM-IV specifies a chronic state of depression that does not meet full criteria for major depression. To qualify, the patient must have depressed (or, for children and adolescents, irritable) mood for most of the day and more days than not for more than 2 years and have two or more of the following six symptoms: (1) poor appetite or overeating, (2) insomnia or hypersomnia, (3) low energy or fatigue, (4) low self-esteem, (5) poor concentration or difficulty making decisions, or (6) feelings of hopelessness. For medically ill patients, this diagnosis could be used, dropping the duration requirement, to specify minor depression. Use of antidepressants is necessary in minor depression after stroke, but there are few if any other studies to guide treatment.

In DSM-IV, it is at last possible to apply the diagnostic criteria for major depression even when the depression follows the medical condition in time (and is therefore secondary). The terminology states that the mood disturbance is "due to," for example, stroke, MI, or HIV infection. The mood can be described as "with depressive features," "with major depressive-like episode," "with manic features," or "with mixed features."

Adjustment Disorder with Depressed Mood

Adjustment disorder with depressed mood (309.00) is probably the most overused diagnosis by consultation psychiatrists. It should not be given to a medical patient unless the depressive reaction is maladaptive, either in intensity of feeling (an overreaction) or in function (e.g., when a despondent patient interacts minimally with caregivers and family).

Bereavement

Bereavement (V62.82) refers to the death of a loved one. In the case of the medical patient, of course, it is the self that is mourned after a narcissistic injury (e.g., an MI). DSM-IV unnecessarily restricts bereavement to loss of a loved one. In acute grief, major depression can be a difficult diagnosis, but when it is present, it requires treatment, perhaps even more than when it is present without acute grief. Clues helpful to determine the presence of major depression include (1) guilt beyond that about actions taken around the time of the death of the loved one; (2) thoughts of death other than wanting to be with the lost person or feeling one would be better off dead—suicidal ideation should count in favor of major depression; (3) morbid preoccupation with worthlessness; (4) marked psychomotor retardation; (5) prolonged and marked functional impairment; (6) hallucinations other than seeing, hearing, or being touched by the deceased person.

Prigerson et al.[111] have developed two useful empirical constructs, bereavement depression (depressive symptoms in wake of a loss) and complicated grief. The first predicts future medical burden of the person, and the latter predicts functional impairment at 18-month follow-up. The symptoms related to the bereavement-depression factor are hypochondriasis, apathy, insomnia, anxiety, suicidal ideation, guilt, loneliness, depressed mood, psychomotor retardation, hostility, and low self-esteem. The symptoms that are the principal components of the complicated grief factor are yearning for, and preoccupation with, thoughts of the deceased, crying, searching for the deceased, disbelief about the death, being stunned by the death, and inability to accept the death. When patients with a Hamilton depression scale score higher than 17 were treated with nortriptyline, at doses that averaged a low but therapeutic level of 68.1 ng/ml, those treated lowered their bereavement-depression scores substantially. This supports our clinical recommendation that any person who meets criteria for major depression should be treated. There is no evidence that antidepressants retard the grieving process.

Despondency Consequent to Serious Illness

Despondency in serious illness appears to be a natural response and is here regarded as the psychic damage done by the disease to the patient's self-esteem. Bibring's[112] definition of depression is "response to narcissistic injury." The response is here called *despondency* and not *depression* because depression is reserved for those conditions that meet the research criteria for primary or secondary affective disorder. In any serious illness, the mind sustains an injury of its own, as though the illness, for example, MI, produces an ego infarction. Even when recovery of the diseased organ is complete, recovery of self-esteem appears to take somewhat longer. In MI patients, for example, although the myocardial scar has fully formed in 5 to 6 weeks, recovery of the sense of psychological well-being seems to require 2 to 3 months.

Management of the Acute Phase of Despondency

A mixture of dread, bitterness, and despair, despondency presents the self as broken, scarred, and ruined. Work and relationships seem jeopardized. Now it seems to the patient too late to realize career or personal aspirations. Disappointment with both what has and has not been accomplished haunts the individual, who may now feel old and like a failure. Concerns of this kind become conscious early in acute illness, and their expression may prompt consultation requests as early as the second or third day of hospitalization.[113]

Management of these illness-induced despondencies is divided into acute and long-term phases. In the acute phase, the patient is encouraged but never forced to express such concerns. The extent and detail are determined by the individual's need to recount them. Many patients are upset to find such depressive concerns in consciousness and even worry that this signals a "nervous breakdown." It is therefore essential to let patients know that such concerns are the normal emotional counterpart of being sick and that even though there will be ups and downs in their intensity, these concerns will probably disappear gradually as health returns. It is also helpful for the consultant to be familiar with the rehabilitation plans common to various illnesses, so that patients can also be reminded, while still in the acute phase of recovery, that plans for restoring function are being activated.

Paradoxically, many of the issues discussed in the care of the dying patient (see Chapter 23) are relevant here. Heavy emphasis is placed on maintaining the person's sense of self-esteem. Self-esteem often falters in seriously ill persons even though they have good recovery potential. Hence, efforts to learn what the sick person is like can help the consultant alleviate the acute distress of a damaged self-image. The consultant should learn any "defining" traits, interests, and accomplishments of the patient so that the nurses and physicians can be informed of them. For example, after learning that a woman patient had been a star sprinter on the national Polish track team preparing for the 1940 Olympics, the consultant relayed this both in the consultation note and by word of mouth to her caregivers. "What's this I hear about your having been a champion sprinter?" became a common question that made her feel not only unique but appreciated. The objective is to restore to life the real person within the patient who has serious organic injuries or impairment.

Few things are more discouraging for the patient, staff, or consultant than no noticeable sign of improvement. When there is no real progress, all the interventions discussed in Chapter 23 are necessary. At other times, progress is being made, but so slowly that the patient cannot feel it in any tangible way. By using ingenuity, the consultant

may find a way to alter this. Many of the following suggestions apply, and a knowledge of the physiology of the illness is essential. Psychological interventions, however, can also be helpful. For example, getting a patient with severe CHF out of bed and into a reclining chair (known for 25 years to produce even less cardiovascular strain than the supine position)[114] can provide reassurance and boost confidence. For some patients with severe ventilatory impairments and difficulty weaning from the respirator, a wall chart depicting graphically the time spent off the ventilator each day (one gold star for each 5-minute period) is encouraging. Even if the patient's progress is slow, the chart documents and dramatizes each progressive step. Of course, personal investment in very ill persons may be far more therapeutic in itself than any gimmick, but such simple interventions have a way of focusing new effort and enthusiasm on each improvement.

Management of Postacute Despondencies: Planning for Discharge and After

Even when the patients are confident their illness is not fatal, they usually become concerned that it will cripple them. As noted, psychological "crippling" is a normal hazard of organic injury. Whether the patient is an employable, uncomplicated MI patient or a chronic emphysematous "panter" with a carbon dioxide tension of 60 mm Hg, only restoration of self-esteem can protect him or her from emotional incapacitation. Even when the body has no room for improvement, the mind can usually be rehabilitated. Arrival home from the hospital often proves to be a vast disappointment. The damage caused by illness has been done, acute treatment is completed, and health professionals are far away. Weak, anxious, and demoralized, the patient experiences a "homecoming depression."[115] Weakness is a universal problem for any individual whose hospitalization required extensive bed rest; in fact, it was the symptom most complained of by one group of post-MI patients visited in their homes.[115] Invariably the individuals attribute this weakness to the damage caused by the disease (e.g., to the heart, lungs, and liver). A large part of this weakness, however, is due to muscle atrophy and to the systemic effects of immobilization. Bed

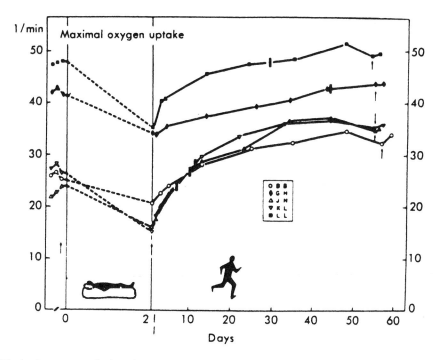

Figure 8-1. Maximal oxygen uptake in sedentary and athletic men after 3 weeks' bed rest.

rest, a disease in itself, includes among its ill effects venous stasis with threat of phlebitis, embolism, OH, a progressive increase in resting heart rate, loss of approximately 10% to 15% of muscle strength per week (owing to atrophy), and reduction of approximately 20% to 25% in maximal oxygen uptake capacity in a 3-week period. This was dramatically illustrated by the study of Saltin et al.[116] of five healthy college students who, after being tested in the laboratory, were placed on 3 weeks' bed rest. Three of the men were sedentary, and two were trained athletes. As shown in Figure 8-1, after the period of bed rest, it took the three sedentary men 8, 10, and 13 days to regain their pre–bed-rest maximal oxygen uptake levels, whereas it took the two athletes 28 and 43 days to reach their initial values. The better the patient's condition, the longer it takes for the recovery of strength. Entirely unaware of the physiology of muscle atrophy, patients mistakenly believe that exercise, the only treatment of atrophy, is dangerous or impossible.

Fear can be omnipresent following discharge from the hospital. The least bodily sensation, particularly in the location of the affected organ,

looms as an ominous sign of the worst recurrence (e.g., MI, malignancy, gastrointestinal bleeding, or perforation), metastatic spread, (another) infection, or some new disaster that will cripple the individual even further. Most of the alarming symptoms felt in the early posthospital days are so trivial that they would never have been noticed before, but the threshold is far lower now, and patients may find any unusual sensation a threat. When the alarm has passed, they may then feel foolish or even disgusted with themselves for being hypochondriacal. It helps to know in advance that such hypersensitivity to bodily sensations commonly occurs, that it is normal, and that it is time-limited. Although there are wide ranges in the time it takes for this problem to disappear, a well-adjusted patient who has an uncomplicated MI requires from 2 to 6 months for these fears to resolve (far more time than the recovery of the myocardium). With specific measures, this time may be shortened.

Whether the person can improve a physical function such as oxygen consumption (e.g., as with MI or gastrointestinal bleeding) or cannot do so at all (e.g., with chronic obstructive pulmonary disease [COPD]), the mental state is basically the same—a sense of imprisonment in a damaged body that is unable to sustain the everyday activities of a reasonable life. The illness has mentally crippled the individual. Horizons have shrunk drastically, so that the person may feel literally unable or afraid to leave the house, to walk across a room, or to stray far from the phone. Moreover, such people are likely to regard routine activities like walking, riding a bike, or raking leaves as too exhausting or dangerous. For some individuals, life comes to a near standstill.

The best therapy for such psychological constriction is a program that emphasizes early and progressive mobilization in the hospital and exercise after discharge. A physician might naturally be wary of prescribing this for a person with severe COPD who is dyspneic while walking at an ordinary pace. For some significantly impaired chronic pulmonary patients,[117] however, objective exercise tolerance can be increased as much as a 1000-fold. The improvement is the result of better limb muscle conditioning. The patient does not have to change pulmonary function at all to experience significantly greater endurance.[118] Several self-imposed restrictions (e.g., never being far from an oxygen tank) are dramatically relieved. The psychiatric consultant should be aware that chronic pulmonary patients considered to have "irreversible" disease can be significantly helped by a specific rehabilitation program.[119–122]

Progress in writing exercise regimens for the recuperation period has been greatly helped by the definition and use of the metabolic equivalent (MET). One MET is defined as the energy expenditure per kilogram per minute of the average 70-kg person sitting quietly in a chair. This amounts to approximately 1.4 calories/min or 3.5 to 4.0 ml of oxygen consumed per kilogram per minute. Table 8-4 lists activities for which measurements in METs have been determined.[123] For example, after recovery from uncomplicated MI, the average middle-aged person is capable of performing at a level of 8 to 9 METs. This includes running at 5.5 miles per hour (jogging slightly faster than 11-minute miles), cycling at 13 miles per hour, skiing at 4 miles per hour, noncompetitive squash and handball, fencing, and vigorous basketball. If, however, less than ordinary activity produces symptoms, the capacity of the postcoronary

patient is nearer 4 METs. Despite obvious impairment, this level of capacity includes swimming the breaststroke at 20 yards per minute; cycling at 5.5 miles per hour; walking up a 5% incline at 3 miles per hour; playing table tennis, golf (carrying clubs), badminton and lawn tennis doubles, and raking leaves. For the patient, these are carefully computed, quantitated capacities. A list of activities quantified in METs is far more concrete and specific than statements such as, "Use your own judgment" or "Do it in moderation." Instead, the patient can be given a list and told to select activities up to a specific level of METs. The physician who wishes to determine a tolerable level can use such devices as the step test, treadmill, and bicycle ergometer for which energy demand in METs at different levels have already been determined. Handy charts can be obtained from the American Heart Association manual.[124]

Activity levels can be gradually increased whenever appropriate. Patients should take responsibility for the extra costs that emotional involvement may require. For example, they could be told, "I am now moving you to a level of activity of 5 METs. You will find at this level all the activities that your heart (or lungs or body) is physically capable of performing. Activities you enjoy are the best. Remember that getting emotionally upset or very competitive during activity increases the energy cost to your heart. If you cannot do some of these things without getting all worked up, you will have to ease off; only you can judge that. But you now know that you are physically capable of performing at 5 METs." In this statement, vagueness remains, but only in the area of subjective emotions. Patients not only experience their emotions physically and mentally, but also should be aware of them, whereas they cannot detect changes in their left-ventricular end-diastolic pressure or arterial oxygen saturation. Moreover, emotional self-control is a fair request to make of patients who, although not responsible for detecting a rising wedge pressure on the tennis court, must try to control rising killer instincts.

Patients with chronic CAD almost always have reduced exercise capacity. Lower maximal stroke volume and heart rate decrease cardiac output and limit maximum oxygen consumption ($VO_{2\ max}$).[125] Yet exercise training increases VO_{2max} for these patients, even when stroke volume cannot

Table 8-4. Energy Expenditure per Kilogram per Minute in the Average 70-kg Person

Activity	MET	Activity	MET
Self-Care		**Housework Activities**	
Rest, supine	1	Hand sewing	1
Sitting	1	Sweeping floor	1.5
Standing, relaxed	1	Machine sewing	1.5
Eating	1	Polishing furniture	2
Conversation	1	Peeling potatoes	2.5
Dressing, undressing	2	Scrubbing, standing	2.5
Washing hands, face	2	Washing small clothes	2.5
Using bedside commode	3	Kneading dough	2.5
Walking, 2.5 mph	3	Scrubbing floors	3
Showering	3.5	Cleaning windows	3
Using bedpan	4	Making beds	3
Walking downstairs	4.5	Ironing, standing	3.5
Walking, 3.5 mph	5.5	Mopping	3.5
Propulsion, wheelchair	2	Wringing by hand	3.5
Ambulation with braces and crutches	6.5	Hanging wash	3.5
		Beating carpets	4
Industrial Activities			
Watch repairing	1.5	**Recreational Activities**	
Armature winding	2.0	Painting, sitting	1.5
Radio assembly	2.5	Playing piano	2
Sewing at machine	2.5	Driving car	2
Bricklaying	3.5	Canoeing, 2.5 mph	2.5
Plastering	3.5	Horseback riding, slow	2.5
Tractor plowing	3.5	Volleyball	2.5
Wheeling barrow, 115 lb, 2.5 mph	4.0	Bowling	3.5
Horse plowing	5.0	Cycling, 5.5 mph	3.5
Carpentry	5.5	Golfing	4
Mowing lawn by hand	6.5	Swimming, 20 yd/min	4
Felling tree	6.5	Dancing	4.5
Shoveling	7.0	Gardening	4.5
Ascending stairs with 1 7-lb load at 27 ft/min	7.5	Tennis	6
Planing	7.5	Trotting horse	6.5
Tending furnace	8.5	Spading	7
Ascending stairs with 22-lb load at 54 ft/min	13.5	Skiing	8
		Squash	8.5
		Cycling, 13 mph	9

MET, Metabolic equivalent.
From Cassem NH, Hackett TP: Psychological aspects of myocardial infarction. *Med Clin North Am* 61:711–721, 1977. Used by permission.

be enlarged (as it is in healthy persons who train). As with the chronic lung patients, the increase in exercise capacity results from changes in the muscles, especially the leg muscles. (β-Blockers, which blunt VO_{2max} improvement in healthy exercisers, do not prevent it in CAD patients. Thompson[126] suggests that CAD patients as well as patients recovering from uncomplicated MI and bypass surgery walk at least 10 minutes per day and add 5 minutes per week to the walk until they are walking 45 or more minutes, four to five times a week. The patients should be instructed to walk briskly but not at a rate that causes dyspnea (which occurs at approximately 50% to 70% VO_{2max}).

Even CHF does not necessarily proscribe exercise. In a group of patients with severely limited left-ventricular function and ejection fractions of 25% or less, Squires et al.[127] were able to produce, without morbidity or mortality, in an 8-week training program, substantial improvement in exercise capacity. Of those fully employed before CHF occurred, more than half returned to full-time work.

In any serious illness in which there are likely to be so many "don'ts" constricting the patient's world, an exercise regimen provides something to do that widens the space of existence. If a patient were limited by a maximum tidal volume of 13 L per minute, an exercise program could not increase it, but it would help the patient to see that even within those limits he or she can increase exercise tolerance, venture further (e.g., away from oxygen), and, one hopes, experience increased freedom. Some patients suffer illnesses in which reserves wax and wane (e.g., the cancer patient with remissions and exacerbations, aplastic anemia patients between transfusions). They may view life energy as a fixed quantity that is used up by activity little by little; thus they fear activity. The psychological benefits of exercise are such that activities should bring some sense of renewed vitality (improved sleep and appetite are common effects) rather than a sense of depletion or exhaustion. As hematocrit level decreases (or blood urea nitrogen level increases), capacity for exercise decreases. To continue exercising, such a person could set as a target a heart rate that was commonly experienced while exercising at his or her prescribed level of MET, or time and distance could be decreased accordingly. When his chronic CHF worsened, one man simply returned to the scene of his exercising, changed into his exercise gear, and sat talking with the regulars before returning home.

Geriatric Implications

Age further compounds the bias against encouraging physical exercise. Contrary to popular myth, vigorous exercise training in youth confers no later cardiovascular health benefits. Moderate exercise (defined as 70% to 80% of maximal heart rate) in later age does so. The trainability of older men has been shown not to depend on whether they trained in youth. Moreover, as a person ages and functional reserve decreases, the size of the training effect becomes relatively greater.[128]

The best measure of the effects of aging on functional activity is the maximum oxygen consumption (VO_{2max}). As one ages, there is a clearly demonstrated decline in VO_{2max}, but it is much steeper for sedentary than for active men. A concrete expression of the difference between the two lifestyles is that by the time the two groups reach the decade of 50 to 59 years of age, there is already a 10-year difference between them. It is literally true, at least in terms of aerobic capacity, that exercise keeps a person younger.

All-cause mortality and physical fitness have been studied in both men and women. When fitness was divided into quintiles, the age-adjusted all-cause mortality rates declined from 64.0 and 39.5/10,000 person-years in the least fit men and women to 18.6 and 8.5/10,000 person-years in the most fit men and women. Higher levels of fitness appeared to delay mortality, primarily owing to lowered rates of cardiovascular disease and cancer.[129]

Even though there is no evidence that exercise in moderation is more hazardous for older adults, how often is it regularly urged for a person of 95? Fiatarone et al.[130] demonstrated that frail, institutionalized volunteer nonagenarians, after only 8 weeks in a supervised weightlifting program for legs only, showed a 174% increase in muscle strength and highly significant gains in muscle mass and walking speed. They concluded, "The potential for reversal of 'age related' muscle weakness has been unexploited."[130] The most important target of conditioning in the geriatric population is the leg muscles. There are no data to prove that better conditioning would prevent falls, one of the most serious causes of morbidity in older persons, but it seems likely that improved muscle strength, tone, balance, and mobility would almost certainly help. Likewise, there may be subtle brain damage that limits an older adult's capacity to perform activities. One measure of this is the number and severity of subcortical hyperintensities seen on MRI scans.[131] Even if these are present, one should never avoid a reconditioning program for an older adult. There are no studies on the effects of these changes on such a program.

Just as the original illness or injury can be demoralizing, so can the seeming snail's pace of recovery. This normal despondency can further retard rehabilitation. Few things heal self-esteem as effectively as regaining the sense of sound body. The consultant who helps the patient grieve those losses beyond restoration, while correcting misconceptions about inactivity and encouraging the patient to shoulder the work of recovery, shortens the convalescence of both body and mind.

References

1. Wells KB, Golding JM, Burnam MA: Psychiatric disorder in a sample of the general population with and without chronic medical conditions, *Am J Psychiatry* 145:976–979, 1988.
2. Weissman MM, Bruce ML, Leaf PJ, et al: *Affective disorders*. In Robins LN, Regier DA, editors: *Psychiatric disorders in America: the Epidemiologic Catchment Area Study*. New York, N.Y., 1991, The Free Press, pp 53–80.
3. Blazer DG, Kessler RC, McGonagle KA, et al: The prevalence and distribution of major depression in a national community sample: the National Comorbidity Survey. *Am J Psychiatry* 151(7):979–986, 1994.
4. Regier DA, Goldberg ID, Taube CA: The de facto U.S. Mental Health Services systems, *Arch Gen Psychiatry* 35:685–693, 1978.
5. Cassem EH: Depression and anxiety secondary to medical illness, *Psychiatr Clin North Am* 13:597–612, 1990.
6. Tufo HM, Ostfeld AM, Shekelle R: Central nervous system dysfunction following open-heart surgery, *JAMA* 212:1333, 1970.
7. Silverstone PH: Depression and outcome in acute myocardial infarction, *BMJ* 294:219–220, 1987.
8. Rabins PV, Harvis K, Koven S: High fatality rates of late-life depression associated with cardiovascular disease, *J Affect Disord* 9:165–167, 1985.
9. Lesperance F, Frasure-Smith N: Depression in patients with cardiac disease: a practical review *J Psychosom Res* 48:379–391, 2000.
10. Pennix BW, Beekman AT, Honig AT, et al: Depression and cardiac mortality: results from a community-based longitudinal study. *Arch Gen Psychiatry* 58:221–227, 2001.
11. DeGroot M, Anderson R, Freedland KE, et al: Association of depression and diabetes complications: a meta-analysis. *Psychosom Med* 63:619–630, 2001.
12. American Psychiatric Association: *Diagnostic and statistical manual of mental disorders*, ed 4, Washington, DC, 1994, American Psychiatric Association.
13. Endicott J: Measurement of depression in patients with cancer, *Cancer* 53(suppl):2243–2249, 1984.
14. Chochinov HM, Wilson KG, Enns M, et al: Prevalence of depression in the terminally ill: effects of diagnostic criteria and symptom threshold judgments, *Am J Psychiatry* 151:537–540, 1994.
15. Ormel J, VonKorff M, Usfun TB, et al: Common mental disorders and disability across cultures, *JAMA* 272:1741–1748, 1994.
16. Michelson D, Stratakis C, Hill L, et al: Bone mineral density in women with depression, *N Engl J Med* 335:1176–1181, 1996.
17. Carney RM, Freedland KE, Eisen SA, et al: Ventricular tachycardia and psychiatric depression in patients with coronary artery disease, *Am J Med* 95:23–28, 1993.
18. Carney RM, Saunders RD, Freedland KE, et al: Association of depression with reduced heart rate variability in coronary artery disease, *Am J Cardiol* 76:562–564, 1995.
19. Frasure-Smith N, Lesperance F, Talajic M: Depression following myocardial infarction: impact on 6-month survival, *JAMA* 270:1819–1825, 1993.
20. Frasure-Smith N, Lesperance F, Talajic M: Depression and 18-month prognosis following myocardial infarction, *Circulation* 91:999–1005, 1995.
21. Yaskin JD: Nervous symptoms as earliest manifestations of carcinoma of the pancreas, *JAMA* 96:1664 1668, 1923.
22. Joffe RT, Rubinow DR, Denicoff KD, et al: Depression and carcinoma of the pancreas, *Gen Hosp Psychiatry* 8:241–245, 1986.
23. Holland JC, Korzun AH, Tross S, et al: Comparative psychological disturbance in patients with pancreatic and gastric cancer, *Am J Psychiatry* 143:982–986, 1986.
24. Atkinson JH, Grant I, Kennedy CJ, et al: Prevalence of psychiatric disorders among men infected with human immunodeficiency virus, *Arch Gen Psychiatry* 45:859–864, 1988.
25. Perry SW: Organic mental disorders caused by HIV: update on early diagnosis and treatment, *Am J Psychiatry* 147:696–710, 1990.
26. Robinson RG, Starr LB, Price TR: A two-year longitudinal study of mood disorders following stroke: prevalence and duration at six months follow-up, *Br J Psychiatry* 144:256–262, 1984.
27. Robinson RG, Bolduc P, Price TR: A two-year longitudinal study of post-stroke depression: diagnosis and outcome at one and two year follow-up, *Stroke* 18:837–843, 1987.
28. Morris PLP, Robinson RG, Beverley R, et al: Lesion location and poststroke depression, *J Neuropsychiatry Clin Neurosci* 8:399–403, 1996.
29. Lipsey JR, Robinson RG, Pearlson GD, et al: Nortriptyline treatment of post-stroke depression: a double-blind study, *Lancet* 1:297–300, 1984.
30. Reding MJ, Orto LS, Winter SW, et al: Antidepressant therapy after stroke: a double blind trial, *Arch Neurol* 43:763–765, 1986.
31. Murray GB, Shea V, Conn DK: Electroconvulsive therapy for poststroke depression, *J Clin Psychiatry* 47:258–260, 1987.
32. Masand P, Murray GB, Pickett P: Psychostimulants in post-stroke depression, *J Neuropsychiatry* 3:23–27, 1991.
33. Robinson RG, Schultz SK, Castillo C, et al: Nortriptyline versus fluoxetine in the treatment of depression

and in short-term recovery after stroke: a placebo-controlled double blind study. *Am J Psychiatry* 157:351–359, 2000.

34. Ross ED, Rush AJ: Diagnosis and neuroanatomical correlates of depression in brain-damaged patients, *Arch Gen Psychiatry* 38:1344–1354, 1981.

35. Zubenko GS, Moossy J: Major depression in primary dementia, *Arch Neurol* 45:1182–1186, 1988.

36. Zubenko GS, Moossy J, Kopp U: Neurochemical correlates of major depression in primary dementia, *Arch Neurol* 47:209–214, 1990.

37. Hachinski VC, Iliff LD, Zilhka E, et al: Cerebral blood flow in dementia, *Arch Neurol* 32:632–637, 1975.

38. Cummings JL, Miller B, Hill M, et al: Neuropsychiatric aspects of multi-infarct dementia and dementia of the Alzheimer type, *Arch Neurol* 44:389–393, 1987.

39. Folstein SE, Abbott MH, Chase GA, et al: The association of affective disorder with Huntington's disease in a case series and in families, *Psychol Med* 13:537–542, 1983.

40. Asnis G: Parkinson's disease, depression, and ECT: a review and case study, *Am J Psychiatry* 134:191–195, 1977.

41. Holcomb HH, Sternberg DE, Heninger GR: Effects of electroconvulsive therapy on mood, Parkinsonism and tardive dyskinesia in a depressed patient: ECT and dopamine systems, *Biol Psychiatry* 18:865–873, 1983.

42. Summergrad P, Peterson B: Binswanger's disease (part I): the clinical recognition of subcortical arteriosclerotic encephalopathy in elderly neuropsychiatric patients, *J Geriatr Psychiatry Neurol* 2:123–133, 1989.

43. Koralnick IJ, Beaumanoir A, Hausler R, et al: A controlled study of early neurologic abnormalities in men with asymptomatic human immunodeficiency virus infection, *N Engl J Med* 323:864–870, 1990.

44. Perry S, Jacobsberg LB, Fishman B, et al: Psychiatric diagnosis before serological testing for human immunodeficiency virus, *Am J Psychiatry* 147:89–93, 1990.

45. Fernandez F, Adams F, Levy JK, et al: Cognitive impairment due to AIDS-related complex and its response to psychostimulants, *Psychosomatics* 29:38–46, 1988.

46. Holmes VF, Fernandez F, Levy JK: Psychostimulant response in AIDS-related complex patients, *J Clin Psychiatry* 50:5–8, 1989.

47. Rabkin JG, Wagner G, Rabkin R: Effects of sertraline on mood and immune status in patients with major depression and HIV illness: an open trial. *J Clin Psychiatry* 55:433–439, 1994.

48. Ferrando SJ, Rabkin JG, deMoore GM, Rabkin R: Antidepressant treatment of depression in HIV-seropositive women. *J Clin Psychiatry* 60:741–746, 1999.

49. Ferrando SJ, Goldman JD, Charness WE: Selective serotonin reuptake inhibitor treatment of depression in symptomatic HIV infection and AIDS: improvements in affective and somatic symptoms. *Gen Hosp Psychiatry* 19:89–97, 1997.

50. Rabkin JG, Wagner GJ, Rabkin R.: Fluoxetine treatment for depression in patients with HIV and AIDS: a randomized, placebo-controlled trial. *Am J Psychiatry* 156:101–107, 1999.

51. Eliot AJ, Uldall KK, Bergam K, et al: Randomized, placebo-controlled trial of paroxetine versus imipramine in depressed HIV-positive outpatients. *Am J Psychiatry* 155:367–372, 1998.

52. Currier MB, Molina G, Kato M: A prospective trial of sustained-release bupropion for depression in HIV-seropositive and AIDS patients. *Psychosomatics* 44:120–125, 2003.

53. Coull DC, Crooks J, Dingwall-Fordyce I, et al: Amitriptyline and cardiac disease: risk of sudden death identified by monitoring system, *Lancet* 2:590–591, 1970.

54. Robinson DS, Barker E: Tricyclic antidepressant cardiotoxicity, *JAMA* 236:1089–1090, 1976.

55. Gray DS, Fujiyoka K, Dewine W, et al: Fluoxetine treatment of the obese diabetic. *Int J Obes* 16:193–198, 1992.

56. O'Kane M, Wiles PG, Wales JK: Fluoxetine in the treatment of obese type 2 diabetic patients. *Diabetic Med* 11:105–110, 1994.

57. Chiasson L, Law DCW, Leiter LA, et al: Fluoxetine has potential in obese NIDDM-multicentre Canadian trial. *Diabetes* 38:154A, 1989.

58. Wise SD: Clinical studies with fluoxetine in obesity. *Am J Clin Nutr* 55:181S-184S, 1992.

59. Kutnowski M, Daubresse JC, Friedman H, et al: Fluoxetine therapy in obese diabetic and glucose intolerant patients. *Int J Obes* 16(suppl 4):S63-S66, 1992.

60. Potter, Van Loon BJ, et al: Fluoxetine increases insulin action in obese non-diabetic and in obese non-insulin-dependant diabetic individuals. *Int J Obes* 16:79–85, 1992.

61. Maheaux P, Ducros F, Bourque J, et al: Fluoxetine improves insulin sensitivity in obese patients with non-insulin-dependant diabetes mellitus independently of weight loss. *Int J Obes Relat Metab Disord* 21:97–102, 1997.

62. Lustman PJ, Griffith LS, Clouse RE, et al: Effects of nortriptyline on depression and glycemic control in diabetes: results of a double-blind, placebo-controlled trial. *Psychosom Med* 59:241–250, 1997.

63. Max MB, Lynch SA, Muir J, et al: Effects of desipramine, amitriptyline, and fluoxetine on pain in diabetic neuropathy. *N Engl J Med* 326:1250–1256, 1992.

64. Peter H, Tabrizian S, Hand I: Serum cholesterol in patients with obsessive compulsive disorder during treatment with behavior therapy and SSRI or placebo. *Int J Psychiatry Med.* 30:27–39, 2000.

65. Olusi SO, Fido AA: Serum lipid concentrations in patients with major depressive disorder *Biol Psychiatry* 40:1128–1131, 1996.

66. Richelson E: Pharmacology of antidepressants, *Psychopathology* 20(suppl 1):1–12, 1987.

67. Richelson E: Pharmacology of antidepressants-characteristics of the ideal drug, *Mayo Clin Proc* 69:1069–1081, 1994.

68. de Boer T: The pharmacologic profile of mirtazapine, *J Clin Psychiatry* 57(suppl 4):19–25, 1996.

69. Greene SL, Reed CE, Schroeter AL: Double-blind cross over study comparing doxepin and diphenhydramine for the treatment of chronic urticaria, *J Am Acad Dermatol* 12:669–675, 1985.

70. Jarvik LF, Read SL, Mintz J, et al: Pretreatment orthostatic hypotension in geriatric depression: predictor of response to imipramine and doxepin, *J Clin Psychopharmacol* 6:368–372, 1983.

71. Stack JA, Reynolds CF, Perel JM, et al: Pretreatment systolic orthostatic blood pressure (PSOP) and treatment response in elderly depressed inpatients, *J Clin Psychopharmacol* 8:116–120, 1988.

72. Roose SP, Glassman AH: Cardiovascular effects of tricyclic antidepressants in depressed patients with and without heart disease, *J Clin Psychiatry Monogr* 7:1–18, 1989.

73. Roose SP, Glassman AH, Siris S, et al: Comparison of imipramine and nortriptyline-induced orthostatic hypotension: a meaningful difference, *J Clin Psychopharmacol* 1:316–319, 1981.

74. Jefferson JW: A review of the cardiovascular effects and toxicity of tricyclic antidepressants, *Psychosom Med* 37:160–179, 1975.

75. Giardina E-GV, Bigger JT: Antiarrhythmic effect of imipramine hydrochloride in patients with ventricular premature complexes without psychological depression, *Am J Cardiol* 50:172–179, 1982.

76. Connolly SJ, Mitchell LB, Swerdlow CD, et al: Clinical efficacy and electrophysiology of imipramine for ventricular tachycardia, *Am J Cardiol* 53:516–521, 1984.

77. Giardina E-GV, Barnard T, Johnson L, et al: The antiarrhythmic effect of nortriptyline in cardiac patients with ventricular premature depolarizations, *J Am Coll Cardiol* 1:1363–1369, 1986.

78. Kulig K, Rumack BH, Sullivan JB Jr, et al: Amoxapine overdose: coma and seizures without cardiotoxic effects, *JAMA* 248:1092–1094, 1982.

79. Pumariega AJ, Muller B, Rivers-Bulkeley N: Acute renal failure secondary to amoxapine overdose, *JAMA* 248:331–341, 1982.

80. Zavodnick S: Atrial flutter with amoxapine: a case report, *Am J Psychiatry* 138:1503–1505, 1981.

81. Murray GB: Atrial fibrillation/flutter associated with amoxapine: two case reports, *J Clin Psychopharmacol* 5:124–125, 1985.

82. Pohl R, Bridges M, Rainey JM Jr, et al: Effects of trazodone and desipramine on cardiac rate and rhythm in a patient with preexisting cardiovascular disease, *J Clin Psychopharmacol* 6:380–381, 1986.

83. Giardina E-GV, Bigger JT, Glassman AH: Comparison between imipramine and desmethylimipramine on the electrocardiogram and left ventricular function, *Clin Pharmacol Ther* 31:230, 1982.

84. Giardina E-GV, Johnson LL, Vita J, et al: Effect of imipramine and nortriptyline on left ventricular function and blood pressure in patients treated for arrhythmias, *Am Heart J* 109:992–998, 1985.

85. Roose SP, Glassman AH, Giardina E-GV, et al: Nortriptyline in depressed patients with left ventricular impairment, *JAMA* 256:3253–3257, 1986.

86. Roose SP, Glassman AH, Giardina E-GV, et al: Cardiovascular effects of imipramine and bupropion in depressed patients with congestive heart failure, *J Clin Psychopharmacol* 7:247–251, 1987.

87. Dec GW, Stern TA: Tricyclic antidepressants in the intensive care unit, *J Intens Care Med* 5:69–81, 1990.

88. Glassman AH, Johnson LL, Giardina E-GV, et al: The use of imipramine in depressed patients with congestive heart failure, *JAMA* 250:1997–2001, 1983.

89. Rosenbaum JF, Fava M, Hoog SL, et al: Selective serotonin reuptake inhibitor discontinuation syndrome: a randomized clinical trial. *Biol Psychiatry* 44:77–87, 1998.

90. Fava M, Mulroy R, Alpert J, et al: Emergence of adverse events following discontinuation of treatment with extended-release venlafaxine. *Am J Psychiatry* 154:1760–1762, 1997.

91. Woods S, Tesar GE, Murray GB, et al: Psychostimulant treatment of depressive disorders secondary to medical illness, *J Clin Psychiatry* 47:12–15, 1986.

92. Tesar GE: The role of stimulants in general medicine, *Drug Ther* 12:186–195, 1982.

93. Krauthammer C, Klerman GL: Secondary mania, *Arch Gen Psychiatry* 35:1333–1339, 1978.

94. Greenberg DB, Brown GL: Mania resulting from brain stem tumor, *J Nerv Ment Dis* 173:434–436, 1985.

95. Harsch HH, Miller M, Young LD: Induction of mania by L-dopa in a nonbipolar patient, *J Clin Psychopharmacol* 5:338–339, 1985.

96. Kwentus JA, Hart RP, Calabrese V, et al: Mania as a symptom of multiple sclerosis, *Psychosomatics* 27:729–731, 1986.

97. Riess H, Schwartz CF, Klerman GL: Manic syndrome following head injury: another form of secondary mania, *J Clin Psychiatry* 48:29–30, 1987.

98. Shukla S, Cook BL, Mukherjee S, et al: Mania following head trauma, *Am J Psychiatry* 144:93–96, 1987.

99. Starkstein SE, Pearlson GD, Boston J, et al: Mania after brain injury: a controlled study of causative factors, *Arch Neurol* 44:1069–1073, 1987.

100. Larson EW: Organic causes of mania, *Mayo Clin Proc* 63:906–912, 1988.

101. Barczak P, Edmunds E, Belts T: Hypomania following complex partial seizures, *Br J Psychiatry* 152:131–138, 1988.

102. Halman MH, Worth JL, Sanders KM, et al: Anticonvulsant use in the treatment of manic syndromes in patients with HIV-1 infection, *J Neuropsychiatry Clin Neurosci* 5:430–434, 1993.

103. Hill RR, Stagno SJ, Tesar GE: Secondary mania associated with the use of felbamate, *Psychosomatics* 36:404–406, 1995.

104. Wellens H, Cats VM, Durren D: Symptomatic sinus node abnormalities following lithium carbonate therapy, *Am J Med* 59:285–287, 1975.

105. Wilson J, Kraus E, Bailas M, et al: Reversible sinus node abnormalities due to lithium carbonate therapy, *N Engl J Med* 294:1222–1224, 1976.

106. Mitchell JE, MacKenzie TB: Cardiac effects of lithium therapy in man, *J Clin Psychiatry* 43:47–51, 1982.

107. Roose SP, Bone S, Haidorfer C, et al: Lithium treatment in older patients, *Am J Psychiatry* 136:843–844, 1979.

108. Richardson HL, Graupner KI, Richardson ME: Intramyocardial lesions in patients dying suddenly and unexpectedly, *JAMA* 195:254–260, 1966.

109. Kemper AJ, Dunlap R, Pietro DA: Thioridazine-induced torsade de pointes, *JAMA* 249:2931–2934, 1983.

110. Wilens T, Stern TA: Ventricular tachycardia associated with desipramine and thioridazine, *Psychosomatics* 31:100–103, 1990.

111. Prigerson HG, Frank E, Kasl SV, et al: Complicated grief and bereavement-related depression as distinct disorders: preliminary empirical validation in elderly bereaved spouses, *Am J Psychiatry* 152:22–30, 1995.

112. Bibring E: *The mechanism of depression*. In Greenacre P, editor: *Affective disorders: psychoanalytic contributions to their study*, New York, 1953, International Universities Press.

113. Cassem NH, Hackett TP: Psychiatric consultation in a coronary care unit, *Ann Intern Med* 75:9–14, 1971.

114. Levine SA, Lown B: "Armchair" treatment of acute coronary thrombosis, *JAMA* 148:1365, 1952.

115. Wishnie HA, Hackett TP, Cassem NH: Psychologic hazards of convalescence following myocardial infarction, *JAMA* 215:1292–1296, 1971.

116. Saltin B, Blomqvist G, Mitchell JH, et al: Response to exercise after bed rest and after training, *Circulation* 38(suppl 7):1–78, 1968.

117. Alpert JS, Bass H, Szucs MM, et al: Effects of physical training on hemodynamics and pulmonary function at rest and during exercise in patients with chronic obstructive pulmonary disease, *Chest* 66:647–651, 1974.

118. Holle RHO, Williams DV, Vandree JC, et al: Increased muscle efficiency and sustained benefits in an outpatient community hospital-based pulmonary rehabilitation program, *Chest* 94:1161–1168, 1988.

119. Unger KM, Moser KM, Hanser P: Selection of an exercise program for patients with chronic obstructive pulmonary disease, *Heart Lung* 9:68–76, 1980.

120. Pardy RL, Rivington RN, Despas PJ, et al: Inspiratory muscle training compared with physiotherapy in patients with chronic airflow limitation, *Am Rev Respir Dis* 123:421–425, 1981.

121. Gift AG, Plaut SM, Jacox A: Psychologic and physiologic factors related to dyspnea in subjects with chronic obstructive pulmonary disease, *Heart Lung* 15:595–602, 1986.

122. Andrews JL Jr: Pulmonary rehabilitation, *Pract Cardiol* 12:127–137, 1986.

123. Cassem NH, Hackett TP: Psychological aspects of myocardial infarction, *Med Clin North Am* 61:711–721, 1977.

124. American Heart Association: Exercise testing and training of individuals with heart disease or at high risk for its development, Dallas, 1975, American Heart Association.

125. Simon HB: *Exercise, health, and sports medicine*. In Dale DC, Federman DD, editors: *Scientific American Medicine 1995: 8. interdisciplinary medicine VII*. New York, 1990, Scientific American.

126. Thompson PD: The benefits and risks of exercise training in patients with chronic coronary artery disease, *JAMA* 259:1537–1540, 1988.

127. Squires RW, Lavie CJ, Brandt TR, et al: Cardiac rehabilitation in patients with severe ischemic left ventricular dysfunction, *Mayo Clin Proc* 62:997–1002, 1987.

128. Larson EB, Bruce RA: Exercise and aging, *Ann Intern Med* 105:783–785, 1986.

129. Blair SN, Kohl HW III, Paffenbarger RS Jr, et al: Physical fitness and all-cause mortality: a prospective study of healthy men and women, *JAMA* 262:2395–2401, 1989.

130. Fiatarone MA, Marks EC, Ryan ND, et al: High-intensity strength training in nonagenarians, *JAMA* 263:3029–3034, 1990.

131. Cahn DA, Malloy PF, Salloway S, et al: Subcortical hyperintensities on MRI and activities of daily living in geriatric depression. *J Neuropsychiatry Clin Neurosci* 8:404–411, 1996.

Chapter 9
Suicidal Patients

Theodore A. Stern, M.D.
Roy H. Perlis, M.D.
Isabel T. Lagomasino, M.D.

The psychiatric consultant is frequently asked to evaluate and treat patients in the general hospital who have contemplated, threatened, or attempted suicide. Although guided by knowledge of epidemiologic risk factors for suicide (Table 9-1), the clinician must rely on a detailed examination and clinical judgment in the evaluation of current suicidal risk.

Epidemiology

Suicide is the eleventh leading cause of death in the United States, accounting for nearly 30,000 deaths each year, and for 1% to 2% of the total number of deaths each year.[1] For every person that completes suicide, approximately 8 to 10 people attempt suicide,[2,3] and for every completed suicide, approximately 18 to 20 attempts are made[4,5]; that is, some individuals make more than one unsuccessful attempt. Approximately 1% to 2% of emergency department visits,[6] 5% of intensive care unit admissions,[7] and 10% of general medical admissions[8] result from failed suicide attempts.

Use of firearms is the most common method of committing suicide for both men and women in the United States, accounting for nearly 60% of completed suicides.[5] Hanging is the second most common method used by men, and drug ingestion is the second most common method used by women.[5] Drug ingestion accounts for approximately 70% of unsuccessful suicides.[9,10]

Demographic Risk Factors

Suicide rates differ by age, sex, and race. Rates generally increase with age; people older than the age of 65 are 1.5 times more likely to commit suicide than are younger individuals.[11] Twenty percent of all suicides occur in the elderly, although they constitute only 13% of the population.[11] One reason for this may be that the elderly appear to make more serious attempts on their lives; one of every four attempts in this group results in a completed suicide.[11,12] Although the elderly have the highest suicide rates, young adults (between the ages of 15 and 24) have manifested a dramatic increase in the rate of suicide. Between 1950 and 1990, completed suicides tripled among adolescents and became the third leading cause of death, following unintentional injuries and homicide.[5,13]

Men are more likely to complete suicide than are women, although women are more likely to attempt suicide than are men. Four times more men than women complete suicide,[1] although three to four times more women than men attempt suicide.[14] The reasons for such disparities have not been established clearly.

Whites are more likely to attempt and complete suicide than nonwhites,[5,15] although Native Americans and Alaskan natives have the highest suicide rates of any ethnic groups.[5] African-Americans and Hispanics have approximately half the suicide rate of whites.[16,17]

Table 9-1. Risk Factors for Suicide

Demographic factors
  Age: elderly, adolescent
  Gender: male
  Race: white
Psychiatric factors
  Depressive disorders
  Alcohol and drug dependence
  Alcohol and drug abuse
  Psychotic disorders
  Personality disorders
  Anxiety disorders
Medical factors
  Acquired immune deficiency syndrome
  Cancer
  Head trauma
  Epilepsy
  Multiple sclerosis
  Huntington's chorea
  Organic brain syndromes
  Spinal cord injuries
  Hypertension
Cardiopulmonary disease
  Peptic ulcer disease
  Chronic renal failure
  Cushing's disease
  Rheumatoid arthritis
  Porphyria
Social factors
  Marital status: widowed, divorced, separated
  Solitary living situation
  Social isolation
  Recent personal loss
  Unemployment
  Financial difficulties
  Legal involvement
  Firearm possession
Familial factors
  Family history of suicide
  Family history of psychiatric illness
  Early parental death
  Early parental separation
  Emotional abuse
  Physical abuse
  Sexual abuse
  Frequent moves
Past and present suicidality
  Prior suicide attempts
  Suicidal ideation
  Suicidal intent
  Hopelessness
Treatment settings
  Recent visit with physician
Status as medical inpatient

Psychiatric Risk Factors

Psychiatric illness is the most powerful risk factor for both completed and attempted suicide. Psychiatric disorders are associated with more than 90% of completed suicides[18–20] and with the vast majority of attempted suicides.[15,21,22] Mood disorders, including major depressive disorder (MDD) and bipolar disorder (BPD), are responsible for around 60% of completed suicides, alcohol and drug abuse for 25%, psychosis for 10%, and personality disorders for 5%.[23,24]

Up to 15% of patients with MDD or BPD complete suicide, almost always during depressive episodes[25]; this represents a suicide risk 30 times greater than that of the general population.[26] True lifetime risk may be somewhat lower, because these estimates (and those for the other diagnoses discussed later) typically derive from hospitalized patient samples.[23] The risk appears to be greater early in the course of a lifetime disorder, early on in a depressive episode,[4,27] in the first week following psychiatric hospitalization,[28] in the first month following discharge,[28] and in the early stages of recovery.[28] The risk may[29] or may not[30] be elevated by comorbid psychosis. A 10-year follow-up study of almost 1000 patients found those who committed suicide within the first year of follow-up were more likely to be suffering from global insomnia, severe anhedonia, impaired concentration, psychomotor agitation, alcohol abuse, anxiety, and panic attacks, whereas those who committed suicide after the first year of follow-up were more likely to be suffering from suicidal ideation, severe hopelessness, and a history of suicide attempts.[30]

Approximately 15% to 25% of patients with alcohol or drug dependence complete suicide,[27,31] of which up to 84% suffer from both alcohol and drug depenence.[31] The suicide risk appears to be greatest roughly 9 years after the commencement of alcohol and drug addiction.[18,32] The majority of patients with alcohol dependence who commit suicide suffer from comorbid depressive disorders,[27,33,34] and as many as one third have experienced the recent loss of a close relationship through separation or death.[35]

Nearly 20% of people who complete suicide are legally intoxicated at the time of their death.[36] Alcohol and drug abuse are associated with more pervasive suicidal ideation, more serious suicidal intent, more lethal suicide attempts, and greater number of suicide attempts.[37] Alcohol and drugs may impair judgment and foster impulsivity.[28]

Roughly 10% of patients with schizophrenia complete suicide, mostly during periods of improvement after relapse or during periods of depression.[34,38] The risk for suicide appears to be increased among young men who are newly diagnosed,[39,40] who have a chronic course and numerous exacerbations, who are discharged from hospitals with significant psychopathology and functional impairment, and who have a realistic awareness and fear of further mental decline.[40] The risk may also be increased with akathisia and with abrupt discontinuation of neuroleptics.[27] Patients who experience hallucinations (that instruct them to harm themselves) in association with schizophrenia, mania, or depression with psychotic features are probably at greater risk for self-harm and should be protected.[41]

Between 4% and 10% of patients with borderline personality disorder and 5% of patients with antisocial personality disorder commit suicide.[42] The risk appears to be greater for those with comorbid depression or alcohol abuse.[43] Patients with personality disorders often make impulsive suicidal gestures or attempts; these attempts may become more lethal if they are not taken seriously. Even manipulative gestures can turn fatal.[41]

As many as 15% to 20% of patients with anxiety disorders complete suicide,[44] and up to 20% of patients with panic disorder attempt suicide.[45] Although the risk of suicide in patients with anxiety and panic disorders may be elevated secondary to comorbid conditions (e.g., major depression and alcohol or drug abuse), the suicide risk remains almost as high as that of major depression, even after coexisting conditions are taken into account.[46] The risk for suicide attempts may be elevated for women with an early onset and with comorbid alcohol or drug abuse.[45]

Medical Risk Factors

Medical illness, especially of a severe or chronic nature, may be a risk factor for completed suicide. Medical disorders are associated with as many as 35% to 40% of suicides[47] and with as many as 70% of suicides in those older than the age of 60.[48]

Acquired immune deficiency syndrome (AIDS), cancer, head trauma, epilepsy, multiple sclerosis, Huntington's chorea, organic brain syndromes, spinal cord injuries, hypertension, cardiopulmonary disease, peptic ulcer disease, chronic renal failure, Cushing's disease, rheumatoid arthritis, and porphyria have each been reported to increase the risk of suicide. Notably, however, few investigations concerning the increased risk for suicide in these populations have controlled for the effects of age, sex, race, psychiatric disorders, other medical disorders, or use of medications.

Patients with AIDS appear to have a suicide risk that is 16 to 66 times greater than that of the general population.[49,50] Testing for antibodies to the human immunodeficiency virus has resulted in an immediate and substantial decrease in suicidal ideation in those who turned out to be seronegative; no increase in suicidal ideation was detected in those who were seropositive.[51] Sexual orientation among men, in and of itself, has not been identified as an independent risk factor for completed suicide.[5,52]

Carrying a diagnosis of cancer may be associated with a suicide rate that is twice as great as that of the general population.[53] Advanced disease, poor prognosis, poor pain control, fatigue, and cancer type (including oral, pharyngeal, gastrointestinal, lung, urogenital, and breast) as well as depression, hopelessness, delirium, disinhibition, prior suicide attempts, recent losses, and a paucity of social supports may place cancer patients at greater risk.[54,55]

Head trauma is associated with a suicide risk that is twice as great as that of the general population.[56] The risk appears to be greater in patients who suffer severe injuries and in those who develop dementia, psychosis, character changes, or epilepsy.[56–58] Patients with epilepsy are five times more likely than those in the general population to complete[59] or to attempt suicide.[60] Sufferers of temporal lobe epilepsy,[61] with concomitant psychosis or personality changes, may be at greater risk.[62]

Individuals with multiple sclerosis may have a slightly greater risk of committing suicide than those in the general population.[58] The risk may be higher for those diagnosed before the age of 40 and within the first 5 years after diagnosis.[63]

Victims of Huntington's chorea appear to have a greater suicide risk than those in the general population.[57] With the advent of biochemical tools to identify disease carriers, the elevated suicide risk may be further increased. In one study, 67 persons with a parent with Huntington's chorea underwent questioning. Approximately 79% wanted to be tested for the disease, 40% revealed they had a family history of attempted or successful suicide, and 11% would consider suicide if they were to test positive for the disease.[64]

Those with organic brain syndromes may be at increased risk for attempted or completed suicides. Delirious and confused patients may suffer from agitation and destructive impulses and be unable to protect themselves from harm.[41]

Victims of spinal cord injuries have a substantially increased risk for suicide.[57] The risk is actually greater for those with less severe injuries.[65,66]

Hypertensive patients[57] and those with cardiopulmonary disease[41] may also have a higher risk for suicide than those in the general population. Although previous reports suggested that β-blockers could contribute to increased risk by promoting depression,[57] recent studies suggest that β-blockers do not increase the risk of developing depression.[67] Patients with peptic ulcer disease may be two to four times more likely to commit suicide than those in the general population.[57] Patients who have undergone surgical treatments and who suffer from comorbid alcoholism may also be at greater risk.[57]

As many as 5% of patients with chronic renal failure who receive hemodialysis die from suicide; those who travel to medical centers for dialysis have a higher suicide rate than those who are dialyzed at home.[3] The risk for suicide among these patients may be as high as 400 times that of the general population.[68]

Cushing's disease is associated with higher rates of suicide and suicide attempts,[34] possibly a consequence of major affective illness, which affects as many as 85% of patients with the disease.[69]

Patients who suffer from rheumatoid arthritis may also have a higher relative risk for suicide (perhaps secondary to use of steroid medications),[57] as do patients with porphyria.[70]

Social Risk Factors

Widowed, divorced, or separated adults are at greater risk for suicide than are single adults, who are at greater risk than married adults.[71,72] Married adults with young children appear to carry the lowest risk.[28,41,47]

Living alone substantially increases the risk for suicide, especially among adults who are widowed, divorced, or separated.[28] Social isolation from family, relatives, friends, neighbors, and co-workers also increases the chance of suicide.[39,47]

Significant personal losses (including diminution of self-esteem or status[47,48]) and conflicts also place individuals, particularly young adults and adolescents at greater risk for suicide.[18,73] Bereavement following the death of a loved one increases the risk for suicide over the next 4 or 5 years, particularly for people with a psychiatric history (including suicide attempts) and for people who receive little family support.[27]

Unemployment, which may produce or exacerbate psychiatric illness or may result from psychiatric illness,[27] increases the likelihood of suicide and accounts for as many as one third to one half of completed suicides.[36,47] This risk may be particularly elevated among men.[27]

Financial and legal difficulties also increase the risk for suicide.[5,28,74] Within prisons, suicide is the leading cause of death.[5,47]

The presence of one or more firearms in the home appears to increase the risk of suicide independently for both genders and all age-groups, even when other risk factors, such as depression and alcohol abuse, are taken into account.[21,73,75] For example, adolescents with a gun in the household have suicide rates between 4 and 10 times greater than other adolescents.[76]

Familial Risk Factors

A family history of suicide, a family history of psychiatric illness, and a tumultuous early family environment have each been found to have an important impact on the risk for suicide.[5,47] As many as 7% to 14% of persons who attempt suicide have a family history of suicide.[77] This increased suicide risk may be mediated through a shared genetic predisposition for suicide, psychiatric disorders, or impulsive behavior, [27,39,78] or through a shared family environment in which modeling and imitation are prominent.[79] A tumultuous early family environment (e.g., with early parental death, parental separation, emotional abuse, physical abuse, sexual abuse, and frequent moves) also increases the risk for suicide.[5,47]

Past and Present Suicidality

A history of suicide attempts is one of the most powerful risk factors for completed and attempted suicide.[5,80] As many as 10% to 20% of people with prior suicide attempts complete suicide.[3,9,81] The risk for completed suicide following an attempted suicide is almost 100 times that of the general population in the year following the attempt, then declines but remains elevated throughout the next 8 years.[27] People with prior suicide attempts are also at greater risk for subsequent attempts and have been found to account for approximately 50% of serious overdoses.[82] The clinical use of past suicide attempts as a predictive risk factor may be limited in the elderly because the elderly make fewer attempts for each completed suicide.[11,12,47]

The lethality of past suicide attempts slightly increases the risk for completed suicide,[27] especially among women with psychiatric illness.[33] The dangerousness of an attempt, however, may be more predictive of the risk for suicide in those individuals with significant intent to suicide and a realization of the potential lethality of their actions.[83]

The communication of present suicidal ideation and intent must be carefully evaluated as a risk factor for completed and attempted suicide. As many as 80% of people who complete suicide communicate their intent either directly or indirectly.[47] Death or suicide may be discussed, new wills or life insurance policies may be written, valued possessions may be given away, or uncharacteristic and destructive behaviors may arise.[47] In one study concerning the communication of ideas about suicide by 134 consecutive cases of completed suicide,[84] as many as 69% communicated their thoughts of suicide to family, friends, co-workers, ministers, or physicians. Approximately 41% specifically stated their intent to commit suicide, 24% expressed that they would be better off dead or that they were tired of living, 22% communicated a desire to die, 22% attempted suicide previously, 18% made reference to methods of committing suicide, and 16% made dire predictions regarding their future.

People who intend to commit suicide may, however, be less likely to communicate their intent to their health care providers than they are to close family and friends.[38] Although 50% of people who commit suicide have consulted a physician in the month before their death, only 60% of them communicated some degree of suicidal ideation or intent to their physician.[18,38] In a study of 571 cases of completed suicide who had met with their health care professional within 4 weeks of their suicide,[85] only 22% discussed their suicidal intent. Many investigators believe that ideation and intent may be more readily discussed with psychiatrists than with other physicians.[85,86]

Hopelessness, or negative expectations about the future, is a stronger predictor of suicide risk than is depression or suicidal ideation[87,88] and may be both a short-term and long-term predictor of completed suicide in patients with major depression.[38]

Treatment Settings

Although nearly half of the people who commit suicide have seen a physician within the month preceding their death,[28,38] only a minority have been diagnosed and treated appropriately in primary care settings.[84,89] Many of these individuals present to their primary care physician with somatic rather with than psychiatric complaints.[90] Fewer than half of those who commit suicide are engaged in active psychiatric treatment.[91]

Some medical and surgical patients in the general hospital commit suicide. Most are male, have severe and chronic illness, suffer from alcohol dependence or organic brain syndromes, have developed depressive or psychotic symptoms in the hours to days preceding their suicide, and are described as demanding and dissatisfied; they are typically not being treated for a recent suicide attempt.[57] Lethal falls account for most deaths in the general hospital; notes or explanations are rarely left.[57] Some inpatients may also make impulsive and unexpected suicide attempts. In one study of 17 attempts over a 7-year period,[92] the majority of patients who made attempts were women with psychiatric disorders who displayed agitation, anger, mood swings, or psychosis in the hours to days before their attempt and who suffered a disruption in their relationship with caregivers. Self-cutting and ingestions accounted for most attempts.

Evaluation of Suicide Risk

The evaluation of suicide risk relies on a detailed clinical examination of the patient who has contemplated, threatened, or attempted suicide (Table 9-2). The thoughts and feelings of the individual must be elicited and placed in the context of known risk factors for suicide. Although useful as a guide to patient populations who may be more likely to commit or attempt suicide, risk factors alone are neither sensitive nor specific in the prediction of suicide. Their pervasive prevalence in comparison with the relatively low incidence of suicide in the general population may also lead to high false-positive rates. A multiple logistic regression model that used risk factors (such as age, sex, psychiatric diagnoses, medical diagnoses, marital status, family psychiatric history, prior suicide attempts, and suicidal ideation) failed to identify any of the 46 patients who committed suicide over a 14-year period from a group of 1906 people with affective disorders.[93]

An evaluation for suicide risk is indicated for all patients who have made a suicide attempt, who have voiced suicidal ideation or intent, who have admitted suicidal ideation or intent on questioning, or whose actions have suggested suicidal intent despite their protests to the contrary. All suicide attempts and suicidal ideation should be taken seriously, regardless of whether the actions or thoughts appear manipulative in nature.

The approach to the patient at potential risk for suicide should be nonjudgmental, supportive, and empathic. The initial establishment of rapport may include an introduction, an effort to create some degree of privacy in the interview setting, and an attempt to maximize the physical comfort of the patient for the interview by perhaps offering to provide a glass of water or adjust the position of the bed.[41] The patient who senses interest, concern, and compassion is more likely to trust the examiner and provide a detailed and accurate history. Often ambivalent about their thoughts and plans, suicidal patients may derive significant relief and benefit from a thoughtful and caring evaluation.[39,41]

The patient should be questioned about suicidal ideation and intent in an open and direct manner. Patients with suicidal thoughts and plans are often relieved and not offended when they find someone with whom they can speak about the unspeakable. Patients without suicidal ideation do not have the thoughts planted in their mind and do not develop a greater risk for suicide.[39,41,94] General questions concerning suicidal thoughts can be introduced in a gradual manner while obtaining the history of present illness. Questions such as "Has it ever seemed like things just aren't worth it?"[41] or "Have you had thoughts that life is not worth living?"[39] may lead to a further discussion of depression and hopelessness. "Have you gotten so depressed that you've considered killing yourself?"[41] or "Have you had thoughts of killing yourself?"[39] may open the door to a further evaluation of suicidal thoughts and plans.

Specific questions concerning potential suicide plans and preparations must follow any admission of suicidal ideation or intent. The patient should be asked when, where, and how an attempt would be made, and any potential means should be evaluated for feasibility and lethality. An organized and detailed plan involving an accessible and lethal method may place the patient at higher risk for suicide.[36] The seriousness of the wish or the intent to die must also be assessed. The patient who has begun to carry out the initial steps of a suicide plan, who wishes to be dead at the present time, and who has no hopes or plans for the future may be at greater risk. The last-mentioned domain (plans for the future) may be assessed by asking questions such as "What do you see yourself doing 5 years from now?" or "What things are you still looking forward to doing or seeing?"[41]

Many clinicians have addressed the issues of lethality and intent by means of the risk/rescue ratio.[95] The greater the relative risk or lethality and

Table 9-2. Evaluation of Suicide Risk

Take suicide attempts and suicidal ideation seriously.
Use a nonjudgmental and supportive approach.
Establish an initial rapport with the patient.
Evaluate suicidal ideation and intent:
    Presence of suicidal thoughts
    Details of suicide plan
    Seriousness of intent
    Risk/rescue ratio
    Precipitants
    Social support
    Degree of impulsivity
Assess for the presence of risk factors.
Perform a mental status examination.
Obtain collateral information.

the lesser the likelihood of rescue of a planned attempt, the more serious the potential for a completed suicide. Although often useful, the risk/rescue ratio cannot be merely applied as a simple formula; instead, one must examine and interpret the particular beliefs of a given patient. For example, a patient may plan an attempt with a low risk of potential harm but may sincerely wish to die and may believe that the plan will be fatal; the patient may thus have a higher risk for suicide. Conversely a patient may plan an attempt that carries a high probability of death, such as an acetaminophen overdose, but may have little desire to die and little understanding of the severity of the attempt; the patient may thus have a lower risk.[36]

The clinician must attempt to identify any possible precipitants for the present crisis in an effort to understand why the patient is suicidal. The patient who must face the same problems and stressors following the evaluation or who cannot or will not discuss potential precipitants may be at greater risk for suicide.[36] The clinician must also assess the social support in place for a given patient. A lack of outpatient care providers, family, or friends may elevate potential risk.[39,47]

The examiner who interviews a patient after a suicide attempt needs to evaluate the details, seriousness, risk/rescue ratio, and precipitants of the attempt. The patient who carries out a detailed plan, who perceives the attempt as lethal, who thinks that death will be certain, who is disappointed to be alive, and who must face unchanged stressors will be at a continued high risk for suicide. The patient who makes a calculated, premeditated attempt may also be at a higher risk for a repeat attempt than the patient who makes a hasty, impulsive attempt (out of anger, a desire for revenge, or a desire for attention) or the patient who is intoxicated.[41]

A thorough psychiatric, medical, social, and family history of the patient who may be at risk for suicide should be completed to evaluate the presence and significance of potential risk factors. Particular attention should be paid to the presence of MDD, alcohol or drug abuse, psychotic disorders, personality disorders, and anxiety disorders. The presence of multiple significant risk factors may confer an additive risk.

A careful mental status examination allows the clinician to detect psychiatric difficulties and assess cognitive capacities. Important aspects to evaluate in the examination include level of consciousness, appearance, behavior, attention, mood, affect, language, orientation, memory, thought form, thought content, perception, insight, and judgment.[96] A psychiatric review of systems aids in the detection of psychiatric disease.

The clinician should interview the family and friends of the patient at risk to corroborate gathered information and obtain new and pertinent data. Families may provide information that patients are hesitant to provide and that may be essential to their care.[36,39,41] Some patients who refuse to discuss an attempt or who insist that the entire event was a mistake may speak in an open and honest manner only when confronted with reports from their family. The evaluation of suicidal risk and the protection of the patient at risk are emergent procedures, which may take precedence over the desire of the patient for privacy and the maintenance of confidentiality in the physician-patient relationship. Concern over a life-or-death situation may obviate obtaining formal consent from the patient before speaking to family and friends.[41]

Treatment of Suicide Risk

The treatment of suicide risk in the general hospital includes stabilization of medical conditions, protection from self-harm, serial assessments of mental status, possible initiation of treatment, and choice of disposition (Table 9-3). Attention to current or potential medical conditions must be

Table 9-3. Treatment of Suicide Risk

Stabilize current or potential medical conditions.
Provide adequate patient safely:
    Detain and restrain
    Remove dangerous objects
    Supervise appropriately
    Use mechanical or chemical restraint
Perform serial assessments of mental status.
Consider initiation of treatment.
Choose a disposition:
    Home with outpatient follow-up
    Admission to medical unit
    Voluntary admission to psychiatric unit
    Involuntary commitment to psychiatric unit

prompt, and medical evaluations must be complete. The severity of the psychiatric presentation should not distract clinicians from their obligation to provide good medical care.[36]

Patient safety must be ensured until the patient is no longer at imminent risk for suicide. Appropriate intervention and the passage of time may aid in the resolution of suicidal ideation and intent.[36,41] Patients who are at potential risk for suicide and who threaten to leave before an adequate evaluation is completed must be detained, in accordance with statutes in most states that permit the detention of individuals deemed dangerous to themselves or others.[97] Patients who attempt to leave nonetheless should be contained by locked environments or restraints.[36]

Potential means for self-harm should be removed from the reach of patients at risk. Sharp objects, such as scissors, sutures, needles, glass bottles, and eating utensils, should be removed from the immediate area. Open windows, stairwells, and structures to which a noose could be attached must be blocked. Medications or other dangerous substances that patients may have brought to the hospital must be confiscated.[36]

Appropriate supervision and restraint must be provided at all times for patients at risk for suicide. Frequent supervision, constant one-to-one supervision, physical restraints, and medications may be used alone or in combination in an effort to protect patients at risk. The least restrictive means that ensures the safety of the patient should be used.

Frequently, physical restraint must be used until the evaluation is completed and the suicidal intent is clarified. Patients who are neither psychotic nor delirious, who can reliably agree not to harm themselves in the hospital, and to alert staff when they are feeling out of control might be managed with frequent supervision, whereas those who cannot contract might require constant one-to-one supervision or physical restraint.[36] Patients with greater size, strength, intent, or impulsivity are likely not to be adequately protected with mere supervision and require physical restraint.[41] Lack of staff availability for supervision also necessitates physical restraint.[23] Those patients who remain out of control even while in physical restraints may require medication to manage agitation. Some actions (such as spitting at staff, attempting to bite staff, or jerking wildly at restraints) endanger both the staff and the patient and usually require use of medication.[36]

Patients who are thought to be at significant risk for suicide and who are admitted to medical and surgical floors should be reassessed on at least a daily basis. The need for supervision and restraint should be continually readdressed.

Pharmacotherapy and, where indicated and available, brief psychotherapy should target the underlying psychiatric illness and emphasize a sense of control by the patient.[53,57] Because pharmacotherapy for depression typically requires several weeks for onset of efficacy, electroconvulsive therapy may be indicated in cases in which suicide risk remains high or antidepressants are contraindicated.[98] Of note, with long-term treatment, only lithium (in affective illness) and clozapine (in schizophrenia) have been shown to decrease suicide risk.[99,100]

Options for disposition following evaluation and treatment in the general hospital include discharge home with a recommendation for outpatient follow-up, treatment on a medical or surgical floor with ongoing psychiatric consultation, voluntary admission to a psychiatric unit, or involuntary commitment to a psychiatric unit. Patients might be discharged home if they are not currently suicidal; if they are able to agree to return if suicidal thoughts or impulses recur; if they are medically stable; if they are not delirious, demented, psychotic, significantly depressed, or intoxicated; if any firearms have been removed from the home; if acute precipitants have been identified and addressed; if social supports are in place; and if outpatient treatment has been arranged and agreed on.[36] A patient should be hospitalized for further evaluation and treatment on a psychiatric unit when the clinician cannot be reasonably certain that the patient is not at imminent risk for suicide. Those who agree to voluntary hospitalization and who cooperate with caregivers may have the highest likelihood of successful treatment.[41] Those who are at high risk for suicide or who cannot control their suicidal urges should be admitted to a locked psychiatric facility. Patients who are at high risk but who refuse hospitalization should be committed involuntarily.

Patients who require hospitalization should be informed of the disposition decision in a clear, direct manner. Possible transfers should proceed as quickly and efficiently as possible because patients may become quite tense and ambivalent about the decision to hospitalize.[47] Transfers to separate psychiatric facilities should be made by ambulance and in restraints.[36]

The clinician should always take a conservative approach to the treatment of suicidal risk and err, if necessary, on the side of excess restraint or hospitalization. From a forensic standpoint, the clinician sued for battery secondary to the use of restraints or to involuntary commitment would be easier to defend than the clinician sued for negligence secondary to a completed suicide. Acting in accordance with good clinical judgment in the best interest of the patient brings little danger of liability.[41] Adequate documentation should include the thought processes behind decisions to supervise, restrain, discharge, or hospitalize.[41]

Difficulties in Assessment of Suicidal Risk

Clinicians may encounter obstacles with certain patients, or within themselves, during the evaluation of suicide risk. They must be adept in the examination of patients who are intoxicated, who threaten, or who are uncooperative, and they must be aware of personal feelings and attitudes (e.g., anxiety, anger, denial, intellectualization, or over-identification) to allow for better assessment and management of the patient at risk.

Patients who are intoxicated may voice suicidal ideation or intent that they frequently retract when sober. A brief initial evaluation while they are intoxicated and their psychological defenses are impaired may reveal the depth of suicidal ideation or the reasons behind a suicide attempt.[41] A more thorough final examination when they are sober must also be completed and documented.[36,41]

Patients who threaten should be evaluated in the presence of security officers and should be placed in restraints as necessary to protect both them and staff.[41] Those who are uncooperative may refuse to answer questions despite all attempts to establish rapport and to create a supportive and empathic connection. Stating "I'd like to figure out how to be of help, but I can't do that without some information from you" in a calm but firm manner might be helpful. Patients should be informed that safety precautions will not be discontinued until the evaluation can be completed and that they will not be able to sign out against medical advice. Their competency to refuse medical treatments should be carefully questioned.[41] Patients who refuse to cooperate until restraints are removed should be reminded of the importance of the evaluation and should be enlisted to cooperate with the goal of removing the restraints in mind. Statements such as "We both agree that the restraints should come off if you don't need them. I am very concerned about your safety, and I need you to answer some questions before I can decide if it's safe to remove the restraints" might be helpful.[41]

Clinicians may experience personal feelings and attitudes toward patients at risk for suicide, which must be recognized and which must not be allowed to interfere with appropriate patient care. Clinicians may feel anxious because of the awareness that an error in judgment might have fatal consequences. They may feel angry at patients with histories of multiple gestures or at patients who have used trivial methods, often resulting in poor evaluations and punitive interventions. Angry examiners may inappropriately transfer a patient with a low risk for suicide to a psychiatric facility or may discharge a patient with a high risk to home.[41]

Some clinicians may be prone to experience denial as they evaluate and treat patients at risk for suicide. They may conspire with the patient or family in the stance that voiced suicidal ideation was "just talk" or that an attempt was "just an accident." Others may practice intellectualization and choose to believe that suicide is "an act of free will" and that patients should have the personal and legal right to kill themselves.[36]

Clinicians commonly overidentify with patients with whom they share personal characteristics. The thought "I would never commit suicide" may become translated into the thought "This patient would never commit suicide," and serious risk may be missed.[41] The examiner may try to assure patients that they will be fine or may try to convince them that they do not feel suicidal. Patients may thus be unable to express themselves fully and may not receive proper evaluation and treatment.

Clinicians who perform evaluations for patients who have made suicide attempts and who have been admitted to general hospital floors have to be aware of their own reactions to the patient as well as to those of the staff. Medical and surgical staff often develop strong feelings toward patients who have attempted suicide and at times wish that these patients were dead. The clinician must diffuse such charged situations, perhaps by holding group meetings for those involved to make them more aware of their negative feelings so that they are not acted out.[101] Such intervention may prevent mismanagement and premature discharge.

Summary

Evaluation and treatment of patients who have contemplated, threatened, or attempted suicide is a common reason for psychiatric consultation in the general hospital. An assessment should include a thorough exploration of suicidal ideation (and the attempt if carried out), a review of relevant risk factors, and a mental status examination. Patient safety should be ensured throughout the evaluation process. Essentially the suicide evaluation is an informed, carefully considered clinical judgment; unfortunately, it has limited long-term predictive reliability. Although suicide evaluations can be complicated by a lack of patient cooperation and by the personal feelings and reactions of the clinician, proper evaluation and treatment can be life-saving.

References

1. Moscicki E: *Epidemiology of suicide. In* Goldsmith S, editor. *Risk factors for suicide*, Washington, DC, 2001, National Academy Press, pp 1–4.
2. Clayton PJ: Suicide, *Psychiatr Clin North Am* 8:203–214, 1985.
3. Hirschfeld RMA, Davidson L: *Risk factors for suicide. In* Frances AJ, Hales RE, editors: *American Psychiatric Press review of psychiatry*, vol 7, Washington, DC, 1988, American Psychiatric Press.
4. Malone KM, Haas GL, Sweeney JA, et al: Major depression and the risk of attempted suicide, *J Affect Dis* 34:173–185, 1995.
5. Moscicki EK: Epidemiology of suicidal behavior, *Suicide Life Threat Behav* 25:22–35, 1995.
6. O'Brien JP: Increase in suicide attempts by drug ingestion: the Boston experience, 1964–1974, *Arch Gen Psychiatry* 34:1165–1169, 1977.
7. Thibault GE, Mulley AG, Barnett GO, et al: Medical intensive care: indications, interventions, and outcomes, *N Engl J Med* 302:938–942, 1980.
8. Kessel N: Patients who take overdoses, *BMJ* 290: 1297–1298, 1985.
9. Weissman MM: The epidemiology of suicide attempts, 1960 to 1971, *Arch Gen Psychiatry* 30:737–746, 1974.
10. Andrus JK, Fleming DW, Heumann MA, et al: Surveillance of attempted suicide among adolescents in Oregon, 1988, *Am J Public Health* 81:1067–1069, 1991.
11. McIntosh JL: Suicide prevention in the elderly (age 65–99), *Suicide Life Threat Behav* 25:180–192, 1995.
12. Richardson R, Lowenstein S, Weissberg M: Coping with the suicidal elderly: a physician's guide, *Geriatrics* 44:43–51, 1989.
13. Berman AL, Jobes DA: Suicide prevention in adolescents (age 12–18), *Suicide Life Threat Behav* 25:143–154, 1995.
14. Moscicki EK: Gender differences in completed and attempted suicides, *Ann Epidemiol* 4:152–158, 1994.
15. Moscicki EK, O'Carroll P, Regier D, et al: Suicide attempts in the epidemiologic catchment area study, *Yale J Biol Med* 61:259–268, 1988.
16. Griffith EEH, Bell CC: Recent trends in suicide and homicide among blacks, *JAMA* 262:2265–2269, 1989.
17. Earls F, Escobar JI, Manson SM: *Suicide in minority groups: epidemiologic and cultural perspectives.* In Blumenthal SJ, Kupfer DJ, editors: *Suicide over the life cycle: risk factors, assessment, and treatment of suicidal patients*, Washington, DC, 1990, American Psychiatric Press.
18. Rich CL, Young D, Fowler RC: San Diego suicide study: young vs. old subjects, *Arch Gen Psychiatry* 43:577–582, 1986.
19. Brent DA: Correlates of medical lethality of suicide attempts in children and adolescents, *J Am Acad Child Adolesc Psychiatry* 26:87–89, 1987.
20. Runeson BS: Mental disorder in youth suicide: DSM III-R Axes I and II, *Acta Psychiatr Scand* 79:490–497, 1989.
21. Brent DA, Perper JA, Goldstein CE, et al: Risk factors for adolescent suicide, *Arch Gen Psychiatry* 45:581–588, 1988.
22. Andrews JA, Lewinsohn PM: Suicidal attempts among older adolescents: prevalence and co-occurrence with psychiatric disorders, *J Am Acad Child Adolesc Psychiatry* 31:655–662, 1992.
23. Mann JJ: A current perspective of suicide and attempted suicide, *Ann Intern Med* 136:302–311, 2002.
24. Isometsa E, Henriksson M, Marttunen M, et al: Mental disorders in young and middle aged men who commit suicide, *BMJ* 310:1366–1367, 1995.
25. Black DW, Winokur G: *Suicide and psychiatric diagnosis.* In Blumenthal SJ, Kupfer DJ, editors: *Suicide over the life cycle: risk factors, assessment, and treatment of suicidal patients*, Washington, DC, 1990, American Psychiatric Press.
26. Roy A: Suicide and psychiatric patients, *Psychiatr Clin North Am* 8:227–241, 1985.
27. Hawton K: Assessment of suicide risk, *Br J Psychiatry* 150:145–153, 1987.
28. Hirschfeld RMA: Algorithm for the evaluation and treatment of suicidal patients, *Primary Psychiatry* 3:26–29, 1996.

29. Black DW, Winokur G, Nasrallah A: Effect of psychosis on suicide risk in 1,593 patients with unipolar and bipolar affective disorders, *Am J Psychiatry* 145:849–852, 1988.

30. Fawcett J, Scheftner WA, Fogg L, et al: Time-related predictors of suicide in major affective disorder, *Am J Psychiatry* 147:1189–1194, 1990.

31. Miller NS, Giannini AJ, Gold MS: Suicide risk associated with drug and alcohol addiction, *Cleve Clin J Med* 59:535–538, 1992.

32. Fowler RC, Rich CL, Young D: San Diego suicide study: substance abuse in young cases, *Arch Gen Psychiatry* 43:962–965, 1986.

33. Appleby L: Suicide in psychiatric patients: risk and prevention, *Br J Psychiatry* 161:749–758, 1992.

34. Buzan RD, Weissberg MP: Suicide: risk factors and prevention in medical practice, *Ann Rev Med* 43:37–46, 1992.

35. Murphy GE, Armstrong JW, Hermele SL, et al: Suicide and alcoholism: interpersonal loss confirmed as a predictor, *Arch Gen Psychiatry* 36:65–69, 1979.

36. Buzan RD, Weissberg MP: Suicide: risk factors and therapeutic considerations in the emergency department, *J Emerg Med* 10:335–343, 1992.

37. Crumley FE: Substance abuse and adolescent suicidal behavior, *JAMA* 263:3051–3056, 1990.

38. Fawcett J, Clark DC, Busch KA: Assessing and treating the patient at risk for suicide, *Psychiatry Ann* 23:244–255, 1993.

39. Hofmann DP, Dubovsky SL: Depression and suicide assessment, *Emerg Med Clin North Am* 9:107–121, 1991.

40. Caldwell CB, Gottesman II: Schizophrenia-a high-risk factor for suicide: clues to risk reduction, *Suicide Life Threat Behav* 22:479–493, 1992.

41. Shuster JL, Lagomasino IT, Okereke OI, et al: *Suicide.* In Irwin RS, Rippe JM, editors: *Intensive care medicine,* ed 5, Philadelphia, 2003, Lippincott-Raven, pp 2162–2170.

42. Goldsmith SJ, Fyer M, Frances A: *Personality and suicide.* In Blumenthal SJ, Kupfer DJ, editors: *Suicide over the life cycle: risk factors, assessment, and treatment of suicidal patients,* Washington, DC, 1990, American Psychiatric Press.

43. McGlashan TH: Borderline personality disorder and unipolar affective disorder, *J Nerv Ment Dis* 175:467–473, 1987.

44. Noyes R: Suicide and panic disorder: a review, *J Affect Dis* 22:1–11, 1991.

45. Weissman MM, Klerman GL, Markowitz JS, et al: Suicidal ideation and suicide attempts in panic disorder and attacks, *N Engl J Med* 321:1209–1214, 1989.

46. Johnson J, Weissman MM, Klerman GL: Panic disorder, comorbidity and suicide attempts, *Arch Gen Psychiatry* 47:805–808, 1990.

47. Mans RW: Introduction, *Suicide Life Threat Behav* 21:1–17, 1991.

48. Conwell Y, Duberstein PR: Suicide among older people: a problem for primary care, *Primary Psychiatry* 3:41–44, 1996.

49. Marzuk PM, Tierney H, Tardiff K, et al: Increased risk of suicide in persons with AIDS, *JAMA* 259:1333–1337, 1988.

50. Plott RT, Benton SD, Winslade WJ: Suicide of AIDS patients in Texas: a preliminary report, *Tex Med* 85:40–43, 1989.

51. Perry S, Jacobsberg L, Fishman B: Suicidal ideation and HIV testing, *JAMA* 263:679–682, 1990.

52. Rich CL, Fowler RC, Young D, et al: San Diego suicide study: comparison of gay to straight males, *Suicide Life Threat Behav* 16:448–457, 1986.

53. Massie MJ, Gagnon P, Holland JC: Depression and suicide in patients with cancer, *J Pain Symptom Manage* 9:325–340, 1994.

54. Breithart W: Suicide in cancer patients, *Oncology* 1:49–53, 1987.

55. Breitbart W: *Suicide in cancer patients.* In Holland JC, Rowland JH, editors: *Handbook of psychooncology: psychological care of the patient with cancer,* New York, 1989, Oxford University Press.

56. Achte KA, Lonnquist J, Hillbom E: Suicides following war brain injuries, *Acta Psychiatr Scand Suppl* 225:3–94, 1971.

57. MacKenzie TB, Popkin MK: Suicide in the medical patient, *Int J Psychiatry Med* 17:3–22, 1987.

58. Stenager EN, Stenager E: Suicide and patients with neurologic diseases: methodologic problems, *Arch Neurol* 49:1296–1303, 1992.

59. White SL, McLean AEM, Howland C: Anticonvulsant drugs and cancer, *Lancet* 2:458–461, 1979.

60. Hawton K, Fagg J, Marsack P: Association between epilepsy and attempted suicide, *J Neurol Neurosurg Psychiatry* 43:168–170, 1980.

61. Barraclough BM: The suicide rate of epilepsy, *Acta Psychiatr Scand* 76:339–345, 1987.

62. Mendez MF, Lanska DJ, Manon-Espaillat R, et al: Causative factors for suicide attempts by overdose in epileptics, *Arch Neurol* 46:1065–1068, 1989.

63. Stenager EN, Stenager E, Koch-Henriksen N: Multiple sclerosis and suicide: an epidemiological investigation, *J Neurol Neurosurg Psychiatry* 55:542–545, 1992.

64. Kessler S: Psychiatric implications of presymptomatic testing for Huntington's disease, *Am J Orthopsychiatry* 57:212–219, 1987.

65. Ducharme SH, Freed MM: The role of self-destruction in spinal cord injury mortality, *Sci Dig* Winter:29–38, 1980.

66. Geisler WO, Jousse AT, Wynne-Jones M, et al: Survival in traumatic spinal cord injury, *Paraplegia* 21:364–373, 1983.

67. Ko DT, Hebert PR, Coffey CS, et al: Beta-blocker therapy and symptoms of depression, fatigue, and sexual dysfunction. *JAMA* 288:351–357, 2002.

68. Abram HS, Moore GL, Westervelt FB: Suicidal behavior in chronic renal patients, *Am J Psychiatry* 127:1199–1204, 1971.

69. Yehuda R, Southwick SM, Ostroff RB, et al: Neuroendocrine aspects of suicidal behavior, *Neurol Clin* 6:83–102, 1988.

70. Roy A: *Suicide*. In Kaplan HI, Sadock BJ, editors: *Comprehensive textbook of psychiatry*, ed 6, Baltimore, 1995, Williams & Wilkins.

71. Smith JC, Mercy JA, Conn JM: Marital status and the risk of suicide, *Am J Public Health* 78:78–80, 1988.

72. Buda M, Tsuang MT: *The epidemiology of suicide: implications for clinical practice.* In Blumenthal SJ, Kupfer DJ, editors: *Suicide over the life cycle: risk factors, assessment, and treatment of suicidal patients*, Washington, DC, 1990, American Psychiatric Press.

73. Brent DA, Perper JA, Allman CJ, et al: The presence and accessibility of firearms in the homes of adolescent suicides: a case-control study, *JAMA* 266:2989–2995, 1991.

74. Heikkinen M, Aro H, Lonnqvist J: Recent life events, social support and suicide, *Acta Psychiatr Scand* 377(suppl):65–72, 1994.

75. Kellermann AL, Rivara FP, Somes G, et al: Suicide in the home in relation to gun ownership, *N Engl J Med* 327:467–472, 1992.

76. Miller M, Azrael D, Hemenway D: Firearm availability and unintentional firearm deaths, suicide, and homicide among 5–14 year olds. *J Trauma* 52:267–274, 2002.

77. Adam KS: Attempted suicide, *Psychiatr Clin North Am* 8:183–201, 1985.

78. Roy A, Segal NL, Centerwall BS, et al: Suicide in twins, *Arch Gen Psychiatry* 48:29–32, 1991.

79. Phillips DP, Cartensen LL: Clustering of teenage suicides after television news stories about suicide, *N Engl J Med* 315:685–689, 1986.

80. Shaffer D, Garland A, Gould M, et al: Preventing teenage suicide: a critical review, *J Am Acad Child Adolesc Psychiatry* 27:675–687, 1988.

81. Roy A: Risk factors for suicide in psychiatric patients, *Arch Gen Psychiatry* 39:1089–1095, 1982.

82. Stern TA, Mulley AG, Thibault GE: Life-threatening drug overdose: precipitants and prognosis, *JAMA* 251:1983–1985, 1984.

83. Beck AT, Beck R, Kovacs M: Classification of suicidal behaviors: quantifying intent and medical lethality, *Am J Psychiatry* 132:285–287, 1975.

84. Robins E, Gassner S, Kayes J, et al: The communication of suicidal intent: a study of 134 consecutive cases of successful (completed) suicide, *Am J Psychiatry* 115:724–733, 1959.

85. Isometsa ET, Heikkinen ME, Marttunen MJ, et al: The last appointment before suicide: is suicide intent communicated? *Am J Psychiatry* 152:919–922, 1995.

86. Isometsa ET, Aro HM, Henriksson MM, et al: Suicide in major depression in different treatment settings, *J Clin Psychiatry* 55:523–527, 1994.

87. Beck AT, Kovacs M, Weissman A: Hopelessness and suicidal behavior: an overview, *JAMA* 234:1146–1149, 1975.

88. Beck AT, Steer RA, Kovacs M, et al: Hopelessness and eventual suicide: a 10-year prospective study of patients hospitalized with suicidal ideation, *Am J Psychiatry* 142:559–563, 1985.

89. Barraclough BM, Bunch J, Nelson B, et al: A hundred cases of suicide: clinical aspects, *Br J Psychiatry* 125:355–373, 1974.

90. Valente SM: Evaluating suicide risk in the medically ill patient, *Nurse Pract* 18:41–50, 1993.

91. Lin EH, Von Korff M, Wagner EH: Identifying suicide potential in primary care, *J Gen Int Med* 4:1–6, 1989.

92. Reich P, Kelly MJ: Suicide attempts by hospitalized medical and surgical patients, *N Engl J Med* 294:298–301, 1976.

93. Goldstein RB, Black DW, Nasrallah A, et al: The predication of suicide: sensitivity, specificity, and predictive value of a multivariate model applied to suicide among 1906 patients with affective disorders, *Arch Gen Psychiatry* 48:418–422, 1991.

94. Blumenthal SJ: Suicide: a guide to risk factors, assessment, and treatment of suicidal patients, *Med Clin North Am* 72:937–971, 1988.

95. Weisman AD, Worden JW: Risk-rescue rating in suicide assessment, *Arch Gen Psychiatry* 26:553–560, 1972.

96. Hyman SE, Tesar GE: *The emergency psychiatric evaluation, including the mental status examination.* In Hyman SE, Tesar GE, editors: *Manual of psychiatric emergencies*, ed 3, Boston, 1994, Little, Brown.

97. Amchin J, Wettstein RM, Roth RH: *Suicide, ethics, and the law.* In Blumenthal SJ, Kupfer DJ, editors: *Suicide over the life cycle: risk factors, assessment, and treatment of suicidal patients*, Washington, DC, 1990, American Psychiatric Press.

98. American Psychiatric Association Task Force: *The practice of electroconvulsive therapy: recommendations for treatment, training, and privileging*, ed 2, Washington DC, 2001, American Psychiatric Association.

99. Tondo L, Hennen J, Baldessarini RJ: Lower suicide risk with long-term lithium treatment in major affective illness: a meta-analysis. *Acta Psychiatr* 104:163–172, 2001.

100. Meltzer HY, Alphs L, Green AI, et al: Clozapine treatment for suicidality in schizophrenia: International Suicide Prevention Trial (InterSePT). *Arch Gen Psychiatry* 60:82–91, 2003.

101. Stern TA, Prager LM, Cremens MC: Autognosis rounds for medical housestaff, *Psychosomatics* 34:1–7, 1993.

Chapter 10

Electroconvulsive Therapy in the General Hospital

Charles A. Welch, M.D.

Electroconvulsive therapy (ECT) remains an indispensable treatment in the general hospital because of the large number of depressed patients who are unresponsive to drugs or intolerant to their side effects. Improvement in drug response rates have resulted from the monitoring of blood levels and the introduction of newer agents, but for 15% to 20% of depressed patients, effective drug treatment is still unattainable. Sustained depression carries a grim prognosis, with a 36% mortality rate at 31 months[1] and an even higher mortality rate in the depressed elderly. Consequently, in the past decade, the use of ECT has increased,[2] and the technique has been refined.[3]

Indications

The symptoms that predict a good response to ECT are those of major depression: anorexia, weight loss, early morning awakening, impaired concentration, pessimistic mood, motor restlessness, increased speech latency, constipation, and somatic or self-deprecatory delusions.[4] The cardinal symptom is the acute loss of interest in activities that formerly gave pleasure. These are exactly the same symptoms that constitute the indication for antidepressant drugs. At the present time, there is no way to predict which patients will ultimately be unresponsive to drugs. The definition of drug failure varies with the individual patient; young, healthy, nonsuicidal patients can safely receive

four or more different drug regimens before moving to ECT, whereas older depressed patients may be unable to tolerate more than one drug trial without developing serious morbidity.

Psychotic illness is the second indication for ECT. The improvement of chronic schizophrenia with ECT is usually incomplete and transient,[5] but case reports suggest that ECT, in combination with a neuroleptic, may result in sustained improvement in up to 80% of drug-resistant chronic schizophrenics.[6–9] A subgroup of young psychotics conforming to the schizophreniform profile (acute onset, affective intactness, and family history of affective disorder) appear to be more responsive to ECT than are chronic schizophrenics and often have a full and enduring remission of their illness with treatment.[10,11]

Mania is also known to respond well to ECT,[5,12] but drug treatment remains the first line of therapy. Nevertheless, in controlled trials, ECT is as effective as lithium or more so,[13] and in drug-refractory mania, more than 50% of cases have remitted with ECT.[14] Preliminary evidence also shows that ECT stabilizes refractory bipolar disorder in adolescents.[15]

Although most patients initially receive a trial of medication regardless of their diagnosis, the following groups are appropriate for ECT as a primary treatment:

1. Patients who are severely malnourished, dehydrated, and exhausted are candidates. Such patients with protracted depressive illness are

medically at risk and should be treated promptly after careful rehydration.

2. Patients with complicating medical illness (e.g., cardiac arrhythmia or coronary artery disease) are candidates. Such patients are often more safely treated with ECT than with antidepressants.

3. Patients with delusional depression are candidates. Most delusionally depressed patients do not improve on an antidepressant alone,[16] but the reported response rate with ECT in delusional depression is 80% to 90%.[17,18] The combination of a tricyclic and an antipsychotic may be effective in some patients,[19] but many patients cannot safely tolerate the side effects of this regimen.

4. Patients who have been unresponsive to medications during previous episodes are candidates.

5. Patients with catatonia are candidates (see Chapter 30). The majority of catatonic patients respond promptly to ECT.[20–22]

Although the catatonic syndrome is most often associated with affective disorder, catatonia may also be a manifestation of schizophrenia, metabolic disorders, structural brain lesions, or systemic lupus erythematosus (SLE). Prompt treatment is essential because the mortality in untreated catatonia is as high as 50%, and even its nonfatal complications (including pneumonia, venous embolism, limb contracture, and decubitus ulcer) are serious. ECT is effective in up to 75% of catatonics, regardless of the underlying cause, and it is the treatment of choice for most catatonic patients.[23] Lorazepam has also been effective for short-term treatment of catatonia,[24] but its long-term efficacy has not been confirmed. Neuroleptic malignant syndrome (NMS) may be clinically indistinguishable from catatonia,[25] although high fever, opisthotonos, and rigidity are more common in the former. ECT has been reported effective in more than 40 cases of NMS,[26] but intensive supportive medical treatment, discontinuation of neuroleptic therapy, use of dantrolene, and use of bromocriptine are still the essential steps of management.

Risk Factors

As the technical conduct of ECT has improved, factors that were formerly considered contraindications have become relative risk factors. The patient is best served by weighing intelligently the risk of treatment against the morbidity or lethality of remaining depressed. The prevailing view is that there are no absolute contraindications to ECT, but the following conditions warrant careful work-up and management.

The heart is physiologically stressed during ECT.[27] Cardiac work increases abruptly at the onset of the seizure initially because of sympathetic outflow from the diencephalon, through the spinal sympathetic tract, to the heart. This outflow persists for the duration of the seizure and is augmented by a rise in circulating catecholamine levels that peak about 3 minutes after the onset of seizure activity.[28,29] After the seizure ends, parasympathetic tone remains strong, often causing transient bradycardia and hypotension, with a return to baseline function in 5 to 10 minutes.

The most common cardiac conditions that may worsen under this autonomic stimulus are ischemic heart disease, hypertension, congestive heart failure (CHF), and cardiac arrhythmia. These conditions, if properly managed, have proved to be surprisingly tolerant to ECT. The idea that general anesthesia is contraindicated within 6 months of a myocardial infarction has acquired a certain sanctity, which is surprising considering the ambiguity of the original data.[30] A more rational approach involves careful assessment of the cardiac reserve, a reserve that is needed as cardiac work increases during ECT.[31] Vascular aneurysms should be repaired before ECT if possible; in practice, they have proved surprisingly durable during treatment.[32,33] Critical aortic stenosis should be surgically corrected before ECT to avoid ventricular overload during the seizure. Patients with cardiac pacemakers are known to tolerate ECT uneventfully, although proper pacer function should be ascertained before treatment.[31,34] Patients with compensated CHF generally tolerate ECT well, although a transient decompensation into pulmonary edema for 5 to 10 minutes may occur in patients with a baseline ejection fraction below 20%. It is unclear whether the underlying cause is a neurogenic stimulus to the lung parenchyma or a reduction in cardiac output because of increased heart rate and blood pressure.

The brain is also physiologically stressed during ECT. Cerebral oxygen consumption approximately doubles, and cerebral blood flow increases several-fold. Increases in intracranial pressure and the permeability of the blood-brain barrier also develop. These acute changes may increase the risk of ECT in patients with a variety of neurologic conditions.[35]

Space-occupying brain lesions were previously considered an absolute contraindication to ECT, and earlier case reports described clinical deterioration when ECT was given to patients with brain tumors.[36] Reports indicate, however, that with careful management patients with meningioma or chronic subdural hematoma may be safely treated.[37–40] Recent cerebral infarction probably represents the most common intracranial risk factor. Approximately 50 case reports of ECT after recent cerebral infarction indicate that in properly performed treatment the complication rate is low.[35] Consequently, ECT is often the treatment of choice for poststroke depression.[41] The interval between infarction and time of ECT should be determined by the urgency of treatment for depression.

ECT has been safe and efficacious in patients with hydrocephalus, arteriovenous malformation, cerebral hemorrhage, multiple sclerosis, SLE, Huntington's disease, and mental retardation. Patients with depression and Parkinson's disease experience improvement of both disorders with ECT, and Parkinson's disease alone may constitute an indication for ECT.[42] Depressed patients with preexisting dementia are likely to develop especially severe cognitive deficits secondary to ECT; fortunately most return to their baseline level after treatment, and many actually improve.[43,44]

The pregnant mother who is severely depressed may require ECT to prevent malnutrition or suicide. Although reports of ECT during pregnancy are reassuring,[45] fetal monitoring is recommended during treatment. The fetus may be protected from the physiologic stress of ECT by nature of its lack of direct neuronal connection to the maternal diencephalon, which spares it the intense autonomic stimulus experienced by maternal end organs during ictus.

Technique

The routine pre-ECT work-up usually includes a thorough medical history and physical examination, with a chest film, electrocardiogram (ECG), urinalysis, complete blood cell count, and determination of blood glucose, blood urea nitrogen, and electrolyte levels. Additional studies may be necessary, at the clinician's discretion. In patients with cognitive deficits, it is sometimes difficult to decide whether a central nervous system work-up is indicated because depression itself is usually the cause of this deficit. A metabolic screen, computed tomography scan, and magnetic resonance imaging are often useful to rule out non–depression-related causes of impaired cognition. Whenever a question of primary dementia arises, neurologic consultation should be requested. Neuropsychological testing is not diagnostically helpful in making the distinction between primary dementia and depressive pseudomentia.[43]

It is essential that the patient's medical condition be optimized before starting treatment. Elderly patients often arrive at the hospital severely malnourished and dehydrated, and ECT should be delayed until they have had several days of rehydration, with alimentation via feeding tube if necessary. Serum levels of digitalis should be in the (middle to low) therapeutic range. Antihypertensive regimens should be optimized before treatment to reduce the chance of a severe hypertensive reaction during treatment. Most diabetic patients are more stable if the morning dose of insulin is held until after their treatment. The insulin requirement usually decreases as a diabetic patient recovers from depression, and blood glucose levels must be monitored frequently during the course of ECT.

Most psychotropic drugs should be discontinued in preparation for ECT. Lithium may cause delirium when used concurrently with ECT, and it should be withheld.[46] Benzodiazepines are antagonistic to the ictal process and should also be discontinued.[47] Even short-acting benzodiazepines may have a long half-life in a sick, elderly person and make effective treatment impossible. For sedation, patients receiving ECT usually do well with a sedating phenothiazine, such as perphenazine (Trilafon), 4 to 8 mg every 6 hours, or a nonbenzodiazepine hypnotic, such as hydroxyzine (Vistaril), 50 to 100 mg, or diphenhydramine (Benadryl), 25 to 50 mg twice daily. Tricyclics make cardiovascular management more difficult and should be discontinued. Monoamine oxidase inhibitors (MAOIs) are typically withheld, although a 10-day washout period before ECT is unnecessary.[48]

In the patient with a preexisting seizure disorder, anticonvulsant treatment should be maintained for patient safety and the elevated seizure threshold overridden with a higher-intensity stimulus.

Because of the profound physiologic disturbances unique to this treatment, ECT should not be performed in conjunction with an anesthesiologist unfamiliar with it. Although ECT was formerly thought to be a trivial exercise in anesthetic management, quite the contrary is true; a careful reading of the pertinent literature is essential for the anesthesiologist.[31,49] All six major complications associated with ECT at Massachusetts General Hospital (MGH) in the past 10 years have occurred in the absence of the regular anesthesiologist.

The use of cardiac monitoring and pulse oximetry on all patients undergoing general anesthesia has been endorsed by the American Society of Anesthesiologists. Existing ECT machines record the ECG only during the treatment itself, but recording of baseline and postictal rhythms is essential, and a separate operating room monitor with paper recording capability is therefore necessary to monitor the ECG adequately.

General anesthesia is induced with methohexital and succinylcholine, each at doses of 0.5 to 1.0 mg/kg. Atropine or glycopyrrolate are not routinely administered because they increase cardiac work during treatment and do not decrease oral secretions.[50] Their use is therefore reserved for patients who are prone to bradycardia.

For patients with coronary artery disease or hypertension, short-acting intravenous (IV) β-blockers effectively reduce stress on the heart. These agents attenuate hypertension, tachycardia, ectopy, and cardiac ischemia, and with proper use they rarely result in hypotension or bradycardia. Esmolol (100 to 200 mg) or labetalol (10 to 20 mg given intravenously) immediately before the anesthetic induction is usually sufficient.[51] Although theoretically these drugs may result in decompensation of CHF, this has not been reported in practice. A second method of reducing cardiac work involves administration of nifedipine (10 mg sublingually 15 minutes before treatment).[52] Nitroglycerine (infused at 0.5 to 3.0 mg/kg/minute) may be used to blunt the hypertensive response of patients who are already receiving β-blockers or calcium channel blockers and who require additional antihypertensives. One must observe for hypotension; if an infusion is used, at least the first treatment should be done with intraarterial blood pressure monitoring.

Treating hypertension adequately before a course of ECT usually reduces the hypertensive response during the treatment itself. Maintenance β-blockers, such as atenolol (25–50 mg orally every day) may render the use of a short-acting antihypertensive during treatment unnecessary.

Conduction system abnormalities during treatment have been reported in 20% to 80% of ECT patients,[53] but they are usually transient. Persistent or severe arrhythmias occasionally require treatment; the approach depends on the type of arrhythmia. Supraventricular tachycardias generally are best treated with calcium channel blockers, whereas ventricular ectopy is most rapidly stabilized with IV lidocaine. Many arrhythmias can be prevented by pretreatment with a short-acting IV β-blocker before subsequent treatments.

Decompensation of CHF is usually treatable with oxygen and elevation of the head. Occasionally, IV furosemide (Lasix) and morphine become necessary, but this is extremely rare. Most patients recompensate within 10 to 15 minutes of the treatment without aggressive intervention.

Cardiac arrest is a rare complication of ECT. Some patients have a period of asystole after the ECT stimulus that may last up to 8 seconds, and this may be mistaken for a true arrest.[27] Patients who receive nonconvulsive stimuli may be especially at risk. Because the intense parasympathetic outflow caused by the stimulus is not counteracted by the sympathetic outflow of the seizure itself, severe bradycardia or arrest may ensue.

The relative efficacy of unilateral and bilateral electrode placement remains unclear, but for most patients, a unilateral stimulus, when performed under optimal conditions, is as effective as a bilateral stimulus.[54,55] Ineffective unilateral ECT is associated with use of threshold stimulus intensity[56] and a short distance between electrodes.[57] Consequently a unilateral stimulus should be at least 50% over threshold with the electrodes placed in the d'Elia position.[56] There is ongoing controversy as to whether unilateral ECT is as effective as bilateral ECT in depressed patients.[58] Nevertheless, at MGH, unilateral nondominant ECT is used in all patients initially, with the exception of patients with treatment-resistant mania. Approximately 5% of depressed patients at this hospital prove refractory to 6 to 12 unilateral treatments and are then switched to bilateral electrode placement.

Brief-pulse waveforms have become the standard of practice in the United States. Although sine wave stimuli were common in the past, the brief-pulse waveform more efficiently induces seizure activity and is associated with less posttreatment confusion and amnesia.[59]

Generalization of the seizure to the entire brain is essential for efficacy.[60] The simplest way to monitor seizure generalization is to inflate a blood pressure cuff on the arm or ankle above systolic pressure, just before injection of succinylcholine. The convulsion can then be observed in the unparalyzed extremity. In unilateral ECT, the cuff is placed on the limb ipsilateral to the stimulus. Most ECT instruments have a built-in, single-channel electroencephalographic monitor, but this is not a reliable indicator of full seizure generalization because partial seizures may also generate a classic seizure tracing.

Following ECT, patients should not be left in the supine position but should be turned on their side to allow better drainage of secretions. They should be monitored carefully by a recovery nurse; vital signs should be taken regularly and pulse oximetry employed. About 1 in 20 patients, typically young, healthy individuals, develop an agitated delirium with vacant stare, disorientation, and automatisms immediately following treatment. This clinical picture is usually due to tardive seizures; it clears promptly with midazolam 2 to 5 mg intravenously, or diazepam 5 to 10 mg intravenously. Posttreatment nausea may be effectively treated with droperidol 1.25 to 2.5 mg intravenously.

The average number of ECT procedures necessary to treat major depression is consistently reported to be between 6 and 12 treatments, but occasional patients may require up to 30. The customary timing is three sessions per week with one full seizure per session. The use of more than one seizure per session (multiple monitored ECT) has no proven advantages. The most objective comparison of single and multiple ECT was performed by Fink,[61] who concluded, "Multiple ECT carried more risks and fewer benefits than conventional ECT for our patients."

Adverse Effects

The most recent data indicate a mortality rate of 0.03% in patients who undergo ECT.[62] Although there is no evidence for structural brain damage as a result of ECT,[63] there are important effects on cognition.[64] Posttreatment confusion varies greatly and is associated with bilateral electrode placement, high stimulus intensity, inadequate oxygenation, and prolonged seizure activity. Difficulty recalling new information (anterograde amnesia) is usually experienced during the ECT series, but it normally resolves within a month after the last treatment. Difficulty remembering events before ECT (retrograde amnesia) is more severe for events closer to the time of treatment.[65] Significant amounts of old information may be irretrievably lost, however, particularly with bilateral ECT. Bilateral ECT causes more memory disturbance than does unilateral ECT, and this is true for both retrograde and anterograde memory function and for both verbal and nonverbal recall.[66] The least memory deficit is seen with a unilateral brief-pulse stimulus.[67]

Severe organic brain syndrome associated with ECT may require discontinuation of treatment. Usually, substantial improvement occurs within 48 hours after the last treatment. If symptoms become more severe with time after cessation of treatment, a full neurologic work-up is indicated to assess whether there is an underlying cause other than ECT.

Maintenance Treatment

Following successful treatment, the risk of relapse is greater than 50% at 12 months without maintenance medication.[68] The only controlled trial of maintenance medication indicates a disappointing efficacy with tricyclics.[69] Patients are probably more likely to remain in remission when taking MAOIs, lithium, bupropion, or fluoxetine, although none of these has been evaluated in a well-controlled trial. Maintenance ECT at one treatment per month, more or less, is widely practiced. Treatment-resistant patients have lower rates of relapse and rehospitalization with maintenance ECT than with maintenance pharmacotherapy.[70–72]

Summary

In recent years, the technique of ECT has become more sophisticated,[73] and this has made the treatment safer in the general hospital setting, where growing numbers of high-risk patients are seen. Increasingly the practice of ECT is regarded as a distinct subspecialty requiring specific training and privileges.[74] In view of its efficacy in patients unresponsive to medication, it is likely that ECT will be an essential part of psychiatry in the general hospital for the foreseeable future.

References

1. Huston PE, Locher LM: Involutional psychosis: course when untreated and when treated with EST, *Arch Neurol Psychiatry* 59:385–394, 1948.
2. Olfson M, Marcus S, Sackheim HA, et al: Use of ECT for the inpatient treatment of recurrent major depression, *Am J Psychiatry* 155:22–29, 1998.
3. American Psychiatric Association: *The practice of electroconvulsive therapy: recommendations for treatment, training, and privileging. A task force report of the American Psychiatric Association*, ed 2, Washington, DC, 2001, American Psychiatric Association.
4. Carney MWP, Roth M, Garside RF: The diagnosis of depressive syndromes and the prediction of ECT response, *Br J Psychiatry* 3:659–674, 1965.
5. Small JG: Efficacy of electroconvulsive therapy in schizophrenia, mania, and other disorders: I. schizophrenia; II. mania and other disorders, *Convuls Ther* 1:263–270, 271–276, 1985.
6. Small JG, Milstein V, Klapper MH, et al: ECT combined with neuroleptics in the treatment of schizophrenia, *Psychopharmacol Bull* 18:34–35, 1982.
7. Gujavarty K, Greenberg LB, Fink M: Electroconvulsive therapy and neuroleptic medication in therapy-resistant positive-symptom psychosis, *Convuls Ther* 3:111–120, 1987.
8. Chanpattana W, Chakrabhand S, Kongsakon R, et al: Short-term effect of combined ECT and neuroleptic therapy in treatment-resistant schizophrenia, *J ECT* 15:129–139, 1999.
9. Tang WK, Ungvari GS: Efficacy of electroconvulsive therapy combined with antipsychotic medication in treatment-resistant schizophrenia: a prospective, open trial, *J ECT* 18:90–94, 2002.
10. Ries RK, Wilson L, Bokan JA, et al: ECT in medication resistant schizoaffective disorder, *Compr Psychiatry* 22:167–173, 1981.
11. Black DW, Winokur G, Nasrallah A: Treatment and outcome in secondary depression: a naturalistic study of 1,087 patients, *J Clin Psychiatry* 48:438–441, 1987.
12. Mukherjee S, Sackheim HA, Schnur DB: Electroconvulsive therapy of acute manic episodes: a review of 50 years' experience, *Am J Psychiatry* 151:169–76, 1994.
13. Mukherjee S, Sackeim HA, Lee C: Unilateral ECT in the treatment of manic episodes, *Convuls Ther* 4:74–80, 1988.
14. Kutcher S, Robertson HA: Electroconvulsive therapy in treatment-resistant bipolar youth, *J Child Adolesc Psychopharmacol* 5:167–175, 1995.
15. Rey JM, Walter G: Half a century of ECT use in young people, *Am J Psychiatry* 154:595–602, 1997.
16. Wheeler Vega JA, Mortimer AM, et al: Somatic treatment of psychotic depression: review and recommendations for practice, *J Clin Psychopharmacol* 20: 504–519, 2000.
17. Kroessler D: Relative efficacy rates for therapies of delusional depression, *Convuls Ther* 1:173–182, 1985.
18. Janicak PG, Easton M, Comaty JE, et al: Efficacy of ECT in psychotic and nonpsychotic depression, *Convuls Ther* 5:314–320, 1989.
19. Petrides G, Fink M, Husain MM, et al: ECT remission rates in psychotic versus nonpsychotic depressed patients: a report from CORE, *J ECT* 17:244–253, 2000.
20. Mann SC, Caroff SN, Bleier HR, et al: Lethal catatonia, *Am J Psychiatry*, 143:1374–1381, 1986.
21. Mann SC, Caroff SN, Bleier HR, et al: Electroconvulsive therapy of the lethal catatonia syndrome, *Convuls Ther* 6:239–247, 1990.
22. Rohland BM, Carroll BT, Jacoby RG: ECT in the treatment of the catatonic syndrome, *J Affect Disord* 29:255–261, 1993.
23. Fink M: Is catatonia a primary indication for ECT? *Convuls Ther* 6:1–4, 1990.
24. Rosebush PI, Hildebrand AM, Furlong BG, et al: Catatonic syndrome in a general psychiatric inpatient population: frequency, clinical presentation, and response to lorazepam, *J Clin Psychiatry* 51:357–362, 1990.
25. Fink M: Neuroleptic malignant syndrome and catatonia: one entity or two? *Biol Psychiatry* 39:1–4, 1996.
26. Davis JM, Janicak PG, Sakkas P, et al: Electroconvulsive therapy in the treatment of the neuroleptic malignant syndrome, *Convuls Ther* 7:111–120, 1991.
27. Welch CA, Drop LJ: Cardiovascular effects of ECT, *Convuls Ther* 5:35–43, 1989.
28. Khan A, Nies A, Johnson G, et al: Plasma catecholamines and ECT, *Biol Psychiatry* 20:799–804, 1985.
29. Liston EH, Salk JD: Hemodynamic responses to ECT after bilateral adrenalectomy, *Convuls Ther* 6:160–164, 1990.
30. Goldman L: Multifactorial index of cardiac risk of noncardiac surgical procedures, *N Engl J Med* 297:845–850, 1977.
31. Drop JD, Welch CA: Anesthesia for electroconvulsive therapy in patients with major cardiovascular risk factors, *Convuls Ther* 5:88–101, 1989.

32. Drop LJ, Bouckoms AJ, Welch CA: Arterial hypertension and multiple cerebral aneurysms in a patient treated with electroconvulsive therapy, *J Clin Psychiatry* 49:280–282, 1988.
33. Viguera A, Rordorf G, Schouten R, et al: Intracranial haemodynamics during attenuated responses to electroconvulsive therapy in the presence of an intracerebral aneurysm, *J Neurol Neurosurg Psychiatry* 64:802–805, 1998.
34. Alexopoulos GS, Frances RJ: ECT and cardiac patients with pacemakers, *Am J Psychiatry* 137:1111–1112, 1980.
35. Hsiao JK, Messenheimer JA, Evans DL: ECT and neurological disorders, *Convuls Ther* 3:121–136, 1987.
36. Maltbie AA, Wingfield MS, Volow MR, et al: Electroconvulsive therapy in the presence of brain tumor: case reports and an evaluation of risk, *J Nerv Ment Dis* 168:400–405, 1980.
37. Fried D, Mann JJ: Electroconvulsive treatment of a patient with known intracranial tumor, *Biol Psychiatry* 23:176–180, 1988.
38. Greenberg LB, Mofson R, Fink M: Prospective electroconvulsive therapy in a delusional depressed patient with a frontal meningioma: a case report, *Br J Psychiatry* 153:105–107, 1988.
39. Malek-Ahmadi P, Beceiro JR, McNeil BW, et al: Electroconvulsive therapy and chronic subdural hematoma, *Convuls Ther* 6:38–41, 1990.
40. Zwil AS, Bowring MA, Price TRP, et al: Prospective electroconvulsive therapy in the presence of intracranial tumor, *Convuls Ther* 6:299–307, 1990.
41. Currier MB, Murray GB, Welch CA: Electroconvulsive therapy for post-stroke depressed geriatric patients, *J Neuropsychiatry Clin Neurosci* 4:140–144, 1992.
42. Fink M: ECT for Parkinson's disease? *Convuls Ther* 4:189–191, 1988.
43. Steif BL, Sackeim HA, Portnoy S, et al: Effects of depression and ECT on anterograde memory, *Biol Psychiatry* 21:921–930, 1986.
44. Nelson JP, Rosenberg DR: ECT treatment of demented elderly patients with major depression: a retrospective study of efficacy and safety, *Convuls Ther* 7:157–165, 1991.
45. Ferrill MJ, Kehoe WA, Jacisin JJ: ECT during pregnancy: physiologic and pharmacologic considerations, *Convuls Ther* 8:186–200, 1992.
46. Mukherjee S: Combined ECT and lithium therapy, *Convuls Ther* 9:274–284, 1993.
47. Greenberg RM, Pettinati HM: Benzodiazepines and electroconvulsive therapy, *Convuls Ther* 9:262–273, 1993.
48. Remick RA, Jewesson P, Ford RWJ: Monoamine oxidase inhibitors in general anesthesia: a reevaluation, *Convuls Ther* 3:196–203, 1987.
49. Folk JW, Kellner CH, Beale MD, et al: Anesthesia for electroconvulsive therapy: a review, *J ECT* 16:157–170, 2000.
50. Bouckoms AJ, Welch CA, Drop LJ, et al: Atropine in electroconvulsive therapy, *Convuls Ther* 5:48–55, 1989.
51. Castelli I, Steiner A, Kaufmann MA, et al: Comparative effects of esmolol and labetalol to attenuate hyperdynamic states after electroconvulsive therapy, *Anesth Analg* 80:557–561, 1995.
52. Kalayam B, Alexopoulos GS: Nifedipine in the treatment of blood pressure rise after ECT, *Convuls Ther* 5:110–113, 1989.
53. Gerring JP, Shields HM: The identification and management of patients with a high risk for cardiac arrhythmias during modified ECT, *J Clin Psychiatry* 43:140–143, 1982.
54. Ottoson JO: Is unilateral nondominant ECT as efficient as bilateral ECT? A new look at the evidence, *Convuls Ther* 7:190–200, 1991.
55. Sackheim HA, Prudic J, Devanand DP, et al: Effects of stimulus intensity and electrode placement on the efficacy and cognitive effects of electroconvulsive therapy, *N Engl J Med* 328.839–846, 1993.
56. McCall WV, Dunn A, Rosenquist PB, et al: Markedly suprathreshold right unilateral ECT versus minimally suprathreshold bilateral ECT: antidepressant and memory effects, *J ECT* 18:126–129, 2002.
57. Pettinati HM, Mathisen KS, Rosenberg J, et al: Meta-analytical approach to reconciling discrepancies in efficacy between bilateral and unilateral electroconvulsive therapy, *Convuls Ther* 2:7–17, 1986.
58. Sackheim HA, Prudic J, Devanand DP, et al: A prospective, randomized, double-blind comparison of bilateral and right unilateral electroconvulsive therapy at different stimulus intensities, *Arch Gen Psychiatry* 57:425–434, 2000.
59. Squire LR, Zouzounis JA: ECT and memory: brief pulse versus sine wave, *Am J Psychiatry* 143:596, 1986.
60. Ottoson JO: Experimental studies on the mode of action of electroconvulsive therapy, *Acta Psychiatr Neural Scand* 35(suppl 145):1–141, 1960.
61. Fink M: *Convulsive therapy: theory and practice*, New York, 1979, Raven Press.
62. Asnis G, Fink M, Saferstein S: ECT in metropolitan New York hospitals: a survey of practice, 1975–1976, *Am J Psychiatry* 135:479–482, 1978.
63. Devanand DP, Dwork AJ, Hutchinson ER, et al: Does ECT alter brain structure? *Am J Psychiatry* 151:957–970, 1994.
64. Calev A, Pass HL, Shapira B, et al: *ECT and memory*. In Coffey CE, editor: *The clinical science of electroconvulsive therapy*, Washington, DC, 1993, American Psychiatric Press.
65. Daniel WF, Crovitz HP: Acute memory impairment following electroconvulsive therapy: I. effects of electrode placement, *Acta Psychiatr Scand* 67:57–68, 1983.
66. Price TRP: Short- and long-term cognitive effects of ECT: Part I: effects on memory, *Psychopharmacol Bull* 18:81–91, 1982.
67. Weiner RD, Rogers HJ, Davidson JRT, et al: Effects of stimulus parameters on cognitive side effects, *Ann NY Acad Sci* 462:315–325, 1986.

68. Sackhim HA, Haskett RF, Mulsant BH, et al: Continuation pharmacotherapy in the prevention of relapse following electroconvulsive therapy: a randomized controlled trial, *JAMA* 285:1299–1307, 2001.

69. Sackeim H, Prudic J, Devanand D, et al: The impact of medication resistance and continuation pharmacotherapy on relapse following response to electroconvulsive therapy in major depression, *J Clin Psychopharmacol* 10:96–104, 1990.

70. Petrides G, Dhossche D, Fink M, et al: Continuation ECT: relapse prevention in affective disorders, *Convuls Ther* 10:189–194, 1994.

71. Schwarz T, Loewenstein J, Isenberg K: Maintenance ECT: indications and outcome, *Convuls Ther* 11:14–23, 1995.

72. Chittaranjan A, Kurinji S: Continuation and maintenance ECT: a review of recent research, *J ECT* 18:149–158, 2002.

73. Welch CA: *ECT in medically ill patients*. In Coffey CE, editor: *The clinical science of electroconvulsive therapy*, Washington, DC, 1993, American Psychiatric Press.

74. Russell JC, Rasmussen KG, O'Connor K, et al: Long-term maintenance ECT: a retrospective review of efficacy and cognitive outcome, *J ECT* 19:4–9, 2003.

Chapter 11
Intensive Care Unit Patients

John Querques, M.D.
Theodore A. Stern, M.D.

Including a chapter on the psychiatric care of patients in an intensive care unit (ICU) runs the risk of proposing that the evaluation of patients is somehow different dependent on their location in the general hospital and that provision of their psychiatric care likewise differs because of that locale. Such a risk recalls the unfortunate appellation "ICU psychosis," with its false suggestion that a psychotic condition could be induced by a patient's mere residence in an ICU, and the absurd, but logical, conclusion that transfer out of that environment is curative. We maintain that patients and their needs transcend geography; however, we also recognize that the critical nature of illnesses treated in ICUs creates a unique environment for patients, staff, and consultation psychiatrists alike. In this chapter, the serial presentation of a typical ICU psychiatric consultation highlights the distinguishing characteristics of this distinctive setting, the common reasons for consultation requests in the ICU, and the clinical approach to consultative practice in the ICU.

The Intensive Care Unit Setting

The chief difference between the ICU and other hospital wards is the severity of the morbidity treated there. Patients are admitted to ICUs when they require life support for organ system failure, close monitoring or treatment for potentially life-threatening complications, or careful observation and treatment that cannot be safely provided elsewhere in the hospital.[1,2] Some of the conditions commonly treated in the ICU include: stroke, myocardial infarction (MI), arrhythmias, severe pneumonia, sepsis, multisystem organ failure, trauma, and burns.

Commensurate with this degree of morbidity, the intensity of the treatment arrayed against these life-imperiling conditions contributes significantly to the ICU ambiance. The numerous "lines"—wires, catheters, and tubes—wending their way to and from critically ill patients attest to the high-technology care rendered in the modern ICU. Patients routinely require mechanical ventilation, which entails endotracheal intubation and sedation and sometimes pharmacologic paralysis; use of vasopressors, cardiac monitors, pacemakers, parenteral nutrition, and several intravenous (IV) antibiotics is frequent. In more severe situations, renal replacement therapies, intraaortic balloon pumps, left ventricular assist devices, and heart-lung machines become necessary. In the center of, and almost eclipsed by, this mechanical mélange lies the patient, usually sedated and still, seemingly lifeless.

The flashing lights, sounding alarms, and constant whirrings of machines in action create an almost surreal, dehumanized atmosphere, difficult for patients, families, and staff to tolerate. It seems odd that human lives hang in the balance in such a mechanized setting, the nature and purpose of which has been indicted for engendering delirium, anxiety, and depression in patients; tension and stress that may progress to fatigue and burn-out in ICU staff; and feelings of hopelessness, helplessness, frustration, despair, and anger in family members, if not also patients and staff. The acuity of illness and potential for rapid changes in clinical status create a tremendous pressure for the staff to stay ahead of the curve and a powerful stimulus for families to remain on high alert. When a patient succumbs to an illness that ultimately proves a foe mightier than the awesome therapeutic forces amassed in the modern ICU, the staff confronts death and their own personal feelings of weakness, imperfection, insecurity, and impotence that may be stimulated by the loss of a patient. Amid their own struggles, they must somehow comfort bereaved family and friends.

The Psychiatrist in the Intensive Care Unit

The psychiatrist called to assess a patient in the ICU approaches the task with all of the preceding in mind. The consultant must brace him or herself for the experience of intense pressure that surrounds the care of critically ill patients, lest she or he be disarmed by it. The consultant is aware of the strain borne by the physicians and nurses who toil in this environment daily and respects that they might be preoccupied or busy with a clinical matter more pressing than the consultant's own. In dealing with families, the consultant is cognizant that their extreme apprehension might color their account of the patient's history and their appraisal of the current situation. Family members may be unimpressed by the need for a psychiatrist when their loved one is seen as barely clinging to life; they may think of such a consultation as superfluous and may even be insulted, annoyed, or angered by what feels like an intrusion. Even staff may not be immune to this reaction to the psychiatrist, feeling that the brain—let alone the psyche—is less important than the "real" problem.

The consulting psychiatrist anticipates the likely moribund state of acutely ill patients, their consequent inability to participate in the usual psychiatric examination, and the need to modify the examination accordingly. Even more than usual, the history from the patient may be vague and spotty, if not entirely nonexistent. The consult-

ant appreciates that the rapidity of clinical change in patients in the ICU necessitates frequent (probably daily, if not twice daily) visits; careful review of clinical developments as discussed with the team, culled from the chart, and gleaned from laboratory results; and a degree of accessibility greater than that required on general medical-surgical floors.

In the account of a psychiatric consultation in the ICU that follows, we highlight each of these characteristics of the ICU setting, and review three common reasons for psychiatric consultation requests in the ICU: depression, altered mental status, and decision-making capacity. The fictitious, but typical, case also demonstrates that the consultee's question often changes as the patient's clinical status changes and that a single consultation in the ICU often is actually several consultations in one. The case is presented in segments, much as a real case frequently unfolds.

Clinical Vignette

Mr. A, a 70-year-old man with diabetes mellitus (DM), hypertension, a prior stroke, and MI, was admitted to the ICU with severe pneumonia. He was febrile, tachypneic, and hypotensive, and the team was concerned about the possibility of sepsis. IV antibiotics were started, and, by the next morning, the chest film and Mr. A's clinical status had improved, although blood cultures were still pending and the possibility of sepsis still loomed. Because Mr. A looked depressed, a psychiatrist was called to evaluate depression. When the psychiatrist arrived at the bedside, Mr. A was diaphoretic and breathing at a rate of 20 respirations per minute. In place were two IV catheters, a cardiac monitor, and a Foley catheter. Because his breathing was so labored, Mr. A initiated no speech and he kept his answers short; they were almost inaudible. At times, he appeared to be drifting off even though he remained awake, and the psychiatrist had to regain Mr. A's attention periodically. Though he was not feeling particularly "joyous," as he said with as much of a laugh as his shallow breath allowed, he denied feeling depressed, sad, or "down in the dumps." Given Mr. A's discomfort, the psychiatrist terminated the interview early; his family was too overwhelmed to talk to the psychiatrist.

The psychiatrist's impression was of delirium, multifactorial in cause (infection and hypotension), perhaps superimposed on dementia, but he could not be sure given the paucity of historical information. In the face of Mr. A's denial of depressed mood; demonstrable, albeit small, affective display; and inattention, a diagnosis of major depression could not be made. Because the delirium was mild and was not associated with agitation, he recommended checking and monitoring "the usual suspects," but not a psychopharmacologic intervention.

Consultation requests to "rule-out depression" are common in the ICU. One reason for this is the notion held by some physicians and nurses that a patient in extreme clinical circumstances *must* be depressed. In this belief, such clinicians consider psychiatric diagnosis to be merely a matter of intuitive common sense, rather than of expert clinical judgment.[3] One expects a patient with a serious illness to have certain feelings about his or her plight (e.g., sadness, anxiety, or anger). However, intuition alone is insufficient to make a diagnosis; careful clinical assessment is required. In this case, the observation that Mr. A looked depressed tipped the scale and prompted the consultation request for a more comprehensive examination and an expert opinion.

Another reason consultations to assess depression are common in the ICU is mistaking *biography* for *history*,[3] as may have occurred if Mr. A had been asked if he was depressed and he answered affirmatively. The syndrome of depression is not just feeling depressed, sad, or "blue," however, but rather a constellation of specific affective, behavioral, and cognitive symptoms and signs. *It is only after a patient's current affective state is embedded in the context of an historical perspective that a diagnosis of major depression can be made.* Under extreme pressure of time and stress, ICU teams often defer to a psychiatrist to elicit the requisite history and to rule depression in or out.

Mr. A's clinical state precluded a thorough elicitation of historical evidence for depression; it highlighted the need for flexibility in modifying the usual clinical examination according to the patient's needs. Faced with a paucity of historical detail, the consultant placed a premium on the mental status examination; most importantly, he noted inattention, which a diagnosis of depression does not readily explain. Some may argue that the consultant should not have ruled out depression because he did not collect the data required by the *Diagnostic and Statistical Manual of Mental Disorders*, fourth edition,[4] and depression may underlie the delirium. Others, as do we, counter

that a diagnosis of depression in the face of delirium is difficult if not impossible to make and that, even if it were feasible, the presence of delirium trumps it. If depression is still suspected after the sensorium clears, the consultant can reinterview the patient and also elicit history from family and friends.

The consultant noted the possibility of dementia underlying the delirium. This suspicion was based on a knowledge of Mr. A's history of DM and hypertension (both of which can cause microvascular changes in the cerebral circulation), as well as prior stroke and MI (evidence of disease in two separate vascular territories) and knowledge that a "bad brain" or an "insulted brain" (a brain affected by age, trauma, structural lesions, extensive substance use, human immunodeficiency virus, or dementia) predisposes to delirium. Given the discomfort of Mr. A and the emotional state of the family at this point, the consultant did not yet have enough data to make this diagnosis definitively. It must await a change in the clinical circumstances.

A discussion of the "usual suspects" invoked by the consultant and the decision to forego pharmacologic treatment is beyond the scope of this chapter; the interested reader is referred to Chapter 13.

> When the consultant returned the following morning, he found that Mr. A had become agitated overnight and had removed both of his IV catheters, thus missing a scheduled dose of antibiotics. Whereas the day before, the consultant believed that Mr. A had a so-called quiet delirium, today he believed that the delirium was an agitated one. After ensuring that serum potassium, calcium, magnesium, and albumin levels as well as the QT interval corrected for heart rate were normal, he recommended haloperidol 1 mg orally twice daily.

This turn of events highlights the importance of frequent visits to the patient in the ICU. Given the interval development of agitation, the diagnosis shifted slightly from a quiet to an agitated delirium, which warranted a change in management (i.e., empiric treatment of the agitation with an antipsychotic). Moreover, the agitation in this case had already jeopardized Mr. A's treatment and would very likely continue to do so if not treated. While the team addressed the underlying causes of the delirium (infection and hypotension), empiric treatment with an antipsychotic was essential to quell the agitation.

Low serum levels of potassium, calcium, and magnesium, and the administration of certain medications (including haloperidol) can cause prolongation of the QT interval, which itself heightens the risk of torsades de pointes (TDP)—a potentially fatal, polymorphic, ventricular tachyarrhythmia. The QT interval varies with heart rate, age, gender, time of day, and a host of other factors. The proper measurement of the QT interval; the most accurate method for its correction for heart rate; and the relationship among QT prolongation, TDP, and antipsychotics are the subjects of considerable uncertainty and disagreement, even among experts. Several reviews of this complicated topic are available,[5–9] to which the interested reader is referred. In short, the administration of haloperidol (or another neuroleptic medication) to an agitated or delirious patient frequently allows necessary medical treatment to proceed uneventfully. This benefit generally outweighs the risk of a cardiac dysrhythmia.

> When the psychiatrist returned later that day, Mr. A's respiratory status had worsened and the team was concerned about needing to intubate him. They had solicited his informed consent, but he had refused to give it. Given his altered mental status, they asked the consultant if Mr. A was competent to refuse intubation and mechanical ventilation.

Again illustrated is the propensity for clinical change in ICU patients, the consequent importance of frequent visits, and the broadening of the consultation question. In this way, the psychiatrist often becomes an integral member of the extended team, much as an infectious-disease or endocrine consultant would in this case.

The team mistook *competency* for *capacity*, the former being a legal notion that can be determined only by a judge. *Capacity*, on the other hand, is a clinical term that refers to a patient's mental capability to understand his situation (the illness, the recommended treatment, alternative treatments, and the risks and benefits of those interventions), and to accept or to refuse a treatment recommendation consistent with his own personal ideals and values.[10] Any physician, regardless of training, is theoretically able to assess a patient's capacity; however, given their special training in examination of affect, behavior, and thinking, psychiatrists are frequently called on to render these opinions.

These consultations often arise only when a patient *refuses* a recommended course of therapy. Paternalistic physicians tend to think the patient's thinking process *must* be impaired if he or she disagrees with the treatment plan; if the patient accepts, his or her capacity is presumed intact. However, this common occurrence belies a fundamental misconception about decision-making capacity; that is, it hinges not on *what* the patient decides but on *how* the patient decides it. Whether the patient opts for the course of treatment recommended by the physician, or the therapy that the doctor would choose for him or herself if the doctor were in the patient's shoes, is irrelevant. Rather, the patient must make a stable choice based on a full understanding of the facts and an appreciation of those facts as they pertain to him or her specifically, and that is consistent with his own goals and values.[10]

A layman's understanding of the medical facts is sufficient. In this case, the consultant wants to assure himself that Mr. A knows and understands the following:

- He may stop breathing because of the pneumonia, an infection of the lungs.
- Should this happen, a machine can breathe for him by means of a tube inserted into his windpipe; without the tube and the machine, he will die.
- Generally, as pneumonia resolves, patients who require a breathing machine eventually resume breathing on their own.
- The risks of the tube include intubation of the food pipe, bleeding, infection, and hoarseness when the tube is removed.
- No alternative treatments exist.

In addition, the consultant must be sure that Mr. A appreciates what these facts mean for him specifically. The following are examples:

- His previous MI renders his heart more vulnerable to the stress of labored breathing and inadequate oxygenation.
- Although small, the risk of infection from the endotracheal tube is greater because he has diabetes.
- Although diabetes compromises his ability to fight the pneumonia, Mr. A does not have a terminal illness and his doctors expect him

to recover, even if he requires mechanical ventilation.

Finally, the consultant looks for evidence that Mr. A's choice coincides with his values and goals. For example, if Mr. A repeatedly indicated that he wanted to live while steadfastly rejecting intubation (without which, as he has been told, he would most assuredly die if he stopped breathing on his own), the consultant would rightly detect an inconsistency between the patient's decision and his desire to live.

Because capacity is not global, a patient may have capacity to make some decisions but not others. The reason for this discrepancy lies in the risk/benefit ratio of the proposed diagnostic or therapeutic intervention.[11] When the benefit of a treatment far outweighs its risk, the standard for capacity to accept is low, but the standard for capacity to refuse is quite high. In Mr. A's case, the relatively small risk of bleeding, infection, and so on, compared with the overwhelming benefit of mechanical ventilation sets a high standard for capacity to refuse.

The psychiatrist offered his opinion that Mr. A did not have the capacity to refuse intubation and mechanical ventilation. When his respirations became even more labored, he was sedated and intubated; mechanical ventilation commenced. He then could not speak and he had no enteral route. The consultant recommended administration of IV haloperidol.

Psychiatric examination and treatment of Mr. A became exceedingly difficult, but not impossible. The psychiatric consultant in the ICU must be creative, resourceful, and ready to accommodate the changing clinical status of the patient. Lack of an oral route is easily circumvented, because medications can be crushed and delivered through a nasogastric tube or delivered parenterally. Although haloperidol is not approved by the Food and Drug Administration for IV use, widespread experience with this agent attests to its safe and effective use by this method in delirious, medically ill patients, with the same caveats that apply to oral use.

Intubated patients can communicate by writing; by mouthing answers; by pointing to letters on a letter board; or by responding to yes-no questions with head nods, eye blinks, or squeezes of the examiner's hand. Requiring practice for both patient and physician, these maneuvers can be quite time-consuming and frustrating, especially when the patient is sedated (which is the rule in intubated patients).

A psychiatric consultant may feel stymied by an obtunded patient's inability to engage in verbal dialogue. However, a host of physical findings can be made by simple observation (e.g., diaphoresis, dry skin, flushing, mydriasis, miosis, tremor, myoclonus, and facial asymmetry). Muscle tone, reflexes (primitive and deep tendon), and pupillary reaction to light are also assessable in a somnolent patient, as are the vital signs. Scoring of verbal, motor, and eye-opening responses according to the Glasgow Coma Scale[12] rounds out the examination of the lethargic patient.

Over the next several days, the pneumonia and the delirium steadily improved. Mr. A was successfully extubated, and haloperidol was discontinued. Now able to speak in full sentences, albeit hoarsely, he provided the consultant with additional history. This information, added to collateral data obtained from the family, allowed the consultant to confirm his preliminary impression of the absence of major depression, but the presence of an underlying dementia.

Conclusion

The successful denouement of this case showcases again the critical importance of flexibility, responsiveness, and resolve on the part of the ICU psychiatric consultant. First and foremost a competent physician, the psychiatric consultant must accept responsibility for the patient's care, see it through from initiation of the consultation to its end, and approach the patient and the family fully aware that the trajectory of each consultation is unique and unpredictable. Patients' beclouded sensoria and family members' taxed emotional states yield information in piecemeal fashion; history emerges only when the bits and pieces are stitched together. Attention to linguistic nuance and "limbic music" take a backseat to keenness of observation and physical and neurologic examination. No place for premature diagnostic closure, the ICU adheres to an unfixed timetable and the clinical state of affairs largely resembles a moving target. In the ICU, one minute's certainty becomes the next minute's wild speculation, and the consultation psychiatrist assigned there must maintain "Condition Red."

References

1. Sekeres MA, Stern TA: On the edge of life. I. Assessment of, reaction to, and management of the terminally ill recorded in an intensive care unit journal, *Prim Care Companion J Clin Psychiatry* 4:178–183, 2002.
2. Daly L: The perceived immediate needs of families with relatives in the intensive care setting, *Heart Lung* 13:231–239, 1984.
3. Kontos N, Freudenreich O, Querques J, et al: The consultation psychiatrist as effective physician, *Gen Hosp Psychiatry* 25:20–23, 2003.
4. American Psychiatric Association: *Diagnostic and statistical manual of mental disorders*, ed 4, Washington, DC, 1994, American Psychiatric Association.
5. Witchel HJ, Hancox JC, Nutt DJ: Psychotropic drugs, cardiac arrhythmia, and sudden death, *J Clin Psychopharmacol* 23:58–77, 2003.
6. Harrison MO, Krishnan KR: Antipsychotic medications and sudden cardiac death, *Psychopharmacol Bull* 36:91–99, 2002.
7. Welch R, Chue P: Antipsychotic agents and QT changes, *J Psychiatry Neurosci* 25:154–160, 2000.
8. Hunt N, Stern TA: The association between intravenous haloperidol and torsades de pointes, *Psychosomatics* 36:541–549, 1995.
9. Moss AJ: Measurement of the QT interval and the risk associated with QTc interval prolongation: a review, *Am J Cardiol* 72:23B–25B, 1993.
10. Appelbaum PS, Grisso T: Assessing patients' capacities to consent to treatment, *N Engl J Med* 319:1635–1638, 1988.
11. Roth LH, Meisel A, Lidz CW: Tests of competency to consent to treatment, *Am J Psychiatry* 134:279–284, 1977.
12. Bastos PG, Sun X, Wagner DP, et al: Glasgow Coma Scale score in the evaluation of outcome in the intensive care unit: findings from the Acute Physiology and Chronic Health Evaluation III study, *Crit Care Med* 21:1459–1465, 1993.

Chapter 12
Delirious Patients

Ned H. Cassem, M.D., S.J.
George B. Murray, M.D.
Jennifer M. Lafayette, M.D.
Theodore A. Stern, M.D.

Life-threatening illness in itself is difficult enough to manage, but the difficulty of management and the jeopardy of the patient can be dramatically increased when the patient develops an abnormal mental state. Agitation, in particular that which threatens indwelling lines, catheters, pacing wires, and other therapeutic or monitoring devices, is one of the most common reasons for requesting a psychiatric consultation in critical care settings or intensive care units (ICUs).[1] On the list of all psychiatric consultations, delirium ranks second only to depression. Awareness of the complicated nature of caring for agitated patients led to the American Psychiatric Association's publication in 1999 of practice guidelines for the treatment of delirium.[2]

Diagnosis

The essential feature of delirium, according to the *Diagnostic and Statistical Manual of Mental Disorders*, fourth edition (DSM-IV), is a disturbance of consciousness accompanied by cognitive deficits that cannot be accounted for by past or evolving dementia.[3] The diagnostic criteria are the following:

1. A disturbance of consciousness (i.e., reduced clarity of awareness of the environment) with reduced ability to focus, sustain, or shift attention

2. A change in cognition (e.g., memory deficit, disorientation, or a language disturbance) or the development of a perceptual disturbance that is not better accounted for by a preexisting, established, or evolving dementia

3. A disturbance that develops over a short period (usually hours to days) and tends to fluctuate during the course of the day

4. Evidence from the history, physical examination, or laboratory findings that the disturbance is caused by the direct physiologic consequences of a general medical condition.

Disturbance of the sleep-wake cycle is also common, sometimes with "sundowning" or even complete reversal of the night-day cycle. Both Chedru and Geschwind[4] and Mesulam et al.[5] regard impaired attention as the main deficit of the acute confusional state. DSM-IV makes no distinction between a patient in an acutely agitated state and one in a lethargic or minimally responsive state. It also emphasizes that delirium is related to a general medical condition and attempts to specify the cause as medical, substance-induced, or caused by multiple factors.

Psychotic symptoms, such as visual or auditory hallucinations and delusions, are common among patients with delirium.[6] Sometimes the psychiatric symptoms are so bizarre or so offensive (e.g., a paranoid patient in a belligerent rage is shouting that pornographic movies are being made in the unit) that diagnostic efforts are distracted. The hypoglycemia of a diabetic can be missed in the emergency department if his or her behavior is threatening, uncooperative, and resembles that of a drunk person. The opposite can happen when one is predisposed to blame bizarre behavior on stress itself or on the technology of a hospital setting.

The term *ICU psychosis* is a popular diagnosis often applied to patients exhibiting abnormal behavior in a critical care setting. Acute functional psychosis in the critical care setting, however, is rare. The term is invoked to imply that the environmental features of critical care settings are themselves capable of inducing psychosis. The rationale given for this is either sensory deprivation or monotony. In fact, the use of this diagnosis usually means that the cause of the patient's delirium is simply unknown. Moreover, this diagnosis has more risks than benefits because it tends to discourage thoughts of differential diagnosis, and it inhibits the search for a specific cause.

There are clinical contrasts between anticholinergic deliria (manifest by tachycardia and by dry, hot skin) and adrenergic deliria, such as those seen with alcohol withdrawal (manifest by sweating and tachycardia). Years of clinical involvement managing acute delirium have led to the hypothesis that an increase in endogenous dopamine (DA) during the stress of surgery can cause postoperative agitation and delusions in the patient. Similarly, a decrease in endogenous acetylcholine can produce disorientation, a memory deficit, and hallucinations. In delirium, the electroencephalogram (EEG) is usually abnormal; most often it shows generalized slowing.[7] In monkeys given intravenous (IV) scopolamine[8] and lower animals given atropine,[9] the EEG shows similar changes. In laboratory studies, stress has been shown to elevate levels of mesocortical DA,[10] whereas a cholinergic deficiency is often present with even mild hypoxia.[11] Clinically, IV haloperidol, a DA-blocking agent, and IV physostigmine, an anticholinesterase agent, have both been used successfully to treat delirium. Occasionally in the delirious state, the EEG shows a predominance of fast activity, as in a confusional state produced by benzodiazepines.

Differential Diagnosis

No treatment can proceed without a careful diagnostic evaluation. Although instincts are impressive when correct, there is no substitute for a systematic search for the specific cause of the delirium. The timing of the events gives the best clues to its potential causes. For example, before a patient extubated himself, he was almost certainly in trouble. When did his mental state actually change? Nursing notes can be studied for the first indication of an abnormality (e.g., restlessness, mild confusion, or anxiety). If the time of onset can be established as a marker, other events can be examined for a possible causal relationship to the change in mental state. Starting a new drug or stopping a drug, the onset of fever or hypotension, or the acute worsening of renal functioning, if near the time of mental status changes, become more likely culprits.

Without a convincing temporal connection, the cause may be discovered by its likelihood in the unique clinical situation of the patient. In critical care settings, as in emergency departments, there are seven states that the clinician can routinely call to mind just to make sure the patient is not suffering from one of them. These are states in which intervention needs to be especially prompt because prolonged failure to make the diagnosis may result in permanent central nervous system (CNS) damage. These conditions are (1) Wernicke's disease; (2) hypoxia; (3) hypoglycemia; (4) hypertensive encephalopathy; (5) intracerebral hemorrhage; (6) meningitis/encephalitis; and (7) poisoning, whether exogenous or iatrogenic. Other, less urgent but still acute conditions requiring intervention include subdural hematoma, septicemia, subacute bacterial endocarditis, hepatic or renal failure, thyrotoxicosis/myxedema, delirium tremens, anticholinergic psychosis, and complex partial status epilepticus. If not already ruled out, these conditions are easy to verify, if present.

Bacteremia commonly clouds mental state. In prospectively studied seriously ill hospitalized patients, the presence of an encephalopathic state correlated with bacteremia.[12] In that study, the mortality of septic patients with delirium was higher than in septic patients with a normal mental state. In an elderly person, regardless of the setting, the onset of confusion should trigger concern about infection. Urinary tract infections (UTIs) and pneumonias are the two most common infections in older patients, and when bacteremia is associated with a UTI, confusion is the presenting feature 30% of the time.[13] Once a consultant has eliminated these basic illnesses as possible causes of the patient's disturbed brain function, there is time enough for a more systematic approach to the differential diagnosis. A comprehensive list of differential diagnoses, similar to the one compiled by Ludwig[14] (slightly expanded in Table 12-1) is recommended. A quick review of this list is warranted even when the consultant is relatively sure of a diagnosis.

To understand the acute reaction of the individual patient, one should begin by reviewing the chart completely. Vital signs may reveal periods of hypotension or fever. The highest temperature recorded will also be key. Operative procedures and the use of anesthesia may also reveal a sustained period of hypotension or unusually large blood loss and replacement. Laboratory values should be scanned for abnormalities that could be related to an encephalopathic state. Postoperative delirium is rather common and occurs in about 30% of patients after cardiac surgery.

The old chart, no matter how thick, cannot be overlooked without risk. Some patients have had prior psychiatric consultations for similar difficulties. Others have had no psychiatric consultations but have caused considerable trouble for their caregivers on prior admissions, much of which may be extensively documented. Similar to the patient's psychiatric history, the family psychiatric history can help make a diagnosis, especially if a major mood or anxiety disorder, alcoholism, schizophrenia, or epilepsy is present.

Table 12-1. Differential Diagnosis of Brain Dysfunction in Critical Care Patients*

General Cause	Specific Cause
Vascular	Hypertensive encephalopathy; cerebral arteriosclerosis; intracranial hemorrhage or thromboses; emboli from atrial fibrillation, patent foramen ovale, or endocarditic valve; circulatory collapse (shock); systemic lupus erythematosus; polyarteritis nodosa; thrombotic thrombocytopenic purpura; hyperviscosity syndrome; sarcoid
Infectious	Encephalitis, bacterial or viral meningitis, fungal meningitis (*cryptococcal, coccidioidal, Histoplasma*), sepsis, general paresis, brain/epidural/subdural abscess, malaria, human immunodeficiency virus, Lyme disease, typhoid fever, parasitic (*toxoplasma, trichinosis, cysticercosis, echinococcosis*), Behçet's syndrome, mumps
Neoplastic	Space-occupying lesions, such as gliomas, meningiomas, abscesses; paraneoplastic syndromes; carcinomatous meningitis
Degenerative	Senile and presenile dementias, such as Alzheimer's or Pick's dementia, Huntington's chorea, Creutzfeldt-Jakob disease, Wilson's disease
Intoxication	Chronic intoxication or withdrawal effect of sedative-hypnotic drugs, such as bromides, opiates, tranquilizers, anticholinergics, dissociative anesthetics, anticonvulsants, carbon monoxide from burn inhalation
Congenital	Epilepsy, postictal states, complex partial status epilepticus, aneurysm
Traumatic	Subdural and epidural hematomas, contusion, laceration, postoperative trauma, heat stroke, fat emboli syndrome
Intraventricular	Normal pressure hydrocephalus
Vitamin deficiency	Deficiencies of thiamine (Wernicke-Korsakoff syndrome), niacin (pellagra), B_{12} (pernicious anemia)
Endocrine-metabolic	Diabetic coma and shock; uremia; myxedema; hyperthyroidism, parathyroid dysfunction; hypoglycemia; hepatic or renal failure; porphyria; severe electrolyte or acid/base disturbances; paraneoplastic; syndrome; Cushing's/Addison's syndrome; sleep apnea; carcinoid; Whipple's disease
Metals	Heavy metals (lead, manganese, mercury); other toxins
Anoxia	Hypoxia and anoxia secondary to pulmonary or cardiac failure, anesthesia, anemia
Depression—other	Depressive pseudodementia, hysteria, catatonia

* Ludwig's[14] differential diagnosis of the confusion-delirium-dementia-coma complex.
Modified from Ludwig AM: *Principles of clinical psychiatry*, New York, 1980, The Free Press.

Examination of current and past medications is mandatory because pharmacologic agents can produce abnormal psychiatric symptoms either from their presence in the patient (even) in therapeutic quantities or in overdose quantities, or in withdrawal. Moreover, these considerations must be routinely reviewed, especially in patients whose drugs have been stopped because of surgery or hospitalization or whose drug orders have not been transmitted during transfer to the ICU. Alcohol as well as barbiturates, narcotics, benzodiazepines, tricyclic antidepressants, neuroleptics, and other psychotropic medications are regularly associated with withdrawal symptoms if abruptly terminated. Steroids, anticonvulsants, psychostimulants, β-blockers, and clonidine are also associated with withdrawal symptoms.[15]

Psychiatric symptoms in medical illness can have other causes. Besides the abnormalities that may arise from the effect of the patient's medical illness or its treatment on the CNS (e.g., the abnormalities produced by systemic lupus erythematosus or high-dose steroids), the disturbance may be the effect of the medical illness on the patient's mind (the subjective CNS), as in the patient who thinks he is "washed up" after a myocardial infarction, quits, and withdraws into a hopeless state. Second, the disturbance may arise from the mind primarily, as a conversion symptom or as malingering about pain to get more narcotics. Finally, the abnormality may be the result of interactions between the sick patient and his or her environment or family (e.g., the patient who has no complaints until his family arrives, at which time he promptly looks acutely distressed and begins to whimper continuously). Nurses commonly identify these sorts of abnormalities, although they may not be documented in the medical record.

The Examination of the Patient

Appearance, level of consciousness, thought, speech, orientation, memory, mood, judgment, and behavior are all assessed. In the formal mental status examination (MSE), one should begin with examination of consciousness. If the patient does not speak, a handy commonsense test is asking oneself, "Do the eyes look back at me?" One could formally rate consciousness by using the

Table 12-2. Glasgow Coma Scale for Scoring

Eye opening (E)	
Spontaneous	4
To verbal command	3
To pain	2
No response	1
Motor (M)	
Obeys verbal command	6
Localizes pain	5
Flexion withdrawal	4
Abnormal flexion (decortication)	3
Extension (decerebration)	2
No response	1
Verbal (V)	
Oriented and converses	5
Disoriented and converses	4
Inappropriate words	3
Incomprehensible sound	2
No response	1
Coma Score = (E + M + V)	Range 3 to 15

From Bastos PG, Sun X, Wagner DP, et al: Glasgow Coma Scale score in the evaluation of outcome in the intensive care unit: findings from the Acute Physiology and Chronic Health Evaluation III study, *Crit Care Med* 21:1459–1465, 1993.

Glasgow Coma Scale (Table 12-2), as modified for the Acute Physiology and Chronic Health Evaluation (APACHE) III study.[16]

If the patient can respond to an examination, attention should be examined first because if this is disturbed, other parts of the examination may be invalid. One can ask the patient to repeat those letters of the alphabet that rhyme with "tree." (If the patient is intubated, ask that a hand or finger be raised whenever the letter of the recited alphabet rhymes with tree.) Then the rest of the MSE is performed. The Folstein Mini-Mental State Examination,[17] which is presented in Figure 12-1, is usually included. Specific defects are more important than the score. Other functions are often abnormal in delirium, such as writing, which Chedru and Geschwind[4] noted as one of the most sensitive indicators of impairment of consciousness.

The patient's problem may involve serious neurologic syndromes as well, although we recommend that the clinical presentation of the patient dictate the examination. In general, the less responsive and more impaired the patient is, the more one is pushed to look for "hard" signs. A directed search for abnormality of the eyes and pupils, nuchal rigidity, hyperreflexia (withdrawal)

Patient _____
Examiner _____
Date _____

"MINI-MENTAL STATE"

Maximum score	Score	
		Orientation
5	( )	What is the (year) (season) (date) (day) (month)?
5	( )	Where are we? (state) (country) (town) (hospital) (floor).

Registration

3   ( )   Name 3 objects: 1 second to say each. Then ask the patient all 3 after you have said them. Give 1 point for each correct answer. Then repeat them until he learns all 3. Count trials and record.

Trials _____

Attention and Calculation

5   ( )   Serial 7's. 1 point for each correct. Stop after 5 answers. Alternatively spell "world" backwards.

Recall

3   ( )   Ask for the 3 objects repeated above. Give 1 point for each correct.

Language

9   ( )   Name a pencil, and watch (2 points)
Repeat the following "No ifs, ands or buts." (1 point)
Follow a 3-stage command:
"Take a paper in your right hand, fold it in half, and put it on the floor" (3 points)
Read and obey the following:

Close your eyes (1 point)

Write a sentence (1 point)
Copy design (1 point)
Total score
ASSESS level of consciousness
along a continuum _____
Alert Drowsy Stupor Coma

Figure 12-1. Mini-Mental State Examination.
From Folstein MF, Folstein SE, McHugh PR: "Mini-mental state." A practical method for grading the cognitive state of patients for the clinician, *J Psychiatr Res*, 12:189–198, 1975. Used by permission.   *Continued*

INSTRUCTIONS FOR ADMINISTRATION OF
MINI-MENTAL STATE EXAMINATION

Orientation

(1) Ask for the date. Then ask specifically for parts omitted, e.g., "Can you also tell me what season it is?" One point for each correct.

(2) Ask in turn "Can you tell me the name of this hospital?" (town, country, etc.). One point for each correct.

Registration

Ask the patient if you may test his memory. Then say the names of 3 unrelated objects, clearly and slowly, about one second for each. After you have said all 3, ask him to repeat them. This first repetition determines his score (0–3) but keep saying them until he can repeat all 3, up to 6 trials. If he does not eventually learn all 3, recall cannot be meaningfully tested.

Attention and calculation

Ask the patient to begin with 100 and count backwards by 7. Stop after 5 subtractions (93, 86, 79, 72, 65). Score the total number of correct answers.

If the patient cannot or will not perform this task, ask him to spell the word "world" backwards. The score is the number of letters in the correct order. E.g., dlrow = 5, dlorw = 3.

Recall

Ask the patient if he can recall the 3 words you previously asked him to remember. Score 0–3.

Language

Naming: Show the patient a wrist watch and ask him what it is. Repeat for pencil. Score 0–2.

Repetition: Ask the patient to repeat the sentence after you. Allow only one trial. Score 0 or 1.

3-Stage command: Give the patient a piece of plain blank paper and repeat the command. Score 1 point for each part correctly executed.

Reading: On a blank piece of paper print the sentence "Close your eyes", in letters large enough for the patient to see clearly. Ask him to read it and do what it says. Score 1 point only if he actually closes his eyes.

Writing: Give the patient a blank piece of paper and ask him to write a sentence for you. Do not dictate a sentence, it is to be written spontaneously. It must contain a subject and verb and be sensible. Correct grammar and punctuation are not necessary.

Copying: On a clean piece of paper, draw intersecting pentagons, each side about 1 in., and ask him to copy it exactly as it is. All 10 angles must be present and 2 must intersect to score 1 point. Tremor and rotation are ignored.

Estimate the patient's level of sensorium along a continuum, from alert on the left to coma on the right.

Figure 12-1. *Continued*

or "hung up" reflexes (myxedema), one-sided weakness or asymmetry, gait (normal pressure hydrocephalus), Babinski's reflexes, tetany, absent vibratory and position senses, hyperventilation (acidosis, hypoxia, or pontine disease), or other specific clues can help verify or reject hunches about causality stimulated by the abnormalities of the examination.

Frontal lobe function may deserve specific attention. Grasp, snout, palmomental, suck, and glabellar responses can be helpful when present. Hand movements thought to be related to the premotor area (Brodmann's area 8) can identify subtle deficiencies. The patient is asked to imitate, with each hand separately, specific movements. The hand is held upright, a circle formed by thumb and first finger ("ok" sign), then the fist is closed and lowered to the surface on which the elbow rests. Second, one hand is brought down on a surface (a table or one's own leg) in three successive positions: extended with all five digits parallel ("cut"), then as a fist, and then flat on the surface. Finally, both hands are placed on a flat surface in front of the patient, one flat on the surface, the other resting as a fist. Then the positions are alternated between right and left hands, and the patient is instructed to do likewise.

For verbally responsive patients, we ordinarily ask their response to the "Frank Jones story" (i.e., I have a friend, Frank Jones, whose feet are so big he has to put his pants on over his head. How does that strike you?). Three general responses are given. Type 1 is normal: The patient sees the incongruity and smiles (a limbic response) and can explain (a neocortical function) why it cannot be done. Type 2 is abnormal: The patient smiles at the incongruity (a limbic connection), but cannot explain why it cannot be done. Type 3 is abnormal: The patient neither gets the incongruity nor can explain its impossibility.

Drugs Associated with Delirium

Of all causes of an altered mental status, use of or withdrawal from drugs are probably the most common. Some, such as lidocaine, are quite predictable in their ability to cause an encephalopathic state, and the relationship is clearly dose-related. Others, such as antibiotics, are much rarer causes

of delirium, and reactions usually cause delirium only in someone whose brain is already vulnerable, as in a patient with a low seizure threshold.[18] Table 12-3 lists some drugs in clinical use that have been associated with delirium.[19–21]

The number of drugs that can be involved either in direct toxic actions or in toxic effects because of drug interactions are numerous, potentially bewildering, and constantly changing. Certain sources provide regular review of published summaries and updates.[20] Although physicians are usually aware of these hazards, a common drug, such as meperidine, when used in doses above about 300 mg/day for several days, causes CNS symptoms because its metabolite, normeperidine, which has a half-life of 30 hours, accumulates and causes "the shakes," myoclonus (the best clue), anxiety, and ultimately seizures.[22] The usual treatment is to stop the drug or reduce the dose. Sometimes this is not possible.

Elderly patients and those with mental retardation or a history of significant head injury are more susceptible to the toxic actions of many of these drugs. Some of those drugs listed in Table 12-3 have been reported to cause delirium only in the elderly (e.g., nonsteroidal antiinflammatory drugs and eye and nose drop preparations).

Specific Management Strategies for Delirium

Thirty years ago, it was routine to administer atropine to newly admitted coronary care unit (CCU) patients who developed bradycardia. Some of these patients, particularly older ones with some preexisting organic brain disease, developed an acute delirium. For such patients, parenteral propantheline bromide (Pro-Banthine), a quaternary ammonium compound that does not cross the blood-brain barrier and is equally effective in treating bradycardia, was substituted. This can still be done, but problems are seldom so simple. Often the drugs that may be causing the delirium, such as lidocaine or prednisone, cannot be changed without possible detriment to the patient. Alternatively, pain may be the cause of agitation in a delirious patient. Morphine sulfate can relieve pain but may be contraindicated by an associated decrease in blood pressure or respiratory rate.

Psychosocial measures are not effective in treating a bona fide delirium of uncertain or unknown

Table 12-3. Drugs Implicated in Delirium

Antiarrhythmics	Anticonvulsants	Interleukin-2 (high dose)
Disopyramide	Phenytoin	L-Asparaginase
Lidocaine	Antihypertensives	Methotrexate (high dose)
Mexiletine	Captopril	Procarbazine
Procainamide	Clonidine	Tamoxifen
Propafenone	Methyldopa	Vinblastine
Quinidine	Reserpine	Vincristine
Tocainide	Antiviral agents	Monoamine oxidase
Antibiotics	Acyclovir	inhibitors
Aminoglycosides	Interferon	Phenelzine
Amodiaquine	Ganciclovir	Procarbazine
Amphotericin	Nevirapine	Narcotic analgesics
Cephalosporins	Barbiturates	Meperidine
Chloramphenicol	β-Blockers	(normeperidine)
Gentamicin	Propranolol	Pentazocine
Isoniazid	Timolol	Podophyllin (topical)
Metronidazole	Cimetidine, ranitidine	Nonsteroidal
Rifampin	Digitalis preparations	antiinflammatory drugs
Sulfonamides	Disulfiram	Ibuprofen
Tetracyclines	Diuretics	Indomethacin
Ticarcillin	Acetazolamide	Naproxen
Vancomycin	Dopamine agonists (central)	Sulindac
Anticholinergics	Amantadine	Other medications
Atropine	Bromocriptine	Clozaril
Scopolamine	Levodopa	Cyclobenzaprine
Tricyclic	Selegiline	Lithium
antidepressants	Ergotamine	Ketamine
Amitriptyline	GABA agonists	Sildenafil
Clomipramine	Benzodiazepines	Trazodone
Desipramine	Baclofen	Mefloquine
Imipramine	Immunosuppressives	Sympathomimetics
Nortriptyline	Aminoglutethimide	Amphetamine
Protriptyline	Azacytidine	Aminophylline
Trimipramine	Chlorambucil	Theophylline
Trihexyphenidyl	Cytosine arabinoside (high dose)	Ephedrine
Benztropine	Dacarbazine	Cocaine
Diphenhydramine	5-Fluorouracil	Phenylpropanolamine
Thioridazine	Hexamethylmelamine	Phenylephrine
Eye and nose drops	Ifosfamide	Steroids, ACTH

ACTH, Adrenocorticotrophic hormone; *GABA*, gamma aminobutyric acid.
From Cassem NH, Lake CR, Boyer WF: Psychopharmacology in the ICU. In Chernow B, editor: *The pharmacologic approach to the critically ill patient*, Baltimore, 1995, Williams & Wilkins; and Drugs that may cause psychiatric symptoms. *Med Letter Drugs Ther* 44:59–62, 2002.

cause. It is commendable to have hospital rooms with a picture window,[23] calendars, clocks, and a few mementos from home on the walls; soft and low lighting at night to help "sundowners"; and, most of all, a loving family in attendance to reassure and orient the patient. Even when present, the psychiatric consultant is summoned because the psychosocial measures have failed to prevent the patient's delirium. Restraints (e.g., poseys, geriatric chairs, "vests," helmets, and locked leather restraints for application to one or more extremities, chest, and [even] head) are also available and quite useful to protect patients from inflicting harm on themselves or others. One or several of these are often in place when the consultant arrives. One hoped-for outcome of the consultation is that the use of these devices can be reduced or eliminated. The unfortunate misnomer, *chemical restraint*, is frequently applied to the most helpful class of drugs for delirium (i.e., neuroleptics). Physicians do not use chemical restraints in the treatment of patients—at least we have never seen the use, or any documentation, of tear gas, pepper spray, mace, or nerve gas employed against agitated patients by their physicians.

When the cause of the delirium seems relatively clear, the treatment is straightforward. A discovered deficiency can be replaced (e.g., blood, oxygen, thiamine, vitamin B_{12}, synthroid, or glucose). Pathologic conditions can be treated (e.g., volume replacement for hypotension, diuretics for pulmonary edema, antibiotics for infection, calcium administration for hypocalcemia, or dialysis for acute lithium toxicity). Implicated drugs, such as meperidine and cimetidine, can be stopped, reduced, or changed, (switched to morphine or to famotidine or sucralfate), respectively. If the offending drug cannot be stopped immediately, the following regimen may be required simultaneously. For example, in a patient with life-threatening ventricular irritability for whom lidocaine at a high rate of infusion seems essential, there may be no way that one can immediately reduce the dosage even though the causal connection with agitation is clear. Treatment of nonspecific delirium, specifically use of IV haloperidol, can proceed while the lidocaine is maintained. The CNS derangement will not cease, however, until the lidocaine is reduced to a nontoxic level or is withdrawn. Once a florid delirium with lidocaine begins, reduction of the dosage to a prior level that was not toxic may not immediately eliminate the delirium. Steroids are similar, in that they may be essential for treatment of the patient's primary illness, and once a disturbance such as psychosis, mania, or depression has begun, reduction in dose may not bring about prompt relief.[24] Again, haloperidol is useful for the management of both psychosis and mania, and for the latter, lithium or divalproex sodium may be added as well.

Specific antidotes are available that can reverse the delirium caused by some drugs. Flumazenil and naloxone reverse the effects of benzodiazepines and opioid analgesics, respectively. Caution is necessary because flumazenil may precipitate seizures in a patient dependent on benzodiazepines, and naloxone can also precipitate withdrawal symptoms in a narcotic-dependent patient.

An anticholinergic psychosis can be reversed by IV physostigmine in doses of 0.5 to 2 mg administered parenterally. Caution is essential for medically ill patients, however, because their autonomic nervous systems are generally less stable than basically healthy patients who have developed an anticholinergic psychosis as a result of a voluntary or accidental overdose. Moreover, if there is a reasonably high amount of an anticholinergic drug on board that is clearing from the system slowly, the therapeutic effect of physostigmine, although sometimes quite dramatic, is usually short-lived. The cholinergic reaction to intravenously administered physostigmine can cause profound bradycardia and hypotension, thereby multiplying the complications instead of reducing them. It should also be noted that a continuous IV infusion of physostigmine has been successfully used to manage a case of anticholinergic poisoning.[25] Because of the diagnostic value of physostigmine, one may wish to use it even though it will make no meaningful therapeutic contribution. If one uses an IV injection of 1 mg of physostigmine, protection against excessive cholinergic reaction can be provided by preceding this injection with an IV injection of 0.2 mg of glycopyrrolate. This anticholinergic agent does not cross the blood-brain barrier and should protect the patient from the peripheral cholinergic actions of physostigmine.

Drug Treatment

Because an agitated critical care patient may harm himself or herself by pulling out pacemaker wires, pumps, sutures, the endotracheal tube, or other therapeutic lifelines, the decrease of agitation is the most common treatment goal against which any drug's effects are titrated. If the patient has a paranoid delusion without agitation, the goal is the reduction or elimination of the delusion. In an ICU patient who cannot communicate, agitation may stem from pain or even shivering caused by hypothermia. Naturally, morphine and diazepam are the respective treatments of choice. These are routinely tried in practice before more complicated sedative regimens are used. Opioids, benzodiazepines, neuroleptics, barbiturates, neuromuscular blocking agents, inhalant anesthetics (such as isoflurane or nitrous oxide), and assorted other agents, such as propofol, ketamine, isoflurane, chloral hydrate, and clonidine, are available to use alone or in creative combinations. Although common sense indicates that the most cost-effective agents, morphine and diazepam, can take care of many patients' sedative requirements, intensivists are regularly challenged by delirious states not managed by these agents alone. The perfect sedation regimen does not yet exist.[26]

Benzodiazepines are often effective in mild agitation and in practice, after morphine, are tried first, as 2.5 mg of IV diazepam or 0.5 to 1 mg of midazolam. Especially in higher doses, these agents can cause or exacerbate confusion in older patients. This occurs much less often with antipsychotics, unless the chosen drug, such as thioridazine, has potent anticholinergic properties.

Neuroleptics are the agent of choice for delirium. Haloperidol is probably the antipsychotic most commonly used to treat agitated delirium in the critical care setting. Its effects on blood pressure, pulmonary artery pressure, heart rate, and respiration are milder than those of the benzodiazepines, making it an excellent agent for severely ill patients with impaired cardiorespiratory status.[3,20,27]

Although haloperidol can be administered orally or parenterally, acute delirium with extreme agitation typically requires parenteral medication. IV administration is preferable to intramuscular (IM) administration because drug absorption may be poor in distal muscles if a patient's delirium is associated with circulatory compromise or with borderline shock. The deltoid is probably better than the gluteus muscle for IM injection, but neither is as reliable as the IV route. Second, the agitated patient is commonly paranoid, and repeated painful IM injections may increase the patient's sense of being attacked by enemy forces. Third, IM injections can complicate interpretations of muscle enzyme studies if enzyme fractionation is not available. Fourth, and most important, haloperidol is less likely to produce extrapyramidal side effects when given intravenously than when given IM or by mouth (PO),[28] at least for patients without a prior serious psychiatric disorder.

In contrast to the immediately observable sedation produced by IV diazepam, IV haloperidol has a mean distribution time of 11 minutes in normal volunteers[29]; this may be even longer in critically ill patients. The mean half-life of IV haloperidol's subsequent, slower phase is 14 hours. This is still a more rapid metabolic rate than the overall mean half-lives of 21 and 24 hours for IM and PO doses. The PO dose has about half the potency of the parenteral dose, so that 10 mg of haloperidol PO corresponds to 5 mg IV or IM.

Haloperidol has not been approved by the Food and Drug Administration (FDA) for IV administration. However, any approved drug can be used for a patient for a nonapproved indication or route and is justified as "innovative therapy." For critical care units desirous of using IV haloperidol, one approach is to present this to the hospital's institutional review board or human studies committee with a request to use the drug with careful monitoring of results based on the fact that it is the drug of choice for the patient's welfare, it is the safest drug, and it is justifiable as innovative therapy. After a period of monitoring, the committee can choose to make the use of the drug routine in that particular hospital.

In Europe, IV haloperidol has been used to treat delirium tremens and acute psychosis and to premedicate patients scheduled for electroconvulsive therapy. Its use has been associated with few side effects on blood pressure, heart rate, respiratory rate, or urine output and has been linked with few extrapyramidal side effects. The reason for the latter is not known. Studies of the use of IV haloperidol in psychiatric patients have not shown that these side effects were fewer. The reason for their more rare appearance after IV administration in medically ill patients may be due to the fact that many of the medically ill patients have other medications on board, especially the benzodiazepines, that are protective or that patients with psychiatric disorder are more susceptible to the side effects.[28]

Before administration of IV haloperidol, the IV line should be flushed with 2 ml of normal saline. Phenytoin precipitates haloperidol, and mixing the two in the same line must be avoided. Occasionally, haloperidol may precipitate with heparin, and because many lines in critical care units are heparinized, the 2-ml flush is advised. The initial bolus dose of haloperidol usually varies from 0.5 to 20 mg; it is usually 0.5 (for an elderly person) to 2 mg for mild agitation, 5 mg for moderate agitation, and 10 mg for severe agitation. The only time when a consultant would use a higher initial dose is when the patient has already been treated with reasonable doses of haloperidol unsuccessfully. To adjust for haloperidol's lag time, doses are usually staggered by at least a 30-minute interval. If one dose (e.g., a 5-mg dose) does not calm an agitated patient after 30 minutes, the next higher dose, 10 mg, should be administered. A calm patient is the desired outcome. Partial control of agitation is usually not adequate, and settling for this only prolongs the delirium or guarantees excessive doses of haloperidol after the delirium is under control.

Haloperidol can be combined every 30 minutes with simultaneous parenteral lorazepam doses (starting with 1 to 2 mg). Because the effects of lorazepam are noticeable within 5 to 10 minutes, each dose can precede the haloperidol dose, observed for its impact on agitation, and increased if it is more effective. Some believe that the combination leads to a lower overall dose of each drug.[30]

After calm is achieved, agitation should be the sign for a repeat dose. Ideally the total dose of haloperidol on the second day should be a fraction of that on day 1. After complete lucidity has been achieved, the patient needs to be protected from delirium only at night, by small doses of haloperidol (1 to 3 mg), which can be given orally. As in the treatment of delirium tremens, the consultant is advised to stop the agitation quickly and completely at the outset rather than barely keep up with it over several days. The maximum total dose of IV haloperidol to be used as an upper limit has not been established, although IV administration of single bolus doses of 200 mg has been used in our institution, and up to 1600 mg total has been used in a 24-hour period.[31] The highest requirements have been seen with delirious patients on the intraaortic balloon pump.[32] A continuous infusion of haloperidol has also been used to treat severe, refractory delirium.[33]

When delirium is not responding and agitation is unabated, how can one tell that the neuroleptic, here haloperidol, is not producing akathisia, which now further complicates the original condition? The best indication is the patient's description of an irresistible urge to move—usually the limbs, lower more often than upper. If dialogue is possi-

ble, even nodding yes or no, provided that the patient understands the question, can confirm or exclude this symptom. If the patient cannot communicate, one knows there are only two options: to decrease the dose or to increase it and judge by the response. In our experience, it is far more common for the patient to receive more haloperidol and to respond with reduced agitation.

Hypotensive episodes following the administration of IV haloperidol are rare and almost invariably are caused by hypovolemia. Ordinarily, this is easily checked in ICU patients who have indwelling pulmonary artery catheters, but because agitation is likely to return, volume replacement is necessary before administering further doses. There are no local caustic effects on veins. IV haloperidol is generally safe for epileptics and patients with head trauma, unless psychotropic drugs are contraindicated by the need for careful neurologic monitoring. Although IV haloperidol may be used without mishap in patients receiving epinephrine drips, after large doses of haloperidol a pressor other than epinephrine (e.g., norepinephrine) should be used to avoid unopposed β-adrenergic activity. IV haloperidol does not block a DA-mediated increase in renal blood flow. It also appears to be the safest agent for patients with chronic obstructive pulmonary disease.

Several centers have discovered IV haloperidol use associated with the development of torsades de pointes (TDP) ventricular tachycardia.[34-38] The reason is not clear, although particular caution is urged in the presence of low levels of potassium and magnesium, a prolonged QT interval, hepatic compromise, or a specific cardiac abnormality (e.g., mitral valve prolapse or a dilated ventricle). Progressive QT widening after haloperidol administration may alert one to the danger. Although the incidence remains small, 4 of 1100 cases in one unit,[35] all reports are recent. Delirious patients who are candidates for IV haloperidol require careful screening. Serum potassium and magnesium should be within normal range and a baseline electrocardiogram checked for the pretreatment QT interval corrected for heart rate (QTc) interval. QT interval prolongation occurs in some patients with alcoholic liver disease and is associated with an adverse outcome, especially sudden cardiac death.[39] History of recent use of other medications that may cause QT interval prolongation (such as droperidol or ziprasidone) is worth inquiry.

In the past, IV droperidol was recommended as an alternative agent to haloperidol in part because it was approved for IV administration by the FDA. Unfortunately, its label was revised to include a black box warning for cases of QT prolongation leading to TDP and death.[40] This has limited its utility and availability.

Other parenteral neuroleptic drugs for the treatment of agitation are perphenazine, thiothixene, trifluoperazine, fluphenazine, and chlorpromazine. Perphenazine is approved for IV use as an antiemetic. Chlorpromazine is extremely effective, but its potent α-blocking properties can be exceedingly dangerous for critically ill patients. When administered intravenously or intramuscularly, it can abruptly decr ease total peripheral resistance and cause a precipitous fall in cardiac output. Nevertheless, IV use in small doses (10 mg) can be both safe and effective in the treatment of delirium.

Occasionally, the psychiatric consultant wishes to choose an orally administered atypical antipsychotic for mild agitation in a delirious patient.[41] PO risperidone 0.5 to 2 mg once or twice daily, olanzapine 2.5 to 10 mg, and quetiapine 12.5 to 50 mg have all been used as starting doses with good effect. As with other medications, start with lower doses in elderly patients. Little is known at this point about the efficacy of PO or IM ziprasidone, particularly with regard to QTc prolongation.[41]

Delirium in Specific Diseases

Critical care patients with human immunodeficiency virus infection may be more susceptible to the extrapyramidal side effects of haloperidol, including a case of neuroleptic malignant syndrome (NMS),[42–45] leading an experienced group to recommend molindone. The latter is associated with fewer of such effects, is available only in PO preparation, and can be prescribed from 5 to 25 mg at appropriate intervals or, in a more acute situation, 25 mg every hour until calm. Risperidone 0.5 to 1 mg per dose is another PO agent recommended. If parenteral medication is required, 10 mg of chlorpromazine has been effective.

Perphenazine is readily available for parenteral use as well, and 2 mg doses can be used.

Patients with Parkinson's disease pose a special problem because DA blockade aggravates their condition. If PO treatment of delirium or psychosis is possible, clozapine, starting with a small dose of 6.25 or 12.5 mg, is probably the most effective agent available that does not exacerbate the disease. Risperidone 0.5 to 1 mg to start is also worthy of trial and requires no monitoring of the patient's leukocyte count.

IV diazepam is used routinely to treat agitated states, particularly delirium tremens, as are IV chlordiazepoxide and lorazepam, and benzodiazepines are probably the preferred drug class for the treatment of alcohol withdrawal.[46] Neuroleptics have been successfully used, and both have been combined with clonidine. IV alcohol is also extremely effective in the treatment of alcohol withdrawal states, particularly if the patient does not seem to respond as rapidly as expected to higher doses of benzodiazepines. The disadvantage is that alcohol is toxic to both liver and brain, although its use can be quite safe if these organs do not show already extensive damage (and sometimes quite safe even when they do). A 5% solution of alcohol mixed with 5% dextrose in water run at 1 ml per minute often brings a calming effect quickly.

Propofol, the newest agent for sedation of critically ill patients, can also be extremely effective in calming agitation.[47–49] It has both moderate respiratory depressant and vasodilator effects, although hypotension can be minimized by avoiding bolus doses of the drug. Impaired hepatic function does not slow metabolic clearance, but clearance declines with age and is significantly slower in the elderly. When it was compared with midazolam as a sedative for postoperative coronary artery bypass graft patients, both drugs, without affecting cardiac output, provided safe and effective sedation and lowered arterial blood pressure and heart rates. The group treated with propofol, however, had significantly lower heart rates during the first 2 hours and significantly lower blood pressures 5 to 10 minutes after the initial dose (mean loading doses for propofol and midazolam were 0.24 mg/kg and 0.012 mg/kg, and maintenance doses 0.76 mg/kg/hour and 0.018 mg/kg/hour). For the propofol group, there was a reduced need for sodium nitroprusside and supplemental opioids.[50]

In a prospective, randomized, crossover, placebo-controlled trial, propofol's affect on critically ill patients' response to chest physiotherapy was studied. Propofol, in an IV bolus dose of 0.75 mg/kg, significantly reduced the hemodynamic and metabolic stresses caused by chest physical therapy.[51] This drug's rapid onset and short duration make it especially useful for treating responses to short periods of stress. When rapid return to alertness from sedation for an uncompromised neurologic examination is indicated, propofol is a nearly ideal agent.[52] However, its use in the treatment of a prolonged delirious state has specific disadvantages.[53] Delivered as a fat emulsion containing 0.1 g of fat per milliliter, propofol requires a dedicated line, and accumulation can lead to a fat overload syndrome, which has been associated with overfeeding with significant CO_2 production, hypertriglyceridemia, ketoacidosis, seizure activity 6 days after discontinuation, and even fatal respiratory failure.[53–55] Obese patients provide an excess volume of distribution, and their doses should be calculated using estimated lean, rather than actual, body mass. If the patient is receiving fat by parenteral feeding, this must be adjusted or eliminated and adequate glucose infusion provided to prevent ketoacidosis. Although no clear association has been demonstrated with addiction, tolerance, or withdrawal, doses seem to require escalation after 4 to 7 days' infusion. The seizures seen after withdrawal activity or muscular rigidity during administration are poorly understood. Expense associated with prolonged infusions is high because propofol costs about three to four times as much as equivalent quantities of midazolam.

Drug infusions may be more effective and efficient than bolus dosing because the latter may intensify side effects, such as hypotension, waste time of critical care personnel, permit more individual error, and so on. The contents of the infusion can address simultaneously multiple aspects of a patient's difficulties in uniquely appropriate ways. The report of the sufentanil, midazolam, and atracurium admixture for a patient who required a temporary biventricular assist device is an excellent example of multiple-drug infusion and creative problem solving.[56,57]

Anxiety that Inhibits Weaning from the Ventilator

In intensive care settings, weaning a patient from a ventilator can appear as a primarily psychiatric problem. Basically the "numbers" (blood gases, oxygen inspired pressure, and ventilator settings) look to the intensivist as though the patient is physiologically able to breathe progressively without the need of the ventilator. At times, such a patient, on examination, may be delirious. When this is so, treatment can proceed according to the aforementioned guidelines. Other factors, however, can hinder a patient's efforts to breathe independently.

No more dramatic and simple lesson has perhaps been delivered than that of Thorens's et al.[58] that the duration of mechanic ventilation in their ICU was inversely related to the number of available ICU nurses. In fact, in the 5 years after onset, duration of mechanical ventilation rose progressively from 7.3 to 38.2 days, whereas the percentage of certified nurses dropped from 64% to 37%. In the sixth year, when nursing personnel were restored to full force, the mean duration of ventilatory support dropped back to 10.1 days. In days when cost priorities supercede those of care, this lesson ranks first when patients are slow to escape the ventilator.

The multimodal treatment of weaning difficulties often begins with a benzodiazepine (like lorazepam) administered before weaning periods or a neuroleptic, such as haloperidol, if the patient appears to be near panic. Droperidol has also been helpful for breaking status asthmaticus, with distinct improvements in pulmonary function.[59] Again, if haloperidol or droperidol is used, the IV route is recommended. Lorazepam 0.5 mg sublingually is not likely to cause significant respiratory depression and is worth trying.

Persons who suffer acute and chronic respiratory failure and therefore require prolonged mechanical ventilation may become so anxious when the weaning process begins that psychiatric assistance is requested. Even though the patient is physically ready for weaning, anxiety can transiently increase metabolic demands and cardiac work until further weaning is contraindicated.

Most behavioral exercises for relaxation encourage the subject to take slow, deep, easy breaths. This is one of the quickest and surest ways of inducing relaxation for most people, but it is precisely what patients with respiratory problems cannot do and precisely what makes them so anxious. The multimodal treatment of this difficulty often begins with a benzodiazepine administered before weaning periods or an antipsychotic, such as haloperidol, if the patient appears to be near panic. The patient can indicate whether a drug is effective and which drug is most helpful. In some cases, it may be possible to use a mixture of nitrous oxide if the respiratory physician or anesthesiologist is present to administer it. Hypnosis or relaxation techniques have often been helpful in distracting the patient from the weaning process. In this case, the instruction to breathe easily is better omitted from the hypnotic suggestion; the patient should be encouraged to concentrate either on a tranquil scene, such as a beach, or on a single concept (mantra). Finally, the patient may be helped by the explanation that the weaning process itself can be expected to produce anxiety. Despondency and anxiety can become problems that impede weaning, so that the remarks in the foregoing section on despondency may apply here as well.

Paralyzed Patients

Patients who require paralysis by neuromuscular blocking agents present a unique challenge to caregivers. The psychological state of such a patient, who cannot communicate at all, can be monitored by changes in heart rate, blood pressure, sweating, or the appearance of tears. Habitually addressing the patient whenever approaching the bedside addresses the need for regular orienting and reassuring. Analgesics should be supplied if there is any risk of pain, and some regular antianxiety agent, usually a benzodiazepine, should be administered. Sublingual or IV lorazepam, oxazepam by nasogastric tube, or a bolus of IV diazepam every 6 hours are all ways of addressing this problem.

Transfer Out of a Critical Care Setting

Even when the patient has not been confused, awareness of having been dangerously ill can cause anxiety when transfer to a less intense setting is announced. Coronary patients, for example, experi-ence a dramatic rise in catecholamine excretion on the day of transfer out of the CCU.[60] Even though the delirious patient cannot recall the events of the intensive care stay, this amnesia itself may be worrisome and the prospect of less monitoring more so. Transfer from an ICU to a step-down or general unit is generally both bad and good news for the patient—bad because it means reduced coverage and observation; good because it means that the patient's condition has improved. Ideally the discharge date should be made definite at least 24 hours in advance. Explicit warnings about less frequent checks and fewer nurses should be accompanied by the assurance that intensive care is no longer necessary. In essence, increased independence should be represented as a reward rather than a hazard.

Summary

Psychiatric contributions to the recovery of critically ill patients begin with relief of behavioral, cognitive, or affective disturbances caused by medical problems. Thus CNS disorders may be alleviated by restoring physiologic equilibrium (e.g., glucose levels or oxygen tensions), or by adding a specific psychopharmacologic agent (e.g., haloperidol for delirium). The mind is then helped to recover by specific diagnosis and treatment of any psychiatric disorder, supportive psychotherapy, behavioral therapy (e.g., hypnosis and relaxation), veterinary or limbic therapy (the "laying-on of hands" or "talking a person down"), and preparation for the transition from the critical care unit to the next phase of hospitalization. The ICU environment is optimized for recovery by addition of windows, clocks, or calendars; changing lighting schedules to approximate day and night; noise reduction; addition of music, photos, or earphones; and the tailoring of visiting schedules to meet the patient's needs. Finally, the patient's family and social network is assessed and, when possible, integrated into the treatment and support of the patient.

The psychiatric evaluation particularly stresses a history of psychiatric disorders in the patient or family as well as historical determinants, such as an anniversary reaction; the meaning of the illness to the patient; recent stresses; the nature of the patient's social support network; the patient's premorbid personality; issues of secondary gain and the profit derived from the symptoms of being sick; and the possibility of other causes such as conversion, malingering, or factitial illness. The therapeutic approach is multimodal and closely integrated with the rest of the patient's critical care.

References

1. Rincon HG, Granados M, Unutzer J, et al: Prevalence, detection and treatment of anxiety, depression, and delirium in the adult critical care unit, *Psychosomatics* 42:391–396, 2001.
2. American Psychiatric Association: Practice guidelines for the treatment of patients with delirium, *Am J Psychiatry* 156(5 Supp):1–20, 1999.
3. American Psychiatric Association: *Diagnostic and statistical manual of mental disorders, (DSM-IV),* ed 4, Washington, DC, 1994, American Psychiatric Association.
4. Chedru F, Geschwind N: Writing disturbances in acute confusional states, *Neuropsychologia* 10:343–353, 1972.
5. Mesulam M-M, Waxman SG, Geschwind N, et al: Acute confusional state with right middle cerebral artery infarctions, *J Neural Neurosurg Psychiatry* 39:84–89, 1976.
6. Webster R, Holroyd S: Prevalence of psychotic symptoms in delirium, *Psychosomatics* 41:519–522, 2000.
7. Engle GL, Romano J: Delirium, a syndrome of cerebral insufficiency, *J Chronic Dis* 9:260–277, 1959.
8. Murray GB, Jasper HH: *The role of mechanisms in the learning of a tactile discrimination in the monkey.* In Woody CD, Alkon DL, McGaugh JL, editors: *Cellular mechanisms of conditioning and behavioral plasticity,* Seattle, 1986, University of Washington Press.
9. Wilder A: Pharmacologic dissociation of behavior and EEG "sleep patterns" in dogs: morphine, *N*-allynormorphine and atropine, *Proc Soc Exp Biol Med* 79:261–265, 1952.
10. Thierry AM, Tassin JP, Blanc G, et al: Selective activation of the mesocortical DA system by stress, *Nature* 263:242–243, 1988.
11. Gibson GE, Pusilnalli W, Blass JP: Brain dysfunction in mild to moderate hypoxia, *Am J Med* 70:1247–1254, 1981.
12. Eidelman LA, Putterman D, Sprung CL: The spectrum of septic encephalopathy, *JAMA* 275:470–473, 1996.
13. Barkham TM, Martin EC, Eykyn SJ: Delay in the diagnosis of bacteraemic urinary tract infection in elderly patients, *Age Aging* 25:130–132, 1996.
14. Ludwig AM: *Principles of clinical psychiatry,* New York, 1980, The Free Press.
15. Adler LE, Bell J, Kirch D, et al: Psychosis associated with clonidine withdrawal, *Am J Psychiatry* 139:110–112, 1982.

16. Bastos PG, Sun X, Wagner DP, et al: Glasgow Coma Scale score in the evaluation of outcome in the intensive care unit: findings from the Acute Physiology and Chronic Health Evaluation III study, *Crit Care Med* 21:1459–1465, 1993.
17. Folstein MF, Folstein SE, McHugh PR: "Mini-Mental State," a practical method for grading the cognitive state of patients for the clinician, *J Psychiatr Res* 12:189–198, 1975.
18. Snavely SR, Hodges GR: The neurotoxicity of antibacterial agents, *Ann Intern Med*, 101:92–104, 1984.
19. Cassem NH, Lake CR, Boyer WF: *Psychopharmacology in the ICU.* In Chernow B, editor: *The pharmacologic approach to the critically ill patient,* Baltimore, 1995, Williams & Wilkins.
20. Drugs that may cause psychiatric symptoms, *Med Letter Drugs Ther* 44:59–62, 2002.
21. Sommer BR, Wise LC, Kraemer HC: Is dopamine administration possibly a risk factor for delirium? *Crit Care Med* 30:1508–1511, 2002.
22. Shochet RB, Murray GB: Neuropsychiatric toxicity of meperidine, *J Intens Care Med* 3:246–252, 1988.
23. Dubois MJ, Bergeron N, Dumont M, et al: Delirium in an intensive care unit: a study of risk factors, *Intensive Care Med* 27:1297–1304, 2001.
24. Sirois F: Steroid psychosis: a review, *Gen Hosp Psychiatry* 25:27–33, 2003.
25. Stern TA: Continuous infusion of physostigmine in anticholinergic delirium: case report, *J Clin Psychiatry* 44:463–464, 1983.
26. Shapiro BA: Sedation for mechanically ventilated patients: back to basics please! *Crit Care Med* 22:904–906, 1994.
27. Sos J, Cassem NH: *The intravenous use of haloperidol for acute delirium in intensive care settings.* In Speidel H, Rodewald G, editors: *Psychic and neurological dysfunctions after open heart surgery,* Stuttgart, 1980, George Thieme Verlag.
28. Menza MA, Murray GB, Holmes VF, et al: Decreased extrapyramidal symptoms with intravenous haloperidol, *J Clin Psychiatry* 48:278–280, 1987.
29. Forsman A, Ohman R: Pharmacokinetic studies on haloperidol in man, *Curr Therap Res* 10:319, 1976.
30. Adams F, Fernandez F, Andersson BS: Emergency pharmacotherapy of delirium in the critically ill cancer patient: intravenous combination drug approach, *Psychosomatics* 27(suppl 1):33–37, 1986.
31. Tesar GE, Murray GB, Cassem NH: Use of high-dose intravenous haloperidol in the treatment of agitated cardiac patients, *J Clin Psychopharmacol* 5:344–347, 1985.
32. Sanders KM, Stern TA, O'Gara PT, et al: Delirium after intra-aortic balloon pump therapy, *Psychosomatics* 33:35–41, 1992.
33. Fernandez F, Holmes VF, Adams F, et al: Treatment of severe, refractory agitation with a haloperidol drip, *J Clin Psychiatry* 49:239–241, 1988.

34. Metzger E, Friedman R: Prolongation of the corrected QT and torsades de pointes cardiac arrhythmia associated with intravenous haloperidol in the medically ill, *J Clin Psychopharm* 13:128–132, 1993.

35. Wilt JL, Minnema AM, Johnson RF, et al: Torsades de pointes associated with the use of intravenous haloperidol, *Ann Intern Med* 119:391–394, 1993.

36. Hunt N, Stern TA: The association between intravenous haloperidol and torsades de pointes: three cases and a literature review, *Psychosomatics* 36:541–549, 1995.

37. Di Salvo TG, O'Gara PT: Torsades de pointes caused by high-dose intravenous haloperidol in cardiac patients, *Clin Cardiol* 18:285–290, 1995.

38. Zeifman CWE, Friedman B: Torsades de pointes: potential consequence of intravenous haloperidol in the intensive care unit, *Intensive Care World* 11:109–112, 1994.

39. Day CP, James OFW, Butler TJ, et al: QT prolongation and sudden cardiac death in patients with alcoholic liver disease, *Lancet* 341:1423–1428, 1993.

40. Kao LW, Kirk MA, Evers SJ, et al: Droperidol, QT prolongation and sudden death: what is the evidence? *Ann Emerg Med* 41:546–558, 2003.

41. Schwartz TL, Masand PS: The role of atypical antipsychotics in the treatment of delirium, *Psychosomatics* 43:171–174, 2002.

42. Fernandez F, Levy JK, Mansell PWA: Management of delirium in terminally ill AIDS patients, *Int J Psychiatr Med* 19:165–172, 1989.

43. Breitbart W, Marotta RF, Call P: AIDS and neuroleptic malignant syndrome, *Lancet* 2:1488–1489, 1988.

44. Caroff SN, Rosenberg H, Mann SC, et al: Neuroleptic malignant syndrome in the critical care unit, *Crit Care Med* 30:2609, 2002.

45. Fernandez F, Levy JK: The use of molindone in the treatment of psychotic and delirious patients infected with the human immunodeficiency virus: case reports, *Gen Hosp Psychiatry* 15:31–35, 1993.

46. Olmedo R, Hoffman RS: Withdrawal syndromes, *Emerg Med Clin N Am* 18:237–288, 2000.

47. Barr J, Donner A: Optimal intravenous dosing strategies for sedatives and analgesics in the intensive care unit, *Crit Care Clin* 11:827–847, 1995.

48. Cohen IL, Gallagher TJ, Pohlman AS, et al: Management of the agitated intensive care unit patient, *Crit Care Med* 30(1 suppl):S97–S123, 2002.

49. Hurford WE: Sedation and paralysis during mechanical ventilation, *Respir Care* 47:334–347, 2002.

50. Higgins TL, Yared J-P, Estafanous FG, et al: Propofol versus midazolam for intensive care unit sedation after coronary artery bypass grafting, *Crit Care Med* 22:1415–1423, 1994.

51. Cohen D, Horiuchi K, Kemper M, et al: Modulating effects of propofol on metabolic and cardiopulmonary responses to stressful intensive care unit procedures, *Crit Care Med* 24:612–617, 1996.

52. Mirski MA, Muffelman B, Ulatowski JA, et al: Sedation for the critically ill neurologic patient, *Crit Care Med* 23:2038–2053, 1995.

53. Valenti JF, Anderson GL, Branson RD, et al: Disadvantages of prolonged propofol sedation in the critical care unit, *Crit Care Med* 22:710–712, 1994.

54. Mirenda J: Prolonged propofol sedation in the critical care unit, *Crit Care Med* 23:1304–1305, 1995.

55. El-Ebiary M, Torres A, Ramirez J, et al: Lipid deposition during the long-term infusion of propofol, *Crit Care Med* 23:1928–1930, 1995.

56. Turnage WS, Mangar D: Sufentanil, midazolam, and atracurium admixture for sedation during mechanical circulatory assistance, *Crit Care Med* 21:1099–1100, 1993.

57. Riker RR, Fraser GL, Cox PM: Continuous infusion of haloperidol controls agitation in critically ill patients, *Crit Care Med* 22:433–440, 1994.

58. Thorens J-B, Kaelin RM, Jolliet P, et al: Influence of the quality of nursing on the duration of weaning from mechanical ventilation in patients with chronic obstructive pulmonary disease, *Crit Care Med* 23:1807–1815, 1995.

59. Prezant DJ, Aldrich TK: Intravenous droperidol for the treatment of status asthmaticus, *Crit Care Med* 16:96–97, 1988.

60. Klein RF, Kliner WA, Zipes DP, et al: Transfer from a coronary care unit: some adverse responses, *Arch Intern Med* 122:104–108, 1968.

Chapter 13
Demented Patients

William E. Falk, M.D.
Roy H. Perlis, M.D.
Marilyn S. Albert, Ph.D.

Years ago, patients were frequently admitted to the hospital for what was termed a *dementia work-up*, lasting a week or more. In the current era of managed care, few patients are admitted to a general hospital solely for such a work-up. Thus requests for evaluation of cognitive changes alone usually occur in the outpatient setting. Comprehensive, multidisciplinary assessments of cognitive function are available in the outpatient clinics of many hospitals.

Acute inpatient hospitalization is still indicated, however, when dangerous behavior or psychiatric symptoms (such as assaultive or self-injurious acts) are associated with a previously diagnosed dementing disorder. Numerous specialized geriatric psychiatric units, which can effectively observe, evaluate, and manage such patients, have been developed over the past few years.

Although certain types of dementia can occur in children and young adults, most dementing disorders have advanced age as a major risk factor. This is true for the most common forms of dementia, dementia of the Alzheimer's type (DAT), and vascular dementia, which singly or in combination account for 75% to 90% of all dementing disorders.[1] Typically the request to see an inpatient on a medical or surgical floor is for a behavioral disturbance associated with a delirium (see Chapter 12), not for cognitive difficulties alone. Nonetheless, a patient who develops delirium in the hospital may have a previously undiagnosed dementing disorder. A patient with such a disorder is more likely to develop an acute confusional state than someone without dementia. For example, a demented patient may become delirious as a result of a urinary tract infection (UTI), whereas a cognitively intact elderly patient probably would not. As a useful rule of thumb, the presence of a delirium in an elderly patient should suggest the coexistence of an underlying dementia until proved otherwise.

Another common request is for evaluation of depressive symptoms associated with dementia. It is a diagnostic challenge to determine whether the mood symptoms are causing, coexisting with, or resulting from cognitive difficulties.[2] Determining the sometimes subtle differences in the history and presentation of delirium, depression, and DAT can be helpful in the diagnosis of these disorders (Table 13-1).

Other presenting problems should also raise the red flag of an underlying dementia. These include poor medication compliance and injuries that could be accounted for by memory impairment. For example, many elderly patients experience burns as a result of cooking in a dangerous manner. Another reason for referral may be difficulty coping with the inpatient setting itself. The patient, despite a gradual cognitive decline, may have functioned adequately in the familiar home setting. In the alien environment of the hospital, however, unfamiliar people provide care on an unusual schedule. As a result, trusted coping mechanisms

Table 13-1. Clinical Features of Delirium, Depression, and Dementia of the Alzheimer's Type

	Delirium	Depression	DAT
Onset	Abrupt	Relatively discrete	Insidious
Initial Symptoms	Difficulty with attention and disturbed consciousness	Dysphoric mood or lack of pleasure	Memory deficits—verbal and/or spatial
Course	Fluctuating—over days to weeks	Persistent—usually lasting months if untreated	Gradually progressive, over years
Family History	Not contributory	May be positive for depression	May be positive for DAT
Memory	Poor registration	Patchy/inconsistent	Recent > remote
Memory Complaints	Absent	Present	Variable—usually absent
Language deficits	Dysgraphia	Increased speech latency	Confrontation naming difficulties
Affect	Labile	Depressed/irritable	Variable—may be neutral

DAT, Dementical of the Alzheimer's type.

may not work; anxiety, dysphoria, agitation, or para-noia can result.

As life expectancy extends, we are likely to observe an epidemic of dementia in the general hospital; the number of cases of DAT may increase four-fold in the coming decades.[3] A major task of the consultation psychiatrist is to assist in the diagnosis and treatment of dementing disorders. A few dementing illnesses are reversible; progression of others can be slowed if identified and managed appropriately. Most dementing disorders, including DAT, are incurable; nonetheless, many can be managed. This chapter provides an overview of dementing disorders and an approach to their identification and management.

Epidemiology

According to the gerontologic literature, until the early 1800s the average life span was fairly constant, ranging from 30 to 40 years. With the advent of public health measures and antibiotics, the average life span began to increase. During the twentieth century, the life expectancy of an American increased by more than 25 years—from 47 years in 1900 to 75 years by 1980. Therefore previously unimagined numbers of people are living to old age. Furthermore, those people who are living beyond the age of 85, the so-called "oldest old," are the fastest-growing segment of the U.S. population.[4]

The significance of the "graying" of the population lies in the fact that age is a risk factor for dementia. Although results of epidemiologic studies vary depending on subjects sampled and method employed, approximately 15% of the population older than 65 years of age suffers from some form of dementia. On this basis, nearly 4 million people in the United States are affected.

The results of autopsy and clinical studies suggest that DAT, alone or in combination with other conditions, accounts for 50% to 70% of dementias seen in the population older than the age of 65. Thus it is estimated that more than 2 million people in the United States suffer from DAT.[5] In one study, the prevalence of DAT increased from 1% in the 65 to 69 age group to 40% or more among those 95 years old or older.[6] In another, the prevalence of DAT approached 50% in a community sample for persons older than the age of 85.[7]

Diagnosis

The definition of dementia in the *Diagnostic and Statistical Manual of Mental Disorders*, fourth edition (DSM-IV)[8] is somewhat different from that in previous editions. It has been simplified to emphasize that memory impairment is a necessary but not sufficient sign of the syndrome. At least one of the following additional findings must also be present: aphasia, apraxia, agnosia, or disturbances of executive function (including the ability to think abstractly, as well as to plan, initiate, sequence, monitor, and stop complex behavior). Impaired judgment, poor insight, and personality change, which previously were considered primary diagnostic features, are now considered associated features.

Table 13-2. Diagnostic Criteria for Dementia of the Alzheimer's Type

A. The development of multiple cognitive deficits manifested by both:
  (1) Memory impairment (impaired ability to learn new information or to recall previously learned information)
  (2) One (or more) of the following cognitive disturbances
    (a) Aphasia (language disturbance)
    (b) Apraxia (impaired ability to carry out motor activities despite intact motor function)
    (c) Agnosia (failure to recognize or identify objects despite intact sensory function)
    (d) Disturbance in executive functioning (i.e., planning, organizing, sequencing, abstracting)
B. The cognitive deficits in criteria A1 and A2 each cause significant impairment in social or occupational functioning and represent a significant decline from a previous level of functioning.
C. The course is characterized by gradual onset and continuing cognitive decline.
D. The cognitive deficits in criteria A1 and A2 are not due to any of the following:
  (1) Other central nervous system conditions that cause progressive deficits in memory and cognition (e.g., cerebrovascular disease, Parkinson's disease, Huntington's disease, subdural hematoma, normal pressure hydrocephalus, brain tumor)
  (2) Systemic conditions that are known to cause dementia (e.g., hypothyroidism, vitamin B_{12} or folic acid deficiency, niacin deficiency, hypercalcemia, neurosyphilis, HIV infection)
  (3) Substance-induced conditions
E. The deficits do not occur exclusively during the course of a delirium.
F. The disturbance is not better accounted for by another Axis I disorder (e.g., major depressive disorder, schizophrenia)

Code based on type of onset and predominant features:
With early onset: If onset is at age 65 years or younger:
  290.11 With delirium: If delirium is superimposed on the dementia
  290.12 With delusions: If delusions are the primary feature
  290.13 With depressed mood: If depressed mood (including presentations that meet full symptom criteria for a major depressive episode) is the predominant feature, a separate diagnosis of Mood Disorder Due to a General Medical Condition is not given
  290.10 Uncomplicated: If none of the previously noted symptoms predominate in the current clinical presentation
With late onset: If onset is after age 65 years
  290.3 With delirium: If delirium is superimposed on the dementia
  290.20 With delusions: If delusions are the primary feature
  290.21 With depressed mood: If depressed mood (including presentations that meet full symptom criteria for a major depressive episode) is the predominant feature, a separate diagnosis of Mood Disorder Due to a General Medical Condition is not given
  290.0 Uncomplicated: If none of the previously noted symptoms predominate in the current clinical presentation

Specify if:
With behavioral disturbance
Coding note: Also code 331.0 Alzheimer's disease on Axis III
HIV, Human immunodeficiency virus.
From American Psychiatric Association: *Diagnostic and statistical manual of mental disorders*, ed 4, Washington, DC, 1994, American Psychiatric Association.

Other associated characteristics may include psychiatric symptoms (e.g., persecutory delusions and hallucinations, particularly visual). Motor disturbances—falls, ataxia, and extrapyramidal signs—as well as dysarthria or slurred speech may be associated with certain dementing disorders.

Additional essential elements for a diagnosis of dementia include a significant impact on social or occupational function and a significant decline from a previous level of function. Finally, the impairment should be present at times when delirium is absent. These final criteria are necessary to rule out age-associated memory impairment, congenital mental retardation, and life-threatening acute confusional disorders.

DSM-IV provides separate diagnostic subsections for DAT (Table 13-2) and vascular dementia (replacing the term multi-infarct dementia [Table 13-3]) which is helpful given the prevalence of these disorders. DSM-IV also includes three

Table 13-3. Diagnostic Criteria for 290.4x Vascular Dementia

A. The development of multiple cognitive deficits manifested by both:
  (1) Memory impairment (impaired ability to learn new information or to recall previously learned information)
  (2) One (or more) of the following cognitive disturbances
     (a) Aphasia (language disturbance)
     (b) Apraxia (impaired ability to carry out motor activities despite intact motor function)
     (c) Agnosia (failure to recognize or identify objects despite intact sensory function)
     (d) Disturbance in executive functioning (i.e., planning, organizing, sequencing, abstracting)
B. The cognitive deficits in criteria A1 and A2 each cause significant impairment in social or occupational functioning and represent a significant decline from a previous level of functioning
C. Focal neurologic signs and symptoms (e.g., exaggeration of deep tendon reflexes, extensor plantar response, pseudobulbar palsy, gait abnormalities, weakness of an extremity) or laboratory evidence indicative of cerebrovascular disease (e.g., multiple infarctions involving cortex and underlying white matter) that are judged to be etiologically related to the disturbance
D. The deficits do not occur exclusively during the course of a delirium.
Code based on predominant features:
290.41 With delirium: If delirium is superimposed on the dementia
290.42 With delusions: If delusions are the predominant feature
290.43 With depressed mood: If depressed mood (including presentations that meet full symptom criteria for a major depressive episode) is the predominant feature, a separate diagnosis of Mood Disorder Due to a General Medical Condition is not given
290.10 Uncomplicated: If none of the previously noted symptoms predominates in the current clinical presentation

---

Specify if:
With behavioral disturbance
Coding note: Also code 436 stroke on Axis III
From American Psychiatric Association: *Diagnostic and statistical manual of mental disorders*, ed 4, Washington, DC, 1994, American Psychiatric Association.

other sections to assist the practitioner when making a specific diagnosis.

Dementia Caused by Other Medical Conditions

These conditions include a broad range of disorders that are causally associated with a dementia: structural lesions; trauma; infections; endocrine, nutritional, and metabolic disorders; and autoimmune diseases. In addition, certain disorders principally affecting brain tissue are included in this section. Dementias caused by frontotemporal dementia, Parkinson's disease, Huntington's disease, and Creutzfeldt-Jakob disease are represented here.

The term *frontotemporal dementia* actually encompasses a spectrum of disorders, including Pick's disease.[9] Whereas most other dementias present initially with cognitive decline, frontotemporal dementias may present insidiously with behavioral changes. Typical presenting symptoms may include decline in personal hygiene, disinhibition, and impaired social awareness, impulsivity, inflexibility,

rigidity, or repetitive behaviors, particularly involving an obsessive focus on certain foods. Typical age of onset for this disorder is between age 40 and 70.

Dementia with Lewy bodies shares clinical features of both Alzheimer's disease and Parkinson's disease.[10] In addition to progressive cognitive decline, the consensus criteria for clinical diagnosis require at least two of the following for a probable diagnosis: recurrent visual hallucinations (which are often well-formed), parkinsonism, and fluctuating cognition, with variation in attention and alertness. In addition, patients with dementia with Lewy bodies may suffer repeated falls and be unusually sensitive to the adverse effects of typical neuroleptics.

Substance-Induced Persisting Dementia

To establish the diagnosis of substance-induced persisting dementia, there must be evidence through history, physical examination, or laboratory data that cognitive deficits consistent with dementia are probably caused by the substance. The term *persisting* is important because the diagnosis cannot be made during a period of acute intoxication or during withdrawal. The most common cause of this type of disorder is chronic alcohol usage, but toxins, poisons, inhalants, sedative-hypnotics, and other medications are included in this section.

Dementia Resulting from Multiple Causes

The final diagnostic section of the DSM-IV, "dementia due to multiple etiologies," serves to emphasize the point that a patient can have more than one cause of cognitive decline. Although many combinations can occur, perhaps the most common example of this is the coexistence of DAT and vascular disease. Some authorities refute this assertion, suggesting that diffuse Lewy body disease is the second most common dementing disorder and that its combination with DAT is not sufficiently recognized.[11] An international conference, however, estimated the prevalence of pure Lewy body disease (in the absence of DAT) at 3% of demented patients.

Scores of specific disorders can cause dementia (Table 13-4). The consultant cannot have in-depth

Table 13-4. Dementia: Diagnosis by Categories with Representative Examples

Degenerative	HIV dementia
	HIV-associated infection
Dementia of Alzheimer's type	Syphilis
Frontal lobe dementia with/without motor neuron disease	Lyme encephalopathy
Pick's disease	Subacute sclerosing panencephalitis
Diffuse cortical Lewy body disease	Creutzfeldt-Jakob disease
Corticobasal degeneration	Progressive multifocal leukoencephalopathy
Huntington's disease	Parenchymal sarcoidosis
Wilson's disease	Chronic systemic infection
Parkinson's disease	Demyelinating
Multiple system atrophy	Multiple sclerosis
Progressive supranuclear palsy	Adrenoleukodystrophy
Psychiatric	Metachromatic leukodystrophy
Depression	Autoimmune
Schizophrenia	Systemic lupus erythematosus
Vascular	Polyarteritis nodosa
Vascular dementia	Drugs/toxins
Binswanger's encephalopathy	Medications
Amyloid dementia	Anticholinergics
Diffuse hypoxic/ischemic injury	Antihistamines
Obstructive	Anticonvulsants
Normal pressure hydrocephalus	β-Blockers
Obstructive hydrocephalus	Sedative-hypnotics
Traumatic	Substance abuse
Chronic subdural hematoma	Alcohol
Dementia pugilistica	Inhalants
Postconcussion syndrome	PCP
Neoplastic	Toxins
Tumor—Malignant—primary and secondary	Arsenic
Tumor—Benign (e.g., frontal meningioma)	Bromide
Paraneoplastic limbic encephalitis	Carbon monoxide
Infections	Lead
Chronic meningitis	Mercury
Postherpes encephalitis	Organophosphates
Focal cerebritis/abscesses	

HIV, Human immunodeficiency virus; *PCP*, phencyclidine.
Adapted from Schmahmann JD: Neurobehavioral manifestations of focal cerebral lesions, presented at the Massachusetts General Hospital course in Geriatric Psychiatry, Boston, 1995.

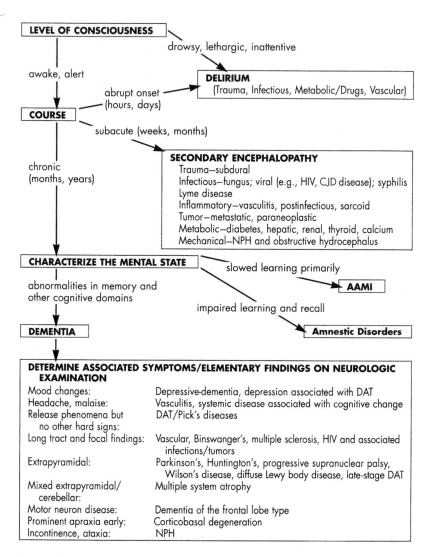

Figure 13-1. An algorithm for dementia diagnosis. *AAMI*, Age-associated memory impairment; *CJD*, Creutzfeldt-Jakob disease; *DAT*, dementia of the Alzheimer's type; *HIV*, human immunodeficiency virus; *NPH*, normal pressure hydrocephalus. (Adapted from Schmahmann JD: Neurobehavioral manifestations of focal cerebral lesions, presented at the Massachusetts General Hospital course in Geriatric Psychiatry, Boston, 1995.)

knowledge of all, but can identify common/typical and rare/unusual presentations. In addition, certain associated findings on examination can direct the consultant to particular diagnoses (Figure 13-1).

Evaluation of Dementia

Brain failure deserves at least as careful an assessment as the failure of any other organ. Only through thoughtful evaluation can remediation of the cognitive decline be possible. Too often, we hear the nihilistic viewpoint that the patient suffers from an "irreversible senility" for which nothing can be done. Although it is true that the majority of dementias are diagnosed as DAT, a disorder that is currently not curable, there is still much that can be done to help these patients and their families. The evaluation requires a reliable history (cognitive, psychiatric, medical, and family), complete medical and neurologic examinations, appropriate laboratory testing, and assessments of the mental status and cognitive function. Although definitive diagnosis of DAT is made only at autopsy with the observation of amyloid plaques and neurofibrillary tangles, a detailed history allows a diagnosis to be made with considerable confidence.

History

A meticulous cognitive history is an extremely sensitive diagnostic tool. Consequently, the patient should never be the sole informant. Onset, course, and associated symptoms must be elicited carefully because these details of history are often the most important diagnostic clues.

Because of time constraints, consultants may be inclined to limit their history-taking to the patient alone. Although some mildly impaired patients may have sufficient capacity to provide an accurate accounting of their deficits, many (owing to their amnesia, agnosia, or failure of insight) do not. To rely solely on the patient's report is unwise; it may be inaccurate and it will be incomplete. The history is best obtained from family members or close friends. It is important to interview informants away from the patient because informants are often uncomfortable discussing evidence of cognitive decline in the presence of the patient. Even a phone call to a family member or a friend can be helpful, as can reviewing old medical records, when available.

A good cognitive history must establish the time at which cognitive changes first became apparent. This information provides important clues regarding the nature of the disorder because some diseases (e.g., Creutzfeldt-Jakob disease) are well known for causing a rapid rate of decline. It also assists the clinician in giving the family some preliminary feedback about the anticipated course of the illness. If time of onset of the disorder is known, the rate of decline can be estimated by seeing how long it has taken the patient to reach the current level of dysfunction. The rate of progression can be only roughly approximated; however, it is helpful to the family to have such estimations to guide them in making plans for the future.

Next, it is important to determine the nature of the behavioral changes that were evident when the disease began. This information can be helpful in the diagnostic process. For example, an early symptom of frontotemporal dementia is a personality change, as manifested by inappropriate behavior, whereas the early symptoms of DAT involve increased passivity and a gradual, progressive decline in the ability to learn new information. Several years after the onset of the disease, when most patients are actually diagnosed, the cognitive symptoms of the two disorders may be quite similar, so information about the initial symptoms may be critical.

It is also important to determine whether the initial symptoms came on gradually or suddenly. If the onset of illness is gradual and insidious, as in DAT, it is often only in retrospect that the family realizes that a decline has occurred. In contrast, a series of small strokes produces a history of sudden onset, even if not evident on computed tomography (CT) or magnetic resonance imaging (MRI) of the head. There is generally an incident (e.g., a fall or a period of confusion) that heralds the onset of the disorder (Table 13-5).[11] Delirium generally has an acute onset as well. If it results from a condition such as a gradually developing drug toxicity, however, onset may be subacute or insidious.

The manner in which symptoms have progressed over time also provides important diagnostic information. Stepwise deterioration characterized by

Table 13-5. Ischemic Score*

Feature	Value, if present	Score
Abrupt onset	2	___
Stepwise deterioration	1	___
Fluctuating course	2	___
Nocturnal confusion	1	___
Relative preservation of personality	1	___
Depression	1	___
Somatic complaints	1	___
Emotional incontinence	1	___
History of hypertension	1	___
History of strokes	2	___
Evidence of associated atherosclerosis	1	___
Focal neurologic symptoms	2	___
Focal neurologic signs	2	___
Total Score		___

*A total score of 5 or greater is suggestive of vascular dementia. From Hachinski VC, Illiff LD, Zilhka E, et al: Cerebral blood flow in dementia, *Arch Neurol* 32:632–637, 1975.

sudden exacerbation of symptoms is typical of vascular dementia. A physical illness (e.g., pneumonia or a hip fracture), in a patient with DAT however, can cause a sudden decline in cognitive function. Thus careful questioning is necessary to determine the underlying cause of a stepwise decline in function.

Accurate cognitive histories are difficult to obtain because most patients and family members are not attuned to the observation and description of subtle behavioral changes. Important aspects of the medical history may not be recognized. For example, the family may state that the first symptoms of the disease were the patient's anxiety and depression about work. Only after further inquiry will family members remember several episodes that preceded the onset of work-related anxiety in which the patient could not remember how to deal with a complex situation or to learn how to use new equipment.

Family members may also have difficulty understanding why certain subtle distinctions are important for diagnosis. For example, they may report that the patient's first symptom was forgetfulness but when asked to provide instances of this forgetfulness may explain that the patient had difficulty installing a new knob in the kitchen or had trouble finding a familiar location. Both features would suggest more spatial difficulty than memory difficulty. In addition, an unwillingness to admit that certain impairments exist may prevent family members from providing accurate information.

Finally, family members can sometimes misinterpret even direct questions. Although a history of gradual, progressive decline is essential to the diagnosis of DAT, informants frequently state that the disorder came on suddenly because they suddenly became aware that something was wrong. This realization on the part of the family often coincides with external events (e.g., a trip to an unfamiliar place prevented the patient from employing over-learned habits and routines, and thus exposed the cognitive decline). The hospital is obviously one such setting; it is not infrequent for family members to state, "He was fine until he got here!" When this misconception appears, it is necessary to determine carefully when subtle symptoms of cognitive change first occurred. Usually, family members can recall episodes that they had previously ignored but that suggest an earlier change in cognitive function.

It is also important to determine the patient's current functional status. This information is best obtained in an informal manner by asking about the patient's typical day. Alternatively, scales, such as the activities of daily living (ADL) scale, have been developed for this purpose. The ADL scale surveys six basic areas of function: bathing, dressing, toileting, transferring, continence, and feeding.[12] The interviewer determines whether the individual can perform these tasks independently or with assistance. The instrumental activities of daily living (IADL) scale provides a sense of a patient's executive functions, including the capacity to use the telephone, ambulate, go shopping, prepare meals, do housework, make home repairs, do laundry, administer medication, and manage money.[13] A substantial discrepancy between the functional and cognitive status of the patient generally suggests the presence of a psychiatric illness. For purposes of comfort, safety, rehabilitation, and determination of appropriate level of care, ADLs and IADLs should be evaluated carefully.

Psychiatric history, looking particularly for reports of past mood or psychotic disorders, may assist in the differentiation of cognitive changes observed in depression from those of a primary dementing disorder. Although cognitive changes can be seen in depression, the history and mental status examination usually allow one to separate depression and dementia or to suggest that both are present. Neurovegetative symptoms of depression may be difficult to link specifically to mood or cognitive disorders because anergia, sleep disturbance, and appetite changes can be seen in both depression and dementia. Thus it is important to modify the questions asked to encompass the possibility of cognitive impairment. For example, if the tasks are simplified and within the capabilities of a nondepressed, demented patient, the patient is typically able to carry them out. Similarly, if food is presented in a manner that the patient can manage, such as meat cut into bite-size pieces, the patient may manifest gusto in his or her eating where none had been seen before (see Table 13-1).

In reviewing medical history, one should consider whether or not surgical procedures (e.g., gastrectomy predisposing to vitamin B_{12} deficiency) or medical illnesses (e.g., hypertension or systemic lupus erythematosus) contribute to the symptoms of cognitive dysfunction. Query regarding blood transfusions (particularly during the early to mid 1980s, when human immunodeficiency virus testing was not readily available) or exposure to toxins (such as lead, other heavy metals, or carbon monoxide), as well as any history of head trauma is crucial. Careful questioning should cover alcohol and drug usage (not just current patterns), including past history of abuse or overuse. Many nonpsychotropic agents, including those sold over-the-counter, can have negative effects on cognition. For example, antihistamines and antispasmodic drugs can cause cognitive difficulties.

The family history portion of the evaluation is helpful for diagnosis. Certain dementing disorders (e.g., Huntington's disease) have definite genetic modes of transmission (e.g., autosomal dominant), whereas for others (e.g., certain vascular dementias), the specific mode of transmission may be unclear, but their prevalence is much higher in affected families than in the population at large. Several familial subtypes of DAT with genetic loci have been identified. An estimated 7% of cases with onset before age 60 are familial, with autosomal dominant inheritance. Several genes, including beta-amyloid precursor protein and presenilin 1 and 2, have been associated with early-onset DAT.[14] The majority of patients with DAT appear to have a complex interaction between genetics and other factors.[15] Variations in the gene for apolipoprotein E, for example, may increase the risk of developing DAT or predispose to earlier onset.[16]

Medical and Neurologic Examination

The consultant should review recent examinations in the medical record to assess their adequacy and accuracy. The cognitive portion of prior examinations may note only that the patient is alert and oriented. Additionally, if notes report "disorientation," it is often unclear from the chart whether the patient could not remember the day of the week or whether he or she was confused or psychotic. Consequently, the psychiatric consultant should look for medical and neurologic findings that are associated with dementing disorders. For example, focal areas of muscle weakness and pyramidal signs may suggest vascular dementia. The presence of extrapyramidal movements may point to

one of the dementias principally affecting subcortical motor areas. Mild-to-moderate DAT, however, may also be associated with extrapyramidal symptoms and other neurologic signs.[17] A comprehensive neurologic examination should include careful assessment of ocular function, as well as the presence of any frontal release signs.

Laboratory Examination

Table 13-6 lists hematologic and other tests that are typically ordered as part of a dementia evaluation. Whenever possible and appropriate, results of prior testing in other settings should be obtained. For example, a chest x-ray examination or CT

Table 13-6. Recommended Laboratory Studies in Dementia Work-up

---

Blood studies
  Complete blood cell count
  Vitamin B_{12}
  Folate
  Sedimentation rate
  Glucose
  Calcium
  Phosphorus
  Magnesium
  Electrolytes
  Liver function tests
  Thyroid-stimulating hormone
  Creatinine, blood urea nitrogen
  Cholesterol (high-density lipoprotein/low-density
    lipoprotein)
  Triglycerides
  Syphilis serology
Urinalysis
Other studies
  Electrocardiogram
  CT or MRI
Representative additional studies based on history and
    physical findings
  Chest x-ray examination
  Electroencephalogram
  Noninvasive carotid studies
  Human immunodeficiency virus testing
  Rheumatoid factor, antinuclear antibody, and other
    autoimmune disorder screens
  Lumbar puncture
  Drug levels
  Heavy metal screening

CT, Computed tomography; *MRI*, magnetic resonance imaging.

scan should not be reordered if one was recently done unless an acute change has occurred. Additional tests (e.g., serum copper and ceruloplasmin for Wilson's disease or serum and urine porphyrins for acute intermittent porphyria) should be requested when history and examination suggest a particular disorder.

Psychiatric Mental Status Examination

The bedside psychiatric examination covers considerable territory but it focuses on assessments of affective and psychotic symptoms and signs. One should probe for mood symptoms, irritability or tearfulness, and nihilistic or suicidal thinking. Depressed elderly patients may, among their somatic complaints, describe decrements in memory. Depressed patients, as opposed to DAT patients, however, may perform better on more difficult memory tasks than on simple ones.

Psychotic symptoms can be present in primary psychiatric disorders, such as psychotic depression or schizophrenia, but they can also be associated signs of delirium or dementia. The prevalence of psychosis in moderate-to-severe DAT is estimated to be in the range of 40% to 80%.[18] Usually, delusions in patients with DAT are of a paranoid nature, often with the mistaken belief that misplaced items have been stolen. With progression of the disease, the patient may come to believe that spouses are parents or that they are actually imposters (i.e., Capgras' syndrome). Illusions and hallucinations, usually of a visual nature, also occur with advanced DAT. For example, some patients describe seeing "little people" entering their homes. Despite their unusual nature, not all hallucinations or delusions are troublesome to the patient. Mood and psychotic symptoms can occur as part of the clinical picture of many dementing disorders. Generally, they are nonspecific. Taken together with other elements of the assessment, however, such symptoms can provide clues as to whether a psychiatric disorder or a dementing disorder is present.

Cognitive Assessment

Domains of cognitive function that require rapid and accurate bedside assessment can be remembered with the mnemonic A CALM VISAGE, the face the consultant would put forward when confronted with a difficult-to-diagnose patient. These include the following: Attention, Conceptualization, Appearance/behavior, Language, Memory, VISuospatial, Agnosia and apraxia, and General intelligence.

Attention is important to consider because simple attentional abilities must be preserved if any other cognitive task is to be performed adequately. If the patient has difficulty concentrating on a task for 1 to 3 minutes at a time, assessment of other areas of function is inadequate. For this reason, attention is often assessed before other cognitive domains have been evaluated. Auditory and visual attention can be assessed easily by means of digit span and letter cancellation tests. With digit span, the patient is asked to repeat a series of numbers spaced 1 second apart. Gradually increasing spans are provided by the examiner; unimpaired individuals are able to repeat five to seven numbers. With letter cancellation, the patient is asked to cross off a particular letter each time it is observed in any series of letters. A gross assessment can be inferred from how well the patient responds to questions during an interview. The physician should note whether there appears to be a fluctuation in the level of arousal or easy distractibility during the interview.

Tasks that examine conceptualization include tests of concept formation, abstraction, set shifting, and set maintenance. Similarities and proverbs are useful in this regard.

Observation of appearance and behavior is helpful in determining whether patients are able to care adequately for themselves. Detecting that a patient's buttons are misaligned, for example, may suggest that he or she has spatial difficulties or apraxias.

Language testing for aphasia should include evaluation of comprehension, repetition, reading, writing, and naming. If aphasia has been ruled out or is not suspected, confrontation naming (e.g., of objects and their parts, such as jacket and lapel) should be included in an assessment of the older individual because declines in naming ability occur with age but are prominent in a number of disorders, including DAT. In addition, alterations in verbal fluency (tested by having the patient name as many animals or words beginning with a certain letter as possible in a minute) are seen in many dementing diseases.[19]

The presence of memory dysfunction is essential for a diagnosis of dementia. The nature and severity of the memory impairment can serve as a guide to diagnosis, but the assessment of memory is complicated by the fact that changes in memory capacity normally occur with aging. Normal elders may require more time to retain new information. Therefore careful testing is important to differentiate normal from pathologic memory performance.

Assessment of visuospatial abilities may be more difficult in the elderly than in the young because of the frequency of visuosensory deficits in the older age group. It is difficult to enlarge certain test stimuli to evaluate this domain; therefore figure copying (e.g., of intersecting pentagons or a cube) is the most useful method of assessment.

When agnosia or apraxia is evident, the patient usually has quite advanced disease. Agnosia is diagnosed when a patient fails to recognize a familiar object despite intact sensory function. With apraxia, the patient's ability to carry out motor tasks is impaired despite intact motor systems and an understanding of the tasks. For example, the patient is unable to mimic the use of common objects (such as use of a toothbrush) or carry out well-learned motor behaviors (such as pretending to blow out a candle). A subtle finding is "organification of praxis" in which the subject, for example, uses a finger as the toothbrush.

In addition to the areas of assessment previously mentioned, the examiners should estimate general intelligence to determine whether the patient has access to previously acquired knowledge. A rough approximation can be inferred from the patient's highest level of education. Alternatively, the vocabulary subtest of the Wechsler Adult Intelligence Scale–Revised can be used to estimate level of intelligence.[20]

Mini-Mental State Examination

Nonstandard testing developed by the clinician can be used to evaluate the cognitive domains noted previously, but a variety of standardized, brief mental status tests can be useful as well. Commonly used screening tests are the Mini-Mental State Examination (MMSE),[21] the Blessed Dementia Scale,[22] and the Short Portable Mental Status Questionnaire.[23] All have high test-retest reliability, and

all are relatively brief, taking 5 to 15 minutes to administer. Of these, the MMSE is most often used in clinical settings (Table 13-7). It is excellent for this purpose because it assesses a broad range of cognitive abilities (i.e., attention, concentration, memory, language, spatial ability, and set shifting) in a simple, straightforward manner. The other screening tests mentioned primarily evaluate memory and orientation. Screening tests may identify cognitive difficulties, but they are not sufficient to establish a diagnosis of dementia.

The wide use of the MMSE in epidemiologic studies has yielded cutoff scores that facilitate the identification of patients with cognitive dysfunction. In addition, the popularity of the MMSE has produced considerable familiarity with its scoring system, facilitating communication among clinicians. Scores on the MMSE range from 0 to 30, with scores greater than 26 generally indicating normal cognitive function. Mildly impaired patients typically obtain MMSE scores of 20 to 26, moderate impairment is reflected in scores of 11 to 20, and severe impairment is indicated by scores of 10 or lower. A cutoff score of 23 is generally recommended as suggestive of cognitive dysfunction; however, the application of this cutoff score must be modified by the knowledge of the educational level of the patient. For example, subjects with a substantial amount of formal education can experience a considerable amount of cognitive decline before a score of 23 is achieved, whereas nondemented persons with little education may obtain a score of 23 at baseline. This effect occurs because some items on the MMSE require at least a minimal educational background. For example, "serial 7s" (a task requiring the patient to subtract 7 from 100, and continue subtracting 7 from the result), which contributes heavily to the score, can be difficult for most elderly persons who have limited education. This difficulty may lower the total score such that, with a few other minor errors, the patient falls below the cutoff point on the test.

Studies offer some guidelines for adjusting the MMSE cutoff scores according to the premorbid education of the patient. Murden and associates[24] reported that a cutoff score of 17 produced a sensitivity of 81% and a specificity of 100% for dementia in geriatric patients with 8 or fewer years of education. Among those with more than 8 years of education, the standard cutoff score of 23 yielded

Table 13-7. Mini-Mental State Examination

Patient _____   Date _____
Examiner _____

Maximum Score	Patient Score	
		Orientation
5	[ ]	What is the (year) (season) (date) (day) (month)?
5	[ ]	Where are we (state) (county) (town) (hospital) (floor)?
		Registration
3	[ ]	Name three objects: Give 1 second to say each, then ask the patient all three after you have said them. Give 1 point for each correct answer, then repeat them until he or she learns all three. Count trials and record, Trials ____
		Attention and Calculation
5	[ ]	Serial 7s: 1 point for each correct. Stop after 5 answers. Alternately, spell *world* backward.
		Recall
3	[ ]	Ask for the three objects repeated in previous test. Give 1 point for each correct answer.
		Language
2	[ ]	Name a pencil and a watch
1	[ ]	Repeat the following: "No ifs, ands, or buts."
3	[ ]	Follow a three-stage command: "Take a paper in your right hand, fold it in half, and put it on the floor." Give 1 point for each part done correctly.
1	[ ]	Read and obey the following: "Close your eyes!"
1	[ ]	Write a sentence. Must contain subject and verb and be sensible.
		Visual-Motor Integrity
1	[ ]	Copy design (two intersecting pentagons). All 10 angles must be present and 2 must intersect.
30		Patients' Total Score

Adapted from Folstein MF, Folstein SE, McHugh PE: Mini-Mental State Exam: a practical method for grading the cognitive state of patients for the clinician, *J Psychiatr Res* 12:189–198, 1975.

a sensitivity of 93% and a specificity of 100%. But even with higher scores, if by history memory is notably affected, further testing is warranted.

Tests for Severe Impairment

The MMSE is a useful screening tool in the assessment of demented patients with mild-to-moderate cognitive impairments, but it is less helpful, in the evaluation of the severely impaired patient. The quantification of cognitive abilities in severely impaired patients can serve a variety of needs, including the ability to follow patients throughout an intervention trial, the assessment of spared abilities (which health care professionals can use in the development of management strategies), and the examination of the relationship between post-mortem neurochemical and neuropathologic findings and cognitive status shortly before death.

The Test for Severe Impairment (TSI) is a useful scale for severely impaired patients that can contribute to improved patient management (Table 13-8).[25] It minimizes the need for the patient to use language skills because severely impaired patients often have minimal intact verbal skills. Nonetheless the TSI can evaluate motor performance, language comprehension, language production, immediate and delayed memory, general knowledge, and conceptualization. Stimulus items needed to administer the TSI are small and commonly available (i.e., five various colored pens, two large paper clips, a key, a comb, and a spool of thread).

With all structured tests, the examiner must not simply look at the total score but rather assess the qualitative areas of low and high function. The pattern of deficits may confirm a diagnostic opinion. Conversely, determining that areas of function have been preserved assists the clinician in making

Table 13-8. Test for Severe Impairment

Name _____   Date _____   Age _____
ID # _____   Rm # _____

Write down all responses verbatim that are different from those on the sheet, If Subject (S) does not hear a question or is distracted, you may repeat the question up to five times to engage Subject's attention.

	Maximum Score	Score
1. Motor Performance		
A. Comb: "SHOW ME HOW TO USE THIS COMB." Hand S comb.		
Correctly demonstrates combing:	1	_____
B. Pen and top: "CAN YOU PUT THE TOP ON THE PEN?" Remove the top of the pen in full view of S, hand the pen and top to S.		
Correctly puts top on pen (not on bottom of pen):	1	_____
C. Pen and paper: "WRITE YOUR NAME." Hand S pen (without the top) and place paper on table in front of S.		
Writes name correctly (first or last name legible):	1	_____
	Total (3)	_____
2. Language—comprehension		
A. "POINT TO YOUR EAR." "CLOSE YOUR EYES."		
Correctly points to ear:	1	_____
Correctly closes eyes:	1	_____
B. Pens—red, blue, green		
"SHOW ME THE RED PEN,. . .THE GREEN PEN." Place the two pens on the table spread out so that they have some space between them.		
Correctly points to red pen:	1	_____
Correctly points to green pen:	1	_____
	Total (4)	_____
3. Language—production		
A. "WHAT IS THIS CALLED?" Point to your nose.		
Correctly identifies nose:	1	_____
B. Pens—red, green		
"WHAT COLOR IS THIS PEN?" One at a time, hold up a (red/green) pen in front of S.		
Correctly names red:	1	_____
Correctly names green:	1	_____
C. "WHAT IS THIS CALLED?" Show S the key.		
Correctly names key:	1	_____
	Total (4)	_____
4. Memory—immediate		
One large paper clip: "WATCH CAREFULLY," Place clip in your hand so S can see. Hold hands out to S.		
A. With hands open—"WHICH HAND IS THE CLIP IN?"		
Correctly points to clip:	1	_____
B. With hands closed—"WHICH HAND IS THE CLIP IN?"		
Correctly points to clip:	1	_____
C. Move hands behind back—"WATCH CAREFULLY. WHICH HAND/SIDE IS THE CLIP IN/ON?"		
Correctly points to hand with clip.	1	_____
	Total (3)	_____
5. General Knowledge		
A. "HOW MANY EARS DO I HAVE?"		
Correctly states two:	1	_____

Continued

Table 13-8. *Continued*

B. "COUNT MY FINGERS AND THUMBS." Place hands in front of S with fingers pointing up, palms toward S. Credit given even if no one-to-one correspondence between fingers and numbers. If S only gives final answer, ask "CAN YOU COUNT TO 10 STARTING AT '1'?"		
Correctly counts to 10:	1	_____
C. "HOW MANY WEEKS ARE IN A YEAR?"		
Correctly states 52:	1	_____
D. "I'M GOING TO SING A SONG. IF YOU KNOW THE WORDS, I WANT YOU TO SING ALONG WITH ME." Softly sing "Happy Birthday."		
Sings most of the words	1	_____
	Total (4)	_____
6. Conceptualization		
A. Two large paper clips, one pen		
"WHICH ONE OF THESE IS DIFFERENT FROM THE OTHER TWO?" Spread objects out on the table.		
Correctly points to pen or states *pen*:	1	_____
B. Two red pens, one green pen		
"PUT THIS NEXT TO THE PEN THAT IS THE SAME COLOR." Place one red and one green pen spread out on the table. Hand S the other red pen.		
Correctly matches pen by color:	1	_____
C. One large paper clip		
Place hands out in front of S. Alternate the clip between the open hands four times. "WATCH ME MOVE THE PAPER CLIP. WHICH HAND WILL I PUT THE CLIP IN NEXT?" After S responds, place clip in correct hand; if S is incorrect, say "I'D PUT THE CLIP IN THIS HAND." Then say, "WHICH HAND WILL I PUT IT IN NEXT?"		
Correctly points to correct hand:	1	_____
	Total (3)	_____
7. Memory—delayed		
Thread, key, paper clip "WHICH ONE OF THESE HAVEN'T WE DONE SOMETHING WITH WHILE YOU WERE HERE WITH ME?" Place objects spread out on table.		
Correctly points to thread:	1	_____
	Total (1)	_____
8. Motor Performance		
"THANK YOU FOR SPENDING TIME WITH ME." Extend hand to shake hands.		
Correctly shakes hands:	1	_____
	Total (1) Grand Total (24)	_____

From Albert M, Cohen C: The test for severe impairment: an instrument for the assessment of patients with severe cognitive impairment, *J Am Geriatr Soc* 40:449–453,1992.

recommendations to the patient and the family for adaptive coping with the dementia.

Treatment Considerations

The approach to treatment of a dementing disorder depends on the specific diagnosis established as well as on the troublesome symptoms and signs that must be managed. Treatment is divided into three broad categories: medical and surgical interventions, behavioral treatments, and pharmacotherapy.

Medical and Surgical Interventions

Some dementing disorders can be helped dramatically by surgical intervention. One example is the benefit achieved by the shunting of cerebrospinal fluid in patients with normal pressure hydrocephalus.[26] Similarly, patients who have frontal subdural hematomas drained can improve their cognition and behavior.

Other reversible medical disorders that cause dementia should be corrected. For example, thyroid repletion in the myxedematous patient improves cognitive functioning. In many conditions, however, damage has already been done, and repletion may provide only marginal improvement. For example, a patient who had deteriorated over several years was found to have an extremely low vitamin B_{12} level. Her dementia was profound, and it did not respond to intramuscular injections of vitamin B_{12}. Further deterioration of her cognition and other nervous system functions, however, may have been prevented by the treatment.

Sometimes the reduction or elimination of drugs can be helpful. For example, patients with Parkinson's disease and psychotic symptoms secondary to use of dopamine agonists may require dosage adjustment to reduce the psychotic symptoms. Other examples are barbiturate-induced cognitive decline, or benzodiazepine-induced memory impairment. Elimination of the sedative is essential because cognitive symptoms caused by the drug are most likely to remit with cessation. Care must be taken, however, to avoid a withdrawal syndrome caused by too abrupt a discontinuation.

Searching for treatable contributors to cognitive decline is important, even when the principal diagnosis is DAT. Identification of coexisting medical conditions that have a deleterious effect on the patient's cognition is critical. For example, the aggressive treatment of a UTI not only improves physical comfort, but also intellectual functioning (because infection in the face of DAT usually causes a delirium). Pain, too, may have a negative effect on cognition. A patient whose DAT was manageable at home became severely aggressive and more confused owing to the discomfort of an impacted bowel. Another patient with presumed vascular dementia showed some improvement in cognition when congestive heart failure was treated.

Behavioral Treatments

Once drug effects and contributing medical conditions are identified and managed, acute behavioral symptoms associated with dementia may subside.

The environmental strangeness of the hospital, however, may be enough to trigger new psychiatric and behavioral problems, such as paranoid thinking and agitation.

Often, behavioral management alone reduces certain symptoms. The basic approaches are well known but bear repeating. Patients with dementia require frequent reorientation to their environment. The addition of clock and calendar assists in this regard. Having the family bring in familiar pictures from the home can be quite reassuring.

The way staff communicates with the patient is also important. Speaking "just loud enough" is a critical first step. Decreased hearing acuity affects all elders, but this does not mean that one has to shout at them. The content of what is said should be simple and to the point. If the patient has considerable expressive language difficulties, questions should be framed so that a yes-no response is adequate. Reassurance and distraction are preferred responses to patients who are easily distressed or become paranoid.[27]

Pharmacotherapy

Pharmacotherapies in dementia generally target both cognitive decline and the behavioral and other psychiatric consequences of disease. Because DAT is associated with cholinergic dysfunction, cholinesterase inhibitors (ChE-Is) have been developed and are now widely used in treatment. A recent meta-analysis concluded that these agents have modest benefit in the neuropsychiatric symptoms and functional impairment in mild to moderate DAT.[28]

The commonly-used ChE-Is in the United States include donepezil, rivastigmine, and galantamine. A fourth agent, tacrine, is no longer widely used because of its association with hepatotoxicity. The ChE-Is differ in their pharmacokinetic and dynamic properties; for example, donepezil is generally administered once daily, whereas the galantamine and rivastigmine are dosed twice daily.

Evidence-based recommendations suggest that treatment with a ChE-I should begin as early as possible in DAT patients.[29] The usefulness of these agents in other forms of dementia is not well studied. The most common side effects include nausea, vomiting and diarrhea; other bothersome adverse effects may include insomnia or vivid dreams, fatigue, muscle cramps, incontinence, and bradycardia or syncope. As a result, these drugs may be contraindicated in cases of bradycardia or sick-sinus syndrome; severe asthma and peptic ulcer disease may also be relative contraindications.

Finally, memantine, an N-methyl-D-aspartate antagonist, reduced clinical deterioration in moderate to severe DAT with few side effects; it is likely to be approved by the U.S. Food and Drug Administration in 2004.[30]

Pharmacotherapy may also be useful for managing disruptive or distressing psychiatric or behavioral symptoms unresponsive to the medical corrections and behavioral interventions noted. Furthermore, certain symptoms are poorly responsive to drug therapies. For example, the motor restlessness and wandering behavior seen in DAT patients are typically nonresponsive to medications; in addition, some treatments (e.g., neuroleptics that cause akathisia) may actually aggravate the problem.[31] When other symptoms, such as visual hallucinations or delusions, cause no distress to the patient and are not dangerous, medication is not required.

When treatment is necessary, the golden rule of geriatric pharmacotherapy is, "Start low, go slowly, but go all the way." This maxim applies whether target symptoms relate to psychosis, depression, agitation, or some combination of these three domains.

Psychotic Symptoms

Hallucinations (particularly visual) and delusions (paranoid, persecutory, somatic, and others) are common in DAT but they can also occur in other primary dementing disorders.[32,33] The first-line treatment of these symptoms is an atypical antipsychotic, of which risperidone is the best studied to date.[34] High-potency neuroleptics, such as haloperidol, trifluoperazine, perphenazine, and thiothixene, are all equally effective in the treatment of psychotic symptoms.[34] Specific guidelines are difficult to provide because patients can differ considerably in their tolerance to neuroleptics. The atypical antipsychotics may be better tolerated than typical high-potency agents because of their relatively benign side effect profile (although some concern

has been recently noted about the rare association of risperidone treatment and cerebrovascular events, particularly in patients with vascular dementia). For example, dosing risperidone at 0.25 mg/day to start, with gradual dose increments, may be quite helpful.[35] In our experience, low-potency agents, such as thioridazine or chlorpromazine, have marginal utility because of their sedative and postural hypotensive side effects, often seen at all but extremely low doses.

Treatment of psychosis associated with Parkinson's disease requires special mention. High-potency neuroleptics may aggravate tremor and bradykinesia; here too, atypical antipsychotics likely cause fewer side effects and have been used with success.[36]

Depression

The depressive component of any dementia should be assessed and treated aggressively. If it is unclear how much affective symptoms are contributing to cognitive dysfunction, a therapeutic trial of an antidepressant should be employed. Choice of an agent is based principally on the side effects it produces; the selective serotonin reuptake inhibitors (e.g., fluoxetine, paroxetine, sertraline, and citalopram) and bupropion have favorable side effect profiles and should be considered, despite a paucity of literature on their use in depression associated with dementia. Nortriptyline has been used effectively in depression following strokes and is generally well tolerated.[37] Tertiary amine tricyclics (such as amitriptyline and imipramine) should be avoided. When anergy or lack of motivation are prominent symptoms with dementia, psychostimulants could be tried.[38] Finally, as long as they are administered in a safe manner, monoamine oxidase inhibitors may be useful in the treatment of depression associated with DAT.[39]

Agitation

Agitation can take the form of motor restlessness, verbal outbursts, or physical aggression. There are no Food and Drug Administration–approved drugs for the treatment of these symptoms in the context of dementia, but many classes of drugs (including neuroleptics, benzodiazepines, antidepressants, β-blockers, and mood stabilizers) have been tried. Before instituting any medication, reversible causes of agitation, such as infection or drug effects, should be investigated.

Neuroleptics are the most widely used agents for agitation[40]; in addition to oral forms, some agents may be administered intramuscularly when required.[41,42] Dosage recommendations are generally the same as for treatment of psychotic symptoms. Usage should be reassessed periodically, particularly because target symptoms may subside with disease progression and tardive movement disorders occur frequently in this population and typically do not resolve spontaneously.[31]

Benzodiazepines have also been used to treat the agitation associated with dementia; however, the risk of worsening cognition and inducing behavioral disinhibition should be weighed, particularly before prescribing a long-acting agent (such as diazepam or clonazepam) or prescribing them for protracted periods.[43] The short-acting lorazepam (in an oral dosage of 0.25 to 1 mg) is often quite helpful when administered before an uncomfortable or potentially frightening procedure, such as lumbar puncture or MRI. Reports of buspirone's treatment of agitation exist, but it usually takes at least a few weeks to achieve a modest benefit with this agent.[44]

Among the antidepressants, trazodone has been the subject of most case reports demonstrating behavioral improvement in agitated, demented patients.[45] In our experience, it has been modestly effective for agitation but quite useful for nocturnal insomnia.[46] Starting at a dosage of 25 to 50 mg/day, trazodone can be increased to as much as 400 mg/day, as tolerated. Sedative effects are usually quite rapidly achieved. Although generally well tolerated, trazodone may induce postural hypotension and priapism.

β-Blockers (e.g., propranolol and pindolol) have been beneficial in treatment of agitation associated with dementias of various causes.[47] The risk of side effects, however, may outweigh potential benefits; a gradual dosage escalation is necessary, particularly with geriatric patients.

Finally, lithium carbonate, carbamazepine, and valproic acid have all been reported to treat agitation associated with dementia.[48–50] Of the three, valproic acid may hold the most promise because doses found effective were low and side effects were minimal and well tolerated. In an open-label study of 10 elderly patients with DAT or vascular dementia, Lott and colleagues[50] observed "moderate" or better improvement in eight, with doses ranging from 250 to 750 mg (yielding levels of 13 to 52 μg/ml).

Conclusions

As the population ages, the number of people with dementing disorders is increasing dramatically; most have DAT or vascular dementia. Although neither is curable, both have treatable components (e.g., with ChE-Is),[51,52] as have all other dementias—whether they are reversible, static, or progressive. The role of the psychiatric consultant in the diagnosis and treatment of dementing disorders is important, particularly in the identification of treatable psychiatric and behavioral symptoms.

Family members are the hidden victims of progressive dementia. They typically appreciate the consultant's communication about the diagnosis and the expected course of the disorder. They can benefit from advice about how best to relate to the patient, how to restructure the home environment, and how to seek out legal and financial guidance if appropriate. Family members also should be made aware of the assistance available to them through such organizations as the Alzheimer's Association.

References

1. Cummings JL, Benson DP: *Dementia: a clinical approach*, ed 2, Boston, 1992, Butterworth-Heinemann.
2. Emory VO, Oxman TE: Update on the dementia spectrum of depression, *Am J Psychiatry* 149:305–317, 1992.
3. Fratiglioni L, Launer LJ, Andersen K, et al, for the Neurologic Diseases in the Elderly Research Group: Incidence of dementia and major subtypes in Europe: a collaborative study of population-based cohorts. *Neurology* 54:S10–S15, 2000.
4. Albert MS, Moss MB: *Geriatric neuropsychology*, New York, 1988, Guilford Press.

5. Jenike MA: *Geriatric psychiatry and psychopharmacology:* a clinical approach, Chicago, 1989, Yearbook Medical Publishers.

6. Hy LX, Keller DM: Prevalence of AD among whites: a summary by levels of severity. *Neurology* 55:198–204, 2000.

7. Evans DA, Funkenstein HH, Albert MS, et al: Prevalence of Alzheimer's disease in a community population of older persons, *JAMA* 262:2551–2556, 1989.

8. American Psychiatric Association: *Diagnostic and statistical manual of mental disorders*, ed 4 (DSM-IV), Washington, DC, 1994, American Psychiatric Association.

9. Kertesz A, Munoz DG: Frontotemporal dementia. *Med Clin North Am* 86:501–518, 2002.

10. Ritchie K, Lovestone S: The dementias, *Lancet* 360:1759–1766, 2002.

11. Beck BJ: Neuropsychiatric manifestations of diffuse Lewy body disease, *J Geriatr Psychiatr Neurol* 8:189–196, 1995.

12. Katz S, Downs TD, Cash HR, et al: Progress in the development of the index of ADL, *Gerontologist* 10:20–30, 1970.

13. Lawton MP, Brody E: Instrumental activities of daily living (IADL) scale: original observer rated version, *Pharmacol Bull* 24:785, 1988.

14. Nussbaum RL, Ellis CE: Alzheimer's disease and Parkinson's disease. *N Engl J Med* 348:1356–1364, 2003.

15. Selkoe DJ: Deciphering Alzheimer's disease: molecular genetics and cell biology yield major clues, *J NIH Res* 7:57–64, 1995.

16. Farrer LA, Cupples LA, Haines JL, et al: Effects of age, sex, and ethnicity on the association between apolipoprotein E genotype and Alzheimer disease: a meta-analysis, *JAMA* 278:1349–1356, 1997.

17. Funkenstein HH, Albert MS, Cook NR, et al: Extrapyramidal signs and other neurologic findings in clinically diagnosed Alzheimer's disease, *Arch Neurol* 50:51–56, 1993.

18. Drevets WC, Rubin EH: Psychotic symptoms and the longitudinal course of senile dementia of Alzheimer's type, *Biol Psychiatry* 25:39–48, 1988.

19. Milberg W, Albert MS: Cognitive differences between patients with progressive supranuclear palsy and Alzheimer's disease, *Exp Neuropsychol* 11:605, 1989.

20. Wechsler D: *The Wechsler Adult Intelligence Scale—Revised*, New York, 1989, Psychological Corporation.

21. Folstein MR, Folstein SE, McHugh PR: Mini-mental state exam: a practical method for grading the cognitive state of patients for the clinician, *J Psychiatr Res* 12:189–198, 1975.

22. Blessed G, Tomlinson BE, Roth M: The association between quantitative measures of dementia and senile changes in the cerebral gray matter of elderly subjects, *Br J Psychiatry* 114:797–811, 1968.

23. Pfeiffer E: SPMSQ: short portable mental status questionnaire, *J Am Geriatr Soc* 23:433–441, 1975.

24. Murden R, McRae T, Kaner S, et al: Mini-mental state exam scores vary with education in blacks and whites, *J Am Geriatr Soc* 117:326–328, 1991.

25. Albert M, Cohen C: The test for severe impairment: an instrument for the assessment of patients with severe cognitive dysfunction, *J Am Geriatr Soc* 40:449–453, 1992.

26. Mamo HL, Meric PC, Porsin JC, et al: Cerebral blood flow in normal pressure hydrocephalus, *Stroke* 18:1074–1080, 1987.

27. Marchello V, Boczko F, Shelkey M: Progressive dementia: strategies to manage new problem behaviors, *Geriatrics* 50:40–43, 1995.

28. Trin N, Hoblyn J, Mohanty S, Yaffe K: Efficacy of cholinesterase inhibitors in the treatment of neuropsychiatric symptoms and functional impairment in Alzheimer disease, *JAMA* 289:210–216, 2003.

29. Cummings J: Use of cholinesterase inhibitors in clinical practice: evidence-based recommendations, *Am J Geriatr Psychiatry* 11:131–145, 2003.

30. Reisberg B, Doody R, Stoffler A, et al: Memantine in moderate-to-severe Alzheimer's disease, *N Engl J Med* 348:1334–1341, 2003.

31. Dubovsky SL: *Geriatric neuropsychopharmacology.* In Coffey CE, Cummings JL, editors: *Textbook of geriatric neuropsychiatry*, Washington, DC, 1994, American Psychiatric Association.

32. Cummings JL, Miller B, Hill MA, et al: Neuropsychiatric aspects of multi-infarct dementia and dementia of the Alzheimer's type, *Arch Neurol* 44:389–393, 1987.

33. Brodaty H, Ames D, Snowdon J, et al: A randomized placebo-controlled trial of risperidone for the treatment of aggression, agitation, and psychosis of dementia, *J Clin Psychiatry* 64:134–143, 2003.

34. Schneider LS, Pollack VE, Lyness SA: A meta-analysis of controlled trials of neuroleptic treatment in dementia, *J Am Geriatr Soc* 38:553–563, 1990.

35. Hillert A, Maier W, Wetzel H, et al: Risperidone in the treatment of disorders with a combined psychotic and depressive syndrome: a functional approach, *Pharmacopsychiatry* 25:213–217, 1993.

36. Musser WS, Akil M: Clozapine as a treatment for psychosis in Parkinson's disease: a review, *J Neuropsychiatry Clin Neurosci* 8:1–9, 1996.

37. Lipsey JR, Pearlson GD, Robinson RG, et al: Nortriptyline treatment of post-stroke depression: a double-blind study, *Lancet* 1:297–300, 1984.

38. Watanabe MD, Martin EM, DeLeon OA, et al: Successful methylphenidate treatment of apathy after subcortical infarcts, *J Neuropsychiatry Clin Neurosci* 7:502–504, 1995.

39. Jenike MA: MAO inhibitors as treatment for depressed patients with primary degenerative dementia, *Am J Psychiatry* 142:763–764, 1985.

40. Sunderland T, Silver MA: Neuroleptics in the treatment of dementia, *Int J Geriatr Psychiatry* 3:79–88, 1988.

41. Altamura AC, Sassella F, Santini A, et al: Intramuscular preparations of antipsychotics: uses and relevance in clinical practice, *Drugs* 63:493–512, 2003.

42. Meehan KM, Wang H, David SR, et al: Comparison of rapidly acting intramuscular olanzapine, lorazepam, and placebo: a double-blind, randomized study in acutely agitated patients with dementia. *Neuropsychopharmacology* 26:494–504, 2002.

43. Salzman C, Fisher J, Nobel K, et al: Cognitive improvement following benzodiazepine discontinuation in elderly nursing home residents, *Int J Geriatr Psychiatry* 7:89–93, 1992.

44. Sakauye KM, Camp CJ, Ford PA: Effects of buspirone on agitation associated with dementia, *Am J Geriatr Psychiatry* 1:82–84, 1993.

45. Aisen PS, Johannessen DJ, Marin DB: Trazodone for behavioral disturbance in Alzheimer's disease, *Am J Geriatr Psychiatry* 4:349–350, 1993.

46. Copeland MP, Falk WE, Gunther J: Trazodone treatment for behavioral symptoms in dementia, presented at the American Association for Geriatric Psychiatry Annual Meeting, New Orleans, 1993.

47. Schneider LS, Sobin PB: Non-neuroleptic medication in the management of agitation in Alzheimer's disease and other dementias: a selective review, *Int J Geriat Psychiatry* 6:691–708, 1991.

48. Holton A, George K: The use of lithium in severely demented patients with behavioral disturbance, *Br J Psychiatry* 146:99–100, 1985.

49. Tariot PN, Erb R, Leibovic A, et al: Carbamazepine treatment of agitation in nursing home patients with dementia: a preliminary study, *J Am Geriatric Soc* 42:1160–1166, 1994.

50. Lott AD, McElroy SL, Keys MA: Valproate in the treatment of behavioral agitation in elderly patients with dementia, *J Neuropsychiatry Clin Neurosci* 7:314–319, 1995.

51. Knapp MJ, Knopman DS, Solomon PR, et al: A 30-week randomized controlled trial of high-dose tacrine in patients with Alzheimer's disease, *JAMA* 271:985–991, 1994.

52. Rogers SL, Friednoff LT, Donepezil Study Group: The efficacy and safety of donepezil in patients with Alzheimer's disease: results of a United States multicenter, randomized, double-blind, placebo-controlled trial, *Dementia* 7:293–303, 1996.

Chapter 14
Psychotic Patients

Donald C. Goff, M.D.
Oliver Freudenreich, M.D.
David C. Henderson, M.D.

Psychosis, broadly defined, is a gross impairment of reality testing. Psychosis may take several forms and can result from a wide range of psychiatric and medical disturbances. The elderly woman lying quietly in bed listening to Satan whisper bears little resemblance to the wildly agitated young man who accuses the nursing staff of trying to poison him. Psychiatric symptoms, which alone or in combination may indicate that the patient has lost touch with reality, generally fall into three categories. Hallucinations, which are sensory perceptions in the absence of an external source, can occur in any sensory modality and may take the form of voices, visions, odors, or even complex tactile perceptions (such as electric shocks or the sensation that one is being fondled). Delusions are firmly held false beliefs. Delusional individuals cling to their beliefs with unfaltering conviction even in the face of overwhelming evidence to the contrary. Delusions range from beliefs that are plausible, albeit unlikely (such as being monitored by the Central Intelligence Agency), to bizarre convictions (e.g., that one's internal organs have been replaced with empty beer cans). The third category of psychotic symptoms comes under the rubric of a formal thought disorder, which refers to a disruption in the form, or organization, of thinking. Patients with a formal thought disorder may be incoherent; they may not be able to make sense of reality or to communicate their thoughts to others.

When called to see a patient with psychosis, the psychiatric consultant can be of immediate help by ensuring that patient and staff are safe; moreover, he or she can demystify this often-frightening condition. Psychosis can best be approached by proceeding with a well-ordered differential diagnosis, which transforms the patient's condition in the eyes of medical staff from insanity, with all its disturbing connotations, to a more comprehensible disorder of brain function.

Diagnostic Evaluation

It cannot be stressed enough that the presence of psychotic symptoms does not always mean that a primary psychiatric disorder like schizophrenia is present. Therefore the diagnostic assessment of a psychotic patient begins with a thorough screening for toxic or medical conditions that can present with psychosis (Table 14-1).[1,2] A medical history, review of systems, family history, and physical examination are crucial elements of this process because most organic causes can be identified on this basis. A bedside examination of cognitive function should be performed with the Mini-Mental State Examination or with a similar screening instrument. Serious deficits in attention, orientation, and memory suggest delirium or dementia rather than a primary psychotic illness. Careful delineation of the temporal course of psychotic

Table 14-1. Medical Conditions Associated with Psychosis

Epilepsy	Neurosyphilis
Head trauma (history of)	Neuroborreliosis (Lyme disease)
Dementias	HIV infection
Alzheimer's disease	CNS-invasive parasitic infections (e.g., cerebral malaria,
Pick's disease	toxoplasmosis, neurocysticercosis)
Lewy body disease	Tuberculosis
Stroke	Sarcoidosis
Space-occupying lesions and structural brain	Cryptococcus infection
abnormalities	Prion diseases (e.g., Creutzfeldt-Jakob disease)
Primary brain tumors	Endocrinopathies
Secondary brain metastases	Hypoglycemia
Brain abscesses and cysts	Addison's disease
Tuberous sclerosis	Cushing's syndrome
Midline abnormalities (e.g., corpus callosum agenesis,	Hyper- and hypothyroidism
cavum septi pellucidi)	Hyper- and hypoparathyroidism
Cerebrovascular malformations (e.g., involving the	Hypopituitarism
temporal lobe)	Narcolepsy
Hydrocephalus	Nutritional deficiencies
Demyelinating diseases	Magnesium deficiency
MS	Vitamin A deficiency
Leukodystrophies (metachromatic leukodystrophy,	Vitamin D deficiency
X-linked adrenoleukodystrophy, Marchiafava-Bignami	Zinc deficiency
disease)	Niacin deficiency (pellagra)
Schilder's disease	Vitamin B_{12} deficiency (pernicious anemia)
Neuropsychiatric disorders	Metabolic disorders (partial list)
Huntington's disease	Amino acid metabolism (Hartnup disease,
Wilson's disease	homocystinuria, phenylketonuria)
Parkinson's disease	Porphyrias (acute intermittent porphyria, porphyria
Friedreich's ataxia	variegata, hereditary coproporphyria)
Autoimmune disorders	GM-2 gangliosidosis
SLE	Fabry's disease
Rheumatic fever (history of)	Niemann-Pick type C disease
Paraneoplastic syndrome	Gaucher's disease, adult type
Myasthenia gravis	Chromosomal abnormalities
Infections	Sex chromosomes (Klinefelter's syndrome, XXX
Viral encephalitis (e.g., herpes simplex, measles	syndrome)
including SSPE, cytomegalovirus, rubella, Epstein-Barr,	Fragile X syndrome
varicella)	VCFS

CNS, Central nervous system; *HIV*, human immunodeficiency virus; *MS*, multiple sclerosis; *SLE*, systemic lupus erythematosus; *SSPE*, subacute sclerosing panencephalitis; *VCFS*, velo-cardio-facial syndrome.

symptoms is of particular importance. One should consider whether the disorder is chronic, episodic, or of recent onset. The pattern of psychotic symptoms should be examined to determine whether a mood disorder, substance abuse, medication use, or medical or neurologic illness is present. Substance abuse, such as intoxication with stimulants, is a frequent and reversible cause of psychosis. Many medications have the potential to cause psychosis; unfortunately, causality is often difficult to prove (Table 14-2). Such drug-induced psychoses should be considered if the psychosis is of new onset, if there is no personal history of psychosis, or if the psychosis starts in the hospital, particularly if a delirium is present. A urine toxicologic screening test might identify unsuspected drug use, but it would not rule out drug-induced psychosis if it were negative, nor would a positive toxicologic screening test necessarily establish a cause for the psychosis, because comorbid substance use and abuse is common in psychotic disorders. Routine testing includes determination of a sedimentation rate, a complete blood cell count, serum electrolytes, urinalysis, levels of calcium,

Table 14-2. Substances Associated with Psychosis

Drugs of Abuse

Associated with Intoxication
Alcohol
Anabolic steroids
Amphetamine
Cannabis
Cocaine
Hallucinogens: LSD, MDMA
Inhalants: glues and solvents
Opioids (meperidine)
Phencyclidine (PCP), ketamine
Sedative-hypnotics (including withdrawal): barbiturates and benzodiazepines
Associated with Withdrawal
Alcohol
Sedative-hypnotics
Medications (Broad Classes with Selected Medications)
Anesthetics and analgesics (including NSAIDs)
Anticholinergic agents and antihistamines
Antiepileptics (with high doses)
Antihypertensive and cardiovascular medications (e.g., digoxin)
Antiinfectious medications (antibiotics [e.g., fluoroquinolones, TMP/SMX], antivirals [e.g., nevirapine], tuberculostatics
    [e.g., INH], antiparasitics [e.g., metronidazole, mefloquine])
Antiparkinsonian medications (e.g., amantadine, levodopa)
Chemotherapeutic agents (e.g., vincristine)
Corticosteroids (e.g., prednisone, ACTH)
Interferon
Muscle relaxants (e.g., cyclobenzaprine)
Over-the-counter medications (e.g., pseudoephedrine, caffeine in excessive doses)
Toxins
Carbon monoxide
Heavy metals: arsenic, manganese, mercury, thallium
Organophosphates

Key Diagnostic Questions to Determine Causality between a Substance and Psychosis
Does the patient have a personal history of psychosis?
Does the patient have a history of illicit drug use?
Did the psychosis start after a medication was started? After the patient came to the hospital?
Is there evidence of delirium?

ACTH, Adrenocorticotrophic hormone; *INH,* isoniazid, *LSD,* d-lysergic acid diethylamide; *MDMA,* methylenedioxymethamphetamine; *NSAID,* nonsteroidal antiinflammatory drug; *TMP/SMX,* trimethoprim-sulfamethoxazole.

glucose, creatinine, and blood urea nitrogen. In addition, liver function tests, thyroid function tests, and syphilis serology (specific, such as the fluorescent treponemal antibody absorption test), are appropriate. Human immunodeficiency virus testing should be recommended. Some have argued that screening for known conditions that can present with schizophrenia-like symptoms is justified because some medical and neurologic disorders present only with psychiatric symptoms.[3] Extended work-ups may include karyotyping for chromosomal abnormalities or urine testing for metabolic disorders.[4] The diagnostic yield from neuroimaging of the brain (magnetic resonance imaging or computed tomography) is low in the absence of localizing neurologic findings. Neuroimaging should be obtained, however, in cases with atypical psychotic symptoms when psychotic symptoms first appear and should be considered even in cases with typical psychotic features because the long-term costs and morbidity of this disorder are potentially quite high in relation to the expense of diagnostic procedures.[5] The electroencephalogram (EEG) is useful when evaluating a confused patient to rule out a delirium or when a history of serious head trauma or symptoms suggestive of a seizure disorder are present.[6,7] An EEG is not helpful if it is employed as a routine screening procedure. Similarly, a lumbar puncture is not necessary for a routine work-up, but it can be life-saving if a treatable central nervous system infection is suspected.

Several neuropsychiatric disorders in particular should be considered during the diagnostic work-up of a patient with psychosis.[1] Huntington's disease is suggested by family history of Huntington's disease, dementia, and choreiform movements; psychotic symptoms may occur before motor and cognitive symptoms become prominent.[8] Neuroimaging may be necessary to establish the diagnosis in some cases. Parkinson's disease also may present with psychosis, along with bradykinesia, tremor, rigidity, and a festinating gait. The diagnosis of Parkinson's disease can be complicated by exposure to neuroleptics—review of the time course of neurologic symptoms in relation to the use of antipsychotics should clarify this diagnostic possibility.[9] Wilson's disease may also present with psychotic symptoms, tremor, dysarthria, rigidity, and a gait disturbance.[10] Kayser-Fleischer rings, which are golden brown deposits that encircle the cornea, are pathognomonic for this disease. The diagnosis can be confirmed by measuring concentrations of ceruloplasmin in the urine and serum. Finally, acute intermittent porphyria is characterized by acute episodes of abdominal pain, weakness, and peripheral neuropathy; this condition may be associated with psychosis. Because this is a hereditary (autosomal dominant) illness, a family history often points to this diagnosis. During acute attacks, levels of δ-aminolevulinic acid and porphobilinogen are elevated in the urine.

After an organic cause has been ruled out, the psychiatric differential diagnosis of psychosis flows from the diagnostic criteria contained in the Psychotic Disorders section of the *Diagnostic and Statistical Manual of Mental Disorders,* fourth edition (DSM-IV).[11] It should be emphasized, however, that these criteria are guidelines for diagnosis; they are to be used only in conjunction with a full understanding of the descriptions of disorders contained in the text (Table 14-3). A clear, longitudinal

view of the illness is necessary to identify affective episodes and to determine whether the patient's level of function has declined. In addition, the range and severity of psychotic and negative symptoms must be determined and a judgment made as to whether delusional beliefs are bizarre or plausible. Psychotic patients are often unable to provide an accurate history; therefore information must be collected from as many sources as possible. In one study, information necessary for diagnosis, such as the presence of persecutory delusions, was missed more than 30% of the time when the assessment was based on the interview only.[12] Concurrent substance abuse is also frequently missed in patients with schizophrenia if toxicologic screening is not performed.[13]

If major depression and mania are not present and have not played a prominent role in the past, the diagnosis is likely to be schizophrenia, delusional disorder, or schizotypal personality disorder

Table 14-3. Psychiatric Disorders That May Present with Psychosis

Continuous Psychosis
Schizophrenia
Schizoaffective disorder, bipolar type (with prominent episodes of mania)
Schizoaffective disorder, depressed type (with prominent depressive episodes)
Delusional disorder (plausible, circumscribed delusions)
Shared psychotic disorder (in which delusions are induced by another person)

Episodic Psychosis
Depression with psychotic features
Bipolar disorder (manic or depressed)
Schizophreniform disorder (<6 mo duration)
Brief psychotic disorder (<1 mo duration)

Key Diagnostic Questions
Has a reversible, organic cause been ruled out?
Are cognitive deficits prominent? (delirium or dementia)
Is the psychotic illness continuous or episodic?
Have psychotic symptoms (active phase) been present for at least 4 weeks?
Has evidence of the illness been present for at least 6 months?
Is there evidence of a decline in level of functioning?
Are negative symptoms present?
Are mood episodes prominent?
Have there been episodes of major depression or mania?
Do psychotic features occur only during affective episodes?

(depending on the severity of the illness). To meet criteria for schizophrenia, the patient must have demonstrated a decline in function and displayed, for at least 4 weeks, symptoms of the active phase, which can consist of either bizarre delusions or typical auditory hallucinations (voices conversing or keeping up a running commentary). If neither of these psychotic symptoms is present, the active phase criteria can also be met by the presence of any two of the following: nonbizarre delusions, less typical hallucinations, disorganized speech, disorganized behavior, or negative symptoms. Negative symptoms of schizophrenia include apathy, affective flattening, social withdrawal, and impoverished thought. The diagnosis of schizophrenia is made only after evidence of the illness has been present for at least 6 months—if symptoms have been present for less than 6 months, the provisional diagnosis of schizophreniform disorder is used. Patients whose psychotic symptoms fully remit within 4 weeks of their onset are diagnosed as having a brief psychotic disorder if no organic cause is identified.

If the patient's condition does not meet the criteria for schizophrenia or schizophreniform disorder, but a nonbizarre (plausible) delusion is present, the diagnosis of delusional disorder is made, provided that the patient does not exhibit severe deterioration in function outside of the circumscribed delusional system. Typical delusions include the belief that one has a physical defect or medical condition or that one is being followed, poisoned, infected, loved by a famous person, or cheated on by a spouse. Patients who do not meet the active phase criteria for schizophrenia but who present with chronic, bizarre, or idiosyncratic thoughts or behaviors are classified as having schizotypal personality, which probably is a less severe form of schizophrenia.

If the patient meets criteria for major depression and has exhibited psychotic symptoms only during episodes of depression, the diagnosis is major depression with psychotic features. If psychotic features characteristic of schizophrenia have also occurred during periods when the patient was euthymic, the illness is classified as schizoaffective disorder, depressed type if depressions have been prominent throughout the course of the illness, or schizophrenia with superimposed depression if depressions have been infrequent. Patients who have experienced manic episodes and who have been psychotic only during affective

episodes are diagnosed as having bipolar disorder. If psychosis has been present between manic and depressive states, the diagnosis is schizoaffective disorder, bipolar type, or schizophrenia with superimposed mood disorder; again, the diagnosis depends on how prominent a role affective episodes have played in the overall course of the illness. The proper psychiatric diagnosis of a patient who is psychotic on a cross-sectional examination requires an intimate knowledge of the patient's longitudinal course, something that is often unavailable during an in-patient admission.

Clinical Pictures and Corresponding Problems on the Medical Ward

It is often surprising to see that psychotic patients do perfectly well when admitted to a medical or surgical service; they tend to require little in the way of special treatment. One survey found that only half of schizophrenic patients admitted to a general hospital required psychiatric consultation.[14] Interestingly, the most common reason for a psychiatric consultation in patients with schizophrenia admitted to the medical service of the Massachusetts General Hospital was "schizophrenia" (30%); there was no specific question. This may reflect a concern that is evoked by managing a patient with schizophrenia.[15] Other referrals revolve around depression (16%), capacity assessment (14%), and help with prescription of psychotropic medications (10%). For patients with psychotic disorders, the role of the consultation psychiatrist in the general hospital can be seen as threefold: conducting conventional consultations with an emphasis on making a correct diagnosis and instituting proper treatment, educating staff about the nature of schizophrenia, and serving as an advocate for the chronically mentally ill so that they can receive standard and comprehensive medical care.[16,17]

The specific form of illness that a schizophrenic patient manifests determines the nature of the staff's concerns as well as the staff's level of comfort. Studies have demonstrated that the symptoms of schizophrenia tend to cluster into at least three groups: reality distortion (e.g., delusions and hallucinations), disorganization (e.g., formal thought disorder and inappropriate affect), and negative symptoms (e.g., apathy, anhedonia, social withdrawal, alogia, and flat affect).[18,19] A fourth symptom domain, cognitive deficits, has been rediscovered.[20] Schizophrenia was once known as dementia praecox because of its prominent cognitive problems. The majority of patients with schizophrenia display symptoms from all four categories and are classified as having an undifferentiated type. Some patients, however, exhibit prominent symptoms from only one category, and the difficulties they encounter in the general hospital are determined by which cluster of symptoms predominates.

In all cases, a question can arise as to whether the patient is competent to make treatment decisions. Some patients may already have a guardian who must be involved in treatment decisions; if not, assessment for competency and initiation of appropriate legal steps may be necessary to ensure proper medical treatment. It is crucial to assess to what degree, if at all, delusions affect the patient's decision-making. The consultant should make it clear that patients with psychosis may have the capacity to make certain decisions, such as weighing risks and benefits of proceeding with or refusing medical treatment, even when their judgment is impaired in other realms. The idiosyncratic speech manifest by some patients may give an exaggerated impression of cognitive impairment, whereas their capacity to understand aspects of their medical condition may be adequate.

The Paranoid or Delusional Patient

Patients with schizophrenia whose symptoms are restricted to complex delusional systems and hallucinations are classified as having the paranoid type, even when their delusions are not persecutory in nature. In the absence of overt disorganization and negative symptoms, the individuals with paranoid schizophrenia may go unnoticed by hospital staff. These patients often conceal all psychiatric symptoms and fail to exhibit the bizarre appearance and speech that attract attention in others with schizophrenia. Patients with paranoid schizophrenia may antagonize nursing staff because of their anger, argumentativeness, or patronizing manner. Nursing staff often appreciate learning that these annoying characteristics are actually common features of the illness. Despite complex and bizarre delusional beliefs, these individuals may elude detection and

complete a medical or surgical hospitalization without incident. Difficulties arise when circumstances in the hospital collide with an individual's delusions. The patient who believes that the Mafia is attempting to kill him may refuse all hospital food for fear of being poisoned. Others become convinced that their physicians are members of the conspiracy that is plotting against them or that the surgeons have implanted a microchip intended to control or monitor their thoughts. To assess safety and to anticipate potential problems with compliance, the psychiatric consultant must understand the full scope of the person's delusional system and the nature of any hallucinatory experiences.

Because paranoid patients usually are reluctant to reveal their delusional beliefs, the consultant must proceed carefully and deliberately. A direct, interrogatory approach often convinces the patient that conspirators sent the interviewer. Because delusional individuals are preoccupied and distressed by their delusional beliefs, it is usually sufficient to engage them in a neutral, nonthreatening discussion about their current interests and activities. Comments that seem out of place or inappropriate to the content may provide clues as to the subject of the delusional system, and these should be explored. Questions should never imply a judgment about psychopathology, but rather they should demonstrate the interviewer's interest and concern. Examples of such questions include, "Are you safe? Have you noticed any strange coincidences? Are you aware of anyone trying to play with your mind? How do you understand what is happening to you? What is it that you overhear from others about this?" The interviewer should neither agree with the delusion nor reality-test—impartial interest and concern are usually a welcome relief to a delusional patient. This technique is sometimes called *partial joining of perspectives*.[21] Ideally, the consultant can serve as an intermediary, listening to the concerns of both the patient and the hospital staff; as a consequence he or she can mediate misunderstandings.

In addition to persecutory delusions, somatic delusions may also pose unique problems for the schizophrenic patient admitted to a medical service. In a retrospective chart survey, McGilchrist and Cutting found that more than half of patients with schizophrenia described somatic delusions.[22] These delusions were typically bizarre (such as the belief that a third arm is growing out of one's chest) and could usually be immediately recognized as delusional. Having heard a patient's somatic delusions, however, medical staff tend to discount other somatic complaints. The consultant may be needed to help sort out which physical complaints merit further investigation by hospital staff and which delusional concerns are best ignored.

The Disorganized Patient

The disorganized patient can be problematic on a medical service. Disordered speech may make communication about medical symptoms difficult and may interfere with discussions about treatment options. If disorganization is subtle, the patient may merely appear stubborn or oppositional, and make routine nursing tasks difficult. One major area of concern for disorganized patients is their lack of judgment and behavioral control. These patients may engage in inappropriate behaviors (such as masturbating or disrobing in public, stealing food, and smoking in restricted areas). Of even greater concern is the occasional violent or self-injurious behavior of an agitated, disorganized patient. These patients typically require aggressive pharmacotherapy and may require physical restraints or round-the-clock attendants. A review of past behavioral problems, which can be provided by outpatient caregivers or family, can help the consultant anticipate behavioral problems that are likely to arise during a medical or surgical hospitalization.

The Patient with Negative Symptoms or Neurocognitive Deficits

Schizophrenic patients who display prominent negative symptoms may encounter unique difficulties when admitted to medical or surgical services. Moreover, negative symptoms are often compounded by cognitive deficits, particularly in the realms of sustained attention, memory, and executive function. Patients may seem indifferent to their medical problems and unappreciative of the care. Nursing staff can easily be put off by the poor hygiene and soiled clothing. Sustaining empathy and enthusiasm for the care of a withdrawn, unmotivated patient can require unusual efforts by nursing staff. This process may be facilitated by the psychiatric consultant, who can explain that poor hygiene, apathy, and deficits in interpersonal skills are symptoms of illness that require management and that should not be interpreted as willful or as a weakness of character. When ongoing treatment or rehabilitation is required after discharge, a comprehensive plan should be developed to provide supervision for avolitional patients, who otherwise would be unlikely to follow through with treatment. If little history about the patient's baseline level of function is available, it is important to rule out other causes of negative symptoms, such as a hypoactive delirium or a seizure disorder.[23]

The Manic Patient

Although psychotic features in patients with schizophrenia are typically bizarre and idiosyncratic, patients who are manic are much more likely to present with grandiose delusions that typically impair judgment and self-esteem. These patients may be difficult to manage because of their boundless energy and their grandiose misinterpretation of their situation. Staff may at first mistake mania for unusually high energy, talkativeness, and positive self-esteem; eventually they turn to the psychiatric consultant when the patient refuses to stop pacing or to stop talking to other patients late at night, or when he or she is belligerent or insists that he or she is free of any medical problems. Patients with irritable or dysphoric mania may present with persecutory delusions and can be superficially indistinguishable from a patient with paranoid schizophrenia. Management of the manic patient should begin with containment and isolation from distracting stimuli and behavioral temptations. Short-term behavioral control can be achieved with use of antipsychotics in combination with benzodiazepines, whereas the ultimate goal of mood stabilization requires a therapeutic blood level of lithium carbonate, valproic acid, or another mood stabilizer.[24]

The Psychotic Depressed Patient

The delusions of the psychotically depressed patient usually reflect ruminative concerns about guilt, worthlessness, or physical decrepitude. These patients may puzzle their medical or surgical caregivers with somatic delusions involving fanciful disease or dysfunction. Their overwhelming sense of hopelessness and sense of being responsible for their plight may also interfere with attempts to involve them in treatment decisions—they may seem more interested in euthanasia. Some psychotically depressed patients withdraw and may become mute. Persecutory delusions also occur in psychotic depression, but these beliefs tend to be less bizarre than those encountered in patients with schizophrenia. In fact, it may be quite difficult to discern whether strangers are actually attempting to break into the patient's house or whether family members are stealing the elderly aunt's savings. Treatment of psychotic depression typically requires either a course of electroconvulsive therapy or the use of an antipsychotic agent, plus an adequate dose of an antidepressant.[25,26]

The Elderly Psychotic Patient

Psychotic symptoms are relatively common among the medically ill or disabled elderly. One survey found that 21% of newly admitted nursing home patients were delusional, and approximately 4% of elderly individuals in the community suffer from persecutory delusions.[27] Isolation and sensory impairment probably contribute to the higher incidence of paranoia and agitation in the elderly. *Late paraphrenia* is an older term still used to describe such patients.[28] In addition, such individuals are at particular risk for a host of organic causes of psychosis, including dementia, medication toxicity, and depression. Late-onset schizophrenia, which occurs after the age of 45 and may first present in old age, usually occurs in women and appears as a paranoid psychosis.[29] Psychotic symptoms are quite common in patients with Alzheimer's disease; approximately one third of patients with Alzheimer's disease develop paranoid delusions or auditory hallucinations.[30] Management of psychosis in the elderly involves a comprehensive screening for organic causes, administration of low doses of an atypical antipsychotic agent (typically risperidone or olanzapine), and supportive measures. Supportive measures should be individualized but include reassurance, visits from family to alleviate isolation, and measures to compensate for

sensory or cognitive deficits, such as providing clear and repeated instructions, orienting aids (such as clocks and calendars), and preserving sleep-wake cycles. Supportive measures alone are usually inadequate to treat the confused, elderly person in the hospital.

Management of Psychotic Patients

General Considerations

As has been emphasized, the first step in approaching the treatment of a psychotic patient is to clarify the diagnosis, along with any prior psychotropic medication use. Delirium, which is characterized by fluctuations in mental status and by confusion, must be recognized and the underlying cause addressed. The pharmacologic management of delirium is described in Chapter 12. Specific information about individual antipsychotic agents and drug-drug interactions is provided in Chapter 18.

Target symptoms for antipsychotics fall into three categories: (1) psychotic symptoms (e.g., hallucinations, delusions, and disorganization), (2) agitation (e.g., distractibility, affective lability, tension, and increased motor activity), and (3) negative symptoms (e.g., apathy, flat affect, social isolation, and poverty of speech). Although agitation usually responds rapidly, psychotic and negative symptoms tend to respond more gradually, over the course of days to weeks, when an adequate dose of an antipsychotic agent is given. Negative symptoms generally are less responsive to treatment than are psychotic symptoms, although atypical antipsychotics may produce modest improvement.[31] The pharmacologic treatment of psychotic symptoms is similar in many ways to the treatment of infection with antibiotics—the clinician needs to choose a proper dose and then await therapeutic results while monitoring side effects.

Psychotic symptoms and agitation usually improve with antipsychotics, regardless of cause. Most causes of organic psychosis, such as stimulant intoxication (e.g., amphetamines and cocaine), respond readily to antipsychotics. The decision whether to use an antipsychotic in cases of organic psychosis should be informed by a weighing of the anticipated duration and severity of the psychosis and the potential side effects of the drug. When time-limited psychoses, such as those produced by psychoactive substances, are treated with an antipsychotic, care should be taken that this medication not be continued indefinitely after the patient is discharged from the hospital, particularly if a conventional neuroleptic is used; the risk of irreversible tardive dyskinesia must be considered.

Drug Selection

Selection of an antipsychotic agent is usually guided by side-effect profiles and available formulations (i.e., tablet, rapidly dissolving wafer, liquid, intramuscular, intravenous, or depot preparations). Conventional antipsychotics, which act by blocking dopamine D_2 receptors, are of similar efficacy and differ primarily in their potency (i.e., the dose required for their clinical effect) and in their side effects.[32] Currently we are in the midst of a remarkable period of antipsychotic drug development, in which a growing number of "atypical" antipsychotics, with fewer or no neurologic side effects, have become available.[33] Superior efficacy compared with conventional antipsychotics has been established most compellingly for clozapine.[34] The potential therapeutic benefits of clozapine are quite broad; these include greater efficacy for psychosis, negative symptoms, agitation or tension, suicidal ideation, and relapse.[35–37] Risperidone and olanzapine also offer potential advantages, including enhanced efficacy in some patients for psychosis, negative symptoms, and relapse prevention, compared to the conventional agents.[38–41] Risperidone and olanzapine are the best studied of these "second generation" agents. Although risperidone and olanzapine are quite effective, these drugs fall short of clozapine in terms of their over-all efficacy. More recently marketed atypical agents (such as quetiapine, ziprasidone, and aripiprazole) also have favorable side effect profiles and efficacy when compared with conventional agents.[33] However, head-to-head efficacy trials involving these newer agents are limited. In response to the rapid introduction of so many new medications, the National Institute of Mental Health has established a large, multicenter trial, "Clinical Antipsychotic Trials of Intervention Effectiveness" (CATIE) to examine the relative effectiveness, tolerability, and economic effect of atypical agents as compared with a representative conventional agent (perphenazine). When completed, results from the CATIE project should be able to help guide treatment selection.

Use of the conventional antipsychotics has rapidly declined during the past decade as experience with the atypical agents has grown. This trend reflects improved tolerability that results in part from the reduction in extrapyramidal side effects as well as the apparent reduction of the incidence of tardive dyskinesia. However, atypical agents are not free of side effects.[42] High-potency conventional agents continue to have their strongest support in the short-term treatment of medically compromised agitated patients; they have been relatively free of serious medical side effects. An additional role for conventional antipsychotics is in the treatment of patients for whom compliance is a problem. Currently only haloperidol and fluphenazine are available in depot (long-acting) intramuscular formulations. As many as 70% of schizophrenic patients do not take their medications as prescribed, in part because of disorganization, side effects, and a lack of insight.[43,44] A long-acting form of an atypical agent (i.e., risperidone microspheres) may soon be available; it will be a valuable addition to the antipsychotic armamentarium.

If a patient has been taking an antipsychotic with good results, it is best not to make changes in the regimen unless medical problems or potential drug interactions necessitate a switch. Exacerbations in otherwise stable patients, particularly if related to stress and accompanied by depressive symptoms, usually improve without altering the medication or raising the dosage.[45]

Conventional Antipsychotics (Neuroleptics)

Low-potency conventional antipsychotic agents (such as chlorpromazine and thioridazine), are often prescribed in doses of 300 to 600 mg/day; they are associated with orthostatic hypotension, anticholinergic side effects, sedation, and weight gain, and they are less readily or safely administered in a parenteral fashion.[42] Thioridazine also produces substantial QT interval prolongation, which may be dangerous in patients with cardiac conduction defects.[46] High-potency conventional agents (such as haloperidol) are more likely to produce extrapyramidal side effects (EPS), such as acute dystonias, parkinsonism, and akathisia (see later discussion), except when administered intravenously. Haloperidol is available for parenteral (including intravenous) administration. In the setting of serious medical illness, particularly if other medications with anticholinergic or hypotensive side effects are being administered, haloperidol is typically the antipsychotic of choice. Although considerable inter-individual variability exists, daily oral doses of haloperidol between 5 and 15 mg are adequate for the vast majority of patients; increasing the dose beyond the dose range may only aggravate side effects without improving antipsychotic efficacy. Intramuscular and intravenous administration tends to require roughly half the dose. In the elderly, 0.5 mg to 2 mg of haloperidol at bedtime may be sufficient. If a patient has not previously received an antipsychotic, it is best to start with a low dose (e.g., haloperidol 2 to 5 mg orally) before increasing it to a standard therapeutic dose.

Extrapyramidal Side Effects and Tardive Dyskinesia

Younger patients (i.e., those younger than 40 years of age) started on high-potency conventional antipsychotics are especially vulnerable to developing an acute dystonic reactions during the first week of treatment.[47] Dystonia, the sudden constriction of muscles, is a frightening and uncomfortable experience; when manifest as a laryngeal spasm, it can be life-threatening. The occurrence of dystonia early in treatment jeopardizes future compliance with antipsychotics; therefore it is important to anticipate and treat this side effect aggressively. Prophylaxis with an anticholinergic agent, such as benztropine 1 to 2 mg twice daily substantially reduces the likelihood of a dystonic reaction even in a high-risk patient.[48] Dystonia is less common with the use of atypical agents than with conventional high-potency agents; moreover, it probably does not occur with either quetiapine or clozapine.

Akathisia is an extremely unpleasant sensation of motor restlessness that is primarily experienced in the lower extremities in patients who receive an antipsychotic medication.[49] For the psychotic patient hospitalized on a medical service, akathisia can make bed rest unbearable. Akathisia substantially increases the risk that a patient will leave the hospital against medical advice, and it has been associated with self-injurious behaviors as well as a worsening of psychosis. Untrained staff frequently mistake akathisia for psychotic agitation, which leads to unfortunate escalations of antipsychotic doses. Dose reduction may improve akathisia; if relief is not obtained, propranolol (10 to 20 mg two to four times daily) is often helpful.[50] Even more effective is a switch to an atypical antipsychotic, which usually resolves the problem.

Antipsychotic-induced parkinsonism can easily be mistaken for depression or for the negative symptoms of schizophrenia.[51] The presence of tremor and rigidity distinguishes this side effect in more severe cases; subtle cases can easily be missed. Parkinsonian side effects commonly improve with a reduction of the neuroleptic dosage or with addition of an antiparkinsonian agent (e.g., benztropine 1 to 2 mg twice daily or amantadine 100 mg twice or three times daily).[52] Because anticholinergic agents impair attention and memory and can produce a vast array of troublesome side effects in the elderly, long-term use of these agents should be avoided.[53] Atypical agents as a class produce substantially fewer parkinsonian side effects; both clozapine and quetiapine are essentially free of EPS, which makes them the drugs of choice for patients with idiopathic Parkinson's disease complicated by psychosis.[54]

Tardive dyskinesia rarely appears after less than 6 months of treatment with an antipsychotic; once present, tardive dyskinesia may be irreversible.[55] Tardive dyskinesia usually takes the form of involuntary, choreiform movements of the mouth, tongue, or upper extremities, although a dystonic form has also been described.[56] Studies suggest that the risk for developing tardive dyskinesia with conventional agents is approximately 5% per year of exposure, with a lifetime risk possibly as high as 50% to 60%.[57] The incidence of tardive dyskinesia is much higher in the elderly, although a substantial proportion of these cases may represent spontaneously occurring dyskinesias.[58] As part of informed consent, patients requiring prolonged antipsychotic treatment with conventional agents should be educated about the risk of developing tardive dyskinesia after their acute psychosis has been treated and before

6 months has elapsed. Preliminary evidence that indicated α-tocopherol (vitamin E), at doses of 400 to 1200 IU daily, improved symptoms of tardive dyskinesia was not supported by a much larger controlled trial.[59] Clozapine has not been linked to tardive dyskinesia; switching a patient from a conventional agent to clozapine increases the likelihood of improvement in tardive dyskinesia.[60] Risperidone and olanzapine have also been associated with substantially lower rates of tardive dyskinesia when compared with conventional agents, and it is expected that the atypical agents as a class will share this advantage.[61,62] Lowering the dose of a conventional antipsychotic or switching to an atypical agent can occasionally produce a "withdrawal dyskinesia," which typically resolves within 6 weeks, or may unmask an underlying dyskinesia that was previously suppressed by the antipsychotic.[63]

Atypical Antipsychotics

Atypical agents as a class are generally better tolerated and produce fewer neurologic side effects (e.g., dystonia, akathisia, and parkinsonism) than the conventional agents; they are also associated with less tardive dyskinesia. Although risperidone is rarely associated with EPS at doses of less than 6 mg daily, at higher doses it may occur. Risperidone is unique among the atypical agents because of its propensity to produce hyperprolactinemia.[64] Several of the atypical agents, particularly clozapine and olanzapine, have been associated with substantial weight gain, which is highly variable and unpredictable.[65] Risperidone and quetiapine are associated with intermediate weight gain and ziprasidone and aripiprazole appear to produce little to no weight gain.[65] Recent attention has focused on possible effects of atypical antipsychotics on glucose metabolism.[66] A large number of cases have been reported of treatment-emergent diabetes mellitus (and diabetic ketoacidosis), which, in some cases, resolved after discontinuation of the atypical antipsychotic.[67,68] Clozapine and olanzapine have been the agents most commonly implicated in these case reports; however, preliminary studies have suggested a reduction in insulin sensitivity with these two agents.[69,70] Large pharmacoepidemiologic studies have not

consistently identified particular agents, but rather have tended to raise concerns about all atypical agents.[71–74] Possible differences between atypical agents in their risk for causing diabetes may be obscured in part by the considerable variability between patients regarding weight gain, the potential delay between initiation of treatment and elevation of glucose levels, as well as an abnormal glucose metabolism associated with schizophrenia (independent of drug treatment).[75] Until this issue is better understood, all patients treated with atypical agents should be monitored for diabetes, with particular attention paid to use of olanzapine and clozapine.[69]

Olanzapine and aripiprazole have few or no cardiac effects, and they can safely be initiated at a full therapeutic dose. Clozapine, risperidone, quetiapine and ziprasidone have alpha-adrenergic effects that necessitate dose titration to avoid orthostatic hypotension. Clozapine produces the most hypotension and tachycardia. Ziprasidone appears to prolong the QT interval more than other atypical agents but less than thioridazine,[46] whereas aripiprazole appears to have no adverse effect on cardiac conduction. Serious cardiac events have been rare in patients treated with ziprasidone (not differing from placebo in registration trials), and reported cases of overdose have been benign.[46] However, ziprasidone's effect on cardiac repolarization may be problematic in the presence of underlying heart disease or when it is added to other agents with similar effects.

Clozapine, although clearly possessing unique antipsychotic efficacy, can produce many bothersome and even potentially lethal side effects, including agranulocytosis (in approximately 1% of patients), sialorrhea, weight gain, hypotension, tachycardia, seizures, impairment of esophageal and bowel motility, and urinary incontinence.[76] Clozapine has also been linked to cardiomyopathy, pericarditis, and pulmonary embolism. Despite the list of potentially serious medical complications, clozapine was found in one study to decrease mortality; this net positive effect on mortality rates probably reflects the magnitude of its protective effect against suicide in contrast to its relatively low frequency of serious adverse effects.[77]

If a patient is to be started or restarted on clozapine, a colleague with experience in the use of this agent should be consulted to clarify the system for monitoring white blood cell counts and to outline strategies for the initiation and optimization of the dosage of this novel agent.[78] Clozapine treatment should not be interrupted when patients are admitted to a medical or surgical service because abrupt discontinuation has been associated with acute worsening of psychosis and cholinergic rebound. If clozapine has been discontinued for more than 4 days, clozapine should be reintroduced at a low dose and titrated upward toward the patient's previous optimal dose.

Treating Agitation

Usual therapeutic doses of antipsychotics do not always treat agitation associated with psychosis successfully. Benzodiazepines can effectively enhance the tranquilizing effect of antipsychotics or be used alone for the treatment of agitation.[79,80] Lorazepam can be combined (in the same syringe) with haloperidol for acute behavioral control—usually 1 mg of lorazepam is given with 5 mg of haloperidol intramuscularly.[79] Once agitation is controlled, the patient can be started on a usually therapeutic dose of an antipsychotic, with a benzodiazepine (e.g., lorazepam 1 to 2 mg) given as needed or as a standing order two to three times daily for as long as is needed. Typically, as the psychotic symptoms improve with use of an antipsychotic, use of a benzodiazepine often becomes unnecessary. Several atypical antipsychotics (i.e., olanzapine and ziprasidone) have been Food and Drug Administration–approved in intramuscular formulations for the control of agitation.[81–83]

Neuroleptic Malignant Syndrome

Neuroleptic malignant syndrome (NMS) is a rare, potentially lethal complication of neuroleptic treatment characterized by hyperthermia, rigidity, confusion, diaphoresis, autonomic instability, elevated creatine phosphokinase (CPK), and leukocytosis. Although the first symptoms of NMS may involve mental status changes, the syndrome may evolve gradually and culminate in fever and an elevated CPK. NMS probably occurs in fewer than 1% of patients who receive conventional antipsychotics, although subsyndromal cases may

be much more common.[84,85] Parallels have been drawn between NMS and malignant hyperthermia (which results from general anesthesia), largely on the basis of common clinical characteristics. Patients with a history of either NMS or malignant hyperthermia, however, do not appear to be at increased risk for developing the other syndrome, and analysis of muscle biopsy specimens has not consistently demonstrated a physiologic link between the two conditions.[84] Lethal catatonia is a spontaneously occurring syndrome that may be indistinguishable from NMS and that has been described in the absence of neuroleptic treatment.[86] In addition, antipsychotic agents may impair temperature regulation and so may produce low-grade fever in the absence of other symptoms of NMS.[87] The clinician's immediate response to NMS should be to discontinue antipsychotic medications and hospitalize the patient to allow for intravenous fluids and cooling. Whether bromocriptine or dantrolene facilitates recovery remains the subject of debate.[88,89] It is important that reinstitution of antipsychotics be delayed until at least 2 weeks after the episode of NMS has resolved.[90] NMS has been associated with use of clozapine and other atypical antipsychotics, but the incidence is probably substantially lower than with conventional agents.[91] It has been suggested that a variant of NMS without rigidity may result from use of atypical antipsychotics, although if such a syndrome occurs, it is probably quite rare.

Drug Interactions with Antipsychotic Agents

Antipsychotic drugs interact with other medications as a result of alterations of hepatic metabolism, and combined use of drugs with additive side effects (such as anticholinergic effects or impairments of cardiac conduction).[92] Most conventional antipsychotics are extensively metabolized by the 2D6 isoenzyme of the hepatic P450 enzyme system, whereas atypical agents generally have more variable hepatic metabolism, typically involving isoenzymes 3A4, 1A2, and 2D6.[93] Fortunately, the therapeutic index (safety/risk ratio) of antipsychotic drugs is quite large, and interactions with agents that inhibit hepatic metabolism are unlikely to be life-threatening, but may increase side effects. Among the atypical antipsychotics, clozapine produces the most serious adverse effects when blood levels are dramatically elevated; obtundation and cardiovascular effects have been associated with inhibition of clozapine metabolism by fluvoxamine or erythromycin.[94,95] Fluvoxamine, a selective serotonin-reuptake inhibitor (SSRI), has been shown to quadruple clozapine plasma concentrations.[94] Some patients experience a doubling of clozapine blood levels when they quit smoking, along with sedation and worsening of other side effects. Addition of 2D6 inhibitors (e.g., SSRIs) to conventional antipsychotics would be expected to increase extrapyramidal side effects, but in one placebo-controlled trial this was not clinically significant despite substantial increases in blood levels of haloperidol and fluphenazine.[96] Drugs that induce hepatic metabolism, such as certain anticonvulsants (e.g., carbamazepine, phenobarbital, and phenytoin), may lower blood concentrations of antipsychotics substantially and cause loss of therapeutic efficacy.[97]

Considerable inter-individual variability exists for the metabolism of antipsychotic drugs, even without the complication of drug interactions. Therapeutic plasma concentrations have been best established for haloperidol because it is the antipsychotic least complicated by active metabolites. Plasma concentrations between 5 and 15 ng/ml have been associated with an optimal therapeutic response.[98] Clozapine has been found to be most effective at serum concentrations of clozapine greater than 350 ng/ml,[99] whereas the risk of toxicity is generally believed to be significant at levels above 1000 ng/ml.

Great care must be taken if low-potency agents (such as chlorpromazine, thioridazine, and clozapine) are combined with other highly anticholinergic drugs because the additive anticholinergic activity may produce confusion, urinary retention, and constipation. In addition, low-potency antipsychotics can depress cardiac function and can significantly impair cardiac conduction when added to class I antiarrhythmic agents (such as quinidine and procainamide). Ziprasidone also significantly affects cardiac conduction and should not be combined with low-potency phenothiazines or with antiarrhythmic agents.[46]

Working with the Patient and the Family

Patients with schizophrenia may be unable to directly express their fears or concerns; instead, they may exhibit anxiety or insomnia and may become increasingly delusional in the face of stress. Efforts to anticipate and answer a patient's unspoken fears about his or her medical status can greatly alleviate other symptoms, although this process may need to be repeated daily. Patients with schizophrenia may also lack the capacity to "filter out" extraneous stimuli in their environment and so may become easily overwhelmed or overly stimulated in a busy, chaotic environment.[100] Placing a patient with schizophrenia in as quiet and orderly a room as possible can help the patient retain a sense of control and foster reality testing. The patient's need for privacy should be respected, and nursing staff should be advised that some patients with schizophrenia do not respond to overly nurturing or seemingly intrusive attention.

Families of patients with schizophrenia can be an invaluable source of information; they can help establish the diagnosis and identify potential behavioral problems. It has also been well demonstrated that educating families about the illness and helping them develop reasonable expectations for their loved one with schizophrenia significantly improves the course of the illness.[101] In addition, one study found that most families of patients with schizophrenia never receive a clear explanation about the illness or a clarification of their prognosis. Although families of young adults who suffer more familiar and readily understood brain insults, such as closed head injury, experience a time-limited period of grief, families of patients with schizophrenia typically suffer from prolonged, unresolved grief reactions as they continually attempt to make sense of their loss. For these families, a clear, medically oriented discussion of the illness and referral to family self-help groups can bring enormous relief.[102] All too often, families burn out after struggling with the patient's disease, leaving the patient alone without family support.

Working with families is always important; it is arguably most important when the patient experiences or is recovering from his or her first psychotic episode. Education about the illness, a discussion about the use of medication, and identification of the early signs of relapse after remission can start in the hospital and help with the transition to outpatient care. Families need to know about the risk for suicide in schizophrenia because they could be the first ones to recognize that a patient is becoming hopeless or disillusioned after discharge.

More Problems in the Care of Psychotic Patients

Assessment of Dangerousness

Several studies have suggested that psychotic patients are at higher risk than those in the general population for committing violent acts, although it is debated whether the data on violence obtained from legal records or from self-reports are reliable. More compelling are studies conducted on individuals who commit homicide in Europe and the United States. The prevalence of schizophrenia in murderers has consistently been 5 to 20 times higher than in the general population.[103] Although assaultive behavior is probably more likely in disorganized patients as a result of impaired control of aggression, violent acts such as homicide, which involve planning or complex behaviors, are much more likely in patients with persecutory or religious delusions (when they are convinced that they have no alternative but to act violently— either to defend themselves or family or to obey God's command). Negative symptoms reduce the risk for violence because afflicted patients are less likely to initiate activity. Command hallucinations appear to increase the risk of violence only when the individual interprets the voices within a delusional system in such a way that the voices cannot be disobeyed.[104] For example, a patient may believe that it is God's voice giving orders to attack someone believed to be possessed by Satan. Although the potential for violence from disorganized or delusional patients is a cause for concern, homicide is actually committed by fewer than 1% of patients with schizophrenia.

Suicide is the main cause of premature death in patients with schizophrenia; 10% of patients with schizophrenia commit suicide and as many as 50% make an attempt. In addition to delusions and hallucinations, depression and substance abuse are important risk factors for suicide. The consultant must explore carefully these risk factors as well as any history of violent or self-injurious behaviors. In patients at high risk for violence or suicide, the antipsychotic clozapine should be considered. Studies have shown a specific protective effect of clozapine on violence that may not be shared by other antipsychotics.[37,105]

Even in patients with schizophrenia and a history of violence, unusual diagnoses of concurrent illness like encephalitis need to be ruled out.[106] Regardless of its cause, in cases in which risk of violence or self-harm is ongoing in the hospital, patients must be monitored continuously. If safe, a sitter is preferred over use of restraints, but some situations require restraints for the safety of the patient, other hospital patients, and staff. However, the indication for restraint must be clear, and restraint has to be part of an overall treatment plan. Inappropriate restraint is not only unjust, but any restraint carries risks, such as deep vein thrombosis and death from pulmonary embolism.[107]

Pain Threshold in Schizophrenia

A large literature suggests that patients with schizophrenia may have dramatically elevated pain thresholds, which can obscure serious medical problems.[108] In one study, 21% of schizophrenic patients did not describe pain associated with a perforated peptic ulcer, and 37% felt no pain during acute appendicitis.[109] It has been estimated that more than 95% of the general public would experience excruciating pain with either condition. The mechanism underlying this often-dramatic analgesic effect remains unclear, but it does not appear to be the result of medication. It is important for the psychiatric consultant to make medical colleagues aware of this characteristic of patients with schizophrenia so that the existence of serious pathologic processes is not dismissed because of an absence of typical manifestations of pain.

Polydipsia (Water Intoxication)

Polydipsia is defined as chronic or intermittent ingestion of large volumes of water; it is reported in 6% to 17% of chronically ill psychiatric patients.

Polydipsia is most frequently diagnosed in patients with schizophrenia, in whom it generally appears 5 to 15 years after the onset of illness.[110] Polydipsia may lead to several complications, including bladder dilatation, enuresis, incontinence, hydronephrosis, renal failure, and congestive heart failure. Approximately 25% to 50% of patients with polydipsia develop hyponatremia within the first 10 years of this condition. Often referred to as *water intoxication*, symptoms of polydipsia with hyponatremia include nausea, vomiting, blurred vision, tremors, cramps, ataxia, confusion, lethargy, seizures, coma, and death. Polydipsia with hyponatremia should be considered a serious complication of psychotic illness that requires careful evaluation and management. Acute care includes supportive treatment, fluid restriction, normal saline, and, in severe cases, use of hypertonic saline. Rapid correction of an abnormal serum sodium level is unwise, however, because it can lead to congestive heart failure and pontine myelinolysis. A medical admission is often necessary until the serum sodium normalizes. Long-term management includes frequent monitoring of serum sodium concentrations and restriction of fluid intake when possible. Switching from conventional neuroleptics to clozapine may significantly improve polydipsia and hyponatremia in some patients.[111]

Cigarette Smoking

An increasingly complex problem for patients with schizophrenia admitted to general hospital services is posed by the restrictions on smoking in the hospital. Surveys have shown that approximately 85% of patients with schizophrenia smoke cigarettes and usually they smoke quite heavily.[112] In addition to enhancing hepatic metabolism of many antipsychotic drugs and thereby reducing blood levels, cigarette smoking may also directly reduce neurologic side effects of antipsychotic drugs and may improve some aspects of cognitive functioning.[113] This has given rise to the view that patients with schizophrenia may in part be self-medicating both their illness and their medication side effects by smoking cigarettes. Use of nicotine dermal patches may provide some comfort to patients with schizophrenia, although care should be taken that they not smoke heavily while wearing the patch.

Although smoking cessation may be a daunting task, it is both desirable and possible for patients with schizophrenia.[114] A hospital admission might provide a window of opportunity to motivate the patient for a quit attempt, particularly if the admission was predicated by smoking.

Medication Adherence and Insight into Illness

One hallmark of schizophrenia is an often striking lack of insight into illness: its symptoms, consequences, and need for treatment.[115] A psychotic patient who has just been involuntarily committed to hospital after fighting with police might report that the reason for the admission was that he came for coffee. Thankfully, this is an extreme example, and many patients have at least some understanding of the role for treatment and can participate meaningfully in decisions regarding use of medication. For some patients, nonadherence to treatment is a major issue. There is little doubt that for the great majority of patients, maintenance antipsychotics must play a pivotal role in preventing psychotic relapse. This is true for patients who have been ill for many years, and for patients who are recovering from their first psychotic episode. In one study of first-episode psychosis patients who discontinued maintenance antipsychotics, 78% and 96% of patients experienced another psychotic episode within 1 and 2 years, respectively.[116] The prevention of further psychotic episodes is paramount because psychotic episodes come at a high cost to the patient: professional lives are interrupted; there is stigma and embarrassment associated with a psychiatric hospitalization; and there is always the danger of violence, accidental injury, and death.[117] On the other hand, hospital staff can be reassured that antipsychotics can usually be held for a brief hospital stay if necessary because relapse is measured in weeks or months, not days.

References

1. Cummings JL: Organic psychosis, *Psychosomatics* 29:16–26, 1988.
2. Fricchione GL, Carbone L, Bennett WI: Psychotic disorder caused by a general medical condition, with

delusions: Secondary "organic" delusional syndromes, *Psychiatr Clin North Am* 18:363–378, 1995.

3. Coleman M, Gillberg C: *The schizophrenias: a biological approach to the schizophrenia spectrum disorders,* New York, 1996, Springer Publishing Company, Inc.

4. Golomb M: Psychiatric symptoms in metabolic and other genetic disorders: is our "organic" work-up complete? *Harvard Rev Psychiatry* 10:242–248, 2002.

5. Weinberger DR: Brain disease and psychiatric illness: when should a psychiatrist order a CAT scan? *Am J Psychiatry* 141:1521–1527, 1984.

6. Bostwick JM, Philbrick KL: The use of electroencephalography in psychiatry of the medically ill, *Psychiatr Clin North Am* 25:17–25, 2002.

7. Sachdev P: Schizophrenia-like psychosis and epilepsy: the status of the association, *Am J Psychiatry* 155:325–336, 1998.

8. Paulsen JS, Ready RE, Hamilton JM, et al: Neuropsychiatric aspects of Huntington's disease, *J Neurol Neurosurg Psychiatry* 71:310–314, 2001.

9. Marsh L: Neuropsychiatric aspects of Parkinson's disease, *Psychosomatics* 41:15–23, 2000.

10. Dening TR, Berrios GE: Wilson's disease. Psychiatric symptoms in 195 cases, *Arch Gen Psychiatry* 46:1126–1134, 1989.

11. American Psychiatric Association: *Diagnostic and statistical manual of mental disorders,* Washington, DC, 1994, American Psychiatric Association.

12. Fennig S, Bromet EJ, Jandorf L, et al: Eliciting psychotic symptoms using a semi-structured diagnostic interview: the importance of collateral sources of information in a first-admission sample, *J Nerv Ment Dis* 182:20–26, 1994.

13. Shaner A, Khalsa E, Roberts L, et al: Unrecognized cocaine use among schizophrenic patients, *Am J Psychiatry* 150:758–762, 1993.

14. Gilmore JH, Perkins DO, Lindsey BA: Factors related to psychiatric consultation for schizophrenic patients receiving medical care, *Hosp Community Psychiatry* 45:1233–1235, 1994.

15. Freudenreich O, Stern TA: Clinical experience with the management of schizophrenia in the general hospital, *Psychosomatics* 44:12–23, 2003.

16. Kontos N, Freudenreich O, Querques J, et al: The consultation psychiatrist as effective physician, *Gen Hosp Psychiatry* 25:20–23, 2003.

17. Koran LM, Sox HC Jr, Marton KI, et al: Medical evaluation of psychiatric patients: I. Results in a state mental health system, *Arch Gen Psychiatry* 47:733–740, 1989.

18. Liddle PF, Barnes TR: Syndromes of chronic schizophrenia, *Br J Psychiatry* 157:558–561, 1990.

19. Andreasen NC: Negative symptoms in schizophrenia: definition and reliability, *Arch Gen Psychiatry* 39:784–788, 1982.

20. Green MF: *Schizophrenia from a neurocognitive perspective: probing the impenetrable darkness,* Boston, 1998, Allyn and Bacon.

21. Havens L: *Forming effective relationships.* In Sabo AN, Havens L, editors: *The real world guide to psychotherapy practice,* Cambridge, Mass, 2000, Harvard University Press, pp 17–33.

22. McGilchrist I, Cutting J: Somatic delusions in schizophrenia and the affective psychoses, *Br J Psychiatry* 167:350–361, 1995.

23. Getz K, Hermann B, Seidenberg M, et al: Negative symptoms in temporal lobe epilepsy, *Am J Psychiatry* 159:644–651, 2002.

24. Sachs G, Printz DJ, Kahn DA: The expert consensus guideline series: medication treatment of bipolar disorder, *Postgrad Med* April:1–104, 2000.

25. Anton R, Burch E: Response of psychotic depression subtypes to pharmacotherapy, *J Affect Disord* 38:125–131, 1993.

26. Kocsis JH, Croughan JL, Katz MM, et al: Response to treatment with antidepressants of patients with severe or moderate nonpsychotic depression and of patients with psychotic depression, *Am J Psychiatry* 147:621–624, 1990.

27. Grossberg GT, Manepalli J: The older patient with psychotic symptoms, *Psychiatr Serv* 46:55–59, 1995.

28. Almeida OP, Howard RJ, Levy R, et al: Psychotic states arising in late life (late paraphrenia): the role of risk factors, *Br J Psychiatry* 166:215–228, 1995.

29. Yassa R, Suranyi-Cadotte B: Clinical characteristics of late-onset schizophrenia and delusional disorder, *Schizophr Bull* 19:701–707, 1993.

30. Flint AJ: Delusions in dementia: a review, *J Neuropsychiatry Clin Neurosci* 3:121–130, 1991.

31. Goff D, Evins A: Negative symptoms in schizophrenia: neurobiological models and treatment response, *Harvard Rev Psychiatry* 6:59–77, 1998.

32. Baldessarini RJ, Cohen BM, Teicher MH: Significance of neuroleptic dose and plasma level in the pharmacological treatment of psychoses, *Arch Gen Psychiatry* 45:79–91, 1988.

33. Miyamoto S, Duncan GE, Goff DC, et al: *Therapeutics of schizophrenia.* In Meltzer H, Nemeroff C, editors: *Psychopharmacology: the fifth generation of progress,* Philadelphia, 2002, Lippincott Williams & Wilkins, pp 775–808.

34. Wahlbeck K, Cheine M, Essali A, et al: Evidence of clozapine's effectiveness in schizophrenia: a systematic review and meta-analysis of randomized trials, *Am J Psychiatry* 156:990–999, 1999.

35. Kane J, Honigfeld G, Singer J, et al: Clozapine for the treatment-resistant schizophrenic: a double-blind comparison with chlorpromazine, *Arch Gen Psychiatry* 45:789–796, 1988.

36. Rosenheck R, Cramer J, Allan E, et al: Cost-effectiveness of clozapine in patients with high and low levels of hospital use: Department of Veterans Affairs Cooperative Study Group on Clozapine in Refractory Schizophrenia, *Arch Gen Psychiatry* 56:565–572, 1999.

37. Meltzer HY, Alphs L, Green AI, et al: Clozapine treatment for suicidality in schizophrenia: International Suicide Prevention Trial (InterSePT), *Arch Gen Psychiatry* 60:82–91, 2003.

38. Marder S, Davis J, Chouinard G: The effects of risperidone on the five dimensions of schizophrenia derived by factor analysis: combined results of the North American trials, *J Clin Psychiatry* 58:538–546, 1997.

39. Davis JM, Chen N: The effects of olanzapine on the 5 dimensions of schizophrenia derived by factor analysis: combined results of the North American and international trials, *J Clin Psychiatry* 62:757–771, 2001.

40. Csernansky JG, Mahmoud R, Brenner R: A comparison of risperidone and haloperidol for the prevention of relapse in patients with schizophrenia, *N Engl J Med* 346:16–22, 2002.

41. Volavka J, Czobor P, Sheitman B, et al: Clozapine, olanzapine, risperidone, and haloperidol in the treatment of patients with chronic schizophrenia and schizoaffective disorder, *Am J Psychiatry* 159:255–162, 2002.

42. Goff DC, Shader RI: Non-neurologic side effects of antipsychotic agents. In Winberger D, Hirsch D, editors: *Schizophrenia*, London, England, Washington, DC, 1995, Blackwell Science, Ltd., pp 566–586.

43. Cramer JA, Rosenheck R: Compliance with medication regimens for psychiatric and medical disorders, *Psychiatr Serv* 49:196–210, 1998.

44. Olfson M, Mechanic D, Hansell S, et al: Predicting medication noncompliance after hospital discharge among patients with schizophrenia, *Psychiatr Serv* 51:216–222, 2000.

45. Steingard S, Allen M, Schooler NR: A study of the pharmacologic treatment of medication-compliant schizophrenics who relapse, *J Clin Psychiatry* 55:470–472, 1994.

46. Glassman AH, Bigger JT Jr: Antipsychotic drugs: prolonged QTc interval, torsade de pointes, and sudden death, *Am J Psychiatry* 158:1774–1782, 2001.

47. Arana GW, Goff DC, Baldessarini RJ, et al: Efficacy of anticholinergic prophylaxis for neuroleptic-induced acute dystonia, *Am J Psychiatry* 145:993–996, 1988.

48. Goff D, Arana G, Greenblatt D, et al: The effect of benztropine on haloperidol-induced dystonia, clinical efficacy and pharmacokinetics: a prospective, double-blind trial, *J Clin Psychopharmacol* 11:106–112, 1991.

49. Adler LA, Angrist B, Reiter S, et al: Neuroleptic-induced akathisia: a review, *Psychopharmacology* 97:1–11, 1989.

50. Fleischhacker WW, Roth SD, Kane JM: The pharmacologic treatment of neuroleptic-induced akathisia, *J Clin Psychopharmacol* 10:12–21, 1990.

51. Van Putten T, May PRA: "Akinetic depression" in schizophrenia, *Arch Gen Psychiatry* 35:1101–1107, 1978.

52. Gelenberg AJ: Treating extrapyramidal reactions: some current issues, *J Clin Psychiatry* 48(suppl):24–27, 1987.

53. Baker LA, Cheng LY, Amara IB: The withdrawal of benztropine mesylate in chronic schizophrenic patients, *Br J Psychiatry* 143:584–590, 1983.

54. Friedman JH, Factor SA: Atypical antipsychotics in the treatment of drug-induced psychosis in Parkinson's disease, *Mov Disord* 15:201–211, 2000.

55. Jeste D, Caligiuri M: Tardive dyskinesia, *Schizophr Bull* 19:303–316, 1993.

56. Cooper SJ, Doherty MM, King DJ: Tardive dystonia: the benefits of time, *Br J Psychiatry* 155:113–115, 1989.

57. Kane J, Woerner M, Weinhold P, et al: Incidence of tardive dyskinesia: five-year data from a prospective study, *Psychopharmacology Bull* 20:39–40, 1984.

58. Khot V, Wyatt RJ: Not all that moves is tardive dyskinesia, *Am J Psychiatry* 148:661–666, 1991.

59. Adler LA, Rotrosen J, Edson R, et al: Vitamin E treatment for tardive dyskinesia, *Arch Gen Psychiatry* 56:836–841, 1999.

60. Lieberman JA, Saltz BL, Johns CA, et al: Clozapine effects on tardive dyskinesia, *Psychopharmacol Bull* 25:57–62, 1989.

61. Tollefson G, Beasley C, Tamura R, et al: Blind, controlled, long-term study of the comparative incidence of treatment-emergent tardive dyskinesia with olanzapine or haloperidol, *Am J Psychiatry* 154:1248–1254, 1997.

62. Jeste DV, Lacro JP, Bailey A, et al: Lower incidence of tardive dyskinesia with risperidone compared to haloperidol in older patients, *J Am Geriatr Soc* 47:716–719, 1999.

63. Munetz MR, Toenniessen L, Scala C, et al: Onset and course of tardive dyskinesia, *Psychosomatics* 30:346–356, 1989.

64. Umbricht D, Kane J: Risperidone: efficacy and safety, *Schizophr Bull* 21:593–606, 1995.

65. Russell JM, Mackell JA: Bodyweight gain associated with atypical antipsychotics: epidemiology and therapeutic implications, *CNS Drugs* 15:537–551, 2001.

66. Henderson D, Cagliero E, Gray C, et al: Clozapine, diabetes mellitus, weight gain, and lipid abnormalities: a five year naturalistic study, *Am J Psychiatry* 157:975–981, 2000.

67. Koller E, Schneider B, Bennett K, et al: Clozapine-associated diabetes, *Am J Med* 111:716–723, 2001.

68. Koller EA, Doraiswamy PM: Olanzapine-associated diabetes mellitus, *Pharmacotherapy* 22:841–852, 2002.

69. Henderson DC: Atypical antipsychotic-induced diabetes mellitus: how strong is the evidence? *CNS Drugs* 16:77–89, 2002.

70. Newcomer JW, Haupt DW, Fucetola R, et al: Abnormalities in glucose regulation during antipsychotic treatment of schizophrenia, *Arch Gen Psychiatry* 59:337–345, 2002.

71. Sernyak MJ, Leslie DL, Alarcon RD, et al: Association of diabetes mellitus with use of atypical neuroleptics in the treatment of schizophrenia, *Am J Psychiatry* 159:561–566, 2001.

72. Gianfrancesco FD, Grogg AL, Mahmoud RA, et al: Differential effects of risperidone, olanzapine, clozapine, and conventional antipsychotics on type 2 diabetes: findings from a large health plan database, *J Clin Psychiatry* 63:920–930, 2002.

73. Caro JJ, Ward A, Levinton C, et al: The risk of diabetes during olanzapine use compared with risperidone use: a retrospective database analysis, *J Clin Psychiatry* 63:1135–1139, 2002.

74. Buse JB, Cavazzoni P, Hornbuckle K, et al: A retrospective cohort study of diabetes mellitus and antipsychotic treatment in the United States, *J Clin Epidemiol* 56:164–170, 2003.

75. Ryan MC, Collins P, Thakore JH: Impaired fasting glucose tolerance in first-episode, drug-naive patients with schizophrenia, *Am J Psychiatry* 160:284–289, 2003.

76. Buchanan RW: Clozapine: efficacy and safety, *Schizophr Bull* 21:579–591, 1995.

77. Walker AM, Lanza LL, Arellano F, et al: Mortality in current and former users of clozapine, *Epidemiology* 8:671–677, 1997.

78. Lieberman JA, Kane JM, Johns CA: Clozapine: guidelines for clinical management, *J Clin Psychiatry* 50:329–338, 1989.

79. Garza-Trevino ES, Hollister LE, Overall JE, et al: Efficacy of combinations of intramuscular antipsychotics and sedative-hypnotics for control of psychotic agitation, *Am J Psychiatry* 146:1598–1601, 1989.

80. Salzman C, Solomon D, Miyawaki E, et al: Parental lorazepam versus parental haloperidol for the control of psychotic disruptive behavior, *J Clin Psychiatry* 52:177–180, 1991.

81. Altamura AC, Sassella F, Santini A, et al: Intramuscular preparations of antipsychotics: uses and relevance in clinical practice, *Drugs* 63:493–512, 2003.

82. Breier A, Meehan K, Birkett M, et al: A double-blind, placebo-controlled dose-response comparison of intramuscular olanzapine and haloperidol in the treatment of acute agitation in schizophrenia, *Arch Gen Psychiatry* 59:441–448, 2002.

83. Lesem MD, Zajecka JM, Swift RH, et al: Intramuscular ziprasidone, 2 mg versus 10 mg, in the short-term management of agitated psychotic patients, *J Clin Psychiatry* 62:12–18, 2001.

84. Addonizio G, Susman VL, Roth SD: Neuroleptic malignant syndrome: review and analysis of 115 cases, *Biol Psychiatry* 22:1004–1020, 1987.

85. Keck PEJ, Sebastianelli J, Pope HGJ, et al: Frequency and presentation of neuroleptic malignant syndrome in a state psychiatric hospital, *J Clin Psychiatry* 50:352–355, 1989.

86. Weller M: NMS and lethal catatonia, *J Clin Psychiatry* 53:294, 1992.

87. Lazarus A: Differentiating neuroleptic-related heatstroke from neuroleptic malignant syndrome, *Psychosomatics* 30:454–456, 1989.

88. Rosebush PI, Stewart T, Mazurek MF: The treatment of neuroleptic malignant syndrome: are dantrolene and bromocriptine useful adjuncts to supportive care? *Br J Psychiatry* 159:709–712, 1991.

89. Sakkas P, Davis JM, Janicak PG, et al: Drug treatment of the neuroleptic malignant syndrome, *Psychopharmacol Bull* 27:381–384, 1991.

90. Rosebush PI, Stewart TD, Gelenberg AJ: Twenty neuroleptic rechallenges after neuroleptic malignant syndrome in 15 patients, *J Clin Psychiatry* 50:295–298, 1989.

91. Levenson JL: Neuroleptic malignant syndrome associated after the initiation of olanzapine, *J Clin Psychopharmacol* 19:477–478, 1999.

92. Goff D, Baldessarini R: Drug interactions with antipsychotic agents, *J Clin Psychopharmacol* 13:57–67, 1993.

93. Ereshefsky L: Pharmacokinetics and drug interactions: update for new antipsychotics, *J Clin Psychiatry* 57(suppl 11):12–25, 1996.

94. Wetzel H, Anghelescu I, Szegedi A, et al: Pharmacokinetic interactions of clozapine with selective serotonin reuptake inhibitors: differential effects of fluvoxamine and paroxetine in a prospective study, *J Clin Psychopharmacol* 18:2–9, 1998.

95. Cohen LG, Chessley S, Eugenio L, et al: Erythromycin-induced clozapine toxic reaction, *Arch Intern Med* 156:675–677, 1996.

96. Goff D, Midha K, Brotman A, et al: Elevation of plasma concentrations of haloperidol after addition of fluoxetine, *Am J Psychiatry* 148:790–792, 1991.

97. Arana GW, Goff DC, Friedman H, et al: Does carbamazepine-induced reduction of plasma haloperidol levels worsen psychotic symptoms? *Am J Psychiatry* 143:650–651, 1986.

98. Van Putten T, Marder S, Wirshing W, et al: Neuroleptic plasma levels, *Schizophr Bull* 17:197–216, 1991.

99. Kronig MH, Munne RA, Szymanski S, et al: Plasma clozapine levels and clinical response for treatment-refractory schizophrenic patients, *Am J Psychiatry* 152:179–182, 1995.

100. Grillon C, Courchesne E, Ameli R, et al: Increased distractibility in schizophrenic patients. Electrophysiologic and behavioral evidence, *Arch Gen Psychiatry* 47:171–179, 1990.

101. Leff J: Working with the families of schizophrenic patients, *Br J Psychiatry* 23:71–76, 1994.

102. McFarlane WR, Lukens E, Link B, et al: Multiple-family groups and psychoeducation in the treatment of schizophrenia, *Arch Gen Psychiatry* 52:679–687, 1995.

103. Taylor PJ, Estroff SE: *Schizophrenia and violence.* In Hirsch SR, Weinberger DR, editors: *Schizophrenia.* Oxford, UK, 2003, Blackwell Science Ltd, pp 591–612.

104. Zisook S, Byrd D, Kuck J, et al: Command hallucinations in outpatients with schizophrenia, *J Clin Psychiatry* 56:462–465, 1995.

105. Frankle W, Shera D, Berger-Hershkowitz H, et al: Clozapine-associated reduction in arrest rates of psychotic patients with criminal histories, *Am J Psychiatry* 158:270–274, 2001.

106. Tardiff K: Unusual diagnoses among violent patients, *Psychiatr Clin North Am* 21:567–576, 1998.

107. Hem E, Steen O, Opjordsmoen S: Thrombosis associated with physical restraints, *Acta Psychiatr Scand* 103:73–76, 2001.

108. Dworkin RH: Pain insensitivity in schizophrenia: a neglected phenomenon and some implications, *Schizophr Bull* 20:235–248, 1994.

109. Marchand W: Occurrence of painless myocardial infarction in psychotic patients, *N Engl J Med* 253:51–55, 1955.

110. Illowsky BP, Kirch DG: Polydipsia and hyponatremia in psychiatric patients, *Am J Psychiatry* 145:675–683, 1988.

111. Henderson D, Goff DC: Clozapine for polydipsia and hyponatremia in chronic schizophrenics, *Biol Psychiatry* 36:768–770, 1994.

112. Hughes JR, Hatsukami DK, Mitchell JE, et al: Prevalence of smoking among psychiatric outpatients, *Am J Psychiatry* 143:993–997, 1986.

113. Goff DC, Henderson DC, Amico E: Cigarette smoking in schizophrenia: relationship to psychopathology and medication side effects, *Am J Psychiatry* 149:1189–1194, 1992.

114. Addington J, el-Guebaly N, Campbell W, et al: Smoking cessation treatment for patients with schizophrenia, *Am J Psychiatry* 155:974–976, 1988.

115. David A, Kemp R: Five perspectives on the phenomenon of insight in psychosis. *Psychiatric Annals* 27:791–797, 1997.

116. Gitlin M, Nuechterlein K, Subotnik KL, et al: Clinical outcome following neuroleptic discontinuation in patients with remitted recent-onset schizophrenia, *Am J Psychiatry* 158:1835–1842, 2001.

117. Lieberman JA, Fenton WS: Delayed detection of psychosis: causes, consequences, and effect on public health (editorial), *Am J Psychiatry* 157:1727–1730, 2000.

Chapter 15
Anxious Patients

Mark H. Pollack, M.D.
Michael W. Otto, Ph.D.
Jerrold G. Bernstein, M.D.
Jerrold F. Rosenbaum, M.D.

The clinical challenges in the diagnosis and treatment of anxiety are endemic to the general hospital setting: discerning normal from pathologic anxiety, differentiating medical from psychiatric causes, and choosing effective therapeutic approaches. In addition to a knowledge of medical and psychiatric differential diagnosis, the clinician may rely on a variety of strategies and interventions, including pharmacologic, cognitive-behavioral, interpersonal, and psychodynamic skills. The ubiquitousness of anxiety and the nonspecific nature of anxiety symptoms can confound the care of the patient. Pathologic anxiety symptoms and behavior may be attributed to other physical causes or, when viewed as "only anxiety," may be prematurely dismissed as insignificant.

Anxiety is indistinguishable from fear except as to cause. The former is the same distressing experience of dread and foreboding as the latter except that it derives from an unknown internal stimulus or is inappropriate to the reality of the current situation. Anxiety is manifested in the physical, affective, cognitive, and behavioral domains. The possible physical symptoms of anxiety reflect autonomic arousal and include an array of bodily perturbations (Table 15-1). The anxious state ranges from edginess and unease to terror and panic. Cognitively, the experience is one of worry, apprehension, and thoughts concerned with emotional or bodily danger. Behaviorally, anxiety triggers a multitude of responses concerned with diminishing or avoiding the distress.

The importance of recognizing and attending to the suffering of the anxious patient is not always easily apparent, given the universality of the experience of anxiety. Anxiety is expected and normal as a transient response to stress and may be a necessary cue for adaptation and coping. Excessive or pathologic anxiety, however, is no more a normal state than is the production of excess thyroid hormone.

Pathologic anxiety is distinguished from a normal emotional response by four criteria: (1) autonomy, (2) intensity, (3) duration, and (4) behavior. *Autonomy* refers to suffering that, to some extent, has a "life of its own," with a minimal basis in recognizable environmental stimuli. *Intensity* refers to the level of distress; the severity of symptoms is such that the patient's level of anguish moves the physician to offer relief. The patient's capacity to bear discomfort has been exceeded. The *duration* of suffering also can define anxiety as pathologic: Symptoms that are persistent rather than transient, possibly adaptive responses indicate disorder and are a call to evaluation and treatment. Finally, *behavior* is a critical criterion; if anxiety impairs coping, if normal function is disrupted, or if behavior, such as avoidance or withdrawal results, the anxiety is of a pathologic nature.

Stereotyped syndromes of pathologic anxiety are represented in the American Psychiatric

Table 15-1. Physical Signs and Symptoms of Anxiety

Anorexia	Muscle tension
"Butterflies" in stomach	Nausea
Chest pain or tightness	Pallor
Diaphoresis	Palpitations
Diarrhea	Paresthesias
Dizziness	Sexual dysfunction
Dry mouth	Shortness of breath
Dyspnea	Stomach pain
Faintness	Tachycardia
Flushing	Tremulousness
Headache	Urinary frequency
Hyperventilation	Vomiting
Light-headedness	

Association's *Diagnostic and Statistical Manual of Mental Disorders*, Anxiety Disorders (Table 15-2).[1] In epidemiologic studies, anxiety disorders were found to be among the most common psychiatric disorders in the general population.[2] This observation predicts that a significant percentage of the general hospital population would also suffer from anxiety symptoms. In addition to those patients who suffer from an anxiety disorder before admission to the hospital for medical care, medical and surgical settings are also associated with the onset of anxiety symptoms as a consequence of hospitalization, medical illness, or its

treatment (e.g., adjustment disorder with anxious mood and organic anxiety disorder).[3]

The Nature and Origin of Anxiety

Despite the protean physiologic manifestations of anxiety, the experience of anxiety can be divided into two broad categories: (1) an acute, severe, and brief wave of intense anxiety with impressive cognitive, physiologic, and behavioral components and (2) a lower-grade persistent distress, quantitatively distinct and with some qualitative differences as well. Pharmacologic and epidemiologic observations suggest a clinically relevant distinction between these two states.

In light of phenomenologic similarities, fear and anxiety likely reflect a common underlying neurophysiology. The first category of anxiety resembles acute fear or alarm in response to life-threatening danger: a cognitive state of terror, helplessness, or sense of impending disaster or doom, with autonomic but primarily sympathetic activation, and an urgency to flee or seek safety. The second type of anxiety corresponds to a state of alertness with a heightened sense of vigilance to possible threats and less intense levels of inhibition, physical distress, and behavioral impairment.

Table 15-2. Anxiety Disorders

Panic disorder: Recurrent panic attacks ranging in severity from severe (experienced as terror, "going to die" or "lose control") to mild (only "limited symptom attacks" or rare panic attack); if complicated by fear of places of restricted or embarrassing escape or where help is unavailable, by travel restriction (or need for a companion), or by endurance of such situations despite intense anxiety, the diagnosis is panic disorder with (mild, moderate, or severe) agoraphobia.

Phobic disorders:
    Simple phobia: Intense fear of and attempt to avoid specific objects or situations (e.g., heights)
    Social phobia: Intense anxiety or discomfort in situations of scrutiny by others with typical fear of embarrassment or humiliation (e.g., stage fright)
    Agoraphobia: (without history of panic disorder)

Generalized anxiety disorder: 6-month history of anxious symptoms but not panic attacks, with cognitive (worry) and autonomic symptoms.

Posttraumatic stress disorder: A syndrome with onset following a traumatic, usually life-threatening, event. The course may resemble panic disorder with the herald attack a real-life threat rather than spontaneous panic. Recurrent images of the original event frequently occur.

Obsessive-compulsive disorder: Recurrent intrusive unwanted thoughts and images as well as compulsive behaviors, such as rituals, characterize this disorder. Panic attacks and generalized anxiety also occur.

The most common form of anxious suffering in a hospital population is most likely transient situational reactions or adjustment disorders with anxiety.

Reprinted with permission from American Psychiatric Association: *Diagnostic and statistical manual of mental disorders*, ed 4, Washington, DC, 1994, American Psychiatric Association.

The two fear states resemble the clinical syndromes of panic attacks and generalized or anticipatory anxiety. As innate responses for protecting the organism and enhancing survival, panic and vigilance are normal when faced with threatening stimuli. As anxiety or psychopathologic symptoms, other factors besides actual physical threat must be implicated as triggers or cause. Of several explanatory models proposed, the biologic model places emphasis on the nervous system, the psychodynamic on meanings and memories, and the behavioral on learning.

Animal and neuronal receptor studies suggest that there are a number of central systems involved in fear and pathologic anxiety.[4,5] The alarm or panic mechanism is likely to have a critical component involving central noradrenergic mechanisms, with particular importance placed on a small retropontine nucleus, the primary source of the brain's norepinephrine, the locus coeruleus (LC). When this key to sympathetic activation is stimulated in monkeys, for example, an acute fear response can be elicited with distress vocalizations, fear behaviors, and flight. Alternatively, destruction of the LC leads to abnormal complacency in the face of threat.[6] Biochemical perturbations that increase LC firing similarly elicit anxious responses in animals and humans that are blocked by agents that decrease LC firing, some of which are in clinical practice as antipanic agents (e.g., antidepressants, alprazolam).[7]

Another critical system involves limbic system structures, including the amygdala and septohippocampal areas. An important role of the limbic system is to scan the environment for life-supporting and life-threatening cues, as well as to monitor internal or bodily sensations, and to integrate these with memory and cognitive inputs in assessing the degree of threat and need for action to maintain safety.[8]

Vigilance or its psychopathologic equivalent, generalized anxiety, most probably involves limbic system activity: limbic alert. Benzodiazepine receptors in high concentration in relevant limbic system structures may play a role in modulating limbic alert, arousal, and behavioral inhibition[9] by increased binding of the inhibitory neurotransmitter gamma aminobutyric acid (GABA).[10] As one might expect, there are neuronal connections between the LC and limbic systems. An increased firing rate of LC neurons may serve as a rheostat to generate levels of arousal from vigilance to alarm.

A number of neurotransmitters are implicated as modulators of both the limbic alert and the central alarm systems. For example, LC firing is regulated by the α_2-noradrenergic autoreceptors as well as by 5-hydroxytryptamine (5-HT), serotonin receptors, GABA-benzodiazepine receptors, opiate, and other receptors. The limbic system also has important GABA-benzodiazepine receptor and serotonergic modulations. Peptides such as cholecystokinin[11] have also been implicated as potential activators of the alarm system and an accruing body of work points to abnormalities in corticotropin-releasing factor and hypothalamic pituitary axis function as critical in the genesis and maintenance of pathologic affective states.[12] As a critical function, the central security system is endowed with redundancy of regulation.

When inappropriately activated, vigilance and alarm (the stereotyped functions of the security system) are manifested as psychopathology: anxiety states. The more sustained, variably intense, but distressing arousal state of vigilance (i.e., preparation for threat) becomes generalized anxiety. The sudden, stereotyped, and intense (but false) alarm response is a panic attack.

Cognitive-behavioral formulations of anxiety disorders, although attending to possible differences in biologic reactivity, focus primary attention on the information processing and behavioral reactions that characterize an individual's anxiety experience. Although anxiety patterns may stem from a variety of experiences, including (mis)information, observational learning, and direct conditioning events with real or perceived trauma, the enduring consequences of such learning can be found in current patterns of behavior. In cognitive-behavioral formulations, emphasis is placed on the role of thoughts and beliefs (cognitions) in activating anxiety as well as the role of avoidance or other escape responses in maintaining both fear and faulty thinking patterns. Faulty cognitions are frequently marked by the overprediction of the likelihood or degree of catastrophe of negative events and may focus on external experiences (e.g., "my colleagues will laugh at me if I ask this question") or internal experiences (e.g., "I am going to lose control if this anxiety gets worse"). Intolerance and catastrophic misinterpretations of the anxiety experience itself play a role in a variety of anxiety conditions and can help propel mild anxiety into a full, intense panic attack. Attempts to neutralize anxious feelings, with avoidance or compulsive behavior, can serve to lock in anxiety reactions and help develop the chronic arousal and anticipatory anxiety that marks many anxiety disorders.

Developmental experiences receive particular emphasis in psychodynamic approaches to anxiety. Although Freud's early writing implied a more physiologic basis for anxiety attacks in terms of undischarged libido, later emphasis was on anxiety as a signal of threat to the ego, signals elicited because of events and situations with similarities (symbolic or actual) to early developmental experiences that were threatening to the vulnerable child (traumatic anxiety), such as separations, losses, certain constellations of relationships, and symbolic objects or events (e.g., snakes, successes). More recent psychodynamic thinking emphasizes object relations and the use of internalized objects to maintain affective stability under stress.

Phobic disorders, whose sufferers may experience panic, anticipatory anxiety, or no anxiety symptoms at all (depending on the success of avoidance behavior), serve to illustrate the differing models of understanding anxiety. The biologic view recognizes the stereotyped nature of phobias. Most of the objects and situations in everyday life that truly threaten us are rarely selected as phobic stimuli; children, who proceed normally through a variety of developmental phobias (e.g., strangers, separation, darkness), rarely become phobic of objects and situations that parents attempt to associate with danger (e.g., electric outlets, roads), and most phobic stimuli have meaning in the context of biologic preparedness and were presumably selected through evolution.[13] Most human phobias are of objects and situations that make sense in the context of enhancing survival before the dawn of civilization: places of restricted escape, groups of strangers, heights, and snakes, for example. Social phobias, for example, fear of scrutiny by others, resemble the intense discomfort elicited in primates introduced into a new colony or in any animal simply being stared at—a glare is a threat. When panic attacks and anticipatory anxiety

heighten the general sense of danger and insecurity, a variety of phobias may become manifested as part of the patient's increased concern with security and safety.

The principal explanatory models in psychiatry of how a normal protective system might become the source of distress and dysfunction include the biologic, with its emphasis on constitutional vulnerability; the cognitive-behavioral, with its emphasis on self-perpetuating patterns of cognitions and behaviors; and the psychodynamic, with its emphasis on meanings, memories, and internal representations derived from developmental experience. The pragmatic and pluralistic modern clinician should not regard these models as mutually exclusive. Potential biologic vulnerabilities, for example, may never become manifested without specific developmental experiences, sustained adversity, or trauma. Accumulating evidence indicates that for anxiety disorders, as with affective and psychotic disorders, biologic systems are responsive to and perturbable by environmental influences. Potentially dysregulated (i.e., anxiety-prone) neurobiologic systems may remain homeostatic until developmental experience, life events, or other stressors disturb them. An integrated model predicts risk for manifested anxiety disorder as a consequence of constitutional vulnerability shaped by developmental experience (whether harmful or protective) and, in later (adult) life, either activated or influenced by environmental factors and maintained by ongoing chains of maladaptive cognitions and avoidance responses.

Anxiety in the Medical Setting

Although some distress from anxiety is expected as a routine consequence of hospitalization, anxiety may also be a significant clinical issue in the treatment of patients in a medical setting. The hospitalized patient encounters a world of both internal and external dangers: assaults on bodily integrity in the form of uncomfortable procedures and forced intimacy with strangers; the atmosphere of illness, pain, and death; and separation from loved ones and familiar surroundings. The patient typically experiences uncertainty about his or her illness and its implications for the patient's capacity to work and maintain social and family relationships. Just as depression has been described as a "psychobiologic final common pathway" of a number of interacting determinants,[14] it is likely that anxiety too represents a multidetermined expression of the variety of psychological, biologic, and social factors having impact on the patient.

The anxious patient can be a diagnostic challenge. The presence of anxiety may represent the patient's reaction to the meaning and implications of medical illness or to the medical setting, a manifestation of the physical disorder itself, or the expression of an underlying psychiatric disorder. The distinction between anxiety as a symptom and anxiety as a syndrome may be difficult to make in the medical setting, where there may be an overlap between normal situational anxiety or fear, anxiety-like symptoms resulting from a variety of organic disease states and their treatments, and the characteristic presentation of anxiety disorders.

Methodological obstacles surface in attempts to identify the nature and prevalence of anxiety in medical patients.[15] Studies of anxiety in the medical setting are often difficult to interpret because of a lack of clarity of case definition and assessment measures, heterogeneity of the study populations, absence of appropriate control groups, and the nonspecific and often transitory nature of the anxiety symptoms themselves.

Approximately 60% of patients with psychiatric conditions are treated by primary practitioners; the most common disorders are depression and anxiety.[16,17] In a study of patients presenting to a group of primary care physicians (PCPs), anxiety was the fifth most common diagnosis overall; others suggest this may be an underestimate.[18,19] Anxiety is the chief complaint of 11% of patients presenting in primary care settings.[20] This prevalence is mirrored by the high rate of prescribing benzodiazepines by PCPs.[21] Panic disorder has a reported prevalence of 1% to 2% in the general population,[22] as compared with 6% to 10% of patients in a primary care setting[23] and 10% to 14% of patients in a cardiology practice.[24] The number of patients with anxiety disorders, furthermore, is but a subgroup of those for whom anxiety is a complicating factor in their diagnosis and treatment in hospital.

In view of the likely frequency of normal anxiety in this setting, there must be special circumstances surrounding those patients identified by primary caregivers as deserving psychiatric attention. Although some overly anxious patients go unrecognized, those who generate concern must have impressed their caregivers in some way by the autonomy, intensity, duration, or behavior associated with their distress. Several typical scenarios of anxiety in the general hospital can be recognized.

Anxiety from the Failure to Cope

For most patients, the potentially overwhelming stressors of hospitalization are mitigated by a variety of coping mechanisms. The sources of threat and the flood of perceptions signaling potential danger are managed by common strategies: rationalization and self-reassurance ("I've come this far," "the doctors know what they're doing," "safest place in the world"), denial and minimization ("the chest pain is just heartburn," "these machines will protect me"), religious faith, support from family and friends, and other strategies determined by the patient's personality style.

Even for those without a preillness anxiety disorder, coping strategies may fail and yield to a sense of fear and vulnerability. A host of factors may be implicated in this failure: personality features with brittleness or a tendency to regress in the face of threat (or paradoxically in a setting that evokes passivity and offers access to nurturance), the suddenness of the onset of threat (acute, life-threatening medical or surgical disease), unavailability of familial or other social support, feelings of aloneness or abandonment, or the unconscious meaning of the particular illness or injury. The patient becomes frightened, trembles, cannot sleep, repeatedly seeks attention and reassurance, registers excessive pain complaints and other physical symptoms, and becomes disruptive and unable to manage the fear. For many, especially the young or those with organic brain syndromes (e.g., mental retardation, dementia), catastrophic emotional responses are more readily triggered.

Case 1

A psychiatric consultation request was received for a 17-year-old high school junior following above-the-knee amputation for osteogenic sarcoma without evidence of metastasis at the time of surgery. He had returned to school with a prosthesis and had done well. Some months later, a pulmonary metastasis was discovered, and he was rehospitalized for surgery and chemotherapy. Although anticipating a favorable outcome at this point, his behavior was unlike that of his prior hospitalization. He raged at caregivers, acted panicky, and withdrew from contact. Consultation was sought for treatment of his anxiety.

He was a tall, handsome, athletic, young man admired by his peers, a "leader" who managed his life with braggadocio and pseudoindependence. For the first time in his illness, he was overwhelmed and frightened. Two critical issues emerged from the interview. In the past, he had a great deal of support from his peers, but lately he had refused their visits. He was embarrassed by hair loss from chemotherapy. Second, during this hospitalization, his father, feeling overwhelmed by this turn of events, had decreased the frequency of visits to his son claiming increased work demands.

Two interventions calmed the acute anxiety. First, effort was made to find a well-suited wig; second, a psychotherapeutic contact with the father helped him to manage his grief adequately to increase the frequency of visits and thereby relieve his son's separation anxiety.

Although the oncologist's request was for an anxiolytic prescription, recognition of the failure of coping ability yielded the appropriate therapy for the acute anxiety.

This case serves to underscore two points: (1) Previously well-adapted individuals can become anxious in the face of serious or life-threatening illness; (2) despite the appropriateness of anxiety in the face of serious illness, other factors, potentially remediable, may be involved in triggering anxious symptoms or behavior. In this case, troublesome behavior was evident; for others, only more subtle physical symptoms may have occurred.

Anxiety Resulting from Traumatic Procedures

In recent years, increasing attention has been paid to the role of serious medical illness and invasive procedures in producing marked anxiety reactions that approach or meet criteria for post-traumatic stress disorder (PTSD). For example, symptoms of PTSD have been documented in patients following myocardial infarction (MI) and coronary artery bypass graft (CABG) surgery[25] and treatment for breast cancer.[26] Estimates of rates of PTSD in these samples of patients range from 5% to 10%,[26] with rates of PTSD in patients hospitalized after traumatic physical injuries as high as 30% to 40%.[27] The emergence of PTSD is considered most likely when a traumatic event is perceived as both uncontrollable and life-threatening[28]; as such, any attempts to help patients regain or maintain a sense of control over their experiences may prevent or reduce emergent distress.

Attention is also being paid to PTSD reactions that may follow surgery performed under inadequate anesthesia.[29] Memory for events during anesthesia has been well documented in controlled trials,[30,31] leading to recommendations that the surgical staff provide reassurance to patients during surgery and monitor their own verbalizations in the presence of anesthetized patients. Postoperative anxiety was a significant predictor of patients who reported recall in a series of 30 patients who underwent CABG surgery, with the proportion of patients recalling intraoperative events ranging between 10% and 23%,[30] although other reports suggest that rates of recall may be far less.[32] One source of this variability may be that some patients do not readily discuss their memories and that memories may emerge some time after discharge.[33] Routine postoperative inquiry about possible awareness has been recommended to ensure that patients have an opportunity to discuss their memories, if present, and to allow assessment of the need for treatment if traumatic reactions are evident.[34]

Reactions to awareness during surgery include generalized anxiety and irritability, repetitive nightmares, and preoccupation with death as well as reluctance to discuss the memory or associated symptoms.[33] More severe reactions have also been documented, including the full emergence of PTSD following experiences of awareness during surgery. Patients who are aware during surgery may face the terrifying experience of pain occurring in conjunction with anesthesia-induced paralysis (ensuring that no overt coping or escape responses are available) and the fear of death. As memories of the trauma emerge, patients may face the full spectrum of PTSD symptoms, including reexperiencing symptoms (intrusive memories, nightmares, and over-responsivity to cues of the surgery), avoidance of reminders of the experience (e.g., avoidance of strong emotions, prone bodily positions or sleep, medical television shows, colors similar to those of surgical scrub suits), and symptoms of pervasive autonomic arousal (e.g., exaggerated startle, sleep difficulties, hypervigilance, and irritability). Timely identification of this syndrome can aid in rapid referral for full psychiatric evaluation and treatment, which may include both cognitive-behavioral and pharmacologic interventions.

Anxiety Interfering with Evaluation or Treatment

A request for consultation may be a consequence of anxiety that interferes with a patient's evaluation or treatment: refusal of work-up or treatment because of fear of pain or discomfort, catastrophic interpretation of physical symptoms or of the planned work-up ("they're looking for cancer") with an excessively fearful response, or the need to minimize or deny a potentially serious condition and its implications limiting cooperation with evaluation.

Case 2

Examination of a 38-year-old woman revealed a large breast lump. Although initially reluctant, she eventually agreed to a mammogram. In the waiting room, she became increasingly anxious and, when her name was called, refused to come in for the test. A psychiatric consultation was called to provide management of the patient's anxiety to permit the mammogram.

An attractive woman, she had stopped working as a teacher 12 years earlier after marrying a successful business executive and having the first of her two children. On interview she spoke of a favorite aunt who had died of breast cancer after disfiguring surgeries and her own fear of a similar lesion. She was plagued by the thought that the loss of a breast would cause her husband to lose interest and abandon her. She had not informed her husband of her current medical situation.

Meeting subsequently with both husband and wife, the psychiatrist gave explicit information about the possibility of malignancy and treatment options. The husband's manifest interest, support, and affection were reassuring; following the mammogram, a benign lump was removed.

Discovery of the meaning to the patient of the illness and procedure permitted an intervention that sufficiently reduced her anxiety to allow evaluation and treatment. As with any situational anxiety, the fear of serious or fatal illness can be managed with education, support, cognitive and behavioral strategies, and at times the short-term use of benzodiazepines.

Review of a patient's conceptualization of his or her medical condition, the procedures the patient faces, and the patient's interpretation of symptoms offers the physician the opportunity to correct quickly cognitive distortions that may needlessly engender anxiety. Care should be taken in discussing symptoms and procedures, with sensitivity to an individual's coping style. The clinician should elicit the patient's conceptualization of his or her condition (or upcoming procedure) and provide corrective information when distortions are encountered.

Additional strategies may be helpful when phobias about select medical procedures are encountered. For example, the enclosed chamber of the magnetic resonance imaging (MRI) scanner presents a phobic challenge to some individuals, engendering fears of overwhelming anxiety because of the inability to "escape" the MRI scanner quickly. For individuals with a history of claustrophobia, panic disorder, or PTSD, pretreatment with medications (e.g., benzodiazepines) or cognitive-behavioral therapy (CBT) may be required. In less severe cases, anxiety may be managed with simple procedures designed to maximize the patient's sense of safety and control. For example, compliance and comfort during MRI may be aided by explaining to the patient the periods when he or she can shift positions or rub his or her hands together, the patient's ability to communicate with the nurse or technician, the patient's understanding of sounds and sensations to be experienced during the procedure, and the patient's ability to terminate the procedure, if need be. Initial practice of being moved in and out of the scanning chamber before the actual experience as well as discussion of normal sensations of heat and anxiety experienced by patients while being scanned can help normalize the experience and prevent catastrophic interpretations. There is evidence from analogue studies that information about the somatic sensations to be experienced during a procedure can help reduce anxiety and panic reactions.[35] Instruction in comforting imagining may also aid the patient in tolerating the procedure.

Anxiety that occurs in patients with a known and potentially fatal illness is more accurately termed *fear* because there is a known danger. Such fear, however, can adversely affect the course of illness and treatment. A study of survivors of MI, for example, indicates that 95% had increased tension and anxiety, and of one group of post-MI patients discharged from the hospital, 40% did not return to work; in 80%, psychological impairment, including anxiety, was the cause.[36] Worry that activity will cause further heart damage or death interferes with rehabilitation and the return to autonomous functioning. Most effective therapeutic approaches for these patients center on education, group discussion, and support and stress management techniques.[37] Anxious patients with a diagnosed serious or fatal illness require treatment that includes education in addition to the possible use of supportive, cognitive-behavioral, or insight-oriented psychotherapy and anxiolytic or antidepressant medications.

Among patients with medical disorders, such as gastrointestinal (GI) disorders or allergies, the course and symptoms of the illness may be exacerbated by anxiety.[37,38] Anxiety, similar to other emotional responses, may adversely affect normal physiologic function; asthma symptoms are exacerbated by emotional arousal or stress, and the increased symptoms generate further anxiety.[39] Psychological and emotional responses and behavior possibly affect the survival of patients with cancer through effects on the immune system.[40]

Medical Illness Mimicking Anxiety Disorder

Anxiety symptoms may be the principal manifestation of an underlying medical illness.[41] Of patients referred for psychiatric treatment, 5% to 42% have been reported as having an underlying medical illness responsible for their distress, with depression and anxiety as frequent complaints.[42,43] Of reported cases of medical illnesses causing anxiety symptoms, 25% have been secondary to neurologic problems; 25% to endocrinologic causes; 12% to circulatory, rheumatoid–collagen vascular disorders and chronic infection; and 14% to miscellaneous other illnesses.[41] A most common organic cause of anxiety may be alcohol and drug use; the anxiety results from either intoxication or, more typically, withdrawal states.[44]

The clinical presentation of anxiety in the medical setting takes many forms: The bewildering array and variable nature of the physical and psychic symptoms reported by anxious patients may lead the physician to overlook symptoms related to another disorder.[45] The relative contribution of situational, psychiatric, and physiologic factors to the presentation of anxiety-like symptoms in a medical patient is often murky. The number of medical illnesses, furthermore, that may generate or exacerbate anxiety symptoms (Table 15-3) obviously renders an exhaustive evaluation for each of them impractical. A thorough yet efficient evaluation of the differential diagnostic possibilities, however, includes the following considerations[41,46]:

1. In a patient with a known medical illness, the condition and its associated complications and treatment should be suspected. For example, in the asthmatic patient, hypoxia, respiratory distress, and sympathomimetic bronchodilators may all contribute to the experience of anxiety. In some patients, risk factors or predisposition, as with a family history of medical illness capable of causing anxiety-like symptoms (e.g., thyroid disease), may be clues to diagnosis.

2. In medical illnesses considered mimics of anxiety, the quality of anxiety symptoms when closely examined may be different from that of primary anxiety disorders. For example, Starkman et al.[47] studied 17 patients with pheochromocytoma and compared their anxiety symptoms with those of a group of 52 patients with anxiety disorders. Most patients with pheochromocytoma did not meet the criteria for panic disorder or generalized anxiety disorder (GAD); none developed agoraphobic symptoms, and their overall severity of symptoms was lower. There was a significant lack of psychological as opposed to physical symptoms of anxiety in most of these patients.

3. Harper and Roth[48] noted that patients with primary anxiety disorders were more likely to have had emotional trauma related to the onset of anxiety, daily symptoms, neurotic features, and gradual resolution of symptoms after an attack and less likely to have a loss of speech or consciousness during an episode of anxiety than were patients with anxiety associated with temporal lobe epilepsy. Thus the lack of a significant

Table 15-3. Medical Causes of Anxiety

Endocrine
  Adrenal cortical hyperplasia (Cushing's disease)
  Adrenal cortical insufficiency
  (Addison's disease)
  Adrenal tumors
  Carcinoid syndrome
  Cushing's syndrome
  Diabetes mellitus
  Hyperparathyroidism
  Hyperthyroidism
  Hypoglycemia
  Hypothyroidism
  Insulinoma
  Menopause
  Ovarian dysfunction
  Pancreatic carcinoma
  Pheochromocytoma
  Pituitary disorders
  Premenstrual syndrome
  Testicular deficiency
Drug-related
  Intoxication
    Analgesics
    Antibiotics
    Anticholinergics
    Anticonvulsants
    Antidepressants
    Antihistamines
    Antihypertensives
    Antiinflammatory agents
    Antiparkinsonian agents
    Aspirin
    Caffeine
    Chemotherapy agents
    Cocaine
    Digitalis
    Hallucinogens
    Neuroleptics
    Steroids
    Sympathomimetics
    Thyroid supplements
    Tobacco
  Withdrawal
    Ethanol
    Narcotics
    Sedative-hypnotics
Cardiovascular and circulatory
  Anemia
  Cerebral anoxia
  Cerebral insufficiency
  Congestive heart failure
  Coronary insufficiency
  Dysrhythmias
  Hyperdynamic β-adrenergic state
  Hypovolemia
  Mitral valve prolapse
  Myocardial infarction
  Type A behavior

Respiratory
  Asthma
  Hyperventilation
  Hypoxia
  Pneumonia
  Pneumothorax
  Pulmonary edema
  Pulmonary embolus
Immunologic-collagen vascular
  Anaphylaxis
  Polyarteritis nodosa
  Rheumatoid arthritis
  Systemic lupus erythematosus
  Temporal arteritis
Metabolic
  Acidosis
  Acute intermittent porphyria
  Electrolyte abnormalities
  Hyperthermia
  Pernicious anemia
  Wilson's disease
Neurologic
  Brain tumors (especially third ventricle)
  Cerebral syphilis
  Cerebrovascular disorders
  Combined systemic disease
  Encephalopathies (toxic, metabolic, infectious)
  Epilepsy (especially temporal lobe epilepsy)
  Essential tremor
  Huntington's disease
  Intracranial mass lesion
  Migraine headaches
  Multiple sclerosis
  Myasthenia gravis
  Organic brain syndrome
  Pain
  Polyneuritis
  Postconcussive syndrome
  Postencephalitic disorders
  Posterolateral sclerosis
  Vertigo (including Ménière's disease and other vestibular dysfunction)
Gastrointestinal
  Colitis
  Esophageal dysmotility
  Peptic ulcer
Infectious disease
  Acquired immunodeficiency syndrome
  Atypical viral pneumonia
  Brucellosis
  Malaria
  Mononucleosis
  Tuberculosis
  Viral hepatitis
Miscellaneous
  Nephritis
  Nutritional disorders
  Other malignancies (e.g., oat cell carcinoma)

emotional experience of anxiety or the occurrence of anxiety only coincidental with particular physical events (e.g., a run of ventricular tachycardia on a cardiac monitor or spike activity on an electroencephalogram) may suggest the presence of an organic anxiety syndrome. Evaluation directed toward the somatic system (e.g., GI or cardiac) most prominently affected by anxiety symptoms may provide the greatest yield from further diagnostic investigations.

4. Characteristic features of anxiety disorders should be systematically considered: an onset of anxiety symptoms after the age of 35 years, a lack of personal or family history of anxiety disorders, negative childhood history of anxiety symptoms, an absence of significant life events heralding or exacerbating anxiety symptoms, a lack of avoidance behavior, and a poor response to standard antianxiety agents all suggest the presence of an organically based anxiety syndrome.[38]

5. Even for the apparently healthy patient, particular scrutiny should be directed at more common conditions associated with anxiety: arrhythmias, thyroid abnormalities, excessive caffeine intake, and other drug use. Anxiety-like symptoms may be the first clue to a withdrawal syndrome in a patient with unreported regular sedative-hypnotic (e.g., ethchlorvynol, glutethimide, a benzodiazepine) or alcohol use before admission to the hospital. Intoxication or withdrawal from prescription or over-the-counter medication or substances of abuse should also be suspected. Up to 3% of individuals have been reported to develop psychiatric symptoms after using prescribed or over-the-counter medication.[49]

Case 3

A psychiatric consultation was requested from the medical service for a 31-year-old female clerk who developed anxiety attacks shortly after learning that she had contracted syphilis from her boyfriend. She had previously experienced spontaneous anxiety attacks in her mid-20s that had remitted early in a 6-month course of imipramine hydrochloride, and she had been symptom-free since. During the interview with the psychiatrist, she manifested anger and sadness about her boyfriend's infidelity and her own victimization as well as anxiety about the future of their relationship. Her anxiety attacks, however, were different from those she had previously experienced: They consisted of blurred vision; dull biparietal headaches, primarily left-sided; numbness in her extremities; and feelings of dizziness. She reported feeling anxious after the onset of these symptoms. On further questioning, the patient described a history of menstrual irregularities over the last 2 to 3 years and galactorrhea. Her prolactin level was found to be elevated, and a computed tomography scan revealed a pituitary adenoma. Surgical resection of the adenoma resulted in resolution of her anxiety attacks, although she elected to pursue psychotherapy to consider issues raised by the difficulties in her relationship.

This case serves to illustrate the following points. The presence of a history of an anxiety disorder or a recent stressor does not eliminate the need to consider medical illness in the differential diagnosis of a new or different presentation of anxiety. The patient's experience of anxiety attacks was primarily somatic, and it was fortuitous that she had a history of more typical anxiety attacks for comparison; the nature of her symptoms led to a careful exploration for neurologic disease and allowed an appropriate and timely intervention.

Anxiety Mimicking Medical Illness

The autonomic arousal associated with anxiety states allows anxiety to present as a great imitator of medical illness. Patients with anxiety disorders repeatedly visit their PCPs or "make the rounds" of a variety of medical practitioners to seek a medical diagnosis to explain their symptoms. Along the way, they may be considered "hypochondriacs," "crocks," or "just nervous" and possibly receive benzodiazepines or reassurance but fail to be offered adequate or definitive treatment. Patients with untreated panic disorder, for example, have increased rates of alcoholism and sedative-hypnotic abuse, presumably in an attempt to self-medicate.[19,50] Sheehan et al.[51] noted that 70% of patients with panic disorder in their series had been to at least 10 medical practitioners without receiving a diagnosis or adequate treatment: They had high somatization scores on the Symptom Checklist-90 that decreased with the treatment of the panic disorder. The majority of these patients met the criteria for somatization disorder and tended to focus on the somatic symptoms of the untreated panic disorder. The nature of a patient's complaints may contribute to missed diagnosis and misdiagnosis. Greater than 90% of panic patients present primarily with somatic complaints.[52] Although 95% of patients with mood or anxiety disorders are correctly diagnosed if the affective symptoms are their presenting complaint, only 48% are accurately assessed if presenting with somatic complaints.[53] Individuals with somatization disorder are nearly 100 times more likely than the general population to suffer from a co-morbid panic disorder.[54] Of 55 patients with panic disorder referred by PCPs in one study, 49 (89%) initially presented with one or two somatic complaints and were misdiagnosed for months to years.[19] The three most common somatic loci of symptoms were cardiac, GI, and neurologic, with 45 (81%) of the 55 patients having a presenting pain complaint. These patients may focus on specific physical symptoms, such as chest pain or diarrhea, thereby obscuring other anxiety symptoms, or may deny affective or cognitive responses to avoid the stigmatization of psychiatric illness. As noted, anxiety may also exacerbate preexisting physical conditions, such as asthma, which then become the focus of attention of both the patient and the physician.

The cost of unrecognized and untreated anxiety disorders in patients is high in terms of continued suffering, inefficient use of medical personnel, and costly repetitive diagnostic procedures. In one study of "high utilizers" of medical services, 58% had a mood or anxiety disorder, including 22% with panic disorder.[55] Clancy and Noyes[56] have documented the high rate of medical specialty consultations and procedures (most commonly cardiologic, neurologic, and GI) requested by patients with panic disorder. In one series of patients with chest pain who were undergoing coronary arteriography, Bass et al.[57] noted that 61% of the patients with insignificant coronary disease had psychiatric morbidity on a standardized interview as opposed to only 23% of those with significant coronary disease. In those with normal coronary arteries, the most common psychiatric diagnosis was anxiety neurosis. Recognition and treatment of the anxiety disorder, in some cases, may have eliminated the necessity for arteriograms. In another study, 30% of patients

admitted to a cardiac care unit (CCU) were determined to have no coronary disease but were subsequently diagnosed with panic disorder.[58] Wulsin et al.[59] noted that 43% of patients presenting in the emergency department with chest pain had panic attacks, and 16% had panic disorder; panic patients presenting in the emergency department with chest pain make more subsequent medical and emergency department visits than those without panic disorder.[60] Richter et al.[61] estimated that the average patient with noncardiac chest pain spends $3500 per year on emergency department, physician, and hospital visits and medications. In one series,[19] panic disorder exacerbated the symptoms of patients with preexisting medical disease and led to multiple hospitalizations—a trend that was reversed with treatment of the panic disorder. Dirks et al.[62] reported that patients with chronic asthma and high levels of anxiety had more hospitalizations than did asthmatic patients with physiologic illness of comparable severity but normal degrees of anxiety.

Anxiety may play an especially important role in intensifying hypochondriacal concerns. Once a fear of disease is activated, that fear provides a context for organizing subsequent experiences, including the experience of anxiety symptoms. The fear of disease helps direct attention to somatic symptoms, including anxiety-related symptoms, and can help engender a self-perpetuating cycle of vigilance, worry, and disease concern.[63] In 1972 Mechanic[64] provided a cogent description of aspects of this pattern in his characterization of "medical student disease":

> Medical school exposes students to continuing stress resulting from the rapid pace, examinations, anxieties in dealing with new clinical experiences, and the like. Students, thus, are emotionally aroused with some frequency, and like others in the population, they experience a high prevalence of transient symptoms. The exposure to specific knowledge about disease provides the student with a new framework for identifying and giving meaning to previously neglected bodily feelings. Diffuse and ambiguous symptoms regarded as normal in the past may be reconceptualized within the context of newly acquired knowledge of disease. Existing social stress may heighten bodily sensations through autonomic activation, making the student more aware of his bodily state, and motivating him to account for what he is experiencing. The new information that the student may have about possible disease

and the similarity between the symptoms of a particular condition and his own symptoms establishes a link that he would have more difficulty making if he were less informed.

Although consideration of the medical differential diagnosis for anxiety is crucial, recognition and treatment of anxiety disorders is essential in preventing inefficient use of medical resources and patient exposure to costly and occasionally dangerous diagnostic and therapeutic procedures. Failure to make the pertinent psychiatric diagnosis may result in a patient continuing to "doctor shop" in the search to discover "what's really wrong with me," with repeated diagnostic procedures resonating with the patient's hypochondriacal concerns. Untreated anxiety can exacerbate symptoms of existing medical pathologic conditions and drive a cycle of escalating help-seeking behavior and hospitalization.

Case 4

An emergency department psychiatric consultation was requested for a 35-year-old man seen acutely by cardiology six times in the past month for chest pain and tachycardia. He had been admitted to the CCU twice, where MIs were ruled out. An extensive negative workup at another hospital had included a cardiac angiogram. After being told "there's nothing wrong with your heart, you're just nervous" and being given a prescription for diazepam, he sought emergency treatment at our institution in the hope that "they'll find out what's wrong." He had refused previous consultations with psychiatry in the fear that he would be dismissed as "a head case," but he finally agreed to evaluation at the insistence of the medical team.

He was an athletic-looking salesman in his 30s, a self-described "take charge kind of guy" without any previous psychiatric or medical history. He had a family history of hypertension and was concerned about potential "inherited heart problems." His electrocardiogram recorded a sinus tachycardia of 120 beats per minute and ST-T wave changes deemed secondary to the elevated rate. The episodic periods of anxiety, chest pain, tachycardia, diaphoresis, and hyperventilation began approximately a year earlier without clear precipitants during highway driving and had caused him to pull off the road and seek emergency medical treatment. He reported anticipating long trips with trepidation lest the episodes of chest pain be repeated.

His diagnosis was panic disorder with mild agoraphobia, and treatment was initiated with alprazolam. He felt reassured that he was not "crazy" and had a definable condition for which treatment was available. The panic attacks remitted shortly thereafter, as did the patient's use of emergency medical services.

Treatment with a number of agents can dramatically relieve the spells and secondary complications of panic disorders, thus underscoring the importance of early diagnosis. Further, because of the physical nature of the symptoms, general medical and emergency department evaluators need to be alert to the clinical phenomena of a panic attack. Patients who describe their symptoms as anxiety or who evolve a major depression may be more likely to be identified as having a psychiatric disorder. Given the dramatic physical complaints in a variety of bodily systems, however, as with depression, in which somatic symptoms may dominate the presentation and mask diagnosis, an analogy may be made with missed or masked panic disorder.

The absent report of the affective, cognitive, or behavioral components of a panic attack can obscure the diagnosis in the face of paroxysmal physical symptoms. One case report[65] describes a patient with a symptom picture suggesting panic attack but who failed to describe the emotional experience of anxiety or panic; alexithymia, or the inability to describe one's emotions, was offered as a possible mechanism for the clinical picture. The predominance of physical symptoms or the absence of cognitive or behavioral responses, however, may not reflect alexithymia or a cognitive impairment, but rather variability in symptom expression. Some patients suffer panic attacks without experiencing a need to flee; others experience panic attacks without a sense of terror or dread but do not necessarily lack the ability to describe their own emotions.

Most patients with clinically significant panic attacks also suffer limited-symptom attacks that feature only one or two physical symptoms. These may be interspersed with major attacks and be either situational or unexpected, consisting, for example, of runs of tachycardia or bouts of flushing, hyperventilation, or dizziness. Panic disorder, in its early stages, may be manifested exclusively by such minor attacks. Similarly, as antipanic therapy is effective, both unexpected and situational limited-symptom attacks may be the last vestige of the disorder or continue to represent a residual disorder.

As stated, patients vary in the primary somatic locus of anxiety distress.[46] For example, predominant panic attack symptoms may appear as cardiovascular symptoms (tachycardia, palpitations), neurologic symptoms (dizziness, paresthesias), respiratory symptoms (dyspnea), GI symptoms (diarrhea), and so forth. Recurrent limited-symptom attacks may therefore be initially indistinguishable from symptoms of a number of disorders in these systems (see Table 15-3).

As noted, limited symptom attacks may be a harbinger of progression to the full syndrome, but in some cases they may also be disabling themselves and progress to such panic disorder complications as persistent anxiety, phobic avoidance, and depression.

Case 5

A 32-year-old married factory supervisor had been out of work for 2 years because of stomach pain, nausea, and vomiting. He described his discomfort as "gnawing pains" that would occur paroxysmally followed by vomiting with little warning. In the previous 5 years, he had had extensive GI workups and medical management, vagotomy and pyloroplasty, and ultimately hemigastrectomy without relief of symptoms. He was totally disabled and was referred for psychiatric evaluation. The following features were noted: (1) His severe pain was paroxysmal with lower-grade persistent symptoms; (2) diazepam helped diminish, but not eradicate his symptoms; (3) he was homebound and described attacks of stomach pain and vomiting only when he left his apartment as, for example, if he were to go shopping; (4) the onset had followed the break-up of a relationship; (5) a major depression had evolved.

On treatment with sertraline (coadministered with diazepam), he experienced complete symptomatic relief in 6 weeks and with maintenance treatment remained symptom-free for 5 years. He sought and found a new job following treatment and has been continuously employed for the past 5 years. He recalls frequently needing to leave school as a child because of a "nervous stomach."

This case reflects a missed or masked diagnosis of panic disorder because of the predominance of a limited-symptom attack resembling a GI syndrome. Clues to a diagnosis of panic disorder were evident, and appropriate treatment led to dramatic improvement in this disabled patient. Features reminiscent of more typical patients with panic disorder were identified before definitive treatment, including severe paroxysmal and lower-grade persistent symptoms, onset with a major life event, agoraphobic features, a childhood history suggesting separation anxiety, partial relief with benzodiazepines, and secondary depression. No family history of panic attacks or agoraphobia was reported in this case.

Panic Disorder Associated with Medical Illness

An association between panic disorder and other medical illnesses has been described. More than a third of patients with chronic obstructive pulmonary disease (COPD) have an anxiety disorder, including 8% to 25% with panic disorder.[66–68] Pollack et al.[69] found an elevated prevalence of panic disorder (11%) among patients referred to a general hospital for pulmonary function testing, including two thirds of those with COPD. Almost half of all patients evaluated reported substantial symptoms of anxiety.

Katon[19] and Noyes et al.[70] report an increased incidence of peptic ulcer and hypertension in patients with panic disorder. Close to a third of patients with irritable bowel syndrome have panic disorder, and 44% of panic patients have irritable bowel syndrome; symptoms of both conditions improve with treatment of the panic disorder.[71]

Retrospective studies by Coryell et al.[72] suggest an increased risk of premature mortality from cardiac disease in men with panic disorder. A relationship also exists between mitral valve prolapse (MVP) and panic disorder. MVP, usually asymptomatic, may predispose to arrhythmias and occurs in roughly 5% to 10% of the population. Although diagnosed much more frequently in patients with panic disorder (30% to 50%) than in normals or those with generalized anxiety,[73,74] the nature of the association between the disorders remains unclear. A proposed genetic linkage remains controversial.[75] Patients with panic attacks and MVP do not differ from those with panic alone in their family history of panic disorder or their response to treatment.[76]

Primary Anxiety Disorders

Patients with a number of primary psychiatric disorders may present with anxiety in the medical setting. A history of psychiatric illness may precede the patient's entry into the medical setting and is exacerbated by the medical condition. For some, however, the onset of symptoms associated with a psychiatric disorder may be provoked by the stress of medical illness. Anxiety disorders include panic disorder with and without agoraphobia, GAD, simple phobia, social phobia, PTSD, and obsessive-compulsive disorder (OCD).[1]

Panic Disorder

A panic attack usually lasts minutes with fairly stereotyped physical, cognitive, and behavioral components. Patients with panic disorder may experience these attacks intermittently over time or in clusters and, as stated, may develop a number of complications, including persistent anxiety, phobic avoidance, depression, alcoholism, or other drug overuse.

Physical symptoms are experienced as if there is a sudden surge of autonomic, primarily sympathetic, arousal, which may include cardiac, respiratory, neurologic, and GI symptoms. Cognitively the patient feels a sense of terror or fear of losing control, dying, or going crazy and behaviorally often feels driven to flee from the setting in which the attack is experienced to a safe, secure, or familiar place or person.

The initial attack that appears to "turn on" the disorder, the herald attack, is particularly well remembered by the patient. Subsequent attacks may be a mixture of spontaneous, unexpected attacks and those preceded by a build-up of anticipatory anxiety; the latter, called situational attacks, occur in settings in which the patient might sense being at risk for panic, such as crowded places. Attacks may be major, with four or more symptoms, or limited-symptom attacks with fewer symptoms.

Panic disorder has its typical onset in early adult life and afflicts women two to three times as commonly as men. More than half of patients with panic disorder have a history of anxiety disorders beginning in childhood.[77] The disorder is clearly familial and likely has a genetic basis, given a higher concordance in monozygotic as compared with dizygotic twins,[78] but it is not clear whether a genetic influence is specific to panic disorder or whether it represents a general anxiety-proneness that may be expressed variably as any of a number of anxiety disorders.

The onset of the disorder in a clinical population typically follows either a major life event, such as a loss, threat of loss, other upheavals in work or home situations, or some physiologic event, such as medical illness (e.g., hyperthyroidism, vertigo) or drug use (marijuana, cocaine). For example, some patients whose first or herald attack appears to be triggered by a physiologic perturbation, such as follows marijuana use, may continue thereafter with persistent or recurrent symptoms without further drug use.

A panic attack, similar to an endogenous "false alarm," appears to turn on a state of vigilance or postpanic anxiety that resembles GAD. Between attacks, patients may remain symptomatic with low-level constant anxiousness and anticipatory anxiety that may crescendo into panic in certain situations or be punctuated by panic unexpectedly.

In this state of vigilance, phobic avoidance may occur as a complication. The patient may develop mild or extensive phobic avoidance, usually of travel or places of restricted escape, immediately following the onset of attacks, after a number of attacks, or never at all. In some cases, the phobic avoidance evolves as a progressive constriction with the cumulative avoidances of settings where attacks have occurred.

Major depressive episodes may also complicate the course of the patient with panic disorder and occur in up to two thirds of cases.[79] The demoralization attending the sustained distress and progressive disability of panic disorder, for some, extends to a typical depression with characteristic signs and symptoms. As noted, the relationship between panic and depression is a complicated one, however. Some patients manifest no depressive symptoms; for others, it is unclear which disorder is primary because symptoms arise concurrently. Alcohol use can temporarily tame the distress of panic disorder but soon yields to rebound symptoms, thereby setting the stage for alcohol overuse.

Generalized Anxiety Disorder

Patients with GAD suffer from chronic worry about a number of life circumstances (e.g., finances or danger to loved ones) that is difficult to control and is present on more days than not for longer than 6 months.[1] These patients are often called "nervous" or "worriers" by family or friends. Their anxiety is accompanied by a number of somatic and cognitive symptoms associated with motor tension and autonomic hyperactivity (e.g., muscle tension, restlessness, difficulties concentrating, sleep disturbances). Although the disorder may be differentiated from panic disorder by the persistent rather than episodic nature of the symptoms, careful questioning often reveals that patients with GAD may experience panic attacks as well.[80,81] Many patients with GAD in the medical setting manifest anxiety in addition to the symptoms of other psychiatric disorders (e.g., panic disorder, depression, or alcohol abuse).[82]

Specific Phobia

Patients with specific phobias are afraid of circumscribed situations or objects (e.g., heights, closed spaces, animals, or the sight of blood).[1] Exposure to the feared stimulus results in intense anxiety and avoidance that interferes with the patient's life. Some patients are so afraid of needles or blood that compliance with procedures in the medical setting is nearly impossible. Acute treatment with benzodiazepines may decrease the patient's anxiety to the point where he or she agrees to treatment. The only consistently effective treatment for specific phobias, however, is behavioral therapy, a technique that involves exposure and desensitization to the feared object or situation.[83]

Social Phobia (Social Anxiety Disorder)

Social phobia, also referred to as *social anxiety disorder*, is diagnosed when the patient perceives that he or she will be the object of public scrutiny and fears that he or she will behave in a way that will be humiliating or embarrassing.[1] This perception leads to persistent fear and avoidance or endurance with intense distress. Circumscribed situations may be feared (e.g., including speaking before a group, performance anxiety, writing or eating in the presence of others, or urinating in public lavatories); many patients experience more global difficulties in which most social interactions are difficult. Again, depression and alcoholism can frequently occur with social phobia.[84,85] Patients with social phobias may have intense anxiety in the hospital because they are under intense scrutiny by others. Long-term treatments include antidepressants with serotonin selective reuptake inhibitors (SSRIs) (fluoxetine, sertraline, paroxetine, fluvoxamine, citalopram, and escitalopram), serotonin-norepinephrine reuptake inhibitors (SNRIs) (venlafaxine) and monoamine oxidase inhibitors (MAOIs) (phenelzine and tranylcypromine) generally being more effective than tricyclic antidepressants (TCAs) (e.g., imipramine, desipramine, and nortriptyline), β-blockers (for performance anxiety rather than generalized social phobia), or CBT. Some reports support the clinical efficacy of high-potency benzodiazepines (HPBs) (e.g., clonazepam[86] and alprazolam[87]) for the treatment of social phobia; when immediate intervention is necessary, the use of these agents is appropriate.

Posttraumatic Stress Disorder

Patients with PTSD have experienced a catastrophic event that would be clearly distressing to anyone (e.g., having faced a serious threat to one's life, having one's home suddenly destroyed, or having witnessed a serious accident or act of violence).[1] Afflicted patients frequently reexperience the traumatic event. They have recurrent dreams or suddenly act or feel like the event is recurring (i.e., a flashback). Individuals with PTSD frequently avoid situations that remind them of the event and may become numb, irritable, or hypervigilant and experience difficulty with sleep or concentration. Although much attention has been directed toward PTSD in combat veterans, PTSD can occur in civilians who suffer life-threatening accidents or assaults or who have survived natural disasters. PTSD is unfortunately common and often unrecognized in the medical setting, with reported rates of PTSD in over a third of patients hospitalized after traumatic injury, such as occurring in motor vehicle accidents, assaults, or fires.[88,89] Injured patients who develop PTSD have increased functional impairment and problem drinking when followed up on a year after surgery.[90]

Acute stress disorder involves the development of dissociation and reexperiencing symptoms along with avoidance, anxiety, increased arousal, and significant distress or impairment lasting up to

4 weeks after a trauma.[1] The presence of acute stress disorder, particularly symptoms of acute numbing, depersonalization, a sense of relieving the trauma, and motor restlessness within a month of a trauma is strongly associated with the development of PTSD.[91]

There is growing interest in whether early intervention in trauma victims can prevent the development of PTSD. Emerging data suggests that whereas single session debriefing after a traumatic event will likely have no benefit and may in fact interfere with the natural recovery process,[92,93] more extensive, multiple session cognitive-behavioral interventions incorporating information, cognitive-restructuring, and exposure elements appear effective.[94,95] Pharmacologic interventions have also demonstrated potential benefit in reducing the morbid sequelae of trauma. One small double-blind randomized trial in burned children demonstrated significant reduction in symptoms of acute stress disorder with imipramine as compared with chloral hydrate treatment.[96] A small placebo-controlled trial demonstrated that a 10-day course of propranolol (40 mg four times daily) initiated within 6 hours of a traumatic event resulted in reduction of PTSD symptoms and physiologic arousal at 3-month follow-up.[97] Although further research in this area is warranted and ongoing, the work to date suggests the potential benefit of some early intervention strategies in reducing the morbid consequences of trauma exposure.

Both CBT[98] and SSRI pharmacotherapy have become first-line interventions for the treatment of PTSD.[99] They are frequently coadministered to improve outcome. Although far from definitive, there is evidence suggesting that benzodiazepine administration may impede the recovery process in traumatized individuals,[100,101] and other agents, including atypical neuroleptics (e.g., risperidone, olanzapine) and anticonvulsants (e.g. lamotrigine, topiramate, tiagabine, and gabapentin) may be useful alternatives as well as having a role in management of the refractory patient.

Obsessive-Compulsive Disorder

Patients with OCD suffer from recurrent, intrusive, unwanted thoughts (i.e., obsessions, such as the fear of hurting a loved one or the fear of contamination) or compulsive behaviors or rituals (such as repetitive hand-washing or checking a door multiple times to make sure it is locked).[1] The obsessions and compulsions are distressing and time-consuming (i.e., they may take more than 1 hour per day) and interfere with the patient's normal function. In the medical setting, the patient with OCD may suffer a marked increase in anxiety if physical disability or hospital routine makes it impossible for him or her to perform compulsive rituals. CBT aimed at reducing the patient's obsessive thoughts and compulsive behavior has demonstrated clear efficacy for OCD. Benzodiazepine therapy may be necessary to control overwhelming anxiety, particularly in acute treatment. Effective long-term treatments include serotonergic antidepressants (e.g., SSRIs and clomipramine) as well as behavioral therapy.

Other Psychiatric Disorders

In addition to primary anxiety disorders, anxiety symptoms may be associated with a number of other psychiatric disorders, such as schizophrenia, depression, and bipolar disorder. Vague uneasiness extending to severe anxiety may either precede or accompany the symptoms of schizophrenia. Patients with significant degrees of anxiety may have a reduced level of functioning and manifest withdrawal that superficially resembles schizophrenia. The presence of hallucinations, delusions, and bizarre and disordered thinking, a marked degree of social withdrawal, and a characteristic premorbid personal and family history usually allows an uncomplicated differentiation of schizophrenia from anxiety disorders.

The relationship between anxiety and depression is complex. Weissman et al.[102] reported an increased prevalence of both panic disorder and depression in the families of probands with both disorders. One estimate holds that one third of patients with panic disorder, with or without agoraphobia, develop a secondary major depression, and 22% have had a major depressive disorder before developing panic disorder.[103] The incidence of a major depressive episode in patients with panic disorder has been reported as ranging between 28% and 90% depending on the diagnostic criteria used.[104] Leckman et al.[105] found that 58% of a group of depressed patients had anxiety symptoms meeting *Diagnostic and Statistical Manual for Mental Disorders*, third edition criteria for agoraphobia, panic disorder, or GAD.

Although this overlap between syndromes can make the distinction between anxiety and depression difficult, a number of clinical considerations may be useful. Psychomotor retardation, persistent dysphoria, early morning awakening, diurnal variation, a sense of hopelessness, and suicidal thoughts are more indicative of depression. Patients with an anxiety disorder have often not lost interest in their usual activities but rather have lost the ability to negotiate them comfortably. They are more likely to report autonomic hyperactivity, derealization, perceptual distortions, and anxious impatience than hopelessness.[44] Advances in neurobiology at this time offer few diagnostic markers for differentiating anxiety and depressive disorders. The sleep of patients with panic disorders differs from the sleep of depressives during all-night polysomnograms.[106] There are also differences in physiologic parameters and platelet receptor binding patterns between anxious and depressed patients.[107,108]

The principal concern in differentiating depression from anxiety is not to overlook treatment with an antidepressant and, in particular, to avoid the common scenario of prescribing only a benzodiazepine for the anxiety component of a depression, thereby leaving the depression untreated. Otherwise, the frequent overlap in clinical presentation between primary depressive and primary anxiety disorders is fortunately mirrored by an overlap in therapeutic considerations. One important consideration, however, regards the possibility that depressed symptomatology may reflect an underlying bipolar ("manic-depressive") disorder. Anxiety disorders are a common comorbidity among bipolar individuals.[109] However, the use of antidepressants in bipolar patients may precipitate mania and provoke greater mood cycling. Bipolar disorder should be considered in the differential of depression particularly in those patients with a history of marked mood instability or a family history of manic-depressive illness, as well as in those individuals who become more agitated or dysphoric after antidepressant administration. For bipolar patients, use of an anticonvulsant may treat both the mood and the anxiety disorder, with use of benzodiazepines, in preference to antidepressants, considered for persistent anxiety in those individuals without a substance abuse diathesis. Although cognitive-behavioral interventions for anxiety and depression differ in both their focus and procedures, it is not unusual for treatment of one condition to extend benefit to the associated disorder. For example, the CBT of panic disorder is associated with improvement in comorbid depression. Nonetheless, comorbidity generally serves as a predictor of worse overall treatment response to CBT, just as it does for pharmacologic approaches.[110]

Treatment

The nature of the medical setting favors expedient interventions, such as drug treatment to ease acute distress because of the time-limited nature of medical and surgical stays (Table 15-4). Nonetheless, as illustrated by case examples, comprehensive assessments, including systematic scrutiny of cognitive and psychosocial factors, may lead to practical interventions short of formal psychotherapy, including CBT. In addition, disrupted relations with family members may be provocative, and family interventions may prove therapeutically expedient.

Pharmacologic Treatment of Panic Disorder

The drug treatment of anxiety essentially involves selecting agents for panic, GAD, or both. As with recognizing the primacy of depression in some anxious patients, if the presence of panic attacks is overlooked, treatment for generalized anxiety only is likely to be inadequate, and patient suffering will continue. Familiarity with panic disorder, its complications, and treatments is a necessary resource in evaluating and caring for anxious patients.

Although early intervention offers the likelihood of preventing complications, many patients come for treatment after years of symptoms and disability. Even in the face of chronicity, however, most patients achieve substantial if not dramatic benefit with available treatments, which include antipanic pharmacotherapy and CBT. Given the apparent primacy of the panic attack in the distress and evolution of complications of the disorder, our usual approach is to initiate antipanic medications for patients who continue to experience panic attacks, with the expectation of regression and remission of complications once the attacks have ceased. For patients with residual phobic avoidance despite the prevention of panic attacks, behavioral and cognitive strategies are employed. For some patients, behavioral and cognitive strategies are employed initially, especially when the frequency and intensity of unexpected panic are minimal, with pharmacotherapy subsequently applied if emergence or exacerbation of panic attends the behavioral program.

Antidepressants

The SSRIs, including fluoxetine, sertraline, paroxetine, citalopram, escitalopram, and fluvoxamine, have become first-line agents for the treatment of panic disorder as well as other anxiety disorders[111,112] because of their broad spectrum of efficacy, favorable side-effect profile, and lack of cardiotoxicity. Although effective, these agents may worsen anxiety for some patients at the initiation of treatment. Thus treatment of panic patients or the anxious depressed should be initiated at half

Table 15-4. Standard Pharmacologic Treatment for Anxiety Disorders

Agent	Usual Initial Dose (mg)	Dosage Range (mg)	Chief Dose Limitations	Disorders
TCA				
(e.g., Imipramine)	10–25	150–300	Jitteriness, TCA side effects	PD, AG, GAD, PTSD,
Clomipramine	25	25–250	Sedation, weight gain, TCA side effects	OCD, PD, AG, GAD, PTSD
MAOI				
(e.g., Phenelzine)	15–30	45–90	Diet, MAOI side effects	PD, AG, SP, ?GAD, OCD, PTSD
SSRIs				
Fluoxetine	10	10–80	SSRI side effects	PD, AG, SP, OCD, PTSD
Sertraline	25	25–200	SSRI side effects	PD, AG, SP, OCD, PTSD
Paroxetine	10	10–50	SSRI side effects	PD, AG, SP, OCD, PTSD
Paroxetine-CR	12.5	12.5–62.5	SSRI side effects	PD, AG, SP, OCD, PTSD
Fluvoxamine	50	50–300	SSRI side effects	PD, AG, SP OCD, PTSD
Citalopram	10	20–60	SSRI side effects	PD, AG, SP, OCD, PTSD
Escitalopram	5	10–20	SSRI side effects	PD, AG, SP, OCD, PTSD
SNRI				
Venlafaxine	37.5	75–225	SSRI side effects, hypertension	PD, AG, SP, OCD, PTSD
Benzodiazepines				
Alprazolam	0.25 qid	2–10/d	Sedation, discontinuation syndrome	PD, AG, GAD, SP, ?SpP
Clonazepam	0.25 hs	1–5/d	Abuse, psychomotor and memory impairment	PD, AG, GAD, SP, ?SpP
Diazepam	2.5	5–30/d		GAD, SpP, PD, SP
Buspirone	5 tid	15–60/d	Dysphoria	GAD
β-Blockers				
(e.g., Propranolol)	10–20	10–160/d (maintenance use)	Depression	SP, ?PD, ?GAD

AG, agoraphobia; *d*, day; *GAD*, generalized anxiety disorder; *hs*, at bedtime; *MAOI*, monoamine oxidase inhibitor; *OCD*, obsessive-compulsive disorder; *PD*, panic disorder; *PTSD*, posttraumatic stress disorder; *qid*; four times daily; *SP*, social phobia; *SpP*, specific phobia; *SSRI*, selective serotonin reuptake inhibitor; *TCA*, tricyclic antidepressant; *tid*, three times daily.

or less of the usual starting dose (e.g., fluoxetine 5 to 10 mg/day, sertraline 25 mg/day, paroxetine 10 mg/day (or 12.5 mg/day of the controlled-release formulation), citalopram 10 mg/day, escitalopram 5 mg/day, and fluvoxamine 50 mg/day) to minimize the early anxiogenic effect. Doses can usually be raised, after about a week of acclimation, to typical therapeutic levels. Although the nature of the dose-response relationship for the SSRIs in panic is still being assessed, typical target doses for this indication are fluoxetine 20 to 40 mg/day, paroxetine 20 to 60 mg/day (25 to 72.5 mg/day of the controlled release formulation), sertraline 100 to 150 mg/day, citalopram 20 to 60 mg/day, escitalopram 10 to 20 mg/day, and fluvoxamine 150 to 250 mg/day, although some patients may respond at lower levels. Patients with OCD and PTSD may require higher doses (e.g., fluoxetine 60 to 80 mg/day) to receive maximal benefit.

Onset of benefit with the SSRIs and other antidepressants usually occurs after 2 to 3 weeks of treatment. Although generally better tolerated for acute and long-term treatment than older available classes of antidepressants, SSRIs may be associated with transient or persistent adverse effects, including nausea and other GI symptoms, headaches, sexual dysfunction, and apathy. Despite their reputation as stimulating agents, sleep disturbance is generally not a persistent or significant problem during SSRI therapy. The SSRIs are usually administered in the morning; emergent sleep disruption can usually be managed by the addition of hypnotic agents.

The extended release SNRI venlafaxine has also demonstrated efficacy for the treatment of panic disorder and the other anxiety disorders. Similar to other antidepressants, it may cause uncomfortable stimulation early in the treatment of anxious patients, so dosing should be initiated with low doses (i.e., venlafaxine 37.5 mg/day). Other newer antidepressants, such as nefazodone and mirtazapine, are also likely effective for the treatment of anxiety disorders, but there is little systematic data supporting their use for these indications. Trazodone appears to be relatively less effective for panic disorder than other agents; studies assessing the effectiveness of bupropion for panic disorder are small and present mixed results.

The TCA imipramine hydrochloride has well-established efficacy in panic disorder.[113] Although other TCAs are probably also effective (e.g., desipramine is frequently employed because of its lower anticholinergic burden), this class of agents has several drawbacks, including a delayed onset of benefit and treatment-emergent adverse effects. In addition to usual TCA side effects, such as dry mouth, constipation, and orthostatic hypotension, panic patients are particularly prone to a sudden worsening of their disorder with the first doses. To minimize the effect of this adverse response, treatment can be initiated with small test doses (e.g., 10 mg of imipramine hydrochloride). If this is well tolerated, standard antidepressant dosing can be pursued; for others, the adverse response typically fades over a few days, thus allowing an upward titration of dose. For a small percentage of patients, this apparent worsening of the disorder does not subside. Mavissakalian and Perel[114] reported that a reasonable target dose of imipramine for treatment of panic disorder and agoraphobia in most patients is approximately 2.25 mg/kg/day (usually between 100 and 200 mg/day for most patients), with a total plasma level of 75 to 150 ng/ml for imipramine and its metabolite, desipramine.

The MAOI phenelzine has stood up well in clinical use and controlled trials,[113] and many clinicians believe that MAOIs are potentially the most comprehensively effective agents for treating panic disorder, blocking panic attacks, relieving depression, and offering a confidence-enhancing effect of considerable value to the patient needing to recover from vigilance and phobic avoidance. Except for postural hypotension, MAOIs are free of most of the early TCA and SSRI side effects, including the anxiogenic response. Unfortunately, as treatment proceeds, a variety of challenging problems emerge, including insomnia, weight gain, edema, sexual dysfunction, nocturnal myoclonus, and other unusual symptoms. Further, many anxious patients are most circumspect about the dietary precautions and instructions about hypertensive crises. Because the SSRIs offer a similar spectrum of efficacy as the MAOIs in terms of treating panic disorder, social phobia, and atypical depressive symptoms with a superior safety and side-effect profile, they are generally used first in most patients. MAOIs, however, may be effective in patients failing to respond to other interventions; thus no patient should be considered truly treatment refractory to pharmacotherapy until the patient has had an MAOI trial.

Benzodiazepines

When treatment refusal, treatment discomfort from side effects, and treatment failure are considered, the need for a better-tolerated and effective antipanic treatment is apparent. In some respects, benzodiazepines, such as alprazolam and clonazepam, fit this need. They have demonstrated antipanic efficacy as well as patient acceptability and a reasonable record of safety. In addition, they provide the speed of action that is desirable in a medical setting. Although it was once believed that higher potency agents, such as alprazolam and clonazepam, were more effective than lower potency agents, such as diazepam, for the treatment of panic, it appears that all benzodiazepines may be effective at equivalent doses (i.e., 4 mg/day of alprazolam and 40 mg/day of diazepam.[115]

The usual dose range for most panic disorder patients receiving alprazolam is 2 to 8 mg/day, with most achieving a benefit around 4 to 6 mg/day. Clinical response is evident early, but lower doses are necessary to initiate treatment so that the patient can accommodate to sedation. Most patients adapt within a few days to the sedating effects, and this allows a stepwise increase in panic-blocking doses. Adaptation to sedation usually occurs without a loss of therapeutic benefit, but some upward adjustment may be required after the first 2 weeks. A small percentage of patients appear particularly sensitive to the drug and experience persisting sedation despite time and careful titration. Alprazolam must be given in divided doses, usually three to four times a day, because of its relatively short duration of action; a recently introduced extended release formulation permits once-a-day dosing. It does not change the elimination half-life or need for a gradual taper with discontinuation.

Despite the ease of administration of alprazolam and frequently dramatic results even in the first days of treatment, clinical drawbacks include concerns about abuse and dependency, rebound symptoms between doses, withdrawal, and early relapse. The abuse potential of alprazolam, like other benzodiazepines, varies widely among clinical populations; patients with a history of alcohol or other substance abuse are most at risk for abusing benzodiazepines. Numerous studies are reassuring that panic patients treated with benzodiazepines do not experience therapeutic tolerance or dose escalation; in fact, doses of benzodiazepines generally decrease over the maintenance period, often despite the presence or persistence of untreated anxiety symptoms.[116] Most well-informed panic and phobic patients who have endured severe distress over time treat their medication with respect and understand the wisdom in maintaining the lowest effective dose; thus, unless there is evidence that a particular patient is at risk, the use of this agent appears generally safe for the disorder under consideration. As with any benzodiazepine, without controlled prescribing for targeted symptoms, inappropriate use may occur. As a relatively short half-life benzodiazepine, the discontinuation of alprazolam therapy, especially after long-term treatment, without a gradual taper tailored to the individual patient's sensitivity to decreasing doses, may be followed by rebound symptoms (worsened anxiety) or a withdrawal syndrome.

With the pharmacokinetic drawbacks associated with a short half-life agent in mind, the longer-acting, HPB, clonazepam, has been effective for those patients who require an HPB. Because of its long half-life (15 to 50 hours), clonazepam is generally administered on a twice-a-day dosage schedule, with patients less likely to experience inter-dose rebound and withdrawal symptoms than on shorter-acting agents.

With a milligram-for-milligram potency approximately twice that of alprazolam, clonazepam's effective dose range for panic patients is between 1 and 5 mg/day when given in morning and bedtime doses. Sedation is the limiting factor in dose titration and is managed by initiating treatment with a low bedtime dose and titrating upward if symptoms persist and sedation resolves. An initial dose as low as 0.25 mg may be used in drug-naive patients or those particularly sensitive to benzodiazepines. Greater doses may be given at bedtime than in the morning if the patient is not readily accommodating to sedation, but many patients function without sedation on equal morning and bedtime doses, as with alprazolam.

The effect of a daily dose on panic attacks and generalized anxiety is apparent within a few days.

Some patients, for unclear reasons, develop depressive symptoms as a treatment-emergent adverse effect when taking alprazolam or clonazepam. Resolution of depressive symptoms typically occurs with the introduction of an antidepressant; benzodiazepine treatment can then be withheld with the expectation of a comprehensive response to the antidepressant. Combined treatment can again be used if anxiety symptoms break through the antidepressant treatment.

Some clinicians initiate combined treatment with an antidepressant and an HPB to obtain the rapid anxiolysis associated with HPB treatment, decrease the activation associated with initiation of antidepressant therapy, and provide antidepressant coverage of comorbid or benzodiazepine-induced depression. For many patients, the HPB can be tapered after a few weeks when the antidepressant begins to exert therapeutic effects; however, some patients remain on combined treatment with benefit and without adverse consequences.

Pharmacologic Treatment of Generalized Anxiety

As noted previously, the SSRIs and the SNRIs have become first-line pharmacologic agents for the treatment of anxiety disorders, including GAD. They are better tolerated than the older classes of antidepressants and have a broad spectrum of efficacy, which is a critical clinical concern given the high rates of comorbidity, particularly depression affecting the generally anxious individual. In addition, SSRIs and SNRIs do not have significant abuse potential, which is an important consideration for generally anxious individuals with a predisposition to substance abuse. However, use of these agents may be associated with side effects, including sexual dysfunction and GI distress, that may adversely affect compliance. The delay in the onset of therapeutic benefit is a relative disadvantage for antidepressants as well as for buspirone; the call to intervene with medication for the anxious patient in the hospital typically requires a response with a more immediate-acting agent. Thus benzodiazepines are usually employed for acute management of anxiety, with antidepressant addition or substitution considered in patients requiring maintenance pharmacotherapy, particularly those with a depressive or substance abuse diathesis.

Benzodiazepines, by dint of their efficacy, tolerability, and rapid onset of effect, have long been the mainstay of anxiolytic pharmacotherapy, although the clinical decision to prescribe these agents for symptom relief is a difficult one. The attitudes of individual physicians toward prescribing may be characterized as falling along a spectrum between pharmacologic Calvinism and psychotropic hedonism, reflecting a personal and moral stance toward prescribing medication for the relief of psychic distress. The abundant literature on antianxiety agents falls short of providing reliable measures for diagnosis and prescribing. Given the ubiquitousness of anxiety in hospital settings, the physician must frequently confront the question of whether to prescribe. The use of a benzodiazepine for the distressed, anxious patient is often a therapeutic act analogous to the provision of pain relief.

When compared with barbiturates and nonbarbiturate sedative and hypnotic agents (meprobamate, ethchlorvynol, glutethimide, methaqualone, and others), the benzodiazepines are more selectively anxiolytic, with less sedation and less morbidity and mortality in overdose and acute withdrawal. Because using a benzodiazepine represents a clinical decision to offer symptomatic relief, the critical clinical assessment is to evaluate the patient's response. The patient's coping should be enhanced in addition to, and as a consequence of relief from, suffering.

Choice of Benzodiazepine

All available benzodiazepines are effective in treating generalized anxiety. Drug selection is based on pharmacokinetic properties, which determine the rapidity of onset of effect, the degree of accumulation with multidosing, the rapidity of offset of clinical effect, and the risk of drug discontinuation syndrome.

For single or acute dosing, the onset of effect is determined by the rate of absorption from the stomach and offset by distribution from plasma into lipid stores. The half-life of a drug predicts the amount of accumulation of drug in plasma with multidosing and the speed of washout on drug discontinuation (and thus the quickness of return of symptoms or the risk of rebound and withdrawal). For example, a rapidly absorbed, lipophilic agent, such as diazepam, given acutely has a rapid but relatively short-lived effect; with repeated dosing, however, plasma levels are higher than a short half-life drug at steady-state. The long half-life offers some tapering effect to help protect against rebound or withdrawal on discontinuation.

The clinician can choose a drug to have a fast onset for greater clinical effect, a slow onset to minimize sedation or confusion, short action to allow rapid clearing, or long action to minimize inter-dose or posttreatment rebound symptoms (Table 15-5). Treatment begins with low doses (e.g., diazepam 5 to 10 mg/day or its equivalent) and upward titration. Doses vary but for usual situational anxiety usually do not exceed 30 to 40 mg of diazepam a day or its equivalent.

For patients in whom benzodiazepine therapy is being prescribed to manage acute situational reactions, patients should expect that treatment will be of limited duration. For specific phobic anxiety (e.g., fear of flying), occasional use is indicated. For generalized anxiety, using anxiolytics for periods of exacerbation may be effective, although increasing recognition of the distress and chronicity associated with persistent anxiety has underscored the observation that many patients often report sustained improvement and improved quality of life with maintenance treatment.

Precautions in Prescribing

A withdrawal syndrome, usually mild but potentially severe depending on the dose and the duration of treatment, may follow abrupt cessation of therapy. For patients receiving usual doses for less than 3 to 4 weeks, during hospitalization for example, without prior use of sedatives, the risk of an abstinence syndrome is less. In general, however, treatment is discontinued by tapering doses, gradually adjusting decrements according to patient response.

Overuse of medication and drug-seeking from multiple sources is a concern for outpatient prescribing, but with the controlled use of drugs in the hospital, particular vigilance is appropriate primarily for the patient with a history of drug or alcohol abuse.

The sedative effects of benzodiazepines are additive with other CNS depressants, and plasma levels are higher with the use of certain drugs, such as cimetidine. A few patients, particularly with higher-potency benzodiazepines, are prone to increased hostility, aggressivity, and rage eruptions.

Pharmacologic Alternatives to Benzodiazepines

Anticonvulsants (including valproate, gabapentin, tiagabine, topiramate, lamotrigine, and levetiracetam) are increasingly being studied and used for a range of anxiety disorders, with some (e.g., gabapentin and tiagabine) administered as alternatives to benzodiazepines because of their sedating properties and tolerability.[117] Although neuroleptics have long been used in clinical practice for the treatment of anxiety, concerns about extrapyramidal effects and tardive dyskinesia have limited this practice. The atypical neuroleptics also appear to have anxiolytic effects across a variety of

Table 15-5. Characteristics of Commonly Used Benzodiazepines

Drug	Half-Life (h)	Dose Equivalent (mg)	Onset	Significant Metabolites	Typical Route of Administration
Midazolam (Versed)	1–12	2.0	Fast	No	IV, IM
Oxazepam (Serax)	5–15	15	Slow	No	PO
Lorazepam (Ativan)	10–20	1.0	Intermediate	No	IV, IM, PO
Alprazolam (Xanax)*	12–15	0.5	Intermediate-fast	No	PO
Chlordiazepoxide (Librium)	5–30	10	Intermediate	Yes	PO, IV
Clonazepam (Klonopin)*	15–50	0.25	Intermediate	No	PO
Diazepam (Valium)	20–100	5.0	Fast	Yes	PO, IV
Flurazepam (Dalmane)	40	15.0	Fast	Yes	PO
Clorazepate (Tranxene)	30–200	7.5	Fast	Yes	PO

IM, Intramuscular; *IV*, intravenous; *PO*, orally.
*Commonly used to treat panic disorder.

conditions and with emerging supportive data are being more widely applied with a less daunting (though not absent) side effect burden than the older generation of agents.[118]

β-Blocking drugs, such as propranolol hydrochloride, have proved useful in alleviating some of the peripheral autonomic symptoms of anxiety, such as tremor and tachycardia. Although of second-line or third-line importance in treating panic attacks or more cognitively experienced symptoms (e.g., worry), β-blockers are often impressively useful in the performance anxiety subtype of social phobia and cases in which persistent peripheral symptoms (somatic anxiety) predominate. Agents, such as atenolol, that are less able to cross the blood-brain barrier than propranolol may have advantages for patients who experience fatigue or dysphoria when taking propranolol. Effective doses vary, and treatment requires upward titration from low initial doses.

Buspirone is a nonbenzodiazepine anxiolytic without sedative and anticonvulsant properties or abuse potential. It interacts with postsynaptic 5-HT (serotonin) receptors as a partial agonist and with dopamine receptors but apparently not with the benzodiazepine-GABA receptor.[119] Buspirone is ineffective in panic disorder, and although clinical trials suggest that it is effective for the treatment of GAD, many clinicians and patients have found it disappointing for this indication as well. For some patients, this may be due in part to a latency of therapeutic response of weeks, similar to the antidepressants, and the presence of a critical beneficial dose threshold. The dosing range is 5 to 20 mg three times a day.

Cognitive-Behavioral Therapy

For patients with persisting anxiety symptoms, cognitive-behavioral strategies similar to those used for ambulatory patients with anxiety disorders may be adapted to the hospitalized medical patient. CBT for anxiety disorders brings to bear an array of cognitive restructuring, exposure, and symptom management techniques that target the core fears and behavioral pattern characterizing each anxiety disorder. Cognitive interventions include a variety of procedures to challenge and restructure the inaccurate and maladaptive cognitions that increase anxiety and help maintain anxiety disorders. Procedures range from informational discussions, self-monitoring, and Socratic questioning to the construction of behavioral experiments in which patients can directly examine the veracity of anxiogenic expectations. A reliance on corrective experiences also lies at the heart of exposure interventions that provide patients with opportunities to extinguish learned fears, by directly confronting (in a hierarchical fashion) feared events and sensations. Symptom management techniques typically include relaxation and breathing retraining procedures to help eliminate anxiogenic bodily reactions. In addition, training in problem-solving or social skills may be necessary to eliminate behavioral deficits that help maintain anxiety disorders. Likewise, couple's sessions may be required to change family patterns that help maintain avoidant or other anxiety-related behaviors.

Cognitive-behavioral treatment centers on the elimination of core features of each disorder, with treatment for panic disorder targeting fears of arousal, anxiety, and panic symptoms; treatment for social phobia targeting fears of negative evaluations by others; and treatment for PTSD targeting fears of cues of the traumatic event, including fears of the memory and anxiety symptoms accompanying the memory of the trauma. Treatment for GAD focuses on the aberrant worry process itself but also includes symptom management procedures, and treatment for OCD focuses on breaking the link between intrusive thoughts, anxiety, and compulsive behaviors using exposure techniques combined with compulsion-response prevention.

The success of these strategies are among the most promising in the treatment literature, with the efficacy of CBT equaling or surpassing alternative treatments.[98,120–124] Nonetheless, referral for CBT may be limited by the availability of clinicians specializing in these methods. In addition, the hospital setting may not allow timely initiation of treatment or the completion of basic treatment packages. Although patients may respond much earlier, basic treatment interventions are commonly delivered in a series of 12 to 16 sessions. For patients unresponsive, uninterested, or unwilling to make the initial time investment required for CBT, pharmacotherapy offers the most efficacious alternative.

References

1. American Psychiatric Association: *Diagnostic and statistical manual of mental disorders*, ed 4, revised (DSM IV-R), Washington, DC, 1994, American Psychiatric Association Press.

2. Robins LN, Helger JE, Weissman MM, et al: Lifetime prevalence of specific psychiatric disorders in three sites, *Arch Gen Psych* 140:949–958, 1984.

3. MacKenzie TB, Popkin MK: Organic anxiety syndrome, *Am J Psychiatry* 140:342–344, 1983.

4. Charney DS, Redmond DE Jr: Neurobiological mechanisms in human anxiety: evidence supporting noradrenergic hyperactivity, *Neuropharmacology* 22:1531–1536, 1983.

5. Insel TR, Ninan PT, Aloi J, et al: A benzodiazepine receptor mediated model of anxiety: studies in non-human primates and clinical implications, *Arch Gen Psychiatry* 41:741–750, 1984.

6. Huang YH, Redmond DE Jr, Snyder DR, et al: Loss of fear following bilateral lesions of the locus coeruleus in the monkey, *Neurosci Abstr* 2:573, 1976.

7. Charney DS, Heninger GR: Noradrenergic function and the mechanism of action of antianxiety treatment, *Arch Gen Psychiatry* 42:458–481, 1985.

8. Gorman JM, Kent JM, Sullivan GM, Coplan JD: Neuroanatomical hypothesis of panic disorder, revised *Am J Psychiatry* 157:493–505, 2000.

9. Gray JA: *Issues in the neuropsychology of anxiety*. In Tuma AH, Maser JD, editors: *Anxiety and the anxiety disorders*, Hillsdale, NJ, 1985, L Erlbaum.

10. Tallman JF, Gallager DW: The GABA-ergic system: a locus of benzodiazepine action, *Annu Rev Neurosci* 8:21–44, 1985.

11. de Montigny C: Cholecystokinin tetrapeptide induces panic-like attacks in healthy volunteers: preliminary findings, *Arch Gen Psychiatry* 46:511–517, 1989.

12. Heim C, Nemeroff CB: The role of childhood trauma in the neurobiology of mood and anxiety disorders: preclinical and clinical studies, *Biol Psychiatry* 49:1023–1039, 2001.

13. Seligman MEP: Phobias and preparedness, *Behav Ther* 2:307–320, 1971.

14. Akiskal MS, McKinney WT: Overview of recent research in depression, *Arch Gen Psychiatry* 32:285–305, 1975.

15. Rodin G, Voshart K: Depression in the medically ill: an overview, *Am J Psychiatry* 143:696–705, 1986.

16. Regier D, Goldberg ID, Taube CM: The de facto US mental health service system, *Arch Gen Psychiatry* 35:685–693, 1978.

17. Goldberg D: Detection and assessment of emotional disorders in a primary-care setting, *Int J Mental Health* 8:30–48, 1979.

18. Marsland DW, Wood M, Mayo F: Content of family practice: a data bank for patient care curriculum and research in family practice: 526,196 patient problems, *J Fam Pract* 3:25–68, 1976.

19. Katon W: Panic disorder and somatization: review of 55 cases, *Am J Med* 77:101–106, 1984.

20. Shurman RA, Kramer PD, Mitchell JB: The hidden mental health network: treatment of mental illness by non-psychiatrist physicians, *Arch Gen Psychiatry* 42:89–94, 1985.

21. Hollister LE: A look at the issues: use of minor tranquilizers, *Psychosomatics* 21(suppl):4–6, 1980.

22. Weissman MM, Merikangas KR: The epidemiology of anxiety and panic disorders: an update, *J Clin Psychiatry* 47(suppl):11–17, 1986.

23. Rice RL: Symptom patterns of the hyperventilation syndrome, *Am J Med Sci* 8:691–696, 1951.

24. Wood P: DaCosta's syndrome (or effort syndrome), *Br Med J* 1:767–773, 1941.

25. Doefler LA, Pbert L, DeCosimo D: Symptoms of post-traumatic stress disorder following myocardial infarction and coronary artery bypass surgery, *Gen Hosp Psychiatry* 16:193–199, 1994.

26. Cordova MJ, Andrykowski MA, Redd WH, et al: Frequency and correlates of post-traumatic-stress-disorder-like symptoms after treatment for breast cancer, *J Consult Clin Psychol* 63:981–986, 1995.

27. Zatzick DF, Kang SM, Muller HG, et al: Predicting posttraumatic distress in hospitalized trauma survivors with acute injuries, *Am J Psychiatry* 159:941–946, 2002.

28. Foa EB, Steketee G, Rothbaum BO: Behavioral/cognitive conceptualizations of post-traumatic stress disorder, *Behav Ther* 20:155–176, 1989.

29. Macleod AD, Maycock E: Awareness during anaesthesia and post-traumatic stress disorder, *Anaesth Intensive Care* 20:378–382, 1992.

30. Goldmann L, Shah MV, Hebden MW: Memory of cardiac anaesthesia, *Anaesthesia* 42:596–603, 1987.

31. Bennett HL, Davis HS, Giannini JA: Non-verbal response to intraoperative conversion, *Br J Anaesth* 57:174–179, 1985.

32. Liu WHO, Thorp TAS, Graham SG, et al: Incidence of awareness with recall during general anaesthesia, *Anaesthesia* 46:435–137, 1991.

33. Blacher RS: On awakening paralyzed during surgery: a syndrome of traumatic neurosis, *JAMA* 234:67–68, 1975.

34. Blacher RS: Awareness during surgery, *Anesthesiology* 61:1–2, 1984.

35. Rapee RM: Psychological factors influencing the affective response to biological challenge procedures in panic disorder, *J Anxiety Disord* 9:59–74, 1995.

36. Wishnie MA, Hackett TP, Cassem NH: Psychological hazards of convalescence following myocardial infarction, *JAMA* 215:1292–1296, 1971.

37. Shuckit MA: Anxiety related to medical disease, *J Clin Psychol* 44:31–36, 1983.

38. Wolf S, Alma TB, Bacharach W, et al: The role of stress in peptic ulcer disease, *J Human Stress* 1:27–37, 1979.

39. Fauman MA: The central nervous system and the immune system, *Biol Psychiatry* 17:1459–1482, 1982.

40. Greer S, Morris T, Pettingale KW: Psychological response to breast cancer: effect on outcome, *Lancet* 2:785–787, 1979.

41. Hall RCW, editor: *Psychiatric presentations of medical illness: somatopsychic disorders*, New York, 1980, SP Medical & Scientific Books.

42. Hall RCW, Gardner ER, Popkin MK, et al: Unrecognized physical illness prompting psychiatric admission: a prospective study, *Am J Psychiatry* 138:629–635, 1981.

43. Cavanaugh S, Wettstein RM: *Prevalence of psychiatric morbidity in medical populations*. In Grinspoon L, editor: *Psychiatric update*, vol 3, Washington, DC, 1984, American Psychiatric Press.

44. Cameron OG: The differential diagnosis of anxiety: psychiatric and medical disorders, *Psychiatr Clin North Am* 8:3–24, 1981.

45. MacKenzie TB, Popkin MK: Organic anxiety syndrome, *Am J Psychiatry* 140:342–344, 1983.

46. Rosenbaum JF: The drug treatment of anxiety, *N Engl J Med* 306:401–404, 1982.

47. Starkman MN, Zelnick TC, Nesse RM, et al: A study of anxiety in patients with pheochromocytoma, *Arch Intern Med* 145:248–252, 1985.

48. Harper M, Roth M: Temporal lobe epilepsy and the phobic-anxiety depersonalization syndrome, *Compr Psychiatry* 3:129–151, 1962.

49. Avant RF: Diagnosis and management of depression in the office setting, *Fam Pract Res* 5(suppl 1):41, 1983.

50. Quitkin F, Rifkin A, Kaplan T, et al: Phobic anxiety syndrome complicated by drug dependency and addiction, *Arch Gen Psychiatry* 27:159–162, 1972.

51. Sheehan DV, Ballenger J, Jacobsen A: Treatment of endogenous anxiety with phobic, hysterical and hypochondriacal symptoms, *Arch Gen Psychiatry* 37:51–59, 1980.

52. Katon W: Panic disorder and somatization: a review of 55 cases, *Am J Med* 77:101–106, 1984.

53. Bridges KW, Goldberg BP: Somatic presentation of DSM-III psychiatric disorders in primary care, *J Psychosom Res* 29:563–569, 1985.

54. Boyd JH, Burke JD, Greenberg E, et al: Exclusion criteria of DSM-III: a study of co-occurrence of hierarchy-free syndromes, *Arch Gen Psychiatry* 41:983–987, 1984.

55. Katon W, Von Korff M, Lin E, et al: Distressed high utilizers of medical care: DSM-III-R diagnoses and treatment needs, *Gen Hosp Psychiatry* 12:355–362, 1990.

56. Clancy J, Noyes R: Anxiety neurosis: a disease for the medical model, *Psychosomatics* 17:90–93, 1976.

57. Bass C, Wade C, Gardner WN, et al: Unexplained breathlessness and psychiatric morbidity in patients with normal and abnormal coronary arteries, *Lancet* 1:605–609, 1983.

58. Carter C, Maddox R, Amsterdam E, et al: Panic disorder and chest pain in the coronary care unit, *Psychosomatics* 33:302–310, 1992.

59. Wulsin LR, Hillard JR, Geier P, et al: Screening emergency room patients with atypical chest pain for depression and panic disorder, *Int J Psychiatry Med* 18:315–323, 1988.

60. Worthington JJ, Pollack MH, Otto MW, et al: *Panic disorder in emergency room ward patients with chest pain*, 147th Annual Meeting of the American Psychiatric Association, 1994, Philadelphia.

61. Richter JE, Bradley LA, Castell DO: Esophageal chest pain: current controversies in pathogenesis, diagnosis, and therapy, *Ann Intern Med* 110:66–78, 1989.

62. Dirks JF, Schraa JC, Brown E, et al: Psycho-maintenance in asthma: hospitalization rates and financial impact, *Br J Med Psychol* 53:349–354, 1980.

63. Warwick HMC, Salkovskis PM: Hypochondriasis, *Behav Res Ther* 28:105–117, 1990.

64. Mechanic D: Social psychologic factors affecting the presentation of bodily complaints, *N Engl J Med* 286:1132–1139, 1972.

65. Jones BA: Panic attacks with panic masked by alexithymia, *Psychosomatics* 25:858–859, 1984.

66. Yellowlees PM, Alpers JH, Bowden JJ, et al: Psychiatric morbidity in subjects with chronic airflow obstruction, *Med J Aust* 146:305–307, 1987.

67. Karajgi B, Rifkin A, Doddi S, et al: The prevalence of anxiety disorders in patients with chronic obstructive pulmonary disease, *Am J Psychiatry* 147:200–201, 1990.

68. Porzelius J, Vest M, Nochomovitz M: Respiratory function, cognitions, and panic in chronic obstructive pulmonary patients, *Behav Res Ther* 30:75–77, 1992.

69. Pollack MH, Kradin R, Otto MW, et al: Prevalence of panic in patients referred for pulmonary function testing at a major medical center, *Am J Psychiatry* 153:110–113, 1996.

70. Noyes R, Clancy J, Moenk PR, et al: Anxiety neurosis and physical illness, *Compr Psychiatry* 19:407–413, 1978.

71. Lydiard RB, Fossey MD, Marsh W, et al: Prevalence of psychiatric disorders in patients with irritable bowel syndrome, *Psychosomatics* 34:229–234, 1993.

72. Coryell W, Noyes R Jr, Howe JD: Mortality among outpatients with anxiety disorders, *Am J Psychiatry* 143:508–510, 1986.

73. Liberthson R, Sheehan DV, King ME, et al: The prevalence of mitral valve prolapse in patients with panic disorder, *Am J Psychiatry* 143:511–515, 1986.

74. Dager SR, Comess KA, Dunner DL: Differentiation of anxious patients by two dimensional echocardiographic evaluation of the mitral valve, *Am J Psychiatry* 143:533–536, 1986.

75. Hickey AJ, Andrew G, Wilcken DEL: Independence of mitral valve prolapse and neurosis, *Br Heart J* 50:333–336, 1983.

76. Gorman JM, Fyer AJ, King D, et al: *Mitral valve prolapse and panic disorders: effect of imipramine.* In Klein DJ, Rabkin JG, editors: *Anxiety: new research and changing concepts,* New York, 1981, Raven Press.

77. Otto MW, Pollack MH, Rosenbaum JF, et al: Childhood history of anxiety in adults with panic disorder: association with anxiety sensitivity and comorbidity, *Harvard Rev Psychiatry* 1:288–293, 1994.

78. Crowe RR: The genetics of panic disorder and agoraphobics, *Psychiatr Dev* 2:171–186, 1985.

79. Ball SG, Otto MW, Pollack MH, et al: Predicting prospective episodes of depression in patients with panic disorder: a longitudinal study, *J Consult Clin Psychol* 62:359–365, 1994.

80. Barlow DH, Blanchard EB, Vermilyea JA, et al: Generalized anxiety and generalized anxiety disorder: description and reconceptualization, *Am J Psychiatry* 143:40, 1986.

81. Katon W, Vitaliano PP, Anderson K, et al: Panic disorder: residual symptoms after the acute attacks abate, *Compr Psychiatry* 28:151, 1987.

82. Breslau N, Davis GC: DSM-III generalized anxiety disorder: an empirical investigation of more stringent criteria, *Psychiatry Res* 14:231, 1985.

83. Roy-Byrne PP, Katon W: An update on treatment of the anxiety disorders, *Hosp Comm Psychiatry* 38:835, 1987.

84. Kushner MG, Sher KJ, Beitman BD: The relation between alcohol problems and the anxiety disorders, *Am J Psychiatry* 147:685–695, 1990.

85. Schneier FR, Johnson J, Hornig CD, et al: Social phobia: comorbidity and morbidity in an epidemiologic sample, *Arch Gen Psychiatry* 49:282–288, 1992.

86. Reiter SR, Pollack MH, Rosenbaum JF, et al: Clonazepam for the treatment of social phobia, *J Clin Psychiatry* 51:470–472, 1990.

87. Lydiard R, Laraia M, Howell E, et al: Alprazolam in the treatment of social phobia, *J Clin Psychiatry* 49:17, 1988.

88. Zatzick DF, Kang SM, Muller HG, et al: Predicting posttraumatic distress in hospitalized trauma survivors with acute injuries, *Am J Psychiatry* 159:941–946, 2002.

89. Ilechukwu ST: Psychiatry of the medically ill in the burn unit, *Psychiatr Clin North Am* 25:129–147, 2002.

90. Zatzick DF, Jurkovich GJ, Gentilello L, et al: Posttraumatic stress, problem drinking, and functional outcomes after injury, *Arch Surg* 137:200–205, 2002.

91. Harvey AG, Bryant RA: The relationship between acute stress disorder and posttraumatic stress disorder: a prospective evaluation of motor vehicle accident survivors. *J Consult Clin Psychol* 66:507–512, 1998.

92. Mayou RA, Ehlers A, Hobbs M: Psychological debriefing for road traffic accident victims: three-year follow-up of a randomised controlled trial, *Br J Psychiatry* 176:589–593, 2000.

93. Suzanna RO, Jonathan BI, Simon WE: Psychological debriefing for preventing post traumatic stress disorder (PTSD), *Cochrane Database Syst Rev* 2: CD000560, 2002.

94. Bryant RA, Sackville T, Dang ST, et al: Treating acute stress disorder: an evaluation of cognitive behavior therapy and supportive counseling techniques. *Am J Psychiatry* 156:1780–1786, 1999.

95. Foa EB, Hearst-Ikeda D, Perry KJ: Evaluation of a brief cognitive-behavioral program for the prevention of chronic PTSD in recent assault victims. *J Consult Clin Psychol* 63:948–955, 1995.

96. Robert R, Blakeney PE, Villarreal C, et al: Imipramine treatment in pediatric burn patients with symptoms of acute stress disorder: a pilot study, *J Am Acad Child Adolesc Psychiatry* 38:873–882, 1999.

97. Pitman RK, Sanders KM, Zusman RM, et al: Pilot study of secondary prevention of posttraumatic stress disorder with propranolol, *Biol Psychiatry* 51:189–192, 2002.

98. Otto MW, Penava SJ, Pollock RA, et al: *Cognitive-behavioral and pharmacologic perspectives on the treatment of post-traumatic stress disorder.* In Pollack MH, Otto MW, Rosenbaum JF, editors: *Challenges in clinical practice: pharmacologic and psychosocial strategies,* New York, 1996, Guilford Press.

99. Davidson JR: Pharmacotherapy of posttraumatic stress disorder: treatment options, long-term follow-up, and predictors of outcome, *J Clin Psychiatry* 61(suppl 5): 52–56, 2000.

100. Gelpin E, Bonne O, Peri T, et al: Treatment of recent trauma survivors with benzodiazepines: a prospective study. *J Clin Psychiatry* 57:390–394, 1996.

101. Mellman TA, Bustamante V, David D, et al: Hypnotic medication in the aftermath of trauma. *J Clin Psychiatry* 63:1183–1184, 2002.

102. Weissman MM, Lechman JF, Merikangas JR, et al: Depression and anxiety disorders in parents and children, *Arch Gen Psychiatry* 41:845–852, 1984.

103. Breier A, Charney DS, Heninger GR: Major depression in patients with agoraphobia and panic disorder, *Arch Gen Psychiatry* 41:1129–1135, 1984.

104. Lesser IM, Rubin RT: Diagnostic considerations in panic disorders, *J Clin Psychol* 47(suppl):6, 1986.

105. Leckman JF, Weissman MM, Merikangas KR, et al: Panic disorder in major depression, *Arch Gen Psychiatry* 40:1055–1060, 1983.

106. Uhde TW, Roy-Byrne P, Gillin JC, et al: The sleep of patients with panic disorder: a preliminary report, *Psychiatry Res* 12:251–259, 1984.

107. Kelly D, Walter CJS: A clinical and physiological relationship between anxiety and depression, *Br J Psychiatry* 115:401–406, 1969.

108. Cameron OG, Smith CR, Hollingsworth PJ, et al: Platelet alpha-2 adrenergic receptor binding and plasma catecholamines in panic anxiety patients, *Arch Gen Psychiatry* 41:1144–1188, 1984.

109. McElroy SL, Altshuler LL, Suppes T, et al: Axis I psychiatric comorbidity and its relationship to historical

illness variables in 288 patients with bipolar disorder. *Am J Psychiatry* 158:420–426, 2001.

110. Otto MW, Gould RA: *Maximizing treatment-outcome for panic disorder: cognitive-behavioral strategies.* In Pollack MH, Otto MW, Rosenbaum JF, editors: *Challenges in clinical practice: pharmacologic and psychosocial strategies,* New York, 1996, Guilford Press.

111. Jobson KO, Davidson JRT, Lydiard BR, et al: Algorithm for the treatment of panic disorder with agoraphobia, *Psychopharmacol Bull* 31:483–485, 1995.

112. Pollack MH, Smoller JW: Pharmacologic approaches to treatment-resistant panic disorder. In Pollack MH, Otto MW, Rosenbaum JF, editors: *Challenges in psychiatric treatment: pharmacologic and psychosocial strategies,* New York, 1996, Guilford Press.

113. Pohl R, Berchou R, Rainey JM Jr. Tricyclic antidepressants and monoamine oxidase inhibitors in treatment of agoraphobia, *J Clin Psychopharmacol* 2:399–407, 1982.

114. Mavissakalian MR, Perel JM: Imipramine treatment of panic disorder with agoraphobia: dose ranging and plasma level-response relationships, *Am J Psychiatry* 152:673–682, 1995.

115. Noyes R Jr, Burrows GD, Reich JH, et al: Diazepam versus alprazolam for the treatment of panic disorder, *J Clin Psychiatry* 57:349–355, 1996.

116. Otto MW, Gould RA, Pollack MH: Cognitive-behavioral treatment of panic disorder: considerations for the treatment of patients over the long term, *Psychiatr Ann* 24:307–315, 1994.

117. Lydiard RB. The role of GABA in anxiety disorders. *J Clin Psychiatry,* 64(suppl 3):21–27, 2003.

118. Stein MB, Kline NA, Matloff JL: Adjunctive olanzapine for SSRI-resistant combat-related PTSD: a double-blind, placebo-controlled study, *Am J Psychiatry,* 159:1777–1779, 2002.

119. Goa KL, Ward A: Buspirone: a preliminary review of its pharmacological properties and therapeutic efficacy as an anxiolytic, *Drugs* 32:114–125, 1986.

120. Clum GA, Clum GA, Surls R: A meta-analysis of treatments for panic disorder, *J Consult Clin Psychol* 61:317–326, 1993.

121. Gould RA, Otto MW, Pollack MH: A meta-analysis of treatment outcome for panic disorder, *Clin Psychol Rev* 15:819–844, 1995.

122. Gould RA, Otto MW, Yap L, et al: *Cognitive-behavioral and pharmacological treatment of social phobia: a meta-analysis,* 28th Annual Meeting of the Association for the Advancement of Behavior Therapy, 1994, San Diego.

123. Hunt C, Singh M: Generalized anxiety disorder, *Int Rev Psychiatry* 3:215–229, 1991.

124. Christensen H, Hadzi-Pavlovic D, Andrews G, et al: Behavior therapy and tricyclic medication in the treatment of obsessive-compulsive disorder: a quantitative review, *J Consult Clin Psychol* 55:701–711, 1987.

Chapter 16

Alcoholic Patients—Acute and Chronic

David R. Gastfriend, M.D.
John A. Renner, Jr., M.D.
Thomas P. Hackett, M.D.

From cases of simple intoxication, when the diagnosis can be made on the basis of breath odor and slurred speech, to the more complicated mental status of withdrawal states, alcohol is responsible for more psychiatric and neuropsychiatric problems in general hospitals than are all other substances combined. One study found that nearly 25% of patients who were hospitalized for injuries were intoxicated at the time of their trauma[1] and estimates of the prevalence of alcohol-related problems in general hospitals range from 12.5% to 30%.[2] Even when problem drinking is not in the immediate picture, a history of alcoholism or of heavy social drinking predisposes a patient to delirium in conjunction with surgery, fever, head trauma, or massive burns. This vulnerability may be related to the neuropathologic changes that have been found in the brains of heavy drinkers and alcoholics. Yet, the Centers for Disease Control and Prevention reports that millions of Americans with drinking problems are still not given advice about how to restrict and control their use of alcohol.[3] Failure to diagnose alcoholism and other substance abuse in hospitalized patients is exceedingly costly in terms of both morbidity and expense. At a major East Coast teaching hospital, when investigators reviewed more than 1000 consecutive admissions during a 23-day period, the actual number of substance abusers admitted was 160, as assessed by an independent evaluator; however, in no cases did physicians document that substance abuse was addressed. Hospital costs for these 160 substance abusers totaled $4.3 million

over a 23-day period.[4] When substance abusers are identified by hospital-based physicians and offered referrals, nearly two thirds accept.[5] Months after referral, these patients report improved outcomes with relation to alcohol problems (e.g., abstinence, duration since last drink, job performance, and personal happiness).[5–7] Controlled studies confirm that even a single, brief, detailed discussion by the physician yields measurable reductions in the consequences of alcoholism.[8–9] Therefore the Institute of Medicine[10] has called for the screening of hospitalized patients for alcohol problems.

A simple, inexpensive screening interview, the CAGE (Table 16-1)[11] offers brevity, as well as low cost, and better sensitivity and specificity for alcohol problems than currently available markers, such as the serum γ-glutamyl transpeptidase, serum transaminases, and the mean corpuscular volume.[12] Laboratory markers, particularly the serum level of carbohydrate-deficient transferrin, can be helpful, however, in tracking decrements in patients' drinking following intervention.[11]

Drunkenness

Inebriation is potentially disruptive and dangerous. Few sights are more frightening than that of a young and powerful man, mindlessly angry, anesthetized to pain, yet in full possession of his motor coordination and muscular power.

Table 16-1. CAGE Questionnaire for Alcohol Problems Screening*

C—Have you felt the need to **C**ut down on your drinking?
A—Have people **A**nnoyed you by criticizing your drinking?
G—Have you ever felt bad or **G**uilty about your drinking?
E—Have you had a drink first thing in the morning to steady your nerves or to get rid of a hangover (i.e., an "**E**ye opener")?

---

*A score of two positive items indicates the need for detailed assessment.[11]

Management

The actions of ethanol on neuronal systems are complex; initially, use of ethanol at low doses produces electric excitability, whereas at higher doses it depresses it. In the emergency room, behavioral disinhibition is mediated by alcohol's action as a γ-aminobutyric acid (GABA) agonist, and its interactions with the serotonin system may account for its association with violent behavior. Blood alcohol concentrations (BACs) as low as 40 mg/dl may impair memory, lead to an alcoholic blackout, with argumentativeness or assaultiveness at 150 to 250 mg/dl and coma or death at 400 to 500 mg/dl. Yet, chronic alcoholics may be fully alert with BACs of more than 800 mg/dl, owing to tolerance.[13] Because these interactions are unpredictable, the first management principle is to *alert the hospital police or security force* before starting an interview with a boisterous drunk. Although seldom required, it is reassuring to have police assistance at the ready, especially if the patient is armed or has a history of combativeness.

The second principle is for staff to *be tolerant and nonthreatening*. People who possess a skill for disarming the abusive drunk seem to have little or no need to express their authority or toughness, even though they may have both qualities in abundance. They tolerate insults, threats, and oaths because they do not take them personally. Conversely, we have observed that individuals who galvanize the alcoholic's anger and mobilize his or her aggression are often autocratic and rigid; their flimsy sense of security is easily punctured by an inebriate's invective. The successful interviewer temporarily accepts the drunk as he or she is; the unsuccessful interviewer rapidly attempts to make the drunk civil. This latter effort usually backfires. When approaching an alcoholic person, a handshake of introduction should be extended. Unless the patient is well-known, the patient should be addressed by his or her proper name, for example, "Mr. or Mrs. Smith." For the time being, no attempt should be made to change the patient's behavior; instead, it is better to listen to a tirade and to make sense of it than to demand that the patient lower his or her voice and to talk temperately. This approach has occasionally uncovered a legitimate grievance or misunderstanding that, once corrected, quickly alleviated the patient's bellicosity.

It is advisable to avoid direct eye contact that lasts for more than a few seconds at a time. More than momentary eye contact is often taken as a challenge; it becomes the prelude to combat for animals as well as for humans. The interviewer should listen intently to what the patient has to say and appear puzzled or perplexed rather than angry or amused if the accusation or complaint is absurd. Above all, it is important to avoid a belligerent posture. A colleague once observed that he patterned his behavior with hostile drunks after the humble-submissive posture assumed by a wolf when bested in battle. Transposed to the human habitus, this physician keeps his eyes downcast, fists unclenched, and shoulders stooped. Once the patient sees that the interviewer is not going to attack, his outburst may quiet and his anger slacken.

The third principle is to *offer food*. Some of the most antagonistic alcoholics have been soothed by an offer of coffee. If the individual is willing to leave the scene with the inducement of coffee, food, and quiet (luring with the promise of a beer is absolutely the last resort), he or she should be escorted to a lobby or foyer where people are within easy calling distance. Many alcoholic persons are claustrophobic and feel trapped in small rooms. Those with underlying homosexual conflicts might associate the closeness of the tiny quarters with the fear of sexual advance. Furthermore, it is discomforting for most physicians to be in an enclosed area with a potentially violent person. The value of offering food, cigarettes, or drink in this case can be justified by empiric evidence only. With food the patient will often lose his or her fight. The next step is to persuade the patient to take a sedative (if alert and agitated) or an antipsychotic (if still ataxic and dysarthric) and to go to bed.

As in handling other conditions of psychotic excitement, it often helps to let the patient know that his or her behavior is frightening. Resolution of intoxication follows steady-state kinetics, so that a 70-kg man metabolizes approximately 10 ml of absolute ethanol or 1.5 to 2 drink equivalents ($^1/_2$ oz whiskey = 4 oz wine = 12 oz beer) per hour.

Case 1

A female psychiatrist was called to the emergency department to see a patient who had leapt from the examining table while a scalp laceration was being repaired. The patient accused the intern of deliberately trying to hurt him, and he accused the entire staff of racism. The patient was a large man with a deep and penetrating voice and a menacing manner. The psychiatrist, a small woman, asked the others to leave, which they did reluctantly. They heard the patient thunder accusations for 3 to 4 minutes. Then quiet reigned. A shattering scream was expected, but not even a breath could be heard. The psychiatrist emerged 5 minutes later, and the patient was lying peaceably on the examining table after having consented to an intramuscular (IM) injection of a sedative. The psychiatric technique was simple. During a pause for breath in his ranting, she told him that she was nearly speechless with fear. She reminded him that she was harmless, that she could do nothing to hurt him, and that she wanted to help him. The tremor in her voice verified her statement. He stared at her for a moment. Then he muttered, "Don't want to scare nobody," and accepted the sedative.

To sedate an intoxicated individual, one must begin with a smaller dose than usual to avoid delirium that results from the cumulative effects of alcohol and the agent used. Once the individual's tolerance has been established, a specific dose can be safely determined. In the patient who is excessively agitated without ataxia or dysarthria, lorazepam (Ativan) 1 to 2 mg offers effective absorption via all routes—orally, intramuscularly, or intravenously; diazepam (Valium) and chlordiazepoxide (Librium) are erratically and slowly absorbed after IM administration unless they are given in large, well-perfused sites. When incoordination suggests that the additive effect of a benzodiazepine have produced excessive sedation, it may be advantageous to use haloperidol 5 to 10 mg orally or intramuscularly. The initial dose

should be followed by a wait of 0.5 to 1 hour before augmenting it. Just being acutely intoxicated does not require hospitalization. If there is no risk of withdrawal, the patient can safely be referred to an alcohol detoxification program. Inpatient detoxification is preferable to outpatient care if the patient is not well known to the team; is psychosocially unstable; has serious medical, neurologic, or psychiatric comorbidity; has previously suffered withdrawal complications; or is undergoing his or her first episode of treatment.[14] Repeatedly undertreated withdrawal may put the patient at subsequent risk for withdrawal seizures and for other neurologic sequelae. This increasing risk is believed to occur through "kindling," a type of electrophysiologic effect[15] and it may be mediated, similar to other neurodegenerative effects of ethanol, via the glutamate excitatory neurotransmitter system.[16]

Alcoholic Coma

Alcoholic coma, although rare, is a medical emergency. It occurs when extraordinary amounts of alcohol are consumed, often in conjunction with another drug. The main goals of treatment are to prevent aspiration by placing the patient on his or her side, to monitor closely for respiratory depression because of the potential need for admission to the intensive care unit, and to be prepared for respiratory arrest with a need for mechanic ventilation (realizing that the GABA antagonist, flumazenil may not reverse ethanol's respiratory depression).[17]

Pathologic Intoxication and Alcoholic Paranoia

In pathologic intoxication, the patient becomes intoxicated on small amounts (as little as 4 oz) of alcohol. There may be subsequent automatic behavior that is violent and for which the patient is totally amnestic. The alcoholic person with a known history of pathologic intoxication should be sedated heavily and confined until sobriety is ensured to avoid possible danger to others.

Pathologic intoxication may last for an hour or for days, and it usually ends after prolonged sleep.

During the episode, the patient is agitated, impulsive, and often aggressive. Delusions and visual hallucinations may occur. Generally the disorder is marked by hyperactivity, anxiety, or depression. Suicide risk is increased during these episodes. It may be more likely in patients with borderline personality disorder or epilepsy or in those individuals who tend toward emotional instability and whose pattern of defense is easily disorganized. Haloperidol 5 to 10 mg orally or intramuscularly decreases agitated or violent behavior with a minimum of sedation and with little likelihood of seizure potentiation; doses may be repeated in 30 minutes, if necessary.[18]

Alcoholic paranoia is somewhat similar to pathologic intoxication. It is a state of cognitive disorganization brought about by use of alcohol that may manifest as strong feelings of jealousy, antagonism, or suspicion.

The prognosis is poor for patients with pathologic intoxication or alcoholic paranoia. Such patients often have a history of violence and aggression with repeated incarcerations. The consultation psychiatrist should be on the watch for emergence of amnesia or for the return of the premorbid behavior after the intoxication has been slept off. Although the premorbid personality of the paranoid alcoholic patient is apt to be somewhat suspicious, it is not nearly as intense or threatening as when under the influence of alcohol.

Alcohol Withdrawal Syndrome

The syndrome of alcohol withdrawal can range from mild discomfort that requires no medication to multiorgan failure that requires intensive care. Uncomplicated withdrawal is surprisingly common and frequently missed. Although more than 90% of alcoholics in withdrawal need nothing more than supportive treatment, those with comorbid illness in the general hospital undoubtedly have a higher rate of complications.[19] The most common features of uncomplicated alcohol withdrawal emerge within hours and resolve after 3 to 5 days as the BAC is descending. Uncomplicated withdrawal symptoms are predictable: Loss of appetite, irritability, and tremulousness are early features. A hallmark of the abstinence syndrome is generalized tremor, fast in frequency and more pronounced when the patient is under stress. This tremor may involve the tongue to such an extent that the patient cannot talk. The lower extremities may tremble so that the patient cannot walk. The hands and arms may shake so violently that a drinking glass cannot be held without spilling the contents. The patient is hypervigilant, has a pronounced startle response, and complains of insomnia.

Less commonly, patients experience hallucinations (without delirium) or seizures associated with alcohol withdrawal. Illusions and hallucinations of a mild variety may appear and produce vague uneasiness. These symptoms may persist for as long as 2 weeks and then clear without developing delirium. Grand mal seizures ("rum fits") may occur, usually within the first 2 days. More than one out of every three patients who suffer seizures develop subsequent delirium tremens (DTs).

Treatment

Rigid adherence to only one protocol for all alcohol withdrawal is unrealistic. Moreover, the failure to individualize treatment may increase costs—an undesirable result in the era of managed and capitated care. Symptom-triggered dosing, in which dosages are individualized and only administered upon the appearance of early symptoms, reduces medication doses by a factor of four and shortens symptom duration by a factor of six,[20,21] although benefits may be less dramatic in medically ill inpatients.[22] Chlordiazepoxide 50 to 100 mg orally should be given initially, and be followed by 50 to 100 mg every 1 to 2 hours until the patient is sedated and the vital signs are within normal limits. Alternatively, diazepam 10 to 20 mg may be given initially, and then repeated every 1 to 2 hours until sedation is achieved. Often a first day's dose of a long-acting benzodiazepine is sufficient for the entire detoxification process because of the self-tapering effect and slow elimination.[23] Patients with impaired liver function are better managed with shorter-acting agents, such as oxazepam or lorazepam 1 to 4 mg orally or intramuscularly, or 0.5 mg/minute slow intravenous (IV) infusion in severe withdrawal), repeated after 1 to 2 hours, with dose tapering by 25% per day over the subsequent 3 to 6 days.

Alcoholic Hallucinations

Diagnosis

Much less common than alcohol withdrawal delirium, but more bizarre, is alcoholic hallucinosis. The onset is usually within 24 to 48 hours after alcohol cessation, but it can occur during active drinking or weeks later. The patient experiences vivid auditory illusions and hallucinations that occur in an otherwise clear sensorium. These hallucinations may become accusatory and threatening. The individual reacts with fear but is fully oriented and realizes that the voices are hallucinations. As the accusations persist, however, the patient develops ideas of persecution. Although hallucinosis is more apt to occur in the setting of alcohol withdrawal, it is by no means uncommon in individuals who continue to drink. Some authors believe that hallucinosis is programmed by a disturbance of the auditory pathways. Tinnitus is found in many patients who report hallucinosis. Curiously, when tinnitus is one-sided, the hallucinatory experience usually occurs only on that side. Olfactory hallucinations may occur with alcoholic hallucinosis, but visual hallucinations seldom occur.

The clinical picture is one in which auditory hallucinations occur in the absence of tremor, disorientation, and agitation. The content may be sexually oriented; for example, a male patient may hear voices accusing him of homosexuality and threatening retaliation, or a woman may hear accusations of promiscuity. Soon after the voices begin, a frightening systematized delusional system develops that may incite the patient to call the police or to arm himself or herself. Then the patient is particularly dangerous. The patient is capable of acting with an otherwise clear mind. Suicide is a distinct danger in this condition and it may occur, as in delirium, without appreciable warning.

Case 2

A 27-year-old merchant seaman had begun listening to a local disc jockey while at a bar the previous evening. His attention was suddenly caught when he heard his name announced as a third-prize winner. He had won 14 sheep, 5 head of cattle, and a strawberry farm in Kansas. A taxi driver who had listened to him for 3 hours and had driven him to multiple radio stations finally insisted on taking him to a hospital. Since this was the early 1950s, the era of the colossal giveaways, the story sounded plausible, especially because the patient told it in a straightforward and reasonable manner. The cab driver was asked by hospital personnel whether he had heard the announcement on the car radio. He exclaimed, "Oh, no! Not you too! They all believe him instead of me. Ask him what else the voices said." When asked, the seaman grudgingly admitted that the disc jockey, along with announcing his name as a winner, had accused him of homosexual acts. As he spoke he became serious and threatening. He clearly believed these voices to be real. He readily agreed, however, to enter the hospital. He seemed certain that the truth of his statement would be quickly discovered if he were hospitalized. A week later, he no longer heard voices and had substantially minimized the experience, just as he forgot that alcohol had caused it.

Paranoid schizophrenia may be confused with alcoholic hallucinosis. The differential diagnosis is apt to be difficult. The predominance of the auditory component of the disorder and a history of alcoholism can aid in the diagnosis of this condition.

Treatment

There is no specific treatment for alcoholic hallucinosis. Generally the condition clears within 30 days, but it may last another month. There are reported instances in which the hallucinosis continued for years. If the individual continues to drink, recurrences are the rule.

The most important aspect of treatment is to determine whether the patient should be in a protected environment. Behavior destructive to the self or to others is common, and it may require commitment to a psychiatric hospital. Sedation with benzodiazepines can be given as needed. Because patients in general feel quite normal after the disappearance of auditory hallucinations, they often insist on being discharged as soon as the voices desist. As in DTs, the course can be intermittent, and the patient should be kept in a hospital until 1 to 2 days have passed without hallucinations. The patient should also be vigorously warned against drinking because the hallucinations are apt to return with a relapse.

Alcohol Withdrawal Seizures

Withdrawal seizures are estimated to occur in only 1% of unmedicated alcoholics undergoing withdrawal, although the prevalence is increased in individuals with prior alcohol withdrawal seizures, seizure disorders, and previous brain injury. Although brain imaging may not be necessary in first-episode patients,[24] seizures during alcohol withdrawal do require careful examination for other causes. Indications for imaging studies include neurologic and other physical findings suggestive of focal lesions, meningitis, and subarachnoid hemorrhage—all of which may occur in patients with prior alcohol withdrawal seizures. Multiple prior detoxifications predispose to withdrawal seizures more than the quantity or duration of a drinking history, implying a kindling cause.[25] Seizures may occur during relative withdrawal or during the 6 to 24 hours after drinking cessation. Generalized seizures typically occur (i.e., in 75% of cases) in the absence of focal findings, and in individuals with otherwise unremarkable electroencephalogram (EEG) findings. Repeated seizures may occur over a 24-hour period; however, status epilepticus occurs in less than 10% of those who seize.

Treatment

In patients without a prior seizure disorder, diphenylhydantoin offers no benefit over placebo, and given the potential for side effects, diphenylhydantoin is therefore not indicated.[25] Also, given that loading with carbamazepine or valproate may not address the rapid time course of withdrawal seizures, the most parsimonious approach remains effective treatment with benzodiazepines. In cases where there is a known seizure disorder, however, conventional management with anticonvulsants is in order.

Alcohol Withdrawal Delirium

DTs, the major acute complication of alcohol withdrawal, has been, renamed *alcohol withdrawal delirium* in the *Diagnostic and Statistical Manual of Mental Disorders,* fourth edition (DSM-IV).[26] Until open heart procedures spawned new postoperative deliria, DTs were by far the most frequently encountered delirium in a general hospital, reportedly occurring in 5% of hospitalized alcoholics.[27] Although it was first described in the medical literature more than 150 years ago and has been frequently observed in general hospitals ever since, DTs still go undiagnosed in a large number of cases. It is missed because physicians tend to forget that alcoholism is rampant among people of all possible backgrounds and appearances in the United States. Physicians also fail to suspect the patient who deliberately or unwittingly minimizes dependence on alcohol and underestimates the amount consumed. Because deaths have occurred in 10% of patients with untreated alcohol withdrawal delirium and in 25% of those patients with medical or concomitant surgical complications, it is imperative to be on the alert for this life-threatening condition.

Prediction

It is difficult to predict who will develop DTs. Until a decade ago, DTs rarely developed in patients younger than the age of 30 years. This is no longer true. Today the condition is frequently observed in young patients who may have had a decade or more of chronic heavy alcohol consumption. The mechanisms may involve N-methyl-D-aspartate (NMDA)-glutamate receptor supersensitivity.[15] Although regarded as a withdrawal syndrome, some heavy drinkers fail to develop delirium after sudden withdrawal of ethanol. Infection, head trauma, and poor nutrition probably contribute factors to delirium. A history of DTs is an obvious predictor of future DTs.

Case 3

A 64-year-old longshoreman entered the hospital with recurrent gout (i.e., 16 episodes during a 3-year period). Each time he became tremulous and disoriented during the second night and went on to develop mild visual and vestibular hallucinations that cleared over 3 days. Large ships would issue though the walls or windows, and the whole room would rock and sway like a wharf in a storm. The pattern was identical, including his insistence that the only alcohol he ever swallowed was a drop or two from his mouthwash.

Diagnosis

The incidence of DTs is approximately 5% among hospitalized alcoholics and about 33% in patients with alcohol withdrawal seizures. If DTs are to occur, they generally do so within 24 to 72 hours after abstinence begins. There have been reports, however, of cases in which the clinical picture of DTs did not emerge until 7 days after the last drink. The principal features are disorientation (to time, place, or person), tremor, hyperactivity, marked wakefulness, fever, increased autonomic tone, and hallucinations. Hallucinations are generally visual but they may be tactile (in which case they are probably associated with a peripheral neuritis), olfactory, or auditory. Vestibular disturbances are common and often hallucinatory. The patient may complain of the floor moving beneath his or her feet or believe that he or she is on an elevator. The hallucinatory experience is always frightening. Animals, typically snakes, are seen in threatening poses. Mice or lice are felt and seen crawling on the skin. Once the condition manifests itself, DTs usually last 2 to 3 days, often resolving suddenly after a night of sound sleep. Should it persist for a longer time, one must suspect an underlying disorder, such as an infection or subdural hematoma. There are, however, a small number of individuals whose course is characterized by relapses with intervals of complete lucidity. These patients offer the consultant the most challenging diagnostic opportunities. As a rule of thumb, it is always wise to include DTs in the list of diagnoses considered whenever delirium appears.

A psychiatric consultant is apt to miss the diagnosis of DTs when the patient's manner, social position, or reputation belies the possibility of alcoholism. For example, the following problem arose after emergency surgery.

Case 4

A 54-year-old woman was admitted to the hospital for a cholecystectomy. She was a society matron; she and her surgeon were neighbors. On her third postoperative day (her fifth day without alcohol), the nurses reported that they could not keep her in bed. She got up and walked about her room in a restless, agitated fashion, constantly gazing back over her shoulders as though she feared she was being followed. Soon her peregrinations included

other patients' rooms as well as the hospital corridor. She resisted violently every attempt to keep her confined to quarters. The surgeon, when called, described her as "fearful, overactive, stubborn, but polite." Although she would not give any reason for her distress, she readily swallowed a 25-mg capsule of chlordiazepoxide hydrochloride. This produced no change in her behavior after 2 hours. She talked to herself while she paced but was able to maintain a shaky semblance of poise when approached by others. Although her physician opposed psychiatric consultation, the nurses prevailed because they feared she might inadvertently hurt herself. When a house officer suggested the possibility of a small stroke because of the patient's long history of hypertension, the physician agreed to request psychiatric advice.

After reviewing the history and noting a bilateral hand tremor while observing the patient, the psychiatrist diagnosed DTs. Although the patient refused to speak with him after he identified himself, the psychiatrist maintained his diagnosis because it was the most likely possibility in the absence of other signs. Her personal physician refused to accept the diagnosis but did follow the recommended regimen of medication (100 mg of chlordiazepoxide each hour) until the patient was able to stay in bed. The medication was then reduced to a maintenance level and supplemented by 50 mg of thiamine daily. Round-the-clock special nurses were also employed. In the morning, following a night's sleep, the patient was her normal self.

The patient subsequently admitted drinking four to seven very dry martinis a day, each about 4 oz. She had been doing so for the last 30 years and had gone through all her maternity confinements without having DTs. She was so frightened by her experience, however, that she agreed to enter treatment for alcohol dependence.

The consultant is also frequently misled when the delirium is intermittent and the patient is examined during a lucid stage.

Case 5

A 52-year-old architect was admitted for hematemesis. The patient readily admitted heavy alcohol intake but had no difficulty in the hospital until the fourth day. He then began to gaze fixedly at a point on the ceiling and to talk in low, menacing tones to an imaginary companion. He sweated, trembled, and thrashed about so wildly that he had to be restrained in bed. He readily described auditory hallucinations of a persecutory nature. These became alarmingly vivid in the evening. The following morning a psychiatrist was called to see him and found him to be fully oriented, lucid, perfectly capable of discussing his hallucinatory experiences of the previous evening, and willing to accept the diagnosis of DTs, although he had been a heavy drinker for many years. The psychiatrist noted a probable episode of DTs but observed that the patient was now lucid and ready for further diagnostic procedures. Restraints were removed. A few hours later the patient leapt out of bed, ran through the ward, upset tables, and screamed that someone was chasing him. Once again he was forcibly restrained, placed in bed, given 8 ml of paraldehyde orally and 50 mg of chlorpromazine intramuscularly. When the psychiatrist returned a few hours later, the patient's mental status was entirely normal, and he could recall the violent episode. He was, in fact, so clear-thinking and his mentation so intact that the psychiatrist once again suggested that the restraints be removed. Within 20 minutes, the patient sprang out of bed, left the ward, and almost left the hospital. After this second unexpected episode, the consultant sent him to a psychiatric hospital where he remained for the next 2 weeks with intermittent episodes of delirium.

Although a course of intermittent episodes is highly atypical for DTs, it does occur. Consultants should be wary of relinquishing restraints or discontinuing private nursing service until the patient has been lucid for 24 hours.

Differential Diagnosis

The differential diagnosis must include the many causes of deliria in a general hospital. Hypoglycemia and alcoholic and diabetic ketoacidosis can co-occur with alcohol withdrawal; these are readily distinguished by their attendant electrolyte and blood glucose abnormalities and by their differential response to emergency treatment. Emergency treatment should include parenteral 50% glucose, thiamine, hydration, and in the case of diabetic ketoacidosis, insulin and potassium. Postoperative and postconcussive deliria occur, as well as other metabolic disorders. Two examples of the latter are (1) impending hepatic coma and (2) acute pancreatitis. A patient with impending hepatic coma may well be disoriented and confused but tends to manifest decreased activity rather than agitation. Usually there are no visual hallucinations. Speech is slow and monotonous, and the face is mask-like. Hyperphagia rather than anorexia is evident in impending hepatic coma. Physical signs, such as jaundice, hepatomegaly, and *fetor hepaticus* from elevation of blood ammonia levels, help determine this diagno-

sis. A delirium sometimes occurs in acute pancreatitis. In this condition, however, there is generally severe abdominal pain with an elevated serum amylase concentration.

Prognosis

The prognosis for DTs is reasonably good if the patient is aggressively medicated, but death can occur as the syndrome progresses through convulsions to coma and death. Death can also result from heart failure, an infection (chiefly pneumonia), or injuries sustained during the restless period. In a small proportion of patients the delirium may merge into Korsakoff's psychosis, in which case the patient may not regain full mentation. This is more apt to happen with closely spaced episodes of DTs in the elderly.

Treatment

Prevention is the key. Symptom-triggered dosing for alcohol withdrawal has been shown to reduce DTs compared to standing benzodiazepine orders, in medically ill inpatients.[22] As in the treatment of any delirium, the prime concern must be round-the-clock surveillance so that the patient cannot harm him or herself or others. This monitoring is essential. Although not necessarily suicidal, delirious patients take terrible unpremeditated risks. Falling from windows, slipping down stairs, and walking through glass doors are common examples of unintended lethal behavior. Restraint should be used only for short periods. As required by law, when four-point restraint is used, the patient must be closely observed, and relief must be provided every hour. Usually, physical restraint can be avoided with aggressive pharmacotherapy.

The patient may require careful rehydration (up to several liters of saline per day), correction of electrolyte imbalance (particularly magnesium, using $MgSO_4$ 1 to 2 g intravenously in 50% solution every 6 hours), hypoglycemia prevention, or correction of hyperthermia with a cooling blanket as well as nutritional supplementation. Concurrent aggravating conditions must be considered, such as sepsis, meningitis, subdural hematoma, hepatic failure, and pancreatitis.

The delayed onset of this hyperarousal state may reflect alcohol's broad effects across multiple neurotransmitter systems, chief among which may be the NMDA-glutamate system.[16] Adrenergic hyperarousal alone appears to be an insufficient explanation so that α-adrenergic agonists (e.g., clonidine and lofexidine) alone are not appropriate. Benzodiazepines may not suffice; in rare cases, we have seen doses in excess of diazepam 500 mg/day prove insufficient. Haloperidol 5 to 10 mg orally or intramuscularly may be added and repeated after 1 to 2 hours when psychosis or agitation is present.

Because the B vitamins are known to help prevent peripheral neuropathy and the Wernicke-Korsakoff syndrome, their use is vital. Thiamine 100 mg should be given intravenously immediately, and 100 mg should be given intramuscularly for at least 3 days until normal diet is resumed. A smaller amount of thiamine may be added to infusions for IV use. Folic acid 1 to 5 mg orally or intramuscularly per day should be included for megaloblastic anemia and peripheral neuropathy. A high-carbohydrate soft diet containing 3000 to 4000 calories a day should be given with multivitamins.

Wernicke-Korsakoff Syndrome

Victor et al.,[27] in their classic monograph *The Wernicke-Korsakoff Syndrome*, state that "Wernicke's encephalopathy and Korsakoff's syndrome in the alcoholic, nutritionally deprived patient may be regarded as two facets of the same disease. Patients evidence specific central nervous system pathology with resultant profound mental changes." Although perhaps 5% of alcoholics have this disorder, in 80% of these, the diagnosis is missed. In all of the cases reported by Victor et al., alcoholism was a serious problem and was almost invariably accompanied by malnutrition. Malnutrition, particularly in the absence of thiamine, has been shown to be the essential factor.

Korsakoff's Psychosis

Korsakoff's psychosis, also referred to as *confabulatory psychosis* and *alcohol-induced persisting amnestic disorder* in DSM-IV,[26] is characterized by impaired memory in an otherwise alert and responsive individual. This condition is slow to start and may be the end stage of a lengthy alcohol-dependence process. Hallucinations and delusions are rarely encountered. Curiously, confabulation, long regarded as the hallmark of Korsakoff's psychosis, was exhibited in only a limited number of cases in the large series collected and studied by Victor et al.[27] Most of these patients have no insight into the nature of their illness, diminished spontaneous verbal output, and a limited understanding of the extent of their memory loss.

The memory loss is bipartite. The retrograde component is the inability to recall the past, and the anterograde component is the lack of capacity for retention of new information. In the acute stage of Korsakoff's psychosis, the memory gap is so blatant that the patient cannot recall simple items, such as the examiner's first name, the day, or the time, even though the patient is given this information several times. As memory improves, usually within weeks to months, simple problems can be solved, limited always by the patient's span of recall.

Patients with Korsakoff's psychosis tend to improve with time. In the series of Victor et al.,[27] 21% of the patients recovered more or less completely, 26% showed no recovery, and the rest recovered partially.[26] During the acute stage, there is, however, no way of predicting who will improve and who will not. The EEG may be unremarkable or may show diffuse slowing, and magnetic resonance imaging (MRI) may show changes in the periaqueductal area and medial thalamus.[13] The specific memory structures that are affected in Korsakoff's psychosis are the medial dorsal nucleus of the thalamus and the hippocampal formations.

Wernicke's Encephalopathy

Wernicke's encephalopathy appears suddenly and is characterized by ophthalmoplegia and ataxia followed by mental disturbance. The ocular disturbance, which is necessary for the diagnosis, consists of paresis or paralysis of the external recti, nystagmus, and a disturbance in conjugate gaze. A global confusional state consists of disorientation, unresponsiveness, and derangement of perception and memory. Exhaustion, apathy, dehydration, and profound lethargy are also part of the picture. The patient is apt to be somnolent, confused, slow to reply, and may fall asleep in midsentence. Once treatment with thiamine is started for Wernicke's encephalopathy, improvement is often evident in the ocular palsies within hours. Recovery from ocular muscle paralysis is complete within days or weeks. In cases reported by Victor et al.,[27] approximately one third recovered from the state of global confusion within 6 days of treatment, another third within 1 month, and the remainder within 2 months. The global confusional state is almost always reversible, in marked contrast to the memory impairment of Korsakoff's psychosis.

Treatment

Administration of the B vitamin, thiamine, IM or IV, should be routine for all suspected intoxicated and dependence cases, directly in the emergency room, or immediately on admission, whichever comes earlier.[28] The treatment for Wernicke's encephalopathy and Korsakoff's psychosis is identical, and both are medical emergencies. Because subclinical cognitive impairments can occur even in apparently well-nourished patients, routine orders should include thiamine, folic acid, and multivitamins with minerals, particularly zinc. Prompt use of vitamins, particularly thiamine, prevents advancement of the disease and reverses at least a portion of the lesions where permanent damage has not yet been done. The response to treatment is therefore an important diagnostic aid. In patients who show only ocular and ataxic signs, the prompt administration of thiamine is crucial in preventing the development of an irreversible and incapacitating amnestic disorder. Treatment consists of 100 mg of thiamine and 1 mg of folic acid given intravenously immediately and 100 mg intramuscularly each day until a normal diet is resumed, followed by oral doses for 30 days. Parenteral feedings and the administration of B-complex vitamins become necessary if the patient cannot eat. If a rapid heart rate, feeble heart sounds, pulmonary edema, or other signs of myocardial weakness appear, digitalization should be started. Because these patients have impaired mental function, nursing personnel should be alerted to the patient's possible tendency to wander, to be forgetful, and to

become obstreperously psychotic. If the last should occur, benzodiazepines can be given.

Memory and Alcohol

Cranial computed tomography (CT) scan, MRI, and neuropsychological tests have demonstrated a loss of brain tissue and cognitive impairments in individuals who are either alcoholics or heavy drinkers, findings that largely escaped notice until the advent of these modern techniques. Abnormalities on the CT scan have been reported in 50% or more of chronic alcoholic subjects. These abnormalities can occur in subjects in whom there is neither clinical nor neuropsychological test evidence of cognitive defects. The limitations of CT technology include its inability to determine whether white or gray matter reductions account for increased cerebrospinal fluid spaces or to quantify lesions in areas such as the mamillary bodies or cerebellum. MRI is free of ionizing radiation, which makes it safe for repeated measurement, and it also provides discrimination between tissue types. In chronic alcoholics, MRI has demonstrated accelerating gray matter loss with age, which is to some extent reversible with abstinence, suggesting that some of these changes are secondary to changes in brain tissue hydration.[29]

Short-term memory, performance on complex memory tasks, visual motor coordination, visual spatial performance, abstract reasoning, and psychomotor dexterity are the areas most seriously damaged. Intelligence scores often do not change, and there is a sparing of verbal skills and long-term memory. As a consequence of this sparing, it is possible for individuals to appear quite intact unless they are administered neuropsychological tests. According to Rinn et al.,[30] subtle impairment of executive function may underlie fixed denial, which inhibits self-awareness of alcohol's damaging effects, impairs learning from counseling, simulates resistance, frustrates caregivers and generates anger toward the patient. These defects, particularly memory disturbances, can be reversed at least in part with abstinence.

For both the cognitive reasons described and emotional reasons, the principal problem encountered in all therapeutic modalities is denial. Many alcoholic patients in the general hospital with problems secondary to drinking have difficulty admitting their addiction to alcohol. Research on substance abuse cessation has demonstrated that most patients do not suddenly leap from denial into active recovery, but rather proceed over time through five *stages of change* (Table 16-2).[31] Each patient must be assessed for his or her current stage regarding substance abuse cessation and assisted to make the transition from the current to the next desired stage in a linear progression. The alternative (e.g., asking a patient in denial to enter intensive treatment immediately) is unrealistic and likely to disappoint both patient and provider. Intervention with the help of a significant other or family members can often make the pivotal difference. Family members often need education about the disease's potential effects on them as well, including the tendency to feel frustrated and hopeless about recovery. A brief meeting that covers the potential benefits of Al-Anon support may have lasting benefits to both family and patient.

Referral after Hospitalization

Brief intervention in general medical practice is a well-developed, effective technique.[9] Even brief contact with a specialist addiction consultant has been shown to yield improvement rates in 30% to 50% of patients months after hospitalization, and this is more effective with those who have no prior psychiatric illness and addiction treatments and good social function and resources.[6] Compared with general consultation psychiatrists specialist addiction nurse consultants were found to double the rate of patient follow-through and completion in rehabilitation (40% versus 88%, p < 0.001).[7] Addiction psychiatry consultation to hospital physicians should assist with diagnosis, intervention, pharmacologic management, and postacute care referral. At the Massachusetts General Hospital (MGH), a centralized intake procedure has been available to conduct objective, multidimensional assessment and protocol-driven referral. Consultants tell each alcoholic patient about the types of treatment programs available in the community. Alcohol dependence causes diverse disruptions in people's self-awareness, communication skills, capacity for relationships, sense of purpose in the life and spirituality of others. Alcoholics Anonymous (AA) and similar approaches that examine the broader character, lifestyle, and spiritual issues have a record of successful accomplishments and accessibility. Visits on the inpatient unit from AA volunteers may be particularly helpful when patients are ambivalent about accepting their physician's recommendation for alcoholism treatment. Such personal contact increases the likelihood that the patient will attend the AA program. Once the community resources have been identified and their differences described, the patient is advised of the optimal choice. Despite the severity of their drinking problem, some alcoholics may often reject intensive approaches as too restrictive or stigmatizing. In this event, a *contingency contract* in which the patient may begin a less intensive treatment is helpful, but if improvement does not follow within 4 to 6 weeks, the

Table 16-2. Stages of Change and Treatment Objectives

Stage of Change	Treatment Objective
Precontemplation (i.e., denial)	Cultivate rapport through repeated contact to promote patient's self-examination
Contemplation (awareness of problem)	Review substance use losses and potential risks (e.g., detailed teaching about hematologic and liver abnormalities and prognostic implications with continued drinking)
Preparation (intends behavioral changes, seeks treatment)	Anticipate treatment benefits, promote sense of self-efficacy and optimism for recovery
Action (cessation and treatment or self-help participation)	Facilitate entry to treatment and contingency plan in the event of dropout
Maintenance (ongoing avoidance of relapse cues)	Plan for relapse prevention via longitudinal treatment and recovery treatment and recovery activity (i.e., self-help group participation)
Relapse (resumption of substance use)	Support rapid reconnection with treatment system

patient agrees to enter the recommended treatment (e.g., inpatient rehabilitation or a halfway house). When this plan is supported by family members, patients often follow through to a successful treatment episode.

Two decades ago, it was common policy at the MGH to insist that the patient make the first contact with the treating agency; however, only approximately one in five patients actually made contact with treatment. After the introduction of a *central intake model,* referral completion rates increased to 58%. Key features of central intake include directly assisting patients with access to treatment, helping patients to call programs, subsidizing transportation to treatment program interviews, obtaining concrete services to diminish treatment obstacles, such as homelessness or lack of child care, and motivational interviewing. The last-mentioned is a model based on neurochemical evidence that chemical addiction is fundamentally a disease of motivation. With this brief technique, the provider assesses the patient's losses and risks in detail, helps the patient recognize the underlying cause as substance abuse, and encourages the patient to believe in the potential value of treatment. By avoiding a threatening style of confrontation about denial, motivational interviewing has been found to enhance motivation for recovery.[32]

Studies of treatment outcome show that up to two thirds of patients who enroll in therapeutic programs improve[33] in terms of abstinence or reduced amount of drinking. Pressures to shorten lengths of stay, while improving patient follow-through, are stimulating creative strategies at the hospital gateway to addictions treatment. Examples include intensive case management, home nursing, and counseling visitation, and predischarge initiation of pharmacotherapies such as disulfiram, naltrexone, or serotonin uptake inhibitors. Disulfiram 125 to 250 mg orally daily, an aversive agent when combined with alcohol, has reduced subsequent drinking days in chronic alcoholics by approximately 50%.[34] If a patient drinks alcohol after taking disulfiram, the disulfiram-ethanol reaction produces flushing, hypotension, headache, nausea, and vomiting. Treatment of severe disulfiram-ethanol reactions may require modified Trendelenburg position and an anticholinergic agent for bradycardia and ascor-

bic acid 1 mg intravenously every 1 to 2 hours. Naltrexone 50 mg orally daily, an opiate antagonist, has no adverse reaction with alcohol and has produced similar reductions in drinking days presumably through diminished reward from alcohol.[35,36] Because both agents have slight hepatotoxic risk themselves in addition to the risks from chronic ethanol use, liver function studies are helpful at baseline and then at 1, 3, and every 6 months thereafter. Selective serotonin reuptake inhibitors (SSRIs) have produced only modest drinking reductions—independent of antidepressant effects—at typical antidepressant doses, presumably through an anticraving effect, which may be more effective in patients with depression and early-onset type alcoholism.[37,38] These agents are gaining renewed interest as adjuncts to a comprehensive psychosocial recovery plan. If corroborated data indicate the existence of a comorbid psychiatric syndrome, and a treatment plan with expected good prognosis for abstinence can be put into place, studies support initiation of an SSRI antidepressant for co-occurring major depression, mood stabilizers for bipolar illness, buspirone for generalized anxiety, and third-generation antipsychotics for schizophreniform disease.[39]

The disposition of individuals with an acute or chronic alcohol syndrome is clinically complicated and increasingly subject to economic pressures because of managed care. This requires multidimensional assessment to optimize the use of treatment resources.[40] The key dimensions of assessment specified by the Patient Placement Criteria of the American Society of Addiction Medicine[41] are the following:

1. Acute intoxication or withdrawal potential
2. Biomedical conditions and complications
3. Emotional/behavioral conditions or complications
4. Treatment acceptance/resistance
5. Relapse potential
6. Recovery environment

These dimensions help determine both acute treatment needs and prognosis, and their use may inform the managed care review process as well.[42] All active problem areas among these dimensions must be addressed in the treatment plan to achieve a good likelihood of success.[43]

References

1. Blondell RD, Looney SW, Hottman LM, et al: Characteristics of intoxicated trauma patients, *J Addict Dis* 21:1–12, 2002.
2. Moore R, Bone L, Geller G, et al: Prevalence, detection, and treatment of alcoholism in hospitalized patients, *JAMA* 261:403–407, 1989.
3. Denny CH, Serdula MK, Holtzman D, et al: Physician advice about smoking and drinking: are U.S. adults being informed? *Am J Prev Med* 24:71–74, 2003.
4. Hopkins T, Zarro V, McCarter T, et al: The adequacy of screening, documentary, and treating the diseases of substance abuse, *J Addict Dis* 13:81–88, 1994.
5. Elvy G, Wells J, Baird K: Attempted referral as intervention for problem drinking, *Br J Addict* 83:83–89, 1988.
6. Alaja R, Seppa K: Six-month outcomes of hospital-based psychiatric substance use consultations, *Gen Hosp Psychiatry* 25(2):103–107, 2003.
7. Hillman A, McCann B, Walker NP: Specialist alcohol liaison services in general hospitals improve engagement in alcohol rehabilitation and treatment outcome, *Health Bull* (Edinb) 59:420–423, 2001.
8. Langenbucher J: Rx for health care costs: resolving addictions in the general medical setting, *Alcohol Clin Exp Res* 18:1033–1036, 1994 (review).
9. Fleming MF: Brief interventions and the treatment of alcohol use disorders: current evidence, *Recent Dev Alcohol* 16:375–390, 2003.
10. Institute of Medicine: *Broadening the base of treatment for alcohol problems: a report of a study by a committee of the Institute of Medicine*, Division of Mental Health and Behavioral Medicine, Washington, DC, 1990, National Academy Press.
11. Ewing J: Detecting alcoholism: the CAGE questionnaire, *JAMA* 252:1905–1907, 1984.
12. Girela E, Villanueva E, Hernandez Cueto C, et al: Comparison of the CAGE questionnaire versus some biochemical markers in the diagnosis of alcoholism, *Alcohol Alcohol* 29:337–343, 1994.
13. Brust JCM: *Neurological aspects of substance abuse*, Boston, 1993, Butterworth-Heinemann.
14. Hayashida M, Alterman A, McLellan A, et al: Comparative effectiveness and costs of inpatient and outpatient detoxification of patients with mild-to-moderate alcohol withdrawal symptoms, *N Engl J Med* 320:358–365, 1989.
15. Booth BM, Blow FC: The kindling hypothesis: further evidence from a U.S. national study of alcoholic men, *Alcohol Alcohol* 28:593–598, 1993.
16. Tsai G, Gastfriend DR, Coyle JT: The glutamatergic basis of human alcoholism, *Am J Psychiatry* 152:332–340, 1995.
17. Suzdak PD, Glowa JR, Crawley JN, et al: A selective imidazobenzodiazepine antagonist of ethanol in the rat, *Science* 234:1243–1247, 1986.
18. Lenehan GP, Gastfriend DR, Stetler C: Use of haloperidol in the management of agitated or violent, alcohol-intoxicated patients in the emergency department: a pilot study, *J Emerg Nursing* 11:72–79, 1985.
19. Castenada R, Cushman P: Alcohol withdrawal: a review of clinical management, *J Clin Psychiatry* 50:278–284, 1989.
20. Saitz R, Mayo Smith MF, Roberts MS, et al: Individualized treatment for alcohol withdrawal: a randomized double-blind controlled trial, *JAMA* 272:519–523, 1994.
21. Daeppen JB, Gache P, Landry U, et al: Symptom-triggered vs fixed-schedule doses of benzodiazepine for alcohol withdrawal: a randomized treatment trial, *Arch Intern Med* 162:1117–1121, 2002.
22. Jaeger TM, Lohr RH, Pankratz VS: Symptom-triggered therapy for alcohol withdrawal syndrome in medical inpatients, *Mayo Clin Proc* 76:695–701, 2001.
23. Sellers E, Naranjo C, Harrison M, et al: Diazepam loading: simplified treatment of alcohol withdrawal, *Clin Pharmacol Ther* 34:822–826, 1983.
24. Schoenenberger RA, Heim SM: Indication for computed tomography of the brain in patients with first uncomplicated generalised seizure, *BMJ* 309:986–989, 1994.
25. Alldredge B, Lowenstein D, Simon R: Placebo-controlled trial of intravenous diphenylhydantoin for short-term treatment of alcohol withdrawal seizures, *Am J Med* 87:645–648, 1989.
26. American Psychiatric Association: *Diagnostic and statistical manual of mental disorders*, ed 4 (DSM-IV), Washington, DC, 1994, American Psychiatric Press.
27. Victor M, Adams R, Collins G, et al: *The Wernicke-Korsakoff syndrome*, Philadelphia, 1971, FA Davis Co.
28. Thomson AD, Cook CC, Touquet R, Henry JA: The Royal College of Physicians report on alcohol: guidelines for managing Wernicke's encephalopathy in the accident and emergency department. *Alcohol Alcohol* 37:513–521, 2002.
29. Pfefferbaum A, Sullivan EV, Rosenbloom MJ, et al: A controlled study of cortical gray matter and ventricular changes in alcoholic men over a 5-year interval, *Arch Gen Psychiatry* 55):905–912, 1998.
30. Rinn W, Desai D, Gastfriend D, et al: Addiction denial and cognitive dysfunction: a preliminary investigation, *J Neuropsych Clin Neurosci* 14:52–57, 2002.
31. Prochaska J, Velicer W, Rossi J, et al: Stages of change and decisional balance for 12 problem behaviors, *Health Psychol* 13:39–46, 1994.
32. Miller W, Rollnick S: *Motivational interviewing: preparing people to change addictive behavior,* New York, 1991, The Guilford Press.
33. Cook CC: The Minnesota model in the management of drug and alcohol dependency: miracle, method, or myth: II. evidence and conclusions, *Br J Addict* 83:735–748, 1988.
34. Fuller R, Branchey L, Brightwell D, et al: Disulfiram treatment of alcoholism, *JAMA* 256:1449–1455, 1986.
35. Volpicelli J, Alterman A, Hayashida M, et al: Naltrexone in the treatment of alcohol dependence, *Arch Gen Psychiatry* 49:876–880, 1992.

36. Froehlich J, O'Malley S, Hyytia P, et al: Preclinical and clinical studies on naltrexone: what have they taught each other? *Alcohol Clin Exp Res* 27:533–539, 2003.

37. Sellers EM, Higgins, GA, Tomkins DM, et al: Opportunities for treatment of psychoactive substance use disorders with serotonergic medications, *J Clin Psychiatry* 52:49–54, 1991.

38. Pettinati HM, Kranzler HR, Madaras J. The status of serotonin-selective pharmacotherapy in the treatment of alcohol dependence. *Recent Dev Alcohol* 16:247–262, 2003.

39. Cornelius JR, Bukstein O, Salloum I, et al: Alcohol and psychiatric comorbidity, *Recent Dev Alcohol* 16:361–374, 2003.

40. Gastfriend DR, McLellan AT: Treatment matching: theoretic basis and practical implications, *Med Clin North Amer* 81:945–966, 1997.

41. Mee-Lee D, Shulman GD, Fishman M, et al: *ASAM patient placement criteria for the treatment of substance-related disorders*, ed 2—revised, (ASAM PPC-2R). Chevy Chase, MD, 2001, American Society of Addiction Medicine, Inc.

42. Gastfriend DR, Lu SH, Sharon E: Placement matching: challenges and technical progress. *Subst Use Misuse* 35:211–213, 2000.

43. Gastfriend DR, Mee-Lee D: The ASAM patient placement criteria: context, concepts and continuing development, *J Addictive Dis* (in press).

Chapter 17
Drug-Addicted Patients

John A. Renner, Jr., M.D.
David R. Gastfriend, M.D.

Unfortunately, the number of patients treated for substance abuse–related problems in the United States has grown steadily in the last decade. Between 1997 and 2002, the number of emergency department visits for drug-related events increased by more than 24%.[1] Clinical presentations in this domain are also becoming more complex. More than 55% of the drug-related problems seen in emergency departments in the first half of 2002 involved use of multiple drugs. In 37% of these cases, drug dependence was identified as the primary problem; 20% of the cases involved individuals seeking drug-induced psychic effects and 20% involved suicide attempts. Successful treatment of this expanding group of patients requires that clinicians improve their skills in the management of substance-related problems. Although most physicians feel comfortable treating the symptoms of substance abuse, it has been our experience that they are often reluctant to deal with the core disease process, and little effort is made to refer the patient for substance abuse treatment. The chronic, relapsing nature of substance abuse is inappropriately thought to imply that substance abuse treatment is not helpful. This leads clinicians to ignore multiple opportunities to intervene in the disease process. Most clinicians fail to appreciate that the relapse rate in other common chronic medical disorders, such as diabetes, hypertension, and asthma, exceeds that for the substance abuse disorders, and, hence, they do not handle substance abuse patients with comparable therapeutic diligence.[2] The policy at the Massachusetts General Hospital (MGH) is to ensure that problems related to substance abuse are addressed with the same degree of compassion and persistence that is directed to other common relapsing medical disorders. This chapter contains material to aid clinicians in the prompt recognition and effective management of patients with drug-related problems. The treatment of concurrent medical and surgical problems should always be seen as an opportunity for intervention in the underlying substance abuse problem.

Cocaine

Abuse

After alcohol, cocaine continues as the leading drug of abuse in terms of frequency of emergency department contacts, general hospital admissions, family violence, and other social problems, although the numbers are down from the peak of 123,300 visits recorded in emergency department data in 1993.[3] Even mature individuals with normal psychological profiles are vulnerable to compulsive cocaine use. Acute users experience intense euphoria often associated with increased sexual desire and improved sexual functioning. These positive rewards are often followed by a moderate-to-severe post-cocaine depression that provides a strong compulsion for further cocaine use.

The signs and the symptoms of acute cocaine intoxication are similar to those of amphetamine abuse. Typical complaints associated with intoxication include anorexia, insomnia, anxiety, hyperactivity, and rapid speech and thought processes ("speeding"). Signs of adrenergic hyperactivity, such as hyperreflexia, tachycardia, diaphoresis, and dilated pupils responsive to light, may also be seen. More severe symptoms, such as hyperpyrexia, hypertension, and cocaine-induced vasospastic events, such as stroke or myocardial infarction, are relatively rare among users, but are fairly common in the emergency department. Patients may also manifest stereotyped movements of the mouth, face, or extremities. Snorting may produce rhinitis or sinusitis and, rarely, perforations of the nasal septum. Free-basing (inhalation of cocaine alkaloid vapors) may produce bronchitis. Grand mal seizures are another infrequent complication. Patients also describe "snowlights," flashes of light usually seen at the periphery of the visual field. Crack is a highly addictive free-base form of cocaine that is sold in crystals that can be smoked.

The most serious psychiatric problem associated with chronic use is a cocaine-induced psychosis manifested by visual and auditory hallucinations and paranoid delusions often associated with violent behavior. Tactile hallucinations, called "coke bugs," involve the perception that something is crawling under the skin. A cocaine psychosis may be indistinguishable from an amphetamine psychosis, but it is usually shorter in duration.

Management

Cocaine abusers can be seen in any medical or surgical setting. The problem became common among affluent young people in the early to mid-1980s, but with the availability of packaged smokable cocaine, or crack, in low-cost doses, all classes and racial groups have become potential users. Occasional cocaine use does not require specific treatment except in the case of a life-threatening overdose. Most lethal doses are metabolized within 1 hour by enzymes in the blood and liver. In the interim, intubation and assisted breath-

ing with oxygen may be necessary. Stroke has been reported, and death can be caused by ventricular fibrillation or myocardial infarction. The cardiac status should therefore be monitored closely. Intravenous (IV) diazepam should be used to control convulsions.

Chronic cocaine use produces tolerance, severe psychological dependency, and physiologic dependence marked by irritability, anhedonia, low mood, and anxiety.[4] Many dependent users follow a cyclical pattern of 2 or 3 days of heavy binge use, followed by a withdrawal "crash." Use is resumed again in 3 to 4 days, depending on the availability of cash and drug. A gradual reduction in use of the drug is almost never possible. Detoxification is accomplished by the abrupt cessation of all cocaine use, usually through restricted access, such as a loss of funds or contacts, or incarceration. Withdrawal symptoms begin to resolve within 7 days, and specific medical treatment is rarely indicated. The value of medication for withdrawal symptoms has yet to be confirmed. Drugs that enhance central nervous system (CNS) catecholamine function may reduce craving, although they are of limited benefit clinically and they have not been proven effective in double-blind placebo-controlled trials. The major complication of withdrawal is a severe depression with suicidal ideation. If this occurs, the patient requires psychiatric hospitalization.

For the cocaine addict, the compulsion to use is overwhelming. We have seen patients who continued dealing from the hospital room after near-fatal injuries or ones who injected cocaine through a region of intensely painful cellulitis that occasioned the admission. For this reason, an active-using, cocaine-dependent patient who has been hospitalized should have a drug screen performed after any behavioral change, particularly after receiving visitors or departures from the floor. Urine should be examined for cocaine metabolites or, preferably, all drugs of abuse.

All cocaine abusers should also be referred for individual or group counseling, and participation in twelve-step self-help programs should be strongly recommended. Similarly, family members or significant others should be referred separately to Al-Anon because they may gain insights that may help them eliminate systemic support for the patient's further drug use. Manual-guided cognitive-behavioral therapy has been shown to be effective in the treatment of cocaine dependence.[5] Once compulsive cocaine use has begun, it is almost impossible for the user to return to a pattern of occasional, controlled use. Such individuals are also likely to develop problems with alcohol and other drugs. For that reason, the goal of treatment should be total abstinence from cocaine and all other drugs.

Amphetamines

Abuse

Stricter federal controls on the production and distribution of amphetamines have greatly reduced the number of amphetamine abusers. Routine medical evaluation may uncover the most common type of amphetamine abuse seen in the inpatient setting. Typically, this involves a patient who began using amphetamines to control obesity and later became a chronic amphetamine abuser. The patient quickly develops tolerance and may use 100 mg or more a day in an unsuccessful effort to control weight. This amphetamine abuse can be treated by abruptly discontinuing usage of the drug or by gradually tapering the dose, whichever is more acceptable to the patient. In either case, the patient should be shown a more appropriate program for weight control.

A more serious problem involves the patient who develops a severe psychological dependence on amphetamines and who may present the same symptoms seen in younger street-drug abusers. Amphetamine and methamphetamine (speed) accounted for a total of 16,215 emergency department visits in the first half of 2002.[1] The signs and symptoms of acute amphetamine intoxication are similar to those described in the section on cocaine abuse.

The other classic syndrome seen in either acute or chronic amphetamine intoxication is a paranoid psychosis without delirium. Although typically seen in young people who use IV methamphetamine hydrochloride, it can also occur in individuals who use dextroamphetamine or other amphetamines orally on a chronic basis. The paranoid psychosis may occur with or without other manifestations of amphetamine intoxication. The absence of disorientation distinguishes this condition from most other toxic psychoses. This syndrome is clinically indistinguishable from an acute schizophrenic episode of the paranoid type, and the correct diagnosis is often made only in retrospect, based on a history of amphetamine use and a urine test positive for amphetamines. Intramuscular (IM) haloperidol is effective in the acute management of this type of substance-induced psychosis.

Treatment

Amphetamines can be withdrawn abruptly. If the intoxication is mild, the patient's agitation should be handled by reassurance alone. The patient should be "talked down," much as one would handle an adverse D-lysergic acid diethylamide reaction. If sedation is necessary, benzodiazepines are the drugs of choice. Phenothiazines should be avoided because they may heighten dysphoria and increase the patient's agitation. Hypertension will usually respond to sedation with benzodiazepines. In severe hypertension, we recommend the use of phentolamine for vasodilation. Beta- or mixed alpha- and beta-adrenergic blockers, such as propranolol or labetalol, are to be avoided because they may exacerbate stimulant-induced cardiovascular toxicity.

Most signs of intoxication clear in 2 to 4 days. The major problem is appropriate psychiatric management of postamphetamine depression. In mild cases, this depression is manifested by feelings of lethargy with the subsequent temptation to use amphetamines again for energy. In more serious cases, the patient may become suicidal and requires inpatient psychiatric treatment. The efficacy of antidepressants in such cases has not been adequately documented. Even with support and psychotherapy, most patients experience symptoms of depression for 3 to 6 months following the cessation of chronic amphetamine abuse.

Club Drugs

In the last decade there has been a significant increase in the abuse of "club drugs," primarily 3,4-methylenedioxy-methamphetamine (MDMA) (Ecstasy), γ hydroxybutyrate (GHB), and ketamine. MDMA has both amphetamine-like and hallucinogenic effects. It was initially used experimentally to facilitate psychotherapy, but its use was banned after it was found to be neurotoxic in animals. In toxic amounts, it produces distorted perceptions, confusion, hypertension, hyperactivity, and potentially fatal hyperthermia. GHB (sodium oxybate) is a CNS depressant that has recently been approved by the Food and Drug Administration (FDA) for the treatment of narcolepsy. In overdose it can produce coma and death; it has also been identified as a "date rape" drug. Ketamine has been used as an anesthetic and it can produce delirium, amnesia, and respiratory depression when abused. The treatment for overdoses of all of these drugs is primarily symptomatic.

Narcotics

There has been a steady increase in heroin-related emergency department visits in the last decade. The abuse of narcotic analgesics, primarily oxycodone (OxyContin), almost doubled between 1997 and 2002.[1] In addition, more than 31% of acquired immune deficiency syndrome cases in the United States are related to a history of injection drug use.[6] As a result, the treatment of opiate dependence is becoming commonplace on medical and surgical units. Proper management of such patients necessitates knowledge of FDA regulations and appropriate techniques for using opiate substitution therapy and community treatment resources.

The classic signs of opiate withdrawal are easily recognized and usually begin 8 to 12 hours after the last dose. The patient generally admits the need for drugs and shows sweating, yawning, lacrimation, tremor, rhinorrhea, marked irritability, dilated pupils, and an increased respiratory rate. More severe withdrawal signs occur 24 to 36 hours after the last dose and include tachycardia, hypertension, nausea and vomiting, insomnia, and abdominal cramps. Untreated, the syndrome subsides in 5 to 10 days. Withdrawal symptoms are similar in patients addicted to methadone, but they may not appear until 24 to 30 hours after the last dose and abate over a period of 2 to 4 weeks. Patients addicted to oxycodone may present a particularly severe and prolonged withdrawal syndrome and may require high doses of opiates for adequate control.

FDA regulations define opiate substitution therapy (either methadone, l-a acetyl methadol [LAAM], or buprenorphine maintenance) as any treatment with an approved opiate that extends beyond 30 days. Maintenance clinics may extend detoxification treatment from 30 to 180 days if the briefer detoxification program is not successful. Addicts cannot be placed in methadone maintenance unless they show physiologic evidence of current addiction (withdrawal signs) and can document a 1-year history of addiction. The only exceptions to this rule are pregnant addicts; addicts who are hospitalized for the treatment of a medical, surgical, or obstetric condition; and formerly addicted individuals who have just been released from incarceration. Under these regulations, the physician has the option of providing opiate substitution therapy to any addict for the duration of the pregnancy or the period of hospitalization required to treat the primary illness. At MGH, we strongly recommend that such treatment be continued until the addict has fully recovered from the presenting illness and that the addict then be referred to a maintenance clinic or for detoxification treatment.

In addition to methadone, other options for opiate substitution therapy include LAAM, a synthetic opiate with a duration of action of 48 to 72 hours; and buprenorphine, a long-acting partial opiate agonist. Patients on LAAM must be monitored for evidence of a prolonged QTc interval. Buprenorphine produces a milder state of opiate dependence, and it can be used in the treatment of addicts who meet *Diagnostic and Statistical Manual for Mental Disorders,* fourth edition, criteria for opiate dependence. When dispensed in a sublingual tablet in combination with naloxone, it has minimal potential for IV abuse and has been demonstrated effective for maintenance treatment.[7] It has been approved for use in the office-based treatment of opiate dependence and provides an attractive alternative to methadone treatment for higher functioning addicts and individuals with short-term histories of opiate dependence.

If a patient is already in an opiate substitution program before admission to the hospital, the methadone, LAAM, or buprenorphine dose should be confirmed by inpatient staff and should not be changed without consultation with the outpatient physician responsible for the patient's treatment. Under no circumstances should such a patient be withdrawn from drugs unless there is full agreement among the patient, the hospital physician, and the outpatient clinic staff on this course of action. Such detoxification is rarely successful, particularly if the patient is under stress from a concurrent medical or surgical condition. Withdrawal from drugs may complicate the management of the primary illness. The option of detoxification should not be considered until the patient has fully recovered from the condition that necessitated hospitalization.

Patients on long-term opiate substitution therapy should continue daily oral methadone treatment while hospitalized. If parenteral medication is necessary, methadone can be given in IM doses of 5 or 10 mg every 8 hours. This regimen should keep the patient comfortable regardless of the previous oral dose. An alternative method is to give one third of the daily oral dose intramuscularly every 12 hours. As soon as oral medication can be tolerated, the original oral dose should be reinstated.[8]

Establishing the appropriate dose of methadone for a street addict is a trial-and-error process. Because the quality of street heroin is never certain, the addict's description of the size of the current habit is of minimal value. The safest guide to dosage is to monitor the patient's pulse, respiration, and pupil size. After the presence of withdrawal is documented, the patient should receive 20 mg of methadone orally. Only if the patient is well known as a heavy user should the starting dose be as high as 30 mg. A relatively young patient or a patient who reports a small habit can begin treatment with 10 mg given orally. If vital signs have not stabilized or if withdrawal signs reappear after 2 hours, an additional 5 or 10 mg can be given orally. It is rare to give more than 60 mg during the first 24 hours. Successful long-term outpatient maintenance treatment generally requires doses in the range of 60 to 120 mg, although lower doses may be adequate to control withdrawal symptoms in the hospital setting.

Case 1

One woman, aged 17 years, was admitted for an evaluation of fever of undetermined origin and associated epigastric distress. She requested large doses of methadone and claimed to have a heroin habit costing $200/day. Further history revealed that she and her husband had been addicted for less than 3 months and both were relatively naive heroin users. After she began to show signs of opiate withdrawal, she was given 10 mg of methadone orally; an additional 5 mg was given 10 hours later when her respiratory rate was again noted to be more than 18 breaths per minute. The following day she remained comfortable after a single dose of 15 mg. Later it was discovered that she had regional enteritis. Given the short history of opiate abuse in this patient, she would likely be an appropriate candidate for office-based detoxification treatment with buprenorphine once her medical problems have been stabilized.

An addict should be maintained on a single daily oral dose that keeps him or her comfortable and that keeps heart rate and respiratory rate within the normal range. The dose should be reduced 5 or 10 mg if the patient appears lethargic. If the street addict is to be withdrawn from drugs immediately, the methadone dose can be reduced by 10% to 20% a day. If the drug habit has been maintained in the hospital for 2 or more weeks or if the patient has been using methadone before admission, detoxification should proceed more slowly. The dose can be reduced by 5 mg/day until 20 mg/day is reached. Further dosage reduction should occur more slowly, if the patient is unable to tolerate the withdrawal symptoms. Clonidine, an alpha-2 adrenergic agonist, suppresses the autonomic symptoms of withdrawal and can be used as an alternative withdrawal medication. The patient should first be stabilized on methadone. Clonidine should not be substituted for methadone until the methadone dose has been reduced to 20 mg/day. After an initial oral dose of 0.2 mg, patients usually require doses in the range of 0.1 to 0.2 mg every 4 hours. The total daily dose should not exceed 1.2 mg. Patients on clonidine should be monitored closely for side effects, particularly hypotension and sedation. In an inpatient setting, the clonidine dose can be reduced to zero over a period of 3 to 4 days.[9,10] A transdermal clonidine patch is often applied on the third day. Supplemental doses of lorazepam can also be used to moderate withdrawal-related anxiety. Because use of clonidine does not adequately suppress the subjective symptoms of withdrawal as does use of methadone and buprenorphine, it is not acceptable to all addicts. Rates for successful completion of opiate detoxification with buprenorphine (see following text) are almost 65% higher than those reported for clonidine.[11]

Buprenorphine has been shown to be effective for the short-term inpatient detoxification of opiate addicts. Patients are stabilized using sublingual doses of 2 to 4 mg and these doses can usually be tapered off over 2 to 4 days. An alternative protocol uses 0.3 to 0.6 mg of IM buprenorphine for 3 to 5 days, with a transdermal clonidine patch applied on the second day.[12] Addicts typically report that a buprenorphine detoxification is more comfortable than detoxification with either methadone or clonidine.

Chances for successful withdrawal treatment are enhanced if the patient is aware of the dose and is able to choose the withdrawal schedule within limits established by the physician. By involving the patient in the treatment process and by using a flexible withdrawal schedule, the physician can keep withdrawal symptoms to a tolerable level. Rigid adherence to a fixed-doing schedule is less likely to achieve success, and it may lead to premature termination of treatment.

Other techniques permit rapid inpatient detoxification from opiates but require more intensive medical management. The addict is first stabilized on clonidine as described previously. On the second treatment day, 12.5 mg of naltrexone is added and then increased later that day and the following days up to a single dose of 150 mg by the fourth day. A supplemental benzodiazepine is also given for agitation and insomnia. At the end of 5 days, there are no further withdrawal symptoms and the patient can be discharged directly to an outpatient naltrexone program.[10,13] A more rapid experimental protocol using high doses of opiate antagonists given under general anesthesia permits completion of detoxification in 24 to 48 hours.[14] This approach has not been adequately evaluated in randomized clinical trials, and it cannot be recommended at this time.

Although techniques that permit a safe, rapid, and medically effective detoxification from opiates seem highly attractive in an era of managed care, clinicians must understand that detoxification alone is rarely successful as a treatment for any addiction. Unless opiate addicts are directly transferred to a long-term treatment program, relapse rates following detoxification are extremely high.

The resulting costs to the patient, to society, and to the health care system far outweigh any saving realized from a rapid "cost-effective" detoxification protocol.

A common problem is determining the appropriate dosage of an analgesic for patients receiving opiate substitution therapy.

Case 2

A 28-year-old woman was hospitalized for the treatment of acute renal colic. Four years earlier she had been hospitalized for similar symptoms that subsided after she passed a kidney stone. During the year before her second hospitalization, the patient was in a maintenance program and was receiving 60 mg of methadone daily. She was doing well in treatment and for the last 6 months was working regularly as a secretary. A psychiatrist was asked to see the patient because she was threatening to sign out of the hospital. She claimed that she was receiving no effective relief for her pain and that she wished to obtain heroin to treat herself. The nurses described her as constantly complaining, demanding, and attempting to get additional doses of narcotics. A review of her chart revealed that she was receiving doses of 5 mg of morphine, approximately half the usual analgesic dose in such situations, with strict orders not to repeat the dose sooner than every 4 hours because of her history of drug abuse. Her physician assumed that she would require lower doses of morphine because she was taking methadone.

After the consultation, the physician accepted the psychiatrist's recommendation that the usual dose of 10 mg of morphine be given every 2 hours as circumstances required because the patient would probably metabolize any narcotic more rapidly than normal. This regimen effectively controlled the patient's pain, and she suddenly became more cooperative. There was no recurrence of her manipulative behavior or other management problems. Two days later, she passed several renal stones; she was discharged several days later. Her physician had not realized hat her "demands and manipulations" were legitimate requests for effective doses of analgesics.

The analgesic effect of methadone is minimal in maintenance patients, and, at best, it lasts only 6 to 8 hours. If pain control is required, addicts should be given standard doses of other narcotics in addition to methadone. Because of cross-tolerance, a patient on maintenance narcotic therapy metabolizes other narcotics more rapidly and may therefore require more frequent administration of analgesics than might a nonaddicted patient. Pentazocine and other partial opiate agonists are contraindicated for such patient. Because of their narcotic antagonist effects, these analgesics produce withdrawal symptoms in opiate addicts. If patients on the buprenorphine/naloxone combination tablet require additional narcotic analgesia treatment, they can be switched to buprenorphine alone. Higher than usual narcotic doses will be required to overcome the partial antagonist action of buprenorphine. Alternatively, such patients can also be switched to methadone and be managed as described previously.

Opiate overdoses are treated with 0.4 mg/ml of IV or IM naloxone. Medication can be repeated every 2 minutes, as needed, up to a total dose of 1 to 2 mg. If the patient does not respond after 20 minutes, he or she should be treated for a combined drug overdose. Because of the long duration of action of methadone and LAAM, overdoses of these drugs often require an IV naloxone drip.

Discharge planning should be initiated as quickly as possible after admission. For patients who are not already in treatment, several weeks may be required to arrange admission to a drug-free residential program or to an opiate substitution therapy program. Because a serious illness usually causes an addict to reexamine his or her behavior and possibly to choose rehabilitation, the physician should emphasize the need for long-term treatment. No addict should be discharged while still receiving methadone unless the addict is returning to a maintenance program or specifically refuses detoxification. Even when a physician discharges a patient for disciplinary reasons, medical ethics necessitate that the patient be withdrawn from methadone before discharge. Hospital physicians cannot legally prescribe addicts methadone, LAAM, or buprenorphine for administration at home.

Benzodiazepines

Patterns of Chronic Use versus Abuse

Benzodiazepines can produce dependence, especially when used in high doses or in prolonged deviation from the usual therapeutic dose. Up to 45% of patients receiving stable, long-term doses show evidence of physiologic withdrawal. Withdrawal symptoms, which are usually the same in both high-dose and low-dose patients, include anxiety, insomnia, irritability, depression, tremor, nausea or vomiting, and anorexia. Seizures and psychotic reactions have also been reported in a few cases. The more common symptoms are similar to those seen during withdrawal from all of the sedative-hypnotic drugs and may often be difficult to distinguish from the symptoms for which the benzodiazepine was originally prescribed. In general, withdrawal symptoms abate within 2 weeks.

Benzodiazepines with a rapid onset of action, such as diazepam and alprazolam, seem to be sought out by drug abusers and are generally presumed to have a greater potential for abuse than benzodiazepines with a slower onset of action. Nonetheless, there is relatively little evidence for the abuse of benzodiazepines when they are prescribed for legitimate medical conditions. Ciraulo et al.[15] found that the use of benzodiazepines, even among former alcoholics, was similar to that of other psychiatric patients. A study of alcoholics conducted at the Addiction Research Foundation of Ontario found that 40% were recent users of benzodiazepines and that there was a 20% lifetime incidence of anxiolytic abuse or dependence.[16] Although these studies suggest that concerns about the abuse of benzodiazepines by alcoholics may be exaggerated, the problem is real. When appropriate, anxiolytics may be prescribed to this population, but they should never be a first-line treatment, and patients must always be monitored carefully. There is no evidence that anxiolytics are effective as a primary treatment for alcoholism.

It is important to distinguish between a drug abuser who uses benzodiazepines primarily to get high, often deliberately mixing them with alcohol and other drugs of abuse, and an individual who takes benzodiazepines appropriately under medical supervision. In both cases, the user may develop physiologic and psychological dependence. Such dependence, in and of itself, is not evidence of drug abuse. Unless there is evidence of dose escalation, deliberate use to produce a high, or dangerous states of intoxication, there is no reason to assume that chronic benzodiazepine users are abusers. Even though clonazepam is the only benzodiazepine with an indication for long-term use, common medical practice supports the merit of the continued use of benzodiazepines in some individuals with chronic medical and psychiatric conditions.

Case 3

> A 68-year-old retired teacher was admitted to the MGH for evaluation of severe gouty arthritis. His internist requested a psychiatric consultation regarding the management of long-term chlordiazepoxide use. The patient had been a heavy drinker before retirement but he had been sober for the last 5 years. Two years after becoming sober, he developed complaints of severe anxiety and he was started on a regimen of chlordiazepoxide 25 mg three times a day. Two efforts had been made to reduce or eliminate the medication, but the anxiety symptoms returned. The patient expressed a strong desire for continued medication, and he became fearful that he might resume drinking. The symptoms were well controlled when regular treatment with chlordiazepoxide was resumed. After reviewing the case, the psychiatrist determined that the patient was dependent on the chlordiazepoxide but that there had been no escalation of dose or other signs of abuse. The medication continued to be effective in controlling his anxiety. It was recommended that he be continued on his current dose of chlordiazepoxide.

Overdose

Flumazenil, a specific benzodiazepine antagonist, reverses the life-threatening effects of a benzodiazepine overdose. An initial IV dose of 0.2 mg should be given over 30 seconds, followed by a second 0.2 mg IV dose if there is no response after 45 seconds. This procedure can be repeated at 1-minute intervals up to a cumulative dose of 5.0 mg. This treatment is contraindicated in individuals dependent on benzodiazepines or those taking tricyclic antidepressants because flumazenil may precipitate seizures in these patients.[17,18] When flumazenil is contraindicated, benzodiazepine overdoses should be handled similarly to other sedative-hypnotic overdoses (see following section).

Withdrawal

In cases in which there is clear evidence of benzodiazepine abuse or when the patient desires to stop use of these medications, it is important that detoxification occur under medical supervision. During the withdrawal process, patients should be warned to expect a temporary increase in anxiety symptoms. The simplest approach to detoxification is a gradual reduction in dose that may be extended over several weeks or months. When a more rapid inpatient detoxification is desired, dosage reduction can be completed within 2 weeks. For some patients, this rapid withdrawal process produces an unacceptable level of subjective distress. An alternate approach is to switch to a high-potency, long-acting benzodiazepine, such as clonazepam. Most patients seem to tolerate detoxification on clonazepam quite well. Because of the prolonged self-taper after completion of detoxification, patients experience a smoother course of withdrawal with a minimum of rebound anxiety.[19,20]

Withdrawal from the high-potency, short-acting benzodiazepines, such as alprazolam, has been particularly problematic. A rapid tapering of these drugs is often poorly tolerated by patients, and a switch to equivalent doses of a long-acting benzodiazepine often allows acute withdrawal symptoms to emerge. We recommend that clonazepam be substituted for alprazolam, at a dose ratio of 0.5 mg of clonazepam for each 1 mg of alprazolam. Clonazepam should then be continued for 1 to 3 weeks. A drug taper is not always required, although abrupt discontinuation of even a long-acting agent, such as clonazepam, can be associated with a withdrawal syndrome that includes seizures, but it tends to occur several days after discontinuation. A 2- to 3-week taper is usually adequate.

Supplemental medication is of little use during benzodiazepine withdrawal; beta-adrenergic blockers (propranolol) and alpha-adrenergic agonists (clonidine) offer no advantage over detoxification using benzodiazepines alone. Although they tend to moderate the severity of physiologic symptoms, they are ineffective in controlling the patients' subjective sense of anxiety, and they do not prevent withdrawal seizures. Buspirone has no cross-tolerance for the benzodiazepines and does not control withdrawal symptoms from this class of drugs.

Sedative-Hypnotics

Abuse

Use of CNS depressants account for high rates of emergency department visits related to suicidal attempts and accidental overdoses (consequent to recreational and self-medication). Although benzodiazepines have become the most commonly abused sedative-hypnotic in the United States, there are still areas where the nonmedical use of barbiturates, such as butalbital (Fiorinal and Esgic), and carisoprodol (Soma), and other sedative-hypnotics, such as methaqualone and glutethimide, causes serious clinical problems.

A person intoxicated by other CNS depressants typically presents with many of the same diagnostic problems that are associated with alcohol intoxication. Slurred speech, unsteady gait, and sustained vertical or horizontal nystagmus, or both, that occur in the absence of the odor of alcohol on the breath suggest the diagnosis. Unfortunately, drug abusers frequently combine alcohol with other sedative-hypnotic drugs. The clinician may be misled by the odor of alcohol. The diagnosis of mixed alcohol-barbiturate intoxication can be missed unless a careful history is taken and blood and urine samples are analyzed for toxic drugs. The behavioral effects of barbiturate intoxication can vary widely, even in the same person, and may change significantly depending on the surroundings and on the expectations of the user. Individuals using barbiturates primarily to control anxiety or stress may appear sleepy or mildly confused as a result of an overdose. In young adults seeking to get high, a similar dose may produce excitement, loud boisterous behavior, and loss of inhibitions. The aggressive and even violent behavior commonly associated with alcohol intoxication may follow. The prescribed regimen for managing an angry alcoholic individual can also be used for the disinhibited sedative-hypnotic abuser.

As tolerance to barbiturates develops, there is not a concomitant increase in the lethal dose, as occurs in opiate dependence. Although the opiate addict may be able to double the regular dose and still avoid fatal respiratory depression, as little as a 10% to 25% increase over the usual daily dosage may be fatal to the barbiturate addict. Thus a barbiturate overdose should always be considered potentially life-threatening, especially for drug abusers.

In overdose, a variety of signs and symptoms may be observed, depending on the drug or the combination of the drugs used; the amount of time since ingestion; and the presence of such complicating medical conditions as pneumonia,

hepatitis, diabetes, heart disease, renal failure, or head injury. Initially the patient appears lethargic or semi-comatose. The pulse rate is slow, but other vital functions are normal. As the level of intoxication increases, the patient becomes unresponsive to painful stimuli, reflexes disappear, and there is a gradual depression of the rate of respiration; eventually cardiovascular collapse ensues. Pupil size is not changed by barbiturate intoxication, but secondary anoxia may cause fixed, dilated pupils. In persons who have adequate respiratory function, pinpoint pupils usually indicate an opiate overdose or the combined ingestion of barbiturates and opiates. Such patients should be observed carefully for increased lethargy and for progressive respiratory depression. Appropriate measures for treating overdoses should be instituted as necessary. Patients should not be left unattended until all signs of intoxication have cleared.

Because there is no cross-tolerance between narcotics and barbiturates, special problems are presented by patients receiving methadone maintenance who continue to abuse sedative-hypnotics. If a barbiturate overdose is suspected, the methadone-taking patient should be given a narcotic antagonist to counteract any respiratory depression caused by methadone. We recommend naloxone hydrochloride (Narcan) 0.4 mg given intramuscularly or intravenously because it is a pure narcotic antagonist and it has no respiratory depressant effect even in large doses. If the respiratory depression does not improve after treatment with naloxone, the patient should be treated for a pure barbiturate overdose. Supportive measures include maintenance of adequate airway, mechanic ventilation, alkalinization of the urine, correction of acid-base disorders, and diuresis with furosemide or mannitol. Severe overdose cases may require dialysis or charcoal resin hemoperfusion.[18]

Withdrawal

The sedative-hypnotic withdrawal syndrome can present a wide variety of symptoms, including anxiety, insomnia, hyperreflexia, diaphoresis, nausea, vomiting, and sometimes delirium and convulsions. As a general rule, individuals who ingest 600 to 800 mg/day of secobarbital for more than 45 days develop physiologic addiction and show symptoms after withdrawal. Minor withdrawal symptoms usually begin within 24 to 36 hours after the last dose. Pulse and respiration rates are usually elevated, pupil size is normal, and there may be postural hypotension. Fever may develop, and dangerous hyperpyrexia can occur in severe cases. Major withdrawal symptoms, such as convulsions and delirium, indicate addiction to large doses (more than 900 mg/day of secobarbital).

Because of the danger of convulsions, barbiturate withdrawal should be carried out only on an inpatient basis. Grand mal convulsions, if they occur, are usually seen between the third and seventh days, although there have been cases reported of convulsions occurring as late as 14 days after the completion of a medically controlled detoxification. Withdrawal convulsions are thought to be related to a rapid drop in the blood barbiturate level. Treatment should therefore be carefully controlled so that barbiturates are withdrawn gradually with minimal fluctuation in the blood barbiturate level. Theoretically, this should decrease the danger of convulsions. Treatment with phenytoin does not prevent convulsions caused by barbiturate withdrawal, although it controls convulsions caused by epilepsy.

Delirium occurs less frequently than do convulsions; it rarely appears unless preceded by convulsions. It usually begins between the fourth and sixth days and is characterized by both visual and auditory hallucinations, delusions, and fluctuating levels of consciousness. The presence of confusion, hyperreflexia, and fever helps distinguish this syndrome from schizophrenia and other nontoxic psychoses.

Treatment for Withdrawal

Several techniques are available for managing barbiturate withdrawal. The basic principle is to withdraw the addicting agent slowly to avoid convulsions. First, the daily dosage that produces mild toxicity must be established. Because barbiturate addicts tend to underestimate their drug use, it is dangerous to accept the patient's history as completely accurate. Treatment should begin with an oral test dose of 200 mg of pentobarbital, a short-acting barbiturate. If no physical changes occur after 1 hour, the patient's habit probably exceeds 1200 mg

of pentobarbital per day. If the patient shows only nystagmus and no other signs of intoxication, the habit is probably about 800 mg/day. Evidence of slurred speech and intoxication but not sleep suggests a habit of 400 to 600 mg/day. The patient can then be given the estimated daily requirement divided into four equal doses administered orally every 6 hours. Should signs of withdrawal appear, the estimated daily dosage can be increased by 25% following an additional dose of 200 mg of pentobarbital given intramuscularly. After a daily dose that produces only mild toxicity has been established, phenobarbital is substituted for pentobarbital (30 mg phenobarbital equals 100 mg pentobarbital) and then withdrawn at a rate of 30 to 60 mg/day (Table 17-1).[21] An alternative method is to treat withdrawal symptoms orally with 30 to 60 mg phenobarbital hourly, as needed, for 2 to 7 days. After the patient has received similar 24-hour doses for 2 consecutive days, the 24-hour stabilizing dose is given in divided doses every 3 to 6 hours. A gradual taper is then instituted as described previously. At MGH, we recommend this latter method because the use of a long-acting barbiturate produces fewer variations in the blood barbiturate level and should produce a smoother withdrawal.

Inpatient Management and Referral

Sedative-hypnotic addicts can present a variety of psychological management problems. Effective treatment requires a thorough evaluation of the

Table 17-1. Equivalent Doses of Common Sedative-Hypnotics

Generic Name	Dose (mg)
Barbiturates	
Phenobarbital	30
Secobarbital	100
Pentobarbital	100
Benzodiazepines	
Alprazolam	1
Diazepam	10
Chlordiazepoxide	25
Lorazepam	2
Clonazepam	0.5–1
Others	
Meprobamate	400

patient's psychiatric problems and the development of long-term treatment plans before discharge. Treatment for withdrawal or overdose presents an opportunity for effective intervention in the addict's self-destructive lifestyle. Drug abuse patients have a reputation for deceit, manipulation, and hostility. They frequently sign out against medical advice. It is rarely acknowledged that these problems are sometimes caused by clinicians who fail to give appropriate attention to the patient's psychological problems. Most of these difficulties can be eliminated by effective medical and psychiatric management. The patient's lack of cooperation and frequent demands for additional drugs are often the result of anxiety and the fear of withdrawal seizures. This anxiety is greatly relieved if the physician thoroughly explains the withdrawal procedure and assures the patient that the staff knows how to handle withdrawal and that convulsions will be avoided if the patient cooperates with a schedule of medically supervised withdrawal.

Physicians sometimes fail to realize that the patient's tough, demanding behavior is a defense against a strong sense of personal inadequacy and a fear of rejection. Addicts have been conditioned to expect rejection and hostility from medical personnel. The trust and cooperation necessary for successful treatment cannot be established unless physicians show by their behavior that they are both genuinely concerned about the patient and medically competent to treat withdrawal. Physicians can expect an initial period of defensive hostility and testing behavior and should not take this behavior personally. Patients need to be reassured that their physician is concerned about them.

If the patient manifests signs of a serious character disorder and has a history of severe drug abuse, the setting of firm limits is necessary to ensure successful detoxification. Visitors must be limited to those individuals of known reliability. This may mean excluding spouses and other relatives. Urine should be monitored periodically for illicit drug use. Family counseling should be started during hospitalization and should focus on the family's role in helping the patient develop a successful long-term treatment program. Hospital passes should not be granted until detoxification is completed; however, passes with staff members as escorts should be used as much as possible. An active program of recreational and physical therapy is necessary to keep young, easily bored patients occupied. Keys to successful inpatient treatment are summarized in Table 17-2.

The story of a 21-year-old man who was hospitalized after having a grand mal seizure illustrates several of the problems that may occur.

Table 17-2. Inpatient Management and Referral

Keys to Successful Inpatient Treatment

Perform psychiatric evaluation.
Develop long-term treatment plan.
Demonstrate explicit concern and expertise.
Expect testing behavior.
Set appropriate limits.
Limit and monitor visitors.
Supervise passes.
Monitor urine for illicit drug use.
Encourage ward activities and recreation.
Initiate family/network therapy.
Treat with respect.

Case 4

The son of an eminent attorney described several years of episodic barbiturate and alcohol use and admitted to 3 months of daily barbiturate use after dismissal from college for failing grades. Three days before the patient's seizure, his father discovered that he had been ingesting secobarbital tablets taken from the medicine cabinet. The patient agreed to stop using barbiturates but did not realize that he was addicted. After admission to the hospital, the patient became a serious management problem. He demanded additional medication and refused to obey hospital regulations. Twice he left the floor without permission, and on one occasion he returned obviously high. A discussion with his physician became an angry shouting match. The patient denied any extra drug use and insisted that he be permitted to leave the ward. He threatened to file a lawsuit for violation of his civil rights. When seen by the psychiatric consultant, the patient was hostile and provocative. He denied having any psychiatric problems and suggested that his physician was trying to have him committed to a psychiatric hospital.

The patient's hostility disappeared after the psychiatrist indicated that he had no interest in committing him but that he was concerned that his arguments with his physician and the nurses were interfering with his medical treatment. Once reassured that the psychiatrist did not think he was crazy, he admitted his fear of having more seizures. He did not know what to expect during detoxification and was too frightened to admit his fears to his physician. He finally admitted that he was meeting friends in the hospital cafeteria and they were giving him extra drugs. A meeting was then arranged between the patient and his physician. The physician explained the detoxification procedure in detail, including possible causes of seizures and the need for diagnostic tests. The patient was relieved to receive this information and readily agreed to appropriate limitations on visitors and hospital passes. The remainder of his hospitalization passed without incident, and he agreed to continue seeing the physician after his discharge.

Because treatment for detoxification or for an overdose rarely cures an addict, referrals for long-term outpatient or residential care should be made early in the treatment process. Ideally the patient should meet the future therapist before discharge. Alcoholics Anonymous and Narcotics Anonymous are useful adjuncts to any outpatient treatment program. If transferring to a halfway house or residential program, the patient should move there directly from the hospital. Addicts are not likely to execute plans for follow-up care without strong encouragement and support.

Mixed-Drug Addiction

Increasing numbers of patients are addicted to varying combinations of drugs, including benzodiazepines, cocaine, alcohol, and opiates. Accurate diagnosis is difficult because of confusing, inconsistent physical findings and unreliable histories. Blood and urine tests for drugs are required to confirm the diagnosis. A patient who is addicted to both opiates and sedative-hypnotics should be maintained on methadone while the barbiturate or other sedative-hypnotic is withdrawn. Then methadone can be withdrawn in the usual manner. Dose equivalents of narcotics are provided in Table 17-3.

Behavioral problems should be dealt with as previously described. Firm limit-setting is essential to the success of any effective psychological treatment program. Some patients who overdose or present with medical problems secondary to drug abuse, such as subacute bacterial endocarditis and hepatitis, are not physiologically addicted to any drug despite a history of multiple drug abuse. Their drug abuse behavior is usually associ-

Table 17-3. Equivalent Doses of Narcotic Pain Medications

Generic Name	Dose (mg)
Morphine	10
Oxycodone (Percocet, OxyContin)	5–10
Hydrocodone (Vicodin, Lortab)	10
Meperidine (Demerol)	100
Hydromorphone (Dilaudid)	2.5
Methadone	5
Heroin	10

ated with severe psychopathology. These patients should receive a thorough psychiatric evaluation and may require long-term treatment.

References

1. U.S. Department of Health and Human Services, Substance Abuse and Mental Health Services Administration, Office of Applied Studies: *Emergency department trends from the drug abuse warning network, preliminary estimates January-June, 2002*, Rockville, MD.
2. O'Brien CP, McLellan AT: Myths about the treatment of addiction, *Lancet* 347:237–240, 1996.
3. U.S. Department of Health and Human Services: *Preliminary estimates from the drug abuse warning network*, Public Health Service, Substance Abuse and Mental Health Services Administration, Advance Report No. 8, 1994, Rockville, MD.
4. Gawin F, Kleber H: Abstinence symptomatology and psychiatric diagnosis in cocaine abusers, *Arch Gen Psychiatry* 43:107–113, 1986.
5. Carroll KM: Relapse prevention as a psychosocial treatment approach: a review of controlled clinical trials, *Exp Clin Psychopharm* 4:46–54, 1996.
6. Centers for Disease Control and Prevention: Reported U.S. AIDS cases by HIV-exposure category—1994, *Morb Mortal Wkly Rep* 44:4, 1995.
7. Ling W, Charuvastra C, Collins JF, et al: Buprenorphine maintenance treatment of opiate dependence: a multicenter, randomized clinical trial, *Addiction* 93:475–486, 1998.
8. Fultz JM, Senay EC: Guidelines for the management of hospitalized narcotics addicts, *Ann Intern Med* 82:815–818, 1975.
9. Charney DS, Sternberg DE, Kleber HD, et al: The clinical use of clonidine in abrupt withdrawal from methadone, *Arch Gen Psychiatry* 38:1273–1277, 1981.
10. Jaffe JH, Kleber HD: *Opioids: general issues and detoxification.* In American Psychiatric Association:

Treatment of psychiatric disorders: a task force report of the American Psychiatric Association, vol 2, Washington, DC, 1989, American Psychiatric Association.

11. Fingerhood MI, Thompson MR, Jasinski DR: A comparison of clonidine and buprenorphine in the outpatient treatment of opiate withdrawal, *Subst Abus* 22:193–199, 2001.

12. Umbricht A, Hoover DR, Tucker MJ, et al: Opioid detoxification with buprenorphine, clonidine, or methadone in hospitalized heroin-dependent patients with HIV infection, *Drug Alcohol Depend* 69:263–272, 2003.

13. O'Connor PG, Waugh ME, Carrol KM, et al: Primary care-based ambulatory opioid detoxification, *J Gen Intern Med* 10:255–260, 1995.

14. Legarda JJ, Gossop M: A 24-h inpatient detoxification treatment for heroin addicts: a preliminary investigation, *Drug Alcohol Depend* 35:91–95, 1994.

15. Ciraulo D, Sands B, Shader R: Critical review of liability for benzodiazepine abuse among alcoholics, *Am J Psychiatry* 145:1501–1506, 1988.

16. Ross HE: Benzodiazepine use and anxiolytic abuse and dependence in treated alcoholics, *Addiction* 88:209–218, 1993.

17. Weinbroum A, Halpern P, Geller E: The use of flumazenil in the management of acute drug poisoning: a review, *Intensive Care Med* 17(suppl 1):S32–S38, 1991.

18. Wiviott SD, Wiviott-Tishler L, Hyman SE: *Sedative-hypnotics and anxiolytics*. In Friedman L, Fleming NF, Roberts DH, et al, editors: *Source book of substance abuse and addiction*, Baltimore, 1996, Williams & Wilkins.

19. Herman JB, Rosenbaum JF, Brotman AN: The alprazolam to clonazepam switch for the treatment of panic disorder, *J Clin Psychopharmacol* 7:175–178, 1987.

20. Patterson JF: Withdrawal from alprazolam dependency using clonazepam: clinical observations, *J Clin Psychiatry* 51:47–49, 1990.

21. Smith DE, Wesson DR: Phenobarbital technique for treatment of barbiturate dependence, *Arch Gen Psychiatry* 24:56–60, 1971.

Suggested Readings

Carroll KM: A cognitive-behavioral approach: treating cocaine addiction. *NIDA Therapy Manuals for Drug Addiction Series* (DHHS Pub No. ADM 98–4308), Rockville, MD, National Institute on Drug Abuse.

Ciraulo DA, Shader RI, editors: *Clinical manual of chemical dependence*, Washington, DC, 1991, American Psychiatric Press.

Galanter M, Kleber HD, editors: *The American Psychiatric Press textbook of substance abuse treatment*, Washington, DC, 1999. The American Psychiatric Press.

Graham AW, Schultz TK, editors: *Principles of addiction medicine*, ed 2, Chevy Chase, MD, 1998, American Society of Addiction Medicine, Inc.

Kosten TR, McCance E: A review of pharmacotherapies for substance abuse, *Am J Addictions* 5(supp 1):S30–S37, 1996.

McNicholas L, Howell EF: *Buprenorphine clinical practice guidelines*, Rockville, MD, Substance Abuse Mental Health Services Administration, Center for Substance Abuse Treatment. Available at http:// buprenorphine.samhsa.gov.

Renner JA: *Biologic approaches to addiction treatment*. In Milkman HB, Sederer LI, editors: *Treatment choices for alcoholism and substance abuse*, Lexington, MA, 1990, Lexington Books.

Smith DE, Wesson DR: *Diagnosis and treatment of adverse reactions to sedative-hypnotics*, Rockville, 1974, U.S. Department of Health, Education, and Welfare Publication No. (ADM) 75–144, National Institute on Drug Abuse.

Chapter 18

Psychopharmacologic Issues in the Medical Setting

Jonathan E. Alpert, M.D., Ph.D.
Maurizio Fava, M.D.
Jerrold F. Rosenbaum, M.D.

Most clinical trials designed to establish the efficacy and safety of psychotropic medications exclude individuals who suffer from unstable nonpsychiatric medical conditions or take nonpsychiatric medications with appreciable central nervous system (CNS) effects. The psychiatrist in the general medical setting, however, typically faces the challenges posed by comorbid medical disorders and concurrent medications that hinder the detection of psychiatric symptoms and alter the effectiveness, tolerability, and safety of psychiatric drug treatment.[1–4] Fortunately, inroads are being created, as controlled multicenter pharmacotherapy trials are gradually extended to individuals with unstable medical illness[5] and large effectiveness trials in psychiatry are designed to allow participation of patients in primary care settings with comorbid medical illness and complex medical regimens.[6] As a guide to making informed decisions about psychotropic medication use in the medical setting, this chapter focuses on principles of psychopharmacologic practice and on the rapidly expanding knowledge base regarding pharmacokinetics and drug-drug interactions. This chapter also reviews some of the important psychiatric uses of nonpsychiatric medications that have emerged.

Principles of Psychopharmacologic Practice

The complicated clinical and psychosocial contexts in which psychotropic medications are often administered in the general hospital call on a sound understanding of basic principles that underlie the practice of psychopharmacology.[7] If pharmacologic efforts fail to achieve their intended goals, a review of these principles frequently helps to uncover potential explanations and to redirect treatment.

Initiating Treatment

The appropriate use of psychotropic medications starts with as precise a formulation of diagnosis as possible. The use of an antidepressant alone for a depressed college student presenting to an emergency department might be appropriate if the diagnosis is of a major depressive episode; less pertinent if the diagnosis is of an adjustment disorder; and seriously inadequate and quite possibly harmful if the diagnosis is of a bipolar disorder, psychotic depression, or cocaine or alcohol abuse (see Chapter 8). As a rule, it is best to defer pharmacologic treatment until a good working diagnosis can be reached. The establishment of a psychiatric diagnosis, however, often requires longitudinal assessment of course and treatment response and symptoms of psychiatric disorders may be obscured or altered by co-occurring medical conditions. Therefore, in acute clinical situations, it is frequently not possible to defer the implementation of psychotropic medications until a diagnosis is fully clarified. In this context, it is particularly crucial to document probable and differential diagnoses, to outline the rationale for selecting a particular treatment over others, and to indicate the kind of information needed to achieve greater diagnostic certainty. When a disorder appears to present in a subsyndromal form, such as minor depression, the rationale for proceeding with psychopharmacologic treatment should be well defined.

The identification of a particular set of target symptoms plays an integral role in establishing a pretreatment baseline and in later efforts to monitor the success of treatment. These symptoms might include anger attacks, insomnia, anhedonia, delusions of reference, racing thoughts, or the frequency and intensity of suicidal longings. The identification of target symptoms serves to focus attention on those symptoms that are causing greatest danger, disability, and distress to the patient while also more fully informing the patient about the core symptoms of his or her illness and the specific goals for which psychotropics have been recommended.

For some conditions, clinician-rated instruments, such as the Brief Psychiatric Rating Scale,[8] the Hamilton Rating Scale for Depression,[9] the Hamilton Rating Scale for Anxiety,[10] and the Young Mania Scale,[11] provide useful, well-studied templates for the serial assessment of relevant symptoms. In addition, the patient and family or other caregivers can be recruited in formal efforts to monitor progress. In the case of episodic or complex presentations, the use of daily mood charts, self-rating scales, such as the Beck Depression Index,[12] or behavioral logs—analogous to patient monitoring of blood pressure or glucose—may reveal temporal patterns (e.g., rapid mood cycling) and associations (e.g., to menstrual cycle or medication changes) that are not apparent cross-sectionally during office or bedside visits.

Along with the assessment of target symptoms, evaluation of current levels of function and subsequent changes with treatment relevant to quality of life are an integral part of good psychopharmacologic practice. Thus, for example, for an outpatient, improvement in work or school function, family, and other social relationships, and use of leisure time or, for an inpatient, progress in the level of independence and reduction in the overall degree of anguish help confirm the adequacy of treatment, whereas a lack of improvement along these dimensions directs attention to residual symptoms or to problems not initially apparent.

The Global Assessment of Function scale, a routine part of *Diagnostic and Statistical Manual of Mental Disorders*, fourth edition (DSM-IV), multi-axial assessment, provides a composite index of symptoms and dimensions pertaining to quality of life, which is useful for documentation of treatment course over time.[13] Some clinicians also make use of the Clinical Global Impression (CGI) scale.[14] This scale, widely used in clinical trials, rates severity of disease on a scale of 1 to 7 (from normal to most extreme) and improvement on a scale of 1 to 7 (from very much improved to very much worse) and provides another simple quantitative means to document overall treatment outcome.

The understanding that a patient's psychiatric condition is influenced by psychosocial factors does not imply that psychotropic medications should be withheld. A major depression evolving in the setting of a spouse's chronic illness or panic attacks emerging in the weeks following the break up of a significant relationship may well be as severe and as responsive to pharmacologic treatment as the same disorders that developed in other patients without similar precipitants. Vague referrals to counseling do not constitute sufficient treatment under such circumstances and may be viewed by patients as dismissive. If psychotherapy is recommended and pharmacotherapy deferred, the referral to psychotherapy—whether, for example, to individual cognitive therapy, couples therapy, or a pain management group (i.e., behavioral treatment)—must be viewed with the same deliberateness as the prescription of medication, and it should include a plan for follow-up. If substantial progress is not made within a clinically appropriate time frame (e.g., no more than 8 to 12 weeks for a moderately severe episode of major depression), the adequacy of the psychotherapy should be reevaluated. Severity, chronicity, and risk of recurrence of symptoms are often more relevant in determining the need for pharmacotherapy of psychiatric conditions than the presence of aggravating life circumstances or a caricatured description of illness as chemical or reactive.

Reciprocally, the expanding range of safe and well-tolerated psychotropic agents, such as the selective serotonin reuptake inhibitors (SSRIs) and other newer antidepressants, does not alter the imperative to explore the use of nonmedication interventions whenever medications are considered. An assessment of a patient for psychiatric medications should include an equally careful evaluation for other targeted interventions instead of, or in addition to, pharmacotherapy or psychotherapy. Often uniquely helpful are judicious referrals to parenting classes; elder care; Alcoholics Anonymous, Narcotics Anonymous, and Al-Anon; vocational assessment and rehabilitation; support groups for the bereaved, separation, and medical disorders (e.g., epilepsy, human immunodeficiency virus [HIV] infection); and psychiatric self-help groups, such as those sponsored by the National Manic Depressive and Depressive Association.

Patient education and informed consent are important legal and ethical imperatives that are also critical to the success of a course of treatment with psychotropic medications. If the capacity of the patient to make his or her own decisions fluctuates or is questionable, the clinician should obtain the patient's permission to include family or other patient-appointed individuals in important treatment decisions. When a patient is clearly not competent to make such decisions, formal legal mechanisms for substituted judgment should be used. Such mechanisms, however, in no way diminish the importance of educating a patient about medications and target symptoms to the fullest extent possible. Following resolution of a psychotic episode, patients not infrequently remember the importance to them, while psychotic, of a clinician's reassuring efforts to provide a better understanding of the illness and its treatment.

When presenting recommendations to a patient about medications, information about diagnosis, target symptoms, treatment options, and anticipated means of follow-up should be included, as well as the medication name, class, and dosing instructions. Side effects that are common (e.g., dry mouth, nausea, tremor, drowsiness, sexual dysfunction, and weight gain) should be reviewed together with side effects that are uncommon but require immediate attention (e.g., a hypertensive crisis on a monoamine oxidase inhibitor [MAOI], dystonia on an antipsychotic, or a rapidly progressing rash on lamotrigine). Patients should be specifically cautioned about the risks of abrupt psychotropic drug discontinuation. Dietary and drug restrictions must be clearly described and, particularly in the case of MAOIs, should be provided in written form as well.

In the context of urgent, life-threatening conditions, such as acute mania, counseling about some potential adverse effects, particularly those not anticipated in the foreseeable future (e.g., tardive dyskinesia or perinatal risks), can be deferred until greater clinical stability is achieved and the risks and benefits of longer-term treatment can be meaningfully addressed.

All too frequently omitted in discussions preceding the initiation of medications is clear information about the anticipated time course of response (whether to anticipate improvement in hours or weeks), the anticipated length of treatment, and the ready availability of strategies to address side effects or lack of efficacy. A patient's reluctance to initiate treatment may arise from a variety of concerns, including the fear that medication will be stigmatizing, may engender physical or psychological dependence, will be "mind altering" or personality transforming, is being used to mask a problem rather than treat it, implies consignment to life-long treatment, or reflects a narrow therapeutic philosophy. The faithfulness of a patient to a recommended course of treatment is invariably strengthened by a physician's dedicated efforts to elicit and address misgivings and potential misunderstandings at the outset. Referral to relevant pamphlets, websites, and books on diagnosis and treatment are often welcomed by patients and family members as a source of more detailed information, particularly when longer-term treatment is anticipated.

Medication Selection and Administration

Fortunately, for the majority of psychiatric disorders, there exist at least several agents within a single class that are known to have roughly equivalent efficacy. Decisions regarding choice of a particular medication for a patient should give considerable weight to previous treatment response and the current feasibility of the medication in terms of cost, tolerability, and complexity of dosing. Anticholinergic, hypotensive, and sedative effects of drugs must be considered carefully, particularly in the prescription of medications to elderly patients or patients who are medically frail.

Once a drug is chosen, the goal should be to achieve a full trial with adequate doses and an adequate duration of treatment. Inadequate dosing and duration count among the principal factors in treatment failure for accurately diagnosed patients. Furthermore, in the service of decisions regarding a patient's care weeks or months later, it is crucial to document whether a trial of medication was successful, failed, or abbreviated because of clinical deterioration, medication side effects, patient noncompliance, or drug abuse. Patient suffering is unnecessarily prolonged and resources are poorly used when medications that were previously ineffective have been tried again because of inadequate documentation of failure or when medications that could have been effective are avoided because previous trials of those medications had not been flagged as having been incomplete.

Medication dosages should be adjusted to determine the lowest effective dose and the simplest regimen. There is significant variability among individuals with respect to response, blood levels, the expression of side effects, and the development of toxicity, such that the recommended dose ranges provide only a general guide. Documentation of a patient's response to a particular dose becomes a much more meaningful reference point for future treatment. As a rule, elderly patients should be started on lower doses than younger patients, and the interval between dosage changes should be longer because the time to achieve steady-state levels is often prolonged. In the elderly, there is also frequently prolonged storage of medication and active metabolites in body tissues. Nevertheless, the goal of reaching an effective dose must be pursued with equal determination in elderly as in younger patients.

For individuals with chronic psychiatric conditions, symptom exacerbations may prompt increases in the dosages of medications or addition of other medications. So too, for patients presenting acutely with severe disorders, medication doses may be titrated up more rapidly than usual or combined with other psychotropic medications at an early point

such that the lowest effective dose and simplest regimen is likely to be unclear. Under these circumstances, reevaluation for cautious dose reduction when an appropriate interval of stability has followed should be routine. When a patient's care is likely to be transferred to another clinician or another setting, such as a chronic care facility or a community health center, it is essential that such a plan be communicated to the accepting clinical staff to avoid committing a patient to long-term treatment with doses or regimens that are excessive.

The attentive management of side effects plays an important role in developing a therapeutic alliance and improving the quality of life for a patient who may be on psychopharmacologic treatment for months or years. Although some adverse events require immediate drug discontinuation (e.g., serotonin syndrome or neuroleptic malignant syndrome [NMS]), most can be addressed initially with a dose reduction, modification in the timing or division of doses, taking the medication with or without food, a change in the preparation of medication (e.g., from valproic acid to divalproex sodium), or guidance about sleep hygiene, exercise, or diet (e.g., caffeine, fluids, or fiber). When such measures prove unhelpful in addressing a side effect that is causing distress or that poses a safety risk, consideration must be given to other measures (e.g., bethanechol for urinary retention on tricyclic antidepressants [TCAs], sildenafil for sexual dysfunction on SSRIs, or support hose for hypotension on MAOIs) or to replacement of the offending medication with a more tolerable agent. For side effects that are likely to be transient and not dangerous, a patient's understanding that a variety of straightforward strategies are available in the case of persistence or worsening may be enough to help the patient endure the side effects until they subside.

It is best to avoid responding to short-term crises with long-term changes in medication. The decision to discontinue a successful antidepressant and substitute another in the setting of despair and insomnia following a traumatic event offers the patient only the prospect of benefit from the new medication weeks hence while currently depriving the patient of active treatment known to have been effective. Although it may seem tempting to respond proportionally to a patient's marked distress with a fundamental change in established treatment, exacerbations that are thought likely to be transient are most reasonably addressed with interventions that are short-term and focused coupled with adequate follow-up.

Approach to Treatment Failure

Lack of improvement, clinical worsening, or the emergence of unexpected symptoms require a concerted reevaluation of diagnosis, dose, drugs, and disruptions.

Diagnosis

Among at least one third of patients with major psychiatric disorders, initial treatment fails to bring about significant improvement despite accurate diagnosis. Nevertheless, treatment failure should motivate a careful review of history, initial presentation, and symptoms that seem incongruous with the provisional diagnosis (e.g., confusion in an individual with a seemingly mild depression; olfactory hallucinations in a patient presenting with panic attacks). A patient with fatigue out of proportion to other depressive symptoms may have a primary sleep disorder, such as obstructive sleep apnea. A depressed and cachectic elderly patient who fails to improve despite a series of adequate courses of antidepressant may turn out to have a psychotic depression, early dementia, carcinoma, or a frontal lobe tumor. An adolescent with obsessive-compulsive disorder who appears increasingly bizarre and erratic on an SSRI may have an undiagnosed bipolar mood disorder exacerbated by the antidepressant.

Dose

Apparent treatment refractoriness is often the result of the prescription of subtherapeutic doses or patient noncompliance, and when treatment fails, the onus is on the clinician to confirm the adequacy of dose. Whenever possible, blood levels of prescribed medications help establish whether a patient is taking the medications and, for medications with established dose ranges (e.g., lithium, anticonvulsants, TCAs, but not generally antipsychotics or SSRIs or other newer generation antidepressants), whether the medication doses are likely to be in a therapeutic range. When adequate doses of a drug prescribed to a conscientious patient fail to achieve consistent blood levels or clinical response, factors that affect drug metabolism (e.g., cigarette smoking, chronic alcohol use, or use of concurrent medications that result in lower levels of the drug) must also be considered, as should the possibility of changes in brand when prescriptions for generic preparations have been refilled causing variation in the bioavailability of the active agent.

Drugs

Patients not infrequently compartmentalize their medication use and forget to mention as-needed or over-the-counter medications or treatments prescribed in different settings. When psychopharmacologic treatments fail, a careful reevaluation of the patient's current nonpsychiatric medication use is warranted. Thus a patient whose panic disorder responds incompletely to full doses of a high-potency benzodiazepine may be unaware that his or her condition is aggravated by use of a β-agonist inhaler or a sympathomimetic decongestant. So, too, a patient with bipolar disorder, previously stabilized on lithium but now presenting with hypomania, may have not realized the importance of reporting the recent initiation of prednisone for a flare of inflammatory bowel disease. It has become increasingly apparent that widely consumed herbal and other natural remedies marketed as dietary supplements (e.g., St. John's wort) may participate in clinically important drug interactions[15,16]; the possibility of such interactions may be easily missed, however, because the use of alternative and complementary therapies is typically reported by patients only on direct inquiry by their clinician. Details of alcohol and illicit drug use must also be carefully elicited as factors that, when excessive, frequently masquerade as and, at the very least, exacerbate other psychiatric disorders and virtually always jeopardize the safety and efficacy of pharmacotherapy.

Disruptions

Although psychosocial stressors are not an excuse for psychopharmacologic nihilism, neither can they be meaningfully ignored as potential impediments to treatment. Incomplete remission of depressive symptoms in a patient living with an alcoholic spouse or of a psychotic exacerbation in a patient with schizophrenia whose community residential treatment facility has recently closed should be met both by aggressive efforts to ensure the adequacy of pharmacologic treatment and by equally determined efforts to develop a plan to address the environmental factors that appear to be compromising a patient's recovery.

Discontinuing Medications

The discontinuation of psychotropics must be carried out with as much care as their initiation. For patients on complicated regimens of psychotropics, periodic review for dose reduction and potential discontinuation must be standard. Because there is a paucity of data providing guidelines for drug discontinuation, the process is often empiric. Thoughtful polypharmacy is widely recognized as appropriate and helpful in the treatment of many complex or treatment-refractory psychiatric conditions. Therefore a patient's use of two or more psychotropic medications ought not to be viewed reflexively as in need of dismantling. One patient may arrive at a precisely adjusted, albeit complicated, regimen through a series of careful trials guided by a single experienced clinician, whereas another may accumulate multiple medications in a haphazard fashion across diverse treaters and settings. For the former patient, even a modest dose change may result in a severe relapse threatening the patient's safety or livelihood, whereas for the latter, a directed plan to taper medications and perhaps even to "start from scratch" is likely to be most helpful. Successful discontinuation therefore relies heavily on a good knowledge of a patient's history together with adequate follow-up.

Assessment of a patient for drug discontinuation involves appreciation of the short-term risks of rebound and withdrawal effects and the long-term risks of relapse and recurrence. Rebound effects refer to the transient return of symptoms for which a medication has been prescribed (e.g., insomnia or anxiety), and withdrawal effects refer to the development of new symptoms characteristic of abrupt cessation of the medication (e.g., muscle spasms, delirium, or seizures following high-dose benzodi-azepine discontinuation; hot flashes, nausea, unusual shocklike sensations, or malaise following antidepressant discontinuation).

To make sound decisions regarding the reinstatement of medications, it is essential to distinguish rebound and withdrawal effects from relapse, which is a persistent rather than self-limited state, typically has a more delayed onset, and represents the clinically significant reemergence of symptoms of the underlying illness in the absence of (or sometimes despite the continuation of) active treatment. Thus the return of daily panic attacks after a several-month remission and an exacerbation of psychosis requiring hospitalization after 2 years of exclusively outpatient treatment are examples of relapse.

For disorders that may present episodically, particularly major depression, the term *relapse* refers more precisely to the recrudescence of symptoms during an initial period of remission, whereas the additional term recurrence refers to symptom return following a defined period of full remission (at least 4 to 6 months) on or off continued treatment. In the case of recurrence, the reappearing symptoms are conceptualized as denoting a new episode rather than a continuation of the one previously treated. In parallel with the concepts of relapse and recurrence, continuation treatment refers to the ongoing use of medication prescribed to consolidate a symptom remission brought about by an initial (acute) phase of treatment to prevent relapse. Maintenance treatment refers to a more extended course of medication thereafter aimed at prophylaxis of recurrences and reserved for individuals with an illness characterized by chronicity, past recurrences, or particular severity. For major depression, acute treatment is typically in the range of 6 to 12 weeks, whereas continuation treatment extends 4 to 6 months beyond that point and maintenance treatment may extend a further 1 to 5 years or more depending on the clinical context. Although antidepressants appear to be more effective than placebo during long-term treatment, the number of controlled antidepressant trials focusing on treatment of depression beyond the first year remains quite limited.[17]

A taper of medications over 48 to 72 hours is typically adequate to minimize the risk of rebound or withdrawal. With respect to relapse or recurrence, however, patients at risk may well benefit from a more protracted, carefully monitored taper of medications. This allows for rapid reinstatement of full-dose treatment at the early signs of worsening to avert a more serious escalation. Moreover, analyses of discontinuation of lithium[18] and antipsychotic agents[19] suggest that too rapid cessation of psychotropic medications may, in fact, increase the risk of relapse when compared with a more gradual taper. Furthermore, sudden discontinuation of lithium may be associated with later nonresponse to lithium among a subset of patients with bipolar disorder.[20] Findings such as these suggest that, for elective discontinuation of psychotropic medications, a taper of at least 2 to 4 weeks' duration should be considered. With patients for whom the consequences of relapse are likely to be severe (e.g., most individuals with bipolar and psychotic disorders), an extended taper with dose reductions of no more than 25% at intervals of no less than 4 to 6 weeks is likely to be a more prudent course. For patients with anxiety disorders maintained on high-potency benzodiazepines, the introduction of a targeted course of therapy (e.g., a cognitive-behavioral panic disorder group) in preparation for a drug taper is likely to reduce further the risks of relapse (see Chapter 15).

Far from being an afterthought, then, decisions regarding the timing and pace of drug discontinuation should be regarded as an integral part of psychopharmacologic management and remain an important topic for further study.

Pharmacokinetics

Pharmacokinetic processes refer to absorption, distribution, metabolism, and excretion, factors that determine plasma levels of a drug and the local availability of drug to biologically active sites. Pharmacokinetics refers to the mathematical analysis of these processes. Advances in analytic chemistry and computer methods of pharmacokinetic modeling[4,21,22] and a growing understanding of the molecular pharmacology of the hepatic isoenzymes responsible for metabolism of most psychotropic medications have furnished increasingly sophisticated insights into the disposition and interaction of administered drugs. Because the pharmacokinetics of a medication are subject to a myriad of influences, including age, genes, gender, diet, disease states, and concurrently administered

drugs, a working knowledge of pharmacokinetic principles is of particular relevance to psychopharmacology in medical settings.

Absorption

Factors that influence drug absorption are generally of less importance in determining the pharmacokinetic properties of psychiatric medications than factors influencing subsequent drug disposition. When relevant, they typically pertain to oral, rather than parenteral, administration, for which alterations in gastrointestinal drug absorption may affect the rate or the extent (or both) of absorption. The extent or completeness of absorption, also known as the fractional absorption, is measured as the area under the curve when plasma concentration is plotted against time. The bioavailability of an oral dose of drug refers, in turn, to the fractional absorption for oral compared with intravenous (IV) administration of the drug when corrected for dose.

Because the upper part of the small intestine is the primary site of drug absorption through passive membrane diffusion and filtration and both passive and active transport processes, factors that speed gastric emptying (e.g., metoclopramide) or diminish intestinal motility (e.g., TCAs or marijuana) may facilitate greater contact with and absorption from the mucosal surface into the systemic circulation potentially increasing plasma drug concentrations. Conversely, antacids, charcoal, kaolin-pectin, and cholestyramine may bind to drugs, forming complexes that pass unabsorbed through the gastrointestinal lumen. Changes in gastric pH associated with food or other drugs alter the nonpolar, unionized fraction of drug available for absorption. In the case of drugs that are very weak acids or bases, however, the extent of ionization is relatively invariant under physiologic conditions. Properties of the preparation administered (e.g., tablet, capsule, or liquid) may also influence the rate or extent of absorption and, for some medications (e.g., lithium, paroxetine, or methylphenidate), preparations intended for slow release are available. Finally, the local action of enzymes in the gastrointestinal tract (e.g., monoamine oxidase [MAO] and cytochrome P450 3A4) may be responsible for metabolism of drug before absorption. This is of critical relevance to the emergence of hypertensive crises that occur when excessive quantities of the dietary pressor tyramine are systemically absorbed in the setting of irreversible inhibition of the MAO isoenzymes for which tyramine is a substrate.

Alterations in absorptive processes may theoretically affect plasma concentrations and the onset and duration of drug action and therefore should be considered in the search for an explanation of unexpected drug reactions and in the treatment of certain clinical populations (e.g., individuals with gastric or ileal disease or motility disorders). Nevertheless, the extent and clinical importance of alterations in absorption to most psychopharmacologic effects is often dwarfed by the influence of alterations in other pharmacokinetic processes.

Following gut absorption but before entry into the systemic circulation, many psychotropics are subject to first-pass liver metabolism. Thus, in addition to their effect on subsequent metabolism of drug, hepatic dysfunction, primary liver disease, and conditions impeding portal circulation (e.g., congestive heart failure) are likely to increase the fraction of drug available for distribution for the majority of psychotropic drugs, which are subject to hepatic metabolism, thereby contributing to clinically significant increases in plasma levels of drug.

Distribution

Drugs distribute to tissues through the systemic circulation. The amount of drug ultimately reaching receptor sites in tissues is determined by a variety of factors, including the concentration of free (unbound) drug in plasma, regional blood flow, and physiochemical properties of drug (e.g., lipophilicity or structural characteristics). For entrance into the CNS, penetration across the blood-brain barrier is required. Fat-soluble drugs, such as benzodiazepines, neuroleptics, and cyclic antidepressants, distribute more widely in the body than water-soluble drugs, such as lithium, which distribute through a smaller volume of distribution. Changes with age, typically including an increase in the ratio of body fat to lean body mass, therefore result in a yet greater volume of lipophilic drug distribution and potentially greater accumulation of drug in adipose tissue in older than in younger patients. Although inadequately studied, a similar potential exists for female compared with male patients because of their generally higher ratio of adipose tissue to lean body mass.[23]

In general, psychotropic drugs have relatively high affinities for plasma proteins (some to albumin but others, such as antidepressants, to α_1-acid glycoproteins and lipoproteins). Most psychotropic drugs are more than 80% protein bound. A drug is considered highly protein-bound if more than 90% exists in bound form in plasma. Fluoxetine, aripiprazole, and diazepam are examples of the many psychotropic drugs that are highly protein-bound. In contrast, venlafaxine, lithium, topiramate, and gabapentin are examples of drugs with minimal protein binding. A reversible equilibrium exists between bound and unbound drug. Only the unbound fraction exerts pharmacologic effects. Competition by two or more drugs for protein-binding sites often results in displacement of a previously bound drug, which, in the free state, becomes pharmacologically active. Similarly, reduced concentrations of plasma proteins in a severely malnourished patient may be associated with an increase in the fraction of unbound drug potentially available for activity at relevant receptor sites. Under most circumstances, the net changes in plasma concentration of active drug are, in fact, quite small because the unbound drug is available for redistribution to other tissues and for metabolism and excretion, thereby offsetting the initial rise in plasma levels. It is important to be aware, however, that clinically significant consequences can develop when protein-binding interactions alter the unbound fraction of previously highly protein-bound drugs that have a low therapeutic index (e.g., warfarin). For these drugs, relatively small variations in plasma level may be associated with serious untoward effects.

An emerging understanding of the drug transport proteins, of which P-glycoproteins are the best characterized, indicates a crucial role in regulating permeability of intestinal epithelia, lymphocytes, renal tubules, biliary tract, and the blood-brain barrier. These transport proteins are thought to account for the development of certain forms of drug resistance and tolerance, but are increasingly seen as likely also to mediate clinically important drug interactions.[4,24] Little is known yet about their relevance to drug interactions involving psychiatric medications; the capacity of St. John's wort to lower blood levels of several critical medications, including cyclosporine and indinavir, is hypothesized to be related, at least in part, to an effect of the botanical agent on this transport system.[15]

Metabolism

Metabolism refers to the biotransformation of a drug to another form, a process that is usually enzyme-mediated and that results in a metabolite that may or may not be pharmacologically active and may or may not be subject to further bio-transformations before eventual excretion. Most drugs undergo several types of biotransformation, and many psychotropic drug interactions of clinical significance are based on interference with this process. A growing understanding of hepatic enzymes, and especially the rapidly emerging characterization of the cytochrome P450 isoenzymes and other enzyme systems including the uridine-diphosphate glucuronosyltransferases and flavin-containing monooxygenases,[4,25–27] has significantly advanced a rational understanding and prediction of drug interactions and individual variation in drug responses.

Phase I reactions include oxidation (e.g., hydroxylation or dealkylation), reduction (e.g., nitro reduction), and hydrolysis, metabolic reactions typically resulting in intermediate metabolites that are then subject to phase II reactions, including conjugation (e.g., glucuronide and sulfate) and acetylation. Phase II reactions typically yield highly polar, water-soluble metabolites suitable for renal excretion. Most psychotropic drugs undergo both phase I and phase II metabolic reactions. Notable exceptions are lithium, which is not subject to hepatic metabolism, and a subset of benzodiazepines (lorazepam, oxazepam, and temazepam), which undergo only phase II reactions and are therefore especially appropriate when benzodiazepines are used in the context of use of concurrent medications, advanced age, or disease states in which alterations of hepatic metabolism is likely to be substantial.

The synthesis or activity of hepatic microsomal enzymes is affected by metabolic inhibitors and inducers as well as distinct genetic polymorphisms (stably inherited traits), which may result in alteration or individual variation in the plasma concentration of active drugs as well as in the absolute and relative concentrations of the various metabolites associated with the drug. Table 18-1 lists enzyme inducers and inhibitors common in clinical settings. Inhibitors impede the metabolism of a concurrently administered drug producing a rise in its plasma level, whereas inducers enhance the metabolism of another drug resulting in a decline in its plasma levels. Although inhibition is usually immediate, induction is typically a more gradual process, such that a fall in plasma levels may not be apparent for days to weeks following introduction of the inducer. This is particularly important to keep in mind when a patient's care is being transferred to another setting where clinical deterioration may be the first sign that drug levels have declined. It should also be remembered, in evaluating unexpected changes in plasma drug levels, that an elevation in plasma drug concentrations could reflect the discontinuation of a prior inducing factor (e.g., cigarette smoking) just as it could the introduction of an

Table 18-1. Commonly Used Drugs and Substances That Inhibit or Induce Hepatic Metabolism of Other Medications[4,26,27]

Inhibitors	Inducers
Antifungals (ketoconazole, miconazole, itraconazole)	Barbiturates (e.g., phenobarbital, secobarbital)
Macrolide antibiotics (erythromycin, clarithromycin, triacetyloleandomycin)	Carbamazepine
Fluoroquinolones (e.g., ciprofloxacin)	Oxcarbazepine
Isoniazid	Phenytoin
Antiretrovirals	Rifampin
Selective serotonin inhibitors (fluoxetine, fluvoxamine, paroxetine, sertraline)	Primidone
Nefazodone	Cigarettes
β-Blockers (lipophilic) (e.g., propranolol, metoprolol, pindolol)	Ethanol (chronic)
Quinidine	Cruciferous vegetables
Valproate	Charbroiled meats
Cimetidine	
Calcium channel blockers (e.g., diltiazem)	
Grapefruit juice	
Ethanol (acute)	

inhibitor (e.g., fluoxetine), and the reciprocal is true for a fall in plasma drug concentrations.

Depending on genetic control over the enzyme, *N*-acetyltransferase involved in phase II metabolism of some drugs (e.g., clonazepam), rapid acetylation is found in a majority of patients, whereas a smaller number are slow acetylators who may require lower doses of compounds undergoing acetylation. Ethnic variations in genetic make-up may place an important role in the activity of certain metabolic enzymes.[28] Using mephenytoin as a probe for cytochrome P450 2C19, nearly 20% of Japanese and African-Americans appear to be poor metabolizers, a three-fold to four-fold higher percentage than among whites. The proportion of frankly poor metabolizers with respect to P450 2D6 appears to be higher among whites (2.9% to 10%) than among Asians (0.5% to 2.9%) and African-Americans (1.9%). The proportion of normal (or extensive) metabolizers, however, who, in fact, have intermediate levels of activity, appears to be higher among the latter two groups, thereby resulting in an overall lower P450 2D6 metabolism for Asians and African-Americans than whites when taken in aggregate.[28,29] In general, individuals who are classified as poor compared with normal metabolizers with respect to a particular cytochrome P450 isoenzyme may have higher plasma concentrations of a drug metabolized by that isoenzyme, thereby requiring lower doses. They may also have higher plasma levels of metabolites that are produced through other metabolic pathways, thereby potentially incurring pharmacologic activity or adverse effects related to these metabolites at unexpectedly low doses of the parent drug. Poor metabolizers are relatively impervious to drug interactions that are based on the inhibition of the particular isoenzyme system for which they are deficient, whereas normal metabolizers are, in effect, converted to poor metabolizers by such interactions.

Current understanding of the clinical relevance of genetic polymorphisms in drug therapy remains rudimentary. Given the many contributions to drug response and side-effects, it is yet unwarranted to assume that patients of a particular racial or ethnic background (e.g., Asian-Americans) will be adequately treated with lower than usual doses of psychotropic medications. Nevertheless, in decisions about initial dosing and titration and in the setting of unexpected plasma levels or unantici-pated side effects not otherwise explained, the possible contribution of a genetic polymorphism should be considered.

The capacity of many of the SSRI antidepressants to inhibit cytochrome P450 isoenzymes fueled great interest in the pattern of interaction of psychotropic and other drugs with these enzymes in the understanding and prediction of drug-drug interactions in psychopharmacology. The cytochrome P450 isoenzymes represent a family of more than 30 related heme-containing enzymes, largely located in the endoplasmic reticulum of hepatocytes (but also present elsewhere, including gut and brain), which mediate oxidative metabolism of a wide variety of drugs as well as endogenous substances, including prostaglandins, fatty acids, and steroids. The majority of antidepressant and antipsychotic drugs are metabolized by or inhibit one or more of these isoenzymes. Table 18-2 summarizes the interactions of psychiatric and nonpsychiatric drugs with a subset of isoenzymes that have been increasingly well characterized (1A2, 2D6, 2E1, 3A4, and the 2C subfamily). In addition to the numerous publications in which these interactions are cited,[4,26,27] several relevant websites are regularly updated, including www.drug-interactions.com and www.mhc.com/Cytochromes. The relevance of these and other interactions is highlighted in a later section of this chapter in which clinically important drug-drug interactions are reviewed.

Excretion

Because most antidepressant, anxiolytic, and antipsychotic medications are largely eliminated by hepatic metabolism, factors that affect renal excretion (glomerular filtration, tubular reabsorption, and active tubular secretion) are generally far less important to the pharmacokinetics of these drugs than to lithium, for which such factors may have clinically significant consequences. Conditions resulting in sodium deficiency (e.g., dehydration, sodium restriction, thiazide diuretics) are likely to result in increased proximal tubular reabsorption of lithium, resulting in increased lithium levels and potential toxicity. Lithium levels and clinical status must be monitored especially closely in the setting of vomiting, diarrhea,

Table 18-2. Selected Cytochrome P450 Isoenzyme Substrates, Inhibitors, and Inducers*[4,26,27]

1A2	Substrates	Acetaminophen, aminophylline, caffeine, clozapine, cyclobenzaprine, haloperidol, mirtazapine, olanzapine, phenacetin, procarcinogens, ropinirole, tacrine, tertiary tricyclic antidepressants, theophylline
	Inhibitors	Fluoroquinolones, fluvoxamine, cimetidine, grapefruit juice
	Inducers	Charbroiled meats, cigarette smoking, cruciferous vegetables, omeprazole
2C	Substrates	Barbiturates, diazepam, fluvastatin, glipizide, glyburide, irbesartan, losartan, mephenytoin, NSAIDs, nelfinavir, phenytoin, propranolol, proguanil, proton pump inhibitors, rosiglitazone, tamoxifen, tertiary TCAs, THC, tolbutamide, warfarin
	Inhibitors	Fluoxetine, fluvoxamine, ketoconazole, modafinil, omeprazole, oxcarbazepine, sertraline
	Inducers	Rifampin
2D6	Substrates	Aripiprazole, atomoxetine, β-blockers (lipophilic), codeine, debrisoquine, dextromethorphan, diltiazem, donepezil, dextromethorphan, encainide, flecainide, haloperidol, hydroxycodone, lidocaine, metoclopramide, mexiletine, mCPP, nifedipine, odansetron, phenothiazines (e.g., thioridazine, perphenazine), propafenone, risperidone, SSRIs, tamoxifen, TCAs, tramadol, trazodone
	Inhibitors	Amiodarone, antimalarials, bupropion, duloxetine, fluoxetine, methadone, metoclopramide, moclobemide, paroxetine, phenothiazines, protease inhibitors (ritonavir), quinidine, sertraline, terbinafine, TCAs, yohimbine
	Inducers	?
3A3/4	Substrates	Alfentanil, alprazolam, amiodarone, amprenavir, aripiprazole, bromocriptine, buspirone, calcium channel blockers, carbamazepine, cisapride, clozapine, cyclosporine, diazepam, disopyramide, efavirenz, estradiol, fentanyl, indinavir, HMG-CoA reductase inhibitors (lovastatin, simvastatin), lidocaine, loratadine, methadone, midazolam, nimodipine, pimozide, prednisone, progesterone, propafenone, quetiapine, quinidine, ritonavir, sildenafil, tacrolimus, testosterone, tertiary TCAs, triazolam, vinblastine, warfarin, zolpidem, zaleplon, ziprasidone
	Inhibitors	Antifungals, calcium channel blockers, cimetidine, efavirenz, indinavir, fluvoxamine, fluoxetine (norfluoxetine), grapefruit juice, macrolide antibiotics, mibefradil, nefazodone, ritonavir
	Inducers	Carbamazepine, modafinil, oxcarbazepine, phenobarbital, phenytoin, rifampin, ritonavir, St. John's Wort

HMG-CoA, Hydroxy-methylglutaryl coenzyme A; *mCPP*, *NSAID*, nonsteroidal antiinflammatory drug; *SSRI*, selective serotonin reuptake inhibitor; *TCA*, tricyclic antidepressant; *THC*, tetrahydrocannabinol.
*www.drug-interaction.com

excessive evaporative losses, or polyuria. Factors, such as aging, that are associated with reduced renal blood flow and glomerular filtration rate (GFR) also reduce lithium excretion. For this reason, as well as for their reduced volume of distribution for lithium because of the relative loss of total body water with aging, elderly patients typically require lower lithium doses than younger patients, and a low starting dose (i.e., 150 to 300 mg/day) is often prudent. Apparently separate from pharmacokinetic effects, however, elderly patients may also be more sensitive to the neurotoxic effects of lithium even at low therapeutic lev-

els. Factors associated with an increased GFR, particularly pregnancy, may produce an increase in lithium clearance and a fall in lithium levels.

Renal excretion may sometimes be exploited in the treatment of a drug overdose. Acidification of the urine by ascorbic acid, ammonium chloride, or methenamine mandelate increases the rate of excretion of weak bases, such as the amphetamines and phencyclidine (PCP). Therefore such measures may be important in the emergency management of a patient with severe PCP or amphetamine intoxication. Conversely, alkalinization of the urine by administration of sodium bicarbonate or acetazolamide may hasten the excretion of weak acids, including long-acting barbiturates, such as phenobarbital.

Mildly to moderately impaired renal function does not typically prompt routine changes in the dose or dosing intervals of psychotropic medications other than lithium. Increased plasma concentrations of hydroxylated metabolites of TCAs have been measured in patients with renal disease and dialysis patients, and more modest increases in TCA plasma levels have been measured in dialysis patients.[30] The clinical significance of these findings, however, appears to be largely limited to suggesting more cautious dose titration and surveillance in the renal patient rather than routine dose adjustments. A similar empiric strategy is prudent for SSRIs as well as for most antipsychotic medications and anxiolytics. In patients with severe renal function impairment, there may be accumulation of metabolites and, to a lesser extent, of the parent compound across repeated doses. An increase in the dose interval and possible reduction in drug dose should therefore be considered in this setting, particularly in the case of chronically administered agents with active metabolites.

Gabapentin, used at present to a limited extent in psychiatry for some patients with anxiety, mood instability, or pain, is not a salt but it resembles lithium in respect to the observation that it is not hepatically metabolized, is not appreciably protein-bound, and is excreted by the kidney largely as unchanged drug. As with lithium, therefore, it is essential to adjust dose according to changes in renal function. Similarly the anticonvulsant, topiramate, under further study for its putative mood-stabilizing and weight reducing effects, is eliminated largely unchanged by the kidneys and requires dose reduction in the setting of renal insufficiency.

Renal excretion is only one contribution to the elimination half-life, a pharmacokinetic construct that refers to the time required for the plasma concentration of a drug to be reduced by one half. The elimination phase (also referred to as the β-phase) reflects all processes that contribute to drug removal, including renal excretion, hepatic metabolism, and, to a much lesser extent, other factors (e.g., loss of drug in sweat or biliary secretions) potentially affecting drug clearance (the volume of blood or plasma cleared of drug per unit time). For the majority of drugs, whose elimination follows first-order kinetics (i.e., their rate of elimination is proportional to the amount of drug in the body rather than equal to a constant amount), steady-state drug levels are reached in four to five elimination half-lives, whereas, on discontinuation, almost all drug is out of the body within five half-lives. For drugs that are administered for their single-dose effects (e.g., an as-needed benzodiazepine) rather than for long-term effects of repeated administration (e.g., antidepressants), the duration of action of the drug depends not only on elimination half-life, but also often more critically on the initial phase of drug redistribution from the systemic circulation to other tissues, such as muscle and fat.

After a single dose of a drug, initial redistribution typically accounts for more rapid and extensive disappearance of drug from plasma than the subsequent phase of elimination, whose slope (on the plot of declining plasma drug concentration versus time) is usually much less steep. Once volume of distribution is saturated (with repeated doses of a drug), however, the slope of the curve reflecting redistribution from the systemic circulation flattens, and the elimination half-life becomes the more critical variable influencing duration of action.

In addition, because duration of action reflects the relationship between plasma concentration and a postulated minimum effective concentration, below which the drug has no clinical activity, the duration of action of a drug also depends on the magnitude of the actual dose of drug administered.

Thus it should be clear that although they are interdependent concepts, excretion is only one process encompassed by the pharmacokinetic construct of elimination and that the half-life of elimination, in turn, is only one factor determining the anticipated duration of action of a drug.

Drug Interactions

An understanding of pharmacokinetics is increasingly seen as important to the understanding and prediction of many drug-drug interactions encountered in psychopharmacology. Nevertheless, drug-drug interactions include not only pharmacokinetic interactions, which result in a change in the plasma level and tissue distribution of drug, but also interactions described as pharmacodynamic, which occur at biologically active (receptor) sites and result in a change in the pharmacologic effects rather than on the concentration of a drug. In addition, there appear to be idiosyncratic interactions, which occur unpredictably in a small number of patients and are unexpected from the known pharmacokinetic and pharmacologic properties of the drug.[31]

The scientific literature on psychotropic drug-drug interactions has grown immensely since first reviewed in *Massachusetts General Hospital Handbook of General Hospital Psychiatry* in 1978.[32] Despite impressive advances in clinical and molecular pharmacology, much of the extensive literature available on drug-drug interactions is based on case reports and uncontrolled studies, extrapolation from animal studies, and inferences drawn from knowledge about the in vitro properties of individual drugs. Fortunately, systematic in vivo drug-drug interaction studies are increasingly becoming an integral part of drug development.

Given the necessity of polypharmacy under many circumstances, the vast literature of reported and potential drug-drug interactions, and the increasingly litigious society in which physicians practice, the physician today is faced with a difficult dilemma when evaluating the potential significance of drug-drug interactions. When reviewing the literature, therefore, it is important to bear in mind that although isolated case reports may serve to flag potential drug-drug interactions that prove to be clinically important, they are also liable to reflect adverse events that are idiosyncratic or multifactorial. Data from controlled pharmacokinetic studies provide the most systematic account of drug-drug interactions, although not infrequently involving healthy volunteers receiving limited doses of the medications under study. Although potential drug-drug interactions are ubiquitous, fortunately the practical affect of many drug-drug interaction are clinically insignificant when compared with the inevitable inter-individual variability in drug levels, responses, and toxicities expected among clinical populations.

Nonetheless, several circumstances common to medical settings require a good knowledge of drug-drug interactions. Such knowledge becomes imperative: when the medications used have a narrow therapeutic index (e.g., lithium, digoxin, or war-farin) or a potentially narrow therapeutic window (e.g., indinavir, nortriptyline, or cyclosporine) such that relatively small alterations in pharmacokinetic or pharmacodynamic behavior may have significant medical consequences; when drug levels are unexpectedly variable or extreme; when a patient on multiple medications presents with a confusing clinical picture; when the introduction of a medication is associated with lack of improvement, clinical deterioration, or unexpected side effects; when a patient is medically frail or elderly, for whom the pharmacokinetics of drugs may be quite altered and the consequences of adverse drug effects more severe; when patients are significant users of alcohol, cigarettes, or illicit drugs; when a patient presents with a drug overdose; and when the consequences of an interaction, although uncommon, could be catastrophic (e.g., ventricular arrhythmias, agranulocytosis, hypertensive crises).

Antipsychotic Drugs

The antipsychotic or neuroleptic drugs used in the treatment of schizophrenia, schizoaffective disorder, organic psychoses, mood disorders with psychotic features, and other conditions, such as Tourette's syndrome, include the phenothiazines (e.g., chlorpromazine, fluphenazine, perphenazine, thioridazine, and trifluoperazine), butyrophenones (haloperidol), thioxanthenes (thiothixene), indolones (molindone), diphenylbutylpiperidines (pimozide), dibenzodiazepines (loxapine), and the newer atypical agents (clozapine, olanzapine, risperidone, quetiapine, ziprasidone, and aripiprazole). As a class, they are generally rapidly, if erratically, absorbed from the gastrointestinal tract after oral administration (peak plasma concentrations ranging from 30 minutes to 6 hours). They are highly lipophilic and distribute rapidly to body tissues with a large apparent volume of distribution. Protein-binding in the circulation ranges from approximately 90% to 98% except for molindone and quetiapine which are only moderately protein-bound. The antipsychotics generally undergo substantial first-pass hepatic metabolism (primarily oxidation and conjugation reactions), reducing their systemic bioavailability when given orally compared with intramuscular administration, the fractional absorption of which nearly approximates that of IV administration. Most of the individual antipsychotics have several pharmacologically active and yet other inactive metabolites. They are excreted primarily by the kidneys. Because of their propensity to sequester in body compartments, the elimination half-life of antipsychotics is quite variable, generally ranging from approximately 20 to 40 hours. For butyrophenones, however, elimination pharmacokinetics appear to be especially complex, and the disappearance of drug from the systemic circulation, and even more so from brain, may take much longer.[7,33] as it does for the newer agent, aripiprazole (and its active metabolite, dehydro-aripirazole), the half-life of which may exceed 90 hours.

The lower-potency antipsychotics (including chlorpromazine, mesoridazine, thioridazine, and clozapine) are generally the most sedating and have the greatest anticholinergic, antihistaminic, and α_1-adrenergic antagonistic effects, whereas the higher-potency antipsychotics (with the exception of the atypical agent, risperidone), including haloperidol, loxapine, molindone, and the piperazine phenothiazines, such as trifluoperazine, are more likely to be associated with an increased incidence of extrapyramidal effects, including akathisia, dystonia, and parkinsonism. The atypical antipsychotics generally have multiple receptor affinities, including antagonism at dopamine D_{1-4} receptors, serotonin 5-hydroxytryptamine (5-HT)$_1$ and 5-HT$_2$ receptors, alpha$_1$ and alpha$_2$ adrenergic receptors, histamine H$_1$ receptors, and cholinergic muscarinic receptors, with variations across agents; thus, for example, clozapine (Clozaril) and olanzapine have notably greater affinity at the muscarinic receptors than the other agents and aripiprazole is actually a partial agonist at the D_2 receptor. The more complex pharmacologic profile of these agents has generally been associated with lower risk of extrapyramidal effects.

With respect to pharmacodynamic interactions,[33,34] lower-potency drugs as well as atypical antipsychotics can produce significant hypotension when combined with vasodilator or antihypertensive drugs related to α_1-adrenergic blockade (Table 18-3). Exceptions are guanethidine and clonidine, whose antihypertensive efficacy may, in fact, be blocked by some phenothiazines, as with some antidepressants because of interference with neuronal reuptake mechanisms. Hypotension can also occur when low-potency antipsychotics and atypical antidepressants are combined with TCA and MAOI antidepressants. Severe hypotension has been reported when chlorpromazine has been administered with the angiotensin-converting enzyme (ACE) inhibitor captopril. Hypotension can develop when epinephrine is administered with low-potency antipsychotics. In this setting, the β-adrenergic stimulant effect of epinephrine, resulting in vasodilation, is unopposed by its usual pressor effect because α_1-adrenergic receptors are occupied by the antipsychotic. A similar effect may result if a low-potency neuroleptic is administered to a patient with a pheochromocytoma. Norepinephrine or phenylephrine, rather than β-agonists, should be considered when vasopressors are needed in a patient on psychotropic drugs that have significant α_1-adrenergic antagonistic effects. Finally, hypotension may develop when low-potency antipsychotics are used in combination with a variety of anesthetics, such as halothane, enflurane, and isoflurane. In addition, the low-potency antipsychotics have quinidine-like effects on cardiac conduction (and may prolong Q-T and P-R intervals). Ziprasidone may also cause Q-T prolongation; although clinically significant prolongation (QTc longer than 500 msec) appears to be rare when administered to otherwise healthy subjects.[35] Significant depression of cardiac conduction, heart block, and life-threatening ventricular dysrhythmias may result from the coadministration of low-potency antipsychotics or ziprasidone with class I antiarrhythmics (quinidine, procainamide, and disopyramide) as well as from the TCAs, which have quinidine-like activity on cardiac conduction, and when administered in the context of other aggravating factors including hypokalemia, hypomagnesemia, bradycardia, or congenital prolongation of the QTc. Pimozide also can depress cardiac conduction as a result of its calcium channel-blocking action and the combination of pimozide with other calcium channel blockers (e.g., nifedipine, diltiazem, and verapamil) is contraindicated. Related to cytochrome P450 isoenzyme inhibition, agents that interfere with P450 2D6, such as fluoxetine or paroxetine, can greatly increase levels of low potency agents, particularly thioridazine, and thus increase the risk of arrhythmia, whereas agents that interfere with P450 3A4, such as erythromycin or nefazodone, entail similar risk when combined with pimozide. These combinations are

Table 18-3. Selected Drug Interactions with Antipsychotic Medications

Drug	Potential Interaction
Antacids (aluminum–magnesium-containing), fruit juice	Interference with absorption of antipsychotic agents
Carbamazepine	Decreased antipsychotic drug plasma levels; additive risk of myelosuppression with clozapine
Cigarettes	Decreased antipsychotic drug plasma levels; reduced extrapyramidal symptoms
Rifampin	Decreased antipsychotic drug plasma levels
TCAs	Increased TCA and antipsychotic drug plasma levels; hypotension, depression of cardiac conduction (with low-potency antipsychotics)
SSRIs	Increased SSRI and antipsychotic drug plasma levels (see Table 18-7)
Bupropion, duloxetine	Increased antipsychotic drug plasma levels (see Table 18-2)
Fluvoxamine, nefazodone	Increased antipsychotic drug plasma levels (see Table 18-2)
β Blockers (lipophilic)	Increased antipsychotic drug plasma levels; reduced akathisia
Anticholinergic drugs	Additive anticholinergic toxicity
Antihypertensive, vasodilator drugs	Hypotension (with low-potency antipsychotics and risperidone)
Guanethidine, clonidine	Blockade of antihypertensive effect
Epinephrine	Hypotension (with low-potency antipsychotics)
Class I antiarrhythmics	Depression of cardiac conduction; ventricular arrhythmias (with low-potency antipsychotics, ziprasidone)
Calcium channel blockers	Depression of cardiac conduction; ventricular arrhythmias (with pimozide)
Lithium	Idiosyncratic neurotoxicity; ? neuroleptic malignant syndrome risk

SSRIs, Selective serotonin reuptake inhibitors; *TCA,* tricyclic antidepressant.

contraindicated. The concurrent administration of P450 3A4 inhibitors with ziprasidone may increase levels and theoretically increase QTc and risk of arrhythmias. When other low-potency to intermediate-potency antipsychotics are used with medications with significant quinidine-like effects, monitoring of the electrocardiogram for conduction delays should be planned. For patients with preexisting cardiac conduction problems who require antipsychotic treatment, the selection of high-potency agents, such as haloperidol, without quinidine-like properties and lower potential for vagolytic and hypotensive effects, should be considered.[36,37] Another pharmacodynamic interaction arises when low-potency antipsychotics, clozapine, or olanzapine are administered with other drugs that have anticholinergic effects (including TCAs, benztropine, and diphenhydramine). When these drugs are combined, there is a greater risk of urinary retention, constipation, blurred vision, impaired memory and concentration, and, in the setting of narrow-angle glaucoma, increased intraocular pressure. With intentional or inadvertent overdoses, a severe anticholinergic syndrome can develop, including delirium, paralytic ileus, tachycardia, and dysrhythmias. With lower affinity for muscarinic cholinergic receptors, the high-potency agents and nonanticholinergic atypical agents (e.g., risperidone) are indicated when anticholinergic effects need to be minimized.

The sedative effects of low-potency agents and atypical antidepressants are also often additive to those of the sedative-hypnotic medications and alcohol. In patients for whom sedative effects may be especially dangerous, including the elderly, the cautious selection and dosing of antipsychotics should always take into account the overall burden of sedation from their concurrent medications. For these patients, starting with a low, divided dose is often an appropriate first step.

Because dopamine receptor blockade is a property common to all antipsychotics, they are all likely to interfere, although with varying degrees, with the efficacy of levodopa in the treatment of Parkinson's disease. When antipsychotic treatment is necessary in this setting, the low-potency antipsychotics, and in more recent years, clozapine and the newer atypical agents have been preferred. Reciprocally, antipsychotics are likely to be less effective in the treatment of psychosis in the setting of levodopa, stimulants (e.g., dextroamphetamine), and direct agonists (e.g., bromocriptine) that facilitate dopamine transmission. Nevertheless, these agents have been combined with antipsychotics in cautious, modestly successful efforts to treat the negative symptoms of schizophrenia, including blunted affect, paucity of thought and speech, and social withdrawal. In addition, elevated prolactin is common when on antipsychotics, particularly higher potency agents and risperidone; it often presents with irregular menses, galactorrhea, diminished libido, or hirsutism. If these agents are necessary to the treatment of the patient and other causes of hyperprolactinemia have been excluded, there is an appropriate role for concurrent use of dopamine agonists, particularly bromocriptine, to lower prolactin.

The risk of agranulocytosis, which occurs rarely with the low-potency antipsychotics, is much higher with clozapine, with an incidence as high as 1% to 3%. For this reason, the combination of clozapine with other medications associated with a risk of myelosuppression (e.g., carbamazepine) should be avoided. Some patients may experience prolonged neuromuscular blockade when succinylcholine is coadministered with phenothiazines, putatively because of neuroleptic-induced reductions in levels of cholinesterase.[38]

Concern has been raised that coadministration of lithium with antipsychotic agents (most notably haloperidol) may be associated, rarely, with potentially irreversible neurotoxicity, characterized by mental status changes, extrapyramidal symptoms, and, perhaps in some cases, cerebellar signs and hyperthermia. Nevertheless, these findings have not been consistently reported.[39,40] Related to this concern is the suggestion, which remains to be confirmed, that lithium coadministration with an antipsychotic may increase the risk of NMS.[41,42] Other clinical variables, including dehydration and poor nutrition, have been more consistently emphasized as putative risk factors for NMS.[7] At present, the evidence is not sufficient to warrant avoidance of the widely used combination of lithium and neuroleptics. Such a

possibility, however, should be considered when a patient receiving these medications presents with neuropsychiatric toxicity of unclear origin.

Pharmacokinetic drug interactions are quite common among the antipsychotic drugs. Plasma levels of the neuroleptics, however, may vary as much as 10-fold to 20-fold between individuals, and, as a class, they have a relatively wide therapeutic index. Therefore factors that alter antipsychotic drug metabolism may not have apparent clinical consequences. Exceptions include those antipsychotics linked to risk of arrhythmia, most notably thioridazine and pimozide, for which close attention to pharmacokinetic interactions is required. Also, for patients with chronic psychotic disorders maintained on the lowest effective doses of a neuroleptic, pharmacokinetic factors resulting in a decline in neuroleptic concentrations in plasma and brain are likely to be clinically relevant risk factors for relapse.

Antipsychotic drug levels may be lowered by aluminum-containing or magnesium-containing antacids, which reduce their absorption and are best given separately. Mixing liquid preparations of phenothiazines with beverages such as fruit juices presents the risk of causing insoluble precipitates and inefficient gastrointestinal absorption. Carbamazepine, known to be a potent inducer of hepatic enzymes, has been associated with reduction of steady-state antipsychotic drug plasma levels by as much as 50%. This effect is especially important to bear in mind as a potential explanation when a neuroleptic-treated patient with bipolar or schizoaffective disorder appears to deteriorate in weeks following the introduction of carbamazepine. Oxcarbazepine may also induce antipsychotic drug metabolism as can a variety of other anticonvulsants, including phenobarbital and phenytoin. Cigarette smoking may also be associated with a reduction in antipsychotic drug through enzyme metabolism.[43] Although not well established, nicotine may exert an independent pharmacodynamic effect and result in reduction in neuroleptic-associated extrapyramidal symptoms in some patients. Because inpatient units and community residential programs have widely become "smoke-free," there are often substantial differences in smoking frequency between inpatient and outpatient settings. Among patients who smoke heavily, consideration should be given to the impact of these changes in smoking habits on antipsychotic treatment.

When an antipsychotic drug is given together with a TCA, the plasma level of each agent may rise, presumably because of mutual inhibition of microsomal enzymes. Reciprocally, when a patient with psychotic depression is tapered off an antipsychotic, it is important to remember that the plasma level of TCAs may also decline. SSRIs and other antidepressants with inhibitory effects on cytochrome P450 isoenzymes may also produce an increase in the plasma levels of a concurrently administered antipsychotic agent (see Table 18-2). Thus increases in clozapine, olanzapine, and haloperidol plasma levels may occur when coadministered with fluvoxamine. Increases in risperidone, aripiprazole, and typical antipsychotic levels may follow initiation of fluoxetine, paroxetine, bupropion, duloxetine, and sertraline. Quetiapine and ziprasidone levels may rise following addition of nefazodone, fluvoxamine, or fluoxetine. Phenothiazine drug levels may be increased when coadministered with propranolol, another inhibitor of hepatic microenzymes. Because propranolol is often an effective symptomatic treatment for neuroleptic-associated akathisia, the combined use of the β-blocker with an antipsychotic drug is common. When interactions present a problem, the use of a water-soluble β-blocker, such as atenolol, which is not likely to interfere with hepatic metabolism, provides a reasonable alternative.

Mood Stabilizers

Lithium

Lithium, used for the treatment of bipolar disorder, refractory depression, and other conditions, including severe aggressive behavior, is absorbed completely from the gastrointestinal tract, and peak plasma concentrations are reached after approximately 1.5 to 2 hours for standard preparations and 4 to 4.5 hours for slow-release preparations. It distributes throughout total body water and, in contrast to most psychotropic drugs, does not bind to plasma proteins and is not metabolized. It is filtered and reabsorbed by the kidneys, and 95% of it is excreted in the urine. Lithium elimination is highly dependent on total body sodium and fluid balance; it competes with sodium for reabsorption in the proximal tubules. To a lesser extent, lithium is reabsorbed also in the loop of Henle but, in contrast to sodium, is not reabsorbed in the distal tubules. Its elimination half-life is approximately 24 hours; clearance is generally 20% of creatinine clearance but is diminished in elderly patients and in patients with renal disease. The risk of toxicity is increased in these patients as well as in patients with cardiovascular disease, dehydration, or hypokalemia. The most common drug-drug interactions involving lithium are pharmacokinetic. Because lithium has a low therapeutic index, such interactions are likely to be clinically significant and potentially serious (Table 18-4).

Among the most well studied of these interactions are thiazide diuretics and drugs that are chemically distinct but share a similar mechanism of action (e.g., indapamide, metolazone, and quinethazone). These agents decrease lithium clearance and thereby greatly increase the risk of toxicity. Thiazide diuretics block sodium reabsorption at the distal tubule, producing sodium depletion, which, in turn, results in increased lithium reabsorption in the proximal tubule. Loop diuretics (e.g., furosemide and bumetanide) appear to interact to a lesser degree with lithium excretion, presumably because they block lithium reabsorption in the loop of Henle, potentially offsetting possible compensatory increases in reabsorption more proximally.[44,45] The potassium-sparing diuretics (e.g., amiloride, spironolactone, ethacrynic acid, and triamterene) also appear to be less likely to cause an increase in lithium levels.[46] The potential impact of thiazide diuretics on lithium levels does not contraindicate their combined use, which has been particularly valuable in the treatment of lithium-associated polyuria. Potassium-sparing diuretics have also been used for this purpose. When a thiazide diuretic is used, a lithium dose reduction of 25% to 50% and close monitoring of lithium levels are required. Monitoring of serum electrolytes, particularly potassium, is also important; hypokalemia enhances the toxicity of lithium, the risk of digitalis intoxication, and the potential for significant arrhythmias. Although not contraindicated with lithium, ACE inhibitors (e.g., captopril) and angiotensin II receptor antagonists (e.g., losartan), can elevate lithium levels and close monitoring of levels is required when these agents are introduced.

Table 18-4. Selected Drug Interactions with Lithium

Drug	Potential Interaction
Aminophylline, theophylline, acetazolamide, mannitol, sodium bicarbonate, sodium chloride load	Decreased lithium levels
Thiazide diuretics	Increased lithium levels; reduction of lithium-associated polyuria
Nonsteroidal antiinflammatory drugs, COX-2 inhibitors, tetracycline, spectinomycin, metronidazole, angiotensin II receptor antagonists, angiotensin-converting enzyme inhibitors	Increased lithium levels
Neuromuscular blocking drugs (succinylcholine, pancuronium, decamethonium)	Prolonged muscle paralysis
Antithyroid drugs (propylthiouracil, thioamide, methimazole)	Enhanced antithyroid efficacy
Antidepressants	Enhanced antidepressant efficacy
Calcium channel-blockers (verapamil, diltiazem)	Idiosyncratic neurotoxicity
Antipsychotic drugs	Idiosyncratic neurotoxicity, neuroleptic malignant syndrome risk

COX-2, Cyclooxygenase-2.

Many of the nonsteroidal antiinflammatory drugs (NSAIDs), including ibuprofen, indomethacin, diclofenac, naproxen, mefenamic acid, ketoprofen, and piroxicam, have been reported to increase serum lithium levels, potentially by as much as 50% to 60%. This may occur by inhibition of renal clearance of lithium by interference with a prostaglandin-dependent mechanism in the renal tubule. The limited available data suggest that sulindac,[47] phenylbutazone,[48] and aspirin[49] are less likely to produce this effect. Because use of the NSAIDs is widespread and some of these agents are now available over-the-counter, patients should be advised of this potential interaction when lithium is prescribed. The COX-2 inhibitors, celecoxib and rofecoxib, may also raise lithium levels 15% to 20%, requiring close monitoring and potential dose adjustment.

A number of antimicrobials are associated with increased lithium levels, including tetracycline, metronidazole, and parenteral spectinomycin. Renal function alterations associated with the ACE inhibitors, such as captopril, enalapril, and lisinopril also appear to carry a risk of lithium intoxication.[50] There is a case report of a lithium-treated patient who experienced increased serum lithium concentrations during the course of marijuana smoking, putatively related to slowed gastrointestinal motility, which allowed for increased lithium absorbtion.[51]

Decreased lithium levels have been observed in patients taking psyllium-containing bulk laxatives during lithium therapy. More importantly, the methylxanthines (e.g., aminophylline and theophylline) can cause a significant decrease in lithium levels by increasing renal clearance; close blood level monitoring when coadministration occurs is necessary. A reduction in lithium levels can also result from alkalinization of urine (e.g., with acetazolamide use or with sodium bicarbonate), osmotic diuretics (e.g., urea or mannitol) or from ingestion of a sodium chloride load, which also increases lithium excretion.

In addition to those concerning the combination of lithium and antipsychotic medications, there exist a variety of case reports of apparently idiosyncratic neurotoxicity, despite normal or inconsistently altered lithium levels, when lithium has been combined with the calcium channel-blockers, verapamil[52] and diltiazem,[53] and when lithium has been administered with the antihypertensive methyldopa.[54]

A potential cardiac effect, presumably the result of an increased effect of lithium on cardiac repolarization mechanisms, has been reported when hydroxyzine and lithium have been combined.[55]

A probable pharmacodynamic interaction exists between lithium and agents used clinically to produce neuromuscular blockade (e.g., succinylcholine, pancuronium, and decamethonium) during anesthesia. Significant prolongation of muscle paralysis can occur when these agents are administered to the lithium-treated patient.[56] Although the mechanism is unknown, the possible inhibition by lithium of acetylcholine synthesis and release at the neuromuscular junction is a potential basis for synergism.

Lithium interferes with the production of thyroid hormones through several mechanisms, including interference with iodine uptake, tyrosine iodination, and release of triiodothyronine (T_3) and thyroxine (T_4).[7] Lithium may therefore enhance the efficacy of antithyroid medications (e.g., propylthiouracil, thioamide, and methimazole) and has also been used preoperatively to help prevent thyroid storm in the surgical treatment of Graves' disease.[57]

There have been isolated reports of increased lithium levels, not explained by known mechanisms, and of neurotoxicity and/or serotonin syndrome, when lithium and SSRIs, venlafaxine, and other serotonergic agents (e.g., tramadol or tryptophan) have been administered concurrently.[58–60] The risks, however, appear to be small, and do not contraindicate the use of lithium as an adjunct to antidepressant pharmacotherapy.

Similarly, in the treatment of refractory bipolar disorder, lithium is frequently administered in conjunction with other mood-stabilizing agents, including valproic acid and carbamazepine. Although some reports indicate sporadically increased lithium levels or neurotoxicity (or both) on the combination of lithium and carbamazepine,[56,61] for most patients, the use of lithium with anticonvulsant mood stabilizers has proved to be a safe, effective strategy. Although the calcium channel-blockers, particularly verapamil, have had limited use for putative mood-stabilizing properties, case reports of neurotoxicity when coadministered with lithium justify additional caution when this combination is considered.

Valproic Acid

Valproic acid is a simple branched-chain carboxylic acid that, in addition to its anticonvulsant properties, has been shown to have significant antimanic properties and has been recently approved by the Food and Drug Administration for this indication. Valproic acid comes in several forms, including syrup and capsule form and, as divalproex sodium, an enteric-coated form that contains equal parts of valproic acid and sodium valproate. Rapidly absorbed after oral administration, peak levels are reached in approximately 1 to 2 hours if taken on an empty stomach and in 4 to 5 hours when taken with food. Divalproex sodium is more slowly absorbed, reaching peak serum concentrations in 3 to 8 hours. Valproic acid is 80% to 95% protein-bound and is rapidly metabolized primarily by hepatic microsomal glucuronidation and oxidation. It has a short elimination half-life of approximately 8 hours.[7] Clearance is essentially unchanged in the elderly and in patients with renal disease, whereas it is significantly reduced in patients with primary liver disease.[62]

In contrast to other major anticonvulsants, valproate does not induce hepatic microsomes. Rather, it tends to inhibit oxidation reactions, thereby potentially increasing levels of coadministered hepatically metabolized drugs (Table 18-5). This includes an elevation of 30% to 40% in plasma phenobarbital levels. Conversely, valproate levels may be reduced by phenobarbital by as much as 25%.[63] A complex pharmacokinetic interaction occurs when valproic acid and carbamazepine are administered concurrently. Valproic acid not only inhibits the metabolism of carbamazepine and its active metabolite, carbamazepine-10,11-epoxide (CBZ-E), but also displaces both entities from protein-binding sites. Although the effect on plasma carbamazepine levels is variable, the levels of the unbound (active) epoxide metabolite are increased with a concomitant increased risk of carbamazepine neurotoxicity.[64] Conversely, coadministration with carbamazepine results in a decrease in plasma valproic acid levels.

Nevertheless, the combination of valproate and carbamazepine has been used successfully in the treatment of patients with bipolar disorder who were only partially responsive to either drug alone.[65] When phenytoin is combined with valproic acid, there is typically a fall in valproate levels because of the enzyme-inducing effects of phenytoin, whereas there may be variable effects on phenytoin concentrations, including a transient elevation of unbound phenytoin owing to protein-binding displacement by valproate.[63] When the metabolism of valproate is induced, a by-product includes 4-ene-valproic acid, which may be a risk factor for hepatoxicity.[4] Unless specifically requested, laboratory evaluations of valproic levels do not include this metabolite. As much as a two- to three-fold increase in lamotrigine levels occurs when valproic acid is added, related to inhibition of glucuronidation of lamotrigine, and the concurrent use of the two anticonvulsants is associated with an increased incidence of rash. Accordingly, the *Physician's Desk Reference*[66] provides guidelines for

Table 18-5. Selected Drug Interactions with Valproate and Carbamazepine

Drug	Interaction with Valproate
Carbamazepine	Decreased valproate plasma levels; increased plasma levels of the epoxide metabolite of carbamazepine; variable effects on plasma levels of carbamazepine
Phenytoin	Decreased valproate plasma levels; variable effects on phenytoin plasma levels
Phenobarbital	Decreased valproate plasma levels; increased phenobarbital plasma levels
Lamotrigine	Increased lamotrigine levels; rash
Aspirin	Increased unbound (active) fraction of valproate
Cimetidine	Increased valproate plasma levels
Fluoxetine	
Clonazepam	Rare absence seizures
Drug	**Interaction with Carbamazepine**
Phenytoin	Decreased carbamazepine plasma levels
Phenobarbital	
Primidone	
Macrolide antibiotics	Increased carbamazepine plasma levels
Isoniazid	
Fluoxetine	
Verapamil, diltiazem	
Danazol	
Propoxyphene	
Oral contraceptives	Induction of metabolism by carbamazepine
Corticosteroids	
Thyroid hormones	
Warfarin, cyclosporine	
Phenytoin, ethosuximide	
Carbamazepine, valproate, lamotrigine	
Tetracycline, doxycycline	
Theophylline, methadone	
Benzodiazepines	
TCAs, antipsychotics	
Thiazide diuretics	Hyponatremia
Furosemide	

TCA, Tricyclic antidepressants.

more gradual dose titration of lamotrigine and lower target doses when introduced in a patient already taking valproate. When valproate is added to lamotrigine, the dose of the latter should typically be reduced.

Administration of aspirin with valproic acid has been associated with an increase in the steady-state free fraction of the latter from 12% to 43%, thereby increasing the risk of valproic toxicity.[67] This interaction appears to be based on protein-binding displacement of valproic acid by salicylates.

Cimetidine, a potent inhibitor of hepatic microsomal enzymes, is also associated with decreased clearance of valproic acid, and dose reductions of valproic

acid may be necessary in the patient starting cimetidine[68]; this effect is not expected with ranitidine, famotidine, or nizatidine, which may be used as alternatives when a histamine 2 (H_2)-receptor antagonist is prescribed. Other inhibitors of hepatic metabolism, including fluoxetine, may also cause valproic acid levels to rise,[69] increasing the risk of valproate toxicity when added and, conversely, the risk of subtherapeutic valproate levels when discontinued.

Although absence seizures have been reported with the combination of clonazepam and valproate,[70] this is likely to be rare, limited to individuals with neurologic disorders, and does not preclude simultaneous use of these medications in the treatment of bipolar disorder.

Carbamazepine

Carbamazepine is an iminostilbene anticonvulsant structurally related to the TCA imipramine. Carbamazepine is slowly and inconsistently absorbed from the gastrointestinal tract; peak serum concentrations are achieved approximately 4 to 8 hours after oral administration. It is only moderately (60% to 85%) protein-bound. It is poorly soluble in gastrointestinal fluids, and as much as 15% to 25% of an oral dose is excreted unchanged in the feces. Its CBZ-E metabolite is active as an anticonvulsant, although its antimanic activity is unknown. Carbamazepine, a potent inducer of hepatic metabolism, can also induce its own metabolism such that elimination half-life may fall from 18 to 55 hours to 5 to 20 hours over a matter of several weeks, generally reaching a plateau after 3 to 5 weeks.[7]

Most drug-drug interactions with carbamazepine occur by pharmacokinetic mechanisms. Drugs whose metabolism is increased by carbamazepine include valproic acid, phenytoin, ethosuximide, lamotrigine, alprazolam, clonazepam, TCAs, antipsychotics, doxycycline, tetracycline, thyroid hormone, corticosteroids, oral contraceptives, methadone, theophylline, warfarin, and cyclosporine.[26,71] The concurrent administration of carbamazepine with any of these drugs can cause significant reductions in plasma levels and may lead to therapeutic failure. In two patients with bipolar disorder, the combination of carbamazepine and bupropion resulted in failure to achieve adequate blood levels of bupropion while causing potentially toxic levels of its metabolite, hydroxybupropion.[72] Among patients taking carbamazepine, the possible induction of dexamethasone metabolism renders the dexamethasone suppression test invalid. In addition, patients of child-bearing potential on oral contraceptives must be advised to use an additional method of birth control.

Several drugs inhibit the metabolism of carbamazepine, including the macrolide antibiotics (e.g., erythromycin, clarithromycin, and triacetyloleandomycin), isoniazid, fluoxetine, valproic acid, danazol, propoxyphene, and the calcium channel-blockers verapamil and diltiazem (but not nifedipine).[26,71] Because of its low therapeutic index, the risk of developing carbamazepine toxicity is significantly increased when these drugs are administered concurrently. Conversely, coadministration of phenytoin or phenobarbital, both microsomal enzyme inducers, can increase the metabolism of carbamazepine, potentially resulting in subtherapeutic plasma levels.

The combination of carbamazepine with thiazide diuretics or furosemide has been associated with severe, symptomatic hyponatremia,[73] suggesting the need for close monitoring of electrolytes when these medications are used concurrently.

Oxcarbazepine appears to be a less potent metabolic inducer than carbamazepine, although it still may render certain important agents, particularly P450 3A4 substrates, less effective because of similar pharmacokinetic interactions. Women of childbearing potential should therefore receive guidance about supplementing oral contraceptives with a second effective form of birth control as with carbamazepine. Similarly, like carbamazepine, oxcarbazepine is also associated with risk of hyponatremia.

Antidepressants

The antidepressant drugs include the TCAs, the MAOIs, the SSRIs, the atypical agents (bupropion, trazodone, nefazodone, and mirtazapine), and the selective serotonin-norepinephrine reuptake inhibitors (SNRIs) duloxetine and venlafaxine. Another class of medications, the psychostimulants, although used primarily for the treatment of attention deficit hyperactivity disorder (ADHD) and narcolepsy, have also been prescribed for more than 50 years for their antidepressant properties. Over the past decade, much systematic attention has been devoted to the study of antidepressant efficacy in the treatment of conditions other than depression, including obsessive-compulsive disorder, social phobia, panic disorder, bulimia, somatoform disorders, impulse control disorders, and ADHD.

Tricyclic Antidepressants

TCAs are thought to exert their pharmacologic action by inhibiting the presynaptic neuronal reuptake of norepinephrine and serotonin in the CNS with subsequent modulation of both presynaptic and postsynaptic β-adrenergic receptors. TCAs also have significant anticholinergic, antihistaminic, and α-adrenergic activity as well as quinidine-like effects on cardiac condition, in these respects resembling the low-potency antipsychotic drugs, which are structurally similar.[74]

TCAs are well absorbed from the gastrointestinal tract and subject to significant first-pass liver metabolism before entry into the systemic circulation, where they are largely protein-bound, ranging from 85% (trimipramine) to 95% (amitriptyline). Peak plasma concentrations are reached approximately 2 to 6 hours after oral administration. They are highly lipophilic with a large volume of distribution. TCAs are extensively metabolized by hepatic microsomal enzymes, and most have pharmacologically active metabolites.[75]

With two methyl groups on the terminal nitrogen of the TCA side-chain, imipramine, amitriptyline, trimipramine, doxepin, and clomipramine are called tertiary amines. The demethylation of imipramine, amitriptyline, and trimipramine yields the secondary amine TCAs, desipramine, nortriptyline, and protriptyline, which are generally less sedating and have less affinity for anticholinergic receptors. The demethylation of imipramine relies on cytochrome P450 isoenzymes 1A2 and 3A3/4, whereas that of amitriptyline appears to rely primarily on 1A2. These tertiary amines as well as their secondary amine offspring are then hydroxylated via cytochrome P450 2D6, a step sensitive to inhibition by a wide variety of other drugs.[2] The hydroxymetabolites of the most commonly prescribed TCAs can be active. Furthermore, the hydroxymetabolite of nortriptyline may block the antidepressant effect of the parent drug,[76] and some hydroxymetabolites of the TCAs may be cardiotoxic.[77]

Additive anticholinergic effects can occur when the TCAs are coadministered with other drugs possessing anticholinergic properties (e.g., low-potency antipsychotics, antiparkinsonian drugs), potentially resulting in an anticholinergic syndrome. SSRIs, atypical antidepressants, and MAOIs are relatively devoid of anticholinergic activity, although the MAOIs may indirectly potentiate the anticholinergic properties of atropine and scopolamine. Additive sedative effects are not uncommon when TCAs are combined with sedative-hypnotics, anxiolytics, or narcotics or alcohol (Table 18-6).

TCAs possess class 1A antiarrhythmic activity and can lead to depression of cardiac conduction potentially resulting in heart block or ventricular arrhythmias when combined with quinidine-like agents, including quinidine, procainamide, and disopyramide as well as the low-potency antipsychotics.[78–80] The antiarrhythmics quinidine and propafenone, inhibitors of cytochrome P450 2D6, may additionally result in clinically significant elevations of the TCAs.[81,82]

TCAs inhibit nerve reuptake of biogenic amines both peripherally and centrally. They may thereby increase myocardial norepinephrine levels; this, in

Table 18-6. Selected Drug Interactions with Tricyclic Antidepressants

Drug	Potential Interaction
Carbamazepine	Decreased TCA plasma levels
Phenobarbital	
Rifampin	
Isoniazid	
Antipsychotics	Increased TCA plasma levels
Methylphenidate	
SSRIs	
Quinidine, propafenone	
Antifungals	
Macrolide antibiotics	
Verapamil, diltiazem	
Cimetidine	
Class I antiarrhythmics	Depression of cardiac conduction; ventricular
Low-potency antipsychotics	Arrhythmias
Guanethidine, clonidine	Interference with antihypertensive effect
Sympathomimetic amines	Arrhythmias, hypertension (e.g., isoproterenol, epinephrine)
Antihypertensives, vasodilator	Hypotension drugs, low-potency antipsychotics
Anticholinergic drugs	Additive anticholinergic toxicity
MAOIs	Delirium, fever, convulsions
Sulfonylurea hypoglycemics	Hypoglycemia

MAOI, Monoamine oxidase inhibitor; *SSRI*, selective serotonin reuptake inhibitor; *TCA*, tricyclic antidepressant.

conjunction with their anticholinergic actions and quinidine-like effects, may give rise to cardiac arrhythmias. Arrhythmias are most often manifested by atrial or ventricular premature beats, which may be unifocal or multifocal, or they may give rise to runs of ventricular tachycardia. The arrhythmogenic effect of a TCA is more likely to occur in an individual with underlying coronary or valvular heart disease, or when a patient has had a recent myocardial infarction; hypokalemia; and is receiving sympathomimetic amines such as isoproterenol, ephedrine, or amphetamine stimulants.[78,79,83]

TCAs also interact with several antihypertensive drugs. TCAs can antagonize the antihypertensive effects of guanethidine, bethanidine, debrisoquine, or clonidine via interference with neuronal reuptake by noradrenergic neurons. Conversely, because TCAs can cause varying degrees of postural hypotension, when coadministered with vasodilator drugs, antihypertensives, low-potency neuroleptics, and possibly risperidone, additive hypotension may occur.

Hypoglycemia has been observed on both secondary and tertiary TCAs, particularly in the presence of sulfonylurea hypoglycemic agents[2]; adequate blood glucose monitoring but not routine dose adjustments of hypoglycemic agents is recommended in this setting.

Pharmacokinetic interactions involving the TCAs are often clinically important. The antipsychotic drugs (including haloperidol, chlorpromazine, thioridazine, and perphenazine) are known to increase TCA levels by 30% to 100%.[84,85] Apart from this pharmacokinetic interaction, the combination of a TCA with an antipsychotic drug is among the best-documented pharmacologic treatments of psychotic depression, with a response rate of 70% to 80%, compared with 30% to 50% when treated with either class of medication alone. Cimetidine can also raise tertiary TCA levels as predicted by microsomal enzyme inhibition,[86] as can methylphenidate, which may also potentiate the antidepressant efficacy of TCAs on a pharmacologic rather than a pharmacokinetic basis. The antifungals (e.g., ketoconazole), macrolide antibiotics (e.g. erythromycin), and calcium channel-blockers (e.g., verapamil and diltiazem) as inhibitors of cytochrome P450 3A4 may also impair the clearance of tertiary amine TCAs, thereby requiring a TCA dose reduction. SSRIs have been associated with clinically significant increases in TCA plasma levels, believed to be the result of inhibition of cytochrome P450 2D6 and potentially 3A4 and 1A2.[21] TCA and SSRI antidepressants have also been used successfully in combination in efforts to augment antidepressant efficacy.[57,87] Augmentation of TCA antidepressants with lithium or thyroid hormone (liothyronine or, less commonly, thyroxine), not generally associated with alterations of TCA levels, is another common strategy in the management of TCA treatment-refractory depression.[57]

Inducers of P450 enzymes can increase the metabolism of TCAs. Thus plasma levels of TCAs may be significantly reduced when carbamazepine, phenobarbital, rifampin, or isoniazid are coadministered or in the setting of chronic alcohol or cigarette use.

SSRIs and Other Newer Antidepressants

The SSRIs (e.g., fluoxetine, sertraline, paroxetine, fluvoxamine, citalopram, and escitalopram) share similar pharmacologic actions, including minimal anticholinergic, antihistaminic, and α_1-adrenergic blocking effects, and potent presynaptic inhibition of serotonin reuptake.[7,88] There are important pharmacokinetic differences, which account for distinctions among them with respect to potential drug interactions (Table 18-7). Nefazodone, similar to trazodone, is distinguished from classic SSRIs by its antagonism of the 5-HT$_2$ receptor (and differs from trazodone in its lesser antagonism of the α_1-adrenergic receptor). Mirtazapine also blocks the 5-HT$_2$ receptor, although it also blocks the 5-HT$_3$ receptor and α_2 adrenergic receptors. Venlafaxine, similar to TCAs, inhibits serotonin and norepinephrine reuptake, but, in contrast to TCAs, is relatively devoid of postsynaptic anticholinergic, antihistaminic, and α_1-adrenergic activity. Similarly, duloxetine is an inhibitor of serotonin and norepinephrine reuptake, although whereas venlafaxine is predominantly serotonergic at low to moderate doses, duloxetine is a potent inhibitor of both the norepinephrine and serotonin transporters across its clinical dose range. Although not an approved antidepressant, the SNRI atomoxetine, indicated for the treatment of ADHD, may have a role in depression pharmacotherapy as single agent or adjunctive treatment. It is neither a significant inhibitor nor inducer of the P450 cytochrome system, but owing to its adrenergic effects, the risk

Table 18-7. Potential Drug Interactions with the Selective Serotonin Reuptake Inhibitors and Other Newer Antidepressants

Drug	Potential Interaction
MAOIs	Serotonin syndrome
Secondary amine TCAs	Increased TCA levels when coadministered with fluoxetine, paroxetine, sertraline, bupropion, duloxetine
Tertiary amine TCAs	Increased TCA levels with fluvoxamine, paroxetine, sertraline, bupropion, duloxetine
Antipsychotics (typical) and risperidone, aripiprazole	Increased antipsychotic levels with fluoxetine, sertraline, paroxetine, bupropion, duloxetine
Thioridazine	Arrhythmia risk with P450 2D6 inhibitory antidepressants
Pimozide	Arrhythmia risk with P450 3A4 inhibitory antidepressants (nefazodone, fluvoxamine)
Clozapine and olanzapine	Increased antipsychotic levels with fluvoxamine
Diazepam	Increased benzodiazepine levels with fluoxetine, fluvoxamine, sertraline
Triazolobenzodiazepines (midazolam, alprazolam, triazolam)	Increased fluvoxamine, nefazodone, sertraline (diazepam)
Carbamazepine	Increased carbamazepine levels with fluoxetine, fluvoxamine, nefazodone
Theophylline	Increased theophylline levels with fluvoxamine
Type 1C antiarrhythmics (ecainide, flecainide, propafenone)	Increased antiarrhythmic levels with fluoxetine, paroxetine, sertraline, bupropion, duloxetine
β-Blockers (lipophilic)	Increased β-blocker levels with fluoxetine, paroxetine, sertraline, bupropion, duloxetine
Calcium channel blockers	Increased levels with fluoxetine, fluvoxamine, nefazodone

MAOI, Monoamine oxidase inhibitor; *SSRI,* selective serotonin reuptake inhibitor; *TCA,* tricyclic antidepressant.

of palpitations or pressor effects is likely to be greater than with serotonergic agents when combined with prescribed and over-the-counter sympathomimetics.

All of the SSRIs are highly protein-bound (95% to 99%) except fluvoxamine (77%), citalopram (80%), and escitalopram (56%). Venlafaxine is minimally protein-bound (20% to 30%). All of them are hepatically metabolized, and all of them except paroxetine have active metabolites. The major metabolites of sertraline and citalopram, however, appear to be minimally active. Elimination half-lives range from 5 hours for venlafaxine and 11 hours for its metabolite, *O*-desmethylvenlafaxine, to 2 to 3 days for fluoxetine and 7 to 14 days for its metabolite, norfluoxetine. Nefazodone, similar to venlafaxine, has a short half-life, with fluvoxamine, sertraline, paroxetine, citalopram, and escitalopram intermediate in the range of 15 to 35 hours.[7] Food may have variable effects on SSRI bioavailability, including an increase for sertraline but a decrease for nefazodone and no change for escitalopram.

The growing knowledge about the interaction of the newer antidepressants with the cytochrome P450 isoenzymes has revealed differences among them in their pattern of enzyme inhibition that are likely to be critical to the understanding and prediction of drug-drug interactions.[4,27]

P450 2D6

Fluoxetine, norfluoxetine, paroxetine, bupropion, duloxetine[89] and, to some degree, sertraline as well as to a lesser extent, citalopram and escitalopram,[4] all inhibit P450 2D6, most notably accounting for their potential inhibitory effect on TCA clearance and the metabolism of other P450 2D6 substrates. Other drugs metabolized by P450 2D6 include the type 1C antiarrhythmics (e.g., encainide, flecainide, and propafenone) as well as β-blockers (e.g., propranolol, timolol, and metoprolol), antipsychotics (e.g., risperidone, haloperidol, aripiprazole, thioridazine, and perphenazine), TCAs, and trazodone. P450 2D6 converts codeine into its active analgesic form. These observations underscore the need to exercise care and to closely monitor when prescribing these SSRIs, bupropion, or duloxetine in the setting of complex medical regimens. Plasma TCA levels do not routinely include levels of active or potentially toxic metabolites, which may be altered by virtue of shunting to other metabolic routes when P450 2D6 is inhibited. Therefore, particularly in the case of patients at risk for conduction delay, electrocardiography as well as blood level monitoring is recommended when combining SSRIs, duloxetine, or bupropion with TCAs. There have been case reports of adverse events, including bradycardia, lethargy, and syncope, when fluoxetine has been coadministered with lipophilic, hepatically metabolized β-blockers, such as metoprolol and propranolol.[90,91] This is less likely to occur, however, on water-soluble β-blockers, such as atenolol or nadolol, which are cleared by the kidney and which therefore bypass P450 2D6 metabolism.

P450 3A4

Fluoxetine's metabolite (norfluoxetine), fluvoxamine, nefazodone, and, probably to a generally clinically insignificant extent, sertraline, desmethylsertraline, citalopram and escitalopram inhibit P450 3A4. All of these agents therefore have the potential for elevating levels of pimozide and cisapride (arrhythmia risks), calcium channel blockers, the "statins," carbamazepine, midazolam, and many other important and widely prescribed substrates.

P450 2C

Serum concentrations of drugs metabolized by this subfamily may be increased by fluoxetine, sertraline, and fluvoxamine. Reported interactions include decreased clearance of diazepam on all three SSRIs, a small reduction in tolbutamide clearance on sertraline, and increased plasma phenytoin concentrations reflecting decreased clearance on fluoxetine. Warfarin is also metabolized by this subfamily. Whether the highly bound SSRIs displace warfarin from plasma proteins is unclear because the SSRIs are largely bound to α_1-acid glycoproteins, whereas warfarin is largely bound to albumin. SSRIs may interact with warfarin by still other, probably pharmacodynamic mechanisms. Thus in one study, paroxetine was observed to increase bleeding when coadministered with warfarin, whereas plasma levels of warfarin were unaffected.[92] The paucity of reports of adverse events on the combination of warfarin and SSRIs is reassuring. Increased monitoring is recommended nevertheless when SSRIs are prescribed with warfarin or phenytoin.

P450 1A

Among the SSRIs, only fluvoxamine appears to be a potent inhibitor of P450 1A2. Accordingly, increased serum concentrations of theophylline, haloperidol, clozapine, olanzapine, and the tertiary amine TCAs including clomipramine, amitriptyline, and imipramine (and not of the secondary amine TCA desipramine) may occur.[4,88] Because theophylline and TCAs have a relatively narrow therapeutic index and because the degree of elevation of antipsychotic blood levels appears to be substantial (e.g., up to four-fold increases in haloperidol concentrations), additional monitoring and consideration of dose reductions are necessary when fluvoxamine is coadministered with these agents.

Additional Interactions

Plasma levels of valproic acid, as is true of carbamazepine, are reported to be increased when valproate is coadministered with fluoxetine, although the nature of this interaction remains to be established.[69] There are several case reports of neurotoxicity when bupropion was introduced following a sustained period of fluoxetine use.[93,94] The extent to which this reflects a pharmacokinetic interaction is unknown. At present, empiric reduction of bupropion dose may be warranted when coadministered with fluoxetine. Nevertheless, the combined use of fluoxetine and other SSRIs with bupropion represents a widely employed strategy for antidepressant augmentation as well as one of several strategies that exist to address SSRI-associated sexual dysfunction.

Mirtazapine, although neither a potent inhibitor nor inducer of the P450 cytochrome isoenzymes, has numerous pharmacodynamic effects including antagonism of the histamine$_1$, alpha$_2$ adrenergic, 5-HT$_2$ and 5-HT$_3$, and muscarinic receptors, creating the possibility of myriad pharmacologic interactions. Thus, for example, the antihypertensive effects of clonidine appeared to be blocked in one case when mirtazapine was added[95] and both

SSRI-related nausea and sexual dysfunction may be attenuated by the presence of mirtazapine.[96]

The serotonin syndrome is a potentially life-threatening condition characterized by confusion, diaphoresis, hyperthermia, hyperreflexia, muscle rigidity, tachycardia, hypotension, and coma.[60] Although this may arise whenever an SSRI is combined with a serotoninergic drug (e.g., L-tryptophan, clomipramine, or venlafaxine) and drugs with serotoninergic properties (e.g., lithium, mirtazapine, dextromethorphan, tramadol, meperidine, and pentazocine), the greatest known risk is associated with the coadministration of an SSRI with an MAOI, which is contraindicated. In view of the long elimination half-life of fluoxetine and norfluoxetine, at least 5 weeks must elapse after fluoxetine discontinuation before an MAOI can be safely introduced. With the other SSRIs, an interval of 2 weeks appears to be adequate. The coadministration of SSRIs with other serotoninergic agents is not contraindicated, but should prompt immediate discontinuation in any patient on this combination of drugs who presents with mental status changes, fever, or hyperreflexia of unknown origin.

Monoamine Oxidase Inhibitors

MAO is an enzyme located primarily on the outer mitochondrial membrane and is responsible for intracellular catabolism of the monoamines. It is found in high concentrations in brain, liver, intestines, and lung. In presynaptic nerve terminals, MAO metabolizes cytoplasmic monoamines. In liver and gut, MAO catabolizes ingested bioactive amines, thus protecting against absorption into the systemic circulation of potentially vasoactive substances, particularly tyramine. Two subtypes of MAO have been distinguished: Intestinal MAO is predominantly MAO-A, whereas brain MAO ispredominantly MAO-B. MAO-A preferentially metabolizes norepinephrine and serotonin. (Phenylethylamine and benzylamine are the prototypic substrates for MAO-B.) Both MAO subtypes metabolize dopamine and tyramine. The currently available MAOIs—phenelzine, tranylcypromine, and isocarboxazid—are nonspecific inhibitors of both MAO-A and MAO-B. Inhibition by phenelzine and isocarboxazid is irreversible, such

that restoration of enzyme activity after the MAOI is discontinued relies on new synthesis of MAO and takes up to 2 weeks. Inhibition of MAO by tranylcypromine may not be entirely irreversible but appears to be slowly reversible such that return of enzyme activity after discontinuation appears to be almost equally delayed. The MAOIs are well absorbed after gastrointestinal absorption, and maximal inhibition of MAO is achieved within 3 to 5 days.[7] MAOIs have been successfully used in the treatment of major depression (including atypical depression) and anxiety disorders, including social phobia and panic disorder. Dietary and medication restrictions must be closely followed to avoid serious interactions. The MAOIs are, therefore, generally reserved for use in responsible or supervised patients when adequate trials of other classes of antidepressants have failed.

The two major types of MAOI drug-drug interaction are the serotonin syndrome and the hypertensive (also called hyperadrenergic) crisis.[97] The hypertensive crisis, a potentially fatal interaction, is perhaps the most well-known drug-drug interaction in psychiatry. The reaction is characterized by an abrupt elevation of blood pressure, severe headache, nausea, vomiting, and diaphoresis; intracranial hemorrhage or myocardial infarction can occur. Prompt intervention to reduce blood pressure with the α_1-adrenergic antagonist, phentolamine, or the calcium channel-blocker nifedipine may be lifesaving. Potentially catastrophic hypertension appears to be due to release of bound intraneuronal stores of norepinephrine and dopamine by indirect vasopressor substances. The reaction can therefore be precipitated by the concurrent administration of vasopressor amines, stimulants, anorexians, and many over-the-counter cough and cold preparations; these include L-dopa, dopamine, amphetamine, methylphenidate, phenylpropanolamine, phentermine, mephentermine, metaraminol, ephedrine, and pseudoephedrine.[98,99] By contrast, direct sympathomimetic amines (e.g., norepinephrine, isoproterenol, and epinephrine), which rely for their cardiovascular effects on direct stimulation of postsynaptic receptors rather than on presynaptic release of stored catecholamines, appear to be safer when administered to individuals on MAOIs.[100]

Hypertensive crises may also be triggered by ingestion of naturally occurring sympathomimetic amines (particularly tyramine), which is present in various food products, including aged cheeses (e.g., stilton, cheddar, bleu cheese, or camembert, rather than cream cheese, ricotta cheese, or cottage cheese), yeast extracts (e.g., Marmite and brewer's yeast tablets), fava (broad) beans, overripened fruits (e.g., avocado), pickled herring, aged meats (e.g., salami, bologna, and many kinds of sausage), chicken liver, fermented bean curd, sauerkraut, many types of red wine and beer (particularly imported beer), and some white wines. Although gin, vodka, and whiskey appear to be free of tyramine, their use should be minimized during the course of MAOI treatment, as with other antidepressants, because of the risk of exaggerated side effects and reduced antidepressant efficacy. Other less stringent requirements include moderated intake of caffeine, chocolate, yogurt, and soy sauce. Because inhibition of MAO by phenelzine and tranylcypromine can persist for 2 weeks following their discontinuation, a tyramine-free diet and appropriate medication restrictions should be continued throughout that period.[98,99,101–104]

The serotonin syndrome, the other major drug-drug interaction involving the MAOIs, occurs when MAOIs and serotoninergic agents are coadministered, particularly the SSRIs and clomipramine.[60] Potentially fatal reactions most closely resembling the serotonin syndrome can also occur with other drugs with less selective serotoninergic activity, most notably meperidine as well as dextromethorphan, a widely available cough suppressant. Both of these medications, similar to the SSRIs and clomipramine, are absolutely contraindicated when MAOIs are used. Other serotoninergic medications (e.g., buspirone and trazodone) are not contraindicated but should be used with care. Other narcotic analgesics (e.g., propoxyphene, codeine, oxycodone, morphine, alfentanil, or morphine) appear to be safer alternatives to meperidine, but, in conjunction with MAOIs, their analgesic and CNS depressant effects may be potentiated, and they should be started at one fifth to one half of the standard doses and gradually titrated upward, with monitoring for untoward hemodynamic or mental status changes.[26,35,105]

Extremely adverse, although reversible, symptoms of fever, delirium, convulsions, hypotension, and dyspnea were reported on the combination of imipramine and MAOIs.[106] This has contributed to avoidance of the once popular TCA-MAOI combinations. Nevertheless, although incompletely studied, the regimen has been observed in some instances to be successful for exceptionally treatment-refractory patients.[107–110] When combined, simultaneous initiation of a TCA-MAOI or initiation of the TCA before but never after the MAOI is recommended as is avoidance of the more serotoninergic TCAs (in addition to clomipramine), including imipramine and amitriptyline.[111,112]

The sedative effects of CNS depressants may be potentiated by MAOIs, including the benzodiazepines, barbiturates, and chloral hydrate. MAOIs often cause postural hypotension, and severe additive effects have occurred when coadministered with vasodilator or antihypertensive medications or low-potency antipsychotics. As is true of the TCAs and low-potency antipsychotics, the MAOIs may block the antihypertensive effects of guanethidine, by an unknown mechanism, and may be dangerous when used concurrently with catecholamine-depleting antihypertensives (e.g., reserpine and methyldopa), which may cause hypertension, confusion, or manic symptoms in this setting.[26]

The MAOIs, similar to the TCAs, have also been observed to potentiate hypoglycemic agents, including insulin and sulfonylurea drugs. The mechanism of this potential interaction remains to be established. The several existing reports justify more frequent glucose monitoring when MAOIs are coadministered with hypoglycemic medications.[26]

Phenelzine has been associated with lowered serum pseudocholinesterase levels and prolonged neuromuscular blockade.[38] When possible, phenelzine may be discontinued 10 to 14 days before elective procedures requiring succinylcholine.[26] Nevertheless, the concurrent use of phenelzine is not a contraindication to surgery or electroconvulsive therapy (ECT).

There are case reports of a hypertensive crisis on propranolol that was presumably related to the combined effect of β-receptor blockade and unopposed α_1-adrenergic stimulation and of bradycardia in two patients on nadolol when phenelzine was added. β-Blockers, nevertheless, may be coadministered with MAOIs, provided that there is close monitoring and cautious dosing.[26]

β-Agonists, including the methylxanthines and inhaled bronchodilators, are not contraindicated, although the potential exists for enhanced β-adrenergic effects including tachycardia, palpitations, and anxiety.[26]

The development of reversible inhibitors of MAO-A, such as moclobemide and brofaromine, and of novel delivery systems, such as transdermal selegiline[113] offers some promise that MAOIs will be devised that provide antidepressant benefits with lesser dietary and medication restrictions. Until the efficacy and safety of these alternative MAOIs is established, however, phenelzine, tranylcypromine, and isocarboxazid continue to serve an important role in the management of depression and anxiety disorders refractory to other treatments.

Stimulants

Psychostimulants have provided an often rapidly effective treatment of depressive symptoms among elderly and medically frail individuals, including those with heart disease or HIV infection, who would be at particular risk from anticholinergic, hypotensive, sedative, or quinidine-like effects of the TCAs.[113–116] Although the broader range of options presented by the newer antidepressants has limited the need for stimulants in these settings, they continue to be recruited as antidepressants and antidepressant adjuncts to the SSRIs, TCAs, and bupropion in the management of treatment-refractory depression. In addition, the cautious combination of methylphenidate and dextroamphetamine with MAOIs has been found to be effective in a subset of treatment-refractory depressed patients[118–119] and in efforts to treat particularly severe postural hypotension on the MAOIs. In view of the high risk of hypertensive crises, the addition of stimulants to MAOIs for antidepressant augmentation should remain an option only in exceptional cases in which other options (e.g., ECT) have been carefully weighed.

A variety of drug-drug interactions involving the psychostimulants have been reported. These include increased plasma levels of TCAs (and possibly other antidepressants); increased plasma levels of phenobarbital, primidone, and phenytoin; increased prothrombin time on anticoagulants; attenuation or reversal of the guanethidine antihypertensive effect; and increased pressor responses to vasopressor drugs.[26]

Although methylphenidate has been implicated in putative drug interactions more often than dextroamphetamine or mixed amphetamine salts, drug interactions involving psychostimulants have been insufficiently studied to draw firm conclusions about their comparative suitability for use among patients on complex medical regimens.[120]

Benzodiazepines

The benzodiazepines are a class of widely prescribed psychotropic drugs that have anxiolytic, sedative, muscle-relaxant, and anticonvulsant properties. Their rate of onset of action, duration of action, presence of active metabolites, and tendency to accumulate in the body vary considerably and can influence both side effects and the success of treatment. Most benzodiazepines are well absorbed on an empty stomach, with peak plasma levels achieved generally between 1 and 3 hours, although with more rapid onset of some (e.g., diazepam and clorazepate) than others (e.g., oxazepam). Duration of action of a single dose of benzodiazepine generally depends more on distribution from systemic circulation to tissue than on subsequent elimination (e.g., more rapid for diazepam than lorazepam). With repeated doses, however, the volume of distribution is saturated, and elimination half-life becomes the more important parameter in determining duration of action (e.g., more rapid for lorazepam than diazepam). A benzodiazepine that is comparatively short-acting on acute administration may therefore become relatively long-acting on long-term dosing. Benzodiazepines are highly lipophilic and distribute readily to the CNS and to tissues. Plasma protein-binding ranges from approximately 70% (alprazolam) to 99% (diazepam).[7]

Of the benzodiazepines, only lorazepam, oxazepam, and temazepam are not subject to phase I metabolism. Because phase II metabolism (glucuronide conjugation) does not produce active metabolites and is less affected than phase I metabolism by primary liver disease, aging, and concurrently used inducers or inhibitors of hepatic microsomal enzymes, the 3-hydroxy substituted benzodiazepines are much preferred in such settings. Under normal circumstances, the triazolobenzodiazepines have metabolites that are minimally active. In contrast to the 3-hydroxy substituted benzodiazepines, however, plasma levels of these benzodiazepines (alprazolam, midazolam, and triazolam) are much more likely to be affected by factors that interfere with hepatic metabolism, particularly those involving cytochrome P450 3A4. The nonbenzodiazepine, sedative-hypnotic agents zolpidem and zaleplon are also substrates of cytochrome P450 3A4, the metabolism of which may be inhibited by nefazodone, fluvoxamine, and other agents and induced by rifampin and carbamazepine to name a few.

Perhaps the most common and clinically significant interactions involving benzodiazepines are the additive CNS-depressant effects, which can occur when a benzodiazepine is administered concurrently with barbiturates, narcotics, or ethanol. These interactions can be serious because of their potential to cause excessive sedation, cognitive and psychomotor impairment, and, at higher doses, potentially fatal respiratory depression. An interesting pharmacodynamic interaction exists between benzodiazepines and physostigmine, which can act as a competitive inhibitor at the benzodiazepine receptor, antagonizing benzodiazepine effects. The specific benzodiazepine antagonist, flumazenil, however, is now more commonly the treatment of choice in managing a severe benzodiazepine overdose. Another pharmacodynamic interaction concerns possible reduction of levodopa efficacy in some patients with Parkinson's disease concurrently treated with benzodiazepines. This is presumably related to the γ-aminobutyric acid facilitatory influence of the benzodiazepines, which may counter dopamine's stimulatory effects of levodopa in the basal ganglia.[26] Orally administered progesterone has been observed to enhance the psychomotor, memory, and sedative effects of triazolam, without affecting benzodiazepine clearance.[120] Although the generality of this finding for other benzodiazepines and steroid hormones is unknown, it would be consistent with in vitro binding studies suggesting that progesterone metabolites, such as 3α-hydroxy-5α-dihydroprogesterone, modulate the $GABA_A$ receptor, thereby potentially altering the pharmacodynamic effects of concurrently administered benzodiazepines.[121]

Pharmacokinetic interactions include a decreased rate of absorption of benzodiazepines but probably not decreased extent of absorption in the presence of antacids or food. This is more likely to be a factor in determining the subjective effects accompanying the onset of benzodiazepine action for single-dose rather than repeated-dose administration. Carbamazepine, phenobarbital, and rifampin may induce metabolism, lowering levels of benzodiazepines that are oxidatively metabolized. In contrast, potential inhibitors of cytochrome P450 3A4, including macrolide antibiotics, antifungals (e.g., ketoconazole and itraconazole), nefazodone, fluvoxamine, and cimetidine, have been associated with decreased clearance of the triazolobenzodiazepines metabolized through this pathway. The metabolism of diazepam depends in part on cytochrome P450 2C19. Decreased diazepam clearance has been reported with concurrent administration of fluoxetine, sertraline, propranolol, metoprolol, omeprazole, disulfiram, low-dose estrogen containing oral contraceptives, and isoniazid.[26]

Psychiatric Uses of Nonpsychiatric Medications

In the general hospital, consideration of the psychiatric complications of nonpsychiatric medications[122] is an integral part of the evaluation of alterations in mood, behavior, or mental status. A selected array of nonpsychiatric medications that are associated with neuropsychiatric symptoms are listed in the this text in the differential diagnosis of mood changes (Chapter 8), delirium (Chapter 12), psychosis (Chapter 14), and anxiety (Chapter 15) in the medical setting. Nevertheless, whether by extrapolation from known in vitro mechanisms or through serendipity, nonpsychiatric drugs have also been found to be useful in the treatment of psychiatric illness. These include medications that ameliorate the side effects of psychotropic drugs as well as the growing number of nonpsychiatric medications studied for the treatment of mood, anxiety, psychotic, substance abuse, attentional, and tic disorders.

Medications for Psychotropic Drug Side Effects

The importance of attentive management of psychotropic drug side effects for the alleviation of patient suffering, the development of a therapeutic alliance, and the likelihood of patient adherence to necessary treatment continues to fuel the search for effective pharmacologic strategies when more conservative measures fail to reduce dangerous or difficult to tolerate side effects.[7,96] Anticholinergic agents (benztropine 1 to 2 mg twice a day, biperiden 1 to 3 mg twice a day, and trihexyphenidyl 1 to 3 mg twice a day) and, less frequently, anticholinergic antihistamines (diphenhydramine 25 to 50 mg twice a day) and amantadine (100 mg two to three times a day) are used widely for the management of the parkinsonian side effects of antipsychotics. Benztropine 2 mg and diphenhydramine 50 mg are also used intramuscularly or intravenously for the acute management of dystonia. Anticholinergic side effects are not uncommon, however, and combination of these drugs with other highly anticholinergic agents (e.g., tertiary amine TCAs) invites the risk of frank toxicity. In this regard, IV physostigmine has been used in the emergency management of the anticholinergic syndrome, which includes delirium and tachyarrhythmias.

β-Blockers (including propranolol starting at 10 to 20 mg one to two times a day or the less centrally active atenolol 50 mg/day) have been useful for akathisia on antipsychotics and antidepressants, for lithium-associated tremor, and, less frequently, for jitteriness on antidepressants. Although the risk of depression on β-blockers is likely to be quite small, it is still reasonable nevertheless to monitor for alterations in mood whenever moderate to high doses of the more lipophilic CNS active agents are used (e.g., propranolol doses above 80 mg/day).[123,124]

Diuretics, including amiloride 5 to 10 mg one to three times a day and hydrochlorothiazide 50 to 100 mg/day, have been successful in the treatment of disruptive polyuria on lithium, albeit requiring potential lithium dose reduction and close monitoring of lithium levels and serum potassium. Anticholinergic side effects, including urinary retention, constipation, blurred vision, and dry mouth, may be treated with bethanechol 10 to 25 mg one to three times a day; dry mouth and blurred vision can also be treated with 1% pilocarpine ophthalmic solution. Excessive sweating on antidepressants is infrequently treated with the α_1-adrenergic agents terazosin (1 mg for every

hour of sleep) and doxazosin (1 to 2 mg for every hour of sleep) as well as with anticholinergic agents, such as benztropine (0.5 to 1.0 once or twice daily) or glycopyrrolate (1 to 2 mg once daily to three times a day).

Pharmacologic attempts to reduce orthostatic hypotension on antidepressants have included caffeine or cautious introduction of T_3 (25 to 50 μg/day), T_4 (50 to 200 μg/day), the mineralocorticoid fludrocortisone (0.05 to 0.5 mg/day), salt tablets (600 to 1800 mg/day), methylphenidate, or dextroamphetamine (5 to 20 mg/day). These measures tend to be used after other measures have failed, including efforts to maximize hydration and to improve venous return from the lower extremities by calf muscle exercises or surgical support stockings.

Nausea or indigestion that is not responsive to change in dosing strategy or a change in preparation has been successfully treated with nizatidine (150 to 300 mg/day), famotidine (20 to 40 mg/day), or metoclopramide (5 to 10 mg one to two times a day). It should be kept in mind that metoclopramide, a cholinergic agonist and dopamine antagonist, has been associated rarely with extrapyramidal and dyskinetic effects, akathisia, and a case of mania, and because it increases gastric motility, it can potentially affect the absorption of coadministered medications. With respect to the H_2 antagonists, although all are capable of producing mood and cognitive changes, including delirium, cimetidine, which has been most closely associated with these effects, is also a potent inhibitor of cytochrome P450 metabolism, rendering it least preferable among these agents for use in patients on multiple psychotropic medications. Similarly, omeprazole, an inhibitor of the gastric proton pump, appears to be both a P450 enzyme inducer (1A2) and inhibitor (2C),[4] and its potential impact on the metabolism of concurrent medications should therefore be considered when it is prescribed. Agents that block 5-HT$_3$ receptors also may be helpful in reduction of nausea related to serotonergic agents. Although odansetron is an option, a less expensive, albeit less selective, alternative for appropriate candidates is mirtazapine.

Diarrhea not responsive to changes in preparation or dosing is often responsive to standard agents, such as loperamide or diphenoxylate.

Acidophilus (1 capsule/meal) and cyproheptadine (2 to 4 mg one to three times a day) have also been used as antidiarrheal strategies.

Weight gain on psychotropic medications is common, distressing, and associated with risk of diabetes and hyperlipidemia. In addition to behavioral strategies for weight reduction, attention has also been directed toward pharmacologic strategies. In recent years, these have included exploratory use of the anticonvulsants topiramate (25 to 100 mg one to three times a day) and zonisamide (up to 600 mg once daily). Both agents have carbonic anhydrase inhibitory properties and have been linked to an increased risk of nephrolithiasis. Topiramate in particular is also associated with the side effects of cognitive dysfunction and sedation, which may be a limiting factor. The H_2 antagonists, including nizatidine (up to 300 mg/day) have also showed promise in curbing weight gain, as have dopaminergic agents and bupropion.

Sexual dysfunction has proved to be a particularly common and troublesome side effect of antidepressants, especially the SSRIs, including diminished libido, erectile dysfunction, ejaculatory delay, and anorgasmia. As an alternative to switching medications (e.g., to bupropion, nefazodone, or mirtazapine), a variety of partly effective strategies have been marshaled for when dose reductions or drug holidays[125] have not been feasible. These include sildenafil (25 to 100 mg/day)[126,127]; yohimbine (2.5 mg as needed up to 5.4 mg three times a day), potentially complicated by jitteriness, dizziness, or irritability; cyproheptadine (4 to 16 mg/day), with the potential, although apparently quite small, risk of interfering with serotoninergic antidepressant efficacy; bethanechol (10 to 25 mg one to three times a day); neostigmine (7.5 to 15 mg/day); and amantadine (100 mg two to three times a day). Psychotropic medications have also been used in an effort to treat sexual dysfunction, including bupropion (75 to 150 mg/day),[128] nefazodone (50 to 200 mg qd), methylphenidate (5 to 10 mg one to four times a day), trazodone (25 to 100 mg/day), buspirone (5 to 20 mg two to three times a day), as have dopamine agonists, such as ropinirole.[129] Improvement may be limited, not only by the lack of more effective pharmacologic strategies, but also by the impact of depressive illness on sexual interest and by the influence of rele-

vant psychosocial factors (e.g., marital conflict) that may accompany the depression.

$α_1$-Adrenergic Antagonists

Prazosin, the $α_1$-adrenergic receptor antagonist used for many years to treat hypertension, has been demonstrated in several open-label trials and a double-blind, placebo-controlled trial[130] to offer possible benefit at doses of up to 10 mg at bedtime in the treatment of core symptoms of posttraumatic stress disorder (PTSD), particularly nightmares, insomnia, and hyperarousal. Side effects include orthostatic blood pressure changes and dizziness, and particular caution docs need to be observed when administered concurrently with other agents with $α_1$-adrenergic blocking properties, including low potency antipsychotics.

$α_2$-Adrenergic Agonists

The antihypertensive clonidine is highly lipophilic and readily crosses the blood-brain barrier, where it stimulates $α_2$-adrenergic receptors. In 1980 it was first reported to be an effective pharmacotherapy for Gilles de la Tourette's syndrome of chronic multiple motor and phonic tics,[131] and, as such, an alternative to antipsychotic drugs (such as haloperidol and pimozide and, more recently, risperidone), which have been the mainstays of treatment for this disabling condition arising in childhood. Clonidine alone or with naltrexone has been useful in suppressing the signs and symptoms of autonomic hyperactivity associated with inpatient detoxification from narcotic substances, including heroin, methadone, narcotic analgesics, and propoxyphene.[132] Although generally more likely to cause sedation and hypotension than other treatments for akathisia (e.g., anticholinergic medications, β-blockers, and benzodiazepines), clonidine has also been used to reduce akathisia refractory to other agents.[133] Finally, clonidine has been shown effective in the treatment of ADHD in children and adolescents,[134] and although its use is limited by side effects, it has been helpful in cases in which there is a marked hyperactive or aggressive component. Although controlled trials are generally lacking, guanfacine, another $α_2$-adrenergic receptor agonist antihypertensive drug, appears to be useful for many of the same indications as clonidine but with the potential advantages of a longer half-life and generally less sedation.[135,136]

β-Blockers

In addition to their role in the treatment of akathisia and tremor, the nonselective β-adrenergic receptor antagonists, which block the β_1-adrenergic receptors in heart and brain and β_2-adrenergic receptors in lung, blood vessels, and brain (including glial cells), have been among the first-line treatments for organically based aggressive behavior.[137] Antiaggressive β-blockers include the lipid-soluble agents propranolol and pindolol and the water-soluble agent nadolol.[138] Doses used are generally high (e.g., propranolol up to about 12 mg/kg/day), and there may be a response latency of as long as 6 to 8 weeks. High doses of propranolol may have modest adjuvant antipsychotic properties[139] and antimanic effects[140]; however, the need for doses as high as 800 to 2000 mg or more has limited the utility of this treatment approach.

Much lower doses of β-Blockers (e.g., propranolol 10 to 40 mg or the equivalent) have been used widely to reduce symptoms associated with performance anxiety[141] and are not uncommonly used for this purpose by musicians and public speakers. β-Blockers are less likely to be effective pharmacotherapy for more generalized forms of social phobia, however, when compared with benzodiazepines, MAOIs, or SSRIs. The β-blockers have also had limited use for treatment of autonomic arousal associated with other anxiety states, including PTSD, generalized anxiety disorder, and panic disorder.

The prescription of β-Blockers is potentially hazardous in a variety of common clinical conditions, including bronchospastic pulmonary diseases, insulin-dependent diabetes, hyperthyroidism, significant peripheral vascular disease, and congestive heart failure. In addition, β-blockers entirely or primarily eliminated by liver (e.g., propranolol, metoprolol, and pindolol) may be inhibitors of, as well as substrates for, hepatic microsomal enzymes and are therefore more likely to be subject to pharmacokinetic drug interactions than β-blockers primarily cleared by kidney (e.g., atenolol, nadolol, and sotalol).[142]

Modafinil

The relatively benign side-effect profile of modafinil, together with its stimulant-like properties but differing mechanism, have motivated efforts to define the potential role in psychiatry of this wakefulness promoting agent currently approved for treatment of narcolepsy. Its success as a treatment for fatigue in neurologic conditions, particularly multiple sclerosis[143] suggests the possibility of usefulness as a treatment for drowsiness related to other causes, including medications, although these uses have not yet been adequately studied. In addition, it has shown some promise in initial studies as an agent, like the psychostimulants, useful for treatment of depression with comorbid medical illness[144] and as an antidepressant adjunct in refractory depression.[145] Likewise, preliminary work has also suggested efficacy for children[146] and adults[147] with ADHD. Clinical and preclinical studies have suggested that modafinil may be less likely than methylphenidate or dextroamphetamine (Dexedrine) to generate euphoria[148]; nevertheless it is a Schedule IV drug and its abuse liability is not yet known to be less than the psychostimulants in real-world clinical settings. In addition, the risks of exacerbating psychosis or unmasking motor tics in predisposed individuals, as can occur on psychostimulants, is not well-defined. Finally, modafinil interacts with the P450 cytochrome isoenzymes as a minimal to moderate inducer of 3A4 and yet inhibitor of the 2C isoforms.[149] Modafinil may thereby engage in drug-drug interactions with common substrates, including oral contraceptives (the levels of which may decrease) and β-blockers and warfarin (the levels of which may increase), which require monitoring and patient education.

References

1. Stoudemire A, Fogel BS, Greenberg DB, editors: *Psychiatric care of the medical patient*, ed 2, New York, 2001, Oxford.
2. Robinson RG, Yates WR: *Psychiatric treatment of the medically ill*, New York, 1999, Marcel Dekker.
3. Joseph R, Kontos N: *Polypharmacy in the medically ill psychiatric patient*. In Ghaemi SN, editor: *Polypharmacy in psychiatry*, New York, 2002, Marcel Dekker.

4. Cozza KL, Armstrong SC, Oesterheld JR: *Drug interaction principles for medical practice*, ed 2, Washington DC, 2003, American Psychiatric Publishing.

5. Glassman AH, O'Connor CM, Califf RM, et al: Sertraline treatment of major depression in patients with acute MI or unstable angina, *JAMA* 288:701–709, 2002.

6. Fava M, Rush AJ, Trivedi MH, et al: Background and rationale for the sequenced treatment alternatives to relieve depression (STAR*D) study, *Psychiatr Clin North Am* 26:457–494, 2003.

7. Arana GW, Hyman SE, Rosenbaum JF: *Handbook of psychiatric drug therapy*, ed 4, Boston, 2000, Lippincott Williams & Wilkins.

8. Overall JE, Gorham DR: The brief psychiatric rating scale, *Psychol Rep* 10:799–812, 1962.

9. Hamilton M: Development of a rating scale for primary depressive illness, *Br J Soc Clin Psychol* 6:278–296, 1967.

10. Hamilton M: Diagnosis and rating of anxiety, *Br J Psychiatry* 3:76–79, 1969.

11. Young RC, Biggs, JT, Ziegler VE, et al: A rating scale for mania: reliability, validity and sensitivity, *Br J Psychiatry* 133:429–435, 1978.

12. Beck AT, Ward CH, Mendelson M, et al: An inventory for measuring depression, *Arch Gen Psychiatry* 4:561–571, 1961.

13. American Psychiatric Association: *Diagnostic and statistical manual of mental disorders*, ed 4, Washington, DC, 1994, American Psychiatric Association.

14. Guy W, editor: *Early Clinical Drug Evaluation Unit assessment manual for psychopharmacology*, Department of Health, Education and Welfare Publ. No. ADM-76-338, Washington, DC, 1976, U.S. Government Printing Office.

15. Markowitz JS, DeVane CL: The emerging recognition of herb-drug interactions with a focus on St. John's Wort (*Hypericum perforatum*), *Psychopharm Bull* 35:53–64, 2001.

16. Fugh-Berman A, Ernst E: Herb-drug interactions: review and assessment of report reliability, *Br J Clin Pharmacol* 52:587–595, 2001.

17. Geddes JR, Carney SM, Davies C, et al: Relapse prevention with antidepressant drug treatment in depressive disorders: a systematic review, *Lancet* 361:653–661, 2003.

18. Faedda GL, Tondo L, Baldessarini RJ, et al: Outcome after rapid vs gradual discontinuation of lithium treatment in bipolar disorders, *Arch Gen Psychiatry* 50:448–155, 1993.

19. Baldessarini RJ, Viguera AC: Neuroleptic withdrawal in schizophrenic patients, *Arch Gen Psychiatry* 52:189–192, 1995.

20. Post RM, Leverich GS, Altshuler L, et al: Lithium discontinuation-induced refractoriness: preliminary observations, *Am J Psychiatry* 149:1727–1729, 1992.

21. Kahn AY, Preskorn SH: *Pharmacokinetic principles and drug interactions*. In Soares JC, Gershon S, editors: *Handbook of medical psychiatry*, New York, 2003, Marcel Dekker, pp 933–944.

22. Wilkinson GR: *Pharmacokinetics: the dynamics of drug absorption, distribution, and elimination*. In Hardman JG, Limbird LE, Gilman AG, editors: *Goodman and Gilman's the pharmacological basis of therapeutics*, ed 10, New York, 2001, McGraw-Hill, pp 3–29.

23. Yonkers KA, Kando JC, Cole JO, et al: Gender differences in pharmacokinetics and pharmacodynamics of psychotropic medication, *Am J Psychiatry* 149:587–595, 1992.

24. Von Moltke LL, Greenblatt DJ: Drug transporters in psychopharmacology—are they important? *J Clin Psychopharmacol* 20:291–294, 2000.

25. Liston HL, Markowitz JS, DeVane CL: Drug glucuronidation in clinical psychopharmacology, *J Clin Psychopharmacol* 21:500–515, 2001.

26. Ciraulo DA, Shader RI, Greenblatt DJ, et al: *Drug interactions in psychiatry*, ed 2, Baltimore, 1995, Williams & Wilkins.

27. DeVane CL, Nemeroff CB: 2002 guide to psychotropic drug interactions, *Primary Psychiatry* 9:28–57, 2002.

28. Ruiz P, editor: *Ethnicity and psychopharmacology*, ed 1, Washington DC, 2000, American Psychiatric Press.

29. Lin KM, Poland RE: *Ethnicity, culture, and psychopharmacology*. In Bloom FE, Kupfer DJ, editors: *Psychopharmacology: the fourth generation of progress*, New York, 1995, Raven Press.

30. Lieberman JA, Cooper TB, Suckow RF, et al: Tricyclic antidepressant and metabolite levels in renal failure, *Clin Pharmacol Ther* 37:301–307, 1985.

31. Alpert JE: *Drug-drug interactions in psychopharmacology*. In Stern TA, Herman JB, Slavin PL, editors: *Massachusetts General Hospital guide to primary care psychiatry*, ed 2, New York, 2004, McGraw-Hill.

32. Bernstein JG: Medical-psychiatric drug interactions. In Hackett TP, Cassem NH, editors: *Massachusetts General Hospital handbook of general hospital psychiatry*, St Louis, 1978, Mosby.

33. Goff DC, Baldessarini RJ: Drug interactions with antipsychotic agents, *J Clin Psychopharmacol* 13:57–67, 1993.

34. Meyer MC, Baldessarini RJ, Goff DC, et al: Clinically significant interactions of psychotropic agents with antipsychotic drugs, *Drug Saf* 15:333–346, 1996.

35. Taylor DM: Antipsychotics and QT prolongation, *Acta Psychiatr Scand* 107:85–95, 2003.

36. Tesar GE, Murray GB, Cassem NH: Use of high-dose intravenous haloperidol in the treatment of agitated cardiac patients, *J Clin Psychopharmacol* 5:344–347, 1985.

37. Risch SC, Groom GP, Janowsky DS: Interfaces of psychopharmacology and cardiology: II. *J Clin Psychiatry* 42:47–59, 1981.

38. Janowsky EC, Risch C, Janowsky DS: Effects of anesthesia on patients taking psychotropic drugs, *J Clin Psychopharmacol* 1:14–20, 1981.

39. Prakash R, Keiwala S, Ban TA: Neurotoxicity with combined administration of lithium with a neuroleptic, *Compr Psychiatry* 23:567–571, 1982.

40. Goldney RD, Spence ND: Safety of the combination of lithium and neuroleptic drugs, *Am J Psychiatry* 143:882–884, 1986.

41. Keck PJ, Pope HG, McElroy SL: Declining frequency of neuroleptic malignant syndrome in a hospital population, *Am J Psychiatry* 148:880–882, 1991.

42. Rosebush P, Stuart T: A prospective analysis of 24 episodes of neuroleptic malignant syndrome, *Am J Psychiatry* 146:717–725, 1989.

43. Desai HD, Seabolt J, Jann MW: Smoking in patients receiving psychotropic medications: a pharmacokinetic perspective. *CNS Drugs* 15:469–494, 2001.

44. Jefferson JW, Kalin NH: Serum lithium levels and long-term diuretic use, *JAMA* 241:1134–1136, 1979.

45. Saffer D, Coppen A: Furosemide: a safe diuretic during lithium therapy? *J Affect Disord* 5:289–292, 1983.

46. Batlle DC, von Riotte AB, Gaviria M, et al: Amelioration of polyuria by amiloride in patients receiving long-term lithium therapy, *N Engl J Med* 312:408–114, 1985.

47. Ragheb M, Powell AL: Lithium interactions with sulindac and naproxen, *J Clin Psychopharmacol* 6:150–154, 1986.

48. Ragheb M: The interaction of lithium with phenylbutazone in bipolar affective patients, *J Clin Psychopharmacol* 10:149–150, 1990.

49. Reinman IG, Diener U, Frolich JC: Indomethacin but not aspirin increases plasma lithium ion levels, *Arch Gen Psychiatry* 40:283–286, 1986.

50. Douste-Blazy P, Rostin M, Livarek B, et al: Angiotensin convening enzyme inhibitors and lithium treatment, *Lancet* 1:1448, 1986.

51. Ratey JJ, Ciraulo DA, Shader RI: *Lithium and marijuana*, J Clin Psychopharmacol 1:32–33, 1981.

52. Price WA, Giannini AJ: Neurotoxicity caused by lithium-verapamil synergism, *J Clin Pharmacol* 26:717–719, 1986.

53. Binder E: Diltiazem-induced psychosis and a possible diltiazem-lithium interaction, *Arch Intern Med* 151:373–374, 1991.

54. Walker N, White K, Tornatore F, et al: Lithium-methyldopa interactions in normal subjects, *Drug Intell Clin Pharm* 14:638, 1980.

55. Hollister LE: Hydroxyzine hydrochloride: possible adverse cardiac interactions, *Psychopharmacol Commun* 1:61–65, 1975.

56. Jefferson JW, Greist JH, Baudhuin M: Lithium: interactions with other drugs, *J Clin Psychopharmacol* 1:124–134, 1981.

57. Takami H: Lithium in the preoperative preparation of Graves' disease, *Int Surg* 79:89–90, 1994.

58. Austin LS, Arana GW, Melvin JA: Toxicity resulting from lithium augmentation of antidepressant treatment in elderly patients, *J Clin Psychiatry* 51:344–345, 1990.

59. Noveske FG, Hahn KR, Flynn RJ: Possible toxicity of combined fluoxetine and lithium, *Am J Psychiatry* 146:1515, 1989.

60. Keck PE, Arnold LM: The serotonin syndrome, *Psychiatric Ann* 30:333–343, 2000.

61. Nolen WA: Carbamazepine: a possible adjunct or alternative to lithium in bipolar disorder, *Acta Psychiatr Scand* 67:218–225, 1983.

62. McElroy S, Keck PE Jr, Pope HG Jr, et al: Valproate in bipolar disorder: literature review and treatment guidelines, *J Clin Psychopharmacol* 12:42S–52S, 1992.

63. Wilder BJ, Willmore LJ, Bruni J, et al: Valproic acid: interaction with other anticonvulsant drugs, *Neurology* 28:892–896, 1978.

64. May T, Rambeck B: Serum concentrations of valproic acid: influence of dose and comedication, *Ther Drug Monit* 7:387–390, 1985.

65. Tohen M, Castillo J, Pope HG Jr, et al: Concomitant use of valproate and carbamazepine in bipolar and schizoaffective disorders, *J Clin Psychopharmacol* 14:67–70, 1994.

66. Orr JM, Abbott FS, Farrell K, et al: Interaction between valproic acid in epileptic children: serum protein binding and metabolic effects, *Clin Pharmacol Ther* 31:642–649, 1982.

67. Webster LK, Mihaly GW, Jones DB, et al: Effect of cimetidine and ranitidine on carbamazepine and sodium valproate pharmacokinetics, *Eur J Clin Pharmacol* 27:341–343, 1984.

68. Sovner R, Davis JM: A potential drug interaction between fluoxetine and valproic acid, *J Clin Psychopharmacol* 11:389, 1991 (letter).

69. Watson WA: Interaction between clonazepam and sodium valproate, *N Engl J Med* 300:678–679, 1979.

70. Ketter TA, Post RM, Worthington K: Principles of clinically important drug interactions with carbamazepine: I and II. *J Clin Psychopharmacol* 11:198–203, 306–313, 1991.

71. Popli A, Tanquary J, Lamparella V, et al: Bupropion and anticonvulsant drug interactions, *Ann Clin Psychiatry* 7:99–101, 1995.

72. Yassa R, Nastase C, Camille Y, et al: Carbamazepine, diuretics, and hyponatremia: a possible interaction, *J Clin Psychiatry* 48:281–283, 1987.

73. Preskorn SH, Irwin HA: Toxicity of tricyclic antidepressants: kinetics, mechanism, intervention: a review, *J Clin Psychiatry* 43:151–156, 1982.

74. Baldessarini RJ: *Drugs and the treatment of psychiatric disorders.* In Gilman AG, Rall TW, Nies AS, et al, editors: *Goodman and Gilman's the pharmacological basis of therapeutics*, ed 8, New York, 1990, Pergamon Press.

75. Potter WZ, Manji HK: Antidepressants, metabolites, and apparent drug resistance, *Clin Neuropharmacol* 13:S43–S53, 1990.

76. Pollock BG, Everett G, Perel JM: Comparative cardiotoxicity of nortriptyline and its isomeric 10-hydroymetabolites, *Neuropsychopharmacology* 6:1–10, 1992.

77. Jefferson JW: Cardiovascular effects and toxicity of anxiolytics and antidepressants, *J Clin Psychiatry* 50:368–378, 1989.

78. Risch SC, Groom GP, Janowsky DS: Interfaces of psychopharmacology and cardiology: I. *J Clin Psychiatry* 42:23–34, 1981.

79. Witchel HJ, Hancok JC, Nutt DJ: Psychotropic drugs, cardiac arrhythmia and sudden death, *J Clin Psychopharmacol* 23:58–77, 2003.

80. Ayesh R, Dawling S, Widdop B, et al: Influence of quinidine on the pharmacokinetics of nortriptyline and desipramine, *Br J Clin Pharmacol* 25:140–141, 1988.

81. Katz MR: Raised serum levels of desipramine with the antiarrhythmic propafenone, *J Clin Psychiatry* 52:432, 1991 (letter).

82. Glassman AH, Roose SP, Bigger JT Jr: The safety of tricyclic antidepressants in cardiac patients: risk-benefit reconsidered, *JAMA* 269:2673–2675, 1993.

83. Nelson JC, Jatlow PI, Bock J: Major adverse reactions during desipramine treatment, relationship to plasma drug concentrations, concomitant antipsychotic treatment, and patient characteristics, *Arch Gen Psychiatry* 39:1055–1061, 1982.

84. Gram LF, Fredricson Overo K, Kirk L: Influence of neuroleptics and benzodiazepines on metabolism of tricyclic antidepressants in man, *Am J Psychiatry* 131:863–866, 1974.

85. Henhauer SA, Hollister LE: Cimetidine interaction with imipramine and nortriptyline, *Clin Pharmacol Ther* 35:183–187, 1984.

86. Nelson JC: Combined treatment strategies in psychiatry, *J Clin Psychiatry* 54:S42–S49, 1993.

87. Richelson E: Pharmacology of antidepressants, *Mayo Clin Proc* 76:511–527, 2001.

88. Skinner MH, Kuan H-Y, Pan A, et al: Duloxetine is both an inhibitor and a substrate of cytochrome P450 2D6 in healthy volunteers, *Clin Pharmacol Ther* 73:170–177, 2003.

89. Walley T, Pirmohamed M, Proudlove C, et al: Interaction of metoprolol and fluoxetine, *Lancet* 341:967–968, 1993 (letter).

90. Drake W, Gordon G: Heart block in a patient on propranolol and fluoxetine, *Lancet* 343:425–426, 1994 (letter).

91. Bannister SJ, Houser VP, Hulse JD, et al: Evaluation of the potential for interactions of paroxetine with diazepam, cimetidine, warfarin, and digoxin, *Acta Psychiatr Scand* 80(suppl 350):102–106, 1989.

92. Preskorn SH: Should bupropion dosage be adjusted based upon therapeutic drug monitoring? *Psychopharmacol Bull* 27:637–643, 1991.

93. van Putten T, Shaffer I: Delirium associated with bupropion, *J Clin Psychopharmacol* 10:234, 1990.

94. Abo-Zena RA, Bobek MB, Dweik RA: Hypertensive urgency induced by an interaction of mirtazapine and clonidine, *Pharmacotherapy* 20:47–478, 2000.

95. Kinrys G, Simon N, Farach FJ, et al: Management of antidepressant-induced side effects. In Alpert JE, Fava M, editors: *Handbook of chronic depression*, New York, Marcel Dekker, in press.

96. Livingston MG, Livingston HM: Monoamine oxidase inhibitors: an update on drug interactions, *Drug Saf* 14:219–227, 1997.

97. Blackwell B: Monoamine oxidase inhibitor interactions with other drugs, *J Clin Psychopharmacol* 11:55–59, 1991.

98. Harrison WM, McGrath PJ, Stewart JW, et al: MAOIs and hypertensive crises: the role of OTC drugs, *J Clin Psychiatry* 50:64–65, 1989.

99. Wells DG: MAOIs revisited, *Can J Anaesth* 36:64–74, 1989.

100. McCabe BJ: Dietary tyramine and other pressor amines in MAOI regimens: a review, *J Am Diet Assoc* 86:1059–1064, 1986.

101. Rabkin JG, Quitkin FM, Harrison W, et al: Adverse reactions to monoamine oxidase inhibitors: I. a comparative study, *J Clin Psychopharmacol* 4:270–278, 1984.

102. Rabkin JG, Quitkin FM, McGrath P, et al: Adverse reactions to monoamine oxidase inhibitors: II. treatment correlates and clinical management, *J Clin Psychopharmacol* 5:2–9, 1985.

103. Gardner DM, Shulman KI, Walker SE, et al: The making of a user-friendly MAOI diet, *J Clin Psychiatry* 57:99–104, 1996.

104. Gratz SS, Simpson GM: MAOI-narcotic interactions, *J Clin Psychiatry* 54:439, 1993.

105. Schuckit M, Robins E, Feighner J: Tricyclic antidepressant and monoamine oxidase inhibitors: combination therapy in the treatment of depression, *Arch Gen Psychiatry* 24:509–514, 1971.

106. Ravaris CL, Robinson DS, Ives JO, et al: Phenelzine and amitriptyline in the treatment of depression, *Arch Gen Psychiatry* 37:1075–1080, 1980.

107. Ranzani J, White KL, White J, et al: The safety and efficacy of combined amitriptyline and tranylcypromine antidepressant treatment: a controlled trial, *Arch Gen Psychiatry* 40:657–661, 1983.

108. Schmauss M, Kapfhammer HP, Meyr P, et al: Combined MAO-inhibitor and tri-(tetra-) cyclic antidepressant treatment in therapy-resistant depression, *Prog Neuropsychopharmacol Biol Psychiatry* 12:523–532, 1988.

109. Tyrer P, Murphy S: Effect of combined antidepressant therapy in resistant neurotic disorder, *Br J Psychiatry* 156:115–118, 1990.

110. White K, Simpson G: Combined MAOI-tricyclic antidepressant treatment: a reevaluation, *J Clin Psychopharmacol* 1:264–282, 1981.

111. Lader M: Combined use of tricyclic antidepressants and monoamine oxidase inhibitors, *J Clin Psychiatry* 44:20–24, 1983.

112. Bodkin JA, Amsterdam JD: Transdermal selegiline in major depression: a double-blind, placebo-controlled, parallel-group study in outpatients. *Am J Psychiatry* 159:1869–75,2002.

113. Kaufmann WM, Murray GB, Cassem NH: Use of psychostimulants in medically ill depressed patients, *Psychosomatics* 23:817–819, 1982.

114. Masand PS, Tesar GE: Use of psychostimulants in the medically ill, *Psychiatr Clin North Am* 19:515–547, 1996.

115. Wallace AE, Kofoed LL, West AN: Double-blind, placebo-controlled trial of methylphenidate in older, depressed medically ill patients, *Am J Psychiatry* 152:929–931, 1005.

116. Breitbart W, Rosenfeld B, Kaim M, et al: A randomized, double-blind, placebo-controlled trial of psychostimulants for the treatment of fatigue in ambulatory patients with human immunodeficiency virus disease, *Arch Intern Med* 161:411–420, 2001.

117. Feighner JP, Herbstein J, Damlouji N: Combined MAOI, TCA, and direct stimulant therapy of treatment-resistant depression, *J Clin Psychiatry* 46:206–209, 1985.

118. Fawcett J, Kravitz HM, Zajecka JM, et al: CNS stimulant potentiation of monoamine oxidase inhibitors in treatment-refractory depression, *J Clin Psychopharmacol* 11:127–132, 1991.

119. Markowitz JS, Morrison SD, DeVane CL: Drug interactions with psychostimulants, *Int Clin Psychopharm* 14:1–18, 1999.

120. McAuley JW, Reynolds IJ, Kroboth FJ, et al: Orally administered progesterone enhances sensitivity to triazolam in postmenopausal women, *J Clin Psychopharmacol* 15:3–11, 1995.

121. Bernstein JG: *Psychiatric side effects and psychiatric uses of nonpsychiatric drugs.* In Bernstein JG: *Drug therapy in psychiatry,* ed 3, Boston, 1995, PSG Inc.

122. Bright RA, Everitt DE: β-Blockers and depression: evidence against an association, *JAMA* 267:1783–1787, 1992.

123. Petrie WM, Maffucci RJ, Woolsey RL: Propranolol and depression, *Am J Psychiatry* 139:92–93, 1982.

124. Rothschild A: Selective serotonin reuptake inhibitor-induced sexual dysfunction: efficacy of a drug holiday, *Am J Psychiatry* 10:1514–1516, 1995.

125. Fava M, Rankin MA, Alpert JE, et al: An open trial of oral sildenafil for antidepressant-induced sexual dysfunction, *Psychother Psychosom* 67:328–331, 1998.

126. Nurnberg HG, Hensley PL, Gelenberg AJ, et al: Treatment of antidepressant-associated sexual dysfunction with sildenafil: a randomized controlled trial, *JAMA* 289:56–64, 2003.

127. Gitlin MJ, Suri R, Altshuler L, et al: Bupropion-sustained release as a treatment for SSRI-induced sexual side effects, *J Sex Marital Ther* 28:131–138, 2002.

128. Worthington JJ, Simon NM, Korbly NB, et al: *Ropinirole for SSRI-induced sexual dysfunction,* New Orleans, 2001, 154th Annual Meeting of the American Psychiatric Association, New Orleans.

129. Raskin MA, Peskind ER, Kanter ED, et al: Reduction of nightmares and other PTSD symptoms in combat veterans by prazosin: a placebo-controlled study, *Am J Psychiatry* 160:371–373, 2003.

130. Cohen DJ, Detlor J, Young JG, et al: Clonidine ameliorates Gilles de la Tourette's syndrome, *Arch Gen Psychiatry* 37:1350–1357, 1980.

131. Charney DS, Heninger GR, Kleber HD: The combined use of clonidine and naltrexone as a rapid, safe, and effective treatment of abrupt withdrawal from methadone, *Am J Psychiatry* 143:831–837, 1986.

132. Adler LA, Angrist B, Peselow E, et al: Clonidine in neuroleptic-induced akathisia, *Am J Psychiatry* 144:235–236, 1987.

133. Hunt RD, Minderaa RB, Cohen DJ: Clonidine benefits children with attention deficit disorder and hyperactivity: report of a double-blind placebo-crossover therapeutic trial, *J Am Acad Child Adolesc Psychiatry* 24:617–629, 1985.

134. Hunt RD, Arnsten AFT, Asbell MD: An open trial of guanfacine in the treatment of attention-deficit hyperactivity disorder, *J Am Acad Child Adolesc Psychiatry* 34:50–54, 1995.

135. San L, Cami J, Pier JM, et al: Efficacy of clonidine, guanfacine and methadone in the rapid detoxification of heroin addicts: a controlled clinical trial, *Br J Addict* 85:141–147, 1990.

136. Yudofsky SC, Silver JM, Hales RE: *Treatment of aggressive disorders.* In Schatzberg AF, Nemeroff CB, editors: *The American Psychiatric Press textbook of psychopharmacology,* Washington, DC, 1995, American Psychiatric Press.

137. Ratey JJ, Sorgi P, O'Driscoll GA, et al: Nadolol to treat aggression and psychiatric symptomatology in chronic psychiatric inpatients: a double-blind, placebo-controlled study, *J Clin Psychiatry* 53:41–46, 1992.

138. Manchanda R, Hirsch SR: Does propranolol have an antipsychotic effect? A placebo-controlled study in acute schizophrenia, *Br J Psychiatry* 148:701–707, 1986.

139. Von Zerssen D: Beta-adrenergic blocking agents in the treatment of psychosis: a report on 17 cases, *Adv Clin Psychopharmacol* 43:491–492, 1972.

140. Liebowitz MR, Schneier FR, Hollander E, et al: Treatment of social phobia with drugs other than benzodiazepines, *J Clin Psychiatry* 52(suppl 11):10–15, 1991.

141. Ratey JJ, McNaughton KL: *β-Blockers.* In Ciraulo DA, Shader RI, Greenblatt DJ, et al, editors: *Drug interactions in psychiatry,* ed 2, Baltimore, 1995, Williams & Wilkins.

142. Rammohan KW, Rosenberg JH, Lynn DJ, et al: Efficacy and safety of modafinil (Provigil) for the treatment of fatigue in multiple sclerosis: a two centre

phase 2 study, *J Neurol Neurosurg Psychiatry* 72: 179–183, 2002.

143. Schwartz TL, Leso L, Beale M, et al: Modafinil in the treatment of depression with severe comorbid medical illness, *Psychosomatics* 43:336–337, 2002.

144. Menza MA, Kaufman KR, Castellanos A: Modafinil augmentation of antidepressant treatment in depression, *J Clin Psychiatry* 61:378–381, 2000.

145. Rugino TA, Copley TC: Effects of modafinil in children with attention-deficit/hyperactivity disorder: an open-label study, *J Am Acad Child Adolesc Psychiatry* 40:230–235, 2001.

146. Taylor FB, Russo J: Efficacy of modafinil compared to dextroamphetamine for the treatment of attention deficit hyperactivity disorder in adults, *J Child Adolesc Psychopharmacol* 10:311–320, 2000.

147. Jasinski DR, Kovacevic-Ristanovic R: Evaluation of the abuse liability of modafinil and other drugs for excessive daytime sleepiness associated with narcolepsy, *Clin Neuropharmacol* 23:149–156, 2000.

148. Robertson P Jr., Hellriegel ET: Clinical pharmacokinetic profile of modafinil, *Clin Pharmacokinet* 42:123–137, 2003.

Chapter 19

Functional Somatic Symptoms and Somatoform Disorders

Arthur J. Barsky, M.D.
Theodore A. Stern, M.D.
Donna B. Greenberg, M.D.
Ned H. Cassem, M.D., S.J.

Although Ms. A was only 26 years old, she had been experiencing abdominal pain for 10 years. Multiple contrast radiographic, ultrasonographic, computed tomographic, endoscopic, and colonoscopic studies and three exploratory laparotomies failed to diagnose an organic cause for her pain. Despite appearing active, energetic, and healthy, she had become progressively incapacitated by her pain. Admitted to the surgical service, Ms. A was referred for psychiatric evaluation with questions about diagnosis, prognosis, advisability of proceeding to another laparotomy, and, above all, recommendations for acute and chronic pain management.

Called by Lipowski[1] "the borderland between medicine and psychiatry," *somatization*, defined here as experiencing and complaining about physical symptoms for which there are no discoverable organic causes, presents a fascinating challenge to the consultation psychiatrist. In an excellent review of functional somatic symptoms, Kellner[2] noted that 60% to 80% of a nonpatient population experiences one or more somatic symptoms in any given week. When a patient approaches a physician with a somatic complaint, no organic cause can be found between 20% and 84% of the time. Commonest among these functional somatic symptoms are palpitations, chest pain, headache, fatigue, and dizziness. For patients who persist in searching for a medical cause for their functional symptoms, the dangers of invasive diagnostic procedures, unnecessary surgery, and misdirected therapeutic drug trials can be life-threatening, and the unwarranted costs of these measures further strain limited medical resources.

Differential Diagnosis of Functional Somatic Symptoms

Asked to evaluate a patient whose somatic symptoms show no causative physical abnormality, or that seem far out of proportion to any abnormalities found, the psychiatrist should not think first of the somatoform disorders. Other psychiatric disorders, such as depression, are found far more often. Indeed, half of all the primary care patients who ultimately receive a psychiatric diagnosis presented initially with exclusively somatic symptoms,[3] and 75% of those with major depression or panic disorder on a diagnostic interview presented to their physicians with exclusively somatic symptoms.[4,5] As with any condition, a systematic differential diagnostic approach is required. Table 19-1 lists the diagnoses most likely to produce somatized complaints.

Table 19-1. Differential Diagnosis of Functional Somatic Symptoms: Diagnosis Producing Somatoform Complaints

Physical Disease	Personality Disorders
Depressive disorders	Dependent
Anxiety disorders	Passive-aggressive
Substance abuse disorders	Antisocial
Psychotic disorders	Borderline
Organic mental disorders	Narcissistic
Voluntary symptom production	Compulsive
Malingering	Histrionic
Factitious disorders	Paranoid
Somatoform disorders	Schizoid
	Schizotypal

The approach to these patients must include a thorough history and examination: medical history, personal and family psychiatric history, psychosocial history, current medications, and current laboratory examination results. In fact, the consultant's first question in differential diagnosis should be, "What organic disease, possibly still undiagnosed, could account for these symptoms?" Even when dealing with functional somatic symptoms, this remains the first question because such symptoms often occur in the context of serious medical disease. Reading both the current and (too often formidable) old chart is an indispensable beginning. Not infrequently, a psychiatrist may end up diagnosing a physical disease because something about the patient (personality, odd affect, behavior, or cognition) has effectively distracted the primary physician and obscured the underlying disease.

Depressive Disorders

Depression with somatoform complaints is far more common than is somatoform disorder. Many of the symptoms (e.g., insomnia, fatigue, anorexia, and weight loss) of major depression are somatic in nature.[6] Moreover, depressed patients have more functional somatic symptoms (aches and pains, constipation, dizziness, and the like) than do other patients. The presence of depression behind a veil of functional somatic symptoms is sometimes betrayed by the patient's attitude toward his or her condition. The depressed patient differs from the patient with a somatoform disorder in

feeling that he or she is not worth treating, does not deserve to feel better, and is hopelessness about improvement. There is good evidence that hypochondriacal preoccupations during depressive episodes increase with age. (For further coverage of affective disorders, see Chapter 8.)

When major depression is diagnosed, it should be treated first. Ordinarily both affective and somatic symptoms improve with treatment, although, as shall be discussed, sometimes only the affective illness remits, leaving functional somatic symptoms still to be managed.

Anxiety Disorders

Symptoms of anxiety intermingle with and pervade functional somatic symptoms. Anxiety biases one's attention toward dangerous and threatening perceptions. It also distorts the cognitive appraisal of somatic symptoms, making them seem more ominous and more alarming. Anxious patients thus tend to catastrophize normal physiologic sensations and trivial ailments. As noted in Chapter 15, many of the symptoms of panic disorder are somatic (e.g., dyspnea, palpitations, chest pain, choking, dizziness, paresthesias, hot and cold flashes, sweating, faintness, and trembling).

Although anxiety is not as likely as depression to escape the notice of the primary physician, panic disorder often goes unrecognized. It is far more prevalent among patients with medically unexplained symptoms than was once thought, especially in cardiology, gastroenterology, and neurology practices.[7,8] Even when panic disorder, phobia, or obsessive-compulsive disorder are diagnosed by the treating physician, patients with these conditions are often placed on benzodiazepines. Because benzodiazepines are not the treatment of choice for these disorders, specific treatment has to be initiated by the consulting psychiatrist. Anxiety is also one of the commonest features of major depression. It is important to remember that when comorbid with pain, anxiety can lower the pain threshold dramatically, causing some caregivers to misinterpret the marked discrepancy between pain complaints and objective findings as an intractable form of somatizing (e.g., drug abuse or personality disorder). Because many of these patients cannot distinguish anxiety from pain ("No, I am not frightened; I hurt!"), diagnosis can be delayed and frustrations intensified. Neuroleptics, not benzodiazepines, are the treatment of choice for this type of anxiety, and a small dose of, for example, haloperidol or fluphenazine (1 mg orally three times a day), may significantly reduce requirements of narcotic analgesics.

Substance Abuse Disorders

Alcohol abuse should always be considered in a patient who continues to have multiple, vague somatic symptoms. Whether the patient consciously tries to conceal his or her disorder or simply fails to make the connection, the diagnosis may be elusive. Information from the patient's family may help ("What he calls headache and chest pains, Doctor, I call a hangover"). Because alcohol abuse systematically disrupts sleep, patients may begin using sedative-hypnotic substances as well. Insomnia, morning cough, pains in the extremities, dysesthesias, palpitations, headache, gastrointestinal symptoms, fatigue, bruises—none are strangers to the alcoholic. (See Chapters 16 and 17 for the diagnosis and treatment of substance abuse disorders.)

Psychotic Disorders

Patients with psychotic depression may have somatic delusions, such as the conviction that one's abdominal organs are decomposing. Such patients are much more likely to be misdiagnosed as having schizophrenia than as having a physical illness. The material in Chapter 14 applies here. The somatic delusions of schizophrenia are generally so bizarre and idiosyncratic (e.g., that foreign bodies are inside an organ or orifice, or that body parts are missing or deformed) as to be easily recognized. But when a patient with schizophrenia complains of a functional symptom that is not of delusional proportions, for example, a headache or weakness, his psychosis may be missed. Making such a diagnosis with a thorough psychiatric history and examination is ordinarily no problem. Schizophrenic patients can present with conversion symptoms, for example, hemiparesis. In such a case the proper diagnosis is of a conversion symptom in a patient with schizophrenia, not "conversion disorder."

Organic Mental Disorders

No organic brain syndrome is known to produce a specific functional somatic symptom (this is another way of saying that somatizing cannot at this time be localized either to a specific brain structure or to a particular neurotransmitter system). However, patients with organic brain disease do have functional somatic complaints. The psychiatric consultant's careful examination will detect cognitive dysfunction that may have gone unnoticed prior to the consultation.

Voluntary Symptom Production

Malingering

Of the two types of voluntary symptom production, malingering, is simple enough: The patient lies about the symptom's presence and/or severity. The false or exaggerated symptom may be somatic (e.g., flashbacks or infection) or psychological. The main criterion for making this diagnosis is that there is an obvious goal or purpose behind the symptom (always presupposing that no organic abnormality can be found or what is found is far out of proportion to the magnitude of the complaint). Excruciating back pain may postpone a trial or court-martial, be the key to disability payments, or be the justification for the patient's requests for narcotic analgesics. The consultant should not be cowed by the pejorative connotations of the diagnosis. The latter does not depend on an analysis of the patient's virtue but on the readily understandable nature of the symptom as a means to an end. In fact, one could say that these patients have a *good* reason for lying—in some cases it is so good that they may almost come to believe their own stories. Whether or not the patient believes his or her story is irrelevant to the diagnosis. Malingering could be part of heroic action, as when a prisoner of war feigns illness as part of a plan to escape.

A high suspicion of malingering should be aroused if any combination of the following four factors is present: (1) a medicolegal context, for example, the patient is referred by his or her attorney for examination; (2) a marked discrepancy between the ostensible distress or disability and the objective findings; (3) a lack of cooperation with the diagnostic evaluation or prescribed treatment regimen, for example, as occurs when a patient refuses psychological testing, physical therapy, or permission to obtain past medical records; and (4) the presence of *antisocial personality disorder*. When the goal is truly obvious (e.g., drugs, money, or disability) there is no point in hiding from the patient that failure to comply with any portion of the evaluation and treatment will almost surely be seen as evidence of malingering.

Factitious Disorders

Factitious illness can be quite complicated. Unlike malingering, where the goal obtained has obvious value to the patient, the simulated or feigned "disease" of the patient with factitious illness confers no obvious advantage. It is best to reserve the term for patients whose psychopathologic condition drives them to sustain their contrivance of illness without apparent self-advantage; in fact, it often places their health at considerable risk. Patients with factitious illness are commonly liars, and, in fact, they exercise remarkable ingenuity in fooling the physicians who care for them. Although they do produce the false symptom voluntarily, their "control" is seldom as complete as that of the malingerer. The woman who takes warfarin sodium, is covered with bruises, and suffers a serious gastric hemorrhage that results in hospitalization, is driven by pathologic motives. A psychiatrist might say that the sympathy she received from telling her associates that she had leukemia is an obvious advantage. It is also obviously sick. Moreover, there is a driven quality to the behavior, and the patient may have little or no insight into the reasons for the self-destructive behavior. In one form of factitious disorder, known as pseudologia fantastica, the lies of the patient form the core of the presenting history. It can be difficult to determine whether the lies are delusions or conscious deceptions.[9] These patients usually have borderline personality disorder.

Ford's review of these disorders is excellent.[10] From the viewpoint of the psychiatrist-consultant, two aspects of diagnosis can be summarized: the detective aspects and the spectrum of psychopathology.

Detection. So inventive are these patients with self-inflicted diseases that an exhaustive list is not possible, but stalwart sleuthing by clinicians in the past leaves us with a few helpful strategies worth listing. Factitious fever is relatively common.[11] Patients warm their thermometers on light bulbs, on radiators, by friction or flame, or with anything convenient. Some keep a supply of "preset" thermometers hidden in the hospital room, ready for substitution after the nurse leaves them alone. To counteract this the nurse may remain with the patient or use an electronic thermometer that registers temperature rapidly. Comparison of a freshly voided urine specimen with simultaneous body temperature is another method.[12] Room search for preset thermometers has been used. Even an electronic thermometer can be outwitted, as by one patient who consistently went to the bathroom prior to having her temperature taken and rinsed her mouth out with hot water. She refused to have a rectal temperature taken.[13] Other patients produce a real fever by infecting themselves, usually by injecting contaminated material (including sputum, feces, tuberculous and other organisms), into their skin or veins. A skin biopsy of such a lesion might be helpful, with culture and microscopic analysis.

Skin is commonly attacked as well, producing any number of dermatitides. Excoriations of all kinds occur. One patient in our hospital applied a blowtorch to his own arm, then maintained a nonhealing wound by reinfecting his grafts. Exposure of the factitious nature of the wound is more difficult, especially because these patients usually improve while in the hospital, only to return with a markedly worsened condition. Subcutaneous tissue has also been damaged to create the appearance of legitimate disease. Air has been injected into the tissues, presenting as an "ulcer" on the forearm, but also raising concern about gas gangrene.[14] Another patient presented with intermittently elevated creatine phosphokinase values (to 1000 units/L or more). X-rays led to the diagnosis of factitious disorder in both cases. In the first, a needle was discovered beneath the skin. In the second an even, circumferential band of compressed adipose tissue (1 inch wide) was found. The patient's muscle had been traumatized by tightening a band around her gastrocnemius muscles. Careful inspection of the bruises on her legs revealed a distribution limited to the lateral surface of the right leg and the medial surface of the left leg—a distribution consistent with an injury caused by a right-handed person.

"Hematologic" disorders have been mentioned and include anemia, usually induced by performing a phlebotomy on oneself, but one patient induced a severe hemorrhage by lacerating her colon with a knitting needle. Blood dyscrasia or leukemia is most commonly simulated by surreptitious self-administration of warfarin or heparin sodium.[15–17] Psychogenic purpura or "autoerythrocyte sensitization" has long been studied by investigators at Case Western Reserve in Cleveland and has been reviewed by Ratnoff.[18] Patients also insinuate blood in other body products, especially sputum, with a classic history for pulmonary embolism; urine, with a classic history for renal stone; and stool. A self-inflicted cut or abrasion is the commonest source of the blood (it is simple to urinate over a cut finger into the specimen cup). These are exceedingly difficult to detect. The blood of one patient who appears to be hemorrhaging was discovered by analysis to be non-human blood.

Of bogus endocrine disorders, hypoglycemia is probably the commonest and is usually produced by injection of insulin or by oral ingestion of sulfonylureas. Scarlett et al.[19] showed that the triad of simultaneous demonstration of low plasma glucose, high immunoreactive insulin, and suppressed C peptide immunoreactivity is pathognomonic of exogenous insulin administration. Because C peptide and insulin are secreted from the pancreatic beta cells in equimolar concentrations, the ability to measure C peptide and produce this diagnostic triad answered prior difficulties of the radioimmunoassay technique posed by the interfering presence of insulin antibodies in insulin-treated diabetics and the difficulty of accepting antibodies, in patients not supposed to be taking insulin, as definite proof of exogenous insulin administration.

When the sulfonylurea ingester presents with a possible diagnosis of insulinoma, either his or her plasma sulfonylurea can be determined or tolbutamide can be administered. If an insulinoma is present, plasma insulin rises. In factitious hypoglycemia it remains the same or falls. Moreover, the inexplicable cases of "brittle diabetes" may sometimes be the result of self-induced difficul-

ties. Schade et al.[13] reported five cases, involving self-injection of insulin, use of watered-down insulin bottles (explaining the "high" insulin requirements), and simulated "shortness of breath" after insulin injections that had been erroneously labeled as "allergy" to purified pork insulin. Their patient was diagnosed when pulmonary function tests were normal. There is recent evidence to suggest that self-administration of insulin in juvenile diabetics, not for glucose regulation, but as a manifestation of psychiatric disorder, may either be more common than realized or as a recourse taken by the patient whose recurrent ketoacidosis has become too closely watched for the patient to secretly cause it any longer.[20]

Ingestion of large amounts of thyroxine can simulate thyrotoxicosis, although determination of thyroxine, triiodothyronine, the ratio of the first to the second, thyroid-stimulating hormone, and serum thyroglobulin are usually sufficient to diagnose excess exogenous ingestion.[21,22] Pheochromocytoma is another endocrine disease that has been simulated; it can be suspected when the elevated urine catecholamines consists only of epinephrine. It was diagnosed when a room search revealed an empty vial of epinephrine.

Factitious asthma has also been reported, and in these cases pulmonary function tests and arterial blood analysis helped demonstrate that the "wheezing" of the patients was self-induced. In the three patients studied, Downing et al.[23] defined blood gas values for an acute asthmatic attack as an oxygen partial pressure less than 80 mm Hg and an alveolar-arterial oxygen tension difference greater than 25 mm Hg. Corresponding pulmonary function values included a 1-second forced expiratory volume (FEV_1), the FEV_1 as a percentage of the vital capacity, and the mid-maximal expiratory flow rate as all less than 80% of the predicted.

Laxative abuse can present with abdominal pain, diarrhea, hypokalemia, acid-base abnormalities, weight loss, vomiting, steatorrhea, and skin pigmentation. It should always be considered when a patient presents with chronic diarrhea of unknown cause. The most helpful test to confirm laxative use is the demonstration of phenolphthalein in the stool.[24] In this test the stool specimen is alkalinized; when present, phenolphthalein causes the solution to turn pink. An informative case from the published records of our hospital illustrates the differential diagnostic and detective work required to solve the chronic diarrhea and weight loss of a 60-year-old laxative abuser.[25]

Self-induced vomiting can cause several metabolic abnormalities, especially hypokalemia. Workups can be extensive. For example, the patient may be thought to have a renal disease, such as Bartter's syndrome. This abnormal behavior is most commonly associated with anorexia nervosa, bulimia, or both. A clue signaling that the patient induces vomiting is the presence of "bulimia calluses," lesions on the dorsal surface of the hand, caused by abrasion by the teeth in the course of inducing emesis.[26] Of course, in the eating disorders self-induced vomiting is often combined with laxative and diuretic abuse, leading most commonly to metabolic alkalosis, hypochloremia, and hypokalemia.[27] One survey found that 13% of adolescents indulge in purging behaviors of this type.[28] The medical complications of anorexia and bulimia can be life-threatening.[29]

A variant, occasionally mistakenly called "post-prandial vomiting," is the more rare *rumination syndrome*, a repeated, effortless regurgitation of gastric contents into the mouth immediately after a meal. Part of the contents is chewed and reswallowed, and part is spit out. This process may continue for up to 4 to 5 hours.[30] The cause is unclear. In 8 of 12 patients the onset of the behavior occurred after an acute illness or event associated with nausea and vomiting. Manometric study showed the motility pattern of this pseudoregurgitation to differ distinctly from that of vomiting.

Factitious renal colic has been mentioned and is one way to obtain narcotic analgesics. Some patients may also present with factitious stones. Stone analysis quickly reveals the nature of the hoax. Yet some of these patients traumatize their urethras as well, inserting the "stone" and then reporting that they heard the sound of it falling into the bedpan or other container. Some have even urinated in the presence of a family member or a nurse, adding authenticity to the appearance of the "stone."

Detective work is an essential feature of most of these evaluations. Consultants at Massachusetts General Hospital (MGH) are usually called before the suspicion of factitious disorder is confirmed. It is intellectually stimulating and occasionally the most enjoyable part of the consultation, especially if symptom production can be unambiguously proven.

Although a room search can be one of the most successful diagnostic procedures, ethical questions can arise about violation of the patient's privacy. Like Ford and Abernethy,[31] we evaluate each case individually and refer the reader to a summary of a conference on this subject. Psychiatrists seldom hesitate to intervene when a patient slices his wrists; self-injection of feces or insulin is no less self-destructive. Room searches are routine for hospitalized suicidal patients.

Factitious disorders can include psychological symptoms, as well as the physical ones described previously. The designation of *factitious disorder with predominantly psychological signs and symptoms* (300.16 in the *Diagnostic and Statistical Manual for Mental Disorders*, fourth edition [DSM-IV]) was apparently used originally to describe those patients formerly thought to have *Ganser syndrome, pseudopsychosis*, or *pseudodementia*. Factitious bereavement, a syndrome in which patients present with depression and suicidal ideation after fabricated deaths,[32] may best fit in the 300.16 category as well. However, many of the patients described also had histories of factitious physical disorders. Ganser syndrome, helpfully reviewed by Whitlock,[33] has a complex history. This diagnosis is far too nonspecific to be helpful. There is no substitute for thorough diagnostic evaluation: When dementia is present it is so labeled, and likewise delirium, depression, malingering, factitious disorder, and the like. An almost humorous variant of factitious disorder with psychological symptoms is the patient who presented himself to a hospital emergency room, demanding immediate hospitalization because he suffered from Münchausen syndrome. The unnecessary surgeries he claimed to have undergone were denied by the physicians and hospitals he cited, and the scars covering his abdomen washed off with soap and water.[34]

Finally, one must realize that there exists a form of "proxy" factitious disorder, in which the patient is usually a child and the author of the sham is usually the child's mother. In one case of "brittle diabetes" the parents had spent more than $80,000 in the year prior to this discovery, including evaluations at three major medical centers in the United States and Canada.[13] The child's mother was injecting heparin into the child's central line. Later the mother injected contaminants, producing recurrent gram-negative sepsis. Reviewing the numerous reports of this variant of child abuse that have appeared since 1977, Ford[10] noted that at least one child died as a result of this pathologic maternal behavior.

Spectrum of Psychopathology.   When confronted with the phenomenon of factitious disorder, the consultant is best served by examining each patient individually, with routine careful diagnostic attention devoted to both axes I and II. Generalizations are therefore difficult when considering the entire spectrum. However, inspection of the reported cases show that the majority of patients are female, younger than 40 years of age, and have invariably gained medical sophistication from being a nurse, a medical technician, or a physician; having a physician-parent; or having had an illness. The milder end of the spectrum includes patients with hypochondriasis and possibly depression. Typical is a 15-year-old boy reported by Reich et al.[35] who repeatedly contaminated his urine with feces. At the age of 2 he had undergone surgery for hypospadias. Convinced that something was genuinely wrong with his bladder that his physicians had thus far failed to discover, he kept contaminating his urine by retrograde injections so that continued medical examinations would reveal an abnormality that could be repaired. When supportively confronted he confessed his action, and this seemed to restore him to his senses. After brief psychotherapy his behavior remained normal and he resumed normal peer relationships.

The more severe forms of factitious disorder are accompanied by extensive Axis II disturbance. Although immature, dependent, passive, masochistic, and histrionic traits are described, patients with factitious disorder of several years' duration are most likely to have borderline personality disorder. In an excellent review of 41 cases of factitious disorder, Reich and Gottfried[36] stressed the likelihood of encountering milder forms of this disorder more often than the most extreme form, Münchausen syndrome. Sepsis, nonhealing wounds, fever, and electrolyte disorder accounted for two thirds of the presentations. Two thirds of the patients worked in the medical profession. Self-contamination, surreptitious medication use, and wound exacerbation were the methods used by 29 of the 41 patients. Fourteen room searches led to ten diagnostic discoveries. No patient was found

to have had a diagnosis of borderline personality disorder.

Our MGH experience has not been so benign. Despite their bland and passive exteriors, many of these patients reveal hostility and intense projected self-hatred. Each patient, of course, must be individually evaluated. Because factitious illness tends to generate anger, it is important to consider this as distinct and to be wary of countertransference feelings that arise in response to the patient.

Münchausen syndrome is an extreme form of factitious disorder, defined on the basis of three principal features: (1) psychological and/or physical symptoms that are produced by, and are apparently under the individual's voluntary control; (2) the symptoms that are produced are not explained by any other mental or physical disorder (although they may be superimposed on one); and (3) the individual's goal is apparently to assume the "patient role" and is not otherwise understandable in light of the individual's environmental circumstance (as in the case of malingering).

Individuals with Münchausen syndrome plagued physicians even before Asher gave the syndrome its name in 1951.[37] Uniformly, patients with this disorder wreak havoc once they have been admitted to a hospital, yet only 50% of them are ever seen by psychiatric consultants.[38] When they are seen, recommendations for psychiatric follow-up care are invariably rejected. Successful treatment is rare, and clear management strategies for dealing with these patients while hospitalized are lacking.

Early efforts in managing patients with Münchausen syndrome were directed toward saving physicians from being duped rather than toward treatment. To this end the methods suggested included the creation of blacklists and a central registry. Although Asher first wondered what might cause these individuals to act as they did, it was not until years later that others postulated dynamic hypotheses to account for the patient's impostureship, *pseudologia fantastica*, itinerant lives, absence of close relationships, and masochistic acceptance of painful procedures.[39,40] Along these lines, a wide range of psychiatric diagnoses have been recorded for these patients: hysterical, psychopathic, masochistic, and borderline personalities; schizophrenia; and malingering.

The following case of a young woman with Münchausen syndrome illustrates the value of psychiatric consultation in preventing needless surgical interventions and decreasing the countertransference hatred of the hospital staff.

Ms. B, a 27-year-old, widowed, full-blooded Navajo Indian was admitted to MGH with a chief complaint of abdominal pain, nausea, vomiting, and watery diarrhea.

Her medical history included childhood asthma, rheumatic fever at 7 years of age, an appendectomy when 20 years old, and an emergency cholecystectomy following a car accident in Colorado. At 21 and 27 years of age she underwent cesarean sections at a New York hospital.

She said she was raised in Brooklyn, New York. Her father died when she was 4 years old. She reported that her husband was killed in a motor vehicle accident during her second pregnancy. She reported coming to Boston 6 weeks prior to admission to find work and to start college. Her two children remained in New York City under the care of her mother. Since her arrival in Boston, she had become engaged to a truck driver, who at the time of her admission was in North Dakota.

On physical examination Ms. B was a thin, white female in considerable abdominal distress. Her temperature was 102° F orally, her pulse was 104 beats per minute, her blood pressure was 160/70 mm Hg, and her respiratory rate 20 per minute. Her abdominal examination was notable for multiple midline scars and for moderate tenderness with guarding over the right upper rectus abdominus muscle. The remainder of her examination was entirely normal.

Ms. B was taken to the operating room for exploratory laparotomy, which, except for numerous adhesions, was normal. Postoperatively, she complained of continued right upper quadrant abdominal pain, and had severe tenderness to mild palpation. She began spiking postoperative fevers to 103° F and on the third hospital day a *Klebsiella* infection in the urine was identified and successfully treated with antibiotics; however, the spiking fevers and abdominal pain persisted. For this pain, Ms. B required intramuscular injections of meperidine hydrochloride. A kidneys-ureter-bladder examination, upright abdominal plain film, ultrasound of the abdomen and pelvis, and computed tomographic scan of her abdomen were all normal. Intravenous pyelography was planned, but she refused, stating that a similar test several years earlier had nearly killed her. Instead, an ultrasound record of the kidneys was obtained and was normal. On the ninth hospital day she underwent cystoscopy with bilateral retrograde ureterograms, which were also normal.

Infectious disease consultants were called in to evaluate Ms. B's nightly fevers. Cultures of her blood, stool, urine, and sputum were all negative. Results of a lumbar puncture were also normal. Her white blood cell count remained normal.

On the eighteenth hospital day, psychiatric consultation was requested. The psychiatrist noted Ms. B was alert, oriented, and without either a formal thought disorder or depression. However, she appeared distant and indifferent to questions or events. She answered questions slowly and occasionally grabbed her right side and moaned, "Oh, the pain." The psychiatrist thought that the patient's presentation was consistent with Münchausen syndrome. Her account was replete with impostureship and pseudologia fantastica (i.e., telephone numbers she gave were false, she had no knowledge of Navajo customs, her work and school history were not verifiable, and the hospitals she claimed to have had surgery in had no record of her). She displayed an equanimity to invasive procedures and a medical sophistication by virtue of previous job experience in medical laboratories. In addition, there was evidence of drug abuse, a poor interpersonal style, and threats to sign out unless her pain medications were increased. Moreover, a review of her behavior within the hospital revealed her to be demanding, evasive, and frequently noncompliant with hospital rules.

The psychiatric consultant planned to administer psychological tests. He informed the staff about the need to set limits on her demands and to supervise temperature taking (to eliminate the possibility of factitious fevers) and warned the staff about the likelihood of her signing out against medical advice. Ms. B refused psychological testing. Over the next 3 days the psychiatrist did not challenge her complaint of pain but confronted her with the staff's impression that her pain had no medical basis. During this time she had been afebrile. Ms. B insisted that her care be transferred to a senior attending surgeon so that she might get a more "experienced work-up." However, she did not deny that she was either misrepresenting or fabricating her pain or fevers.

The senior surgeon was consulted and agreed with the need for further psychiatric treatment, but the patient declined; no further medical or surgical care was indicated. Discharge was then urged so that the patient would not further harm herself and require a longer hospitalization; she was escorted out of the hospital by security personnel.

This case presents essentially all of the features generally associated with Münchausen syndrome. Despite the anger of staff toward the patient, psychiatric consultation was delayed until the eighteenth hospital day. Once the possibility of Münchausen syndrome was raised, detective work carried out, and the dynamics discussed with the staff, unproductive struggles with the patient decreased. The patient's discomfort could be addressed, and she could be confronted in a supportive context. Although the patient failed to take advantage of psychiatric follow-up, further invasive treatments were prevented. Without an awareness of the diagnosis and of the physician's countertransference feelings, the percentage of successful psychiatric referrals is low, and the patient continues to be at risk from her or his illness.

Treatment. Treatment for factitious disorder depends on an accurate and specific diagnosis. One needs to consider how best to confront the patient with the evidence or the opinion that the disorder is self-induced. The primary physician may prefer to do this alone or with the consultant present. The option should always be offered. As Reich and Gottfried indicate,[36] these patients, whatever their motives, seek medical care and, at least in the beginning, enlist their physicians as allies rather than as adversaries. One can begin the confrontation with a list of the patient's strengths and his or her long history of suffering; but it is also clear because of the evidence compiled that there is a serious emotional problem present. The patient does not need to admit to inflicting the symptoms upon himself or herself. The best stance is to adopt the quiet conviction that this is unnecessary because its truth is already known. The physician can, after the patient has been given an opportunity to discuss the situation, stress that the focus remains on what is best for the patient, namely, psychiatric treatment.

If present, the psychiatrist should secure some agreement from the patient while the primary physician is still there, offering to remain to discuss this or to return. The more severe the patient's disorder, the more likely he or she is to reject offers of help, express indignation at the physicians' lack of trust, and leave the hospital. Any anger in or by the confronting physician increases the likelihood of this reaction. At the heart of the confrontation is the concern for self-inflicted wounds, dangerous diagnostic or therapeutic measures, and whatever help the patient needs to replace destructive with constructive behaviors. Each of the patient's efforts to precipitate an angry encounter about the "accusation" of factitious disease should be quietly countered with a reminder of how reassuring it is that there is no untreatable infection, malignancy, or other life-threatening illness, and how important it is to help him or her with the genuine psychiatric difficulty that remains.

Personality Disorders

Although included in the differential diagnostic list of Table 19-1, personality disorders do not "cause" functional somatic symptoms. Rather, for the patient with an Axis II disturbance, the somatic symptom is a means to an end. For the *antisocial personality*, pain may be a means to get narcotics, to get out of work, to escape trial, and so on. For the dependent personality, functional weakness gains the attention and nurturance of others.[41] The borderline patient's somatic symptoms are the focus about which the physicians and nurses engage in a sadomasochistic struggle, beginning with a helping relationship and ending with the disappointed and outraged patient accused of wrongdoing and being rejected. The "end" for this patient is the emotionally charged (usually hostile) relationship, and the failure to palliate his or her symptoms means that the physician simply does not care enough about him or her. Somatic symptoms are exaggerated by patients with histrionic personality and may be so intensely fixated on by those with compulsive, paranoid, schizotypal, and schizoid personalities as to make these patients take on a hypochondriacal character, reinforcing their symptoms by their personality styles.

The Somatoform Disorders

The somatoform disorders are characterized by bodily symptoms which suggest a physical disorder but for which there are no demonstrable organic causes or known physiologic mechanisms that are severe enough to result in significant distress or functional impairment; there is also a strong presumption that the symptoms are linked to psychological factors or to conflict.

Conversion Disorder

Conversion disorder is perhaps the classic somatoform disorder. It involves a loss or change in sensory or motor function that is suggestive of a physical disorder but that is actually caused by psychological factors. Common symptoms include paralysis, aphonia, seizures, gait or coordination disturbances, blindness, tunnel vision, and anesthesia. The primary evidence for the psychological cause consists of a temporal relationship between symptom onset and psychologically meaningful environmental precipitants or stressors. A patient who developed conversion blindness, for instance, may have seen her husband with another woman before she complained of being unable to see. The conversion symptom is not under voluntary control, although the patient may to some extent modulate its severity, as in the patient with a functional gait disturbance or weak arm who, with intense concentration, can demonstrate slightly better control or strength. DSM-IV has eliminated pain and sexual dysfunction as conversion symptoms. Reviewing conversion, Ford and Folks[42] recommended that it be considered clinically as a symptom rather than as a primary diagnosis.

The gender ratio is equal in children who present with conversion symptoms, whereas in adults two to five times more women are seen than are men. Predisposing factors are important for both diagnosis and treatment. A prior medical illness is a common source for the symptom. If a viral illness is accompanied by vertigo while a patient is under stress, the illness may "rescue" him or her from the stress and bring attention and support from loved ones. At a later time, when stress recurs, the symptom of vertigo may recur, this time as a conversion symptom. By definition, the symptom is not intentionally produced or feigned. Patients with seizures, especially complex partial seizures (in which consciousness is preserved), are repeatedly exposed to a phenomenon that instantaneously removes them from responsibility for what they are doing and may evoke sympathy and help from a loved one. Pseudoseizures commonly coexist with true seizures and can be exceedingly hard to discriminate, particularly when the electroencephalogram fails to demonstrate spiking activity or shows only nonspecific slowing.

Preexisting psychopathology is another factor that predisposes to the development of a conversion symptom. The most common Axis I disorders associated with conversion are depression, anxiety, and schizophrenia. Axis II personality disorders (especially histrionic personality disorder, passive-dependent personality disorder, and passive-aggressive personality disorder) are common in these patients.

Conversion symptoms may be precipitated by exposure to others with conversion symptoms. Such "figures of identity" may be psychologically important people in the patient's life (such as a parent who has just died), or they may be strangers whose symptoms the patient observes under extreme and sudden stress, as occurs in mass psychogenic illness ("epidemic hysteria"). Indeed, extreme psychosocial stress may be the most important of all precipitating factors. The presence of this in the history provides stronger and more reliable evidence for the diagnosis of conversion than either escaping responsibility or gaining nurturance as a result of the symptom. This is particularly true because these secondary gains can occur in the wake of serious organic illness as well. Some authors have presented evidence for a predominance of conversion symptoms, when unilateral, on the nondominant side in females.[43,44]

The diagnosis of conversion cannot rest comfortably only on the absence of organic disease. Caution in diagnosing conversion symptoms is based on the reports that 13% to 30% of those with this diagnosis go on to develop an organic condition that, in retrospect, was related to the original symptom.[45] For this reason, one usually hopes to demonstrate that function is normal in the symptomatic body part. Electromyograms, evoked responses of vision and hearing, slit lamp examinations, funduscopic examinations, retinoscopic examinations, pulmonary function tests, and barium swallows are examples of tests that should be normal. This negative phase is critical; it requires meticulous review by the psychiatrist. Positive evidence includes not only the psychological data but also any demonstration of normal function in the supposedly disabled body part. Detective work begins with close observation of the patient, including times when he or she is unaware of the observer's presence. In part, one is trying here to discriminate the malingerer. If the patient moves his or her arm normally when unaware of being observed and displays a frail arm when watched, he or she is most likely malingering. Interest has grown in functional brain imaging of the patient with conversion disorder; there have been reports of functional neuroanatomical abnormalities in patients with conversion (i.e., sensorimotor loss).[46]

Conversion symptoms are usually sustained, but sometimes only for a certain activity. The patient who cannot lift his leg adequately in walking may be observed to cross it over his good one during conversation. Deviation of the eyes toward the ground, no matter which side the "semicomatose" patient lies on, is functional and sometimes demonstrates lack of an organic disorder.[47] One may lead the patient with functional blindness around obstacles like chairs; the conversion patient usually avoids them (a malingerer is more likely to bump into them). Carefully watching the "blind" patient's eyes and face while taking a roll of money out of one's wallet, or suddenly menacing (careful to avoid creating a draft or noise) or making a face at him or her is another way to assess vision. Sensory testing on the patient in both prone and supine positions checks for consistency. A malingerer is more likely to become hostile and uncooperative during the examination, probably in the hope of shortening it.

Prognosis and Treatment.   The literature supports an optimistic outlook for these patients, at least in the first few years. From 50% to 90% of patients have recovered by the time of hospital discharge, with Folks et al.[48] recording a 50% complete remission rate by discharge in those with conversion disorder in a general hospital. However, the long-term course is less favorable, because a sizable fraction of these patients develop recurrent conversion symptoms (20% to 25% within 1 year), other forms of somatization, or eventually meet criteria for somatization disorder.

The commonest form of treatment is to suggest that the conversion symptom will gradually improve. This ordinarily begins with reassuring news that tests of the involved body system show no damage and therefore that recovery is certain. Predicting that recovery will be gradual, with specific suggestions (e.g., vague shapes will become visible first; weight bearing will be possible and then steps with a walker; standing up straight will come before full steadiness of gait; strength in squeezing a tennis ball will be followed by strength at the wrist and then elbow joints; feeling will return to the toes first) usually succeeds, provided that the diagnosis is conveyed with serene confidence and the suggestions provided with supportive optimism. Lazare[45] pointed out that the psychiatrist

should also discuss the patient's life stresses and try to detect painful affects to assess the nonverbal interpersonal communication embodied by the symptom.

Confrontation is seldom helpful. However, some patients may ask what the psychiatrist thinks caused their condition and others sense a relationship between the stressful psychosocial conditions and the conversion symptomatology. An approach that has been acceptable to some of these individuals has been to say that the body, mysterious in many ways, can be smarter than we are. It may help us before we realize we need help. When the stress in our lives becomes excessive, especially when our nature is more to overlook it or to grit our teeth and prevail, our body, by its symptoms, may blow the "time-out" whistle, forcing us to stop, to take a rest, and to get some help. This approach invites the patient to greater insight. It may not be necessary. However, if the conversion symptom persists, if the precipitating stress is chronic, or if there is massive secondary gain, then resolution of the situation becomes a target of the intervention. Because the stresses are often social, couples or family therapy may be instrumental in achieving a final resolution.

Some hospitalized patients fail to improve with suggestion. Because they occupy a nonpsychiatric bed, they must be told that if they insist that they are not well enough to leave the hospital, then transfer to a psychiatric hospital or to a psychiatric unit will be arranged. Symptoms that have not responded to earlier suggestion that then improve sufficiently to permit discharge. One would have to entertain in such a patient the possibility that the correct diagnosis is malingering. In general, a favorable outcome depends more on the patient's psychological strengths and on the absence of other psychopathology than on the specific nature of the conversion symptom itself.

Somatoform Pain Disorder

The predominant feature of somatoform pain disorder (termed simply *Pain Disorder* in DSM-IV) is chronic, severe, and preoccupying pain that has no adequate medical explanation. Either there is no medical disease at all, or the patient's pain is grossly disproportionate to demonstrable histopathologic findings. The pain is severe enough to warrant clinical attention and to impair role functioning. It is constant, and is often inconsistent with known neuroanatomic innervation. Psychological factors must be judged to play a significant role in the precipitation, maintenance or exacerbation of the pain, but it is neither intentionally produced nor feigned. Pain is the subject of Chapter 21.

Patients with somatoform pain disorder are often severely disabled by their symptoms; they live like invalids and work infrequently. They have long histories of medical care and many surgical interventions. They are often completely preoccupied with their pain, and view it as the sole source of all their difficulties. Depression is commonly comorbid with somatoform pain disorder; major depression occurs in 25% to 50% of them, and dysthymia or depressive symptoms are reported in 60% to 100%.

Typical was the man who developed a painful exacerbation of an old back injury the day after his wife attended a birthday party to which the patient had not been invited; a neighborhood bachelor gave it in her honor. Physical, neurologic, and radiologic examinations showed either normal function or no change from his baseline. No immediate knowledge of this association was in evidence and it was gained only when the patient was questioned independently about his relationship with his wife (which he said was "excellent"), and asked specifically if she had ever seen another man. He readily admitted feeling angry and hurt. It was only when he was asked the date of his wife's birthday that the consultant noted it was the day before his symptoms began. When asked whether there might be a connection, the patient said sincerely he was sure that no relationship existed—even though he could see why the consultant might see a causal relation. Results of a Minnesota Multiphasic Personality Inventory (MMPI) suggested conversion symptomatology. Projective testing revealed many concerns about dependency and nurturance, and included a story of marital infidelity and other fears of loss of love.

Treatment. The spectrum of reactions of these patients is likely to mimic that for conversion. The same therapeutic approach is recommended, with the reassurance that the body parts in question appear to be normal or no worse and the suggestion that the pain will gradually subside. Some patients can accept their manifest need to resolve the stress that has been uncovered (and can be told that it is worth working on even if it is not at all related to the pain). Use of their own productions in the psychological testing can be presented to them as helpful evidence of the existence of concern in their subconscious or unconscious minds. The "wisdom" of their body in warning them about their stress, by means of pain, may be helpful as well. Early treatment of patients with this disorder is usually limited to individual, marital, or family therapy. If it has continued for a longer time, multimodal, behavioral, and more comprehensive approaches, including relaxation response training, transcutaneous electrical nerve stimulation, and physical therapy are indicated. Much more clinical and epidemiologic information must be gathered on this new diagnostic category.

Somatization Disorder

Originally termed *hysteria* or *Briquet's syndrome* and now given the DSM-IV designation of *somatization disorder*, this condition has been solidly established as clinically and epidemiologically distinct. It is a chronic syndrome of recurring multiple somatic symptoms that are not explainable medically and are associated with psychosocial distress and with medical help-seeking. The disorder is much more common in women than in men, and it tends to occur in those of low socioeconomic, often nonwhite and rural, status, at a prevalence rate of 0.4% in the general population.[49] Of first-degree female relatives, 10% to 20% suffer the same disorder, whereas male relatives show an increased incidence of alcoholism and sociopathy.

Women with this disorder tend to have histories as children of missing, disturbed, or defective parents, and of sexual or physical abuse.[50] They marry sociopathic males more often than chance would predict, and they tend to be poor parents themselves.[51–55] Given these unfortunate circumstances, and their roughly 75% chance of having one or more additional psychiatric diagnoses (the commonest being affective disorder, anxiety disorder, and drug and alcohol abuse[56]), it is no surprise that marital discord and unsatisfactory work histories are also the rule.

DSM-IV diagnostic criteria have been simplified and now include at least the following: (1) four different pain symptoms (e.g., headache; back, joint, extremity or/chest pain; painful urination, intercourse, or menstruation); (2) two gastrointestinal symptoms (e.g., nausea, bloating, diarrhea, and food intolerance); (3) one sexual symptom (e.g., menstrual symptoms, erectile or ejaculatory dysfunction, or sexual indifference); (4) one pseudoneurologic symptom other than pain (e.g., deafness, paralysis, a lump in the throat, aphonia, fainting, anesthesias, or blindness). The symptoms must be disproportionate to demonstrable medical disease and severe enough to result in medical attention or significant role impairment. The diagnostic symptoms are numerous and can be cumbersome for the busy clinician. Othmer and DeSouza[57] have attempted to deal with the first problem by developing an abbreviated list of seven symptoms that can be employed to screen for the disorder. If two or more of the symptoms in their clever mnemonic (Table 19-2) are present, there is a high likelihood of somatization disorder. The presence of three symptoms accurately identified 91% of the patients with somatization disorder with a sensitivity of 87% and a specificity of 95%. However, despite this list of symptoms, the clinical diagnosis almost always requires review of past records; these tend to be voluminous, scattered among a host of hospitals, lost, or a combination of the three. In the absence of the chart, contact with prior treating physicians or family members may help in establishing the symptom count. Notoriously poor historians, these patients will be unable to recall past admissions or clinic visits, and they will deny a history of a symptom that the chart lists as a chief complaint on a past visit. Goodwin and Guze[58] have suggested that menstrual difficulties and sexual indifference are so common in these patients that the diagnosis should be made with caution if the menstrual and sexual histories are normal.

During the interview, the patient usually presents her or his complaints in a histrionic fashion ("Why I bled so much—I've never seen so much blood!!—that I passed out on the bed and my family said I was in a coma for 3 days!"), with symptoms so exaggerated that a psychogenic cause may be suspected from the outset. The other consistent trait these patients possess is a peculiar communication style. Histories are vague and details are either elusive or downright inconsistent. Efforts at clarification may be fruitless and frustrating. ("Is your pain worse in the morning?" "Yes, and it's worse in the afternoon, too.") Emotional distress is openly expressed ("I'm not getting *anywhere*, Doctor! No one can tell me anything! What's happening to me?"), but if one tries to identify the emotion, for example, telling the patient she seems very anxious, that emotion is more likely to intensify ("Well, wouldn't anybody be? It's been a whole month and nobody—nobody, Doctor—knows what's going on with me!"). This type of response tends to drive the physician back to a cognitive search—onset, duration, radiation, intensifying or relieving factors—only to encounter once again the fogbound and trackless wastes of imprecision, inconsistency, and lapsing memory.

Contemporary medicine's shift from clinical to economic priorities has only heightened attention to somatization disorder. Smith et al.[59] have documented that the typical patient with this disorder spends an average of 7 days per month sick in bed

Table 19-2. Seven-Symptom Screening Test for Somatization Disorder

Mnemonic	Symptom	System
Somatization	Shortness of breath	Respiratory
Disorder	Dysmenorrhea	Female reproductive
Besets	Burning in sex organ	Psychosexual
Ladies	Lump in throat (difficulty swallowing)	Pseudoneurologic
And	Amnesia	Pseudoneurologic
Vexes	Vomiting	Gastrointestinal
Physicians	Painful extremities	Skeletal muscle

From Othmer E, DeSouza C: A screening test for somatization disorder (hysteria), *Am J Psychiatry* 142:1146–1149, 1985.

(compared with 0.48 day for the average person), and accrues (mostly unnecessary) annual hospital care expenditures of $2382, physician services of $1721, and total care charges of $4700—charges that are roughly 6 times, 14 times, and 9 times higher, respectively, than those of the average person in the population between the ages of 15 and 64 years. This happens despite their remarkably stable clinical course, with a 90% probability of not developing a new medical or psychiatric disorder in the subsequent 6 to 8 years following diagnosis.

There is now substantial clinical and research evidence that somatization disorder patients constitute a distinct and discrete group.[51] In an effort to clarify their distinctive verbal patterns, Oxman et al.[59] compared samples of free speech from 11 patients with somatization disorder with samples from patients with major depression, paranoid disorders, and medical disorders. The pattern revealed by content analysis was that of a confused, negative self-identity. The authors noted two major factors. The first was a sort of unrelenting negativism, "the relentless modification of objects and actions by their negative attitude." The second centered on self-identification patterns, which the authors likened to pathologic narcissism with impoverished interpersonal relations and deficient empathy, or a bogus empathy manifested as a pseudodependence on others. Yet there appeared to be little of the ambition, exploitativeness, and dependency on admiration and acclaim commonly associated with narcissism.

When extensive neuropsychological testing of these patients was compared with that of patients with psychotic depression, schizophrenia, and normal controls, Flor-Henry et al.[59a] demonstrated bifrontal hemispheric impairment of cognitive processes with greater global impairment of the nondominant hemisphere. The nondominant abnormalities were postulated by the authors to be responsible for depression, psychogenic pain, asymmetric conversion symptoms, and the histrionic pattern, whereas dominant hemisphere abnormalities were seen to mediate the subtle impairment of verbal communication, peculiar incongruity of affective responsiveness, and abnormal sensory motor integration and mobility control.

Treatment.   The management of somatization disorder has been formulated by Murphy.[60] It is best carried out by primary care physicians according to a conservative plan based on (1) being a consistent care provider, (2) preventing unnecessary or dangerous medical procedures, and (3) inquiring in a supportive manner about the areas of stress in the patient's life. The last occurs during the physical examination, without inferring that the real cause for the increase in the patient's somatic complaints was psychosocial stress (which is what most authors believe). The basic goal is to help the patient cope with his or her symptoms rather than to eliminate them completely. In short, the aim is palliation rather than outright cure. Psychotropic medication and prescription analgesics generally are not very helpful, except when used to treat a clear-cut, comorbid psychiatric condition, such as major depression or panic disorder.

Smith et al.[61] codified treatment recommendations in a letter to the primary care physicians of somatization disorder patients. These included regularly scheduled appointments (e.g., every 4 to 6 weeks); a physical examination performed at each visit to look for true disease; the avoidance of hospitalization, diagnostic procedures, surgery, and the use of laboratory assessments, unless clearly indicated; and advice to avoid telling patients, "It's all in your head." In a randomized controlled trial, this intervention reduced quarterly health care charges by 53%, largely as a result of decreases in hospitalization.[62,63] Neither the health of the patients nor their satisfaction with their care was adversely affected by implementation of the advice.

Undifferentiated Somatoform Disorder

The diagnostic criteria for somatization disorder are quite restrictive, and most chronic somatizing patients in medical practice do not cross this stringent threshold. Several researchers, including Kroenke et al.[64] and Escobar et al.,[65,66] have sought to define a more inclusive entity that requires fewer somatic symptoms than are required for somatization disorder, but that nonetheless identifies patients who have the clinical and behavioral features characteristic of the disorder. This entity has been termed "abridged somatization disorder" and "multisomatoform disorder." It has, for example, been shown that patients with four to six somatization disorder symptoms are marked by having significant levels of disability, have psychological impairment and elevated rates of psychiatric comorbidity, and manifest maladaptive illness behaviors, such as undue use of medical care.

In an attempt to provide a diagnostic home for such patients (other than the residual wastebasket diagnosis *Somatoform Disorder Not Otherwise Specified*), DSM-IV now includes the entity *Undifferentiated Somatoform Disorder*. This diagnosis requires one or more physical symptoms that persist for at least 6 months and are medically unexplained. Although this diagnosis will certainly prove more popular and be endorsed more often than somatization disorder, little is known empirically about the patients who will be so diagnosed.

Hypochondriasis

Although continued investigation has brought considerable unity to the concept of somatization disorder, the nosologic status of hypochondriasis remains much less clear. Excessive concern about one's health is common, and it can be difficult to determine the point at which this becomes a psychiatric disorder; many people are transiently hypochondriacal to at least some degree. In addition, it remains unclear how often psychopathologic hypochondriasis is a primary disorder in its own right and how often it is a nonspecific, secondary symptom of another underlying psychiatric disorder. Finally, some have argued that it is better thought of as a personality disorder and placed on Axis II rather than on Axis I.[67]

DSM-IV singles out as the predominant feature of hypochondriasis a preoccupation with the fear or belief of having a serious disease, based on a misinterpretation of benign physical signs or sensations as evidence of disease. Other diagnostic criteria include the absence of a physical disorder that accounts for the patient's symptoms or for his interpretation of them; the persistence of the disease fear or belief despite appropriate medical reassurance; clinically significant distress or role impairment; and a duration of at least 6 months.

Hypochondriasis is fundamentally an overconcern about illness, a fearful attitude toward one's health, and a way of thinking about one's body. Afflicted patients are preoccupied with their symptoms and absorbed by their bodies. Their physical health is an important facet of their sense of self, a nonverbal language used for communicating with others, and a way of reacting to life's stresses and demands. It is these beliefs and attitudes that distinguish hypochondriasis from somatization disorder. Moreover, the cognitive style of hypochondriacal patients tends to be obsessive, whereas that of somatization disorder patients tends to be histrionic. Compulsive traits are common. The diagnosis is made with equal frequency in males and females. The course of the disorder is generally thought to be chronic and long-standing.

The origins of hypochondriasis are not understood, but disease in the patient at an early age or disease in a family member, childhood adversity including neglectful or abusive parents,[68] and other conditioning factors have been noted. The first onset of the syndrome may occur in the context of a physical illness or after the death of a loved one. When a patient has a myocardial infarction, for example, it is normal for bodily preoccupation with the chest area to be heightened in the ensuing 2 to 3 months. Is this hypochondriacal? If so, it is probably of little clinical significance unless it is abnormally prolonged. Yet one would be hard-pressed to define the normal limits of duration. There is some evidence that hypochondriacal patients tend to amplify and augment somatic and visceral sensations more than nonhypochondriacal patients.[69,70]

When confronted with a patient with exaggerated disease fears, unfounded disease beliefs, and bodily preoccupation, the consultant should systematically search for an affective disorder, anxiety disorder, or obsessive-compulsive disorder—and treat them if present. These specific diagnoses are associated with hypochondriasis, and when they are treated the hypochondriasis may disappear or diminish significantly. In addition, clinical lore suggests that many hypochondriacs have a significant Axis II disorder,[68] including hostile, obsessive, compulsive, masochistic, and paranoid traits—none of which facilitate the treatment process.[71]

Prognosis and Treatment. The prognosis of these patients generally has been considered poor. Kenyon,[72] for example, found that among hospitalized patients with primary hypochondriasis, only 21% were judged recovered or much improved at the time of discharge, and 40% were either unchanged or worse than when they were admitted. On the other hand, Kellner[73] finds reason to be optimistic, especially when the illness has lasted less than 3 years and there is no personality disorder.

The primary care physician's goals in managing hypochondriacal patients are three-fold.[74] First, to avoid unnecessary diagnostic testing and to obviate overly aggressive medical and surgical intervention. Second, to help the patient cope with and tolerate his or her symptoms, rather than trying to eliminate them completely. And third, the physician tries to build a durable relationship with the patient, based on the physician's interest in the patient as a person and not just in the patient's symptoms. The primary physician needs to appreciate that these patients have psychological and psychosocial reasons for being symptomatic and that no medical intervention can cure the *need* to feel sick. Once the physician understands his task as palliative rather than curative, the relationship with the patient becomes less contentious and adversarial. And conversely, the patient cannot begin to loosen his grip on his symptoms until he feels that the physician has acknowledged and accepted them.

Several practical measures may be helpful. The physician can demonstrate his interest in the patient as a person by paying attention to the social and personal history, and by providing regularly scheduled appointments rather than appointments on an as-needed basis, because the latter means that the patient can only see his physician if he is symptomatic. It is also important to compliment the hypochondriacal patient on his perseverance and ability to endure in spite of great discomfort. Because hypochondriacs tend to develop complications, iatrogenic illnesses, and treatment side effects, they are more often harmed by overaggressive than underaggressive medical management. This has given rise to the clinical maxim, "Don't just do something, stand there"; as much as possible, the physician prescribes himself or herself. The best medical interventions are modest, simple, and benign: heating pads, ointments, frequent physical examinations, and vitamins, for example. Tangible evidence of the patient's discomfort and of the physician's active interest, such as a cane, brace, or elastic bandages, can also be helpful.

The most successful psychiatric interventions with hypochondriacal patients are probably cognitive, behavioral, and educational.[75-77] Although primary hypochondriasis has generally been thought to be unresponsive to psychotropic agents, there have recently been a few reports suggesting a role for serotonin reuptake inhibitors.[78-81]

Monosymptomatic Hypochondriasis and Body Dysmorphic Disorder

Monosymptomatic hypochondriasis refers to several distinct syndromes characterized by a single, fixed, false belief that one is diseased. The disease conviction is generally delusional,[82] and grossly disproportionate to any objective disease or deformity. This belief is tightly circumscribed, no other thought disorder is present, and the remainder of the patient's personality remains intact and unaffected.[83,84] *Body dysmorphic disorder* (BDD), formerly termed *dysmorphophobia*, is one of the commonest of these syndromes and it is singled out in the DSM-IV as a separate diagnosis. The patient with this disorder believes he or she is physically misshapen and unattractive, although his objective appearance is unremarkable.[85] Other forms of monosymptomatic hypochondriasis include the delusional belief that one is infested with a parasite or insect and the delusion that one emits an offensive odor (olfactory reference syndrome).

The patient with BDD imagines some defect or deformity in his or her appearance, most commonly of the face, breasts, or genitals.[84] The average age of onset for these patients is younger than age 20, with males and females equally represented. Typical males present to plastic surgeons with the conviction that their noses are too large or disfiguring. The typical female, convinced that her facial skin is "scarred," making her appearance grotesque, will seek a plastic surgery or dermatologic consultation. BDD is commonly accompanied by a mood disorder (including atypical depression with rejection sensitivity), social phobia, obsessive-compulsive disorder (OCD), and substance use disorders.

Patients with delusions of infestation believe that parasites, insects, or vermin are under their skin, and as a consequence they have often severely excoriated themselves. These individuals tend to be in their mid-50s at onset and approximately two thirds are women. They may complain of itching or tickling sensations and frequently produce bits of skin or hair as evidence of their infestation.

In olfactory reference syndrome, the patient is falsely convinced he emits a foul odor, for example halitosis, which offends others. The patient engages in elaborate rituals, such as frequent bathing and changes of clothing, and the excessive use of perfume and deodorants. Olfactory reference syndrome is more common in men than women and the typical patient is in his mid-20s.

These three forms of monosymptomatic hypochondriasis share certain clinical characteristics. Despite the encapsulation of their thought disorder, these patients are profoundly anguished about their symptoms and their lives are severely disrupted. Their lives are completely devoted to the pursuit of medical and surgical remedies, and they tenaciously resist psychiatric referral or treatment. They are intensely ashamed and feel that they are under constant scrutiny and derision. This generally leads to profound social withdrawal and disability. Severe anxiety, paranoia, and depression are prevalent. Alcohol abuse is common, especially in younger males.

Treatment. Selective serotonin reuptake inhibitors (SSRIs) and clomipramine are the agents of choice in the treatment of BDD, with doses in the upper therapeutic range. BDD often remits along with major depression. Electroconvulsive therapy (ECT) has also been used successfully when the patient was frankly delusional.

These patients are difficult to treat, in part because they are so ashamed of their appearance and resistant to psychiatric help. Psychopharmacologic agents may be effective, but the patients are frequently unwilling to take them. They do not believe that a psychotropic could correct a physical defect, or once begun on an agent, they may stop taking it without informing their physician.

Pimozide (Orap) can be effective in suppressing the symptoms (e.g., delusions of infestation).[86] A single morning dose is administered daily, starting with 2 mg and moving up in 2-mg increments every 3 days or so. Munro and Chmara[86] noted that one seldom needs to exceed 12 mg/day. Antiparkinsonian agents can be given if dystonic symptoms are experienced. Complete or partial improvement occurred in about 80% of cases, usually within 2 weeks, although treatment failure should not be accepted before a 6- to 8-week course of the drug has been completed.

Maintenance therapy is generally necessary.[84] Even with successful pharmacotherapy, most patients retain some concern about their problem, but its intensity is blunted sufficiently to permit them to lead more normal lives. One may never be able to get some patients to acknowledge the delusional nature of their symptom, even after significant improvement. Hard-pressed to justify the recommendation of a neuroleptic, the physician may even tell the patient that these insects or odors are best "cleansed" from within the system, hence the need for a drug. On the other hand, a few patients will accept the notion that the body is more vulnerable to parasitic infestation or odor generation during times of greater stress. When major depression is present in BDD, medication is more readily accepted.

Functional Medical Syndromes

Although somatoform disorders are characterized by complaints that seem far out of proportion to any abnormalities found, common functional medical syndromes also lack laboratory confirmation. Like the diagnoses in DSM-IV, these diagnoses depend on consensus criteria, description of symptoms, and a natural course of illness. There is substantial overlap in the phenomenology, epidemiology, and co-occurrence of these various syndromes, and they share a great many characteristics.[87,88]

Chronic fatigue syndrome (CFS), fibromyalgia (FM), and irritable bowel syndrome (IBS) are three of the functional medical syndromes, named for the dominant symptom complex. Once the patient acquires a functional diagnosis either by strict research criteria or by looser clinical criteria, that diagnosis is granted greater authority and legitimacy than a comorbid psychiatric diagnosis. Physician and patient often collude to focus attention only on the somatic syndrome. A symptom like disturbed sleep can be seen either as part of a medical or a psychiatric diagnosis. Whether the patient is diagnosed with a functional medical condition, mood disorder, or somatoform disorder, depends on whether the key symptoms are attributed to the physical or psychiatric realms.[89] The fact that the patient carries a functional medical diagnosis should not limit aggressive treatment of comorbid psychiatric diagnoses.

When compared with community residents who have the same symptoms but who never seek out a physician, those patients who seek medical care for functional medical syndromes are more distressed, depressed, and under more life stress. In the medical setting, comorbid psychiatric diagnoses often go unrecognized. The principles of care for somatoform disorders apply here as well. Rule out organic disease. Diagnose and treat affective disorder, substance abuse and the other psychiatric diagnoses. Knowing the patient, listening with respect for his or her suffering, setting limits, and keeping an ear for changes in medical complaints remain pivotal concepts. Cognitive and behavioral therapy are emerging from a number of rigorous intervention trials as effective treatments for many of these syndromes.[90,91] The status of antidepressant pharmacotherapy for them has been systematically reviewed.[92]

Chronic Fatigue Syndrome

Many more patients complain of chronic fatigue without a medical cause than meet formal criteria for CFS. Fatigue itself is a vague symptom that requires exploration of exacerbating factors, timing, mood, and meaning. Patients with major depressive disorder have fatigue that is worse in the morning and they have difficulty initiating activity, as do patients with Parkinson's disease. Sometimes fatigue actually turns out on exploration to be agoraphobic avoidance of leaving home, or a tendency to avoid the risk of social embarrassment. Fatigue may also mean daytime sleepiness, seen in sleep apnea. Fatigue with dysphoria is central to a mood disorder. Apathy—lack of motivation and lack of dysphoria—is more characteristic of a neurologic disorder or hypothyroidism. Patients who value their productivity and strength are especially frustrated by fatigue, and its personal meaning will exacerbate the symptom.

By consensus, CFS is defined as (1) self-reported, clinically evaluated, unexplained, persistent or relapsing chronic fatigue with a definite onset, that lasts more than 6 months; it is not due to exertion or relieved by rest, but it substantially reduces the patient's activities; and (2) four or more of the following symptoms, which came after onset of fatigue: impaired memory or concentration, sore throat, tender cervical or axillary lymph nodes, muscle pain, multijoint pain without joint swelling or redness; new headaches; unrefreshing sleep; and postexertional malaise lasting more than 24 hours.[93]

The formal diagnosis of CFS, like that of a somatoform disorder, requires exclusion of the common psychiatric diagnoses. Patients, according to the most recent research criteria, do not qualify if they have a fatiguing medical condition that has not yet resolved or if they use fatiguing prescription medications. A formal diagnosis of past or current major depressive disorder with psychotic or melancholic features, bipolar mood disorder, schizophrenia, delusional disorder, dementia, substance abuse within the previous 2 years, and anorexia nervosa or bulimia precludes formal diagnosis of CFS.

The patient may have formal CFS and also have a comorbid anxiety disorder, somatoform disorder, nonmelancholic depression, neurasthenia, multiple chemical sensitivity disorder, or FM. The challenge for the consultation psychiatrist is to treat what can be treated using either psychopharmacologic or psychological approaches. Anxiety disorders and nonmelancholic depression remain potentially fatiguing aspects of the syndrome. The psychiatrist should consider the role of personality disorder or the possibility of bipolar disorder, a diagnosis not easily ascertained by history, especially when seen between flagrant episodes. Exploration of the description and meaning of the most prominent symptom is indicated.

Although fatigue may follow a viral infection, no single virus has been shown to cause persistent, debilitating CFS. In the primary care setting, patients with postinfectious fatigue after 6 months are more likely to have had fatigue and psychological distress before the infection.[94] A history of dysthymia and more than eight medically unexplained symptoms not already listed in CFS criteria, may predict prolonged disability in CFS patients.[95]

Suggested screening laboratory tests include a complete blood count, a sedimentation rate, liver and renal function tests, calcium, phosphate, glucose, thyroid stimulating hormone, and urinalysis. Further tests, like a magnetic resonance imaging scan of the head to search for multiple sclerosis, should be guided by clinical findings. Lyme disease, for instance, is unlikely to present with fatigue as the only finding.[96] Acute mononucleosis in adolescence might produce a similar picture, but it is not likely later on in life. The acute diagnosis could be documented by antibody evidence of recent infection.

There is no specific medical treatment for formal CFS. The choice of antidepressant[92] for comorbid mood disorder depends on its capacity to improve sleep but limit sedation. Graduated aerobic exercise programs are important to improve physical conditioning. Cognitive-behavioral programs increasingly appear to have established their effectiveness.[91,97] The goal is to help the patient to achieve maximal function.[98]

Fibromyalgia

FM is a syndrome of generalized muscle pain and tenderness at specific trigger points, detected by physical examination.[99] To make the diagnosis, pain must be bilateral, above and below the waist, and include the axial-cervical spine, chest, or lower back. Criteria require 11 of 18 (9 bilateral) trigger points. Secondary FM occurs with rheumatoid arthritis and Lyme disease.

Affective disorders are common among FM patients who seek out rheumatologists. The diagnosis of FM, originally associated with chronic fatigue and sleep disorder, now only includes pain and trigger points, according to the American College of Rheumatology[99a]; however, patients with FM, fatigue, and unrefreshing sleep may meet diagnostic criteria of CFS.

For FM, amitriptyline and cyclobenzaprine (both tricyclic antidepressants) to relieve pain and improve sleep seem to work at least briefly in some fraction of patients.[100] Doses of 25 to 50 mg/day of amitriptyline are titrated as tolerated.

Irritable Bowel Syndrome

Functional gastrointestinal disorders are recurrent medical syndromes without known biochemical or structural abnormalities. Irritable bowel symptoms occur in 15% to 20% of the population, but the small subset that seek medical help compose a major component, 25% to 50%, of referrals to gastroenterologists.[101]

The international criteria for IBS include continuous or recurrent symptoms (for at least 3 months) of abdominal pain or discomfort relieved by defecation, or associated with a change in stool frequency or consistency *and* an irregular pattern of defecation at least 25% of the time (three or more of the following): (1) altered stool frequency; (2) hard, loose, or watery stool; (3) straining, urgency, or feeling of incomplete evacuation; (4) passage of mucus; (5) bloating or a feeling of abdominal distention.[102]

Those who visit physicians have more severe symptoms and are more likely to have comorbid psychiatric diagnoses than those who do not. Mood disorder,[103] panic with agoraphobia (especially fear of leaving the house because of diarrhea),[104] and a history of childhood abuse are more prevalent among patients than among the general population.[105]

Again, diagnosis depends on criteria, natural history of illness, and absence of laboratory confirmation of another diagnosis. The clinical approach to IBS is similar to that for the somatoform disorders: Rule out organic and psychiatric diagnoses. In the context of a relationship in which the physician continues to learn about the patient, the physician chooses somatic treatments that target the predominant symptom of pain, constipation, or diarrhea. A tricyclic antidepressant that tends to cause constipation may be preferable for a patient with recurrent diarrhea. An SSRI like fluoxetine seems the better choice for comorbid panic disorder or OCD, particularly in patients with constipation. If the patient tends to diarrhea, loperamide, a constipating agent, may be useful. Fiber and dietary adjustments may relieve constipation.[101] The principles of pain management in IBS parallel the principles of management in somatoform pain disorder.

IBS might be characterized as "a career woman's disease": Patients seem compulsive, overconscientious, dependent, sensitive guilty, worried, neurotic, unassertive, and often victimized earlier in life. They have an especially high need for social approval. Flatus or staining are humiliating. Cognitive-behavioral treatment appears effective[106] and includes desensitization. Education about amplification of visceral symptoms and the vicious circle of anxiety, increased vigilance for symptoms, and resultant increase in symptoms and pain; relaxation training; and stress management techniques are all helpful to both individuals and groups.

Conclusions

When one thinks of somatizers, the somatoform disorders may be the first diagnostic category to come to mind. But among general hospital inpatients and outpatients, other psychiatric diagnoses (particularly major affective disorders, the anxiety disorders, and organic mental syndromes) are more likely to be discovered at the end of the history and examination. These require specific treatment, and when the psychiatric disorder remits, the somatic symptoms usually subside. The diagnostic tests we find helpful are the MMPI, an excellent screening device for conversion, somatoform, and Axis II parameters; projective tests, to help both physician and patient understand conflicts in the patient's life that may not be in the patient's awareness; and full neuropsychological test batteries, which delineate precise areas of cognitive deficiency (see Chapter 6).

The treatment, as discussed, depends on the diagnosis. When the diagnosis is somatization disorder or hypochondriasis, treatment guidelines are hard to find and controlled studies rare (exceptions being the demonstration by Smith et al.[62] that an intervention with the primary physician significantly reduced costly and potentially harmful medical interventions without compromising the health or satisfaction of these patients, and by Clark et al.[77] regarding the effectiveness of cognitive-behavioral treatment). General clinical guidelines, however, do exist.[2,10,60,107]

References

1. Lipowski ZJ: Somatization: the concept and its clinical application, *Am J Psychiatry* 145:1358–1368, 1988.
2. Kellner R: Functional somatic symptoms and hypochondriasis, *Arch Gen Psychiatry* 42:821–833, 1985.
3. Goldberg D: Detection and assessment of emotional disorders in a primary care setting, *Intl J Ment Health* 8:30–48, 1979.
4. Kirmayer LJ, Robbins JM: Three forms of somatization in primary care: prevalence, co-occurrence and sociodemographic characteristics, *J Nerv Ment Dis* 179:647–655, 1991.
5. Goldberg G, Bridges K: Somatic presentations of psychiatric illness in primary care settings, *J Psychosom Res* 32:137–144, 1988.
6. Wittenborn JR, Buhler R: Somatic discomforts among depressed women, *Arch Gen Psychiatry* 36:465–471, 1979.
7. Katon W: Panic disorder: epidemiology, diagnosis, and treatment in primary care, *J Clin Psychiatry* 47(suppl 10):21–27, 1986.
8. Goldberg R, Morris P, Christian F, et al: Panic disorder in cardiac outpatients, *Psychosomatics* 31:168–173, 1990.
9. Snyder S: Pseudologia fantastica in the borderline patient, *Am J Psychiatry* 143:1287–1289, 1986.
10. Ford CV: *The somatizing disorders: illness as a way of life*, New York, 1983, Elsevier Biomedical.
11. Aduan RP, Fauci AS, Dale DC: Factitious fever and self-induced infection, *Ann Intern Med* 90:230–242, 1979.
12. Murray HW, Tuazon CU, Guerrero IC: Urinary temperature: a clue to early diagnosis of factitious fever, *N Engl J Med* 296:23–24, 1977.
13. Schade DS, Drumm DA, Eaton RP: Factitious brittle diabetes, *Am J Med* 78:777–784, 1985.
14. Kusumi RK, Plouffe JF: Gas in soft tissues of forearm in an 18-year-old emotionally disturbed diabetic, *JAMA* 246:679–680, 1981.
15. O'Reilly RA, Aggeler PM: Covert anticoagulant ingestion: study of 25 patients and review of world literature, *Medicine* 55:389–399, 1976.
16. Schmaier AH, Carabello J, Day HJ: Factitious heparin administration, *Ann Intern Med* 95:592–593, 1981.
17. Kim HC, Kosmin M: Heparin and factitious purpura (letter), *Ann Intern Med* 96:377, 1982.
18. Ratnoff OD: Psychogenic bleeding. In Ratnoff OD, Forbes CD, editors: *Disorders of hemostasis*, Philadelphia, 1991, WB Saunders Co, pp 552–553.
19. Scarlett JA, Mako ME, Rubinstein AH: Factitious hypoglycemia. Diagnosis by measurement of serum C-peptide immunoreactivity and insulin-binding antibodies, *N Engl J Med* 297:1029–1032, 1977.
20. Orr DP, Eccles T, Lawler R: Surreptitious insulin administration in adolescents with insulin-dependent diabetes mellitus. *JAMA* 256:3227–3230, 1986.
21. Mariotti S, Martino E, Cupini C: Low serum thyroglobulin as a clue to the diagnosis of thyrotoxicosis factitia, *N Engl J Med* 307:410–412, 1982.
22. Pearce CJ, Himsworth RL: Thyrotoxicosis factitia (letter), *N Engl J Med* 307:1708–1709, 1982.
23. Downing ET, Braman SF, Fox MJ: Factitious asthma, *JAMA* 248:2878–2882, 1982.
24. Devore CD, Ulshen MH, Cross RE: Phenolphthalein laxatives in factitious diarrhea, *Clin Pediatr* 21:573–574, 1982.
25. Falchuk ZM, Butterfly LF, Stern TA: A 60-year-old woman with chronic diarrhea and weight loss, *N Engl J Med* 313:1341–1364, 1985.
26. Winn DR, Martin MJ: A physical sign of bulimia (letter), *Mayo Clin Proc* 59:722, 1984.
27. Mitchell JE, Pyle RL, Eckert ED: Electrolyte and other physiological abnormalities in patients with bulimia, *Psychol Med* 13:273–278, 1983.

28. Killen JD, Taylor CB, Telch MJ: Self-induced vomiting and laxative and diuretic use among teenagers, *JAMA* 255:1447–1449, 1986.
29. Brotman AW, Rigotti N, Herzog DB: Medical complications of eating disorders: outpatient evaluation and management, *Compr Psychiatry* 26:258–272, 1985.
30. Amarnath RP, Abell TL, Malagelada JR: The rumination syndrome in adults: a characteristic manometric pattern, *Ann Intern Med* 105:513–518, 1986.
31. Ford CV, Abernethy V: Factitious illness: a multidisciplinary consideration of ethical issues, *Gen Hosp Psychiatry* 3:329–336, 1981.
32. Phillips MR, Ward NG, Ries RK: Factitious mourning: painless patienthood, *Am J Psychiatry* 140:420–425, 1983.
33. Whitlock FA: *The Ganser syndrome and hysterical pseudo-dementia.* In Roy A, editor: *Hysteria*, New York, 1982, John Wiley and Sons, Inc., pp 185–209.
34. Gurwith M, Langston C: Factitious Münchausen's syndrome (letter), *N Engl J Med* 302:1483–1484, 1980.
35. Reich P, Lazarus JM, Kelly MJ: Factitious feculent urine in an adolescent boy, *JAMA* 238:420–421, 1977.
36. Reich P, Gottfried LA: Factitious disorders in a teaching hospital, *Ann Intern Med* 99:240–247, 1983.
37. Asher R: Münchausen's syndrome, *Lancet* 1:339–341, 1951.
38. Stern TA: Münchausen's syndrome revisited, *Psychosomatics* 21:329–336, 1980.
39. Cramer B, Gershberg MR, Stern M: Münchausen syndrome: its relationship to malingering, hysteria, and the physician-patient relationship, *Arch Gen Psychiatry* 24:573–578, 1971.
40. Ford CV: The Münchausen syndrome: a report of four new cases and a review of psychodynamic considerations, *Psychiatr Med* 4:31–45, 1973.
41. Kahana RJ, Bibring GL: *Personality types in medical management.* In Zinberg N, editor: *Psychiatry and medical practice in a general hospital*, New York, 1965, International University Press, pp 108–123.
42. Ford CV, Folks DG: Conversion disorders: an overview, *Psychosomatics* 26:371–383, 1985.
43. Galin D, Diamond R, Braff D: Lateralization of conversion symptoms: more frequent on the left, *Am J Psychiatry* 134:578–580, 1977.
44. Stern DB: Handedness and the lateral distribution of conversion reactions, *J Nerv Ment Dis* 164:122–128, 1977.
45. Lazare A: Conversion symptoms, *N Engl J Med* 305:745–748, 1981.
46. Vuilleumier P, Chicherio C, Assal F, et al: Functional neuroanatomical correlates of hysterical sensorimotor loss, *Brain* 124:1077–1090, 2001.
47. Henry JA, Woodruff GHA: A diagnostic sign in states of apparent unconsciousness, *Lancet* 2:920–921, 1978.
48. Folks DG, Ford CV, Regan WM: Conversion symptoms in a general hospital, *Psychosomatics* 25:285–295, 1984.
49. Swartz M, Blazer D, George L, et al: Somatization disorder in a community population, *Am J Psychiatry* 143:1403–1408, 1986.
50. Morrison J: Childhood sexual histories of women with somatization disorder, *Am J Psychiatry* 146:239–241, 1989.
51. Swartz M, Blazer D, Woodbury M, et al: Somatization disorder in a US Southern community: use of a new procedure for analysis of medical classification, *Psychol Med* 16:595–609, 1986.
52. Guze SB: The validity and significance of the clinical diagnosis of hysteria (Briquet's syndrome), *Am J Psychiatry* 132:138–141, 1975.
53. Cloninger CR, Reich T, Guze SB: The multifactorial model of disease transmission: III. Familial relationship between sociopathy and hysteria (Briquet's syndrome). *Br J Psychiatry* 127:23–32, 1975.
54. Coryell W: A blind family history study of Briquet's syndrome, *Arch Gen Psychiatry* 37:1266–1269, 1980.
55. Zoccolillo M, Cloninger CR: Parental breakdown associated with somatisation disorder (hysteria), *Br J Psychiatry* 147:443–446, 1985.
56. Liskow B, Othmer E, Penich EC: Is Briquet's syndrome a heterogeneous disorder? *Am J Psychiatry* 143:626–629, 1986.
57. Othmer E, DeSouza C: A screening test for somatization disorder (hysteria), *Am J Psychiatry* 142:1146–1149, 1985.
58. Goodwin DW, Guze SB: *Psychiatric diagnosis*, ed 2, New York: Oxford University Press, 1979.
59. Oxman TE, Rosenberg SD, Schnurr PP, Tucker GJ: Linguistic dimensions of affect and thought in somatization disorder, *Am J Psychiatry* 142:1150–1155, 1985.
59a. Flor-Henry. P, Fromm-Arch D, Tapper M, et al: A neuropsychological study of the stable syndrome of hysteria, *Biol Psychiatry* 16(7) 601–626, 1981.
60. Murphy GE: The clinical management of hysteria, *JAMA* 247:2559–2564, 1982.
61. Smith GR, Jr., Monson RA, Ray DC: Psychiatric consultation in somatization disorder: a randomized controlled study, *N Engl J Med* 314:1407–1413, 1986.
62. Smith GR, Rost K, Kashner TM: A trial of the effect of a standardized psychiatric consultation on health outcomes and costs in somatizing patients, *Arch Gen Psychiatry* 52:238–243, 1995.
63. Kashner TM, Rost K, Smith GR, Lewis S: An analysis of panel data: the impact of a psychiatric consultation letter on the expenditures and outcomes of care for patients with somatization disorder, Med Care 30: 811–821, 1992.
64. Kroenke K, Spitzer RL, deGruy FV, et al: Multisomatoform disorder: an alternative to undifferentiated somatoform disorder for the somatizing patient in primary care, *Arch Gen Psychiatry* 54:352–358, 1997.
65. Escobar JI, Waitzkin H, Silver RC, et al: Abridged somatization: a study in primary care, *Psychosom Med* 60, 466–472. 1998.

66. Escobar JI, Gara M, Silver RC, et al: Somatisation disorder in primary care, *Br J Psychiatry* 173:262–266, 1998.

67. Tyrer P, Fowler-Dixon R, Ferguson B: The justification for the diagnosis of hypochondriacal personality disorder, *J Psychosom Res* 34:637–642, 1990.

68. Noyes R, Langbehn DR, Happel RL, et al: Personality dysfunction among somatizing patients, *Psychosomatics* 42:320–329, 2001.

69. Barsky AJ, Wyshak G: Hypochondriasis and somatosensory amplification, *Br J Psychiatry* 157:404–409, 1990.

70. Barsky AJ, Klerman GL: Overview: hypochondriasis, bodily complaints, and somatic styles, *Am J Psychiatry* 140:273–283, 1983.

71. Murray GB: *Hypochondriasis.* In Manschreck TC, editor: *Psychiatric medicine update*, New York, 1979, Elsevier Biomedical, pp 125–134.

72. Kenyon FE: Hypochondriasis: a clinical study, *Br J Psychiatry* 110:478–488, 1964.

73. Kellner R: Prognosis of treated hypochondriasis, *Acta Psychiatry Scand* 67:69–79, 1983.

74. Barsky AJ: The patient with hypochondriasis, *N Engl J Med* 345:1395–1399, 2001.

75. Warwick HMC, Salkovskis PM: Hypochondriasis, *Behav Res Ther* 28:105–117, 1990.

76. Salkovskis PM: *Somatic problems.* In Hawton K, Salkovskis PM, Kirk JW, et al, editors: *Cognitive-behavioral approaches to adult psychiatric disorders: a practical guide*, Oxford, 1989, Oxford University Press, pp 235–276.

77. Clark DM, Salkovskis PM, Hackmann A, et al: Two psychological treatments for hypochondriasis, *Br J Psychiatry* 173:218–225, 1998.

78. Fallon BA, Schneier FR, Marshall R, et al: The pharmacotherapy of hypochondriasis, *Psychopharm Bull* 32:607–611, 1996.

79. Noyes R Jr., Happel RL, Muller BA, et al: Fluvoxamine for somatoform disorders: an open trial, *Gen Hosp Psychiatry* 20:339–344, 1998.

80. Kjernisted KD, Enns MW, Lander M: An open-label clinical trial of nefazodone in hypochondriasis, *Psychosomatics* 43:290–294, 2002.

81. Fallon BA, Liebowitz MR, Salmán E, et al: Fluoxetine for hypochondriacal patients without major depression, *J Clin Psychopharmacol* 13:438–441, 1993.

82. Thomas CS: Dysmorphophobia: a question of definition, *Br J Psychiatry* 144:513–516, 1984.

83. Phillips KA: Body dysmorphic disorder: clinical aspects and treatment strategies, *Bull Menninger Clin* 62(4 suppl A):A33–A48, 1998.

84. Phillips KA, Crino RD: Body dysmorphic disorder, *Curr Opin Psychiat* 14:113–118, 2001.

85. Phillips KA: Body dysmorphic disorder: the distress of imagined ugliness, *Am J Psychiatry* 148:1138–1149, 1991.

86. Munro A, Chmara J: Monosymptomatic hypochondriacal psychosis: a diagnostic checklist based on 50 cases of the disorder, *Can J Psychiatry* 27:374–376, 1982.

87. Wessely S, Nimnuan C, Sharpe M: Functional somatic syndromes: one or many? *Lancet* 354, 936–939, 1999.

88. Barsky AJ, Borus JF: Functional somatic syndromes, *Ann Intern Med* 130:910–921, 1999.

89. Johnson SK, DeLuca J, Natelson BH: Assessing somatization disorder in the chronic fatigue syndrome, *Psychosom Med* 58:50–57, 1996.

90. Sharpe M: Cognitive behavioural therapies in the treatment of functional somatic symptoms. In Mayou R, Bass C, Sharpe M, editors: *Treatment of functional somatic symptoms*, Oxford, England, 1995, Oxford University Press, pp 122–143.

91. Kroenke K, Swindle R: Cognitive-behavioral therapy for somatization and symptom syndromes: a critical review of controlled clinical trials, *Psychother Psychosom* 69:205–215, 2000.

92. O'Malley PG, Jackson JL, Santoro J, et al: Antidepressant therapy for unexplained symptoms and symptom syndromes, *J Fam Pract* 48:980–990, 1999.

93. Fukuda K, Straus SE, Hickie I: The chronic fatigue syndrome: a comprehensive approach to its definition and study, *Ann Intern Med* 121:953–959, 1994.

94. Wessely S, Chalder T, Hirsch S, et al: Postinfectious fatigue: prospective cohort study in primary care, *Lancet* 345:1333–1338, 1995.

95. Clark MR, Katon W, Russo J: Chronic fatigue: risk factors for symptom persistence in a two and a half year follow-up study, *Am J Med* 98:187–195, 1995.

96. Reik L: Lyme disease and fatigue. In Dawson DM, Sabin TD, editors. *Chronic fatigue syndrome*, Boston, 1993, Little, Brown & Co., pp 161–177.

97. Deale A, Chalder T, Marks I, et al: Cognitive behavior therapy for chronic fatigue syndrome: a randomized controlled trial, *Am J Psychiatry* 154:408–414, 1997.

98. Butler S, Chalder T, Ron M, et al: Cognitive behavior therapy in chronic fatigue syndrome, *J Neurol Neurosurg Psychiatry* 54:153–158, 1991.

99. Wolfe F, Smythe HA, Yunus MB: The American College of Rheumatology 1990 criteria for classification of fibromyalgia: report of the multi-center criteria committee, *Arthritis Rheum* 33:160–172, 1990.

99a. Wolfe F, Smythe HA, Yunus MB, et al: The American College of Rheumatology 1990 criteria for classification of fibromyalgia: report of the multi-center criteria committee, *Arthritis Rheum*, 33:160–172, 1990.

100. Carette S, Bell MJ, Reynolds J: Comparison amitriptyline, cyclobenzaprine, and placebo in the treatment of fibromyalgia: a randomized double-blind clinical trial, *Arthritis Rheum* 37:32–40, 1994.

101. Drossman DA, Thompson WG: The irritable bowel syndrome: review and a graduated multicomponent treatment approach, *Ann Intern Med* 116:1009–1016, 1992.

102. Drossman DA, Funch-Jenson P, Janssens J, et al: Identification of subgroups of functional bowel disorders, *Gastroenterol Int* 3:159–175, 1990.

103. Tollefson GB, Tollefson SL, Pederson M: Comorbid irritable bowel syndrome in patients with generalized anxiety and major depression, *Ann Clin Psychiatry* 3:215–222, 1991.

104. Lydiard RB, Fossey MD, Marsh W: Prevalence of psychiatric disorder in patients with irritable bowel syndrome, *Psychosomatics* 34:229–234, 1993.

105. Drossman DA, Leserman J, Nachman G, et al: Sexual and physical abuse in women with functional or organic gastrointestinal disorders, *Ann Intern Med* 113:828–833, 1990.

106. van Dulmen AM, Fennis JFM, Bleijenberg G: Cognitive-behavioral group therapy for irritable bowel syndrome: effects and long-term follow-up, *Psychosom Med* 58:508–514, 1996.

107. Barsky AJ: Clinical crossroads: a 37-year-old man with multiple somatic complaints, *JAMA* 278:673–679, 1997.

Chapter 20
Difficult Patients

James E. Groves, M.D.

The medical equivalent of war is the difficult patient. Doctors soldier steadily on through all kinds of clinical chores, arduous schedules, and "administrivia," but when they get to the types of patients variously called "obnoxious,"[1] "needy," "crocky,"[2] "malignant," and even "hateful,"[3] they fight the worst battles of their careers, become prone to clinical blunders, mess up their personal lives, violate boundaries, and get sued. The good news is that—almost without exception—the "difficult patient" situation makes the consulting psychiatrist more useful to treating physician and patient alike than in any other medical encounter. Harrowing though such situations may temporarily be, it is just this kind of consultation that earns the trust and respect of the physician consultee and generates more consultation requests later on. (And, really, there are few better ways for a psychiatrist starting out to build a practice than by becoming a specialist on the difficult patient.) Before turning to management strategies, it is worth reviewing the presentations of difficult patients.

Types of Difficult Patients

Delirious patients may be assaultive. Guilty, bereaved spouses can be litigious. Temporal lobe epileptics are often clingy and viscous. Manic patients are emotional cyclones. Celebrities at times generate anxiety in their caregivers. Schizophrenics can be noncompliant. Anyone when ill can become angry, dependent, and hypochondriacal. Somehow none of these difficult situations necessarily produces "difficult patient" scenarios.

Difficult patients are almost always individuals with personality disorders—with one exception: Only patients with addictions seem to contradict the difficult-patient-equals-personality-disorder rule (if one includes individuals with eating disorders—thinness addicts). There has been a state-versus-trait debate about whether substances elicit a "true" or "underlying" personality ("*in vino veritas*") as opposed to the idea of substances sickening or "poisoning" the true self (intoxication, dipsomania). Personality disorders lie closer to trait because they so seldom change much, and addictions and eating disorders lie closer to state because when they do change, it can be rather dramatic. Every experienced physician can think of a patient with an addiction who was not typically difficult, and occasionally some "really bad actor" will go to Alcoholics Anonymous, get sober, and a year or two later look and act like a real *mensch*. In the *Diagnostic and Statistical Manual of Mental Disorders* (DSM-IV),[4] personality disorders are defined by clusters of traits, and addictions are states that the substance gives rise to. (For the purposes of management later on in this chapter, however, we will tend to think of excess alcohol as a personality disorder in a bottle.)

Not all individuals with personality disorders are difficult patients. Looking at "pure types" through the lens of DSM-IV, those not necessarily belonging to the difficult patient paradigm are paranoid, schizoid, and schizotypal personality disorders (cluster A); likewise, avoidant, dependent, and obsessive-compulsive personality disorders (cluster C) do not necessarily belong to the difficult patient paradigm. It is not impossible to find the individual with schizotypal or paranoid personality that gets along well with the treating physician. Even the individual with dependent personality—if not angry but merely clinging—can be someone the physician enjoys working with. Although some of these may be difficult patients, it is really when we look into DSM-IV cluster B disorders that a pit of despair opens—antisocial, borderline, and narcissistic. (For the sake of this discussion, histrionic individuals are grouped with borderlines because, as difficult patients, they are almost indistinguishable.)

With these three diagnoses, there is almost a complete overlap between difficult patients and personality disorders. It is not Axis I or Axis III conditions that make for typically difficult patients, but the cluster B subset of Axis II disorders, the "dramatic/emotional/erratic" cluster. DSM-IV defines them as the following:[4]

Antisocial personality disorder involves a pattern of disregard for, and violation of, the rights of others.

Borderline personality disorder is characterized by a pattern of instability in interpersonal relationships, poor self-image, dysphoric affects, and marked impulsivity.

Narcissistic personality disorder is embodied by a pattern of grandiosity, a need for admiration, and a lack of empathy.

The key word here is *pattern*. Personality traits lead to personality disorder "only when they are inflexible, maladaptive, and persisting and cause significant functional impairment or subjective distress."[4] These traits are "enduring" for most of the life span; they are "pervasive" (i.e., they color most of the individual's personal and social interactions). They deviate "markedly" from the expectations of the individual's culture. Finally, they do not result from another mental or physical disorder, such as depression or head trauma.

Antisocial and Narcissistic Personality Disorders

Individuals with antisocial personality disorder display the defining trait of disregard for the rights of others. The disorder satisfies the general criteria

for the other personality disorders and consistently manifests at least three of the following traits[4]: (1) rule-breaking, (2) lying, (3) impulsivity or poor planning, (4) belligerence, (5) recklessness, (6) irresponsibility or faithlessness, and (7) a lack of conscience or empathy.

Narcissistic personality disorder[4] defines itself in the grandiosity and lack of empathy shown by at least five of the following traits: (1) arrogance; (2) a lust for power through beauty, love, brilliance, or money; (3) convictions of "specialness"; (4) a hunger for admiration; (5) entitlement; (6) exploitation and manipulativeness; (7) stunted empathy (an inability to "feel into" the other person); (8) envy; and (9) displays of contemptuousness.

Antisocial personality disorder and narcissistic personality disorder are similar in terms of selfishness but different in terms of social destructiveness. One could think of the difference as that between criminality and shabby ethics. Whether these two entities differ more in degree or in kind is a question perhaps better left to religion or philosophy, yet in psychiatry one view has been that the personality disorders have similar ego defects (except in degree) and similar underlying psychic organizations[5–7] or even a common one called *borderline personality organization*.[8] If it is true that a change in social context (e.g., incarceration) brings out borderline personality in individuals that otherwise look antisocial, as some have claimed,[9] there may be some utility to the notion of a core personality disorder called *borderline with several variant presentations*. At any rate, the management strategies discussed subsequently work for borderlines and for other personality disorders alike, given a rigorous application and a sufficiently strong social structure.

The concept of an underlying or "core" borderline personality organization is a metaphor that has considerable utility in the "difficult patient" discussion. In the medical setting, antisocial and narcissistic individuals are difficult only when they are acting like borderlines. The idea is that the underlying good/bad split or fragmented borderline personality organization is "held together" by the self-promoting program of the antisocial person and the grandiosity of the narcissist. Antisocial and narcissistic individuals who believe their physicians' interests parallel their own are unctuous and undifficult ("prison sincerity"). When the psychopathy and grandiosity are punctured by illness or injury and thwarted by medical treatment, the "underlying" fragmented, rageful, splitting, attacking borderline "comes out." In the discussion that follows, therefore, borderline personality is the referent paradigm of difficulty, to be discussed more at length and used interchangeably with difficult patient.

Borderline Personality Disorder

Borderline personality is so named[10] because it seemed to psychoanalysts to "lie between" the psychoses and the neuroses. Borderline patients are dreaded for their impulsivity, swings from love to hate, and maddening irrationality. They split the world into exaggerated dichotomies of good and evil. An interpersonal middle ground does not exist. These patients, by some combination of innate rage and inept parenting, cannot find a moderate position in any aspect of mental life.[11]

Borderline patients have a multifaceted personality disorder, "without a particular behavioral specialty."[12] Subtypes range from "bordering on psychosis," in which the patient is chaotic or irrational, to "bordering on neurosis," in which the patient desperately clings to others to feel real.[8,13] A few borderline patients cope with an inadequate sense of self by adapting like chameleons to the environment of the moment (the as-if personality).[14] The core borderline patient has the characteristics shown in Table 20-1, the current official diagnostic criteria.[4]

In the past, borderline personality was sometimes held to be a subset of biologic depressive illness[15–17] or a variant of traditional diagnoses, such as hysteria, sociopathy, or alcoholism.[18,19] Because up to 90% of some samples of borderline patients have comorbid conditions, some researchers questioned the construct validity of the borderline diagnosis, whereas others defended it[20–26]: As many as half of some borderline populations suffer a major depressive episode on Axis I; conversely, some 13% of Axis I alcoholics have comorbid borderline personality. On Axis II, at least 20% of borderline patients receive an additional personality disorder diagnosis. Of these Axis I-plus-Axis II patients, some have remission of borderline symptoms when their affective disorder is treated, or when active alcohol abuse stops—again confusing the validity of the diagnosis. (Because it is more closely related to management, differential diagnosis is discussed in a later section.)

Regardless of subtype or comorbid diagnosis, however, borderline patients can abruptly flee treatment or develop psychotic transference and delusions about their caregivers.[27–29] Short, circumscribed episodes of delusional thinking in unstructured situations and when under stress are almost pathognomonic.[13,29–31] Borderlines display a signature trait, poor observing ego[32] (i.e., dense

Table 20-1. DSM-IV Criteria for Borderline Personality Disorder

A pervasive pattern of instability of interpersonal relationships, self-image, and affects and marked impulsivity beginning by early adulthood and present in a variety of contexts, as indicated by 5 (or more) of the following:

1. Frantic efforts to avoid real or imagined abandonment; note: do not include suicidal or self-mutilating behavior covered in criterion 5
2. A pattern of unstable and intense interpersonal relationships characterized by alternating between extremes of idealization and devaluation
3. Identity disturbance: markedly and persistently unstable self-image or sense of self
4. Impulsivity in at least two areas that are potentially self-damaging (e.g., spending, sex, substance abuse, reckless driving, binge eating); note: do not include suicidal or self-mutilating behavior covered in criterion 5
5. Recurrent suicidal behavior, gestures, or threats or self-mutilating behavior
6. Affective instability due to a marked reactivity of mood (e.g., intense episodic dysphoria, irritability, or anxiety usually lasting a few hours and only rarely more than a few days)
7. Chronic feelings of emptiness
8. Inappropriate, intense anger or difficulty controlling anger (e.g., frequent displays of temper, constant anger, recurrent physical fights)
9. Transient, stress-related paranoid ideation or severe dissociative symptoms

From American Psychiatric Association: *Diagnostic and statistical manual of mental disorders*, ed 4, Washington, DC, 1994, American Psychiatric Association.

denial of vital aspects of reality and irrationality to a degree that almost has to be seen to be believed). Although the relation of borderline personality to schizophrenia has long been debated,[14,33-35] it is likely that if there is a border with a biologic illness, it is closer to affective illness[36-39] without being completely tangential to it.[40]

Heredity plays a crucial role in the cause of borderline personality. Innate intolerance to anxiety and a constitutional tendency toward rage are accepted even by psychoanalytic theorists regarding borderline personality.[41] The disorder resembles aspects of traits long thought to run in families, and evidence suggests that borderlines cluster in families with affective disorders—38% of borderline patients have first-degree relatives with some affective disorder[42]—and impulsivity and affective instability generally cluster in some families with borderline members even when depression does not.[43]

Theories of the nonbiologic component also focus on the family of origin.[44,45] Psychoanalysts view borderline personality as arising from failure by the individual's mother to foster coherent self-object differentiation in the first 18 months of life,[46,47] leading to the development of pathologic ego defenses (discussed later, under Management). The individual does not learn to tolerate negative affects associated with separation[48,49]; this continues the child's clinging into adulthood, as if others were desperately needed parts of the self.[8,50,51] The borderline's adult relationships are called *transitional* after the transitional object.[52-54] The patient's mother (probably borderline herself[55]) apparently feared fusion with (and destruction of or by) the child. She could not let the child separate because of her own fears of being alone. On rapprochement, she tended to reject the child for "deserting" her.[52-58] She mostly saw the child as her own transitional object and—used as the imaginary playmate of the mother—the child never grew into an emotionally separate human being.

In borderline personality, the boundaries between the self and others are blurred, so that closeness seems to threaten fusion. Sexuality and dependency are confused with aggression. Needs are experienced as rage. Long-term relationships disintegrate because of an inability to find optimal interpersonal distance. Because of inadequate ego mechanisms of defense, there is little ability to master painful feelings or to channel needs or aggression into creative outlets. Ambivalence is poorly tolerated. Impulse control is dismal. The patient has a fragmented mental picture of the self and views others as all bad and simultaneously all potent, a chaotic mixture of shameful and grandiose images.[11]

In addition to the literature on inadequate parenting, there has been an avalanche of reports linking borderline personality with parental abuse, particularly sexual abuse.[59] The line of reasoning often put forth is that the child victim of sexual abuse (especially of chronic abuse[60]) used dissociation[61] as a defense against massive psychic trauma, and the dissociation became habitual, undermining ego integration. This association with sexual abuse is seen as variously explaining phenomena ranging from a propensity toward dissociative psychotic-like episodes, rage, sexual disorders, psychotic/erotic transferences in psychotherapy, and self-mutilation all the way to the comorbidity of borderline personality with multiple personality and with eating disorders. The literature on abuse does have the important effect of spotlighting the relationship between borderline phenomena and dissociation, something the older literature underemphasized. Although the linkage to childhood sexual abuse is still being worked out, it is clear that a significant number of borderline patients, when asked give a history of such abuse, do so (up to 33% of nonclinical populations and 57% of borderline psychiatric inpatients[59]); this has to be taken into account in management.[62]

Borderline personality is relatively rare; it occurs in perhaps 1% to 5% of the population.[63] Despite its small size, the borderline cohort stands out in the general hospital because of its florid presentation and poor prognosis,[64,65] and because of the feelings of anger and helplessness stirred up in the caregivers.[66] These patients make themselves medical outcasts because they ruthlessly destroy the care they crave.

Difficult Behaviors and the Consultee

The previous discussion about the DSM-IV diagnoses of difficult patients must be leavened with a simple fact: It is not the diagnoses of these patients that make them difficult for the consultee—it is their behaviors. The relationship of these behaviors to other aspects of mental life is schematized in Figure 20-1.

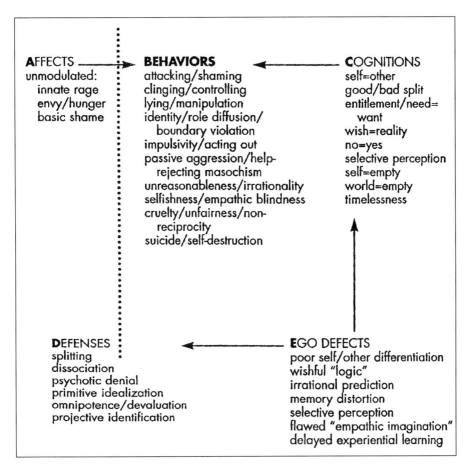

Figure 20-1. Difficult patient's problem behaviors.

Such patients have abnormally intense affects, poorer than average neutralizers of affect, or both. In any case, raw rage, naked dependency, and ontologic shame are present and are frequently found on the surface. The cognitive structures that ordinarily temper intense affects are distorted and primitive. The ego weakness of the patient is shown by the absence of higher-level defenses and by the primitive nature of the ones that are present.

Under pressure of intense affect (rage/terror/shame), the patient uses dissociation to a greater or lesser extent and enters the dreamlike state that individuals ordinarily enter only in extreme emergencies. In this dissociated state (which is probably present much of the time to some degree), the individual is distracted, numb, and difficult to reach. The pervasiveness of dissociation is one feature of borderline personality that is insufficiently discussed in the literature; however, it can contribute drastically to the pathologic cognitions

of borderlines and place a distorting lens of unreality between them and the real world.

Besides dissociation, the borderline individual uses denial of major aspects of reality to cope. This mythification of the external, threatening world is displayed in defenses called primitive idealization, omnipotence, and devaluation. As the names imply, these are metaphors for the dreamy, wishful, mythified world the difficult patient inhabits, a world of black and white and good and evil. These maladaptive defenses may be all too visible in the medical setting, but they are even more troubling than are two others with which such patients try unsuccessfully to manage their extreme negative affects—splitting and projective identification.

Splitting is by definition a rigid separation of positive and negative thoughts or feelings. Normal persons are ambivalent and can experience two contradictory feeling states at one time; the borderline personality characteristically shifts back and forth, entirely unaware of one feeling state while in another. Sometimes one state is rigidly held while its opposite is projected onto the environment. The cause of splitting is unknown; it is said to protect the patient from the anxiety of reconciling contradictory extremes (at the expense of the already unstable personality). In social systems,[67–71] borderlines can split the staff into warring "good" and "bad" factions that unwittingly act out the patient's internal world.

Projective identification[72–76] is said to consist of taking an unwanted aspect of the self, such as cruelty or envy, and wholly ascribing it to ("projecting it into") another. The patient then unconsciously pressures that person to own the projected attribute. Unaware that a self-fulfilling prophecy is being set up, the recipient complies with the projection and acts it out. These two mechanisms can complement each other, with projective identification being used to "confirm" one side of a polarized, split view of the world.[11]

Although the long-term psychotherapy of the borderline patient may involve therapeutic undoing of these defenses,[8,77] it is dangerous to confront such defenses in brief encounters in the medical setting. It is crucial, however, to be aware of their presence. For example, awareness of borderline splitting prepares the consultant to deal with the division of the medical staff into "good ones" and "bad ones." Recognition of the patient's primitive idealization, of a physician for instance, may help the consultant prepare for the furious devaluing that is to follow.

Helping the Consultee

The medical setting is a social system with its own history, boundaries, hierarchy, customs, and taboos. The introduction of a difficult patient into this culture sometimes places such stress on the system as to cause malfunctions in caregiving or outright extrusion of the patient, a situation that active psychiatric consultation can prevent.[78–80] Difficult patients are exquisitely vulnerable to caregivers' ordinary imperfections in communication and consistency, and they are often remarkably attuned to their caregivers' normal negative feelings of anxiety, shame, anger, and depression. Such patients are especially vul-

nerable to feelings of rejection by caregivers,[81] and their shaky defenses are even more compromised than usual by the stresses of illness and treatment.

After initial diagnosis and treatment of the patient, the consultant's next priority should be to gauge the amount of distress the staff is under. A psychologically naive medical staff may regress to a helpless or vengeful position in response to the patient's ingratitude, intractability, impulsivity, manipulativeness, dependency, entitlement, and rage. Regression in any social system may emerge as disagreement among staff; it may take the form of inappropriate confrontation of the patient, or it may manifest itself as a deterioration in the patient's behavior.[11] Regression seems to occur when there exists a large disparity between what is expected and what is found.[82] Troublesome dissonance of this sort between patient and staff may generally occur in any or all of three dimensions: (1) perception of reality, (2) values governing control and aggression, and (3) rules about interpersonal closeness (Table 20-2).

The earliest clue to the nature of the dissonance lies in the consultation request.[83] Its tone, covert messages, intensity, timing, and route by which it reaches the consultant all can reflect the dissonance between patient and staff expectations. (In this sense, the consultation request resembles the chief complaint in the history, often the first, best clue to the problem.) Consultation is sought when the patient is out of touch with the staff's reality. Such dissonance may range from mild (when the patient is from a different culture) to severe (when the patient is psychotic). When the patient is docile, the request is matter-of-fact; when the patient manifests grotesquely sexual or aggressive behavior, the consultant may receive a shrill, disorganized call for help.

Consultation is sought when the patient's aggression violates staff expectations. The staff expects to be in control of the patient, who is expected to be grateful, compliant, and nondestructive. Dissonance in this dimension may range from mild, when the patient sulks, to severe, when the patient is violent or self-destructive. The tone of such a consultation request ranges from irritation to anger or outright fear, depending on the kind of aggression the patient displays.

Table 20-2. Consultation Management of Staff and Difficult Patient Dissonance in the Medical Setting

Type of Dissonance: Consultation Request	Patient's Problem Behaviors	Consultant's Work with the Consultee	Consultant's Work with the Patient
Dissonant reality: vague, confusing request for help; puzzled tone to request	Inappropriate to realities of illness or hospital; denial and demandingness	Explains patient's reality to staff; models "reality testing"	Diagnosis of any cognitive disorders; gives medication and reality testing
Aggressive dissonance: request to control or remove patient; fearful or angry tone	Menacing, self-destructive, or suicidal	Recommends social, chemical, or physical restraints necessary for safety	Evaluates potential violence; searches for source of patient's panic
Staff/patient dissonance regarding interpersonal distance: request consultant to take over care of patient; depressed, guilty tone to consultation request	Dependent	Gives permission to say no to patient's unrealistic, excessive demands	Clarifies for patient that some but not all needs can be realistically met
	Rejecting	Diminishes guilt and depression by stating impossibility of entirely satisfying patient	Allows patient some distance; repeatedly appeals to patient's "entitlement" and autonomous side
	Manipulative (dependent and rejecting)	Serves as forum for hatred toward patient; voices hateful feelings but behaves nonsadistically	Bargains; sets firm, noninterpretive limits on manipulation; clarifies patient's self-interest

Consultation is sought when the patient's need for closeness is different from what the staff deems appropriate. The staff expects the patient to be involved with the caregivers but to keep a certain distance. When the patient asks for repeated reassurances or when the patient makes inexhaustible or contradictory demands, a depressed, guilty request often ensues. Arrogant, peremptory consultation requests often herald a hostile-dependent-manipulative patient; depressed, tired requests may foretell an empty, clinging patient.

The primitive defenses[8,41,72–76,84] of the difficult patient may stimulate staff disagreement (Table 20-3). To cope with deep feelings of self-loathing, the patient may see the staff as loathsome—otherwise why would they care (projective identification)? Or the patient may see the staff as magically all good, to keep all the badness in the world away (primitive idealization). To make sense of a world in which people are both good and bad, such a patient may choose some people on the staff to be "all good" and some to be "all bad" (splitting). This "explains" for the patient "why" things always go wrong: The patient is caught between good and bad forces outside the self and therefore they are not the fault of the self. When the patient views the staff through the defense of splitting, the staff may eventually behave as if it were so. The patient will tell an "all good" staff member what terrible things an "all bad" staff member has done, said, or thought and then swear the "good" one to secrecy. As less

Table 20-3. Manifestations of Primitive Ego Defenses: The Difficult Patient in the Medical Setting

Splitting: Keeping completely apart two opposite ideas and their associated feelings. Staff are divided into "good ones" and "bad ones," reflecting the patient's incapacity to achieve ambivalence enough to see that caregivers have human limits, with "good" and "bad" qualities at the same time.

Projective identification: The tendency to see some staff as "bad" as the patient feels. This gets translated into behavior based on the following kind of "logic": "I'm bad and you take care of me, which means you're rotten as I am, otherwise you wouldn't care for me." This perception is so powerfully held that the staff receiving it tend to act it out unconsciously.

Primitive denial: The alternating expungement from consciousness of first one and then another perception of opposite quality (in which it is called *splitting*) or a wish so powerful that it obliterates crucial aspects of reality contradicting that wish. For instance, fear may cause the patient to deny a serious condition and flee the hospital where it could be treated.

Primitive idealization: The tendency to see some staff as totally "good" to protect the patient from "bad" staff or from the patient's medical condition.

Omnipotence and devaluation: A shift (splitting) between the need to establish a relationship with a magical, powerful staff (primitive idealization) versus the conviction of omnipotence in the self that makes all others impotent by comparison (primitive idealization of the self). Omnipotent caregivers are supposed to deliver the patient perfect care to protect against disease, and when this does not happen, the staff is seen as impotent and hateful. (Splitting makes the perception shift dramatically, whereas projective identification causes the staff to buy into the patient's primitive projections, making them come true).

Adapted from Groves JE: Management of the borderline patient on a medical or surgical ward: The psychiatric consultant's role, *Int J Psychiatry Med* 6:337–348, 1975.

and less communication takes place and as the patient escalates demands, the "good" staff and "bad" staff begin to disagree about the care of the patient because the borderline patient may be "good" with "good" staff and vice versa. The remedy for this depends on reestablishing open staff communication, even if it is hostile, to enable staff to get a well-rounded view of the patient. Firm, nonpunitive limit setting[67,69] (Table 20-4) is crucial for inpatient treatment because it must be made clear that the patient cannot destroy the caregiving system or be destroyed by it, no matter how intense the wishes or fears may be.

It is a natural human instinct to confront such patients angrily, but caregivers should exercise precautions during confrontations. Avoiding a confrontation of narcissistic entitlement is as important

Table 20-4. Rules for Confrontation of the Difficult Patient

Acknowledge the real stresses in the patient's situation.
Avoid breaking down needed defenses.
Avoid overstimulation of the patient's wish for closeness.
Avoid overstimulation of the patient's rage.
Avoid confrontation of narcissistic entitlement.

Adapted from Adler G, Buie DH: The misuses of confrontation with borderline patients, *Int J Psychoanal Psychother* 1:109–120, 1972.

as it is difficult.[85] Such patients exude an offensive sense of deservedness that is always tempting for an overworked staff to confront angrily and suddenly. Often the difficult patient has only this sense of entitlement to keep a fragmented personality together during the stresses of hospitalization. Entitlement for the narcissist is what hope and faith are to normal individuals. Preserving it requires a deliberate effort. Taken together, what Tables 20-2 to 20-4 show is that such behaviors of the difficult patient (e.g., manipulativeness and entitled demanding)—obnoxious though they may be—sometimes function as defenses at a relatively high level for that patient. Stripping them away makes the patient fall back on even lower-level defenses, such as psychotic denial and dissociation, or—worse—be defenseless, panic, or explode.

Setting limits, avoiding confrontation, and avoiding overstimulation of the desire for closeness and rage are difficult to arrange in the fast-paced medical milieu. Prevention of staff splitting is especially difficult because of the various subcultures in medicine. If, for instance, the patient chooses the nurses to be "all bad" and the physicians to be "all good," the nurses may displace anger to the physicians but be unable to express it directly because of role-induced sanctions, and the physicians may see the nurses as incompetent and unable to comprehend their treatment plan for the patient. Such situations are fertile ground for the splitter and require concerted effort toward open communication.

Pathologic dependency presents in one of its extremes as manipulativeness—an intense, covert, contradictory, self-defeating attempt to get needs met.[3,84] It is the behavioral manifestation of a need by the patient to get close but at the same time maintain a safe distance from sources of emotional support. (Occasional patients feel so empty that, paradoxically, getting their needs met threatens them with engulfment; they are so famished that closeness may actually make them feel merged with someone else and therefore not really alive.) Such patients seem to have a deathly fear of what they most crave.

In limit-setting confrontations with manipulative, entitled patients, the consultant may have to model for the staff firmness, repetition, and an appeal to the patient's sense of entitlement (rather than an assault on it): "You deserve the best medical care we can give, and that's why we're recommending X, Y, and Z." The consultant has to keep uppermost in mind the appeal to the entitlement and not get drawn into logical or illogical arguments. Moreover, it is important to avoid interpreting the resistance to cooperation as a fear of dependency, a tactic that would at best leave the patient somewhat bewildered. Repetition is crucial. Encounters to engage compliance often have to be repeated two or three times at varying intervals before the patient agrees, for instance, to take medication.

Dependent, manipulative patients stir up sadism in the caregivers, which inhibits the setting of effective limits. The consultant supports the staff's self-esteem and performance by reinforcing strengths rather than by pointing out weaknesses, by teaching, by lending a conceptual framework to mitigate anxiety, by modeling interactions, and, most of all, by matter-of-factly stating that such patients stir up hatred even in the best of caregivers. Whenever the staff brings even a hint of negative reference to the patient, the consultant can say something like, "Yeah, these patients are manipulative and irritating as hell!" Or, "Everybody hates this kind of patient—I know I do." This personalization, juxtaposed with the consultant's own nonsadistic behavior toward the patient, legitimizes hostility toward the patient, but shares it among staff rather than inflicting it on the patient.

In general, the earlier in the hospitalization the consultant is called, the more overt is the reason for the consultation and the more effective will be the intervention because the difficult patient has had less time to project into the staff the intense, seemingly inborn shame such patients possess in great abundance. Late in the hospitalization, the consultant may be urgently called in to see the patient for vague reasons and arrive to find the situation in a shambles, the patient in restraints, the staff ashamed and in bitter conflict—and nobody either willing or able to say what has been going on.

Consultant's Role

The consultant's role in the management of the difficult patient consists of a specialized type of consultee-oriented approach in which countertransference hatred and fear are drawn away from the patient and strategically metabolized within the staff-consultant relationship. The consultant should actively promote a behavioral management practicum[84] placed in the medical chart for reference and as a symbol of the psychiatrist's helping presence. This "recipe" discusses (1) communicating clearly with the patient and among staff; (2) understanding the patient's need for constant personnel; (3) dealing with entitlement without confronting needed defenses; and (4) setting firm limits on dependency, manipulativeness, rage, and self-destructive behaviors.

Generally the consultant's approach should first lead directly to the consultee. The request should be elicited in person or at least on the phone because the written record never reveals all of the problems in the management of the difficult patient. Then the consultant goes to the head nurse to get a history of the patient's response to hospital routine. Next, the consultant reads the chart and compares medication orders with records of medication actually administered. The consultant will have generated some hypotheses and is now ready to test them in the examination of the patient. As the consultant proceeds through these steps, an orderly plan emerges (Table 20-5).

One helpful approach is the consultee-oriented model of consultation,[86] which involves thinking of the patient and staff as a single entity and dealing as

Table 20-5. Order of Priorities for the Difficult-Patient Consultation in the Medical Setting

1. Rapidly evaluate the most pressing psychiatric problems—beginning with physical or social restraints if the patient appears about to lose control of violent or self-destructive impulses.
2. Create a differential diagnosis of the difficult patient, with an explicit biopsychosocial formulation of the predominant conflicts and stressors.
3. Identify staff-patient dissonance and formulate a plan of action to reduce it (see Table 20-2).
4. Provide treatment recommendations—psychological and pharmacologic (see Box 20-1), short-term and long-term— taking into account the ongoing medical regimen and implicitly addressing staff-patient dissonance while explicitly addressing the patient's conflicts.
5. Educate the consultee and staff to reduce dissonance and to lend a conceptual framework for dealing with future difficult patients.
6. Actively participate without grandstanding or actually taking over the total psychological care of the patient.
7. Follow-up and be involved in disposition planning for the medical and psychiatric needs of the patient.

Adapted from personal communications with TP Hackett, AD Weisman, NH Cassem, AW Alonso, TD Stewart, K Nobel, JA Renner, OS Surman, and many others.

much as possible with the strong, healthy part. The entity consists of two parts. One part, the difficult patient, has problems with object relations, pathologic behaviors exacerbated under stress, and several self-defeating and infuriating defenses, especially splitting. To prevent being split, the consultant should try to deal mainly with the healthy part, the staff. Because the staff is often closely linked in an unwilling, hateful, and guilty alliance with the patient and its collective self-esteem is already damaged by encounters with the patient, the consultant should not damage it further by interpreting the staff's pathology.

The attempt to ally with staff rather than the patient is destined to encounter several kinds of resistance at the outset. First, the patient is eager to engage the consultant to find out whether the consultant is "all good" or "all bad." Second, the staff, needing distance from its sense of failure, wants the consultant to take over the care of the patient completely. Third, neither the staff nor the patient has the energy to understand what is going on; they are in pain and want relief now, preferably by removal of the patient.

The alliance with the staff depends to a large extent on previous experience with the consultant, how long it takes to answer the consultation request, and how much sense the advice makes. The alliance with the difficult patient is dramatically less important in terms of outcome than the alliance with the staff. Such patients are incapable of forming a real alliance, and their "alliances" are mostly primitive idealization. Ideally, the patient should be seen only briefly if there are enough

data from other sources, and the staff is told that the consultant will work mainly with staff and see the patient infrequently.

Visiting the patient should be reserved in the early stages for the specific purpose of the consultant's alliance with the staff. Following the initial patient interview, the consultant goes to see the patient (1) when a magical gesture of "taking over" is needed to comfort a desperate staff, (2) when staff members feel that the consultant does not know how much they are suffering, and (3) when the staff needs a specific model for carrying out recommendations on limit-setting or reality testing.

The consultation note, by its tone, specific information, and description of the patient in a way the staff can immediately recognize, remains in a medical record day and night as a tangible symbol of the consultant's helping presence. It outlines the request, history, mental status at the hour of the examination, and the psychiatric history. It is explicit about medications, and the potential for suicide and for violence. It includes specific, concrete management recommendations. For example, this was the conclusion of a consultation note for a difficult patient who had been spitting in her hyperalimentation line:

Impression: Ms. B is thought to have a chronic, severe personality disorder sometimes called borderline, meaning that she lies on the border of psychosis diagnostically and has only marginal social adjustment.

Recommendations: (1) Continue haloperidol 2 to 10 mg orally twice a day as needed. (2) Have brief, daily staff conferences to compare notes and reach a consensus about her surgical treatment plan. (3) Try to have the same staff members work with Ms. B each day; bear in mind that she tends to panic at each change of shift. (4) Set firm limits on her multiple and contradictory demands. She is quick to rage when her demands are not met and may threaten suicide. Do not imply that Ms. B does not deserve the things she demands, but rather say over and over again that you understand what she is asking, but because you feel she deserves the best possible care, you are going to continue to recommend the course dictated by your experience and judgment. If she continues spitting in her hyperalimentation line, assure her that physical restraint will ensue. (These limits do not mean that she should not be allowed to complain, but you need not tolerate more than twice as much as you would from the average patient.) (5) Suicide precautions. Search her luggage.

The consultant addresses dissonance arising from the patient's version of reality; tendency to act out; and demandingness, neediness, and rage. The consultant gives a mandate for open communication and daily staff conferences to prevent staff splitting, and to provide a supportive environment. Firm limits, without challenging the patient's sense of entitlement, are set forth explicitly. The task now becomes one of seeing that recommendations are effected. There is nothing more frustrating than laboring to devise a treatment plan to find that it is not carried out. When this happens, the consultant often finds that the source of resistance is still-unresolved staff-patient dissonance (see Table 20-2).

Nowhere in the previous discussion is the unconscious motivation of the patient or of the staff brought to the attention of either. This is what is meant by *noninterpretive intervention.* Psychoanalytic interpretations foster a temporary regression and have no place in the consultation with the disruptive medical/surgical patient.[84,87] Instead the consultant analyzes and reduces dissonance by speaking of its behavioral roots and consequences while resisting the temptation to illuminate interesting unconscious processes.

Medication

The psychopharmacologic management of difficult patients is quite complex and uncertain, again suggesting that borderline personality disorder (the referent paradigm of difficulty) is not simply a "border on" depressive disease. The relation of depression to borderline personality is "surprisingly weak and nonspecific,"[40] a bit of a retreat from the consensus of a decade or so ago. Target symptoms, first of all,

do not reliably predict response during symptomatic exacerbations, and haloperidol may sometimes give a better response than tricyclics, even with affective symptoms; similarly, fluoxetine and carbamazepine may work better for rage and behavioral dyscontrol in borderlines than with the affective dysregulation they ameliorate in nonborderline individuals with affective disorders.

Although borderline patients are often maintained on antidepressants, there is no clear evidence of efficacy for the long-term maintenance with neuroleptics and only a questionable benefit from maintenance with monoamine oxidase inhibitors, not surprising because there are few blind-controlled studies, even of the short-term treatment of such patients.[88] Newer compounds, such as the selective serotonin reuptake inhibitors (SSRIs)[89,90] and risperidone, appear to be at least as effective as the tricyclic antidepressants and phenothiazines—for whatever indication; in addition, they are safer and easier to use (and there is some suggestion that the SSRIs are much better than tricyclics for many borderlines, especially with anger and hostility).

In terms of specific recommendations to the consultee, a trial of medication can be quite helpful in particular instances. Box 20-1 sketches some current thinking. With chaotic, inappropriate, negative, hostile, and labile patients, antipsychotic medication may be life-saving. The target-symptom approach seemed more elegant than the trial-and-error method, but it must be admitted that the gist of the newer literature[40,88–90] (somewhat in contrast to the older, symptom-focused literature[11,91–94]) is that trial-and-error treatment with antidepressants and antipsychotic agents may sometimes be of value in any difficult patient regardless of the symptom profile. It is ironic that literature linking symptoms with specific neurotransmitters is converging on serotonergic sensitivity,[95–97] whereas clinical experience is diverging a bit from target symptoms.

Miscellaneous medications, ranging from methylphenidate to levodopa, have been reported to help difficult patients,[11] and there seem to exist single case reports touting almost any conceivable drug.[108] Given the present state of knowledge, it seems well for the consultant to remember that mind and body are not separate, and that many seemingly insoluble problems respond to a search for and aggressive treatment

---

BOX 20-1
Psychopharmacologic Treatment of the Difficult Patient

MAOIs

MAOIs were touted in the literature for avoidant, phobic, and "hysteroid dysphoric"[94,98] (exquisitely rejection-sensitive) patients, but most clinicians try SSRIs first, then tricyclics, before MAOIs because of the toxicity of MAOIs in overdosage and because of the dietary restrictions they entail.

SSRIs, Tricyclics

SSRIs and tricyclic antidepressants are useful, probably even in patients without a prominent neurovegetative component or comorbid affective condition.[99,100] Drug and dosage are empirically determined. (Difficult patients' target symptoms are not very good "targets" for pharmacology, and much of the drug management is trial-and-error.) SSRIs are increasingly preferred over tricyclics because of their great relative safety in overdosage and evidence of their having an especially potent effect on symptoms of anger and hostility in borderline patients. (One relative contraindication to the use of antidepressants is a history suggestive of a bipolar illness, which increases the risk of precipitating a manic episode[94,101] or worsening the violence-prone patient.)

Trazodone

Not an excellent antidepressant, trazodone in low doses is popular in some venues for sleep-disordered borderline patients (usually only women, because of the risk of priapism trazodone poses).

Lithium

Lithium carbonate may be useful for mood swings, irritability, affective instability, and attempts to control violence,[94] but, again, a trial-and-error approach is necessary in the absence of controlled studies. (Clinicians sometimes use lithium to augment mood elevators, even at maintenance serum levels, despite the potential toxicity of the drug to thyroid and kidney and potential lethality in overdosage.)

Carbamazepine

The anticonvulsant and mood stabilizer carbamazepine[94,102] was initially much less popular than lithium because of the need to monitor the patient for carbamazepine-induced neutropenia, but carbamazepine is now used with increasingly greater frequency. (Another antiseizure agent, valproate, does not seem to have penetrated much into this literature, but its indications should be the same as for carbamazepine and its safety profile greater. On an historical note, neurologists for years have used phenytoin for behavioral control of their difficult patients.)

Neuroleptics

Low doses are used, usually of haloperidol or thioridazine, for brief psychotic episodes.[103,104] After the episode, some patients continue neuroleptics as maintenance (perhaps only because the drama of such events is painful to the clinician). Also there is currently an argument that neuroleptics are specifically useful for affective symptoms, which, if true, would make neuroleptics appropriate for maintenance treatment. Note: extrapyramidal side effects: Worsening depression on neuroleptics may stem from subtle akinesia, and worsening agitation or even suicidal ideation may be traced to the insidious onset of akathisia.

Clozapine

There is one study of clozapine in patients with personality disorders,[105] but as yet no indicated use beyond the treatment of schizophrenia.[106]

Risperidone

The lore is that some clinicians like risperidone for the general management of borderline patients, usually a low dose at the patient's bedtime, but there is no significant literature on risperidone in personality-disordered patients.

Sedative Hypnotics

Most experienced clinicians try to avoid benzodiazepines, especially diazepam and alprazolam,[107] because of abuse potential (and their possibly greater disinhibiting, rage-producing effects), but some clinicians may try clonazepam as maintenance or lorazepam as needed. There is no apparent role for triazolam, which has been reported to be associated with cognitive distortions and affective instability, particularly risky in the borderline patient. One possible alternative, if neuroleptic or trazodone is not useful, is antihistamines for sedation.

MAOI, Monoamine oxidase inhibitor; *SSRI,* selective serotonin reuptake inhibitor.

of comorbid psychiatric conditions, especially affective disorders and substance abuse. Common and uncommon medical conditions mimic personality disorders (just for illustration, three random instances in the recent literature are narcolepsy, Wolfram syndrome, and Addison's disease[109–111]). Also, over the lifetime of any given patient, the relationship with a supportive physician is as healing as any drug.

Psychiatrist's Work with the Patient

Although design and promotion of the behavior management protocol and consultation with the staff are the initial work of the consultant, the psychiatrist performs the following tasks with the patient directly:

1. The psychiatric mental status examination, differential diagnosis, and formulation (including the use of observations of transference and countertransference)
2. Assessment of suicide potential
3. Assessment of present need for control of violence (as opposed to making a prediction of dangerousness)
4. Assessment of, and recommendations around, substance abuse and other "dysfunctional," addicted, or "codependent" patterns (e.g., inept parenting, eating disorders, spousal abuse, or obsessive-compulsive disorder)
5. Rarely a highly focused, brief (one- or two-session) tactical psychotherapeutic intervention.

Differential Diagnosis

If the consulting psychiatrist does not do it, there will not be a good mental status examination, psychiatric history, or biopsychosocial formulation in the medical record. However skilled or willing other specialists may be, only the psychiatrist has an understanding of the minute-to-minute fluctuations of transference and counter-transference that occur early, even in a single interview. (Countertransference is so important as to be almost a diagnostic discriminator of borderline personality.[112]) Also, there is a kind of rigor and discipline that the experienced psychodiagnostician brings to these

situations: No one else in the medical setting is, for instance, going to perform a Mini-Mental State Examination, ask about earliest memories, a history of sexual abuse, the content of dreams and fantasies, sexual worries, religious and spiritual concerns, disordered thoughts, and suicidal ideation—all in one interview—and then put them together into a differential diagnosis and formulation.

Differential diagnosis is crucial because comorbidity is almost a hallmark of the difficult patient, and it is surprising (if not impossible) to encounter a cluster B patient who does not also have at least one of the following diagnoses:

1. Another personality disorder
2. Substance abuse disorders
3. Affective disorders
4. Anxiety disorders (especially panic and phobias)
5. Eating disorders
6. Obsessive-compulsive disorder
7. Posttraumatic stress disorders
8. Adult attention deficit hyperactivity disorder
9. Impulse control disorders
10. Other disorders

Suicide Assessment

The gravest predictors of a suicide attempt[113–118] by the difficult patient are the following:

1. History of previous attempts, especially with high risk or a low chance of being rescued, and other violence
2. Standard demographic predictors (advanced age, being single, and the like; see also Chapter 9 on suicide)
3. Comorbidity, especially substance abuse and affective disorders
4. Marginalized socioeconomic and cultural status

These predictors are the same whether the patient is in the medical setting or out of it, but there are other predictors specific to the medical setting: Recent worsening in the medical condition along with perceived rejection by caregivers[81] adds considerably to the risk of suicide. Suicide attempts in medical and surgical settings correlate not so much with depression in serious illness, such as cancer, but rather with anger over the loss of social supports.

The large majority of suicide attempts occur in a clinical setting in which the patient's experience is of being abandoned—during failing treatment, at times of imminent discharge, in conjunction with disputes with the staff, or staff holidays.

Some factors are poor predictors, notoriously the psychiatrist's countertransference.[118,119] Also, it is false to think that individuals with antisocial personality or without clinical depression never kill themselves. Depression and the type of personality disorder are much less predictive of suicide than are punctured defenses and a "no-exit" situation, one the patient deems totally hopeless and inescapable. A good short mnemonic for immediate risk is the "3H rule"—hate, humiliation, and hopelessness. Strongly predictive are self-hate fused with hatred of another (often a spouse who has left), loss of face with extreme shame, and being trapped in a bad situation with no apparent prospect of escape.

Assessment of Potential for Violence

Problems arising when the patient has difficulty controlling aggression are helped when the consultant defines for the staff the range of responses, from supporting the sulking patient or even giving in to a mildly overcontrolling patient, to absolute limits on violence. The medical staff fear overreacting, and the consultant reduces anxiety by defining the management of varying degrees of aggression. Disruptions are mostly born of self-protective or fearful impulses in the confused or delirious patient. Rarely, however, a patient becomes dangerous. In those instances, the most common warning is fear; someone becomes scared of the patient. Staff almost never fear delirious behavior, controllable anger, or senile pique, but they do tend to become wary, then edgy, then frightened. This intuition in the caregivers is often the only warning the consultant gets before an explosion. Ominous signs in the patient are these:

1. Rapidly increasing demandingness
2. More frequent and intense anger, especially with abusive language
3. Mounting agitation and paranoia

The general feeling in the medical setting of an implacable crescendo of menace surrounding the patient is another ominous sign.

Before any decision about physical restraint of the patient is made, hospital security guards should be standing by on the ward. This is a first step in the decision-making process. Security can always be dismissed with thanks after standing by, but to delay summoning help until after such a decision is made risks panicking the patient, who may have an uncanny ability to sense an impending confrontation.

Such ideas refer to control of violent behavior in the immediate situation. Occasionally, however, the consultant is asked about the long-range "dangerousness" of the patient. This is an opinion that involves extrapolating from present behavior in a known, observed situation to a guess about the individual's interaction with a different milieu, one that may contain drugs, weapons, and situations beyond the psychiatrist's ken. Medicine is about healing, not social control. Dangerous individuals (e.g., the man with schizophrenia and a gun, the individual with an antisocial personality who commits rape) may in some sense be "difficult patients," but in these situations, they are not patients at all but criminals.

Psychiatric opinions outside the medical purview violate an important boundary and feed the fallacy that all bad behavior is somehow psychiatric, and that mentally ill individuals have no personal responsibility for their behavior. What the psychiatrist can do, however, is document medical history from the consenting individual about drugs, access to weapons, felony convictions, and the like. Surprisingly often, such an individual discloses useful information in the context of a skillfully elicited childhood history of enuresis, fire-setting, and cruelty to animals. ("Were you ever accused of setting fires? Did anybody ever say you were mean to the neighbor's pets?") Such individuals can be oddly eager to resurrect old denials and often are still indignant about them. They then sometimes go on to give themselves away and provide information needed to protect caregivers and other patients in the medical setting.

Substance Abuse

Substance abuse is the area in which the consultant can be most useful to individuals with primitive personality problems. Substance abuse is such an issue for a significant proportion of difficult patients that excess alcohol can be thought of as a "personality disorder in a bottle." More than half of some samples of borderline individuals—two thirds in one study—abuse substances. Of these, perhaps up to a fourth have such a good response to abstinence that they no longer meet diagnostic criteria for the disorder.[22]

If one adds to the number of patients with substance abuse various other addictive, codependent, or dysfunctional problems (e.g., eating disorders, "sex and love addicts," or incest survivors), it is not implausible that almost any difficult patient would qualify for some sort of 12-step or "recovery" program. Such self-help groups have not excited much interest or research in psychiatry (and have even occasionally inspired disdain because of their focus on spirituality), but there are several conceptual reasons (based on Fig. 20-1) why 12-step programs are ideal for difficult patients: Tenets of the "recovery" movement are essentially antipsychological in their nature, and given the lack of observing ego of borderline patients, this is a benefit, not a deficit. Many borderline patients have such dramatic regressions when involved in psychological treatments that observers have suggested that much of their pathologic behavior is iatrogenic,[120,121] a reaction to too much empathy and psychoanalytic interpretation. Furthermore, such programs have two ingredients well known to help primitive character pathology—an emphasis on taking responsibility for oneself (as opposed to cultivating the victim role) and a highly structured series of steps and methods. Not least in importance, there are myriads of such groups meeting at almost any hour of the day or night in every location in the urban United States.

Not surprisingly, it requires great skill to persuade a difficult patient to identify with one of the 12-step programs. First, there is almost always dense denial of the abuse problem, along with a need to see the self as powerless and victimized. Splitting patients and narcissists see themselves as "better than" individuals in Alcoholics Anonymous, for example, and are so vulnerable to shame that they hesitate to take on another attribute they see as shameful. Also, the general culture outside such programs has little real information about what they can accomplish, so the patient is not only ashamed, but also usually ignorant of these resources.

There is an art to getting a difficult patient to consider that a problem with addiction, "codependency," or the like may be the root of much of the suffering the patient endures. Practicing this art involves accumulating knowledge about such programs and having familiarity with some individuals helped by them. It involves the ability to discern when the patient might be receptive, first to acknowledging an addictive problem and, second to considering such a program. It involves knowing how to elicit information in a nonshaming way ("Do you find yourself drinking more than you really want to be drinking?"), presenting the condition as a disease and "not the person's fault," and introducing the ideas gradually in a nonthreatening way. ("Did your mom ever turn to Al-Anon for help with your father's drinking?" "Did you ever get help from the Adult Children of Alcoholics program or something like that?")

No difficult patient is ever educated easily, and it usually requires multiple inputs from numerous sources over many months even to begin to get some of these options accepted by the individual. The consulting psychiatrist is ideal to introduce such ideas and, given the relapse rate of difficult patients, may get another opportunity with the same patient in the future. The consultant can at least start the educational process without making the patient feel ashamed.

Brief Tactical Psychotherapy

Psychotherapy is a risky proposition, and the consultant is wise to resist the temptation to do much. Rarely, however, the crisis of an illness provides a unique chance for insight and growth for the patient with a primitive personality. This lucid interval is incidentally produced when an illness and treatment cut through the veils of dissociation surrounding such patients, their maladaptive projective defenses, and their habitual externalization of responsibility. In this context, sometimes the patient asks not only the superficial "why me," but also the deeper question, "Who am I that this is happening to?" In a certain sense, catastrophe throws the primitive individual into a developmental crisis in which there may be the potential for recouping a bit of the developmental lack of progress in the first 2 years of life—the maturation from the paranoid position to the depressive position—along with a capacity for grieving and the developing empathy for others that such maturational steps entail.

A study[122] of changes in pathologic narcissism in a cohort of individuals followed for several years found that a majority of them had improved significantly and that the improvement related to life achievements, new durable relationships, and disillusionment. These individuals displayed decreased grandiosity and deeper empathy for others as evidenced by better relationships. The disillusionment related to these improvements, moreover, had occurred at a critical juncture in the individual's development and was of a certain type—challenging but not devastating. Rather than questioning the construct validity of narcissistic personality disorder (as was done in this study), the findings plausibly support the idea that certain painful, constructive real-life experiences help individuals change their primitive pathology. (That brief therapeutic interventions can further this process, even in primitive patients, is shown in some of the therapies detailed by Malan, Budman, Strupp, Bloom, Horowitz, and especially Winnicott.[123])

This is the rationale for a certain brief, tactical intervention by the psychiatric consultant who encounters the difficult patient during a medical or surgical crisis: how to keep the disillusionment from being completely devastating and help the individual make sense of it in terms of personal identity. (As Fig. 20-1 shows, a vague sense of personal identity underlies much of the pathology of the difficult patient.) The patient is in a process of trying to adapt to the illness or injury, to work it through, to grieve losses, and to contain fears. In this context, the psychiatrist's aim is not merely to help further this grieving or adjusting process, but to accomplish a deeper, more lasting goal: using the illness or injury process as a template or map for other life changes, using the crisis of the moment to help the patient learn new ways of thinking about the self, and coping with rage, terror, and shame.

The tactical brief therapy of the difficult patient falls into two types of maneuvers—containment and intervention. Containment involves control of uncontrolled affect, distorted cognition, and destructive behavior. Intervention consists of correcting the misdirection of the patient's trajectory, previously determined by pathologic affect, distorted cognition,

and self-defeating behavior. Containment and intervention roughly correspond to the two parts of traditional psychotherapy, the frame (scheduling, vacations, fee, phone calls, limits on acting-out, confidentiality) and the content (symptoms, history, development, associations, discourse, dreams, fantasies, defenses, adaptation, transference, countertransference, and other nonframework components of therapy). This "moment" of brief tactical psychotherapy assumes the patient in the medical situation is temporarily contained and already in a dialogue with the psychiatrist about the illness or injury that brought the patient to this place at this time.

The therapist's first task—and therapist is what the consultant becomes at this moment—is to listen to see whether the patient is asking for intervention. The patient signals such readiness by not only addressing the impact of the illness or injury, but also by mentioning the overall meaning of the patient's life, the patient's "story," the overarching narrative that helps any human being make sense of the world. If the tactical intervention is to be helpful, the patient must be the one to push for it. The therapist's experience at this point is of being passively drawn into the patient's turbulent material, yet actively steering the discussion away from affects too intense on the one side and cognitions that are psychotically distorted on the other.

So up to this point, the therapist's job has been careful listening and containment. If the patient is ready, the patient will introduce these two themes—the overall story of the patient's life and its meaning, and the meaning of the illness or injury that is serving as the focus of the tactical psychotherapeutic moment. The patient will tend to see the medical crisis as thematically pertinent to the meaningful life story—for instance, just another in a long series of persecutions, a punishment for something bad the patient has done or is. The life story is generally a standard narrative of a search for perfect safety and love, a quest for power so the patient will never again be scared—there are seldom any major surprises at this point.

The therapist's first active step in the tactical intervention occurs now: labeling the life story; labeling the symbolic, metaphoric meaning of the illness or injury; and labeling the pain that is at the interface of the two. This is almost like offering a "title" for the story. ("All your life you've been a survivor—now you wonder if you can survive this terror.") The idea here is that, to survive, individuals have to construct a meaningful narrative of the crisis. Under pressure of converting experience into symbols and then into meaning, the primitive individual may be forced to construct a more realistic life narrative (and hence a more coherent sense of personal identity).

If the patient continues to be receptive to tactical intervention, two things happen at this point—first, production of deeper material in symbolic form (mention of a fantasy or recurrent dream, some external, cultural symbol or icon, a movie or a television character) and, second, a rather pointed question for the therapist about what to do (an acceptance by the patient of the therapist as a relatively separate, helpful person). This turning point requires careful listening because the key organizing theme of the patient's life (as the patient sees it) is presented in this one moment of symbol formation along with the rather concrete question that follows directly after.

Here the therapist does not answer the patient's question about what to do with the illness assaulting the meaning in the patient's life. The therapist labels the assault, points out the crisis in meaning, and thematically throws the question back to the patient. ("In a way you're asking how to cope with this thing, but in a deeper way you're saying that you're Scarlett O'Hara, since you just mentioned her. How would Scarlett handle what you're going through?")

What the patient says next reveals whether the tactical linking of the two meanings/two stories seemed useful to the patient. If so, the patient produces more details of the life story, again asking the therapist what to do about the illness or injury. Again the therapist throws responsibility back to the patient, labeling meaningfulness issues and the importance of the illness or injury to it. ("You just mentioned losing your husband—like Scarlett O'Hara—and now you're asking how to cope with your boyfriend's reaction to your mastectomy. Scarlett fell back on Tara and her own resources. What resources do you have to draw on?")

This working-through cycle of question/deflection continues as long as the therapist has time and the patient has strength to bear the rage, terror, or shame of the moment. Usually the patient soon fatigues and moves the subject back to some specific entitled demand, such as getting more pain medica-

tion. This signals that the therapy part of the encounter is now over and that the consultant is once again back to management of the difficult patient.

Termination

Preparation of the difficult patient for discharge from the hospital is fraught with hazard. The patient may not only intensify disruptive behavior to prolong the hospital stay, but also simultaneously try to leave prematurely. The patient may secretly infect dressings or intravenous lines with saliva or feces and develop a fever while threatening to leave the hospital against advice. Or the patient may increase suicidal gestures, such as wrist slashing, to manipulate (get close to/stay distant from) the staff. Firm limits on sabotage and elopement should be discussed with the staff. Around termination, they should be more observant of the patient and more visible and firm. A specific discharge date should be firmly adhered to[124] despite a predictable worsening in the patient's psychological status.

After the patient has left, it is good for the consultant to touch base with the staff and consultee once more to review the treatment and share some of the consultant's own feelings. In this way, the consultant not only "terminates" with the staff, but also prepares the way for future work with the next difficult patient who comes to the general hospital.

References

1. Martin PA: *The obnoxious patient.* In Giovacchini PL, editor: *Tactics and techniques in psychoanalytic therapy, vol 2, countertransference,* New York, 1975, Jason Aronson.
2. Lipsitt DR: Medical and psychological characteristics of "crocks," *Int J Psychiatry Med* 1:15–25, 1970.
3. Groves JE: Taking care of the hateful patient, *N Engl J Med* 298:883–887, 1978.
4. American Psychiatric Association: *Diagnostic and statistical manual of mental disorders,* ed 4, Washington, DC, 1994, American Psychiatric Association.
5. Meissner WW: *Treatment of patients in the borderline spectrum,* Northvale, NJ, 1988, Jason Aronson.
6. Kernberg OF: *Aggression in personality disorders and perversions,* New Haven, CT, 1995, Yale University Press.
7. Searles HF: *My work with borderline patients,* Northvale, NJ, 1994, Jason Aronson.

8. Kernberg OF: *Borderline conditions and pathological narcissism*, New York, 1975, Jason Aronson.

9. Vaillant GE: Sociopathy as a human process, *Arch Gen Psychiatry* 32:178–183, 1975.

10. Stern A: Psychoanalytic investigation of and therapy in the border line group of neuroses, *Psychoanal Q* 7:467–489, 1938.

11. Groves JE: Current concepts in psychiatry: borderline personality disorder, *N Engl J Med* 305:259–262, 1981.

12. Mack JE: *Afterword.* In Mack JE, editor: *Borderline states in psychiatry*, New York, 1975, Grune & Stratton.

13. Grinker RR, Werble B, Drye R: *The borderline syndrome: a behavioral study of ego-functions*, New York, 1968, Basic Books.

14. Deutsch H: Some forms of emotional disturbance and their relationship to schizophrenia, *Psychoanal Q* 11:301–321, 1942.

15. Klein DF: Psychopharmacology and the borderline patient. In Mack JE, editor: *Borderline states in psychiatry*, New York, 1975, Grune & Stratton.

16. Stone MH: *The borderline syndrome: constitution, personality, and adaptation*, New York, 1980, McGraw-Hill.

17. Fyer MR, Frances AJ, Sullivan T, et al: Comorbidity of borderline personality disorder, *Arch Gen Psychiatry* 45:348–352. 1988.

18. Guze SB: *Differential diagnosis of the borderline personality syndrome.* In Mack JE, editor: *Borderline states in psychiatry*, New York, 1975, Grune & Stratton.

19. Welner A, Liss JL, Robins E: Personality disorder: II. follow-up, *Br J Psychiatry* 124:359–366, 1974.

20. Nace EP, Saxon JJ, Shore N: A comparison of borderline and nonborderline alcoholic patients, *Arch Gen Psychiatry* 40:54–56, 1983.

21. Pope HG, Jonas J, Hudson J, et al: The validity of DSM-III borderline personality disorder, *Arch Gen Psychiatry* 40:23–30, 1983.

22. Dulit RA, Fyer MR, Haas GL, et al: Substance use in borderline personality disorder, *Am J Psychiatry* 147:1002–1007, 1990.

23. Oldham JM, Skodol AE, Kellman HD, et al: Comorbidity of Axis I and Axis II disorders, *Am J Psychiatry* 152:571–578, 1995.

24. Akiskal HS, Yerevanian BI, Davis GC, et al: The nosologic status of the borderline personality: clinical and polysomnographic study, *Am J Psychiatry* 142:192–198, 1985.

25. Barasch A, Frances A, Hurt S, et al: Stability and distinctness of borderline personality disorder, *Am J Psychiatry* 142:1484–1486, 1985.

26. Nurnberg HG, Raskin M, Levine PE, et al: The comorbidity of borderline personality disorder and other DSM-III-R Axis I personality disorders, *Am J Psychiatry* 148:1371–1377, 1991.

27. Gunderson JG, Singer MT: Defining borderline patients: an overview, *Am J Psychiatry* 132:1–10, 1975.

28. Kolb JE, Gunderson JG: Diagnosing borderline patients with a semistructured interview, *Arch Gen Psychiatry* 37:37–41, 1980.

29. Gunderson JG, Kolb JE: Discriminating features of borderline patients, *Am J Psychiatry* 35:792–796, 1978.

30. Chopra HD, Beatson JA: Psychotic symptoms in borderline personality disorder, *Am J Psychiatry* 143:1605–1607, 1986.

31. Anselm G, Soloff PH: Schizotypal symptoms in patients with borderline personality disorders, *Am J Psychiatry* 143:212–215, 1986.

32. Sterba R: The dynamics of the dissolution of the transference resistance, *Psychoanal Q* 9:363–379, 1940.

33. Knight RP: Borderline states, *Bull Menninger Clin* 17:1–12, 1953.

34. Gunderson JG: The relatedness of borderline and schizophrenic disorders, *Schizophr Bull* 5:17–22, 1979.

35. Modell A: Primitive object relationships and the predisposition to schizophrenia, *Int J Psychoanal* 44:282–292, 1963.

36. McGlashan TH: The borderline syndrome, is it a variant of schizophrenia or affective disorder? *Arch Gen Psychiatry* 40:1319–1323, 1983.

37. Stone MH: Borderline syndromes: a consideration of subtypes and an overview, directions for research, *Psychiatr Clin North Am* 4:3–24, 1981.

38. Akiskal HS: Subaffective disorders: dysthymic, cyclothymic, and bipolar II disorders in the "borderline" realm, *Psychiatr Clin North Am* 4:25–60, 1981.

39. Carroll BJ, Greden JF, Feinberg M, et al: Neuroendocrine evaluation of depression in borderline patients, *Psychiatr Clin North Am* 4:89–100, 1981.

40. Gunderson JG, Phillips KA: A current view of the interface between borderline personality disorder and depression, *Am J Psychiatry* 148:967–975, 1991.

41. Kernberg OF: Structural derivatives of object relationships, *Int J Psychoanal* 47:236–253, 1966.

42. Soloff PH, Millward JW: Psychiatric disorders in the families of borderline patients, *Arch Gen Psychiatry* 40:37–44, 1983.

43. Silverman JM, Pinkham L, Horvath TB, et al: Affective and impulsive personality disorder traits in the relatives of patients with borderline personality disorder, *Am J Psychiatry* 148:1378–1385, 1991.

44. Walsh F: *Family study 1976: 14 new borderline cases.* In Grinker RR, Werble B, editors: *The borderline patient*, New York, 1977, Jason Aronson.

45. Gunderson JG, Kerr J, Englund DW: The families of borderlines: a comparative study, *Arch Gen Psychiatry* 37:27–33, 1980.

46. Valenstein AF: Pre-oedipal reconstructions in psychoanalysis, *Int J Psychoanal* 70:433–442. 1989.

47. Mahler MS: *On human symbiosis and the vicissitudes of individuation,* New York, 1968, International Universities Press.

48. Zetzel (Rosenberg) E: Anxiety and the capacity to bear it, *Int J Psychoanal* 30:1–12, 1949.

49. Winnicott DW: The capacity to be alone, *Int J Psychoanal* 39:416–420, 1958.

50. Robbins M: Primitive personality organization as an interpersonally adaptive modification of cognition and affect, *Int J Psychoanal* 70:433–459, 1989.

51. Kernberg OF: The treatment of patients with borderline personality organization, *Int J Psychoanal* 49:600–619, 1968.

52. Winnicott DW: *Playing and reality,* New York, 1971, Basic Books.

53. Horton PC, Louy JW, Coppolillo HP: Personality disorder and transitional related-ness, *Arch Gen Psychiatry* 30:618–622, 1974.

54. Arkema PH: The borderline personality and transitional relatedness, *Am J Psychiatry* 138:172–177, 1981.

55. Masterson JF: The borderline adult: therapeutic alliance and transference, *Am J Psychiatry* 135:437–441, 1978.

56. Zweig FH, Paris J: Parents' emotional neglect and overprotection according to the recollections of patients with borderline personality disorder, *Am J Psychiatry* 148:648–651, 1991.

57. Mahler MS: Rapprochement subphase of the separation-individuation process, *Psychoanal Q* 41:487–506, 1972.

58. Bezirganian S, Cohen P, Brook JS: The impact of mother-child interaction on the development of borderline personality disorder, *Am J Psychiatry* 150:1836–1842, 1993.

59. Nigg JT, Silk KR, Westen D, et al: Object representations in the early memories of sexually abused borderline patients, *Am J Psychiatry* 148:864–869, 1991.

60. Silk KR, Lee S, Hill EM, et al: Borderline personality disorder symptoms and severity of sexual abuse, *Am J Psychiatry* 152:1059–1064, 1995.

61. Shearer SL: Dissociative phenomena in women with borderline personality disorder, *Am J Psychiatry* 151:1324–1328, 1994.

62. Gunderson JG, Chu JA: Treatment implications of past trauma in borderline personality disorder, *Harvard Rev Psychiatry* 1:75–81, 1993.

63. Vaillant GE, Perry JC: *Personality disorders.* In Kaplan HI, Freedman AM, Sadock BJ, editors: *Comprehensive textbook of psychiatry,* ed 3, Baltimore, 1989, Williams & Wilkins.

64. Gunderson JG, Zanarini MC: Current overview of the borderline diagnosis, *J Clin Psychiatry* 48 (suppl I): 5–l4, 1987.

65. McGlashan TH: The Chestnut Lodge follow-up study: III. long-term outcome of borderline personalities, *Arch Gen Psychiatry* 43:20–30, 1986.

66. Adler G: Helplessness in the helpers, *Br J Med Psychol* 45:315–326, 1972.

67. Mac Vicar K: Splitting and identification with the aggressor in assaultive borderline patients, *Am J Psychiatry* 135:229–231, 1978.

68. Main TF: The ailment, *Br J Med Psychol* 30:129–145, 1957.

69. Adler G: Hospital treatment of borderline patients, *Am J Psychiatry* 130:32–35, 1973.

70. Burnham DL: The special-problem patient: victim or agent of splitting? *Psychiatry* 29:105–122, 1966.

71. Stanton AH, Schwartz MS: *The mental hospital,* New York, 1954, Basic Books.

72. Kernberg O: Borderline personality organization, *J Am Psychoanal Assoc* 15:641–685, 1967.

73. Ogden TH: On projective identification, *Int J Psychoanal* 60:357–373, 1979.

74. Goldstein WN: Clarification of projective identification, *Am J Psychiatry* 148:153–161, 1991.

75. Kernberg O: *Neurosis, psychosis and the borderline states.* In Kaplan HI, Freedman AM, Sadock BJ, editors: *Comprehensive Textbook of Psychiatry, ed 3,* Baltimore, 1980, Williams & Wilkins.

76. Nadelson T: Borderline rage and the therapist's response, *Am J Psychiatry* 134:748–751, 1977.

77. Kernberg O: Structural interviewing, *Psychiatr Clin North Am* 4:169–195, 1981.

78. Reding GR, Maguire B: Nonsegregated acute psychiatric admissions to general hospitals—continuity of care within the community hospital, *N Engl J Med* 289:185–189, 1973.

79. Meyer E, Mendelson M: Psychiatric consultation with patients on medical and surgical wards: patterns and processes, *Psychiatry* 24:197–220, 1961.

80. Lipowski ZJ: Consultation-liaison psychiatry: an overview, *Am J Psychiatry* 131:623–630, 1974.

81. Reich P, Kelly MJ: Suicide attempts by hospitalized medical and surgical patients, *N Engl J Med* 294:298–301, 1976.

82. Festinger L: *A theory of cognitive dissonance,* New York, 1957, Row, Peterson.

83. Kucharski A, Groves JE: The so-called "inappropriate" consultation request on a medical or surgical ward, *Int J Psychiatry Med* 7:209–220, 1976–1977.

84. Groves JE: Management of the borderline patient on a medical or surgical ward: the psychiatric consultant's role, *Int J Psychiatry Med* 6:337–348, 1975.

85. Adler G, Buie DH: The misuses of confrontation with borderline patients, *Int J Psychoanal Psychother* 1:109–120, 1972.

86. Caplan G: *The theory and practice of mental health consultation,* New York, 1970, Basic Books.

87. Gordon C, Beresin E: Conflicting models for the inpatient management of borderline patients, *Am J Psychiatry* 140:979–983, 1983.

88. Cornelius JR, Soloff PH, Perel JM, et al: Continuation pharmacotherapy of borderline personality disorder with haloperidol and phenelzine, *Am J Psychiatry* 150:1843–1848, 1993.

89. Norden MJ: Fluoxetine in borderline personality disorder, *Prog Neuro-Psychopharmacol Biol Psychiatry* 13:885–893, 1989.

90. Markovitz PJ, Calabrese JR, Schultz SC, et al: Fluoxetine in the treatment of personality disorders, *Am J Psychiatry* 148:1064–1067, 1991.

91. Klerman GL: *Atypical affective disorders.* In Kaplan HI, Freedman AM, Sadock BJ, editors: *Comprehensive textbook of psychiatry*, ed 3, Baltimore, 1980, Williams & Wilkins.

92. Cole JO: Drug therapy of borderline patients, *McLean Hosp J* 5:110–125, 1980.

93. Klein DP: *Psychopharmacological treatment and delineation of borderline disorders.* In Hartocollis P, editor: *Borderline personality disorders: the concept, the syndrome, the patient*, New York, 1977, International Universities Press.

94. Cowdry RW, Gardner DL: Pharmacotherapy of borderline personality disorder, *Arch Gen Psychiatry* 45:111–119, 1988.

95. Siever EJ, Davis KE: A psychobiological perspective on the personality disorders, *Am J Psychiatry* 148:1647–1658, 1991.

96. Hollander E, Stein DJ, DeCaria CM, et al: Serotonergic sensitivity in borderline personality disorder: preliminary findings, *Am J Psychiatry* 151:277–280, 1994.

97. Simeon D, Stanley B, Frances A, et al: Self-mutilation in personality disorders: psychological and biological correlates, *Am J Psychiatry* 149:221–226, 1992.

98. Liebowitz MR, Klein DF: Interrelationship of hysteroid dysphoria and borderline personality disorder, *Psychiatr Clin North Am* 4:67–88, 1981.

99. Fava M, Rosenbaum JF, Pava JA, et al: Anger attacks in unipolar depression: I. clinical correlates and response to fluoxetine treatment, *Am J Psychiatry* 150:1158–1167, 1993.

100. Salzman C, Wolfson AN, Schatzberg A, et al: Effect of fluoxetine on anger in symptomatic volunteers with borderline personality disorder, *J Clin Psychopharm* 15:23–29, 1995.

101. Soloff PH, George A, Nathan RS, et al: Paradoxical effects of amitriptyline on borderline patients, *Am J Psychiatry* 143:1603–1605, 1986.

102. Gardner DE, Cowdry RW: Positive effects of carbamazepine on behavioral dyscontrol in borderline personality, *Am J Psychiatry* 143:519–522, 1986.

103. Brinkley JR, Beitman BD, Friedel RO: Low-dose neuroleptic regimens in the treatment of borderline patients, *Arch Gen Psychiatry* 36:319–326, 1979.

104. Soloff PH: Neuroleptic treatment in the borderline patient: advantages and techniques, *J Clin Psychiatry* 48(suppl):26–30, 1987.

105. Frankenburg FR, Zanarini MC: Clozapine treatment of borderline patients: a preliminary study, *Compr Psychiatry* 34:402–405, 1933.

106. Baldessarini RJ, Frankenburg FR: Drug therapy: clozapine, *N Engl J Med* 324:746–754, 1991.

107. Rosenbaum JF, Woods SW, Groves JE, et al: Emergence of hostility during alprazolam treatment, *Am J Psychiatry* 141:792–793, 1984.

108. Richmond JS, Young JR, Groves JE: Violent dyscontrol responsive to d-amphetamine, *Am J Psychiatry* 135:365–366, 1978.

109. Aldrich MS: Narcolepsy, *N Engl J Med* 323:389–394, 1990.

110. Swift RG, Perkins DO, Chase CL, et al: Psychiatric disorders in 36 families with Wolfram syndrome, *Am J Psychiatry* 148:775–779, 1991.

111. Keljo DJ, Squires RH: Clinical problem-solving: just in time, *N Engl J Med* 334:46–48, 1996.

112. Zanarini MC, Gunderson JG, Frankenburg FR, et al: Discriminating borderline personality disorder from other axis II disorders, *Am J Psychiatry* 147:161–167, 1990.

113. Paris J: Completed suicide in borderline personality disorder, *Psychiatr Ann* 20:19–21, 1990.

114. Kernberg OF: Suicidal behavior in borderline patients: diagnosis and psychotherapeutic considerations, *Am J Psychother* 47:245–254, 1993.

115. Stone MH: Paradoxes in the management of suicidality in borderline patients, *Am J Psychother* 47:255–272, 1993.

116. Beresin EV, Falk WE, Gordon C: *Borderline and other personality disorders.* In Hyman SE, editor: *Manual of psychiatric emergencies*, Boston, 1994, Little, Brown.

117. Kjelsberg D, Eikeseth PH, Dahl HH: Suicide in borderline patients—predictive factors, *Acta Psychiatr Scand* 84:283–287, 1991.

118. Maltsberger JT, Buie DH: Countertransference hate in the treatment of suicidal patients, *Arch Gen Psychiatry* 30:625–633, 1974.

119. Maltsberger JT, Lovett CG: *Suicide in borderline personality disorder.* In Silver D, Rosenbluth M, editors: *Handbook of borderline disorders*, Madison, CT, 1992, International Universities Press.

120. Friedman HJ: Psychotherapy of borderline patients: the influence of theory on technique, *Am J Psychiatry* 132:1048–1052, 1975.

121. Dawson DF: Treatment of the borderline patient, relationship management *Can J Psychiatry* 33:370–374, 1988.

122. Ronningstam E, Gunderson J, Lyons M: Changes in pathological narcissism, *Am J Psychiatry* 152:253–257, 1995.

123. Groves JE, editor: *Essential papers on short-term dynamic therapy*, New York, 1996, New York University Press

124. Grunebaum HU, Klerman GL: Wrist slashing, *Am J Psychiatry* 124:527–534 1967.

Chapter 21
Pain Patients

Menekse Alpay, M.D.

Of all human experience, pain is, as long as it lasts, the most absorbing; it is the only human experience that when it comes to an end, automatically confers a sense of relief and joy. Moreover, by its very nature it is solitary. However, the oddest thing about pain is that, despite its intensity and its unequalled power over mind and body, it is difficult to recall when it is over.[1]

Psychiatric Consultation

The International Association for the Study of Pain (IASP) has defined pain as "an unpleasant sensory and emotional experience associated with actual or potential tissue damage or described in terms of such damage."[2] This definition recognizes the fact that pain has both an acute nociceptive aspect and an emotional-psychiatric dimension; these factors suggest that psychiatrists have a role in the treatment of the pain patient. Conceptualizing pain in this manner underscores the fact that pain is an important and complicated sensation, one that may present in a multitude of ways. Physicians and patients alike seek knowledge, order, and relief when dealing with pain's chameleon-like manifestations; some of the common reasons pain patients or treating physicians seek consultation and treatment from psychiatrists include:

- To separate functional from organic factors. Unfortunately the request to separate psyche from soma is often vexing. Through such consultations some physicians wish to absolve themselves of further responsibility.
- To assess the patient for depression, anxiety, or some Diagnostic and Statistical Manual of Mental Disorders[3] (DSM-IV) comorbid disorder and its relation to the experience of pain.
- To satisfy the referring physician's personal desire to punish a "hateful" patient, one who will not take yes or no for an answer and who interferes with normal medical decision-making.
- To address a patient's or physician's fear or misunderstanding of narcotics (e.g., use of high-dose narcotics, toxicity, and maintenance treatment).
- To resolve inconsistencies between symptoms and physical findings (or the lack thereof): "No anatomic lesion could account for this." The referring physician wonders if a psychiatric disorder or central nervous system (CNS) pain is present or if he or she is missing something.
- To determine if psychotropics might help alleviate pain and suffering.

Challenges Facing the Psychiatrist

When asked to evaluate a patient with pain, the psychiatric consultant must be prepared to meet specific challenges. These include using language that is common and precise for communication about pain, knowing how to measure pain, and understanding the genesis and characteristics of different types of pain.

Pathophysiology of Pain

To understand pain one needs to know about the pathophysiology of nociception and to realize that the threshold, intensity, quality, time course, and perceived location of pain are determined by CNS mechanisms.[4] For example, neurosurgeons have shown that interruption of the specific pain pathways often does not eliminate pain; numbness does not confer analgesia. Peripheral nerve damage may result in changes in the receptive fields and recruitment of neurons at multiple levels of the nervous system (from the dorsal horn to the brainstem, and to the thalamus and cortex). Somatic therapies directed only at nociceptive input may be ineffective.[5]

Detection of noxious stimuli (i.e., nociception) starts with the activation of peripheral nociceptors (somatic pain) or with the activation of nociceptors in bodily organs (visceral pain). Somatic pain is usually well localized, attributable to certain structures or areas, and described as stabbing, aching, or throbbing. In contrast, visceral pain may be poorly localized, not necessarily attributable to the involved organ (i.e., as is the case with referred pain), and is characteristically described as dull and crampy.

Tissue injury stimulates the nociceptors by the liberation of prostaglandins, arachidonic acid, histamine, and bradykinin. Subsequently, axons transmit the pain signal to the spinal cord (to cell bodies in the dorsal root ganglia; Figure 21-1).

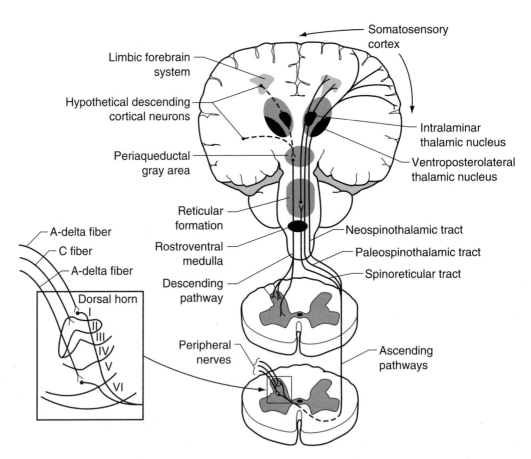

Figure 21-1. Schematic diagram of neurologic pathways for pain perception. (From Hyman SH, Cassem NH: *Pain*. In: Rubenstein E, Fedeman DD, eds. *Scientific American medicine: current topics in medicine. Subsection II*. New York, Scientific American; 1989. Originally from Psychiatry Update and Board Preparation, Stern TA, Herman JB, (eds). McGraw-Hill, 2004.)

Three different types of axons are involved in the transmission of a painful stimulus from the skin to the dorsal horn. A-β fibers are the largest and most heavily myelinated fibers that transmit awareness of light touch. A-Δ fibers and C fibers are the primary nociceptive afferents. A-Δ fibers are 2–5 micrometers in diameter and are thinly myelinated. They conduct immediate, rapid, sharp, and brief pain (first pain) with a velocity of 20 m/second. C fibers are 0.2–1.5 micrometers in diameter and are unmyelinated. They conduct prolonged, burning, and unpleasant pain (second pain) at a speed of 0.5 m/second. A-Δ and C fibers enter the dorsal root and ascend or descend one to three segments before synapsing with neurons in the lateral spinothalamic tract (substantia gelatinosa in the gray matter).

Substance P, an 11 amino acid polypeptide that is the major pain neurotransmitter, is released from the fibers at many of these synapses. Capsaicin, which is extracted from red, hot peppers, inhibits nociception by inhibiting substance P. Inhibition of nociception in the dorsal horn is functionally quite important. Stimulation of the A-Δ fibers not only excites some neurons but also inhibits others. This inhibition of nociception through A-Δ fiber stimulation may explain effects of acupuncture and transcutaneous electrical nerve stimulation (TENS). The lateral spinothalamic tract crosses the midline and ascends toward the thalamus. At the level of the brainstem more than half of this tract synapses in the reticular activating system (in an area called the spinoreticular tract), in the limbic system, and in other brainstem regions (including centers for autonomic nervous system). Another site of projections at this level is the periaqueductal gray (PAG; Figure 21-2), which plays an important role in the brain's endogenous analgesia system. After synapsing in the thalamic nuclei, pain fibers project to the somatosensory cortex, located posterior to the Sylvian fissure in the parietal lobe (Brodmann's areas 1, 2, and 3).[6]

Recent developments in imaging technology have been helpful in understanding the relationship between pain pathways and cortical and limbic areas. These findings may help explain the relationship between emotions, cognition, and pain modulation that we observe in clinical practice as heightened pain perception in depressed patients and high rates of depression in those with chronic pain. In a recent positron emission tomography (PET) study it was shown that acute traumatic nociceptive pain activates the hypothalamus and the PAG in addition to the prefrontal cortex (PFC), insular cortex, anterior cingulate cortex (ACC), posterior parietal cortex, primary motor/somatosensory areas, supplementary motor area (SMA), and cerebellum.[7] Additionally, PET and functional magnetic resonance imaging (fMRI) studies have helped clinicians understand cognitive and emotional modulation of pain perception. Rainville and colleagues[8] have shown that with hypnotic suggestion the activity in the ACC is dependent on the intensity of the suggestion (i.e., same stimulus with the suggestion of "highly unpleasant" induces significantly more ACC activation than when suggestions are less unpleasant).[8] In another study when subjects were distracted during a painful stimulus, pain perception was attenuated in somatosensory regions and the PAG.[9] Another interesting study showed that a short-acting opioid, remifentanil, as well as placebo analgesia, activated the ACC, which is rich in opioid receptors.[10] It is of interest that analgesia induced by both opioids and placebos were reversed with the opioid antagonist naloxone.[11] These findings suggest that cortical areas may exert control over lower brain areas involved in opioid analgesia.[12]

Endogenous analgesic systems involve at least 18 endogenous peptides with opiate-like activity in the CNS (e.g., endorphins, enkephalins, and dynorphins). Different opiate receptors are involved in different effects of opiates.

Mu (μ)-receptors are involved in the regulation of analgesia, respiratory depression, constipation, and miosis. Mu receptors (located in the PAG, rostral ventral medulla, medial thalamus, and dorsal horn of the spinal cord) are the receptors that are mainly responsible for supraspinal analgesia.

Kappa (κ)-receptors are involved in spinal analgesia, sedation, and miosis. They are located in the dorsal horn (spinal analgesia), deep cortical areas, and other locations; pentazocine preferentially acts on these receptors.

Delta (Δ)-receptors, like κ-receptors, mediate spinal analgesia, hypotension, and miosis. Enkephalins have a higher affinity for these receptors than do opiates. They are located in the limbic system, the dorsal horn, and other locations unrelated to pain.

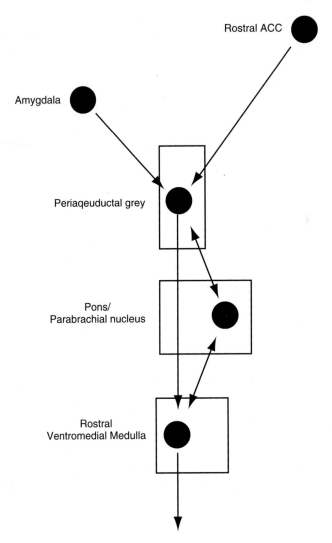

Figure 21-2. Endogenous opioid systems.
(From Petrovic P, Ingvar M: Imaging cognitive modulation of pain processing. *Pain*, 95:1–5, 2002.)

Δ-receptors also mediate psychotomimetic effects (i.e., psychosis) in the CNS. Their effects are not reversed by naloxone, an opiate antagonist.[6]

In terms of anatomic organization, the centers involved in endogenous analgesia include, in addition to PAG, the rostral ACC, amygdala, parabrachial plexus in the pons, and rostral ventromedial medulla.[12]

The descending analgesic pain pathway starts in the PAG (which is rich in endogenous opiates), projects to the rostral ventral medulla, and from there descends through the dorsolateral funiculus of the spinal cord to the dorsal horn. The neurons in the rostral ventral medulla use serotonin to activate endogenous analgesics (enkephalins) in the dorsal horn. This effect inhibits nociception at the level of the dorsal horn since neurons that contain enkephalins synapse with spinothalamic neurons.

Additionally, there are noradrenergic neurons that project from the locus ceruleus (the main noradrenergic center in the CNS) to the dorsal horn and inhibit the response of dorsal horn neurons to nociceptive stimuli. The effect of tricyclic antidepressants (TCAs) and other newer antidepressants is thought to be related to an increase in serotonin and norepinephrine that inhibits noci-ception at the level of the dorsal horn.[6]

Pain Terminology

Acute pain is usually related to an identifiable injury or to a disease; it is self-limited, and resolves over hours to days or in a time frame that is associated with healing. Acute pain is usually associated with objective autonomic features (e.g., tachycardia, hypertension, diaphoresis, mydriasis, or pallor).

Chronic pain (i.e., pain that persists beyond the normal time of healing or lasts longer than 6 months) may have a neurologic origin, involving lowered firing thresholds for spinal cord cells that modulate pain (triggering pain more casily); anatomic plasticity and recruitment of a wide range of cells in the spinal cord (so that touch or movement causes pain); convergence of cutaneous, vascular, muscle, and joint inputs (where one tissue refers pain to another); or aberrant connections (electric short-circuits between the sympathetic and sensory nerves that produce causalgia). Muscle pains often add to the pain experience. Vascular and other visceral mechanisms share features with neurologic mechanisms (for a review, see Meller and Gebhart).[13] The mechanisms involved are not mutually exclusive.[14] Table 21-1[15–34] summarizes the clinical implications of the origins of chronic pain. Characteristic features include vague descriptions of pain and an inability to describe the pain's timing and localization. Unlike acute pain, chronic pain lacks signs of heightened sympathetic activity. Depression, anxiety, and premorbid personality problems are common in this patient population. Usually the major issue is a lack of motivation and incentive to improve. It is usually helpful to determine the presence of a dermatomal pattern (Figure 21-3), determine the presence of neuro-pathic pain, and assess pain behavior.

Continuous pain in the terminally ill tends to originate from well-defined tissue damage due to terminal illness (e.g., cancer). It is a variant of nociceptive pain. Stress, sleep deprivation, depression, and premorbid personality problems may exacerbate this pain.

Neuropathic pain is caused by an injured or dysfunctional central or peripheral nervous system;

it is manifest by spontaneous, sharp, shooting, or burning pain that is usually distributed along dermatomes (see Figure 21-3). Neuropathic pain is often referred to as deafferentation pain, reflex sympathetic dystrophy (RSD), diabetic neuropathy, central pain syndrome, trigeminal neuralgia, or postherpetic neuralgia.

Terms commonly used to describe neuropathic pain include: hyperalgesia (an increased response to stimuli that are normally painful); hyperesthesia (an exaggerated pain response to noxious stimuli [pressor or heat]); allodynia (pain with a stimulus not normally painful [e.g., light touch or cool air]); and hyperpathia (pain from a painful stimuli with a delay and a persistence that is distributed beyond the area of stimulation).

RSD is a syndrome of sympathetically maintained pain, or a complex regional pain syndrome in an extremity that is mediated by sympathetic overactivity. The syndrome is usually caused by injury; however, the cause is unknown in approximately 10% of cases. Either microtrauma or macrotrauma, such as a sprain, a fracture, or a contusion, may cause it; iatrogenic causes include amputation, lesion resection, myelography, and intramuscular (IM) injections. RSD may be disease-related (e.g., due to myocardial infarction, shoulder-hand syndrome, herpes zoster, cerebrovascular accidents, diabetic neuropathy, disc herniation, degenerative disc disease, neuraxial tumors or metastases, multiple sclerosis, or poliomyelitis). It commonly involves four features:

1. A sensory component that includes spontaneous pain and evoked pain in the affected extremity.
2. Autonomic changes (e.g., marbled hyperemic to cyanotic skin color, and edema), changes in blood flow, and asymmetric skin temperatures and perspiration in the affected limbs.
3. Motor changes with decreased strength and range of motion, tremor, hypotonia, atrophy, and dystonias.
4. Trophic changes in approximately 30% of cases that rarely occur within the first 10 days of initial symptoms. These changes include disturbed nail growth, increased hair growth, palmar/planter fibrosis, thin glossy skin, hyperkeratosis, and distal osteoporosis.

The clinical course (which may last up to 6 months) starts with an acute phase that involves

Table 21-1. Chronic Pain: Nervous System Pathophysiology[15–34]

Neurologic Mechanisms	Physiologic Effect	Clinical Implications
Neuroplasticity[15–17]	Recruitment of cortical and subcortical neurons so wide dynamic range cells can be activated by low-threshold mechanoreceptors Allodynia Allaesthesia	Early, concurrent, multimodal treatment of nociceptive, central, vascular, sympathetic and psychiatric aspects of the pain ? Block glutamate, substance P Early use of anticonvulsants, membrane stabilizers, sympatholytics NMDA antagonists
NMDA excess and glutamate-GABA imbalance[18–25] Glutamate up, GABA down	Morphine tolerance Central hyperalgesia Hyperexcitability of peripheral and central pain cells	Normally nonpainful light touch, muscle and joint movements are painful Treatment options: benzodiazepines, baclofen, anticonvulsants, substance P antagonists, or other NMDA antagonists (e.g., ketamine), GABA agents
Neurotoxins[26]	Excitotoxic (e.g., quinolonic acid) Neuropathy	AIDS pain: ? anticonvulsants, ? serotoninergic agents, ? free radical scavengers
Opioid "off" mechanisms[27,28] Off celis in the medulla Morphine 3G/morphine up Side effect intolerance	Hyperalgesia as narcotics increase (particularly intrathecal) Tolerance as morphine 3G increases Side effects greater than benefit	Maintain steady blood levels of narcotics, or decreased narcotic may increase pain Switching to a different narcotic if one does not work Trial off narcotics if narcotics not working
Sympathetic pain[15]	Mechanoallodynia, swelling Dystrophic changes	Sympathetic blockade and/or α-blocking drugs may be useful in RSD, trauma, facial pain, arthritis
Monoamines (5-HT, NE, dopamine)[29–34]	5-HT increase lessens opiate analgesia 5-HT1 dysregulation leads to vascular pain 5-HT1 involved in affective disorders/ suffering of pain	Full dosage, early use of antidepressant drugs, including tricyclics, SSRIs, and dopamine agonists, alone or in combination NE reuptake inhibitors (e.g., desipramine, venlafaxine) useful for pain whether depressed or not Pergolide and methylphenidate (Ritalin) are useful adjuvants
Psychiatric illness	Decreased sleep Decreased muscle relaxation Alienation, anxiety	Differential diagnosis of psychiatric conditions and appropriate treatments

NMDA, *N*-methyl-D-aspartate; GABA, γ-aminobutyric acid; RSD, reflex sympathetic dystrophy; 5-HT, 5-hydroxytryptamine; NE, norepinephrine; SSRIs, selective serotonin reuptake inhibitors.

pain, edema, and warm skin. Subsequently dystrophic changes dominate the picture with cold skin and trophic changes (3–6 months after the onset of the untreated acute phase). Irreversible atrophic changes (atrophy and contractures) eventually occur. There may be symptom improvement with inhibition of sympathetic output; sympathetic blockade may be both diagnostic and therapeutic.[6,35,36]

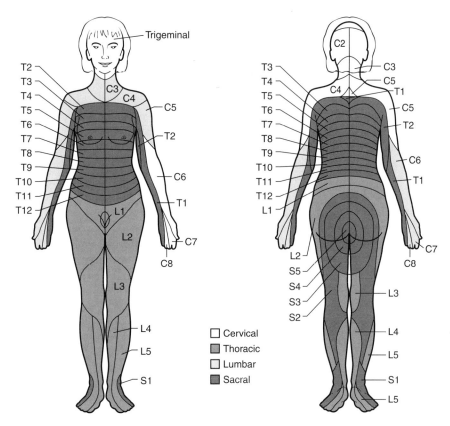

Figure 21-3. Schematic diagram of segmental neuronal innervation by dermatomes. (From Hyman SH, Cassem NH: *Pain*. In: Rubenstein E, Fedeman DD, eds. *Scientific American medicine: current topics in medicine. Subsection II*. New York, Scientific American; 1989. Originally from Psychiatry Update and Board Preparation, Stern TA, Herman JB, (eds). McGraw-Hill, 2004.)

Idiopathic pain, previously referred to as "*psychogenic pain*," is poorly understood. The presence of pain does not imply or exclude a psychological component. Typically, there is no evidence of an associated organic etiology or an anatomical pattern consistent with symptoms. Symptoms are often grossly out of proportion to an identifiable organic pathology.

Jurisigenic pain results from perceived physical or emotional damage related to medical, personal, work, or product injury. Patients with this pain syndrome usually maintain the sick role for as long as possible to maximize financial return. It is important to recognize the existence of a conflict and to educate patients and attorneys; maintenance of a helping and neutral posture is critical.

Phantom pain refers to severe and excruciating pain after amputation; it often presents a major obstacle to the treatment of the amputee. The pain is usually localized to the distal amputated limb, and it tends to vanish 2 to 3 years after the amputation. The pathophysiology of this pain is poorly understood. The chaotic innervation of the amputation site, along with supraspinal mechanisms (e.g., attention and stress) may contribute to this pain syndrome. Consistent with the impact of the psyche on pain, one study showed that it is possible to induce pain in an amputee with hypnotic suggestion.[37]

Myofascial pain can arise from one or several of the following problems: hypertonic muscles, myofascial trigger points, arthralgias, and fatigue with muscle weakness. Myofascial pain is generally used to describe muscle and connective tissue sources of pain. Myofascial pain can be a primary diagnosis (e.g., fibromyalgia) or, as more often is the case, a comorbid diagnosis (e.g., with vascular headache or with a psychiatric diagnosis). Psychiatric symptoms are common in patients with muscle pain; other symptoms often involve decreased energy, impaired sleep, and changes in psychomotor activity. Myofascial pain syndromes may involve muscle trigger points, hypersensitive skin, a subjective sense of swelling and numbness, somatoform pain dis-order, affective and anxiety disorders, nonrestorative sleep, as well as pain of the head and neck. The diagnosis should be considered if there are multiple muscle trigger points in the temporalis, sternocleidomastoid, rhomboids, or trapezius muscles; if the person cannot get at least 5 hours of uninterrupted sleep; and if chronic fatigue is present.[38–41] Deficient stage 4 sleep is thought to underlie the lack of deep muscle relaxation, aching muscles, arthralgias, and general malaise.[42]

Pain Measurement

The experience of pain is always subjective. Objective measurements of the patient's subjective response, however, are possible. Several sensitive and reliable clinical instruments for pain measurement are available. These include:

1. *The pain drawing.* This involves having the patient draw the anatomic distribution of the pain as it is felt in his or her body. The patient draws the outline of the body, labels where the pain is, and keeps this document as part of the medical record. The drawing serves as a clue to the anatomy of the problem, to the psychological state of the patient, and to the patient's level of knowledge.
2. *The visual analog scale.* A 100-mm visual analog scale (with a 0 signifying no pain and 10 representing severe pain) is readily understood by most patients. It is also exquisitely sensitive to change; consequently the patient can mark this scale once a day or even hourly during treatment trials, if desired. Two separate scales can be kept for the least and the greatest pain. Concurrent scales for mood,

overall progress, and pain allow for comparison of the relationship of pain to the total clinical picture, thereby rounding out the psychiatrist's understanding of the patient's syndrome.
3. *Categorical rating scales. Ad hoc* categorical rating scales may be devised that comprise three to five categories for the ranking of pain severity.

The Psychiatrist as Pain Physician

The psychiatrist begins with a clarification of the reason for the consultation, creates some initial hypotheses, and examines the patient. If possible, the psychiatric consultant should be brought into the case early on and introduced as a member of the medical team. The referring physician should take care to ensure that the patient does not interpret the referral as a sign that he or she is not believed, and the physician should state that a psychiatrist is routinely asked to evaluate patients with long-standing pain. When the referring physician is comfortable using the services of a psychiatrist, the patient typically accepts the examination without protest. When the psychiatrist is called in at the end of a long and frustrating stand-off, the patient typically balks.

Gathering Important Preliminary Information

The psychiatric consultant's job begins by answering five questions: (1) Is the pain intractable because of nociceptive stimuli (e.g., from the skin, bones, muscles, or blood vessels)? (2) Is the pain maintained by non-nociceptive mechanisms (i.e., have the spinal cord, brainstem, limbic system, and cortex been recruited as reverberating pain circuits)? (3) Is the complaint of pain primary, as occurs in disorders such as major depression or delusional disorder? (4) Is there a more efficacious pharmacologic treatment? (5) Have pain behavior and disability become more important than the pain itself? Answering these questions allows the mechanism(s) of the pain and suffering to be pursued. Table 21-2 is a useful guideline to organize the questions, to test hypotheses, and to determine diagnosis.

Table 21-2. Questions to Ask When Pain Persists

Pain Syndromes: What Is the Problem?	Selected Diagnostic Considerations	Consider
Is there an ongoing physical disease? (e.g., infection, cancer)	MRI for anatomic pathology Gallium scan for infection ESR for infection, cancer PSA, CEA, p24 testing Pelvic, breast, prostate, gastrointestinal examination	Progression of disease Metastatic disease Visceral pain: adhesions, referred pain, central pain
Is there a problem with the use and response to narcotics? (misuse, lack of efficacy)	Central pain Narcotics masking a DSM-IV problem Narcotic dosing error or inconsistency Narcotic toxicity	Intravenous Antidepressants, anxiolytics, or sleep prescription Narcotic potency P450 2D6 codeine or oxycodone/SSRI interaction Meperidine toxicity
Is there a psychiatric disorder associated with pain? Depression Anxiety Somatoform disorder Psychosis	Loss of all pleasure and mid-late insomnia Panic depersonalization, benzodiazepine failure, anxiety not relieved by analgesics Hypochondriasis	Depression often masked by narcotics or anxiolytics Comorbid somatoform, mood, or anxiety disorders Pain drawing and explanation helpful for diagnosis
Does CNS pain exist? (e.g., neuropathic pain)	Increased sensory threshold, decreased pain threshold Nondermatomal distribution of pain Hyperpathia Allodynia, often narcotic-resistant	Sharp sensation perceived as light touch is common Light touch is painful and sustained and has a delayed crescendo Tuning fork/moving a hair examinations detect allodynia best
Is it a pain behavior syndrome?	Pain disorder (somatoform) rule out masked depression, drug abuse, physical/sexual abuse, missed physical disorder	Anger and anxiety: denied Counterdependent, demanding style Passive and endearing
Is the patient faking? Malingering Factitious disorder	Malingering for drugs/disability Factitious deception to maintain the sick role	Malingering or factitious disorders with physical symptoms are rare, much more likely to be something else
Is an unusual problem responsible for pain? Myofascial pain Porphyria Gastrointestinal pain Pelvic-visceral pain Neuropathic pain Sexual pain disorder	Muscle trigger points absent, deep sleep Laxative abuse, anorexia/bulimia Adhesions Hypoesthesia, allodynia Wasting illness, subcortical deficits/AIDS Conversion symptom, especially pelvic, gastrointestinal head pain	Myofascial pain often comorbid with other pain syndrome Visceral pain is diffuse, nondermatomal, with sympathetic symptoms and may mimic DSM-IV Physical/sexual abuse antidote pain

MRI, magnetic resonance imaging; ESR, erythrocyte sedimentation rate; SSRI, selective serotonin reuptake inhibitor.

Physical Examination

A psychiatrist's physical examination of the pain patient includes examination of the painful area, muscles, and sensation to pinprick and light touch (Table 21-3). The examination is essential to the psychiatric evaluation for pain and serves three purposes. First, examination of the patient allows for better history-taking, therapeutic alliances, and integration of data; it also helps to eliminate

Table 21-3. General Physical Examination of Pain by the Psychiatrist

Physical Finding	Purpose of Examination
Motor deficits	Does the patient give-way when checking strength?
	Does the person try?
	Is there a pseudoparesis, astasia-abasia, or involuntary movements suggesting a somatoform disorder?
Trigger points in head, neck, shoulder, and back muscles	Are any of the common myofascial trigger points present suggesting myofascial pain?
	Presence of evoked pain (such as allodynia, hyperpathia, or anesthesia) suggests neuropathic pain
Evanescent, changeable pain, weakness, and numbness	Does the psychological complaint preempt the physical?
Abnormal sensory findings	Detection of lateral anesthesia to pinprick ending sharply at the midline
	Presence of topographic confusion
	Presence of nondermatomal distribution of pain and sensation suggests either a somatoform or CNS pain disorder
	Presence of abnormal sensation suggests neuropathy or CNS pain
Sympathetic or vascular dysfunction	Detection of swelling, skin discoloration, or changes in sweating or temperature suggests a vascular or sympathetic element to the pain
Uncooperativeness, erratic responses to the physical examination	Detection of an interpersonal aspect to the pain, causing abnormal pain behavior, as in somatoform disease

the physical-mental dichotomy, which, left unspoken, often contributes to the patient's defensiveness. Second, the psychiatrist can search for signs of different types of pain and distinguish them from symptoms of a conversion disorder. Third, inconsistent findings suggestive of a somatoform disorder may be uncovered. Because patients with an extensive history of pain often delight in regaling the examiner with their odysseys through clinics, spas, and hospitals, we often ask them to write detailed accounts of their pain from its onset to the present. We explore the patient's past and present mental state and consider the family history and ethnic beliefs. Open-ended questions may include: Have you ever suffered like this before? What do you do think about in the early morning hours when you cannot sleep? What do others think is the nature of the problem?

Psychiatric Examination

Interviewing the patient with chronic pain demands close attention to both what was said and what was not said, as well as to mindfulness of the patient's style of discourse. We take a detailed history of when and how the pain began, and we inquire about the various treatments received and the patient's relationships with other physicians. Throughout the history, we look for fluctuations in the course of the pain. Why did it improve? Did the medication help, or was it some other factor that proved palliative? The psychiatrist also plays an important role in the treatment of the pain by his or her ability to recognize psychiatric conditions that may present with pain.

Depression

Major depressive illness can be diagnosed by DSM-IV or similar research criteria in approximately 25% of patients who suffer from chronic pain. Recurrent affective illness, a family history of depression, and psychiatric comorbidity (with anxiety and substance use) are often present. More often than not, depression predates the pain; overall, 60% to 100% of pain patients have depressive symptoms. Although some depressive syndromes are secondary to pain itself (e.g., adjustment disorder with affective symptoms), many patients have major depression masked by denial or by medications that promote sleepiness. Denial of affect, particularly anger, is observed in nearly half of chronic pain patients referred to the Massachusetts General Hospital (MGH) Psychiatric Consultation Service. Diagnosing an affective illness when affect is minimized by the patient may be difficult, but the following tactics can be used to help ferret out affective disorders.

Ask questions about neurovegetative symptoms. Examples of questions to be posed include: How often do you wake from sleep at night? How long does it take you to return to sleep? Do you have early-morning awakening? When was the last time you really enjoyed yourself? Does food taste the same as it always has? Do you enjoy eating? What do you do for fun? Can you still smile? Do you have an interest in people, such as your grandchildren or friends? Do you have difficulty with decision-making? What do you do when you are angry? Do you sometimes feel you would rather be dead?

Evaluate the person's limbic (i.e., genuine and uncensored) response to emotionally charged stimuli. Look for denial of any strong emotion, particularly anger or sadness, and note if the patient answers affective questions with affective responses or only with avoidance and denial. Denial, displacement, or suppression of emotions suggests psychopathology. One could ask questions, such as, "Can you laugh at a joke at your own expense? Can you acknowledge anger at yourself and others?" The Minnesota Multiphasic Personality Inventory (MMPI) may be of particular use in refining the differential diagnosis when denial or repression is suspected. Covert hostility is typically elevated, which adds some validity to the label of denier. The so-called "conversion V" is present in about half of pain patients studied at MGH, and it occurs more often among those in denial. Patients with other chronic illnesses are more likely to have an "inverted V" configuration.

Anxiety Disorders

In the pain patient, denial of fear, worry, or nervousness is a more ominous sign than is the mere expression of modulated fear or worry about pain.

Given that it is normal to worry about a painful threat to the body and the mind, pathologic denial of any anxious affect may be suggestive of psychosis, hypochondriasis, conversion, factitious disorder, or personality disorder. Accordingly, DSM-IV provides criteria to recognize anxiety of sufficient intensity that can trigger or exacerbate pain. Questions, such as the following, may help glean important information: "Does the pain make you panic? Do you feel your heart beating fast, have an overwhelming feeling of dread or doom, or experience a sense of sudden high anxiety that overwhelms you?"

Anxiety disorders occur in approximately 30% of intractable pain patients (usually in the form of generalized anxiety or panic disorder). More than 50% of patients with anxiety disorders also have a current or past history of major depression or another psychiatric disorder. Alcohol and substance abuse are the most common comorbid diagnoses; consequently, recognition and treatment of comorbid depression and substance abuse are critical to long-term treatment outcome.

A variety of agents, including TCAs, selective serotoninreuptake inhibitors (SSRIs), nefazodone, mirtazapine, and clonazepam, alone or in combination, improve panic, anxiety, and depression as well as neuropathic pain, muscle tension, and sleep. Anxiety that results from disruptions of bodily integrity, sense of self, or attachment to caregivers occurs in one third to half of chronic pain patients. This narcissistic injury can block efforts at physical and emotional rehabilitation and requires a pragmatic psychodynamic treatment. Anger is often linked to anxiety, although it is typically denied and expressed in terms of nervous somatic symptoms. One can provoke affect quickly by holding up a clenched fist and asking the patient what he or she would do with it. The response will often be telling regarding denied anger. SSRIs are helpful with anger, anxiety, and mood disorders. Existential anxiety may increase when cancer is first diagnosed, when death nears, or when pain engenders feelings of helplessness. Spending time with the person, telling the truth, accepting the situation, and reconnecting with family members (parents and children) often decreases existential anxiety.

Somatization Disorder

The somatoform disorders (see Chapter 19) comprise a group of disorders in which complaints and anxiety about physical illness are the predominant clinical features. These complaints exist in the absence of sufficient organic findings to explain the pain. There are four somatoform disorders in which pain may be present: somatization disorder (300.81), conversion disorder (300.11), hypochondriasis (300.70), and pain disorder (307.80). Somatoform disorders occur in 5% to 15% of treated chronic pain patients, and somatizers account for 36% of all cases of psychiatric disability, as well as 48% of all sick leave occasions.[43]

Among somatizers, pain in the head or neck, epigastrium, and limbs predominates. Visceral pains from the esophagus, abdomen, and pelvis are associated with psychiatric comorbidity, especially somatoform disorders that can be challenging to diagnose.[44] Missed ovarian cancers, central pain following inflammatory disorders, and referred pain are often overlooked because of the nonspecific presentations of visceral pain. Moreover, in one study 64% of women with chronic pelvic pain reported a history of sexual abuse.[45] The two most common comorbid conditions associated with somatoform disorders among MGH pain patients are major depressive disorder (MDD) and anxiety disorders. Surprisingly, drug and alcohol abuse and personality disorders are not significantly associated with somatoform disorders. Patients with somatization disorder consume health care resources at nine times the rate of the average person in the United States.[46]

Sufferers from somatoform disorders often have painful physical complaints and excessive anxiety about their physical illness. Most of their pain complaints to physicians do not have a well-defined cause, and a psychiatric diagnosis is often particularly difficult to establish (Table 21-4).

Conversion Disorder

Conversion disorder may be manifest as a pain syndrome with a significant loss or alteration in physical functioning that mimics a physical disorder. Conversion symptoms may include paresthesia, numbness, dysphonia, dizziness, seizures, globus hystericus, limb weakness, sexual dysfunction, or pain. If pain or sexual symptoms are the sole complaints, the diagnosis is pain disorder or sexual pain disorder rather than conversion disorder. Pain, numbness, and weakness often form a conversion triad in the pain clinic.

Psychological factors are judged to be etiologic for the pain when a temporal relationship between the symptoms and a psychosocial stressor exists—the person must not be intentionally producing their symptom. A mechanism of primary or secondary gain needs to be evident before the diagnosis can be confirmed. *La belle indifference* and histrionic personality traits have little value in making or excluding the diagnosis of conversion. A conversion V on the MMPI denotes the hypochondriacal traits and relative absence of depression that accompany conversion. Evoked responses, electromyogram (EMG), electroencephalogram (EEG), MRI, PET scans, and repeated physical examinations are useful for identification of patients who had been diagnosed erroneously as hysterical.[47]

Hypochondriasis

Hypochondriasis involves the persistent belief that one has a serious illness. Generalized anxiety disorder and depression are the common causes of hypochondriasis-like presentations.[48] Head and orofacial pains, cardiac and gastrointestinal pains, and feelings of pressure, burning, and numbness are common hypochondriacal concerns. Therefore, attention to head and neck pathology, cancer, visceral pains, degenerative disorders, and CNS syndromes should be ongoing.

Care of the hypochondriac begins with a comprehensive differential diagnosis. This care of the patient is longitudinal, and the persistence of vague complaints helps to rule out the most serious diseases, and to set the stage for an alliance with the patient by demonstrating an open, critical mind. A pain drawing may help reveal psychotic somatic beliefs. The psychiatrist should reassure and not reject the patient; one should label behavior as maladaptive or dangerous that will produce more symptoms and openly discuss psychodynamic factors.

Table 21-4. Somatoform and Related Disorders

Disorders	Diagnostic Tips
Somatization disorder	Review the diagnostic criteria
Conversion disorder	Real disease and conversion symptoms co-occur
	An undiagnosed medical condition may underlie the psychiatric diagnosis
	Deciding if psychological factors are causative or a response is often impossible in chronic pain patients
	Culturally determined stress responses, numbness, total body pain, weakness, astasia-abasia, fainting, voices, and pseudoseizures are transient and not included as conversion disorders
Hypochondriasis	Transient hypochondriasis is particularly common in the elderly
	Psychosis and depression may be concealed because of the patient's fears
Pain disorder	Pain is enmeshed in Axis II problems and complicated by drugs (narcotics, , benzodiazepines, or alcohol)
	Central and visceral pain, especially pelvic pain, may mimic somatoform disorders
	Pain can improve with psychotropic drugs or psychological techniques without having a psychiatric diagnosis
Malingering/factitious disorder	Pseudomalingering with dissociative features (Ganser syndrome) presents with malingering, but also underlies real psychiatric illness. Some classify it as a conversion, dissociative, or factitious disorder

Pain Disorder

Pain disorder is defined in DSM-IV as a syndrome in which the focus of the clinical presentation is pain that causes significant impairment in occupational or social functioning, or marked distress or both. Organic pathology, if present, does not explain the pain or the associated social and occupational impairment. Pain disorder has three diagnostic subtypes:

1. Psychological, in which psychological factors play an important role in the onset, severity, exacerbation, or maintenance of the pain.
2. Nonpsychiatric pain associated with a general medical condition. If psychological factors are present, they play only a minor role in the genesis of pain. This medical pain disorder is coded as an Axis III diagnosis.
3. Combined type.

Pain disorder, as it is presently known, has been variously named during different epochs. Examples of such labels include psychogenic pain disorder, somatoform pain disorder, and pain behavior.[49] When behavioral disability predominates, chronic pain syndrome is the behavioral description of this same syndrome. The meander-

ing history of nomenclature is best understood as reflecting the mix of pain behaviors, as well as interpersonal and affective characteristics, that emphasize disability and entreat attention from others.

Psychological antecedents of this syndrome may include a history of physical abuse, counterdependent personal relationships, a family history of alcoholism, and a personal developmental history of attachment problems. Comorbid diagnoses should be sought—particularly, depression, anxiety, and substance abuse. Treatment must address the triad of self-defeating behavior, affective dysfunction, and psychodynamic conflicts, which causes poor coping, disability, and disruptive rehabilitation efforts. Common treatments and their reasons for possible failure are outlined in Table 21-5.

Factitious Disorder with Physical Symptoms

Factitious disorder with physical symptoms involves the intentional production or feigning of physical symptoms. Onset is usually in early adulthood with successive hospitalizations forming the lifelong pattern. The cause is a psychological need

Table 21-5. Treatment and Failures of Pain Disorder

Problem	Reasons (Not Mutually Exclusive)	Treatment
Physical diagnosis	Ignorance, transference, narcissistic fears, or dishonesty Drug abuse	Clarify which demands are and are not ignored/sidelined/mistreated consistent with good practice Refer, if at any impasse Possible drug abuse
Behavior is abnormal	Axis I DSM-IV not applied Relaxation, yoga, physical rehabilitation methods have not been used No common ground/treatment plan agreed to	Reassure the patient about normal suffering, coping, rehabilitation, and distinguish from Axis I symptoms, ensuring treatment
Self-esteem hurts more than the body	Coping methods have not been addressed The physician-patient relationship has not been acknowledged as a treatment aspect Locus of control is thought to be external	Address the muted anger Identify denial, avoidance, rationalization, projection Interpret the unrequited wish for dependency versus self-control
High affective suffering	Major depression or mood disorder complicating general medical condition may not get addressed because of the somatic focus and the patient's fear of being psychiatrically dismissed	Treat the covert depression Is this the hateful patient's psychodynamics?

to assume the sick role, and as such, the intentional production of painful symptoms distinguishes factitious disorder from somatoform disorders, in which intention to produce symptoms is absent. Renal colic, orofacial pain, and abdominal pain are three of the common presenting gambits in factitious disorder; of these, abdominal pain and a scarred belly herald the diagnosis most often. Despite the seeming irrationality of the behavior, those with factitious disorder are not psychotic.

Pain may be described as occurring anywhere in the body, and the patient often uses elaborate technical detail to intrigue the listener with *pseudologica fantastica*. Narcotic seeking, multiple hospitalizations under different names in different cities, inconclusive invasive investigations and surgery, lack of available family, and a suave truculence are characteristic of this disorder. An assiduous inquiry into the exact circumstances of the previous admission and discharge leads to a sudden outraged discharge against medical advice. There is typically no effective treatment. If the patient were willing to receive

care, however, psychotherapy would be the treatment of choice.

Malingering

In malingering, the patient fakes a complaint, although no pain is felt, because of an external incentive, such as obtaining money, drugs, or privilege, or the avoidance of work. The conscious manipulation by malingerers precludes much diagnostic help from Amytal interviews or hypnosis because of the willful withholding of information by the patient. Even the MMPI can be skewed to normality by the clever malingerer, although differences (>7) between obvious and subtle scale scores and high L, F, K scale scores (T >70) may be suggestive nonetheless. The malingerer typically refuses psychological tests; this raises suspicion even before a diagnosis is made. The mnemonic for suspicion of the diagnosis is WASTE (Withholding of information; Antisocial personality; Somatic examination inconclusive and changeable; Treatment erratic with noncompliance and vagueness; E̲xternal incentives exist, such as occur in a medicolegal context). The psychiatrist's familiarity with the neurologic examination is always useful, but it is of critical importance for the diagnosis of malingering when nonanatomic findings arise. Once an organic etiology has been ruled out, careful scrutiny of old records and a few calls to previous physicians may unearth evidence of similar behavior in the past. Similar to lying, malingering tends to be a character trait used in times of stress from early adolescence through the senium. Once revealed, psychotherapy can be offered; unfortunately, noncompliance is typical.

Dissociative States

Dissociation is caused by psychological trauma, and it involves a disturbance or alteration in the normally integrative functions of identity, memory, or consciousness. Pelvic pain, sexual pain disorders, headache, and abdominal pain are the most common pain complaints in developmentally traumatized individuals. Walker et al.[50] reported that in 22 women with chronic pelvic pain, 18 experienced childhood abuse. Of the 21 women selected as controls (i.e., without pelvic pain), 9 had childhood abuse (P < .0005). Dissociation, somatic distress, and general disability were more frequent in the group with pain. Denial makes the diagnosis of dissociative disorders in pain patients a longitudinal process, because truth is shared slowly with the physician only when the patient can tolerate it. Signs of an underlying dissociative disorder are periods of amnesia, nightmares, and panic as well as anxious intolerance of close personal relationships.

Psychosis

Pain can also be a symptom of psychosis. This is a problem of misreporting a delusional symptom as a physical ailment, hence demonstrating the need for assiduous screening of delusional thinking. The diagnostic problems are fourfold: (1) DSM-IV profiles of schizophrenia, affective psychoses, and organic psychoses are not typical presentations for psychosis with pain. Covert delusional thinking and anomie may be the only symptoms; (2) psychotic thinking may be masked by denial, rationalization, concrete thinking, and fear. Historical anamnesis is the last thing the patient wants; (3) the last person the patient wants to see is a psychiatrist because the patient knows the pain "is not in my head;" and (4) the pain belief is misattributed to hypochondriasis. The psychiatrist must always consider pain as a delusional symptom when there is a bizarre, variable distribution to the symptom (best proven by getting the patient to draw a picture of pain); when the patient is not eager to have the discomfort removed; and when the patient complains persistently with vagueness and a flat affect. The question "What have you learned from the other doctors" leads to no useful information.

General Principles of Pain Therapy

Pain Is Not Psychological by Default

The patient should not have his or her pain called psychological or "supratentorial" merely because it is not understood or because it is unresponsive to treatment. The physician should assure the patient that there is no question about the degree of suffering involved. Furthermore, psychological factors may play a role, but this by no means diminishes either the quality or the quantity of pain the patient endures. Education about the close relation of "psyche and soma" in CNS is often useful to establish a doctor-patient relationship.

Long-standing pain is difficult to assess largely because what we learn about pain is based on our concept of acute pain. The patient with acute pain moans, writhes, sweats, begs for help, and gives every appearance of being in great distress. Those nearby someone in acute pain typically feel an urge to help. When pain persists over days and weeks, the individual adapts to it, often without realizing. The patient becomes able to sit in the physician's examining room and complains of agonizing pain while giving little or no evidence of actually being in agony. This adaptation means that the pain has become bearable, although there seems to be no change in intensity. This may be accounted for by several explanations: The sensation may become intermittent; the CNS inhibits the pain, or the sufferer becomes more capable of using distraction. It is ironic that the capacity to adapt to severe pain is often the patient's undoing because it causes the examiner to doubt the patient's veracity. The sufferer now is in the position of having to prove that he or she is in pain. The patient feels himself or herself to be on trial. To counter this end, the physician must know the pathophysiology of pain and employ the full range of neurologic, pharmacologic, and psychological therapies available.

Care Does Not Only Involve Symptom Management

An important principle of pain management is to assure the patient that treatment will continue even if there is no immediate improvement. The physician should also guard against being affected by the patient's sense of discouragement. One of the fears expressed by many patients who suffer from chronic pain is that of abandonment; they believe that if they do not improve, the physician will no longer see them. In this case, an endless series of medications, without continuing examination, psychodynamic care, or critical thinking, is tantamount to noninvolvement or to abandonment. Education about relaxation techniques, yoga, acupuncture, TENS, ultrasound, and massage all have their place in the therapeutic armamentarium. The value is not only in soothing the pain but also in helping the person to feel more in control, that is, less of a victim, and to become an active, educated participant while under the physician's care.

Caveats in Using Placebos

Few phenomena are as misunderstood as the placebo trial. A placebo trial shows whether or not the patient is placebo-positive; it does not prove that the pain is not real or that the person is either an addict or a malingerer. Similarly, it does not

demonstrate that the patient would not benefit from an active medication. The trial is of no assistance in separating psychogenic from organic pain because the placebo response cannot be linked with any type of psychopathology. In fact, patients with depression, somatoform disorder, or other varieties of emotional disturbance are no more apt to be placebo-responders than are so-called normal people.

Whether the pain is from a metastatic lesion or is part of a major affective disorder, relief is experienced by the placebo-responder. Following surgery, about one patient out of three obtains pain relief from saline or from some other inert substance and is therefore considered placebo-positive. For instance, Evans and Hoyle[51] used sodium bicarbonate to treat individuals suffering from angina pectoris. In 38% of their subjects, they found this agent to be as effective as nitroglycerin.

The time-worn custom of slipping in a few saline shots for morphine and calling the deception a placebo trial only demonstrates the ignorance of the perpetrator. If a shot of sterile saline is substituted for a dose of narcotics and the patient responds by obtaining relief, the nature of his or her pain will be questioned even though relief is based on the conditioned response. Moreover, placebo effect and true effects are not independent. The mechanism for the placebo response is possibly the endogenous opioid pain-inhibiting system and is therefore coinfluenced by psychological expectation. Placebo analgesia is reversed with the opioid antagonist naltrexone.[11]

In a valid placebo trial, the inert substance must be given to the patient in a randomized manner along with the usual narcotic under double-blind conditions. Without this control, the placebo trial is useless. The only place for a placebo trial is an informed blinded experiment in which both the patient and the physician have discussed the intention and methodology and are in agreement to find the best treatment for a patient's pain disorder. One of the chief hazards of placebo use is that the patient may feel tricked if he or she discovers that a placebo has been administered to him or her. In this case, it is natural for the patient to feel on trial and wrongly accused, and there is no psychiatric fix for this error once it has happened. The physician who ordered the placebo needs to discuss it with the patient.

Deafferentation Surgery Is Usually Not the Answer

An abiding principle in the treatment of chronic pain is to avoid surgery whenever possible. Few surgical procedures on the CNS are persistently definitive in the cure or control of pain, and most carry with them a tax that is sometimes worse than the pain itself. In particular, CNS pain is notoriously refractory to surgery that interrupts afferent pain pathways. The pain is often made worse by procedures, such as neurectomies, rhizotomies, tractotomies, and cordotomies. Surgery, with the one exception of cingulotomy, is not a treatment for depression that manifests as pain. A central procedure, such as cingulotomy performed stereotactically using radiofrequency lesions, may be useful for intractable pain, especially because it has a low risk of psychiatric and physical morbidity. Personality changes, mental dulling, and memory impairment are rare. Unfortunately, even when pain is reduced with cingulotomy, it can return within 3 to 6 months. To exemplify this multiform plasticity of pain, consider the following account of an extraordinary case.

Case

RC, a 28-year-old mechanic, was thrown from his motorcycle en route to his wedding. Injury occurred to his brachial plexus and arm, requiring an amputation at the shoulder. He then developed severe phantom limb pain. Six months later, the stump was revised and a neurectomy performed; the pain, however, remained unaltered. The nerve was then severed further into the stump with similar result. An unsuccessful rhizotomy was then performed, followed by a chordotomy with the same outcome. The patient was then put in individual psychotherapy for a year, but there was no improvement. After six sessions of electroconvulsive therapy (ECT), the pain was only intensified. A higher cervical chordotomy was performed without success, and then a mesencephalic tractotomy but again with no relief. He next had both dorsomedial thalamic nuclei ablated using stereotactic electrocautery. He emerged from this procedure with his personality intact but still with his original pain. Then electrolytic lesions were made bilaterally in

the inferior mesial quadrant of the frontal lobe in stages, but still the pain remained. Following this, he had a left radiofrequency amygdalotomy followed by a left cingulotomy. Nonetheless, the pain continued as before. The pain remained for 4 years after the accident, as pristine as it was 2 week

Talking and Listening

A strategy to evaluate the feelings and behaviors observed in the pain patient is as necessary as the strategy for evaluating physical aspects of the pain. The skill required is not only a matter of diagnosing the major psychiatric illnesses that can present with pain—these patients often have a maladaptive style of interaction that requires a different kind of interpretive skill—but also a question of the physician's ability to relate to the long-suffering pain patient who shows poor judgment of surgical risk, denies anger, and rapidly alternates between idealizing and denigrating the medical caretaker. The fluctuations of both mood and cooperation frequently encountered in the clinical interview are symptomatic of the patient's damaged self-esteem or his or her injured narcissism. Chronic pain patients invariably feel damaged not only in the body part afflicted with discomfort, but also in self-image and spirit—a phenomenon known as narcissistic injury.[52] The techniques for interviewing the narcissistically injured pain patient are designed to establish a diagnostic working relationship. They allow for an accurate medical history to be elicited, mistrust between physician and patient to be avoided, an effective treatment plan to be developed, and the outcomes through compliance and education to be enhanced.

The interviewer should allow the patient to tell his or her own story. An initial degree of catharsis may be helpful in decreasing the patient's anxiety and in giving the physician a sense of the patient's character. The physician must actively facilitate an alliance with the patient while still maintaining neutrality and avoiding misplaced sympathy. The patient's underlying feelings of fear, anger, resentment, and mistrust are best uncovered by asking how others view the situation, essentially a counterprojective method. This approach sometimes bares unpleasant affects without the use of intrusive questions from the physician. Labeling overt and covert roles assigned by the patient to the physician is an important early intervention. Specifically, this means that the physician should point out when the patient is attributing unrealistic curative powers to him or her or appears to believe that the physician is indifferent to the patient's suffering. The longer one waits to confront these fantasies, the less effective any intervention will be. Expression of affect should be encouraged, and the physician should help the patient express the feelings he or she is having but does not want to acknowledge. The physician's assertive pursuit of the patient's true feelings avoids giving the appearance of unqualified support to feelings that need expression. Too much support not only bypasses psychological problems but also may actually increase conflicted feelings over withholding, control, dependence, and frail self-esteem. The physician's kindness should not be allowed to become a problem for the patient.

Optimal care of intractable pain patients requires the ability to process neurologic and psychiatric data while delineating and responding to the phrase-by-phrase manifestations of suffering and pain behavior. In essence, being able to get patients to talk about what they are angry about is just as important as discussing their insomnia or disc herniation. Progress occurs with these needy, angry patients only when there is clear processing and separation of the reality-based facts of the case from unrealistic expectations. In that way, every clarification of an unrealistic idea can be an introduction to a more realistic alternative. The overall goal is to improve the patient's self-awareness and capacity for insight, thereby gaining control.

Medication for Pain: Analgesia and Adjuvants

Judicious and effective use of medicine in patients with chronic pain rests on the concise evaluation of the four main components of the pain complaint: nociceptive pain, CNS mechanisms of pain, suffering, and pain behavior. In its most elemental form, the medical management of these four components employs opioids, anticonvulsants, antidepressants, and behavioral treatment. Nonsteroidal antiinflam-

matory drugs (NSAIDs), aspirin, and nerve blocks are often helpful in the early stages of these illnesses. Opioids are, however, the most effective medicine for these pains when the severity increases.

Nonsteroidal Antiinflammatory Drugs

The World Health Organization (WHO) has established a three-step guideline for pain treatment (Figure 21-4). Step 1 involves the use of NSAIDs, aspirin, or acetaminophen. Step 2 adds codeine to the NSAID, with other adjuvants. Step 3 employs narcotics with adjunctive medication. Conceived for cancer pain, and reporting efficacy in 90% of cancer patients, the three steps are a useful template for many kinds of acute pain, adjusted for the particular pain mechanism being treated. NSAIDs are useful for acute and chronic pain, such as inflammation, muscle pain, vascular pain, and posttraumatic pain, or when the physician wants to use a potent nonnarcotic analgesic.

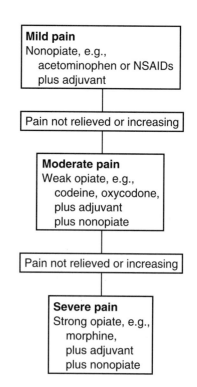

Figure 21-4. The analgesic ladder.
(From Borsook D, Lebel AA, McPeek B [1995]. MGH handbook of pain management. Boston, MA, Little Brown).

NSAIDs are generally equally efficacious and have similar side effects.[53]

Side Effects

Most NSAIDs can cause bronchospasm in aspirin-sensitive patients, induce gastric ulcers, interact with angiotensin converting enzyme (ACE) inhibitors (thereby contributing to renal failure), precipitate lithium toxicity, and impair renal function in the long term. NSAIDs can elevate blood pressure in patients treated with β-blockers and diuretics. The exception to this general rule is the nonacetylated (nonaspirin) salicylates that do not inhibit the synthesis of prostaglandins. These include choline magnesium trisalicylate (Trilisate) and diflunisal (Dolobid); these agents do not cause bronchospasm in aspirin-sensitive patients, precipitate renal failure, or inhibit platelet aggregation. Certain NSAIDs, however, have features that make some preferable over others in particular situations. The recent discovery of the enzyme cyclooxygenase (COX) isoforms (1 and 2) led to the discovery of selective COX-2 inhibitors. COX-2 tends to facilitate the inflammatory response selectively and the use of new agents (rofecoxib and celecoxib) may increase gastrointestinal safety.[54]

Special Features

Synergistic combinations of acetaminophen, aspirin, and caffeine (e.g., Excedrin) are the cornerstone for temporary relief of pain (e.g., headaches and muscle pain) and potentiation of the effects of narcotics. They do, however, have a limit on dosing and have only moderate potency; they are also not well tolerated by those who are very sick. NSAID variations then need to be considered. Choline magnesium trisalicylate (1000 to 1500 mg) is safe in aspirin-sensitive patients, and it does not prolong bleeding. Misoprostol can reduce gastrointestinal erosions in patients on maintenance NSAIDs, but its use can be limited by diarrhea, pain, and flatulence in about one third of patients. Ibuprofen (800 mg) is a rapid-release agent that produces higher blood levels over the first half hour than the other preparations at equal dosage. Ketorolac (up to 30 mg every

6 hours) intramuscularly followed by oral dosing has a rapid onset and a high potency, enabling it to be substituted for morphine (N.B.: 30 mg of ketorolac is equivalent to 10 mg of morphine). It should be used for no more than 5 days. Extended-release preparations can be useful when long, steady analgesia and simple dose regimens are needed (e.g., nabumetone [Relafen], oxaprozin [Daypro], ketoprofen [Oruvail], piroxicam [Feldene]). Naproxen (EC-Naprosyn) (375 to 500 mg twice a day with enteric-coated, delayed-release tablets) can be well tolerated over time. Ketoprofen (200 mg) extended-release tablets can be taken once a day, but they are not intended for patients with renal disease or for those over 75 years of age. Ibuprofen works well as a narcotic adjuvant for bone pain. Naproxen (up to 1500 mg a day), but not flurbiprofen, has also had positive results for bone pain. The newer COX-2 inhibitors (celecoxib and rofecoxib) may cause fewer gastrointestinal problems compared to other NSAIDs. Celecoxib does not impair platelet function. Rofecoxib is currently FDA-approved for osteoarthritis. For a list of NSAIDs, see Table 21-6.

Opioids

Opioids help some cancer patients as well as those with non–cancer related chronic pain.[55,56] Cancer pain is the most common indication for maintenance narcotics.[57] Acute, severe and unremitting pain also requires opioid treatment, as outlined in the WHO analgesic ladder. At times, narcotics may be the only effective treatment for chronic, nonmalignant pain, such as the pain associated with postherpetic neuralgia, degenerative disorders, and vascular conditions.[58] Bouckoms et al.[59] demonstrated that nonmalignant pain treated with long-term oral narcotics provides effective pain relief in about two thirds of those treated. Nociceptive pain, absence of depression, and absence of any drug abuse were all significantly associated with long-term narcotic treatment efficacy. Patients with neuropathic pain or major depression fared especially poorly; a bad outcome was four times more likely than a good outcome. Even when patients were carefully selected (i.e., lack of previous addiction or gross personality

Table 21-6. Properties of Aspirin and Nonsteroidal Antiinflammatory Drugs

Drug	Dose (mg)	Dosage Interval (h)	Daily Dose (mg/day)	Peak Effect (hr)	Half-Life (hr)
Aspirin	81–975	4	4500	0.5–1	0.25
Celecoxib	100–200	12	1200	1	11
Diclofenac	25–75	6–8	200	2	1–2
Diflunisal	250–500	12	1500	1	13
Etodolac acid	200–400	6–8	1600	1–2	7
Fenoprofen	200	4–6	3200	1–2	2–3
Flurbiprofen	50–100	6–8	300	1.5–3	3–4
Ibuprofen	200–400	6–8	3200	1–2	2
Indomethacin	25–75	6–8	200	0.5–1	2–3
Ketoprofen	25–75	6–8	300	1–2	1.5–2.0
Ketorolac*					
Oral	10	6–8	40	0.5–1	6
Parenteral	60 load, then 30	6–8	120	0.5	6
Meclofenamic acid	500 load, then 275	6–8	400	1	2–4
Mefanamic acid	500 load, then 250	6	1250	2–4	3–4
Nabumetone	1000–2000	12–24	2000	3–5	22–30
Naproxen	500 load, then 250	6–8	1250	2–4	12–15
Naproxen sodium	550 load then 275,	6–8	1375	1–2	13
Oxaprozin	60–1200	24	1800	2	3–3.5
Phenylbutazone	100	6–8	400	2	50–100
Piroxicam	40 load, then 20	24	20	2–4	36–45
Refocoxib	12.5–25	24	50	1	17
Sulindac	150–200	12	400	1–2	7–18
Tolmetin	200–400	8	1800	4–6	2

*Use no longer than 5 days.
Source: Adapted from Borsook D, Lebel AA, McPeek B. *MGH Handbook of Pain Management*, Boston, 1995, Little, Brown Publishers.

disorder), one third of patients developed abuse, tolerance, or addiction over a 3-year period. Even so, drug abusers with chronic pain may still benefit from physician-prescribed narcotics for their physical pain if it stops them from turning to illicit supplies. These patients may require specific nonnarcotic prescriptions for their neuropathy and depression if gains are to be made.

Narcotic Potencies

Codeine is a good narcotic for mild to moderate pain, but it has limited efficacy for severe pain. Morphine is the narcotic of choice for acute and chronic pain because it is well known and has a good safety profile. Beyond these starting points, the basic principles of narcotics are as outlined in Table 21-7.

Principles of Narcotics Administration

Potency and Administration.   Potency and administration are consistent with the characteristics of the drug, its half-life, and absorption by different routes; such knowledge helps to ensure that the dosage schedule is consistent with these parameters.

Oral Potency.   Oral potency must be high so that parenteral use can be avoided if possible. Methadone is a good first choice because of its oral potency and relatively slow clearance. Morphine, hydromorphone, and levorphanol may be useful alternatives for initial treatment. Once oral doses have been initiated and titrated to a satisfactory level (e.g., 4-hourly dosing of morphine or methadone), the analgesic effect needs to be sustained by minimizing fluctuations in blood levels and the variable effects of dosing schedules.

Table 21-7. Narcotic Potencies and Special Features

Drug	Parenteral (mg equivalent)	Oral (mg)	Duration (hr)	Special Features
Morphine	10	30	4	Morphine sulfate controlled release has 12-h duration
Codeine	120	200	4	Ceiling effect as dose increases, low lipophilic
Oxycodone	4.5	30	4	Every 12 h oxycontin (10, 20, 40 slow release mg)
Hydromorphone	2	8	5	Suppository 6 mg = 10 mg parenteral morphine
Levorphanol	2	4	4	Low nausea and vomiting, low lipophilic
Methadone	5	10	2	Cumulative effect; day 3–5 decrease respiration
Meperidine	100	300	3	κ, proconvulsant metabolite, peristaltic slowing and sphincter of Oddi decrease
Fentanyl	0.1	25 μg SL	1 (patch 72 hr)	50 μg patch = 60 mg/day morphine IM/IV
Sufentanil	Not recommended	15 μg SL	1	High potency with low volume of fluid
Propoxyphene	Not available	325	4	High dose leads to psychosis
Pentazocine	60	150	3	κ, σ agonist-antagonist, nasal 1 mg q1–2h
Butorphanol	2	Not available 3 (IM), 2 (NS)	μ, κ, σ, agonist-antagonist, nasal 1 mg q1–2h	
Buprenorphine	0.3	Not available	4–6	Partial agonist
Tramadol	Not available	150	4	μ agonist, decreased reuptake 5-HT and NE, P450 metabolism
Nalbuphine	10	Not available	3	Agonist-antagonist

SL, sublingual; IM, intramuscular; IV, intravenous; 5-HT, 5-hydroxytryptamine; NE, norepinephrine; NS, nasal.

Morphine sulfate controlled release (MSC) is ideal for this homeostasis because it is released more slowly than conventional oral morphine. Furthermore, morphine's effect is not significantly affected by minor hepatic disease. Fifty percent of the morphine in MSC reaches the CNS after 1.5 hours, three times longer than it takes conventional oral morphine to reach the CNS. Steady-state is reached with MSC in about 1 day. A steady-state with MSC at any fixed dose and dosing interval has a lower maximum blood concentration than does conventional morphine, thereby reducing fluctuations in blood levels. Note that MSC does not release morphine continuously and evenly, so that a dosing schedule of every 12 hours has more peaks and troughs than conventional oral morphine given every 4 hours. It is also important to be aware that chewing or crushing MSC further increases erratic release. MSC should not be given less than every 12 hours.

Avoid As-Needed Dosing. A steady-state of narcotic blood level requires approximately four half-lives to achieve consistency, and a steep dose-response curve makes pain relief erratic (e.g., if one dose is missed, it can take 23 hours to return to therapeutic analgesia). Dosing on an as-needed basis makes steady relief impossible. It also predisposes the patient to drug-respondent conditioning and to subsequent behavior problems.

Toxicity. Morphine and dihydromorphone uncommonly cause toxicity and hence are prescriptions of choice. Even so, when glomerular filtration rate is poor and morphine or hydromorphone doses are high, toxicity may occur, even when equivalent doses of morphine are used without signs of toxicity. Meperidine hydrochloride should be avoided in difficult cases because of its short duration of action (2 to 4 hours) and because even at normal doses its principal metabolite (normeperidine) can cause irritability, auditory and visual hallucinations, agitation, confused thinking, disorientation, hypomania, paranoia, and muscle twitches, in addition to partial and generalized seizures.[60-62] This CNS excitement is more likely to occur in patients with malignancy or renal impairment or when the drug is given intravenously and the dose exceeds 300 mg/day for more than 4 days—all conditions in which there may be significant accumulation of the proconvulsant normeperidine with repeated dosing. Methadone, safe and effective for analgesia on day 2, can accumulate and cause significant respiratory depression by day 5. Troubleshooting checklists for opioids may be required when the basic principles mentioned have not worked.[63]

Are Opioids the Drugs of Choice in This Case?

Unduly long clinical trials and ongoing patient suffering may be avoided by giving the patient 10 mg of IV morphine as a single-blinded test dose. This is a diagnostic procedure designed to determine if narcotics will relieve the pain. If there is a positive result with relief of pain, one concludes that morphine works well enough to continue its use. A negative outcome might result in a repeat dose of morphine at 20 mg to ensure that it was not just tolerance that failed to produce a benefit at 10 mg. In a doubtful case, one can give 0.4 mg of IV naloxone to confirm the lack of an opioid effect on pain. If there is neuropathic pain, for example, opioids may not produce a good enough response at normal doses. In about 50% of patients with intractable pain, opioids do not have a good enough analgesic effect. In a minority, it is the anxiolytic effect rather than the analgesic effect that is helpful.

Dosing. Prescriber fear and ignorance are the usual reasons that analgesics are given at inadequate dosage and frequency. Appropriate dosing requires knowledge of the potency and half-life of the drug. Common errors that occur at critical moments include failure to adjust the dosage when switching from parenteral to oral use (e.g., not tripling the dose of morphine when switching from IM to oral dosing); failure to administer the drug at longer intervals than its half-life (e.g., methadone's analgesic half-life is 6 hours; consequently, methadone is needed at least four times a day when it is given for pain, not once a day as when it is given for opioid addiction); and underdosing when beginning MSC or fentanyl patches because both require at least 24 hours to reach steady-state (supplementary opioids are required for the first 24 hours).

Drug Delivery. An important question to bear in mind is whether the method of administration and type of opioid have been optimized. The most common problem in severe pain is the threefold to eightfold variability of IM absorption. This can be decreased by using agents that are hydrophilic (e.g., morphine and hydromorphone) rather than lipophilic (e.g., fentanyl, methadone, and meperidine). When more lipophilic agents, such as methadone, are used intramuscularly, injections into the deltoid rather than the gluteus muscle are preferable. If an erratic response occurs, it might be due to inconsistent drug delivery. Alternative methods include delivery of the drug intravenously, sublingually, intrathecally, ventricularly, or transdermally. For example, Kunz et al[64] described the innovative use of sublingual sufentanil, 25 mg every 3 minutes (for three doses) for severe but episodic pain. The drug and route were preferable to patient-controlled analgesia (PCA) fentanyl sublingually or MSC because the volume of fluid was small, speed of onset was within 1 minute, and the half-life was short (and therefore not sedating the rest of the day); in addition, the cost was comparable to PCA, albeit more expensive than sublingual fentanyl. The patient could get out of bed and remain alert and comfortable with a low-tech intervention that is ideal for hospice or for home care.

Tolerance or Excessive Sedation. The age of the patient is an important factor in the efficacy of the drug. The duration of effect may double as age increases; as it does so does the analgesic effect in a 70-year-old versus a 20-year-old. Opioid adjuvants (e.g., methylphenidate) may decrease or increase (e.g., with antidepressants) sedation.

Mixed Agonists-Antagonists. Pentazocine and butorphanol are commonly used opioids because of their mixed antagonist-agonist properties. Not only are they less potent than standard opioids, but also if combined with them during a period of transition, they may cause the patient to develop withdrawal symptoms, an acute confusional state, or even psychosis. Older people are particularly susceptible. Avoidance of mixing agonist opioid drugs with agonist-antagonist agents obviates this problem.

Addiction. The risk of opioid addiction in a general population of medically ill patients is approximately 0.3%. Therefore, considering the patient as an addict on the basis of difficulties with managing narcotics should be done cautiously. Acute sympathetic symptoms from drug withdrawal or tolerance are more likely to be the problem than addiction per se. Rather than addiction, unrecognized depression alone or comorbid with anxiety is a more frequent, immediate explanation for the excessive need for opiates.

Recently, oxycodone has attracted significant attention in the media due to its addiction potential. Clinical practice and research trials show that it is a good medication for pain due to its efficacy, fairly good side-effect profile, and short-onset of action. In patients who cannot tolerate or respond to other opioids it remains a good option.[65]

Opioid Adjuvants. Opioid adjuvants are indicated when toxic or pharmacokinetic factors limit further increases in the patient's opioid dosage or when pain remains uncontrolled by opioids in combination with other secondary treatments, such as decompression surgery, nerve blocks, or anxiolytic drugs. The choice of adjuvant should be individualized; one should aim for the simplest and most potent combination of drugs. The selection of the adjuvant depends on the symptoms associated with the pain; the character of the pain; and the physician's knowledge of any special issues, risks, drug interactions, or special mechanisms (Table 21-8).

Guidelines for Narcotic Maintenance Adjuvants.

- Maintenance narcotics should be considered only after other methods of pain control have been proven unsuccessful. Alternative methods vary from case to case but typically include NSAIDs; oral, transdermal, intravenous, intrathecal, or epidural opioids; membrane-stabilizing drugs; monoaminergic agents and local nerve blocks; nerve stimulation; and physical therapy.
- Narcotics should not be prescribed for addicts unless there is a new major medical illness with severe pain (e.g., cancer or trauma). In such cases, a second opinion from another physician is suggested for all narcotics used for longer than 2 months.
- If narcotics are prescribed for longer than 3 months, the patient should have a second opinion consultation, plus a follow-up consultation at least once per year.
- There should be one pharmacy and one prescriber designated as exclusive agents.
- Narcotic dosage should be defined, as should expectations of what will happen if there are deviations from it. For example, abuse leads to rapid tapering of the drug and a detoxification program, if necessary. There should be no doubt that the physician will stop the drug.
- Informed consent as to the rationale, risks, benefits, and alternatives should be documented.
- The course of treatment (in particular, the ongoing indications, changes in the disease process, efficacy, and the presence of abuse, tolerance, or addictive behavior) should be documented.

Justification for maintenance narcotics, given the mixed benefits and risks, involves humanitarian and public health principles. If narcotics are the only effective treatment for intractable suffering, they should be used for humanitarian reasons. The risk of episodic abuse may be justified in marginally reliable people with drug abuse histories and chronic pain, if use of narcotics lessens disability and illicit drug use. For example, an IV drug addict with chronic pain may benefit from a methadone maintenance program for pain; furthermore, it may be an effective public health means of reducing the risk of acquired immunodeficiency syndrome (AIDS).

Table 21-8. Narcotic Adjuvants

Agent	Dosage	Indications	Special Issues
Prostaglandin inhibitors	Variable, limited by side effects and medical comorbidity	Metastatic bone pain Inflammation Vascular pain	NSAID risks: gastrointestinal bleeding, renal impairment
Neuroleptics Phenothiazines Butyrophenones	Antipsychotic dopamine 2 receptor blocking doses	Postherpetic pain Cancer pain Diabetic neuropathy Adjunct to TCAs Comorbid anxiety or delirium	Haloperidol binds to σ opioid receptors Membrane stabilizing
Stimulants Methylphenidate Dextroamphetamine Pergolide	5–50 mg/day (t½: 2–7 hr) 5–20 mg/day (t½: 4–21 hr) 0.05 mg tid (t½: 6–72 hr)	Postoperative pain and pain in pediatric and cancer patients respond well to analgesic stimulant combinations	Stimulants decrease pain and sedation Appetite and cognition improve methylphenidate shows better long-term efficacy than does amphetamine
Steroids Prednisone Methylprednisolone	15 + mg/day PO 15 mg/kg IV boluses	Bone metastases Brain swelling Spinal cord compression Anorexia and pain Sickle cell pain	Risks: mood lability, withdrawal, anxiety, insomnia, gastrointestinal upset
Peptides Calcitonin Somatostatin Capsaicin crème	100–200 IU SC bid nasal 200 IC/day 500 μg .075%	Paget's, metastatic, and myeloma pain Vascular headaches Neuralgia, cancer pain Hyperalgesia, postherpetic neuralgia, cluster headache, RSD, inflammatory dermatoses, itching secondary to dialysis, psoriasis	Intrathecal, nasal, and SC are used. Somatostatin inhibits SP Capsaicin effect peaks 4–6 wk, for diabetic, postmastectomy and arthritic pain
Antihistamines Diphenhydramine Hydroxyzine	150 mg 100 mg	Narcotic adjunct	Decreased inflammation, 5-HT, NE, dopamine, SR spasm, opiate clearance Increased opiate binding
Radiation therapy External beam Strontium-89 Phosphorus-39	Metastatic bone pain	70% effective after a single dose	
Chemotherapy Hydroxyurea	500 mg tid (20–80 mg/kg)	Sickle cell crises	Less narcotic

NSAID, nonsteroidal antiinflammatory drug; TCAs, tricyclic antidepressants; IV, intravenous; SC, subcutaneous; SP, substance P; RSD, reflex sympathetic dystrophy; 5-HT, 5-hydroxytryptamine; NE, norepinephrine.

Analgesic Adjuvants

Pain may be refractory despite the most judicious application of traditional antinociceptive measures, such as surgery, nerve blocks, and opioids. Stimulants, neuroleptics, tricyclic monoaminergic agents, benzodiazepines, anticonvulsants, antihistamines, peptides, and prostaglandin inhibitors also have roles as non-narcotic pain treatment adjuvants[66] (Table 21-9). The type of pain is as important as its cause in guiding the choice of an adjuvant. The pain may be characterized as a constant aching somatic pain, as in a fracture, or as a paroxysmal burning deafferentation sensation, as in phantom limb pain. The primary cause of the pain, however, does not necessarily determine its type or character. For example, the pain of metastatic cancer may be either neuropathic or somatic (and may or may not respond well to NSAIDs). Neuropathic pain is often refractory to opioids, and it covers a diverse group of conditions, which range from herpetic neuralgia to atypical facial pain. Patients suffering from this type of pain may respond to anticonvulsants or TCAs. In the most difficult or ambiguous cases, a valuable technique is to use an IV dose of the drug to gain a rapid and accurate assessment of its effectiveness for the long-term. Intravenous morphine, lidocaine, and lorazepam can be used in this way to see whether or not any of these classes of drugs are worth pursuing.

Antidepressants for Pain

The mechanisms of action of TCAs are multiple and probably comodulate the pain-relieving effect.[67] First, they have an effect in augmenting the descending periaqueductal spinal inhibitory control of pain mediated by serotonin and norepinephrine. In the spinal cord, the dorsolateral funiculus is a serotoninergic inhibitory descending spinal pain pathway that modulates 80% of the spinal analgesic effect of opiates. Second, they potentiate naturally occurring or administered opiates. For example, desipramine, 8-OH-amoxapine, and imipramine are twice as potent as amitriptyline and four times as potent as trazodone and clomipramine at binding to opiate receptors. Third, antihistamine and α-receptor effects may be important. Fourth, there may be membrane-stabilizing anesthetic, antikindling anticonvulsant

Table 21-9. Analgesic Adjuvants

Medication	Dosage	Indications	Special Issues
Benzodiazepines			
Clonazepam	1–4 mg/day	Adjuvant tricyclics	Not a substitute for diagnosis
Lorazepam	2–16 mg/day	Allodynia	of depression or substance abuse
Anticonvulsants			Paroxysmal pains
Valproate	500–2000 mg/day	Central pain	respond best to
Gabapentin	900–1800 mg/day	Neuropathy	anticonvulsants
Carbamazepine	400–1600 mg/day	Headaches, neuralgia	
Lamictal	100–300 mg/day	Migraine headaches	
Tricyclics	25–300 mg/day	Neuropathy	Burning
Desipramine		Postherpetic neuralgia	Deafferentation pains
Imipramine			respond best to the tricyclic drugs
			Amitriptyline has more side effects
MAOIs		Atypical facial pain	Stage 4 sleep, atypical
Phenelzine (Nardil)	60–90	Myofascial pain	depression helped by
Tranylcypromine (Parnate)	40 mg	Headaches	MAOIs
Famciclovir	500 mg 3 times/day for 7 day	May shorten duration of postherpetic neuralgia	Start within 48 hr of rash
Cytokine blockers		Arthritic pain	Blocks cytokine TNF-α

MAOIs, monoamine oxidase inhibitors; TNF-a, tumor necrosis factor-a.

effects, which may give secondary symptom relief of insomnia or anxiety.

The pain relief obtained from antidepressants is often independent of their effects on mood or the alleviation of major depression.[68,69] In fact, the greatest response to antidepressants in patients with pain may occur in those who are not depressed.[70] Antidepressants as analgesics are best thought of as monoaminergic cell stabilizers rather than just antidepressants. Serotonin, norepinephrine, and dopamine all modulate pain via their actions in the periphery to the CNS.

Serotonin presents a paradox because more serotonin is not necessarily better, yet function must be intact for pain to be inhibited. One type of peripheral serotonin receptor, 5-HT_{ID}, is found in cerebral blood vessels. Sumatriptan, a selective 5-HT_{ID} antagonist, acts to produce vasoconstriction and migraine headache relief. The raphe and mesolimbic structures are important sites of subcortical serotonin receptors, mainly types 1A, 2A, and B. These sites modulate pain and mood—the behavioral sites of action. Despite the important role serotonin plays in pain, there are a number of exceptions to the simplistic notion of more serotonin, less pain.[71] For example, buspirone, fluoxetine (Prozac), and trazodone have all been shown to be ineffective in attenuating certain pain syndromes.[72–74]

Norepinephrine-modulating drugs also have value in treating chronic pain. Venlafaxine, a norepinephrine and serotonin reuptake inhibitor, has reported efficacy in postherpetic neuralgia and neuropathy (at a dose of 25 to 75 mg twice a day). Diamond's retrospective chart review of treatment for refractory vascular and tension headaches using venlafaxine found that 37% of patients improved, 45% displayed no change, and 18% were worse.[75,76] Desipramine (average dose, 200 mg/day) similarly relieved pain in diabetic neuropathy, in both nondepressed and depressed patients,[27] and it also relieved postherpetic neuralgia.[28] Two problems emerge, however, when trying to draw specific conclusions from this research. The first is that no antidepressant is purely specific to norepinephrine. The second is that in a group of sympathetically maintained pain patients, presumably ones who were norepinephrine sensitive, only 28% responded with increased pain when norepinephrine was injected into the skin. One explanation that might help to resolve these

inconsistencies is the possibility that norepinephrine works through comodulation with other neuromodulators or that the sensitivity of norepinephrine may vary over time.[77]

Reviews of Efficacy

Earlier reports of Lindsey and Wycoff[78] showed an efficacy of 70% to 80% for antidepressants for the treatment of chronic pain patients with depression. Stein et al.[79] reported that amitriptyline (150 mg/day) was more effective than acetaminophen 2 g/day in a controlled, double-blind study, with mild depression being one of the predictors of pain relief at the end of the 5-week study. Blumer and Heilbronn[80] showed twice the improvement (60%) in outcome and a halving of the dropout rate (25%) in those pain patients treated with antidepressants.

Pain syndromes that may be responsive to antidepressants include those associated with cancer, postherpetic neuralgia, arthritis, vascular and tension headaches, and facial pain. The literature reports a wide range of generally positive but poorly designed studies.[68,81] Feinman[68] reviewed the reviewed the 11 largest and best-designed studies on pain relief from antidepressants when depressive symptoms were present. TCAs (amitriptyline hydrochloride) and MAOIs (phenelzine sulfate) were used. The results demonstrated that antidepressant drugs were beneficial in the treatment of chronic pain associated with depression.

Goodkin's et al.[82] review found that 37 of 53 trials (70%) of heterocyclic antidepressant drugs for chronic pain syndromes failed to meet minimum criteria for adequate design. Of the remaining 16 trials that met design and protocol criteria, 7 evaluated headache pain and documented positive effects with low-dose regimens. Smaller than typical antidepressant doses were used in many studies. Goodkin et al.[82] reviewed another nonrandom series of 17 studies (selected for key words *pain* and *antidepressants*) published since 1987. Of the 17, 5 (29%) met minimum design and protocol criteria (i.e., clear protocol, placebo-controlled, and defined outcome measurements), and only two of the five trials showed positive results. One study was for low-dose amitriptyline in mixed pain syndromes, and the other study was for desipramine in postherpetic neuralgia. Max[83] found that in 13 well-designed, randomized trials, antidepressants reduced pain in diabetic neuropathy and postherpetic neuralgia, particularly the mixed serotonin and norepinephrine agents (e.g., imipramine, desipramine, and amitriptyline).

Although some patients may respond to low doses of antidepressants for pain, a complete trial of antidepressants in pain patients requires a full dose of an antidepressant, the same as used in major depression. An effort to extract meaning from the pain-antidepressant data was undertaken by Onghena and Van Houdenhove,[84] who reported a meta-analysis of 39 controlled trials of antidepressants for nonmalignant pain. Twenty-eight studies showed a statistically significant difference between active drug and placebo. Overall the average chronic pain patient who received an antidepressant had less pain than 74% of those who received a placebo. Body location and pain type in Onghena and Van Houdenhove's review of studies of head, face, tension, and central pain yielded an antidepressant treatment that had a mean response significantly higher (about twice) that of other body regions. Rheumatologic pain, the pain type most studied (10 studies), derived the smallest benefit. For neuropathic pain, imipramine, amitriptyline, clomipramine, desipramine, and nortriptyline were effective.[85–89] In Onghena and Van Houdenhove's meta-analytic review,[84] the analgesic effect of antidepressants was not explainable by higher or lower doses. The placebo-controlled study of McQuay et al.[90] found that low doses of antidepressants (25 mg of amitriptyline) did not have the efficacy of higher doses.

When is it worth trying a monoaminergic agent? A trial of an antidepressant medication is useful in any intractable pain condition whether or not depression is present, because analgesic effects are at least partly independent from antidepressant effects. Furthermore, the size of the analgesic effect does not differ significantly in the presence of depression.

There is no clear evidence for the superiority of any one antidepressant over any other. Amitriptyline, desipramine, and doxepin hydrochloride have been used most often in the clinical studies. Even though sedating and non sedating properties of drugs have no significant association with analgesic effect, the antihistaminic profile of an antidepressant correlates with effect.[84] Potent serotonin reuptake blockade is not essential to pain relief; moreover, there is doubt about the efficacy of purely serotoninergic drugs for neuropathic pain (e.g., fluoxetine, zimeldine, and trazodone).[91,92] Buspirone does not appear to relieve pain. With the exception of paroxetine, all antidepressant drugs studied in placebo-controlled trials of neuropathic pain have some inhibition of norepinephrine reuptake (i.e., amitriptyline, desipramine, nortriptyline, imipramine, and maprotiline).[88] Venlafaxine has some agonist-antagonist opiate activity as well as norepinephrine, 5-hydroxytryptamine, and dopamine-reuptake effects, but it has yet to be rigorously proven as an analgesic.

MAOIs may be particularly helpful in the attenuation of atypical pain associated with atypical depression. Both MAOIs and TCAs, however, may require a trial of at least 6 weeks for the full benefit to be evident.

Low-dose antidepressants (i.e., those below the normal therapeutic range for depression) may be helpful for pain treatment. The best results in the largest number of people are obtained, however, when the usual antidepressant dosage of drug is used (e.g., 300 mg/day of imipramine hydrochloride or its equivalent). Other pointers include:

- Maintenance treatment for 3 to 6 months is usually necessary for the best results.
- Education of the patient as to the rationale for antidepressant treatment is advised for good compliance.
- Treatment of the depressed pain patient is no different than treatment of any other depressed patient.
- Depression should not be rationalized as appropriate.

Dopamine agonists can augment analgesia. Dopamine has been associated with pain for clinical and experimental reasons, and dopamine has been shown to comodulate opiate and substance P effects in the CNS. Low levels of dopamine and homovanillic acid (HVA) have been measured in the CSF of pain patients.[29] TCAs and SSRIs upregulate mesolimbic dopamine. Methylphenidate and pergolide can relieve the suffering of pain.

Monoaminergic agents in combination with clonazepam (Klonopin), divalproex (Depakote), or narcotics (for cancer pain) are often safe and desirable.

Anticonvulsants

Partial seizures may be comorbid with pain, but this is not the only reason to use an anticonvulsant agent. Blocking abnormally high-frequency and spontaneous firing in afferent neurons, in the dorsal horn, and in the thalamus are the putative mechanisms for the efficacy of anticonvulsants with regard to pain. The consequence of blocking the hyperexcitability of low-threshold mechanoreceptive neurons in the brain lead to pain relief.[16] Carbamazepine, clonazepam, gabapentin, divalproex, and phenytoin are agents used to treat pain. These drugs have a number of shared cellular effects, which include antagonism of excitatory amino acids, γ-aminobutyric acid (GABA)-benzodiazepine-like activity, antagonism of adenosine, benzodiazepine receptor activity, and sodium and calcium pump stabilization. Indirectly, they all antagonize the effects of excitatory amino acids, which are believed to kindle hyperexcitability of CNS neurons.

Lamotrigine is the only direct glutamate/aspartate antagonist in the United States that also inhibits sodium channels. In addition, it can ablate the pain of chronic hyperalgesia more than carbamazepine or phenytoin,[92] although skin rash and a need to escalate the dose slowly may be limiting factors. Gabapentin (100 to 600 mg three times a day) has had considerable anecdotal success for pain, and it is well tolerated. Somnolence, dizziness, and nystagmus can occur at higher doses, but these effects can be minimized if one goes from a low dose to a higher dose over the course of 3 days. Benzodiazepines have been controversial in the alleviation of pain, but they do have a definite place as safe and effective agents.[93] Clonazepam, in doses of 1 to 4 mg orally, is particularly useful because it has few side effects, it decreases allodynia, and it is compatible with other agents, such as antidepressants or opioids. Stimulation of the GABA-benzodiazepine receptor decreases pain transmitted along A-Δ fibers.[94,95] Other possible mechanisms of action for the analgesia of clonazepam are synergistic interaction between μ and GABA receptors in the

spinal cord and a primary weak antinociceptive effect on dorsal horn neurons, which is reversible by flumazenil. Serrao et al.[96] have shown that intrathecal midazolam is effective for chronic low (mechanical) back pain.

Combinations of benzodiazepines with antidepressants or opiates are clinically useful. Intravenous lorazepam was superior to morphine, lidocaine (Xylocaine), and placebo in a single-blind study of neuropathic pain.[97] Orally, clonazepam is the drug of choice. It binds more slowly to central than to peripheral benzo-diazepine receptors, and it is synergistic with serotoninergic pain mechanisms, a factor that distinguishes it from other benzodiazepines. A useful diagnostic test for benzodiazepine-sensitive pain (BSP) is to administer lorazepam 2 mg IV in a single-blind manner evaluated by visual analog scale (VAS) monitoring. Positive results (>3 cm decrease in VAS) signifies relief of ongoing pain. If positive results are achieved, it is recommended to give sequential IV lorazepam doses to break the pain cycle (in severe cases) or clonazepam (e.g., 2 to 4 mg orally at bedtime, and 1 mg twice a day).

Phenytoin has been shown effective in alleviating pain associated with various neuropathies, particularly trigeminal, diabetic, and poststroke pain. Sharp, shooting, lancinating pain has been shown to respond especially well to this drug. It has more behavioral toxicity, however, and is less effective than carbamazepine, thus making it a second choice for analgesia.

Carbamazepine is generally superior to phenytoin for pain. Carbamazepine has been effec-tive for trigeminal neuralgia, postherpetic pain, postsympathetic pain, diabetic neuropathy, multiple sclerosis, and assorted neuralgias.[98] Higher levels (8 to 12 μg/L) are typically necessary for optimal efficacy. The mechanism does not involve the opiate receptors; rather, it concerns multiple effects that involve excitotoxins, GABA-benzodiazepine, adenosine antagonists, benzodiazepine-like activity, calcium stabilization, and weak aspartate, glutamate, and sodium-blocking effects.

Additionally, valproate has been shown to decrease postherpetic neuralgia, episodic and chronic cluster headaches, migraine, and postoperative pain, as well as various neuralgias.[99–102] It has also been demonstrated that valproate is effective in treating migraine headaches in two double-blind, placebo-controlled trials.[102,103] These demonstrations of efficacy in pain reduction are in addition to the traditional place for valproate in the treatment of psychiatric disorders (bipolar and schizoaffective disorders). Depakote sprinkles, in particular, are well tolerated and can substitute for carbamazepine and lithium in pain states, although no head-to-head comparisons have been completed. Valproate is distinctive in that it does not affect adenosine the way that carbamazepine does; however, the clinical significance of this remains unclear.

Membrane-Stabilizing Agents

Mexiletine (150 to 400 mg three times a day) and lidocaine are also used to treat neuropathic pain. Lidocaine-sensitive pain (LSP) is best diagnosed by giving a 100 mg IV bolus or 4 mg/kg over half an hour and then monitoring the analgesic effect by the use of a VAS. Diabetic neuropathy and other deafferentation neuralgias often respond as well.[104] In a double-blind study, topical lidocaine gel has been shown to be effective acutely.[105] Verapamil (80 to 120 mg three times a day) and nimodipine (30 to 90 mg three times a day) may also be useful as calcium channel blockers.

a-Blockers and Sympathetically Maintained Pain

Sympathetically maintained pain—regardless of whether it is due to RSD, opiate tolerance, hyperalgesia, inflammation, vascular headache, postherpetic neuralgia, trauma, facial pain, or arthritis—can respond to sympathetic blockade.[106] The clinician can consider the early use of sympathetic blockade in any chronic pain syndrome with features of sympathetic dysfunction, α-blocking drugs (e.g., phentolamine, α-blocking antidepressants, and clonidine) given with or without opiates, are all potentially useful in patients with chronic pain. Phenoxybenzamine may be a useful oral agent if given early in the course of illness but is probably less useful than a Hannington-Kiff regional α-block. Intrathecal, epidural, and systemic administration of clonidine also produce analgesia.[107] Clonidine is often useful in patients who have developed tolerance to opiates and who have some types of vascular or neuropathic pain.[108] Transdermal clonidine (0 to 3 mg/day) is sometimes useful in neuropathy, although the results on the treatment are mixed.

β-Blockers are not efficacious in the treatment of sympathetically maintained pain except in their use for alleviating migraine headaches. The ischemic regional block (Hannington-Kiff block) is probably the most useful method for treating sympathetically maintained pain. Guanethidine, bretylium, reserpine, and phentolamine have been used successfully to produce a chemical sympathectomy.[109,110] One method is to infuse 500 ml of one-half normal saline before putting phentolamine into an ischemic regional block, then administer phentolamine 10 mg IV over a 10-minute period. A positive test result is marked by relief of evoked pain stimulated by light touch or a tuning fork.[111,112]

Treatment of Neuropathic Pain States

The clinical hallmark of central pain is that it persists without an obvious nociceptive stimulus; the physiologic goal of treatment is to stabilize hyperexcitable neurons.[24] Table 21-10 outlines some clinical approaches to central pain.

Carbamazepine has been shown to be among the most effective agents for some facial neuralgias, which can be so agonizing that some patients actually look forward to death. Within 24 hours of attaining steady-state, it is effective in 80% of patients with trigeminal neuralgia, making it clinically superior to phenytoin. Other types of lancinating pain, such as postherpetic neuralgia, post-sympathectomy pain, and post-traumatic pain, may also respond to anticonvulsants. Intravenous trials offer a quick, definitive way of identifying drug responders in complex or pressured situations. For routine CNS pain, clonazepam is the best-tolerated anticonvulsant for pain syndromes, especially when allodynia is present. It facilitates both presynaptic and postsynaptic inhibition, increases recurrent inhibition, and decreases the firing rate of normal and epileptic neurons in the brain; it also enhances sleep, relaxes muscles and blood vessels, and treats panic. It is the drug that exemplifies the need to select prescriptions based not only on their efficacy and tolerability but also on their mechanisms of action for disease pro- cesses that have multiple pathophysiologies.

Table 21-10. Pain Treatment

Pain Characteristics	What Treatment Is Next?	Comments
Nociceptive element present?	Nerve block for diagnostic and therapeutic reasons Imaging; MRI, looking for lesion	Even in pain that appears central (e.g., trigeminal neuralgia), nociceptive triggers can initiate pain and peripheral deafferentation
Allodynia present? (vibration, cold, or light touch)	Low-dose clonazepam (1–4 mg/day) if the person can tolerate benzodiazepines alone or in combination with desipramine 50 mg at bedtime (up to 300 mg eventually, if necessary) Mexelitine 150–400 mg tid	Allodynia predicts response to clonazepam Clonazepam relaxes muscles, improves sleep and anxiety Membrane stabilizers useful but cardiotoxicity needs to be checked Peptides useful
Paroxysmal attacks? (lightning-like)	Anticonvulsants Carbamazepine 400–1600 mg/day (serum 8–12 μg/L) Divalproex (Depakote) 500–2000 mg/day Gabapentin 300–1200 mg tid Lamictal 100–300 mg/day	Clonazepam should usually be tried first, but works well synergistically with the anticonvulsants listed Depakote for vascular headache Gabapentin: few drug interactions
Central pain—full house? Allodynia Paroxysmal attacks Sharp perceived as light touch Decreased pain threshold Nondermatomal distribution of pain Hyperpathia	Definitive trial is a single-blind random assignment of IV lorazepam (2–4 mg) vs lidocaine (100 mg) vs morphine 10 mg, rated on a VAS pain IV amitriptyline 25 mg infusion as test dose with VAS pain	Careful physical examination essential Is sharp perceived as light touch? Light touch is painful, sustained, and has a delayed crescendo Tuning fork/moving a hair examination best for allodynia
Comorbid central pain? Vascular and myofascial pain	Depakote 250–2000 mg/day Physical therapy Monoaminergic prescription antidepressants Nasal calcitonin 200 IU/day Capsaicin 4–6 week trial Topical preparation (Zostrix)	Common in head, neck, and face pain Mixed results with SSRIs Rule out sympathetically maintained pain
DSM-IV psychiatric diagnosis? Rule out or treat	Comorbid psychiatric and CNS pain: consider prescription with dual effects for pain and psychiatric diagnosis Benzodiazepine for allodynia and anxiety Antidepressants for neuropathy, depression, and anxiety Neuroleptics for neuralgia, anxiety, psychosis, and nausea Anticonvulsants for lancinating pain and mood stabilizers	Rule out depression and anxiety, consider mimics of central pain, such as somatoform, factitious, or psychotic disorders Pain drawing by the patient is a good tool to uncover psychosis and myofascial pain Rule out akathisia, restless leg syndrome

MRI, magnetic resonance imaging; IV, intravenous; VAS, visual analog scale; SSRIs, selective serotonin reuptake inhibitors.

ECT has been used in long-standing pain accompanied by depression. The rationale is that treating the depression eases the suffering associated with pain. Unfortunately, ECT is effective for major depression, but it does not relieve pain. The assumption that there must be chronic depression with chronic pain and that it will be amenable to ECT is usually untenable.

Treatment of Pain Behavior and the Use of Multidisciplinary Pain Clinics

Guidelines

Medicare guidelines offer one set of standards for multidisciplinary pain management. The pain must be at least 6 months in duration (resulting in significant life disturbance and limited functioning), it must be attributable to a physical cause, and it must be intractable to the usual methods of treatment. Desirable characteristics for pain treatment facilities and standards of care in pain management have now been published (in response to skepticism about cost, quality, control, and diversity of pain treatment facilities).[112] Quality control guidelines developed by the Commission on Accreditation of Rehabilitation Facilities (CARF), under the umbrella of the Joint Commission on Accreditation of Healthcare Organizations (JCAHO), have led to the certification of more than 100 chronic pain management programs nationwide. Behavioral treatments, however, are not primarily for pain relief; they merely extinguish the behaviors associated with pain.[113] Furthermore, proof of the cost effectiveness of inpatient multidisciplinary treatment is nascent and consequently still ill defined.

Reasons for Referral to an Inpatient Multidisciplinary Pain Clinic

Inpatient multidisciplinary pain clinics should be considered in the following circumstances:

- When the diagnosis of the physical and psychiatric pathology is already complete or is so obscure that intensive observation is necessary (e.g., malingering).

- When consultation from an independent physician who is an expert in the treatment of chronic pain is necessary to confirm that no single modality of outpatient treatment is likely to work.
- When the patient has already obtained maximum benefit from outpatient treatments (such as NSAIDs, nerve blocks, antidepressants, and simple physical and behavioral rehabilitation).
- When intensive daily interventions are required, usually with multiple concurrent types of therapy, such as nerve blocks, physical therapy, and behavior modification.
- When the patient exhibits abnormal pain behavior and agrees to the goals of improved coping, work rehabilitation, and psychiatric assessment.
- When medications for pain relief are so complex or compliance management so difficult that direct supervision of medical therapy is necessary.
- When a self-medication program is required (typically with a written schedule of medications, a contract, and strategies mutually acceptable for patient and physician).

Hypnosis

The use of hypnosis in chronic pain syndromes is well known. Self-hypnosis is particularly helpful, but only about one in four subjects is able to achieve a state of concentration of sufficient magnitude for lasting pain control. Hypnosis is a method worth looking into, provided that the physician knows its limitations and how to apply it to the individual patient's needs.

Rehabilitation

Rehabilitation of patients who have chronic pain syndromes may require some combination of psychiatry, physical therapy, physiatry, behavioral psychology, and neurology. It is important to bear in mind that no special therapy, including exercise therapy, spinal manipulation, bed rest, orthoses, acupuncture, traction therapy, back schools, and epidural steroids, works well. Successful rehabilitation aims to decrease symptoms, increase independence, and allow the patient to return to work. A positive, rapid return to light-normal activities and work is essential if disability is to be minimized. Psychologically, this is the key to coping with acute trauma. Even with patients who experience low back pain, 50% of whom have a recurrence within 3 years of the initial episode, there is no evidence that a return to work adversely effects the course of the pain syndrome.[114]

Treatment of myofascial pain syndromes may be challenging. It involves restoration of stage 4 sleep, aerobic conditioning (which could include physical therapy or yoga), and avoidance of drugs, such as caffeine and alcohol. Trigger point analgesia, behavioral modification of maladaptive sleep habits, and the treatment of anxiety and depression may be necessary if chronic muscle pain is to be relieved. Monoamine oxidase inhibitors (MAOIs) are often effective. TCAs (e.g., desipramine and imipramine) may also be effective and are easier to use than MAOIs because dietary restrictions are not needed. Response to SSRIs has been unpredictable for myofascial pain, at times provoking muscle spasms and not helping the myofascial pain.[115] Cyclobenzaprine and S-adenosylmethionine (SAMe), however, have resulted in some modest adjunctive efficacy.[116] Nefazodone, related to the hypnotic trazodone, is of theoretic interest because of its hypnotic effect, but it still takes 4 to 8 weeks to see the maximum hypnotic effect as measured by total sleep time or by self-report of sleep. Eight weeks is the duration of an optimal trial for any of these agents.

Education

Education is needed for the caregivers as well as the patient. In the past, medical professionals, be they physicians or nurses, viewed the patient who is in constant need of pain medication with suspicion. Physicians often underestimated the medication's effective dose, overestimated the medication's duration of action, and had an exaggerated notion of the danger of addiction. Rarely were physicians told to vary the amount of drug prescribed based on the patient's body weight, renal function, and previous

tolerance for the drug. The physician's *ennui* with failure, suffering, and death could also have led to flight from pain. When the amount of medication a patient requires for the management of pain becomes a *cause celebre* on the ward, the consulting psychiatrist should call a meeting of the house-staff, attendings, and nurses, so that all biases and suspicions can be brought into the open. Medical personnel are far more apt to underestimate the amount of narcotic required for a given pain than to overestimate it. In either case, their opinions are usually based more on misinformation or folklore than on fact. Once these judgments are aired, the patient usually benefits.

Cognitive and Behavioral Therapies

Hypnosis and imagery conditioning to induce relaxation and pain control are consistently found to be more effective than cognitive-behavioral training.[117,118] Traditional hypnosis, autogenic exercises, yoga methods, and meditation are all useful paths to achieve those goals.

Coping and Psychotherapy

Coping with chronic pain always threatens two fundamentals of survival: attachment behaviors and intrapsychic defenses. To cope means to have people of quality around to fortify one's courage and to have adaptive defense mechanisms to negotiate the thoughts and feelings that arise in one's head. Helping the patient develop cognitive-behavioral coping skills is more effective for decreasing pain and psychological disability than is education alone.[119] Coping is also context dependent and is most effective when the focus includes the couple or family.[120,121]

The psychodynamic aspects of coping involve conflicts over autonomy and care. Old conflicts about nurturance suggest there may be mixed feelings about recovery. Shame may mimic depres-sion, trigger conservation-withdrawal, and produce counterdependent behavior. Regression, some of which is normal, can be manifest as noncompliance, help-rejecting complaining, and behaviors akin to the metaphorical "cutting off your nose to spite your face." The hateful patient and the hateful physician are often compatriots in partnership with chronic pain, and a task of the psychiatrist is to clarify how these problems become played out in the physician-patient relationship. One should understand that the physician is a protective figure who is the recipient of both idealized and angry feelings when a cure is not forthcoming. Modern health care, with its fragmentation, multiple care-givers, and bureaucracies, guarantees rifts in the physician-patient relationship. To help the patient cope, the psychiatrist must be sensitive to the unconscious feelings of the patient and be prepared to manage denial and to employ family counseling, relaxation, exercise, physical rehabilitation, and pharmacotherapy, while still functioning as a teacher and physician. Wisdom, medicine, time, and hope are the professional's charge.

Acknowledgements

The author acknowledges the contribution of Steffany Fredman in preparing this manuscript for publication.

References

1. Fleming P: *My aunt's rhinoceros and other reflections*, New York, 1958, Simon & Schuster.
2. IASP Subcommittee on Taxonomy: Pain terms: a list with definitions and notes on usage, *Pain* 6(3):249–252, 1979.
3. American Psychiatric Association: *Diagnostic and statistical manual of mental disorders,* ed. 4. Washington, DC, 1994, American Psychiatric Press.
4. Wall PD: The prevention of postoperative pain, *Pain* 33(3):289–290, 1988.
5. Wall PD, McMahon SB: The relationship of perceived pain to afferent nerve impulses, *Trends Neurosci* 9:254–255, 1986.
6. Hyman SH, Cassem NH: *Pain*. In: Rubenstein E, Fedeman DD, eds. *Scientific American medicine: current topics in medicine. Subsection II*. New York, Scientific American; 1989.
7. Hsieh JC, Stahle-Backdahl M, Hagermark O, et al: Traumatic nociceptive pain activates the hypothalamus and the periaqueductal gray: a positron emission tomography study. *Pain* 64(2):303–314, 1996.
8. Rainville RK, Hofbauer T, Paus GH, et al: Cerebral mechanisms of hypnotic induction and suggestion. *J Cogn Neurosci* 11:110–125, 1999.
9. Petrovic KM, Petersson PH., Ghatan S, et al: Pain-related cerebral activation is altered by a distracting cognitive task. *Pain* 85:19–30, 2000.
10. Petrovic P, Kalso E Petersson KM, et al: Shared processing in the rostral ACC during opioid and placebo treatment (Abstract). *Neuroscience* 120:10, 2001.
11. Levine D, Gordon NC, Fields HL: The mechanism of placebo analgesia, *Lancet* 2:654–657, 1978.
12. Petrovic P, Ingvar M: Imaging cognitive modulation of pain processing., *Pain*, 95:1–5, 2002.
13. Meller ST, Gebhart GF: Nitric oxide (NO) and nociceptive processing in the spinal cord, *Pain* 52(2):127–136, 1993.
14. Fields HL, Liebeskind JC, editors: Pharmacological approaches to the treatment of chronic pain: new concepts and critical issues, *Progress in pain research and management*, vol 1, Seattle, 1994, IASP Press.
15. Baringa M: The brain remaps its own contours, *Science* 258:216–218, 1992.
16. Coderre TJ, Katz J, Vaccarino AL, et al: Contribution of central neuroplasticity to pathological pain: review of clinical and experimental evidence, *Pain* 52(3):259–285, 1993.
17. Fields HL: Editorial comment, *Pain* 49(2):161–162, 1992.
18. Dubner R: Pain and hyperalgesia following tissue injury: new mechanisms and new treatments, *Pain* 44(3):167–171, 1991.
19. Baringa M: Playing "telephone" with the body's message of pain, *Neuroscience* 258:1085, 1992.
20. Woolf CJ, Thompson SWN: The induction and maintenance of central sensitization is dependent on N-methyl-d-aspartic acid receptor activation: implications for the treatment of post-injury pain hypersensitivity states, *Pain* 44(3):293–299, 1991.
21. Fromm GH: Physiological rationale for the treatment of neuropathic pain, *APS* 2(1):1–7, 1993.
22. Basbaum AI: Insights into the development of opioid tolerance, *Pain* 61(3):349–352,1995.
23. Cherry DA, Plummer JL, Gourlay GK, et al: Ketamine as an adjunct to morphine in the treatment of pain, *Pain* 62(1):119–121, 1995.
24. Mao J, Price D, Mayer D: Mechanisms of hyperalgesia and morphine tolerance: a current view of their possible interactions, *Pain* 62(3):259–274, 1995.
25. Trujillo KA, Akil H: Inhibition of morphine tolerance and dependence by the NMDA receptor antagonist MK-801, *Science* 251(4989):85–87, 1990.
26. Heyes MP, Saito K, Crowley JS, et al: Quinolinic acid and kynurenine pathway metabolism in inflammatory and non-inflammatory neurological disease, *Brain* 115:1249–1273, 1992.
27. Holloway M: No pain, no gain? *Science* 248(4961): 1313, 1990.
28. Paix A, Coleman A, Lees, J, et al: Subcutaneous fentanyl and sufentanil infusion substitution for morphine intolerance in cancer pain management, *Pain* 63(1):263–269, 1995.
29. Ardid D, Guilband G: Antinociceptive effects of acute and "chronic" injections of tricyclic antidepressant

drugs in a new model of mononeuropathy in rats, *Pain* 49(2):279–287, 1992.

30. Fasmer OB, Hunskaar S, Hole K: Antinociceptive effect of serotonergic reuptake inhibitors in mice, *Neuropharmacology* 28(12):1363–1366, 1989.

31. Gomez-Perez FJ, Rull JA, Dies H, et al: Nortriptyline and fluphenazine in the symptomatic treatment of diabetic neuropathy: a double-blind cross-over study, *Pain* 23(4):395–400, 1985.

32. Max MB, Kishore-Kumar R, Schaefer SC, et al: Efficacy of desipramine in painful diabetic neuropathy: a placebo controlled trial, *Pain* 45(1):3–9, 1991.

33. Kishore-Kumar R, Max MB, Schafer SC, et al: Desipramine relieves postherpetic neuralgia, *Clin Pharmacol Tier* 47(3):305–312, 1990.

34. Bouckoms AJ, Poletti CH, Sweet WH, et al: Trigeminal facial pain: a model of peptides and monoamines in intracerebral cerebrospinal fluid, *Agressologie* 32(5):271–274, 1991.

35. Arner S, Meyerson BA: Lack of analgesic effect of opioids on neuropathic and idiopathic forms of pain, *Pain* 33(1):11–23, 1988.

36. Janig W: Experimental approach to reflex sympathetic dystrophy and related symptoms, *Pain* 46(3):241–245, 1991.

37. Willoch F, Rosen G, Tolle TR, et al: Phantom limb pain in the human brain: unraveling neural circuitries of phantom limb sensations using positron emission tomography. *Ann Neurol* 48:842–849, 2000.

38. Travell JG, Simons DG: *Myofascial pain and dysfunction: the trigger point manual*, Baltimore, 1983, Williams & Wilkins.

39. Fricton J, Awad E: *Advances in pain research and therapy*, New York, 1990, Raven Press.

40. Osterweis M, Kleinman A, Mechanic D: *Institute of Medicine's Committee on Pain, Disability, and Chronic Illness Behavior*, Washington, DC, 1987, National Academy Press.

41. Wolfe F, Cathey M: The epidemiology of tender points: a prospective study of 1520 patients, *J Rheumatol* 12(6):1164–1168, 1985.

42. Moldofsky H, Scarisbrick P, England R, et al: Musculoskeletal symptoms and non-REM sleep disturbances in patients with "fibrositis syndromes" and healthy subjects, *Psychosom Med* 37(4):341–351, 1975.

43. Sigvardsson S, von Knorring A, Bohman M, et al: An adoption study of somatoform disorders, *Arch Gen Psychiatry* 41(9):853–859, 1984.

44. McDonald J: What are the causes of chronic gynecological pain disorders? *APS Bulletin* 5(6):20–23, 1995.

45. Walker E, Katon W, Harrop-Griffiths J, et al: Relationship of chronic pelvic pain to psychiatric diagnoses and childhood sexual abuse, *Am J Psychiatry* 145:75–80, 1988.

46. Smith GR, Monson RA, Ray DC: Psychiatric consultation in somatization disorder: a randomized controlled study, *N Engl J Med* 314(22):1407–1413, 1986.

47. Reed JL: The diagnosis of "hysteria," *Psychol Med* 5(1):13–17, 1975.

48. Barsky A, Wool C, Barnett M, et al: Histories of childhood trauma in adult hypochondriacal patients, *Am J Psychiatry* 151(3):397–401, 1994.

49. Fordyce WE: *Behavioral methods for chronic pain and illness*, St. Louis, 1976, Mosby.

50. Walker EA, Katon WJ, Neraas K, et al: Dissociation in women with chronic pelvic pain, *Am J Psychiatry* 149(4):534–537, 1992.

51. Evans W, Hoyle C: The comparative value of drugs used in the continuous treatment of angina pectoris, *J Med* 2:311–338, 1933.

52. Elton NH, Hanna MM, Treasure J: Coping with chronic pain: some patients suffer more, *Br J Psychiatry* 165(6):802–807, 1994.

53. Panel APMG: *Acute pain management: operative or medical procedures and trauma—clinical practice guideline*, Washington, DC, 1992, Agency for Health Care Policy and Research, Public Health Care Policy and Research, Public Health Service, U.S. Department of Health and Human Services.

54. Bertram G., Katzung BG: *Basic & Clinical Pharmacology*, Chapter 39. Furst DE, Munster T. McGraw Hill, 2001.

55. Arkinstall W, Sandier A, Goughnour B, et al: Efficacy of controlled-release codeine in chronic non-malignant pain: a randomized, placebo-controlled clinical trial, *Pain* 62(2):169–178, 1995.

56. Ventafridda V, Tamburini M, Caraceni A, et al: A validation study of the WHO method of cancer pain relief, *Cancer* 59(4):850–856, 1987.

57. Portenoy RK, Foley KM: Chronic use of opioid analgesics in non-malignant pain: report of 38 cases, *Pain* 25(2):171–186, 1986.

58. Gourlay GK: Long-term use of opioids in chronic pain patients with nonterminal disease states, *Pain Rev* 1(1):62–76, 1994.

59. Bouckoms AJ, Masand PS, Murray GB, et al: Non-malignant pain treated with long term oral narcotics, *Ann Clin Psychiatry* 4:185–192, 1992.

60. Kaiko RF: Narcotics in the elderly, *Med Clin North Am* 66(5):1079–1089, 1982.

61. Bruera E, Schoeller T, Montejo G: Organic hallucinosis in patients receiving high doses of opiates for cancer pain, *Pain* 48(3):397–399, 1992.

62. Jellema JG: Hallucinations during sustained-release morphine and methadone administration, *Lancet* 2:392, 1987.

63. Hill RG: Pharmacological considerations in the use of opioids in the management of pain associated with nonterminal disease states, *Pain Reviews* 1(1):47–61, 1994.

64. Kunz KM, Thiesen JA, Schroeder ME: Severe episodic pain: management with sublingual sufentanil, *J Pain Sympt Manage* 8(4):189–190, 1993.

65. Rischitelli DG, Karbowicz SH: Safety and efficacy of controlled-release oxycodone: a systematic literature review. *Pharmacotherapy* 22:898–904, 2002.

66. Murphy TM: Psychoactive drugs for pain control, *Pain Reviews* 1(1):9–14, 1994.

67. Garattini S, Samanin R: Biochemical hypotheses on antidepressant drugs: a guide for clinicians or a toy for pharmacologists? *Psychol Med* 18(2):287–304, 1988.

68. Feinman NC: Pain relief by antidepressants: possible modes of action, *Pain* 23(1):1–8, 1985.

69. Godefroy F, Butler SH, Weil-Fugazza J, et al: Do acute or chronic tricyclic antidepressants modify morphine antinociception in arthritic rats? *Pain* 25(2):233–244, 1986.

70. Max MB, Culnane M, Schafer SC, et al: Amitriptyline relieves diabetic neuropathy pain in patients with normal or depressed mood, *Neurology* 37(4):589–596, 1987.

71. Lance JW: 5-Hydroxytryptamine and its role in migraine, *Eur Neural* 31(5):279–281, 1991.

72. Bragin E, Korneev A, Vasilenko G: Buspirone effect on the development of antinociceptive reactions, *Pain* 36(2):257–261, 1989.

73. Kishore-Kumar R, Schafer SC, Lawlor BA, et al: Single doses of the serotonin agonists buspirone and m-chlorophenylpiperazine do not relieve neuropathic pain, *Pain* 37(2):223–227, 1989.

74. Davidoff G, Guarracini M, Roth E, et al: Trazodone hydrochloride in the treatment of dysesthetic pain in traumatic myelopathy: a randomized, double-blind, placebo-controlled study, *Pain* 29(2):151–161, 1987.

75. Galer BS: Neuropathic pain of peripheral origin: advances in pharmacologic treatment, *Neurology* 45(12 suppl 9):S17–S25, 1995.

76. Diamond S: The management of migraine and cluster headaches, *Compr Ther* 21(9):492–498, 1995.

77. Torebjork E, Wahren L, Wallin G, et al: Noradrenaline-evoked pain in neuralgia, *Pain* 63(1):11–20, 1995.

78. Lindsey P, Wycoff M: The depression-pain syndrome and its response to antidepressants, *Psychosomatics* 22:571–577, 1981.

79. Stein D, Peri T, Edelstein E, et al: The efficacy of amitriptyline and acetaminophen in the management of acute pain, *Psychosomatics* 37(1):63–70, 1996.

80. Blumer D, Heilbronn M: Chronic pain as a variant of depressive disease: the pain-prone disorder, *J Nerv Ment Dis* 170(7):381–406, 1982.

81. Getto CJ, Sorkness CA, Howell T: Issues in drug management: I. Antidepressants and chronic nonmalignant pain: a review, *J Pain Symptom Manage* 2(1):9–18, 1987.

82. Goodkin K, Vrancken MA, Feaster D: On the putative efficacy of antidepressants in chronic, benign pain syndromes, *Pain Forum* 4(4):237–247, 1995.

83. Max MB: Thirteen consecutive well-designed randomized trials show that antidepressants reduce pain in diabetic neuropathy and postherpetic neuralgia, *Pain Forum* 4(4):20–23, 1995.

84. Onghena P, Van Houdenhove B: Antidepressant-induced analgesia in chronic non-malignant pain: a meta-analysis of 39 placebo-controlled studies, *Pain* 49(2):205–219, 1992.

85. Kvinesdal B, Molin J, Froland A, et al: Imipramine treatment of painful neuropathy, *JAMA* 251(13):1727–1730, 1984.

86. Sindrup SH, Ejlertsen B, Froland A, et al: Imipramine treatment in diabetic neuropathy: relief of subjective symptoms without changes in peripheral and autonomic nerve function, *Eur J Clin Pharmacol* 37(2):51–53, 1989.

87. Max MB, Schaefer SC, Culnane M, et al: Amitriptyline, but not lorazepam, relieves postherpetic neuralgia, *Neurology* 38(9):1427–1432, 1988.

88. Max MB, Lynch SA, Muir J, et al: Effects of desipramine, amitriptyline, and fluoxetine on pain in diabetic neuropathy, *N Engl J Med* 326(19):1250–1256, 1992.

89. Watson CPN, Chipman M, Reed K, et al: Amitriptyline versus maprotiline in postherpepetic neuralgia: a randomized, double blind, crossover trial, *Pain* 48(1):29–36, 1992.

90. McQuay HJ, Carroll D, Glynn CJ: Low dose amitriptyline in the treatment of chronic pain, *Anaesthesia* 47(8):646–652, 1992.

91. Watson CPN, Evans RJ: A comparative trial of amitriptyline and zimeldine in postherpetic neuralgia, *Pain* 23(4):387–394, 1985.

92. Gourlay GK, Cherry DA, Cousins MJ, et al: A controlled study of a serotonin reuptake blocker, zimelidine, in the treatment of chronic pain, *Pain* 25(1):35–52, 1986.

93. Nakamura-Craig M, Follenfant RL: Effect of lamotrigine in the acute and chronic hyperalgesia induced by PGE2 and in the chronic hyperalgesia in rats with streptozotocin-induced diabetes, *Pain* 63(1):33–37, 1995.

94. King SA, Strain JJ: Benzodiazepines and chronic pain, *Pain* 41(1):3–4, 1990.

95. Clavier N, Lombard MC, Besson JM: Benzodiazepines and pain: effects of midazolam on the activities of nociceptive non-specific dorsal horn neurons in the rat spinal cord, *Pain* 48(1):61–71, 1992.

96. Serrao JM, Marks RL, Morley SJ, et al: Intrathecal midazolam for the treatment of chronic mechanical low back pain: a controlled comparison with epidural steroid in a pilot study, *Pain* 48(1):5–12, 1992.

97. Bouckoms AJ: *Intravenous lorazepam for pain relief of intractable neuralgia*, In 5th World Congress of Pain in Hamburg, Germany, 1987.

98. Maciewicz R, Bouckoms AJ, Martin JB: Drug therapy of neuropathic pain, *Clin J Pain* 1:39–45, 1985.

99. Bowsher D: Acute herpes zoster and postherpetic neuralgia: effects of ayclovir and outcome of treatment with amitriptyline, *Br J Gen Pract* 42(359):244–246, 1992.

100. Hering R, Kuritzky A: Sodium valproate in the treatment of cluster headache: an open clinical trial, *Cephalalgia* 9(3):195–198, 1989.

101. Martin C, Martin A, Rud C, et al: Comparative study of sodium valproate in the treatment of postoperative pain, *Annales Francoises D Anesthesie Et De Reanimation* 7(5):387–392, 1988.

102. Hering R, Kuritzky A: Sodium valproate in the prophylactic treatment of migraine: a double-blind study versus placebo, *Cephalalgia* 12(2):81–84, 1992.

103. Mathew NT, Saper JR, Silberstein SD, et al: Migraine prophylaxis with divalproex, *Arch Neurol* 52(3):281–286, 1995.

104. Marchettini P, Lacerenza M, Marangoni C, et al: Lidocaine test in neuralgia, *Pain* 48(3):377–382, 1992.

105. Rowbotham MC, Davies PS, Fields HL: Topical lidocaine gel relieves postherpetic neuralgia, *Ann Neurol* 37(2):246–253, 1995.

106. Gracely RH, Lynch S, Bennett GJ: Painful neuropathy: altered central processing maintained dynamically by peripheral input, *Pain* 51(2):175–194, 1992.

107. Coombs DW, Saunders RL, Fratkin JD, et al: Continuous intrathecal hydromorphone and clonidine for intractable cancer pain, *J Neurosurg* 64(6):890–894, 1986.

108. Eisenach JC, DuPen S, Dubois M, et al: Epidural clonidine analgesia for intractable cancer pain, *Pain* 61(3):391–399, 1995.

109. Bonelli S, Conoscente F, Movilia PG, et al: Regional intravenous guanethidine vs. stellate ganglion block in reflex sympathetic dystrophies: a randomized trial, *Pain* 16(3):297–307, 1983.

110. Hyden JLK, Thomas DA, Dubner R: Inflammation-induced thermal hyperalgesia is sensitive to spinal opioids: possible involvement of noradrenergic mechanisms, *Pharmacologist* 32:115, 1990.

111. Campbell JN, Meyer RA, Raja SN: Is nociceptor activation by alpha-1 adrenoreceptors the culprit in sympathetically maintained pain? *APS J* 1:3–12, 1992.

112. Fishbain DA, Rosomoff HL, Steele-Rosomoff R, et al: Types of pain treatment facilities and referral selection criteria: a review, *Arch Fam Med* 4(1):58–66, 1995.

113. Fordyce WE, editor: *Back pain in the workplace: management of disability in nonspecific conditions,* Seattle, 1995, International Association for the Study of Pain.

114. Nachemson A: Work for all: for those with low back pain as well, *Clin Orthop* 179:77–85, 1983.

115. Norregaard J, Volkmann H, Samsoe-Danneskiold B: A randomized controlled trial of citalopram in the treatment of fibromyalgia, *Pain* 61(3):445–449, 1995.

116. Carette S, Bell MJ, Reynolds WJ, et al: Comparison of amitryptyline, cyclobenzaprine, and placebo in the treatment of fibromyalgia: a randomized, double-blind clinical trial, *Arthr Rheum* 37(1):32–40, 1994.

117. Syrjala KL, Donaldson GW, Davis MW, et al: Relaxation and imagery and cognitive-behavioral training reduce pain during cancer treatment: a controlled clinical trial, *Pain* 63(2):189–198, 1995.

118. Spiegel D, Bloom JR: Group therapy and hypnosis reduce metastatic breast carcinoma pain, *Psychosom Med* 45(4):333–339, 1983.

119. Keefe FJ, Williams DA: A comparison of coping strategies in chronic pain patients in different age groups, *J Gerontol* 45(4):161–165, 1990.

120. Manne SL, Zautra AJ: Couples coping with chronic illness: women with rheumatoid arthritis and their healthy husbands, *J Behav Med* 13(4):327–342, 1990.

121. Kopp M, Richter R, Rainer J, et al: Differences in family functioning between patients with chronic headaches and patients with chronic low back pain, *Pain* 63(2):219–224, 1995.

Chapter 22
Legal Aspects of Consultation

Ronald Schouten, M.D., J.D.
Rebecca W. Brendel, M.D., J.D.

Legal issues arise commonly in the practice of medicine. The response of physicians to these legal issues varies. Some ignore them, believing that the law has no business in the physician-patient relationship. Others, although recognizing the extent to which legal issues can be involved in clinical practice, hope that these matters will not require direct action and will resolve spontaneously. Still others have allowed concerns about malpractice and legal requirements to dominate their professional lives, to the detriment of their clinical work.

Although it is true that legal issues are ever-present in medicine, they exist as a background set of requirements and considerations. On those occasions when specific legal issues do arise, medical and surgical physicians often turn to the consultation psychiatrist for assistance. It is unclear why colleagues have accorded psychiatrists the position of legal authority. Perhaps it is because those legal issues that arise most commonly, such as competency and treatment refusal, have to do with mental functions and abnormalities of behavior. Whatever the reason, the psychiatric consultant may be drawn into a turbulent atmosphere in which medical and surgical staff are suddenly confronted with a legal issue. The well-prepared consultant can be invaluable in these matters.

The first and perhaps most important service provided by the consultant is to remind the consultee that the physician's safest haven within the law are the principles of good faith, common sense, and the highest standard of care for the patient. Consultants must be familiar with relevant legal concepts, and must use this knowledge to diminish consultees' anxiety and help them perform their jobs. The challenge for the psychiatric consultant is to ease the burden of the consultee by providing clinical insight and legal information and to know when and how to use the input of the hospital attorney.

Medicine has advanced rapidly in the twentieth century. Concurrently, physicians have confronted a variety of medicolegal issues. These issues are reflected in questions asked by residents and staff alike. How do I determine whether a patient is incompetent? If the patient is competent and making an irrational decision, does that decision have to be honored? What is my liability exposure as a consultant? If a managed care company refuses continued hospitalization or admission to a psychiatric facility for a patient, can the physician be held liable if the patient commits suicide? If the patient has expressed a desire to hurt someone else, what are my obligations to that third party? What obligations do I have if my patient is human immunodeficiency virus (HIV)-positive and refuses to inform his or her sexual partner?

This chapter cannot provide definitive answers to these and all the other medicolegal questions that arise in the practice of general hospital psychiatry. Rather, this chapter outlines general principles that apply in almost all jurisdictions. Because state statutes and case law vary considerably on these medicolegal matters, hospital counsel and legal representatives of medical organizations and insurers should be consulted. They are excellent sources of information about legal aspects of general hospital psychiatry.

Physicians' Rights and Obligations

Malpractice Liability

Malpractice, negligence, and *liability* are three terms that engender great concern and are often misunderstood. Malpractice law is a type of personal injury or tort law that concerns itself with injuries allegedly caused by the treatment activities of professionals. To establish a claim of malpractice, a plaintiff (the complaining party) must prove four things. First, it must be proved that the defendant physician owed a duty to the injured party. Where the injured party is the patient, the duty is to perform up to the standards of the average physician in the community practicing in that specialty. Failure to practice in accordance with that standard, unless there is some justification, constitutes the second element: negligence. The third and fourth elements are closely tied to the first two: The negligent behavior has to be shown to have been the direct cause of actual damages. In the event that all four elements are proved, the defendant may be held liable (responsible for the damage) and ordered to pay compensation to the plaintiff, either directly or through his or her insurer.[1-4] The four elements of malpractice are often summarized as the four Ds: duty, dereliction of duty, direct causation, and damages.

The liability exposure of consultants can be a concern for psychiatric consultants and others. Treating clinicians have the primary duty of care for the patient. Consultants, who by definition are brought in to provide advice to the treating clinicians, do not have the same duty to the patient. The consultant's duty of reasonable care is owed to the consultee, not the patient. This rule does not hold, however, where the consultant steps out of the purely consultative role and assumes direct responsibility for some aspect of the treatment relationship. For example, the consultant who evaluates a patient and then advises the treating physician that a course of antidepressant treatment is appropriate is not liable for an adverse outcome from the treatment. If, however, the consultant writes the prescription and monitors the treatment course, he or she has

assumed the status of treating physician and may be held responsible for any adverse outcomes.[5,6]

Liability and Managed Care

Managed care and liability for injury when coverage is denied have been important issues ever since managed care arrived in force on the health care scene. The basic problem can be seen in this hypothetical example.

> Mr. A was admitted to the trauma unit after leaping off a bridge into the river. After open reduction and internal fixation of his bilateral femoral fractures, the psychiatric consultant saw him. Mr. A was found to be suffering from major depression as well as alcohol abuse. He was believed to be at a moderate to high risk for suicide, and suicide precautions were instituted on the floor. Mr. A was begun on a course of antidepressants, but these had not yet begun to work when he was deemed surgically ready for discharge. The consultant recommended transfer to an inpatient psychiatry unit where Mr. A could undergo treatment for both his depression and substance abuse. Mr. A's mental health coverage had been carved out from his medical-surgical coverage. The utilization reviewer for his medical-surgical coverage insisted that he be discharged from the hospital and scheduled for outpatient physical therapy with visiting nurse coverage. The mental health management company sent its own psychologist reviewer to evaluate Mr. A. The reviewer agreed that Mr. A was depressed but denied authorization for psychiatric hospitalization. The reviewer opined that Mr. A was not acutely suicidal, did not need inpatient substance abuse treatment, and could be managed as an outpatient. He was given the names of the three psychiatrists in his town who were authorized under his plan and was able to get an appointment scheduled for 2 weeks after discharge. Mr. A was discharged from the hospital, over the objections of the consultant. The consultant had found that the patient was still significantly depressed and at risk of drinking again but not committable because he was not imminently suicidal. Ten days later, the visiting nurse found him hanged in his apartment. The death was ruled a suicide. Mr. A's family brought a malpractice action against the hospital, the treating physicians, the consultant, and the managed care company.

What liability does the managed care company have in a case like this, in which the denial of care results in harm to the patient? Would the managed care company's liability supersede that of the physicians? The answers to these questions are still unclear. There have been a series of legal cases addressing these issues, and the law is still evolving. At present, there is a possibility that managed care companies may be held liable in these situations if the company exerted such control over the decision-making process that the physician's judgment was overridden. In other words, for the physician to avoid liability, he or she must protest the denial of care, appeal it to the highest level that the insurer provides, and take other reasonable steps to ensure the patient's safety. Depending on the facts, the liability may be assigned entirely to the managed care company, to the physician, or be shared.[7–10]

However, under federal law, there are limits on managed care companies' liability for denial of care. Most often, decisions made by managed care organizations to limit care are subject only to limited legal remedies under the Employee Retirement Income Security Act (ERISA) of 1974. ERISA limits most employees of private companies to suing their health plans for the cost of the care denied by the managed care organization only, and not for recovery of losses that result from the denial of care or for punitive damages. ERISA's protection of managed care plans from liability for the consequences of their decisions is increasingly seen as unfair given the level of control over treatment decisions exercised by some plans. As a result, several court cases have begun to erode the prohibition on damages under the law. These cases represent only small gains and it remains to be seen whether lawmakers will amend this provision. For the time being, in the face of bad outcomes, patients may try to shift liability to physicians and hospitals to recover losses.[2]

Confidentiality and Privacy

Confidentiality is the clinician's obligation to keep matters revealed by a patient from the ears of third parties.[2,4] It is usually demanded and protected by statute and custom. A variety of exceptions to confidentiality exist, usually where the courts or the legislature determine that maintenance of confidentiality will result in more harm than good from a societal standpoint. This rationale provided the basis for the California court's decision in *Tarasoff v. Board of Regents*,[11] in which the court held that psychotherapists have a duty to act to protect third parties where the therapist knows or should know that the patient poses a threat of

serious risk of harm to the third party.[12,13] In looking at the public policy issue, the court stated,

> The Court recognizes the public interest in supporting effective treatment of mental illness and in protecting the rights of patients to privacy. But this interest must be weighed against the public interest in safety from violent assault.[11]

Although not all states have adopted this view, the majority have. A number of states have enacted statutes dealing with this fertile area of malpractice liability.[14] The consultant should be familiar with the relevant statutory and case law concerning this issue in his or her jurisdiction. The consultant should also be aware that liability can arise when medical or surgical colleagues fail to breach confidentiality and do not warn family members or other contacts about the potential for contagion from an infectious disease.[15] In fact, liability for such failure set the stage for the court's decision in Tarasoff.[11]

Although infectious disease has been the subject of duty to protect cases in the past, infection with the HIV has been treated somewhat differently than other infectious diseases. Controversy persists about the obligation of a physician to warn the partner of an HIV-positive patient when the patient refuses to do so. Many states have statutes that address this issue, with varied approaches, adding to the confusion and highlighting the controversial nature of the issue. The psychiatric consultant should learn the requirements of the jurisdiction in which he or she practices. Several articles and book chapters have addressed this controversial issue, some of which are cited in the references at the end of this chapter.[16–20]

In addition to situations in which disclosure is mandated to protect a third party, such as in *Tarasoff*[11] and infectious disease situations, other breaches of confidentiality may be mandated by statute or case law to protect vulnerable third parties. For example, all 50 states in the United States have statutes that require specific individuals, including physicians, to report suspected child abuse or neglect to state social service agencies. Many states also require that known or suspected abuse or neglect of the elderly or disabled be reported. Failure to comply with these requirements can result in substantial penalties. More recently, some states have begun requiring physicians and others to report known or suspected cases of domestic violence to law enforcement or designated agencies. Mandatory reporting statutes serve an important societal purpose, but they are not without controversy. Every clinician should become aware of the specific requirements in his or her jurisdiction.[21]

Patient health information is also subject to regulation under a federal law known as the Health Insurance Portability and Accountability Act (HIPAA) of 1996. As of mid-2003, institutions and individual providers are required to comply with HIPAA rules. Although the impact of this law on confidentiality is not yet known, HIPAA has already begun to affect hospital practice by requiring distribution, in writing, of the institution's privacy policy to all patients and by mandating physicians to undergo training on privacy and disclosure provisions. The rules are too complex to review in full; however, several salient points stand out for psychiatrists.

Among the most relevant provisions of HIPAA is the treatment of medical records and the distinction between general psychiatric records and psychotherapy notes. Patients are entitled to a copy of their medical records; they also have the explicit right to request changes in the record. Whether or not the applicable staff person amends the contested information, the involved correspondence becomes part of the record. Although HIPAA affords special status to psychotherapy notes and allows psychiatrists not to disclose these notes to patients, this exception is narrow. To qualify for protection under the psychotherapy notes provision, the notes must be kept separate from the patient's medical record. However, even if kept in a separate psychotherapy record, specific types of information are not subject to the psychotherapy notes exclusion; these include medications prescribed, test results, treatment plans, diagnoses, prognosis, and progress to date.[22,23] It should be noted, however, that these notes are considered to be part of the medical record in the event that a subpoena is received for medical records in the course of litigation.

The practical implications of HIPAA regarding psychiatric record-keeping remain to be seen. Nonetheless, consulting psychiatrists should consider documentation of sensitive therapy material carefully because it will be treated like the rest of the medical record unless the psychotherapy notes are kept in a separate file.

Like patients, health insurance companies' access to psychotherapy records is restricted. Health insurance companies cannot demand access to information contained in psychotherapy notes as a requirement of payment for care. If, in a particular circumstance, psychotherapy notes are released to an insurance company, patient consent is required. This consent requirement is in sharp contrast to the disclosure rules for the general medical and general psychiatric record for insurance purposes; HIPAA does not require consent for disclosure of this information to insurance companies for the purpose of obtaining payment for treatment—medical or psychiatric. There are 11 other circumstances in which disclosure is permitted without patient consent, including emergencies and mandated reporting zsituations, such as child abuse—which are generally already part of current medical practice. But other situations may be more concerning, including exceptions for law enforcement and attorney requests.[22] The implications of the disclosure without consent provisions of HIPAA remain to be determined.

Refusal to Treat Patients

Refusal to treat patients, in or out of the hospital, is a right that is rarely invoked by physicians. The physician-patient relationship is, at heart, contractual in nature. Both parties have the same right to enter, or to refuse to enter, the relationship as they do with other contracts. Once the physician offers to treat and the patient accepts, the contract is established and the physician's right to refuse or withdraw is limited in certain ways. For example, maintaining a walk-in clinic or emergency department can be construed as an implicit offer to treat on an emergent basis. The patient's presentation at the clinic or emergency department is an acceptance of the offer, creating a contract. It does not necessarily create an obligation to provide ongoing care, so long as the walk-in or emergency nature of the services is clear and appropriate information is provided regarding ongoing care. In a situation in which a prospective patient discusses his or her history with a physician, it may be difficult to assert that no relationship has been established, particularly if the patient is under the impression that a treatment relationship exists. Physicians should clarify at the outset of the treatment encounter that they may or may not accept a case. It is usually helpful to explain at the first visit that this is an initial evaluation to determine whether or not it is appropriate for the physician to take this particular individual as a patient. Clearly, this principle does not include the emergent, or even urgent, medical problem. In the event that no physician-patient relationship has been created in the initial contact, referral of such a patient to a health care facility, such as a walk-in clinic, demonstrates concern for the patient without necessarily creating an obligation to treat.[24-26]

When the physician elects not to treat an individual, the physician should make every effort to provide an alternative course to avoid claims of abandonment.[1,2] Abandonment is the unilateral severance of the relationship by the physician, leaving the patient without needed medical care. The optimal care of the patient is the first consideration. Whenever a physician desires to transfer the patient to another physician, the transferring physician must take steps to ensure continuity of care by specific arrangement with the physician who is going to treat the patient. The physician may terminate the treatment relationship with a patient for a variety of reasons, including nonpayment, repeated failure to keep appointments, or threatening behavior. In such cases, the patient should be notified of the decision, the available treatment options (including a specific referral, if possible), and available sources of emergency care. The course pursued and the reasons and indications for the transfer or termination should be documented in the medical record.[2,3]

The physician's right to refuse to provide care for patients may be restricted where the refusal is based on the patient's specific illness or inherent characteristics. The refusal to care for patients of certain races, religions, ethnic origins, or disease type (e.g., acquired immunodeficiency syndrome) raises significant ethical concerns as well as potential liability under the Americans with Disabilities Act. These are beyond the scope of this chapter. The general rule, however, is that physicians and other clinicians may be charged with unethical conduct and in some situations with violation of patients' civil rights, when treatment is refused on this basis.[27,28]

The issue of terminating the physician-patient relationship usually arises when some conflict has developed between physician and patient over the course of treatment or as a result of noncompliance.[29] Knowing about the physician's right not to treat is important for consultants. Often the knowledge that a physician can stop treating a particular patient allows enough "give" in a confrontation so that the consultee's anxiety diminishes and negotiation can begin.

End-of-Life Care and Advance Directives

Care of the dying and hopelessly ill patient continues to generate difficult questions, staff conflicts, and requests for help from physicians who find themselves faced with these clinical, ethical, and legal dilemmas.[30,31] Controversy and turmoil are generated when the patient loses the capacity to participate in the decision-making process. The decision of a competent patient to refuse life-sustaining treatment yields similar results. The general rule is that every competent adult has the right to make his or her own decisions about medical care, based on personal preference, even if that choice conflicts with what a majority of others would choose under similar circumstances. An important distinction must be drawn between the competent patient's request that treatment be withheld or withdrawn and requests that the physician take some active, independent step to terminate the patient's life. The former are generally regarded as being within the realm of the patient's right to make treatment decisions. The original illness, rather than the withholding or withdrawal of treatment, is regarded as the cause of death in such situations. Active steps taken to end a patient's life are considered euthanasia; in many states, the complying physician could be subjected to criminal prosecution.[31,32] In fact, in two 1997 cases, the United States Supreme Court upheld two state laws prohibiting physician-assisted suicide after physicians challenged the constitutionality of the laws.[33,34] Currently, only Oregon has legalized physician-assisted suicide.

The treatment requests of the dying patient have not always been taken seriously, especially when the patient's choice is to terminate care. Physicians struggle when faced with a patient who refuses further treatment, especially when there is some hope of improvement. Physicians often find it difficult to give up the fight even at the request of the patient. Consulting psychiatrists in such circumstances should be concerned with determining whether the patient's request to forgo heroic efforts stems from depression or pain and whether or not the patient is capable of understanding the nature of the request. In other words, is the patient's refusal of further treatment informed? If so, the next challenge is working with the treatment team so that they can accept the patient's decision.

When minor children suffer terminal conditions, in the absence of any overriding legal requirements, parents are generally permitted to make decisions regarding continuation of extraordinary efforts.[21,35,36] The consulting psychiatrist is urged to seek the advice of the hospital's general counsel when confronted with these issues. The maze of governmental regulations, statutes, and case law in this area combined with the emotionally charged nature of the situation demand expert legal input. Nevertheless, the larger challenge for the consultant and the treatment team lies in helping the child's parents with the turmoil at hand and the grief ahead.

The psychiatrist should do what he or she can to ensure the comfort of the patient, such as seeing that treatment of clinical depression and alleviation of tractable pain are not overlooked in the anxiety that surrounds the dying patient (see Chapter 23. Development and documentation of written guidelines for the management of these difficult situations can be helpful in ensuring rational constancy in approach. Such attention to the relief of suffering decreases conflict between patient, family, and staff. In turn, this helps avoid legal involvement in the situation.

The status of the patient's right to refuse life-sustaining treatment varies among the states. In 1990 the U.S. Supreme Court handed down its opinion in *Cruzan v. Director, Missouri Department of Public Health*.[37] The Court held that all competent individuals have a constitutionally protected right to refuse life-sustaining treatment. When a patient is incompetent, however, the court held that the state can assert its interest in preserving life and require clear and convincing evidence of the now-incompetent patient's preferences in such matters before a surrogate decision-maker will be allowed to refuse the treatment on the patient's behalf. In most jurisdictions, surrogate decision-makers, whether family members or guardians, are allowed

greater freedom in drawing conclusions about the patient's preference.

Many states have statutes that allow competent individuals to issue advance directives concerning future medical care in these situations. All states have statutes providing for durable powers of attorney, an instrument that can be used to delegate decision-making authority to another person in the event of incapacity. All physicians should be aware of what prior directives are valid in their jurisdictions and encourage their patients to explore these issues with them and with their legal representatives. Under the Patient Self Determination Act of 1990, all health care facilities, nursing homes, and health maintenance organizations must inquire on admission or enrollment whether a patient has an advance directive. If not, the patient must be offered information on the subject and an opportunity to create a directive.[38–40]

Rights of Patients

It is no news that the relationship between physician and patient has changed considerably over the years. The pendulum has swung between the extremes of paternalism and total patient autonomy. More recently, the impact of restrictions on patient choice imposed by managed care has been added to the equation. Most physicians and their patients operate on some middle ground between the extremes of complete patient autonomy and medical paternalism. The fundamental principle is that it is the patient, not the physician, who makes the ultimate choice regarding treatment. This ethical concept has been operationalized by legal decisions and by legislation. Although some physicians still view these changes as dangerous to patient care and as intrusions into their domain of clinical judgment, they represent much-needed measures for protection of the rights of mentally and medically ill patients. Nevertheless, food and drug laws, restrictions on new and experimental treatments and procedures, and commitment and restraint laws—all modified in recent years—trigger anxiety for physicians who previously concerned themselves with only consent, competency, and refusal of treatment against medical advice (AMA).

Informed Consent and Evaluation of Competency

Informed consent issues and the evaluation of competency are major components of the medicolegal workload. Informed consent has been an essential feature of medical practice since the 1960s. It is a process by which the patient agrees to treatment, in which the consent is based on adequate information, and it is voluntarily given by a patient who is competent to do so.[41] The term *informed consent* is somewhat misleading; we are as concerned with informed refusal as we are with informed consent. Bowing to convention, the term informed consent is used with the understanding that the same standards apply to informed refusal.

Informed consent is required before the initiation of any medical treatment, but exceptions do exist. Informed consent need not be obtained in an emergency in which delay would seriously threaten the well-being of the patient. In such cases, the physician is under an obligation to use his or her best judgment and to act in good faith. Such behavior is unlikely to result in litigation, especially if the physician documents (immediately after the emergency passes) the events and the reasons for the steps taken. Other exceptions to informed consent have been found where the patient waives the right to receive information, where the patient is incompetent, or where providing the information needed for informed consent would cause the patient's physical or mental health to deteriorate (known as *therapeutic privilege*). The therapeutic privilege is problematic; it is mentioned here because it has been invoked in the past and was for many years a mainstay of medical paternalism (e.g., patients who were treated for carcinoma without being told the diagnosis for fear it "would just upset them" and worsen their overall condition). Situations in which the therapeutic privilege can be justifiably invoked are rare. The fact that providing the information might lead the patient to refuse treatment or would cause the patient considerable anxiety does not justify invoking therapeutic privilege. The situation must be one in which the informed consent process itself would cause risk of grave harm. The physician who forgoes the informed consent process under the name of therapeutic privilege does so at his or her own risk.[41–43]

An essential feature of modern consent is that it be informed. Simple consent, in which the patient gives the physician blanket permission to take care of the problem, is not deemed adequate, unless the patient has made a specific decision to waive informed consent. The amount and type of information to be provided to the patient or the surrogate decision-maker vary somewhat among jurisdictions.[2] The two basic standards are the professional standard and the patient-oriented standard. In the former, the physician is required to give that amount of information that the average physician in that specialty would provide under the circumstances. In other words, it looks to the standard of care. In other states, the amount of information to be provided is determined by what the patient would require to make an informed decision. This is also known as the materiality standard. In some states, the materiality standard is applied on the basis of what the average patient would require to make a decision, whereas in other states it is assessed in terms of what the specific patient would require. In either case, the physician who covers the following information, taken from a leading Massachusetts case,[44] with the patient will generally be held to have provided adequate information:

- The diagnosis and condition to be treated
- The nature of the proposed treatment
- The nature and probability of the material risks of the treatment
- The benefits that may be expected from the treatment
- The inability of the physician to predict results
- The irreversibility of the procedure, if that is the case
- The likely results of forgoing treatment
- The likely results, risks, and benefits of alternative treatments

The second requirement for informed consent is that the consent be given voluntarily. Coercion is often in the eye of the beholder; the fact that coercion ostensibly occurs in the service of the best interests of the patient does not justify it from the ethical standpoint or qualify it as an element of informed consent. The line between persuasion and coercion often appears both narrow and vague. Generally speaking, if some negative contingency (including an exaggerated prediction of a poor prognosis) is attached to the patient's refusal of treatment, there is coercion, and any subsequent consent is technically invalid.

Competency is the threshold issue in the informed consent process. The term is familiar to all physicians; typically, it is used imprecisely. Competency is defined as the legal capacity of an individual to perform either a specific function or a wide range of functions; before such a determination by a judge, all adults are presumed to be competent. Only a judge can declare a person incompetent for specific functions or for all activities (global incompetence). The psychiatric consultant can only make a clinical assessment of the patient's capacity to function in certain areas. That assessment is usually, but not always, accepted by the court in its determination of incompetence.[2,41] What then of the numerous requests received by the consultation psychiatrist to determine the competency of medical and surgical patients? The use of competency as a shorthand term is justifiable so long as the consultant and the consultee are clear that the most the consultant can do is to assess the patient's capacity to engage in the activity in question. The change in the patient's legal status must be left to a judge.

Competency is usually task specific and defined in relation to a specified act: to make a will (testamentary capacity), to testify in court (testimonial capacity), to consent to or to refuse treatment (decision-making capacity), and the like. Being competent to perform one act does not mean that one is necessarily competent to perform another. Hence, the consultant called to evaluate a patient's competency must first determine the specific type of competency in question and be aware of the applicable judgment criteria. Once the consultant has determined the type of competency in question, the judgment hinges on the patient's understanding of three things: the illness (that something is wrong and to some degree how wrong), the treatment (what is proposed and why it is relevant to what is wrong), and the consequences of the decision. Although a variety of means of assessing decision-making capacity have been proposed, Appelbaum and Grisso have suggested the following four criteria that are particularly useful and straightforward[45]:

1. Does the patient manifest a preference? A patient who is unable or unwilling to express a preference presumably lacks the capacity to make a choice. It does not necessarily follow, however, that a patient who expresses a choice is competent.
2. Is the patient capable of attaining a factual understanding of the situation (nature of the illness, treatment options, prognosis with and without treatment, risks and benefits of treatment, and so on)? The patient need not possess this level of understanding at the time of admission; he or she need only be able to receive the factual information and retain it in some reasonable form during the decision-making process.
3. Does the patient have an appreciation of the significance of the facts presented? Appreciation, in contrast to factual understanding, indicates a broader level of understanding related to the significance of the facts presented and the implications these facts hold for the patient's future.
4. Is the patient able to use the information presented in a rational fashion to reach a decision, that is, to weigh the facts presented in a logical manner? The focus here is not on the rationality of the ultimate decision, but on the rationality of the thought processes leading to the decision.

When a substitute decision-maker is deciding on behalf of an incompetent patient, the same elements of capacity to make a decision apply. The patient's health care agent has the responsibility to express the patient's choice, with an awareness of the facts and appreciation for their significance, thinking through the material in a logical fashion before making a decision.

Competency is not an all-or-nothing proposition, and the same level of competence is not required for all medical decisions. Most experts agree that the strictness of the competency test should vary as the risk/benefit ratio changes. In essence, there is a sliding scale for the level of competence needed before a person can be deemed competent to make medical decisions.[46] The more favorable the risk/benefit ratio, the lower the standard for competence to consent and the higher the standard for competence to refuse. For example, the patient who agrees to accept incision and drainage of an obvious wound abscess would not have his or her competence subjected to rigorous assessment. Refusal could not be taken so lightly; the more serious the abscess, the more intense the examination of competency would have to be. If the risk/benefit ratio were unfavorable to the patient (e.g., extensive surgery to remove a slow-growing brain tumor in a 94-year-old), refusal would not have to be challenged as meticulously as would consent. Although some criticize this approach as being too open to manipulation by a paternalistic physician, it accurately reflects professional obligations to ensure that patients make a truly informed decision based on a rational weighing of the risks and benefits involved. A similar approach was endorsed by the President's Commission for the Study of Ethical Problems in Medicine and Biomedical and Behavioral Research.[47,48]

Dementia, delirium, and psychosis are the conditions most often cited as causes of incompetence.[49–52] The consultant should always consider the possibility of a mood disorder as a basis for impaired competence to make medical decisions. The following example demonstrates some of the complexities of these evaluations.

A psychiatric consultant was asked to assess the competency of a 62-year-old man who presented to the emergency department with a massive subdural hematoma that he had suffered in repeated falls owing to bradycardia. He had a profound expressive aphasia; despite the size of the subdural hematoma, the patient was medically stable and intermittently lucid. Nevertheless, neurosurgical staff were anxious to evacuate the subdural hematoma for fear of increased intracranial pressure. During his lucid intervals, the patient was verbally abusive to his physicians and to the consultant, stated clearly that he did not want surgery, and demanded to be discharged. The limited duration of his lucid intervals and his general irritability prevented the consultant from conducting a more complete mental status examination and determining the degree of his cognitive impairment, if any. An interview with his family members revealed that he had been drinking and becoming more depressed, with marked suicidal ideation, in the previous weeks. He had refused to see a physician about his bradycardia, stating that he would prefer to die. Based on this information, his mental status examination, and the risk/benefit ratio of the proposed treatment, the consultant determined that the patient lacked the capacity to give an informed refusal. An emergency court hearing was held with an "on-call" judge.

The judge ruled that the patient was incompetent to refuse the planned procedure and appointed a family member to be his guardian. The guardian then consented to evacuation of the subdural. The patient tolerated the procedure well; on recovering from surgery and anesthesia, he informed the staff in a clear voice that he was going to sue all of them. The appointment of a guardian and receipt of informed consent by the guardian deprived the patient of any basis for a malpractice action.

Although depression must be considered as a possible cause of impaired judgment and incompetence, caution must be exercised. Just as a patient with schizophrenia is not automatically considered incompetent, a patient with major depression may also retain the ability to make rational decisions. Studies have found that medical decision-making capacity is altered by severe depression but not by depression of lesser severity.[53]

Patients may make decisions in one moment and change those decisions minutes or hours later. This can cause significant disruption of treatment for that patient and for others. Frequent shifts in patient choice can be the basis for questioning the patient's competence. Ideally the patient makes a competent choice before suffering a shift in mental status. Family members should be included in this process so they can assist the treatment team in the event of a subsequent change in the patient's decision.

The cause of incompetence may be treatable. Intense pain may lead a patient to refuse a needed procedure; treatment with adequate doses of analgesics may resolve the problem. Treatment of depression, when it is a factor, may be attempted with psychostimulants, which may act within 1 to 2 days. This can restore the patient's perspective so that the decision to refuse or accept is competently made. Delirium and agitation often interfere with treatment decisions and should be treated with a neuroleptic if no specific cause of the confusional state can be found. The consultant should not determine that the patient is permanently incompetent until these medications have been given an adequate trial, and other potential causes of the confusional state have been addressed. It must be remembered that even psychotic patients may have clear, rational reasons for refusing a treatment. Conversely, the refusal may be the result of voices telling the patient to leave the hospital, that they do not deserve treatment, or that the surgeon is a Federal Bureau of Investigation agent sent to spy on them.[54]

Occasionally, psychiatric consultants are asked to assess a patient's testamentary capacity, competency to execute a contract, financial competency, or the like. Such questions are unlikely to arise in the course of the usual medical consultation but instead are asked by an attorney or the courts, in anticipation, or as a result, of a challenge to the patient's competency to engage in these activities. In the case of testamentary capacity, for example, a psychiatrist may be asked to assess the mental status of a patient to determine whether he or she meets the legal standards for testamentary capacity and to provide documentation of this mental status in the event that the will is challenged after the patient's demise. To do so, the psychiatrist must possess both clinical skills and knowledge of the legal standards: The patient knows that he or she is executing a will, knows the extent of his or her estate, and knows the "natural objects of his or her bounty" (who would normally inherit). Because these assessments involve the application of specific legal requirements to clinical situations, the evaluation should be performed only after consultation with the referring attorney or court representative and with adequate knowledge of the legal standard. For this reason, many psychiatric consultants refer such consultations to colleagues who specialize in consultation to the legal system.[55]

To give consent, the patient must be able to make an informed judgment on the matter at hand. Patients with deficits in this area owing to communication difficulties (foreign language, deafness, or aphasia) or ignorance of important aspects of their care cannot technically give consent, whether or not they are competent. The physician who performs a procedure on a passive, confused, or fearfully mute patient who seems compliant or willing does so at his or her own peril; the physician risks a suit for battery. There is little protection in the ancient maxim *Qui tacet consentire videtur* ("silence gives assent").

The patient's capacity to give consent, understanding, and judgment should be documented in the chart or in office notes of the physician, along with the mental status examination and any specific questions asked about the proposed treatment. Impairment of intellect, memory, attention, or consciousness can limit the patient's understanding; impairment in reality testing, sense of reality, impulse control, and formal logic can influence judgment. The presence or absence of any or all of these should be documented clearly in the chart, along with their relationship to the illness and to the decision-making process.

The general rule in obtaining consent for treatment of minor children is that parents have both the obligation to provide care and the right to make treatment decisions. There are a number of complicating issues in this area, however. First, the age of majority varies by state. Second, minors' rights and the legal ability to consent vary according to the type of treatment being contemplated. Massachusetts, for example, permits minors to give consent for the treatment of drug addiction and sexually transmitted diseases without seeking parental authorization. Virginia allows minors to consent to psychotherapy without parental consent. Third, the law is open to examination of the reason for the parents' denial of consent, rather than upholding it automatically. For example, denial of life-saving treatment because of the parents' religious beliefs will not be upheld. Finally, the law recognizes the concept of the emancipated minor. This is a minor child who is free of parental control and dominance and is therefore deemed competent to consent in the eyes of the law, regardless of age. Informed consent by an emancipated minor, carefully documented in the record, usually protects the physician's action from criticism by the parent or guardian of that minor. Treating clinicians and consultants should learn the rules of their specific states concerning consent by minors.[35,36]

New drugs, treatments, and procedures should not be used without informed consent by patients (or the appropriate surrogate decision-maker) and proper authorization from hospital and government agencies. Although physicians have generally been given considerable freedom in prescribing medications and in doing procedures for off-label (not approved by Food and Drug Administration [FDA]) purposes, this freedom is constrained by federal and state regulations, the standard of care (enforced through malpractice actions), and the patient's right to be informed about the proposed treatment. Use of carbamazepine for treatment of bipolar disorder is a common example of this. As a matter of policy, patients should be informed that the medicine prescribed has not been given FDA approval for that particular purpose and informed about the rationale for prescribing it.[24]

Civil Commitment and Restraint

Civil commitment and physical restraint are commonly encountered but poorly understood by patients and many nonpsychiatric physicians. Civil commitment is a process by which the power of the state is used to remove an individual from society and place him or her in an institutional setting. Originally the mentally ill were confined to institutions to protect the rest of society. As the approach toward the mentally ill became more enlightened, the goal of confinement was to provide treatment and protection. Under this approach, the state was fulfilling its role as protector of its citizens, much as a parent would act on behalf of a child. Hence, this is known as the state's *parens patriae* interest. With the blossoming of the civil liberties movement in the 1970s and the emphasis on individual autonomy, the individual's interest in personal freedom and privacy was given priority over the state's *parens patriae* interest. During the 1970s, the best interest or *parens patriae* approach to civil commitment was replaced by the dangerousness approach in most jurisdictions. This approach, based on the state's police powers, allows an individual to be involuntarily committed to a mental institution only if the individual poses a danger to himself or herself through direct injury, if there is a direct threat of physical harm to others, or if the individual is gravely disabled and unable to care for himself or herself in the community.[2,3,56]

In a general hospital, if a medical or surgical patient is psychiatrically committable but requires further medical or surgical treatment, the wisest course is to initiate commitment procedures and request that a local mental health facility accept the patient but allow the patient to remain in the general hospital for care. Budgetary concerns, insurance issues, and the general reluctance of both state and private psychiatric hospitals to take medically ill patients often make it difficult to place such patients. It behooves the consultation psychiatrist to learn how to anticipate the need for further psychiatric care and begin the search early. The need

for commitment should be reassessed throughout this process and the process halted if appropriate.

This search for inpatient psychiatric placement increasingly requires negotiation with managed care companies to obtain permission for the hospitalization. Often, the interaction with health insurance companies occurs through the process of precertification, which requires the transferring hospital to gain approval for transfer and inpatient care from the insurer before the patient can be transferred and admitted to the receiving psychiatric facility. Because of frequent differences in general medical and psychiatric benefits within health plans, the same precertification process may be required even when a patient is transferred from a medical ward to a psychiatric unit in the same hospital. It is now commonplace for insurance plans to "carve out" or subcontract mental health benefits to a subsidiary or a different company with procedures and guidelines distinct from those of the parent company.

The psychiatric consultant often encounters questions regarding the restraint of patients on medical and surgical floors. Delirium, dementia, acute or chronic psychosis, or severe anxiety or panic can lead a patient to assault staff, to wander off the ward, or to fall. The suicidal patient being treated on an unlocked medical floor poses the risk of elopement and successful fulfillment of suicidal urges. Many hospitals have policies that allow the patient to be restrained before the psychiatric consultant is called. When this occurs, the role of the consultant is to provide management recommendations and approval for the restraint. Usually, the psychiatric consultant is asked to decide whether the restraints can be discontinued.

The legal aspects of restraint of patients on a medical or surgical ward vary among jurisdictions.[4,24] Generally speaking, a patient may be restrained for the purpose of protecting the patient or other patients and staff, for the purpose of allowing examination during an emergency, or for the purpose of treatment in situations in which the patient appears to lack the capacity to make treatment decisions and is refusing care. In this latter situation, no forced treatment should be initiated in the absence of an emergency unless surrogate consent has been obtained. In handling these situations, physician and staff are required to use the least restrictive alternative available. Thus where a sitter or observer is available for a potentially suicidal patient, that option is more appropriate than four-point restraints. Family members often ask whether they can substitute for a sitter. Although this may be possible in some situations, it requires careful clinical judgment that takes into account the type of pathology, the degree of impulsivity, the overall degree of risk, and the relative ability of the sitter to act objectively. Restraint is uncomfortable for the staff as well as for the patient and family, and there may be a tendency to avoid it whenever possible for some types of patients and a tendency to overuse it with others. Again, careful clinical assessment is essential so that protection is provided for those patients who need restraint without zealously overprotecting and restricting those who do not. The justification for restraint, including history and formal mental status examination, should be clearly documented in the medical record, along with the psychiatric differential diagnosis, treatment, and management recommendations.

The restraint of patients gives rise to two potential sources of liability: battery and false imprisonment.[1] A battery is defined as the touching of another person without his or her consent (expressed or implied) or justification. False imprisonment may be charged where an individual is denied the right to move about freely by real or perceived methods of confinement. Failure to restrain a patient with a tendency to wander who is subsequently injured may result in a charge of professional negligence.

Malpractice claims based on battery or false imprisonment are rarely successful if the use of restraint is reasonable under the circumstances, the reasons for the measures are documented in the medical record, proper technique is used, and hospital policies are followed. Failure to restrain when indicated and improper restraining technique carry greater risks of harm to the patient and of malpractice claims.

Right to Refuse Treatment

The right to refuse a specific form of treatment or procedure has a long history and is firmly established in medicine. This right, based on the philosophical principle of autonomy, has been operationalized through the common law (case law), by legislation, and in state and the U.S. constitutions.[57–60] Although widely acknowledged, the right to refuse treatment is not absolute. It may be limited when it is in conflict with legitimate state interests of preserving life, preventing suicide, protecting the interests of third parties, or protecting the integrity of the medical profession.[61] Generally the decision of a competent patient to end treatment presents a difficult dilemma for the treatment team. If the issue ever reaches court, the competent patient's preference is rarely overridden. With the advent of advance directives (e.g., health care proxies and durable powers of attorney), the wishes of the patient, expressed when competent, can be honored after the onset of incompetence. The path to this conclusion is not as smooth as this might suggest. Consider the following example.

A 22-year-old woman was admitted to the hospital after sustaining severe head injuries in a motor vehicle accident. After emergency evacuation of a subdural hematoma, her condition stabilized. She was unresponsive to verbal stimuli, did not track, but did withdraw to pain. She showed decorticate posturing. The treatment team urged aggressive measures, arguing that the injury was recent and the ability to predict ultimate outcome was limited. Tube feedings were begun and an early pneumonia treated with antibiotics. The patient's family told the treatment team that the patient would never want to be kept alive under such circumstances. The patient's mother explained that the patient's cousin had been in a motor vehicle accident 5 years earlier and had lingered in a persistent vegetative state for 3 years until her death. The family had to engage in a costly legal battle to get permission to terminate supportive care. When this occurred, the patient (who was a nursing student at the time) vowed that she would never allow this to happen to her or to her family. She told her family that she would want to be free of life-sustaining measures in the event of a serious injury if there were "no chance of recovery." In addition, she executed a health care proxy naming her mother as her agent for medical decision-making in the event of her incapacity. Her mother believed that the patient would have refused care if able to do so and insisted that the tube feedings be stopped. The treatment team resisted, arguing that there was hope for some recovery. After a series of meetings, the family acquiesced to the recommendations of the team and the patient was transferred to a rehabilitation facility, still posturing and not responding. Two weeks after transfer, she was returned to the hospital with septicemia. This time, the treatment team yielded to the family's preferences and the patient died peacefully.

As this example suggests, there are often no perfect answers to these problems. Both the treatment team and the family were well-meaning and tried to do what they believed was right for the patient. Meetings between the treatment team and the family, facilitated by the consultants to the unit, allowed a process to develop that gave the patient some chance at early recovery but allowed all concerned to allow nature to take its course. Although difficult, the decision-making process was conducted with dignity, with the aim of maintaining the patient's autonomy and ensuring that the decision was informed and with concern for the ethical integrity of her caretakers. In a more contentious setting, the family could have charged the treatment team with battery. Under the law in that state, the agent appointed by the health care proxy (the mother in this case) had the same authority to make decisions as the patient would have if competent, including refusal of permission for further treatment. The treatment team could have raised legal challenges to the exercise of the proxy, arguing that it was not evident that there was "no chance of recovery." In some states, an argument would be made that shutting off the life support constituted murder or assisted suicide or that the state's interest in preserving life and preventing suicide outweighed the individual's expressed wish. The likelihood of such arguments being made or succeeding is much less in light of the Cruzan decision.[37] Finally, if the physicians or the institution had been ethically opposed to the termination of treatment, the request might have been denied and the patient transferred to the care of another physician or facility. The best solution to these challenging problems lies in the sharing of information and concerns between the family and the treaters. Immediate resort to legal posturing hardens positions and shuts off communications in most cases, to the detriment of all concerned.

The requirement of informed consent and the right to refuse treatment do not automatically apply in emergencies. In emergencies that appear to endanger the patient, or in acute situations that threaten the safety of the staff and other patients, the physician who acts in good faith while administering a treatment or procedure is generally not liable for failure to obtain informed consent. Good faith is in doubt, however, when the patient has made his or her preferences regarding treatment in the event of an emergency clearly known before the emergency and the physician chooses to disregard these preferences. For example, the physician who agrees to perform surgery on a Jehovah's Witness with the stipulation that there be no transfusions, even in an emergency, is hard pressed to plead good faith should he or she violate that agreement in the event of a sudden hemorrhage. Some institutions have adopted policies specific to such situations. In the case of chronic medical conditions, ongoing situations, and prolonged heroic measures to sustain life, the emergency exception loses its applicability, and decisions regarding treatment must be returned to the competent patient or to an appropriate surrogate.

Leaving treatment AMA is the prerogative of any competent, nonconsenting patient.[62] The threat to leave AMA, similar to most other medicolegal conflicts, usually represents a clinical problem disguised as a legal dispute. The consultant called to evaluate the patient threatening to leave AMA must evaluate whether the patient is competent to make that decision. In the course of the evaluation, it is common to find that the patient is angry over a perceived lack of caring or dissatisfaction with the amount of information provided by the physician. The consultant who can restore communication between physician and patient may be successful in getting the patient to complete the course of treatment. If the patient does leave, the consultant may then have to calm the staff in preparation for the patient returning at a later date.

From a legal standpoint, if patients possess the capacity to make decisions and do not pose a risk of harm to themselves or others, they cannot be held against their will. A patient requesting to sign out AMA may be deemed to have the requisite capacity (competence) to do so if he or she understands the nature of the illness, the recommended treatment, the alternative treatments available, and the prognosis with or without treatment and is able to use this information in a rational manner to reach a decision. If the patient meets these criteria, he or she can leave against advice, whether or not the form is signed. In the event that the patient refuses to sign the form, the discussions before release and the fact that the patient refused to sign the form should be documented in the medical record.

Conclusion

This chapter began with a discussion of the role of the psychiatric consultant in helping consultees deal with medicolegal issues. It is appropriate to close it with a few cautionary words about the temptations present for those who undertake this task. Consultants are often tempted to meet the needs of their consultees by telling them what they want to hear. Nowhere is this more true than in the assessment of a patient's competency to consent to, or to refuse, treatment. This is compounded by the consultant's own inclinations, as a physician, to seek an outcome that is in the best clinical interests of the patient. In performing competency assessments and other consultations on medicolegal issues, such temptations must be strongly resisted. The assignment of the consultant is to be objective and focused on the issue at hand, rather than on what the consultant or consultee sees as the best overall clinical outcome. Such isolation of purpose is often difficult, but it is essential if the consultant is to serve the consultee and the patient. The consultant must also keep in mind that he or she is just that: a consultant whose job it is to advise, not to decide. The treating physician may choose to disregard the consultant's assessment that a patient is incompetent to make treatment decisions and proceed with treatment. The treating physician assumes both the legal and moral liability of his or her own actions. The consultant can serve only as a guidepost and only then by being both knowledgeable and objective. This task is made easier by taking the following approach to consultation on these highly charged medicolegal issues:

1. Know what you are being asked to do. That is, understand both the overt request and any covert agenda that may exist.
2. Know the clinical facts of the consultation.
3. Know, or find out, the salient legal requirements involved.
4. Determine the presence of any apparent conflict between good clinical care and the law.
5. Get to know the hospital attorney; share information and attempt to develop a multidisciplinary team approach to patient care.
6. Try to move all parties away from a crisis mentality to gain some time to resolve conflicts and to encourage compromise. Avoid

ultimatums. Pushing back deadlines for procedures, treatment, leaving the hospital AMA, and the like decreases time pressures and allows people to think more clearly.
7. Understand the personalities of the physician and the patient.
8. Know the patient's next of kin, their understanding, fears, biases, personalities, and the probabilities of obtaining informed consent from them.
9. Act as a go-between so as to diminish anxiety and communication gaps among physician, patient, and family and try to find areas for compromise and agreement.
10. Search out covert disagreements and hidden fears in the physician and patient; try to find commonsense measures that would remedy these, and search for loopholes and areas in which conflicts can be mended or avoided.
11. Provide detailed documentation in the patient's medical record (or chart) of the patient's understanding, judgment, capacity to give consent, and clinical and psychiatric status as well as the course pursued.
12. Maintain an objective point of view while remaining mindful that the consultant's responsibility is to assess as accurately as possible the patient's capacity to give an informed consent and that truth is a higher goal than scheduling concerns of the consultee and ward staff.
13. Use such consultations to teach physicians that they have little to fear from the law and to teach patients that they have little to fear from their physicians.

References

1. Keeton WP, Keeton DB, Keeton RE, et al: *Prosser and Keeton on torts*, ed 5, St Paul, MN, 1984, West Publishing.
2. Appelbaum PS, Gutheil TG: *Clinical handbook of psychiatry and the law*, ed 3, Philadelphia, 2000, Lippincott Williams & Wilkins.
3. Simon RI: *Clinical psychiatry and the law*, Washington, DC, 1987, American Psychiatric Association Press.
4. Spring RL, Lacoursiere RB, Weissenberger G: *Patients, psychiatrists and lawyers: law and the mental health system*, Cincinnati, 1989, Anderson Publishing.

5. Garrick TR, Weinstock R: Liability of psychiatric consultants, *Psychosomatics* 35:474–484, 1994.

6. Schouten R: *Malpractice in medical-psychiatric practice.* In Stoudemire A, Fogel BS, editors: *Medical-psychiatric practice*, vol 2, Washington, DC, 1993, American Psychiatric Press.

7. Appelbaum PS: Legal liability and managed care, *Am Psychol* 48:251–257, 1993.

8. Hall RC: Legal precedents affecting managed care, *Psychosomatics* 35:105–117, 1994.

9. Hall RC: Social and legal implications of managed care in psychiatry, *Psychosomatics* 35:150–158, 1994.

10. Schouten R: Legal liability and managed care, *Harvard Rev Psychiatry* 1:189–190, 1993.

11. *Tarasoff v. Board of Regents of the University of California*, 17 Cal. 3d 425 1976.

12. Beck JC: Violent patients and the Tarasoff decision in private psychiatric practice, *J Psychiatry Law* 13: 361–376, 1985.

13. Hemlinski F: Near the conflagration: the wide duty to warn, *Mayo Clin Proc* 68:709–710, 1993.

14. Appelbaum PS, Zonana H, Bonnie R, et al: Statutory approaches to limiting psychiatrists' liability for their patients' violent acts, *Am J Psychiatry* 146:821–828, 1989.

15. *Bradshaw v. Daniel*, 854 S.W. 2d 865 Tennessee, 1993.

16. Closen ML, Isaacman SH: The duty to notify private third parties of the risks of HIV infection, *J Health Hosp Law* 21:295–303, 1988.

17. Dickens BM: Legal limits of AIDS confidentiality, *JAMA* 259:3449–3451, 1988.

18. Ensor JC: Doctor-patient confidentiality versus duty to warn in the context of AIDS patients and their partners, *M Law Rev* 47:675–700, 1988.

19. Gostin L, Curran WJ: AIDS screening, confidentiality, and the duty to warn, *Am J Public Health* 77:361–365, 1987.

20. Rosmarin D: Legal and ethical aspects of HIV disease. In *A psychiatrist's guide to AIDS and HIV disease*, Washington, DC, 1990, American Psychiatric Association.

21. Schouten R: *Legal responsibilities with child abuse and domestic violence.* In Jacobson JL, Jacobson AM, editors: *Psychiatric secrets*, Philadelphia, 1995, Hanley & Belfus.

22. Appelbaum PS: Privacy in psychiatric treatment: threats and responses, *Am J Psychiatry* 159:1809–1818, 2002.

23. Maio JE: HIPAA and the special status of psychotherapy notes, *Lippincotts Case Manag* 8:24–29, 2003.

24. Miller R: *Problems in hospital law*, ed 5, Rockville, 1986, Aspen Publishers.

25. Mayer D: Refusals of care and discharging "difficult" patients from the emergency department, *Ann Emerg Med* 19:1436–1446, 1990.

26. Sparr LF, Rogers JL, Beahrs JO, et al: Disruptive medical patients: forensically informed decision-making, *West J Med* 156:501–506, 1992.

27. American College of Physicians: Ethics manual. I. history of ethics, the physician and the patient, the physician's relationship to other physicians, the physician and society. II. research, other ethical issues, recommended readings, *Ann Intern Med* 101:129–137, 263–274, 1984.

28. Emanuel EJ: Do physicians have an obligation to treat patients with AIDS? *N Engl J Med* 318:1686–1690, 1988.

29. Appelbaum PS, Roth LH: Patients who refuse treatment in medical hospitals, *JAMA* 250:1296–1301, 1983.

30. Gostin L, editor: The care of the dying: a symposium on the case of Betty Wright, *Law Med Health Care* 17:205–264, 1989.

31. Wanzer SH, Federman DD, Adelstein SJ, et al: The physician's responsibility toward hopelessly ill patients: a second look, *N Engl J Med* 320:844–849, 1989.

32. Weinstock R, Leong GB, Silva JA: Competence to terminate life-sustaining care, *Am J Geriatr Psychiatry* 2:95–105, 1994.

33. *Washington v. Glucksberg*, 521 U.S. 702 (1997).

34. *Vacco v. Quill*, 521 U.S. 793 (1997).

35. Schetky DH, Benedek EP: *Emerging issues in child psychiatry and the law*, New York, 1985, Brunner/Mazel.

36. Schouten R, Duckworth KS: Medicolegal and ethical issues in the pharmacologic treatment of children. In Werry JS, Aman MG, editors: *Practitioner's guide to psychoactive drugs for children and adolescents*, New York, 1993, Plenum Medical.

37. *Cruzan v. Director*, Missouri Department of Public Health, 110S. Ct. 2841 1990.

38. Emanuel EJ, Emanuel LL: Proxy decision-making for incompetent patients, *JAMA* 267:2067–2071, 1992.

39. Emanuel LL, Emanuel EJ: The medical directive: a new and comprehensive advance care document, *JAMA* 261:3288–3293, 1989.

40. White BD, Siegler M, Singer PA, et al: What does Cruzan mean to the practicing physician? *Arch Intern Med* 151:925–928, 1991.

41. Appelbaum PS, Lidz CW, Meisel A: *Informed consent: legal theory and clinical practice*, New York, 1987, Oxford University Press.

42. Schouten R: Informed consent: resistance and reappraisal, *Crit Care Med* 17:1359–1361, 1989.

43. Drane JF: Competency to give an informed consent, *JAMA* 252:925–927, 1984.

44. *Harnish v. Children's Hospital Medical Center*, 387 Mass 152, 439 NE 2d 240 1982.

45. Appelbaum PS, Grisso T: Assessing patients' capacities to consent to treatment, *N Engl J Med* 319:1635–1638, 1988.

46. Roth LH, Meisel A, Lidz CW: Tests of competency to consent to treatment, *Am J Psychiatry* 134:279–284, 1977.

47. *President's commission for the study of ethical problems in medicine and biomedical and behavioral research:*

deciding to forego life-sustaining treatment, Washington, DC, 1983, US Government Printing Office.

48. *President's commission for the study of ethical problems in medicine and biomedical and behavioral research: making health care decisions: a report on the ethical and legal implications of informed consent in the patient-practitioner relationship*, Washington, DC, 1982, US Government Printing Office.

49. Appelbaum PS, Roth LH: Clinical issues in the assessment of competency, *Am J Psychiatry* 138:1462–1467, 1981.

50. Farnsworth MG: Competency evaluations in the general hospital, *Psychosomatics* 31:60–66, 1990.

51. Ganzini L, Lee MA, Heintz RT, et al: The effect of depression on elderly patients' preferences for life-sustaining therapy, *Am J Psychiatry* 151:1631–1636, 1994.

52. Gutheil TG, Bursztajn H: Clinicians' guidelines for assessing and presenting subtle forms of patient incompetence in legal settings, *Am J Psychiatry* 143:1020–1023, 1986.

53. Sullivan MD, Youngner SJ: Depression, competence, and the right to refuse life-saving medical treatment, *Am J Psychiatry* 151:971, 1994.

54. Katz M, Abbey S, Rydall A, et al: Psychiatric consultation for competency to refuse medical treatment: a retrospective study of patient characteristics and outcome, *Psychosomatics* 36:33–41, 1995.

55. Baker FM: Competent for what? *J Natl Med Assoc* 79:715–720, 1987.

56. Appelbaum PS: Civil commitment and liability for violating patients' rights, *Psychiatric Services* 46:17–18, 1995.

57. Ende J, Kazis L, Ash A, et al: Measuring patients' desire for autonomy: decision-making and information-seeking among medical patients, *J Gen Intern Med* 4:24–30, 1989.

58. Massachusetts General Laws Chapter 111, Sec. 70E *Patients' and residents' rights*; amended 1989.

59. Sprung CL, Winick BJ: Informed consent in theory and practice: legal and medical perspectives on the informed consent doctrine and a proposed reconceptualization, *Crit Care Med* 17:1346–1354, 1989.

60. Swartz M: The patient who refuses medical treatment: a dilemma for hospitals and physicians, *Am J Law Med* 11:1–46, 1985.

61. Wear AN, Brahams D: To treat or not to treat: the legal, ethical and therapeutic implications of treatment refusal, *J Med Ethics* 17:131–135, 1991.

62. Albert HD, Kornfeld DS: The threat to sign out against medical advice, *Ann Intern Med* 79:888–891, 1973.

Chapter 23

End of Life Issues: Principles of Care and Ethics

Ned H. Cassem, M.D., S.J.
Rebecca W. Brendel, M.D., J.D.

Advances in medical technology and practice have extended the human life span. As a result, opportunities and conflicts are emerging at the end of life. Physicians now face multiple challenges when dealing with the dying patient, from issues of care, diagnosis, and treatment, to larger ethical and legal considerations. Medical and surgical colleagues often seek psychiatric consultation for assistance in caring for patients who are nearing death. The unique skills, knowledge, and nurturance of physicians are extremely important in caring for the dying patient. Psychiatrists may be uniquely effective in helping dying patients by ensuring optimization of palliative care and by assisting the patient and the family in the dying process.

Medical specialists and subspecialists regularly face management of the dying patient and have seen every variety of emotional reactions. Therefore, the request for psychiatric consultation usually comes for a patient with the most difficult problems. This chapter provides an overview of central principles of care, diagnosis, and treatment of the dying patient from the perspective of the psychiatric consultant. It also examines current concepts in ethics and legal precedents that surround this changing area in medicine.

Questions for the Psychiatric Consultant

The most common issues leading to psychiatric consultation in the care of the dying patient turn out to be major depression with hopelessness, withdrawal, and the wish to be dead (but rarely active suicidality); delirium and organic brain syndromes with or without cerebral metastases or known metabolic (e.g., hypercalcemia) or paraneoplastic disorders; personality disorders, involving splitting, hostility, treatment rejection, litigation threats, substance abuse, or outrage at having the illness; treatment-resistant continuous pain syndromes; and despondencies, involving grieving, giving up long before the illness seems terminal, and having life plans shattered. Also found are denial, the inability to accept diagnosis or treatment, unrealistic hopes for miracles, or persistent questions, such as why there is no improvement; anxiety, often extreme, with near panic and unspecifiable fears about dying; ambivalence and guilt (e.g., the ambivalence of the daughter with vaginal cancer on learning that the diethylstilbestrol her mother took during pregnancy is implicated and the guilt felt by her mother); and unrelated bad news (e.g., whether a dying person should be told of a relative's death when ability to tolerate another trauma is seriously questioned).

The physician requesting the consultation may or may not be able to specify the disorder. An occasional request may read: "Very difficult situation for unfortunate 32-year-old father of two with widely metastatic adenocarcinoma of unknown origin; please evaluate. Any suggestions appreciated." Nurses make routine observations about the patient, family, and visitors and their interactions. This information provides an invaluable perspective on patient and family problems.

The family of the dying person may be included in or be made the specific subject of the consultation. When a patient is dying, the entire family is the appropriate focus for medical treatment. A family member may be the first to notice a difficulty (such as a personality change) and therefore serves as an indispensable historian. Or a family member may have more difficulty coping with the illness than the patient and because of his or her own needs irritates caregivers, distracts them from the patient, says the patient—not the family member—is anxious, causes isolation of physicians from the family (visits are made to the patient so as to avoid the family), and seriously jeopardizes treatment and the chance to make death meaningful and dignified.

Modern medicine's obsession with money makes it easier to caricature physicians as cold, uncaring, mechanical, and mercenary. The psychiatric consultant who believes that psychiatry is that specialty of medicine with a unique claim on humanitarian perspective, compassion, and ethical principles is headed for deserved trouble. Referring physicians, too, may retain a distorted view of psychiatry as a discipline of good bedside manner and interpersonal relations. In such a case, consultation may represent a sense of guilt over failure to meet the responsibilities of the primary care physician, a deficiency that the consultant will see and possibly rebuke after evaluating the patient. Sensitivity to these pressures on the referring physician helps to preserve this relationship with the patient, a factor essential to the patient's continued well-being.

Confronted by this array of clinical and sociocultural pressures, the consultant can take consolation from knowing that the job is no different with the terminally ill than with any other patient: diagnosis and treatment. Psychiatrists neither work miracles nor have answers for all questions. No matter how tragic and devastating the fatally ill person's predicament, the psychiatric consultant is always willing to see the patient so that the consultant may do what he or she does for other patients: diagnose the patient's conditions and prescribe appropriate treatments. Using the cancer patient as an example of a person with a terminal illness, an approach to diagnosis and treatment of com-

mon problems can be created.[1] In addition to the specifics of psychiatric diagnosis and treatment already mentioned, several practical considerations for management are added to support the goals of treatment.

Caregivers and the Dying Person

Most of the psychosocial information about dying persons comes from them and their families. In the area of experiential reality, the patients are the teachers, and those who care for them always have something further to learn. Over the years, observations made by patients on various aspects of their management have helped in the formulation of essential features in the care and management of the dying patient[2] (Table 23-1). These qualities are competence, concern, comfort, communication, children, family cohesion and integration, cheerfulness, consistency and perseverance, and equanimity.

Competence

In an era in which some discussions of the dying patient seem to suggest that love covers a multitude of sins, it would be unfortunate to encourage the misconception that competence in physicians and nurses is of secondary importance to dying patients. Competence is reassuring, and when one's life or comfort depends on it, personality considerations become secondary. Being good at what one does brings emotional as well as scientific benefits to the patient. For example, no matter how charming physicians, nurses, or technicians may be, the person who is most skillful at venipuncture brings the greatest relief to a patient who is anxious about having blood drawn.

Concern

Of all attributes in physicians and nurses, none is more highly valued by terminal patients than compassion. Although they may never convey it precisely by words, some physicians and nurses are able to tell the patient that they are genuinely touched by his or her predicament. A striking

Table 23.1. Psychiatric Problems of the Dying Patient

Depression
  Risk increased in more severely ill and in hospitalized patients
  Suicide risk: small increase, possibly only in men
  Diagnosis and treatment: same as in primary depression
Delirium
  Second commonest consultation problem in the hospital
  Associated factors: drugs, brain metastases, hypercalcemia, hyponatremia, hyperviscosity, carcinomatous meningitis,
    limbic encephalopathy (paraneoplastic syndrome), leukoencephalopathy, complex partial seizures
Drugs with psychiatric side effects
  Corticosteroids
  Other hormones: tamoxifen, aminoglutethimide, megestrol acetate, leuprolide
  Procarbazine
  L-Asparaginase
  Cytabarabine
  5-Fluorouracil
  Methotrexate (especially high-dose intravenous or intrathecal administration)
  Vincristine
  Vinblastine
  Ifosfamide
  Interferon
  Interleukin-2 with or without lymphocyte-activated killer cells
Anxiety
  Anticipatory nausea (conditioned anxiety)
  Claustrophobia preventing scans, especially magnetic resonance imaging (MRI)
  Panic attacks
  Withdrawal from alcohol or benzodiazepines
  Akathisia from antiemetic neuroleptics
Anorexia
  From chemotherapy, radiation, gastritis, gastroparesis, hypercalcemia
Weakness
  From bed rest, neuropathy, myopathy, anemia, depression, liver disease
Pain
  From bone pain caused by metastases
  Use steroids for swelling
  Use as adjunctive to analgesics
    A nonsteroidal antiinflammatory drug (NSAID)
    A bisphosphanate
  For bone pain in renal transplant patients on cyclosporine, use extended-release nifedipine
Sexual dysfunction
  Treatment-related infertility
  Hormonal deficiency
  Vascular impairment: Delayed effect of pelvic irradiation prevents normal congestion,
    erection; in women, also vaginal stenosis and decreased lubrication
  Central nervous system (CNS) abnormalities
  Depression
  Partner's anticipatory grief, aversion, hostility, fear of injury
Importance of psychoeducational group treatment

example came from a mother's description of her dying son's pediatrician: "You know, that doctor loves Michael." Compassion cannot be feigned. Although universally praised as a quality for a health professional, compassion exacts a cost usually overlooked in professional training. This price of compassion is conveyed by the two Latin roots, *com-*, "with," and *passio*, from *pati*, "to suffer," which together mean "to suffer with" another person. One must be touched by the tragedy of the patient in a literal way, a process that occurs through experiential identification with the dying person. The process of empathy, when evoked by a person facing death or tragic disability, ordinarily produces uncomfortable, burdensome feelings to which internal resistance can arise defensively. Who can bear the thought of dying at the age of 20? It is not perverse but natural for us to discourage discussion of such a topic by the individual facing it. Also, students are sometimes advised to guard against involvement with a patient. When a patient becomes upset, a hasty exit or avoidance is likely.

Few things infuriate patients more than contrived involvement. For this reason, the patient may excuse even an inability to answer direct questions when the inability stems from genuine discomfort on the physician's part. One woman preferred to ask her physician as few questions as possible, even though she wanted more information about how much longer she could expect to survive with stage IV Hodgkin's disease. "Whenever I try to ask him about this, he looks very pained and becomes very hesitant. I don't want to rub it in. After all, he really likes me."

Involvement—real involvement—is not only unavoidable, but also necessary in the therapeutic encounter. Patients recognize it instantly. As a hematologist percussed the right side of his 29-year-old patient's chest, his discovery of pleural effusion brought the realization that a remission had abruptly ended. "Oh shit!," he muttered. Then, realizing what he had said, he added hastily, "Oh, excuse me, Bill." "That's all right," the young man replied. "It's nice to know that you care."

Comfort

With the terminally ill patient, comfort has a technology all its own. Comfort measures never indicate that less attention should be paid to the patient's needs. In fact, ensuring the comfort of a terminally ill person requires meticulous devotion to myriad details, great practical knowledge, and continual exercise of creative ingenuity. It must be an aggressive effort and can be technically complicated (see Axis III, later).

Communication

Talking with the dying is a paradoxic skill. The wish to find the right thing to say is a well-meaning but misguided hope among persons who work with terminally ill patients. Practically every empiric study has emphasized the ability to listen over the ability to say something. Saunders[3] summarizes it best when she says, "The real question is not, 'What do you tell your patients?' but rather, 'What do you let your patients tell you?'" Most people have a strong inner resistance to letting dying patients say what is on their minds. If a patient presumed to be 3 months from death says, "My plan was to buy a new car in 6 months, but I guess I won't have to worry about that now," a poor listener would say nothing or, "Right. Don't worry about it." A better listener might say, "Why do you say that?" or, "What do you mean?"

Communication is, however, more than listening. Getting to know the patient as a person is essential. Learning about significant areas of the patient's life—such as family, work, or school—and chatting about common interests are the most natural if not the only way the patient has of coming to feel known. After a 79-year-old man of keen intellect and wit had been interviewed before a group of hospital staff members, one of the staff said, "Before the interview tonight I just thought of him on the ward as another old man in pain." It is not necessary to talk about esoteric things to a dying person. Similar to anybody else, these individuals get self-respect from a sense that others value them for what they have done and for their personal qualities. Allowing dying persons to tell their own stories helps to build a balanced relationship. The effort spent getting to know them does them more psychological good than trying to guess how they will cope with death.

The physician can help dissolve communication barriers for staff members by showing them the uniqueness of each patient. Comments such as, "She has 34 grandchildren," or, "This woman was an Olympic sprinter," convey information that helps the staff find something to talk about with the patients. Awkwardness subsides when a patient seems like a real person and not merely "a breast cancer." This rescue from anonymity is essential to prevent a sense of isolation.

Communication is more than verbal. A pat on the arm, a wave, a wink, or a grin communicates important reassurances, as do careful back rubs and physical examinations.

Patients occasionally complain about professionals and visitors who regard them as "the dying patient," not as a unique individual. A wise precaution is to take conversational cues from the patient whenever possible.

> A woman in her early 50s with breast cancer that had metastasized to bone, brain, lungs, and liver entered the hospital for a course of chemotherapy. During her entire 6-week stay, she was irascible, argumentative, and even abusive to the staff members. To their surprise, she got a good response with a substantial remission and left the hospital. She later told her oncologist, apologizing for her behavior: "I know that I was impossible. But every single nurse who came into my room wanted to talk to me about death. I came there to get help, not to die, and it drove me up a wall."

Had staff members tuned in to this patient as an individual with a courageous attitude toward her illness instead of treating her as "a dying patient," their efforts to comfort would not have backfired.

Children

All investigators have learned that the visits of children are as likely to bring consolation and relief to the terminally ill patient as any other intervention. A useful rule of thumb in determining whether a particular child should visit a dying patient is to ask the child whether he or she wants to visit. No better criterion has been found.

Family Cohesion and Integration

A burden shared is a burden made lighter. Family members must be helped to support one another, although this requires that the physician get to know each member of the family as well as the patient. Conversely, when a patient is permitted to give support to his or her family, the feeling of being a burden is mitigated.

The often difficult work of bringing the family together for support, reconciliation, or improved relations can prevent disruption when death of the patient begins the work of bereavement. The opportunity to be present at death should be offered to family members as well as the alternative of being informed about it while waiting for the news at home. Flexibility is the rule, and the wishes of the family and patient are paramount. After the patient has died, family members who wish to should be offered a chance to see the body before it is taken to the morgue. Parkes and Weiss[4] have documented the critical importance to grief work of seeing the body of the dead person. Lest one get the idea that simple common sense gives predictive power, intensive studies of families of chronically ill dialysis patients have given evidence that patients from families that appeared to have the stronger bonds died significantly sooner than those in apparently "weaker" families.[5]

Cheerfulness

Dying persons have no more relish for sour and somber faces than anybody else. The possessor of a gentle and appropriate sense of humor can bring relief to all parties involved. "What do they think this is?" said one patient of his visitors. "They file past here with flowers and long faces like they were coming to my wake." Patients with a good sense of humor do not enjoy dead audiences either. Their wit softens many a difficult incident. After an embarrassing loss of sphincter control, one elderly man with a tremor said, "This is enough to give anybody Parkinson's disease!"

Wit is not an end in itself. As in all forms of conversation, the listener should take his or her cue from the patient. Forced or inappropriate mirth with a sick person can increase feelings of distance and isolation.

Consistency and Perseverance

Progressive isolation is a realistic fear of the dying patient. A physician or nurse who regularly visits the sickroom provides tangible proof of continued support and concern. Saunders[3] has emphasized that the quality of time is far more important than the quantity. A brief visit is far better than no visit at all, and the patient may not be able to tolerate a prolonged visit in any case. Patients are quick to identify those who show interest at first but gradually disappear from the scene. Staying power requires hearing complaints.

Praising one of her nurses, a 69-year-old woman with advanced cancer said, "She takes all my guff, and I give her plenty. Most people just pass my room, but if she has even a couple of minutes she'll stop and actually listen to what I have to say. Some days I couldn't get through without her."

Equanimity

The capacity to be comfortable with a dying person is another valued quality.

> A 68-year-old woman with two primary pulmonary malignancies fought, as did her physicians, a steadily losing battle against shortness of breath. She often complained that death would be preferable. Nevertheless, she also worried that her criticisms and unanswerable questions placed an unfair burden on her physicians. After making this observation to one of her physicians, she suddenly fixed her piercing blue eyes on him and said, "You know, you're just like an old shoe—comfortable."

Equally prized by the physician, equanimity not only greatly contributes to, but also is produced by, enriching encounters with the terminally ill.

Goals of Treatment

Deutsch[6] observed from his clinical sample of dying patients that the decline in vital processes is accompanied by a parallel decline in the intensity of instinctual aggressive and erotic drives. With the reduction of these drives, fear of dying is also reduced. The illness could be viewed by the patient as a hostile attack by an outside enemy, such as God or fate, or as a punishment for being bad. Because patients could complicate their conditions by reacting with increasing hostility toward outside objects or with self-punitive actions to offset guilt, Deutsch's therapeutic objective is a "settlement of differences." The ideal stage is reached when all guilt and aggression are dissipated.

The main forces in the psychiatrist's supportive relationship with his or her patients are the ability to share the patients' defenses and to develop a strong admiration for the patients' inner strength, beauty, intelligence, courage, and honesty. Kübler-Ross[7] described the unfinished business of the dying—reconciliations, resolution of conflicts, and pursuit of specific remaining hopes. Saunders[3] has stated that the aim is to keep patients feeling like themselves as long as possible. For her, dying is also a "coming together time" when patient, family, and staff help one another share the burden of saying appropriate good-byes. The LeShans[8,9] have deliberately chosen not to focus on dying (the minor problem) but to search aggressively with patients for what they wish to accomplish in living (the major problem). Weisman and Hackett[10] have coined the term "appropriate death." To achieve this, patients should (1) be relatively pain-free, (2) operate on as effective a level as possible within the limits of their disability, (3) recognize and resolve residual conflicts, (4) satisfy those remaining wishes that are consistent with their conditions and ego ideals, and (5) be able to yield control to others in whom they have confidence. Perhaps more important than any other principle is that the treatment be individualized. This can be accomplished only by getting to know the patient, responding to his needs and interests, proceeding at his pace, and allowing him to shape the manner in which those in attendance behave. There is no one "best" way to die.

Hospice Care of the Terminally Ill

Saunders[11] traces the notion of hospice therapeutics back to a treatise entitled "The Care of the Aged, the Dying and the Dead," written by a family physician for Harvard Medical School students. Using the work in pain control at St. Luke's Hospital in London, St. Joseph's Hospice continued development of the hospice concept. St. Christopher's opened in 1967 with Saunders as medical director, dedicated to enabling a patient, in her words, "to live to the limit of his or her potential in physical strength, mental and emotional capacity, and social relationships. . . . It is the alternative to the negative and socially dangerous suggestion that a patient with an incurable disease likely to cause suffering should have the legal option of actively hastened death, i.e., euthanasia."[11]

Lynn[12] provides a contemporary view of hospice; hospice provided home nursing, support of the family, spiritual counseling, pain treatment, medication, medical care, and some inpatient care for approximately 340,000 dying persons in 1994, of whom 80% had cancer. The average patient is enrolled about 1 month before death. Current hospice programs are not well adapted to meet the needs of patients who are dying from cardiovascular and pulmonary diseases, stroke, dementia, or chronic organ failure—largely because the timing of death is less predictable, and their final phases are less suited to hospice treatment.[12] Medicare requires that 80% of the hospice care days be spent at home, which means that dying patients, to qualify, must have a home and a family capable of providing care. The more intensive the supportive services required for this, the less affordable it will be. Lynn[12] advocates "a care delivery system . . . designed around the important priorities: relief of pain and other symptoms, maintenance of function and control, support of family and personal relationships, avoidance of impoverishment, trustworthiness and continuity, attentiveness to meaningful activities, and spiritual issues." Such a system would decrease priorities on medical treatment and increase them on caring.

The essential features of hospice care for cancer patients are described by Billings.[13] These techniques can be applied more widely to include patients dying from conditions other than cancer and acquired immune deficiency syndrome (AIDS). However, while hospice care is now an ideal that is strongly recommended,[14] it remains to be seen if it can be broadly applied given the fiscal constraints of contemporary health care.

Care and Management: Preliminary Considerations

Breaking Bad News

Because so many reactions to the news of diagnosis are possible, it is helpful to have some plan of action in mind ahead of time that will permit the greatest variation and freedom of response. When the diagnosis is made and it is time to inform the patient, it is best to begin by sitting down with the patient in a private place. Standing while conveying bad news is regarded by patients as unkind and expressive of wanting to leave as quickly as possible. The patient should be informed that when all the tests are completed, the physician will sit down with him or her again. The patient's spouse and family can be included in the discussion of the findings and the treatment. As that day approaches, the patient should be warned again. This permits those patients who wish to have no or minimal information to say so.

If the findings are unpleasant (e.g., a biopsy positive for malignancy), how can it best be conveyed? A good opening statement is one that is (1) rehearsed, so that it can be delivered calmly, (2) brief (three sentences or less), (3) designed to encourage further dialogue, and (4) reassuring of continued attention and care. A typical delivery might go as follows: "The tests confirmed that your tumor is malignant [the bad news]. I have therefore asked the surgeon [radiotherapist, oncologist] to come by to speak with you, examine you, and make recommendations for treatment [we will do something about it]. As things proceed, I will be by to discuss them with you and to figure out how we should proceed [I will stand by you]." Silence and quiet observation at this point yield more valuable information about the patient than any other part of the exchange. What are the emotional reactions? What sort of coping is seen at the start? While observing, one can decide on how best to continue with the discussion, but sitting with the patient for a period of time is the most valuable part of this initial encounter with a grim reality that both patient and physician will continue to confront together, possibly for a long time.

Telling the Truth

Without honesty, human relationships are destined for shipwreck. If truthfulness and trust are so obviously interdependent, how can there be so much conspiracy to avoid truth with the dying? The paradox is that for terminally ill patients, the need for both honesty and the avoidance of the truth can be intense. Osler is reputed to have said, "A patient has no more right to all the facts in my head than he does to all the medications in my bag." For example, a routine blood smear has just revealed that a 25-year-old man has acute myelogenous leukemia. If he were married and the father of two small children, should he be told the diagnosis?

Is the answer obvious? What if he had two prior psychotic breaks with less serious illnesses? What if his wife says he once said he never wanted to know if he had a malignancy?

Most empiric studies in which patients were asked whether or not they wanted to be told the truth about malignancy overwhelmingly indicated desire for truth. When 740 patients in a cancer detection clinic were asked before diagnosis if they wanted to be told their diagnosis, 99% said they did.[15] Another group in this same clinic was asked after the diagnosis was established, and 89% of them replied affirmatively, as did 82% of another group who had been examined and found to be free of malignancy. Gilbertsen and Wangensteen[16] asked the same questions of 298 survivors of surgery for gastric, colonic, and rectal cancers and found 82% wanted to be told the truth. The same investigators questioned 92 patients who had advanced cancer and were judged by their physicians to be preterminal and found that 73 (79%) of the patients thought they should be informed of their diagnosis.

The effects of blunt truth-telling have been studied empirically in both England and the United States. Aitken-Swan and Easson[17] were told by 7% of 231 patients who were explicitly informed of their diagnosis that the frankness of the consultant was resented. Gilbertsen and Wangensteen[16] observed that 4% of a sample of surgical patients became emotionally upset at the time they were told and appeared to remain so throughout the course of their illness. Gerle et al.[18] studied 101 patients that were divided into two groups. Members of one group were told, along with their families, the frank truth of their diagnoses. In the other group, an effort was made to maintain a conspiracy of silence, with family and physician excluding the patient from discussion of the diagnosis. At first, greater emotional upset appeared in the group in which patient and family were informed together, but the investigators observed in follow-up that the emotional difficulties of the families of those patients shielded from the truth far outweighed those of the patients and families that were told the diagnosis simultaneously. In general, empiric studies support the idea that truth is desired by terminally ill patients and does not harm those to whom it is given. Honesty sustains the relationship with a dying person rather than retarding it.

Dr. Hackett saw in consultation a 57-year-old housewife with metastatic breast cancer, now far advanced. She reported a persistent headache which she attributed to nervous tension and asked why she should be nervous. Turning the question back to her, he was told, "I am nervous because I have lost 60 pounds in a year. The priest comes to see me twice a week, which he never did before, and my mother-in-law is nicer to me even though I am meaner to her. Wouldn't this make you nervous?". . . [He] said to her, "You mean you think you're dying." "That's right, I do," she replied. He paused and said quietly, "You are." She smiled and said, "Well, I've finally broken the sound barrier; someone's finally told me the truth."[19]

Not all patients can be dealt with so directly. A nuclear physicist greeted his surgeon on the day following exploratory laparotomy with the words, "Lie to me, Steve." Individual variations in willingness to hear the initial diagnosis are extreme, and diagnosis is entirely different from prognosis. Many patients have said they were grateful to their physician for telling them they had a malignancy. Few, however, reacted positively to being told they are dying. In my experience, "Do I have cancer?" is a common question, whereas "Am I dying?" is a rare one. The question about dying is more commonly heard from patients who are dying rapidly, such as those in cardiogenic shock.

Physicians today generally prefer to tell cancer patients their diagnoses. Oken's 1961 study[20] documented that 90% of responding physicians preferred not to tell patients the diagnosis. When Novack et al.[21] repeated this questionnaire in 1979, 97% of responding physicians indicated a preference for telling the cancer patient the diagnosis. All of the physicians said that patients had a right to know.

Honest communication of the diagnosis (or of any truth) by no means precludes later avoidance or even denial of the truth. In two studies, patients who had been explicitly told their diagnosis (using the words *cancer* or *malignancy*) were asked 3 weeks later what they had been told. Nineteen percent of one sample[17] and 20% of the other[16] denied that their condition was cancerous or malignant. Likewise, Croog et al.[22] interviewed 345 men 3 weeks after myocardial infarction and were told by 20% of them that they had not had a heart attack. All had been explicitly told their diagnosis. For a person to function effectively, truth's piercing voice must occasionally be muted or even excluded from awareness.

In 4 consecutive days, for example, a man who had a widely spread bone cancer exhibited the following answers regarding his diagnosis. On the first day, he said he did not know what he had and did not like to ask questions. The second day, he said he was "riddled with cancer." On the third day, he didn't really know what ailed him. The fourth day, he said that even though nobody likes to die that was now his lot.

Truth-telling is no panacea. Communicating a diagnosis honestly, although difficult, is easier than the labors that lie ahead. Telling the truth is merely a way to begin; but because it is an open and honest way, it provides a firm basis on which to build a relationship of trust.

A Multiaxial Approach to Palliation

A comprehensive approach to palliative care includes attention to psychiatric, psychosocial, and spiritual suffering as well as to medical illness. The World Health Organization (WHO) defines palliative (or hospice) care as "The active total care of patients whose disease is not responsive to curative treatments."[23] This definition does not mention death, an acknowledgment of how this so upsets some patients that they will not accept hospice care even when it is desperately needed. This commonly presents an impasse to care. One may have to implore the patient to accept hospice care for the benefit of their family, and occasionally the physician and family may request hospice care despite the patient's opposition. The goals of palliative care can be simply expressed as aggressive minimization of the patient's burdens and maximization of quality of life. The latter generally is an effort to maximize independence and the number of options available for the dying person as well as an intense effort to make the most of the person's relationships. Although most understand palliation as aimed at physical comfort, this is gravely inadequate, and palliation of psychiatric, psychosocial, and spiritual suffering requires formal consideration and effort.

Some persons, faced with death, come to regard suicide or euthanasia as the most appealing option. Why? The most frequent reasons euthanasia is requested in the Netherlands are loss of dignity, 57%; pain, 46% (but when pain is the only reason, this was 5%); unworthy dying, 46%; being dependent on others, 33%; and being tired of life, 23%.[24] A recent study of Oregon hospice caregivers showed that patients requested assisted suicide to control death, to die at home (because continued life seemed pointless), and to be ready to die.[25] These reasons are all ultimately psychosocial. Psychosocial suffering as we see from this, is even worse than physical suffering, and it requires aggressive palliation. To cover all forms of psychosocial suffering, the multiaxial system of *The Diagnostic and Statistical Manual of Mental Disorders (DSM-IV)*[26] is useful and is employed here for that purpose.

Bereavement

Pending separation by death should focus the efforts of the patient and everyone significant on loss. The basic therapeutic message of the LeShans[8,9] is to remind the patient that "Death is the minor problem, what you do until then is a major problem, and we can work on that." In the realm of relationships, the core work of the dying person is what has to be done to help those who love him or her accept and integrate his or her loss. Each relationship needs to be examined for unfinished business. A young mother of three, even though stricken with a fatal illness, remains her children's mother. Caring and planning for them can preoccupy her constructively, giving her concrete goals to attain and a way to sustain self-esteem in her efforts.

Likewise, the core task for those who love the dying person is what they can do to make the time more comfortable and meaningful, and they must examine their relationships to the dying person. Cassell[27] has observed that an individual life lived is a work of art: what sort of ending can be fitting and expressive of this person's life, what death can he or she be proud of, and what preparation will begin for a memorial with which the bereaved can live comfortably. What frightens most when death is announced on the horizon is the loss of a loved one, although other relationships may also be threatened. Help that rallies all to strengthen and improve their relationships addresses the most frightening aspect of death, loss that feels like abandonment.

Axis I

Major Depression

The more seriously ill a person becomes, the more likely the person is to develop major depression.[28] Because few forms of human suffering match or exceed major depression, careful vigilance for its appearance is necessary, as is aggressive treatment when it appears. Suicidal ideation, rather than accepted immediately as understandable, requires the same thoughtful examination demanded in any other circumstance. Weisman[29] formulated the wish to die as an existential signal that the person's conviction "that his potential for being someone who matters has been exhausted." Ganzini et al.[30] documented that severely depressed patients make more restricted advance directives when depressed and change them after they reach remission. At Memorial Sloan Kettering Hospital, Breitbart and Holland[31] compared terminally ill cancer and AIDS patients with suicidal ideation to similar patients without suicidal ideation. The primary difference was the presence of depression in the patients with suicidal thoughts. Chochinov[32] in a Winnipeg palliative care unit studied the patients who wished that death be hastened. Sixty-two percent met diagnostic criteria for major depression.

Anxiety

Anxiety disorders may or may not intensify during a terminal illness, but clearly they require psychiatric attention when they do. Impending death can generate severe anxiety in the patients facing it, in their families and their friends, and in those who take care of them. When panic, phobia, generalized anxiety, and the other conditions listed in the differential diagnostic outline of Chapter 15 have been sought by the consultant and not found, the four most common fears associated with death are (1) helplessness or loss of control, (2) being bad (guilt and punishment), (3) physical injury or symbolic injury (castration), and (4) abandonment.[6,33]

In the clinical examination, a severely anxious patient usually does not know what it is about death that is so frightening. Memories of someone who died of the same illness or associations to the illness may produce specific material (e.g., it will be painful or disfiguring). Truly disruptive anxiety states are usually related to the patient's developmental history: defective ability to trust or unresolved dependency conflicts (e.g., the fear of helplessness and the loss of control). Conflicts over guilt and castration are lifelong. The worst anxiety encountered may be that associated with defective maternal bonding, in which abandonment appears to be the object of fear. Characteristic would be the dying daughter, now overwhelmed by anxiety she can neither pinpoint nor understand, for whom separation from her mother had always been a major unresolved issue. Where the mother is available and willing, therapy of both simultaneously can be helpful, but because death's separation seems so irreversibly final, considerable discomfort may remain throughout the time left for treatment.

Increased anxiety may be associated with specific memories and associations to the death of parents or to others one identifies with (as the woman whose family members died of breast cancer or the AIDS patient who tended to a lover dying of it), in which the patient pictures the same fate for himself or herself (e.g., agonizing pain or a violent scenario with excessive use of technology). Such stories may not come to light without explicit questions.

Delirium and Dementia

Cognitive difficulties are common. Concomitant confusion, wandering, sundowning, agitation, and belligerence add significant distress for everyone involved. Successful control of these difficulties (see Chapters 12 and 13) makes an invaluable contribution to the care of the dying.

Axis II

Individual traits are defining and taken for granted. Some complicate relationships, and during the last phase of life they may pose serious obstacles, at least to some onlookers, to harmonious relations and quality of life. One skilled in handling traits such as dependency, passive aggressiveness hostility, and a histrionic style can provide useful advice for caregivers and family that lighten the burdens of everyone. When the traits reach the realm of personality disorder, care may be halted until professional intervention comes to the rescue.

Dependency on others is hard for many to tolerate. It was third on the list of reasons why those in the Netherlands requested euthanasia. One of the demands of maturity is to accept help from those we trust. Yet resolves like, "If I have to be dressed and diapered by someone else, that is where I draw the line," are not uncommon when persons think about the end of life. It is perhaps inevitable that we fear being a burden to others, especially those we love. Nevertheless, it may be helpful to ask the patient who objects to the work imposed by the illness on family whether they feel that this is an unacceptable burden or an opportunity to give something back to the dying person. As such, it may be one of life's more meaningful activities.

Among the most unfortunate of dying persons are those in the severely narcissistic or borderline range of personality, as well as some persons with a history of severe physical and sexual abuse. For such a person, a fatal illness is but one more act of brutal victimization. Unfortunately, it may be difficult to believe that any physician, nurse, or caregiver will do anything to them but victimize them further. Help is therefore hard if not impossible to accept and trust. Only a professional with superior psychodynamic diagnostic and treatment skills may help such a person accept palliative care.

Axis III

Palliation of the effects of the medical illness is a complex challenge requiring extensive expertise. Freedom from pain is basic to every care plan and should be achievable in 90% of cases. Pain control for the cancer patient is described in detail in Chapter 21. Unfortunately, palliation is often equated simply with pain control. Even though pain control in itself is so simple in concept that any medical student can master the principles in a few days, physicians are repeatedly indicted for undertreatment of pain, whether for outpatients with metastatic cancer,[34] terminal AIDS patients,[35] or patients dying in prominent academic center intensive care units (ICUs).[36] The same deficiencies are reported in house staff[37] and nurses,[38] although nurses with more education know significantly more.[38] In his presidential address to the annual meeting of the Society of Critical Care Medicine, Hoyt[39] said the ICU study "suggested that ICU physicians did not listen to families. They did not know when to stop treatment. They did not relieve pain and suffering." Fear of addiction and harsh regulatory threats continue to be cited as reasons for this perplexing failure.[40,41] Guidelines for cancer pain management are widely publicized and available.[42,43]

Palliative care includes a vast number of problems more complicated than analgesia for nociceptive pain and is the subject of several texts.[14,44-46] Table 23-2 presents a list of the practical problems commonly found in the care of the terminally ill. This subject is covered in detail by Billings.[13] If one claims to be committed to keeping the terminally ill person comfortable until death comes, one must be prepared, at the very least, to manage common difficulties. The American Board of Internal Medicine has made available an educational resource document on palliative care for all physicians.[47]

Table 23.2. Practical Problems of the Terminally Ill

Pain control
Nausea and vomiting
Hiccoughs
Anorexia and nutritional care
Constipation, diarrhea, gastrointestinal problems
Incontinence, obstruction, hepatic encephalopathy
Mouth problems and dysphagia
Dyspnea, cough, respiratory symptoms, and death rattle
Urinary tract symptoms
Incontinence, indwelling catheters, renal failure and obstruction
Skin problems
Pruritus, pressure sores
Fungating tumors and ulcerating wounds
Odor, bleeding, drainage, and fistulas
Fluid accumulation
Edema, ascites, and pleural/pericardial effusions
Dehydration
Neuropsychiatric symptoms and brain tumors
Weakness and fatigue
Spinal cord compression and spasticity
Infections, fevers, and sweats
Anemia and transfusions
Emergencies
Superior vena cava syndrome and pathologic fractures

Adapted from Billings JA: *Outpatient management of advanced cancer,* Philadelphia, 1985, JB Lippincott.

Axis IV

In the *DSM-IV*, Axis IV is used to categorize psychosocial stressors, and in this section the focus is on the specific relationships that the dying person has with the psychosocial environment.

Family

For family and close friends, a fatal illness may be the only reality important enough to resolve long-standing conflicts. Comments to children such as, "No mother wants to die with the thought that her children will never speak to one another again," may motivate individuals to rally to their mother and cooperate to ease her last months. Reconciliation may also result. Likewise, the psychiatrist can say to the family gathered around the patient, "I hope many years from now none of you will think 'If only I had told Dad/Bill this or that.' You have time for that now." When conflicts are apparent, direct comments can be made. Making peace should be high on the agenda. Specific plans for the family are important: wills, a correct family history, what sort of a funeral or memorial service to have, and so on.

The end of life is an opportunity to give a gift to the younger generation. When they are included in all the planning, the meetings, the discussions, the activities, the care, and the final attendance at death, children learn that death need not be violent or terrifying and that the answer to being threatened is contained in the loss itself, when all loved ones rally to put finishing touches on the relationships that are threatened. We face our losses best together.

Occupation and Work

Work has been critical for the self-esteem of many persons. The relationships made in the course of one's occupation should be activated so that self-esteem can be maintained and the sense given of a life lived meaningfully. The dying person is often too disabled to get around easily; hence, mobilization of friends, especially friends who have been out of touch, needs deliberate attention. Many begin to feel less valuable when work ceases or they retire. For them, the end of life may intensify a sense of failure. Seeing old friends can remind a dying person who he or she is, what he or she accomplished, and that he or she is still remembered and respected regardless of the illness.

Role of Religious Faith and Value Systems

Investigation of the relationship between religious faith and attitudes toward death has been hampered by differences in methodology. Lester[48] and Feifel[49] have reviewed much of the conflicting literature on the relationship between religious faith and the fear of death. Other research has tried to clarify the way belief systems function within the individual. Allport[50] contrasted an extrinsic religious orientation in which religion is mainly a means to social status, security, or relief from guilt, with an intrinsic religious orientation, in which the values appear to be internalized and subscribed to as ends in themselves. Feagin[51] provided a useful 21-item questionnaire to distinguish between these two types of believers. Experimental work[52] and clinical experience indicate that an extrinsic value system, without internalization, seems to offer no assistance in coping with a fatal illness. A religious commitment that is intrinsic appears to offer considerable stability and strength to those who possess it.

One way of examining personal faith is to regard it as another personal relationship, this time with God. Although psychiatric training has often made practitioners suspicious of, hostile to, or uncomfortable with anything associated with religion, people who have a strong internalized faith possess a resource that helps significantly to negotiate a fatal illness. Exploration of this area is mandatory.

Many patients are grateful for the chance to express their own thoughts about their faith. Faith is simply framed in a psychological perspective as a relationship between the person and God. The patient is asked about God with the same questions used to assess the quality of relationship with a parent, friend, or any significant other. For you, what sort of a person is God? Do you picture God? Where? In what historical context was God introduced to you? Warm, secure, pleasant? Cold, scrutinizing, punitive? Does God regard you as a favorite? A black sheep? What sort of trust is there, you for God and vice versa? Does this sense of relationship give you confidence that God truly exists? What is the most powerful sense you have had of God's presence? Do you doubt? When you doubt, how is the sense of relationship affected? In general, the person's ability to tolerate doubt is a good index of the maturity of faith. If we knew, faith would be unnecessary. Doubt, as Baum said, is the shadow cast by faith.

Do you communicate with God? Do you pray? Do you feel heard? Is communication a two-way process? Do you have any sense of God speaking to you? How? Do you get answers or ever feel certain of getting a message in return? Do you (ever) feel "in touch?" Cared about? Do prayers ever feel like "dead letters" sent to an unoccupied address? What then?

Discussing the terminal illness provides an excellent chance to inquire about the patient's view of the age-old problem of evil. Given such a severe or life-threatening illness, just where does God stand in this? Sympathetic? If all good and loving, how could God permit it to happen to you? Do you feel supported? Punished? Justly punished? Betrayed? Are you still able to pray? How has all this affected your prayer or dialogue with God?

When conversation touches on death, it is an opportunity to ask about afterlife. Is there anything after? Do you ever picture it? Does this comfort you somehow or in any way ease some aspects of this illness? In general, those persons who possess a sense of a benign personal presence of God, of being cared for and watched over, will continue to do so, and it will help to maintain tranquillity in their struggle with terminal illness. Firm religious convictions signal that a consultation with the chaplain should be discussed with the patient. The patient's own minister or rabbi, if available, usually can provide many valuable facts and insights about the patient and family and help uniquely to smooth the overall course before death.

Religious persons ordinarily have a community of believers who can be unusually thoughtful and generous in providing support. They may not have been informed of the patient's plight and they need to be contacted. Does the person feel some need of reconciliation to God or to the community? Should the personal clergyperson be contacted?

For those without religious ties, strong convictions about life and values may be coded in a philosophy of life. What is important? What principles or guidelines have you tried to live by? Is there anything worth dying for? What are you proudest of? These issues are the material out of which a dying person may confirm a sense of a life lived well enough. If important persons have rallied to the patient, there may also be the sense of living on in their memories as an intact and valued person.

Recreational Activities Shared with Others

Isolation can be painful and a source of suffering itself. The detailed personal information about a patient at the end of life should include the groups he or she joined to pursue interests or recreation. From bridge and bingo, to sports as participant or fan, to political activism, travel, and the local "haunts" of the individual, activities generate clues to persons or groups who may be able to contribute meaning to the patient's last days. Having a serious illness is itself justification for forming new relationships, and self-help groups have been exceptionally helpful for all kinds of sufferers.

Society

A dying person may be burdened by shame for actions censored or disapproved of by others. A person who has committed a crime, hurt a loved one, abandoned a family, or been disabled by a chronic disease may feel disowned by society. The intense work with caregivers and friends to get through the end of life with courage and graciousness can establish in such a person a sense of being respected as a worthwhile, even admirable, human being.

Psychoeducational Group Treatment

Cancer patients who participate in a psychoeducational treatment group gain significant advantages, including improvement in mood, reduction in anxiety, and knowledge about more adaptive coping skills. The most dramatic benefit demonstrated so far is the significant prolongation of life demonstrated for patients with both breast cancer[53] and melanoma.[54]

Axis V

In *DSM-IV*, Axis V is an estimate of global function. Here function is used as synonymous with the goals of palliative care: that quality of life be maximized with it and to the extent that a person can function as he or she wishes, the work of others provides the critical assistance.

When things go well, care of the dying is a process of mutual growth. Just as the deterioration of another trapped by a fatal disease can be threatening (we feel both horrified at the prospect of the same happening to us and helpless to assist), the response of the dying person to the challenge may be not only edifying but also an invaluable lesson in coping.

Nonabandonment is one of the most important principles in this work. Despite frustration, seemingly unsolvable problems, and relentless deterioration, one must learn that presence itself is of value. Most patients who have lost the ability to communicate have a period when they can still hear or perceive those in attendance. Although the patient may never be able to tell us how important that time is, an occasional incident does so dramatically, as when a supposed unconscious person suddenly smiles appropriately or even speaks. At those times, one's knowledge of the person makes conversation with the family easy or, when the patient is alone for the regular visit, makes conversing possible (e.g., by reporting on something in the news known to be of interest, such as "The Red Sox are only one game out of first place"). It is hoped that this mutual work at the end of life will have ratified the dying person's sense of self and helped the family, friends, and caregivers have a sense they have provided good care and safe passage.

Difficulties of Those Who Care for the Dying

First in psychological importance among the caregiver's responsibilities to the dying person is to understand. To do this, as Saunders[55] says, is "above all to listen." What is the experience like? A suffering person often wants to communicate how awful a fatal illness is. Words are often irrelevant. "When no answers exist," says Saunders, "one can offer silent attention."

The best way to recognize and acknowledge the person's worth is to get to know those features of their history and their nature that make them unique. The empathic effort takes its toll most often by the insights the patients give us about ourselves. Their needs and vulnerabilities bring us face-to-face with our own. The relentless approach of death for a patient with cancer or AIDS may leave the patient with feelings of terror, hopelessness, and despair, which tend to be contagious, intensifying our feelings of impotence

At this point, caregivers' own helplessness and despair may endanger the patient, causing the caregiver to avoid or neglect the patient, retreat, or even, feeling the patient would be better off dead, convey to him or her how burdensome he or she is to caregivers. This could be devastating to the helpless person who looks to his or her physician or nurse for some sense of hope. Hence, the greatest psychological requirement for caregivers is learning to live with these negative feelings and resist the urge to avoid the patients—actions that convey to the patient, not that it is difficult for the caregivers, but that the patient no longer matters. Fortunately, most patients, feeling that they are acceptable to their caregivers no matter how scared, disfigured, or miserable they are, find resources within and make what they can of each day. That sort of shared experience is an opportunity to grow for both persons.

Certain traits make these empathic difficulties hazardous for some caregivers. Dependent persons who expect patients to appreciate, thank, love, and nurture them are unconsciously prone to exhaust themselves regularly because they "can't do too much," a pattern that may be sustainable for a patient with the capacity to nurture the caregiver but that has a disastrous outcome when the patient is completely depleted or intractably hostile. The harder the caregiver strives, the less rewarding the work. Exhaustion and demoralization follow. Some caregivers want to please every physician they consult and come to similar exhaustion because many of these patients cannot improve.

Ethical Decisions at the End of Life

Seven years after the automobile accident that left her in a persistent vegetative state, Nancy Cruzan's feeding tube was removed. She died 12 days later. Her parents' request that the tube be removed initiated a journey that took them through the Missouri and Federal courts, to the U.S. Supreme Court, and, ultimately, back to the original Missouri trial court, which once again authorized removal of the tube. Within an hour of the trial court's decision, the hospital administrator, Donald C. Lamkins, tried unsuccessfully to move her elsewhere. When she died a few weeks later, three dozen armed guards patrolled the hospital premises to guarantee control at the scene where there were unsuccessful legal attempts of several antieuthanasia groups to force reinsertion of the tube. Shortly before the sixth anniversary of Nancy Cruzan's death, another tragic note was sounded by the suicide of her father, Joseph.

The Supreme Court's decision in Cruzan's case reaffirmed most of the major lower court decisions that have helped patients, families, physicians, and hospitals resolve decisions about treatment for incurable illness,[56] specifically: First, competent patients have the right to refuse treatment. Second, forgoing nutrition and hydration is no different from forgoing other medical treatment, such as artificial ventilation or pressor agents. Third, Missouri (and other states) could require "clear and convincing evidence" that the patient, while still competent, had rejected the idea of life-sustaining treatment under such circumstances. But states are also free to adopt less rigorous standards.

The Cruzan decision does not alter any of the standards, laws, or clinical practices that have evolved since the Quinlan case in 1976.[57] During this time, guidelines and principles have been established that enable patients, families, and physicians to reach medically sound, ethical treatment decisions in cases of irreversible illness. As a result, and despite widespread physician feeling to the contrary, these treatment decisions are almost devoid of litigation danger. Nevertheless, physicians should work with their hospital attorneys to clarify the status of legislation and case law on these issues in their particular jurisdiction.

Principles of Ethics at the End of Life

A brief discussion of principles is not intended to supplant the need for concrete individualized judgments for every patient. Principles provide anchor points from which clinical reasoning can proceed, specifically when limitations or stoppage of life-supporting treatment is proposed.

First Principle

The primary obligation of the physician to the patient in traditional medical ethics has been expressed in both positive and negative terms. The negative goal, always referred to as first, is not to harm the patient *(primum non nocere)*. The positive obligation is to restore health or relieve suffering, or both. Our contemporary dilemma, as Slater[58] has pointed out, arose because we now have many situations in which these two aims come into conflict (i.e., the more aggressive the efforts to reverse an incurable illness, the more suffering is inflicted on the patient). If a 70-year-old man with large cell cancer of the lung presents himself for treatment and is found to have metastatic spread of the disease to the other lung and to his liver, any treatment of the cancer is guaranteed to make him feel even worse and probably not even extend his survival. This first principle sums up the medical ethics of the 1950s and 1960s: Do what is best for the patient.

Second Principle

The principle of autonomy has sometimes been stated: Let the will of the patient, not the health of the patient, be the supreme law. This principle guarantees any competent patient the right to refuse any treatment, even a life-saving one. This was the emphasis of the medical ethics of the 1970s and 1980s and focused on refusing life-prolonging treatment, such as mechanical ventilation, and more recently, nutrition and hydration. Honoring such refusals presupposes that the patient is competent (see Chapter 22).

Forgoing versus Stopping.   Patients and families need to know that treatments, such as mechanical ventilation, may actually clarify just how good the chances of recovery are, can be tried until that is clear, and then can be stopped when it is clear that health (or the extent of recovery acceptable to the patient) cannot be restored. Generally, it is psychologically more difficult to stop such a treatment once it is started, but what justified its use in the first place was its relationship to recovery. The ventilator was used because the physician thought the patient might get better. Once it is clear that the patient will not recover, it is no longer necessary.

When the patient is not competent, there are several ways to resolve treatment decisions. The most help is provided when the patient has left a living will or advance directive or appointed a durable power of attorney or a health care proxy to help make decisions should the patient become incompetent. Even when such clarity is not present, common sense should be followed, and the incompetent patient's next of kin should be asked to provide a substituted judgment about what the patient would have wanted.

When Should Treatment Be Limited?   Whenever the risks or burdens of a treatment appear to outweigh the benefits, use of that treatment should be questioned by both physician and patient. The amputation of a poorly vascularized foot, for example, would ordinarily be postponed by patient and physician until life with the foot seems more burdensome than life without it.

Ordinarily, limitation of life-prolonging treatment is reserved for three categories of patients. First, patients whose illness is judged irreversible and who are moribund need to be protected from needlessly burdensome treatments. This is widely accepted for patients who will die with or without treatment, such as the patient with advanced metastatic cancer or the patient with end-stage cardiomyopathy in whom a transplant is not possible. Because of the right to refuse treatment, competent patients who are not moribund but who have an irreversible illness have also been allowed to have life-sustaining treatments stopped. (Competent patients with a reversible illness have the right to refuse any treatment, including life-saving treatments.)

Irreversible Coma.   When irreversible coma has been established, the standard medical recommendation to the next of kin or surrogate would be to stop all life-sustaining treatment, including nutrition and hydration. Even were there are no family or next of kin for the patient with irreversible coma, standard medical practice would allow the patient to die, acknowledging the inevitability of death and the futility of any treatment to prevent it.

Persistent Vegetative State.   Typically, the patient in a persistent vegetative state develops coma, as after a cardiac arrest or severe head trauma, then enters a state of permanent unconsciousness with restoration of periods of wakefulness and physiologic sleep.[59] The eyes may open spontaneously but do not track. The patient has a functioning brain stem with total loss of cortical function.[60,61] The standard of medical practice remains less fully formed for this medical condition. The American Academy of Neurology has taken a position, adopted by us, based on the pathophysiology of the condition and recommends that all life-sustaining treatment, "because it is of no medical benefit to the patient," be withdrawn.[60] The recommendation to withdraw treatments includes nutrition and hydration. The American Medical Association's Council on Scientific Affairs and Council on Ethical and Judicial Affairs provided a statement with diagnostic criteria and data supporting them that maintains the balance between patient preferences and the accuracy of the diagnosis, concluding that even if death is not imminent, "it is not unethical to discontinue all means of life-prolonging medical treatment."[62] Judging when to limit treatment may seem impossible at times. An aortic valve replacement for a suddenly decompensated 80-year-old man in otherwise good health is usually imperative. If he has impaired renal and pulmonary function, both he and his physician may begin to wonder whether a decision to operate will only condemn him to a nightmare of suffering that will end in death. If the patient has widely disseminated large cell cancer of the lung, valve replacement would be unethical and inhumane; the sudden cardiac decompensation would provide a merciful death. Abstract principles cannot solve clinical dilemmas. Rather, principles serve as points about which relevant clinical judgments and patient preferences become more sharply focused. Will benefit exceed suffering? Or does one condition (e.g., cancer, acute respiratory distress syndrome, or AIDS) so overshadow another (e.g., gangrene, aortic insufficiency, or pneumonia) that the benefits of a treatment (e.g., amputation, valve replacement, or use of antibiotics) are negated?

Decisions to Maintain, to Limit, or to Stop Life-Prolonging Treatment.   The guidelines for the framework that follows were developed through more than 25 years of experience by the Optimum Care Committee (OCC) of the Massachusetts General Hospital (MGH).[63] Over the past 20 years, a massive consensus has developed on the ethics of forgoing life-sustaining treatments in the severely ill. From the President's commission statement of 1983,[64] and continuing with input from the Task Force on Ethics of the Society of Critical Care Medicine,[65] a core set of principles governing decisions about life-prolonging treatments has emerged.

Hospital Admission.   On admission to the hospital, patient and family can be assured that any device or technology available to restore health will be used to its fullest potential. Yet, aware that hospitals and intensive care units are often criticized for pursuing treatments that cause more harm than good, patients can be reassured that the hospital's and the physicians' policy is to protect patients from treatments that will not make them better but will only make them suffer more.

Clinical Judgment on Irreversibility.   At what point is the physician clinically sure that the patient is now going to die whether treatment continues or not? When is treatment only going to prolong dying? These are the questions that cause great concern to patients and to families. These prognostic judgments are fallible clinical conclusions, but all turn to the physician to make them. At what point in recovery from coma is it clear that the chance of regaining significant cognitive function is virtually nonexistent? For the AIDS patient battling *Pneumocystis carinii* pneumonia, when does it become likely that resorting to mechanical ventilation, once started, will become permanently essential for continued breathing? (This patient can be reassured that if he or she accepts the recommendation of a ventilator, the patient can indicate that it should be withdrawn once there is clinical certainty that he or she cannot live without it.) The physician on whom this judgment falls experiences heavy responsibility. Reassurance is sometimes necessary, with the reminder that the questioner realizes nothing can be foretold with 100% accuracy in clinical medicine. Unfortunately, where families are angry or litigation is feared, physicians with this responsibility may feel too vulnerable or intimidated to say what they think. The best clinical judgments of patient prognosis should be documented in the medical record. As they change, so should the documentation.

Consultation.   Specialty consultation may be required to clarify further prognostic judgments. Sometimes patients or families ask for a second opinion. These consultants also need encouragement to be explicitly honest and state in the record that in their experience chances of recovery from an illness this severe are unprecedented, or virtually nil, or essentially nonexistent (e.g., "in my experience, neurologic damage of this extent is not compatible with recovery of cortical function").

Autonomy and the Patient's Preferences.   Balancing the physician's judgment are the patient's view of acceptable risks, definition of quality of life, and attitudes toward pain. In the course of battling metastatic cancer with adjuvant chemotherapy, how many treatments will the patient accept, especially if the oncologist has begun to express reservations about the degree of response? One person might grasp at any chance of halting tumor spread no matter how debilitating the treatment. Another might, on hearing the oncologist's reservation, express relief at the chance to back off because of how unacceptable the side effects of treatment are. In this way, patients and physicians together work out the risk-benefit calculus, which results in the final clinical decision about maintaining or forgoing treatment. Because patient attitudes can change, ongoing dialogue is indispensable for clarifying understanding on both sides.

Autonomy applies to accepting or refusing appropriate medical treatment. Just as a patient cannot demand that a surgeon amputate a disease-free leg, a patient does not have the right to demand a treatment that the physician regards as inappropriate. Such a conflict can be painful. When an oncologist, discovering progressive cancer spread and severe treatment side effects, can no longer in conscience prescribe the treatment, this is conveyed to the patient. Many patients have expressed acute dismay and protest, some continuing despite physician avowals that the chemotherapy can do nothing at this time but harm. Some physicians have resolved this by lowering the dose to a nontoxic level but find this unsatisfying because they believe it is dishonest. Usually, such patients believe that stopping anticancer treatment is stopping the fight against cancer, that it is "giving up," that without chemotherapy or radiation there "will be no hope." It is often beneficial to give such patients time (e.g., overnight) to consider what has been said, then to encourage them to describe exactly what it is that has kept them going satisfactorily to this point. Whatever it is, it has helped the patients even when chemotherapy seems to have been impotent against the tumor, causing only unwanted effects. In talking to those who say there will be no hope, our favorite question has been, "Hope for what?" Often, such patients have then reviewed what has been told them from the beginning (e.g., that the malignancy cannot be cured, but that with aggressive palliation the best possible existence for them would be the goal to maintain).

Competent patients can make irrational choices.[66] On hearing that a patient refuses a simple and routine life-saving procedure, physicians are obliged to explore further. It may be a Jehovah's Witness, legitimately refusing a blood transfusion. It could also be a patient who completely misunderstands or has irrational fears of the treatment. More common is the occasional patient who insists on cardiopulmonary resuscitation (CPR) and does not agree to a do-not-resuscitate (DNR) order. Most of these patients do not understand the implications of the DNR order, thinking that after a cardiac arrest a simple procedure will restore them completely. Others may be overwhelmed and unable to process the conversation. Time, discussion with the patient and family together, psychiatric consultation, and recourse to an ethics committee can help resolve these dilemmas.

The Incompetent Patient. Conflict in discussions about forgoing treatment arises most often when the patient is incompetent. When a patient has no advance directive about life-sustaining treatment, surrogates may feel insecure, which makes decisions about life-prolonging treatments difficult. Conflicts tend to rise in such uncertainty and can arise within the treatment team (e.g., nurses regard the treatments as inhumane, whereas physicians wish to pursue them), between the team and the primary physician, between specialties (e.g., anesthesia and surgery), between family members, and between family members and the team. When decisions about life-prolonging treatment reach an impasse of intense conflict, most commonly the family is angry and distrustful of the caregiver team. Such a family, if discussion cannot resolve the tension, can be asked to select a person they

trust (e.g., family physician, clergyperson, or attorney) to confer with the team. This person may help clarify and resolve misunderstandings. The team members may consult other specialists about alternate treatment options for the patient, or they can consult an ethics committee (at the MGH that committee is the OCC).

Process for Resolving Conflicts Over the Use of Life-Prolonging Treatments. It is important that the treatment team knows what its recommendation is and determines the source of the conflict. (1) A meeting is held with the entire family (especially if the conflict is primarily with the designated spokesperson and other family members that may have differing opinions), the team, essential consultants, ethics committee representatives (if invited), and the family's trusted person (if existent). Some partial agreement may occur and another meeting scheduled, as long as there appears to be progress. (2) If there is no resolution, the family can be informed that the care of the patient can be transferred to another physician in the same hospital or to another hospital, if the family wishes that. If the family does not wish such a transfer or the patient cannot be transferred (e.g., the other institution refuses to accept the patient, or the patient is too sick), the family members can be informed that they can have recourse to the Probate Court for a determination. If the team remains clear about its treatment recommendation, there is no reason for the team to consult the Probate Court now; if uncertain, the team should have done so earlier.

Futile Treatment. Conflicts that require the measures previously mentioned often center on treatments that either the family or the treatment team regards as futile, but agreement cannot be reached. In many cases, when a patient is irreversibly ill and dying, resuscitation is simply not an option and is futile.[65,67–69] For example, for a patient whose glioblastoma has advanced to the point at which the patient is semicomatose and he or she will die with or without treatment, CPR is not a medical option. Application of it is contrary to the standards of medical practice, unethical, and inhumane. The family who asks that CPR and all life-saving treatments be withheld or withdrawn from such a patient should be obeyed by the physician inclined to provide it. Likewise, in such a case, the physician does not have a duty to consult anyone before writing a DNR order. We recommend that the physician take the opportunity to remind the family just how severe the illness is and that appropriate attention is being given to the needs of the patient: "It is important for you to know that your father's condition has reached the point where he will die with treatment or without it. We will direct every effort to maintaining his comfort and dignity. Treatments like resuscitation or countershock would only brutalize him and he has been protected from them by specific written order."

Defining futility is currently a major goal of medical ethics.[70] The negative right of refusal has become transformed by some into a positive right to demand any life-sustaining treatment. Others argue that physicians have a duty not to offer or provide treatments that are ineffective.[71] Because most risk/benefit considerations of life-prolonging treatment involve value judgments, and since the principle of autonomy requires that the patient's values come first, some argue that objective standards for futility are impossible to formulate and physicians should make no such judgments.[72] For patients in irreversible coma, and increasingly for those in a persistent vegetative state, however, life-prolonging treatments are seen as futile. For example, more than 90% of neurologists and medical directors responding to a 1996 survey thought that patients in the persistent vegetative state would be "better off dead" and almost 50% thought patients in the persistent vegetative state should be considered dead.[73]

No physician is required to provide harmful treatments to a patient; the principle of beneficence obligates the physician not to do so. No physician is required to provide useless treatments either. CPR for the above-mentioned moribund patient with a glioblastoma is useless (and harmful because it violates the patient's dignity). If a moribund patient with breast cancer had metastasis-riddled ribs and disseminated intravascular coagulopathy, CPR is harmful because it would probably kill her (by causing fatal hemorrhage). Even if the patient were competent, a physician should not offer CPR if harm without resuscitation is the outcome judged clinically likely.

Informed consent is not necessary for either a useless or a harmful treatment. One could even argue that asking for consent (or enlightened refusal) could be itself harmful. The patient is likely to be confused as to why he or she was presented with a treatment that the physician considered useless or harmful. So, too, one could argue that no substituted judgment is required when the treatment is either useless or harmful. One judge of the Massachusetts Superior District Court ruled that for a terminally ill patient who was going to die with or without treatment within a short time, life-prolonging treatments are futile.

These controversial questions about defining treatments as futile will most likely be resolved as the Houston citywide consortium of hospitals has done, setting up a panel of experts to judge on the futility of a treatment, after hearing all evidence presented by family, team, and others.[74]

Documentation. The medical record should be explicit and complete about the judgment of irreversibility and the prognosis, documenting that the patient or family or both have been informed and their reactions and wishes, the limitation of treatment and its reasons, and any discussion or dissent and how it was resolved. Orders in the order book should also be explicit about treatments to be stopped or not started. The latter is particularly necessary to guide house staff, nurses, and others who may be called on in the absence of the primary physician to attend the patient in the event of acute worsening or cardiopulmonary arrest.

Agreement. Once agreement occurs, decisions can be made. If life-sustaining treatment is to be forgone, it is important to chart for the family the consequences of this omission. If no ventilator will be used should the *P. carinii* pneumonia worsen in an AIDS patient, a morphine intravenous infusion will be started as soon as there is sign of respiratory distress, and it will be increased enough to suppress breathlessness or any sense of suffocation. Of course, that may produce loss of consciousness, but if that is necessary, it is routinely done without hesitation. No further transfusions will be given to halt hemorrhage from a metastatic colon cancer lesion. But hemorrhage is one of the gentlest ways to die, and comfort can usually be assured without difficulty. Hydration can be cruel if maintained in the vegetative patient for whom feeding and all curative treatments have been stopped; hydration alone can prolong dying by 2 or 3 weeks. Hospice care avoids intravenous feeding in helping patients die at home; moisture for the mucous membranes is what is needed for comfort. The point is to detoxify the concept of death, so often traumatic or violent in the minds of patients or families.

New Therapeutic Goals.   Whenever a decision is made to limit treatment, the new goal must be clearly articulated (i.e., the relief of suffering and aggressive efforts to make the patient's living as dignified and becoming as possible). Foremost in this are the intensive nursing efforts that provide comprehensive, compassionate attention to breathing, secretions, pressure sores, turning, bathing, odors, and numerous other challenging problems for which such impressive remedies exist. All medical orders must be reexamined in light of the comfort goal. Dressing changes that are unnecessarily painful, venipuncture for laboratory tests, diagnostic procedures, antibiotics, and indwelling lines may be removed if not contributing. Pressor infusions may be stopped or maintained but not increased. Monitors may be removed unless their help in forecasting an arrhythmic death is wanted.

Death is now inevitable. The family needs must also be examined and addressed. Even though time of death cannot be predicted accurately, do family wish to be present at that moment? Do they wish clergy to be notified? If family members do not wish to be present, they may want to know that they will be quickly informed when the patient worsens or dies.

Request for Assisted Suicide or Euthanasia. Sprung,[75] reviewing trends in critical care and reactions to them in 1990, concluded that active euthanasia programs will arise in the United States in the near future. Indeed, since then, the issue of physician-assisted suicide has become a prominent legal and political issue. The call for physician involvement in ending life can be viewed as the public's condemnation of at least two things: the way hospitals and physicians excessively treat the sick in their last days, making death a painful mockery, and medicine's inadequate and ineffective treatment of suffering. It is also a demand for more control in decisions about the end of life.

When a patient requests a prescription for enough medication to commit suicide or that his or her death be hastened, the physician first seeks to learn why. What is it that now makes death seem a better option than life? What was the last straw? What is it that must be avoided or escaped? Is the patient depressed? At what point does the patient specify that his or her potential for being someone who matters has been exhausted? These questions are critical when a nonterminal patient asks for pills to commit suicide. A terminal patient should not be excluded from the same sympathetic, gentle but extensive search of his or her despair, self-esteem, and feelings of being valued by others. Are there financial considerations? Does the patient fear that he or she will become either a financial burden or a burden to care for, or both? Has any of this been discussed with the family? Where does the family stand in this regard? How would they understand the patient's requests and be affected by them? How would the family be affected by suicide? If the patient considers his or her life devoid of value and meaning for himself or herself, does it have meaning for certain others? Does this affect the patient? Has the patient made any effort to achieve consensus so that his or her death could actually be a meaningful, shared family experience?

Physicians and the public are now debating the legalization of physician-assisted suicide in the United States. The numbers for and against appear roughly even in number. All but 2 of 12 experts in a 1989 consensus report believed "that it is not immoral for a physician to assist in the rational suicide of a terminally ill person."[76] The public debate recognizes a careful distinction between euthanasia, or active mercy-killing by physicians, and physician-assisted suicide, where physicians may prescribe medication to help end life but patients actually administer the medication. Mercy killing (euthanasia) is a crime in all 50 states and the District of Columbia. Even in the Netherlands, where physicians are allowed to practice euthanasia and do so commonly, it remains a criminal offense.[77]

However, after a series of court challenges and two state wide votes, in 1997 Oregon became the first state to legalize physician-assisted suicide for competent terminally-ill patients[78] and remains the only state where physician-assisted suicide is legal. Between 1998 and 2001, 91 Oregonians died by ingesting medication prescribed by physicians for the purpose of ending life.[25] Although the law has been in effect for more than 5 years, it is still undergoing challenges to its legitimacy. The Death with Dignity Act most recently came under challenge in 2001 when the Bush Administration sought to indirectly invalidate the law by prohibiting the dispensing of controlled substances to assist suicide under the federal Controlled Substances Act. The state of Oregon challenged this action in federal court and prevailed in 2002.[79] Oregon's court victory allows physician-assisted suicide to continue in Oregon—at least for the time being. The Bush Administration appealed the case and it is currently under review by the Ninth Circuit Court of Appeals.

In upholding the right of Oregon to legalize physician-assisted suicide in this latest challenge, the federal district court in Oregon relied heavily on an earlier Supreme Court Decision that had the opposite effect—to uphold a Washington law that prohibited physician-assisted suicide.[80] In this case, the Supreme Court held that Washington had a legitimate interest in banning physician-assisted suicide but also explicitly left open the possibility that other states could reach different conclusions regarding the legality of physician-assisted suicide: "Throughout the Nation, Americans are engaged in an earnest and profound debate about the morality, legality, and practicality of physician assisted suicide. Our holding permits this debate to continue, as it should in a democratic society."[79] Indeed, the debate over the legality of physician-assisted suicide remains active and is likely to undergo further development at the state and federal levels over time. But, no matter one's side in the debate over physician-assisted suicide, every physician must be willing to identify and to try to palliate the psychosocial and spiritual suffering that makes a sick person feel so bad that death seems like the best option.

Fear of Legal Reprisal. When the physician makes a reasonable clinical judgment of irreversible illness and clarifies the wishes of the patient, or if the patient is incompetent, the patient's proxy or surrogates who reasonably represent the patient's wishes concur that life-sustaining treatment is to be forgone or stopped, fear of litigation is neither reasonable nor a legitimate excuse not to proceed. The courts have made it quite clear over the last 15 years that these decisions are valid and should not be brought to court. It is irrational to demand guar-

antees that no litigation will follow. It is hoped that physicians' energies will be spent doing the best they can for the patient, in accordance with the patient's wishes. Should litigation follow an action taken in accord with the above-mentioned guidelines, they will be well prepared to defend their decisions in court.

Conclusion

Caring for the dying patient is a multidimensional endeavor. Psychiatric consultants often play an important role in palliative care at the end of life for patients as well as their families. This chapter began with an overview of questions often posed to psychiatric consultants and the qualities sought in caregivers of the terminally ill. The goals of treatment and a comprehensive approach to palliation were discussed. Palliation involves not only medical conditions but also comorbid psychiatric illness and psychosocial stressors. This chapter also introduced basic principle of medical ethics, since end-of-life treatment often raises ethical concerns and challenges. Finally, legal considerations regarding end-of-life care were briefly explored.

References

1. Greenberg DB: *Psychiatric consultation in the cancer patient*, Massachusetts General Hospital Psychosomatic Conference, Boston, 1997.
2. Cassem NH, Stewart RS: Management and care of the dying patient, *Int J Psych Med* 6:293–304, 1975.
3. Saunders C: *The moment of truth: care of the dying person*, In Pearson L, editor: *Death and dying*, Cleveland, OH 1969, Case Western Reserve University Press.
4. Parkes CM, Weiss RM: *Recovery from bereavement*, New York, 1983, Basic Books.
5. Reiss D, Gonzalez S, Kramer N: Family process, chronic illness, and death, *Arch Gen Psychiatry* 43:795–804, 1986.
6. Deutsch F: Euthanasia, a clinical study, *Psychoanal Q* 5:347–368, 1933.
7. Kübler-Ross E: *On death and dying*, New York, 1969, Macmillan Publishing.
8. LeShan L, LeShan E: Psychotherapy and the patient with a limited life span, *Psychiatry* 24:318–323, 1961.
9. LeShan L: *Psychotherapy and the dying patient*. In Pearson L, editor: *Death and dying*, Cleveland, OH, 1969, Case Western Reserve University Press.

10. Weisman AD, Hackett TP: Predilection to death: death and dying as a psychiatric problem, *Psychosom Med* 23:232–256, 1961.

11. Saunders C, editor: *The management of terminal illness*, Chicago, 1978, Year Book Medical Publishers.

12. Lynn J: Caring at the end of our lives, *N Engl J Med* 335:201–202, 1996.

13. Billings JA: *Outpatient management of advanced cancer*, Philadelphia, 1985, JB Lippincott.

14. Council on Scientific Affairs, American Medical Association: Good care of the dying patient, *JAMA* 275:474–478, 1996.

15. Kelly WD, Friesen SR: Do cancer patients want to be told? *Surgery* 27:822–826, 1950.

16. Gilbertsen VA, Wangensteen OH: Should the doctor tell the patient that the disease is cancer? Surgeon's recommendation. In *American Cancer Society: The physician and the total care of the cancer patient*, New York, 1962, American Cancer Society.

17. Aitken-Swan J, Easson EC: Reactions of cancer patients on being told their diagnosis, *Br Med J* 1:779–783, 1959.

18. Gerle B, Lunden G, Sandblom P: The patient with inoperable cancer from the psychiatric and social standpoints, *Cancer* 13:1206–1217, 1960.

19. Hackett TP, Weisman AD: The treatment of the dying, *Curr Psych Ther* 2:121–126, 1962.

20. Oken D: What to tell cancer patients: a study of medical attitudes, *JAMA* 175:1120–1128, 1961.

21. Novack DH, Plumer R, Smith RL, et al: Changes in physicians' attitudes toward telling the cancer patient, *JAMA* 241:897–900, 1979.

22. Croog SH, Shapiro SD, Levine S: Denial among male heart patients, *Psychosom Med* 33:385–397, 1971.

23. World Health Organization (WHO): *Cancer pain relief and palliative care: report of a WHO expert committee*, Geneva, 1990, WHO.

24. Van der Maas PJ, van Delden JJM, Pijnenborg L, et al: Euthanasia and other medical decisions concerning the end of life, *Lancet* 338:669–674, 1991.

25. Ganzini L, Harvath TA, Jackson A, et al: Experiences of Oregon nurses and social workers with hospice patients who requested assistance with suicide, *N Engl J Med* 347:582–588, 2002.

26. American Psychiatric Association: *Diagnostic and statistical manual of mental disorders*, ed 4, Washington, DC, 1994, American Psychiatric Press.

27. Cassell EJ: *The nature of suffering*, New York, 1991, Oxford University Press.

28. Cassem NH: Depression and anxiety secondary to medical illness, *Psych Clin North Am* 13:597–612, 1990.

29. Weisman AD: Personal communication.

30. Ganzini L, Lee MA, Heintz RT, et al: The effect of depression treatment on elderly patients' preferences for life-sustaining medical therapy, *Am J Psychiatry* 151:1631–1636,1994.

31. Breitbart W, Holland JC, editors: *Psychiatric aspects of symptom management in cancer patients*, Washington, DC, 1993, American Psychiatric Press.

32. Chochinov HM: *Management of grief in the cancer setting*. In Breitbart W, Holland JC, editors: *Psychiatric aspects of symptom management in cancer patients*, Washington, DC, 1993, American Psychiatric Press.

33. Freud S: *The ego and the id*. In Strachey J, translator/editor: *Standard edition, vol 19*, London, 1961, Hogarth Press.

34. Cleeland CS, Gonin R, Hatfield AK, et al: Pain and its treatment in outpatients with metastatic cancer, *N Engl J Med* 330:592–596, 1994.

35. Kimball LR, McCormick WC: The pharmacologic management of pain and discomfort in persons with AIDS near the end of life: use of opioid analgesia in the hospice setting, *J Pain Sympt Manage* 11:88–94, 1996.

36. The SUPPORT Principal Investigators: A controlled trial to improve care for seriously ill hospitalized patients, *JAMA* 274:1591–1598, 1995.

37. Sloan PA, Donnelly MB, Schwartz RW, et al: Cancer pain assessment and management by housestaff, *Pain* 67:475–481, 1996.

38. Brunier G, Carson G, Harrison DE: What do nurses know and believe about patients with pain? Results of a hospital survey, *J Pain Sympt Manage* 10:436–445, 1995.

39. Hoyt JW: Critical care in 1996: Doing too much? Doing too little? Keeping the patient in focus during a time of smoke and fire, *Crit Care Med* 11:88–94, 1996.

40. Hill CS Jr: The barriers to adequate pain management with opioid analgesics, *Semin Oncol* 20(suppl):1–5, 1993.

41. Reidenberg MM: Barriers to controlling pain in patients with cancer, *Lancet* 347:1278, 1996.

42. Jadad AR, Browman GP: The WHO analgesic ladder for cancer pain management: stepping up the quality of its evaluation, *JAMA* 274:1874–1880, 1995.

43. Jacox A, Carr DB, Payne R, et al: *Management of cancer pain: clinical practice guideline No. 9*, Rockville, Md., 1994, U.S. Public Health Service, Agency for Health Care Policy and Research, AHCPR publication 94–0592.

44. Walsh TD, editor: *Symptom control*, Cambridge, 1989, Blackwell Scientific Publications.

45. Woodruff R: *Palliative medicine*, Melbourne, Australia, 1993, Asperula Pty Ltd.

46. Doyle D, Hanks GWC, MacDonald N, editors: *Oxford textbook of palliative medicine*, Oxford, 1993, Oxford University Press.

47. *Care for the dying: identification and promotion of physician competency*, Educational resource document, Philadelphia, 1996, American Board of Internal Medicine.

48. Lester D: *Religious behaviors and attitudes toward death*. In Godin A, editor: *Death and presence*, Brussels, 1972, Lumen Vitae.

49. Feifel H: Religious conviction and fear of death among the healthy and the terminally ill, *J Sci Study Religion* 13:353–360, 1974.

50. Allport G: *The nature of prejudice*, New York, 1958, Doubleday & Co.

51. Feagin JR: Prejudice and religious types: focused study, Southern Fundamentalists, *J Sci Study Religion* 4:3–13, 1964.

52. Magni KG: *The fear of death.* In Godin A, editor: *Death and presence*, Brussels, 1972, Lumen Vitae.

53. Spiegel D, Bloom JR, Kraemer HC, et al: Effect of psychosocial treatment on survival of patients with metastatic breast cancer, *Lancet* 2:888–891, 1989.

54. Fawzy FI, Fawzy NW, Hun CS, et al: Malignant melanoma: effects of an early structured psychiatric intervention, coping, and affective state on recurrence and survival 6 years later, *Arch Gen Psychiatry* 50: 681–689, 1993.

55. Saunders C: *Foreword.* In Kearney M: *Mortally wounded*, Dublin, 1996, Marino Books.

56. Annas GJ, Arnold B, Aroskar M, et al: Bioethicists' statement on the U.S. Supreme Court's Cruzan decision, *N Engl J Med* 323:686–688, 1990.

57. Annas GJ: Nancy Cruzan and the right to die, *N Engl J Med* 323:670–673, 1990.

58. Slater E: New horizons in medical ethics, *Br Med J* 2:285–286, 1973.

59. Plum F, Posner JB: *The diagnosis of stupor and coma*, ed 3, Philadelphia, 1980, FA Davis.

60. Position of the American Academy of Neurology on certain aspects of the care and management of the persistent vegetative state patient. Adopted by the Executive Board, American Academy of Neurology, April 21,1988. *Neurology* 39:125–126, 1989.

61. Munsat TL, Stuart WH, Cranford RE: Guidelines on the vegetative state: commentary on the American Academy of Neurology statement, *Neurology* 39:123–124, 1989.

62. Council on Scientific Affairs and Council on Ethical and Judicial Affairs: persistent vegetative state and the decision to withdraw or withhold life support, *JAMA* 263:426–430, 1990.

63. Optimum care for hopelessly ill patients: a report of the Critical Care Committee of the Massachusetts General Hospital, *N Engl J Med* 301:404–408, 1976.

64. *Deciding to forgo life-sustaining treatment: a report on the ethical, medical and legal issues in treatment decisions.* President's commission for the study of ethical problems in medicine and behavioral research, Washington, DC, 1983, U.S. Government Printing Office.

65. Consensus report on the ethics of forgoing life-sustaining treatments in the critically ill. Task Force on Ethics of the Society of Critical Care Medicine, *Crit Care Med* 18:1435–1439, 1990.

66. Brock DW, Wartman SA: When competent patients make irrational choices, *N Engl J Med* 322:1595–1599, 1990.

67. Taffet GE, Teasdale TA, Luchi RJ: In-hospital cardiopulmonary resuscitation, *JAMA* 260:2069–2072, 1988.

68. Murphy DJ: Do-not-resuscitate orders, *JAMA* 260: 2098–2101, 1988.

69. Tomlinson T, Brody H: Futility and the ethics of resuscitation, *JAMA* 164:1276–1280, 1990.

70. Pellegrino ED: Ethics, *JAMA* 270:202–203, 1993.

71. Jecker NS, Schneiderman LJ: The duty not to treat, *Camb Q Health Care Ethics* 2:151–159, 1993.

72. Truog RD, Brett AS, Frader J: The problem with futility, *N Engl J Med* 326:1560–1564, 1992.

73. Payne, K, Taylor RM, Stocking C, et al: Physician's attitudes about the care of patients in the persistent vegetative state: a national survey, *Ann Intern Med* 125:104–110, 1996.

74. Halevy A, Brody BA: A multi-institution collaborative policy on medical futility, *JAMA* 276:571–574, 1996.

75. Sprung CL: Changing attitudes and practices in forgoing life-sustaining treatments, *JAMA* 263:2211–2215, 1990.

76. Wanzer SH, Federman DD, Adelstein SJ, et al: The physician's responsibility toward hopelessly ill patients, *N Engl J Med* 320:844–849, 1989.

77. De Wachter MAM: Active euthanasia in the Netherlands, *JAMA* 262:3316–3319, 1989.

78. Oregon Death with Dignity Act, Oreg. Rev. Stat. §§127.800–127.897, 1994.

79. Oregon *v.* Ashcroft 192 F Supp 2d 1077 (D.) Oregon 2002.

80. Washington *v.* Glucksberg, 521 U.S. 702,1997.

Chapter 24
Consultation with Children

Annah N. Abrams, M.D.
Anna C. Muriel, M.D., M.P.H.
Paula K. Rauch, M.D

Psychiatric consultants are called on to respond to a diverse set of needs originating with the child, the family, and the hospital staff. In addition to consulting directly with patients who are children and their families, the child psychiatric consultant, in a liaison capacity, may be called on to assist medical or nursing staff cope with difficult feelings of sadness or anger aroused by treating sick children, to assist with managing the needs and demands of difficult parents, and to help a divided treatment team understand divisive dynamics and unite around common goals of quality care.

Stocking et al.[1] found that 64% of children on their pediatric wards had emotional problems that warranted psychiatric consultation, even though only 11% were referred for such consultation. In a more recent study of pediatricians, Burket and Hodgin[2] found that more than half of the pediatric staff stated that they rarely or never referred to child psychiatry, yet these same pediatricians estimated that more than 30% of their patients had emotional problems. Fritz and Bergman[3] surveyed more than 1000 members of the American Academy of Pediatrics; they questioned pediatricians about their experiences with psychiatric consultation during residency training. They found that 68% of those who had had an interaction with a psychiatrist remembered the consultation as helpful. However, if the experiences were positive and the need identified as substantial, it is curious that half of the pediatricians rarely consulted psychiatry. Another interesting finding in the

Burket and Hodgin[2] study was that the pediatric house staff reported referring to child psychiatry somewhat more often than did their attending staff. This pattern suggests that younger staff have less discomfort with initiating psychiatric consultation, and that as pediatric clinicians gain experience they feel more competent to handle psychosocial problems without the assistance of other disciplines.

There are many potential barriers to psychiatric consultation for the pediatrician. Availability of child psychiatry is limited in many pediatric hospitals. With decreasing length of hospital stays, early identification of children in need of consultation as well as access to consultants become crucial. One way of adapting to the demand for earlier identification is to establish routine psychiatric consultation for specific diagnoses (such as cancer, diabetes, cystic fibrosis, and failure to thrive), as well as for protracted or frequent hospital stays, noncompliance, and psychosocial dysfunction. A psychosocial screening tool, such as the Pediatric Symptom Checklist, may have a role in identifying these high-risk patients.[4] Once consultation has been initiated, pediatricians highly value accessibility and timeliness of child psychiatry consultants. Also important are close follow-up, liaison work, and provision of specific recommendations.[2]

The consultant needs to be attuned not only to the needs of the child and the family, but also to the dynamics of the pediatric ward. Assessing how the child's situation is experienced by the ward team requires awareness of the patient mix on the unit, recent deaths or other traumas, and attitudes toward certain diseases, such as acquired immunodeficiency syndrome or severe disability, as well as identification of psychologically vulnerable team members who may need referral for additional support.[5]

The consultant is challenged to make assessments and treatment plans more quickly (highlighting accessibility and timeliness), to facilitate rapid high-quality communication between members of the health care delivery team, and to create seamless transitions from inpatient to outpatient care (follow-up and specific recommendations). Achieving these goals requires establishing a relationship between the consultant and the pediatricians, learning the community resources, and appreciating and helping others appreciate each medical challenge from within the child's developmental frame of reference.[6,7]

Developmental Approach to Consultation

In assessing a hospitalized child, the consultant must appreciate the child's phase of development, and recognize that the child's presentation can be understood only in the context of his or her previous level of functioning and behavior. The task for the consultant is to place what is learned specifically about an individual child and his or her family into a general context and to understand the developmental challenges faced by all children at that particular developmental level.

For the hospitalized infant, the key developmental challenge is to maintain the quality of attachment between parent and child. The parental component of attachment begins while anticipating the infant's birth or adoption. An infant is a parent's most personal production, embodying the hopes that the child will ultimately possess the strengths and values the parent most values in himself or herself, and the wish that the child will have capacities that offset the perceived parental narcissistic deficits. No infant can meet all the conscious and unconscious fantasized expectations, yet most infants are accepted and loved when they enter the world. Parents adapt to the reality of the infant and embark on the lifelong process of attachment that enables child and parent to weather the stresses and strains of caretaking and growing up while remaining committed and connected.

Parents with affective illness (including postpartum depression), anxiety disorders, psychotic disorders, character pathology, or intense guilt may have difficulty achieving the attunement that is necessary for attachment. The psychiatric consultant may be called on to differentiate between depression, character pathology, or anxious adjustment in the setting of inadequate parental attachment. Infants with medical conditions that interfere with feeding, limit access to holding and soothing, affect appearance, or cause irritability present special challenges to the process of attachment. These infants require that the parent be more mature because the unexpected circumstances may leave a parent feeling incompetent or unloved by the newborn. The medical staff can play a crucial role in successfully supporting new parents through this difficult early phase.

Infants and toddlers are nonverbal, and rely on a small, consistent number of caretakers who know them well enough to be attuned to their nonverbal communications. Therefore the infant's experience of the stress of hospitalization is exacerbated by separations from the mother or primary caretaker. Bowlby's classic work on attachment[8] describes the three phases of separation anxiety seen in infants:

1. Protest: The infant acutely, vigorously, loudly, and thrashingly attempts to prevent departure of the mother or rapidly attempts to recapture her. In the older child, this phase may appear as clinging, nagging, or bargaining as a parent is about to leave.
2. Despair: The infant is less active, may cry in a monotone with less vigor, begins to withdraw, and appears hopeless. Sometimes the withdrawal phase is mistakenly seen as a good adjustment because the infant is quieter.
3. Detachment: The infant seems more alert and accepting of nursing care. These new attachments are superficial, however, and the infant concomitantly shows a loss of affect or positive feeling when the mother appears. With chronic disease that requires numerous prolonged hospitalizations, the infant or young child may make many brief, inconsistent attachments and suffer numerous losses if the primary caretaker is regularly absent and many different surrogate

caretakers interact with the infant. Spitz[9] referred to the overwhelmed infant's state as *hospitalism*.

Tronick et al.[10] found antecedents of Bowlby's more pronounced phases of separation occurring over minutes if the mother is unresponsive to the infant's attempts at relating. In response to these findings of short-term and long-term consequences of maternal separations, hospitals are increasingly encouraging mothers to stay overnight with children and to participate in their child's care.[11,12] In addition, nursing departments have instituted a primary nursing model to limit the number of nurses who care for each child.

Medical conditions in the preschool phase (ages 2.5 years to 6 years) are affected by three important aspects of the child's emotional and cognitive development: egocentricity, magical thinking, and body image anxiety. Egocentricity is the child's perception that all life events revolve around him or her. The child can imagine only that every person sees the world from his or her vantage point. Magical thinking is the creative weaving of reality and fantasy to explain how things occur in the world. The combination of egocentricity and magical thinking may lead the preschool-aged child to imagine that medical conditions are punishment for the child's own bad thoughts or deeds. For example, a 4-year-old with leukemia reported he got his "bad cells" from eating too many cookies. The young child needs ongoing support from family and medical staff to understand that the medical condition is not punishment or secondary to some unrelated experience. Without this support, the child's anxiety is likely to be much greater and be expressed as either inhibition and withdrawal, or as behavioral outbursts. One understanding of the cause of body image anxiety comes from the preschooler's cognitive development, which leads the child to envision the body as a shell (skin) filled with blood, food, and stool, which could ooze out of any hole in the skin. This concept of the body being like a tire or water balloon that can be punctured with dire results may explain the preoccupation with bandages at this age, as well as fear of needle sticks and surgical procedures that seem to exceed what can be explained by painful experiences alone.

Some regression is to be expected in the stressed preschooler.[11,12] This may take the form of enuresis in a previously toilet-trained child, increased dependence on parents for help with dressing or eating, and episodes of unwillingness to use words to express wishes or use of baby talk. Each of these regressed behaviors serves to engage parents and nursing staff in a style of caretaking that may be more commonly associated with a baby or toddler.

Treatment approaches can assist the preschooler with adjustment to medical illnesses and interventions and can minimize regression. Pain should be controlled or eliminated whenever possible, even when it is not the fastest way to proceed. Procedures should be explained in simple terms to the child. The child needs to hear in the most basic terms what will be done, why it is needed, and what parts will be uncomfortable or painful. They will want to know where their parents will be before, during, and after the procedure. Interventions should be performed in designated locations, such as treatment rooms, and there should be safety zones, usually the child's hospital room and the playroom, in which no procedures are done. It is crucial for children of all ages to have safe places within the hospital setting, so that they are not on "high alert" at all times. Similarly, warning children about impending procedures may lead to protest acutely, but over time allows children to relax and not be constantly anticipating an unpleasant "surprise attack."

Latency is characterized by a host of new and developing skills in many arenas—academic, athletic, and artistic. The world outside the family becomes more important with the advent of best friends and status in friendship or interest groups. In the context of medical illness, the age-appropriate investment in mastery of skills may lead to improved coping with a better understanding of medical illnesses (although still rudimentary), pride in learning to anticipate regular treatments, medications, and procedures, better capacity to verbalize their needs, and establishment of relationships with nursing staff and physicians. Children with premorbid competencies may weather the stress of illness somewhat better than their less capable peers. The stress of medical conditions, however, routinely leads to regression in all age-groups, so the improved coping skills of latency may not be present at a given time. Regression is common early in a chronic illness, with the potential for developing better coping after there has been time for adjustment. The level of functioning fluctuates according to the individual stressors (e.g., mood, malaise, pain, procedures, and prognostic changes) and family functioning. Offering age-appropriate activities (such as board games, video games, computers, puzzles, arts and crafts), and school tutors, helps children to function closer to their premorbid levels and serves as a counterweight to the regressive pull of dependency, helplessness, and loss of control that often accompanies hospitalization. Later in a chronic illness, flexible denial can be a healthy component of coping. Flexible denial denotes the child's ability to suppress thoughts about the illness and invest in an array of activities, without abandoning the appropriate measures necessary for treatment of the illness.

It is common for latency-age and older children to have distorted or magical notions of the cause of the illness, which are typical of the thinking of younger children. It is helpful to invite all questions—by saying things like "I like to hear what children wonder about" or "There is no such thing as a silly question"—and invite fantasies about the medical condition by direct questions such as "What do you think might have caused your cancer?" Some children may be uncomfortable expressing themselves in a direct dialogue but may be willing to draw a picture of their cancer or to write a story about a child with an illness. Any outlet for expression can be helpful to elucidate the fears that underlie the child's anxiety.

In chronic illness, the latency-age years offer a less conflicted opportunity to foster positive health care behaviors. The child should be able to give a simple, accurate explanation of the illness. The child should be learning the names of medications, their purpose, and when they are to be taken. At this age, a partially independent relationship with the treating physician can be developed. Psychiatric intervention is warranted if the child is resistant to learning about the illness, if the child is regressed, if parents are noted to be intrusive or overinvolved in the health care regimen, or if noncompliance has become a means of fighting between child and parent. Allowing these patterns to proceed into adolescence will likely increase risk of dysfunction and make intervention more difficult.

The adolescent, similar to an adult, enters the medical setting with the capacity to understand the meaning of an illness, including its possible ramifications. Developmentally, adolescents are venturing out with a more independent posture and leaving behind the intense dependency on parents that is seen in younger children. This brings with it a particular sensitivity and vulnerability. The cognitive maturity to appreciate the multiple demands of hospitalization (including deciphering the meaning of diagnoses and treatments and bearing the physical discomfort, limitations, pain, impact on appearance, and fears about the present and future), may overwhelm the adolescent's newly acquired independence.

The physical limitations imposed by illness may put adolescents at risk for major depression, especially when the illness interferes with activities that are key to the adolescent's emerging self-image.[13]

The assault on the teenager's autonomy may be particularly difficult to bear because it coincides with the strong developmental pull to individuate from parents and to establish an independent identity. Often the illness occurs at a time when other tensions between the adolescent and parent make relying on the parents uncomfortable or unacceptable. Faced with this emotionally complex dilemma, some teens become sullen, aggressive, noncompliant, or withdrawn, whereas others are able to negotiate the discomfort of returning to a more dependent, supportive relationship with parents.

Interview styles should respect the adolescent's wish for autonomy. One should engage the adolescent first before looking to the parents for their input. Adolescents should also be offered private time to share information that may not be easily shared in the company of parents. Sexual experiences or concerns and worries about parental coping or even death may not be voiced without privacy. The risks and benefits of treatments need to be presented to the adolescent with the recognition that his or her compliance is central to the success or failure of any treatment plan.

In general, the maturity of a child's defensive style may help in coping with anxiety; however, defensive patterns are complex. The defenses of denial, isolation of affect, and intellectualization may be adaptive in the modulation of anxiety.[14] An example of useful denial is the 10-year-old with metastatic cancer who is invested in completing his schoolwork and getting promoted to the fifth grade. Another example is the teenager with cystic fibrosis who uses isolation of affect and intellectualization to competently discuss the parameters for needing lung transplantation. Use of an array of defenses that permit compliance with the health care regimen and facilitate investment in age-appropriate activities should be supported. Some children and families have greater capacities to grieve the illness and to invest in the present simultaneously; however, this is a theoretical ideal for many. Denial, particularly in a withdrawn child, can sometimes mask psychopathology and prevent referral.[12] The consultant must use a developmental perspective, an understanding of temperament and premorbid personality, in conjunction with an appreciation of the family's functioning to evaluate the child's behavior, emotional state, and defensive style.

The child cannot be understood separately from the family. Serious or chronic illness in a child is a family crisis. The parents must cope with the uncertainty and the highs and lows associated with hospitalization. Abnormal laboratory results, adverse reactions, life-threatening crises, limitations on the child's future, and the specter of death suddenly become their reality. They observe their child in distress and they often feel fundamentally unable to protect the child. The hospital environment brings with it a host of medical professionals with as many personalities as there are consultants and caretakers; often, each seems to hold a crucial piece of the puzzle. Small nuances in the presentation of data or differing styles of optimism or pessimism among staff may radically shift the family's mood. There is rarely much privacy and sometimes none at all, whether in a shared room or an intensive care unit. Parental anxiety negatively affects the child's capacity to cope and to expect a parent to be other than anxious is unthinkable.[15,16] Parents are the child's most trusted and valuable resource; therefore strategies to support the parents are crucial. Most parents evoke staff empathy and appreciate the skill and compassion of the treatment team. Certain parents are particularly challenging to support because of a combination of personality difficulties and coping style. Their distress, often fueled by a sense of helplessness, is typically expressed either as devaluing staff or as apparent insensitivity to the sick child's needs. The consultant helps the team of caregivers understand the psychological meaning of the parents' troubling behavior so they can continue to provide optimal care.[17,18]

Siblings are often the forgotten sufferers in the context of chronic or life-threatening illness.[19] They not only have worries about the sick sibling, but also they often lose the support of their parents. The parents may be physically absent, spending time at the hospital with the ill child and attempting to meet at least minimal work demands to support the family financially. They are often emotionally absent, depressed, or drained by the emotional demands of the sick child. Many parents feel angry at the well siblings for making any demands and for not selflessly understanding the seriousness of the ill child's predicament. This compounds the well siblings' guilt at the expectable feelings of resentment and jealousy toward the ill child who is receiving so much attention and so many gifts. If the illness results in death, the feelings of guilt and responsibility may become overwhelming.

Reasons for Consultation Requests

Consultation may be requested for assessment and treatment planning of (1) primary psychiatric disorders, (2) psychosomatic illness, (3) psychiatric factors affecting a medical illness, (4) behavioral difficulties contributing to hospitalization, (5) behavioral difficulties during hospitalization that compromise optimal medical care, (6) mental status assessments, (7) child abuse in the form of physical or sexual abuse or Münchausen syndrome by proxy, and (8) supportive interactions in children and families who must cope with life-threatening or chronic illness.[6,7]

Primary Psychiatric Illnesses

Depression

Depression is a frequent disorder in hospitalized children. It may be a secondary response to acute or chronic illness, or it may be the primary diagnosis and present with somatic symptoms or behavior problems. One of the resistances to making the diagnosis of depression in the hospitalized child is the misconception that the child's dysphoric mood is appropriate to the stress of the situation and therefore does not deserve to be called depression. To the contrary, stress increases the likelihood that depression will occur; it does not invalidate the diagnosis.

Depression may be used to refer to a mood, symptom, or a syndrome. As a syndrome, depression in childhood is characterized by a persistent mood disorder, dysfunctional behavior, and, in older children, by self-deprecatory ideation. These symptoms or behaviors should represent a significant change in the child's premorbid functioning and not be a long-standing temperamental trait. The *Diagnostic and Statistical Manual of Mental Disorders*, fourth edition[20] (DSM-IV), criteria for depression are defined as prolonged depressed or irritable mood, the loss of interest in all or almost all activities, and associated symptoms. Although the criteria are the same for children and adults, there are some differences. Associated symptoms that are particularly frequent in prepubertal children with an episode of major depression are separation anxiety, somatic complaints, irritability, or behavior problems.[21] Making the diagnosis of depression is difficult in children who are sick because many of the symptoms they exhibit (e.g., decreased energy or loss of appetite) may be attributed to their illness.[22] Also, children who are sick often use denial as a coping mechanism and underreport their symptoms of depression.[23] Prepubertal children cannot give an accurate self-assessment of sustained mood, so dysphoria must be observed by caretakers over a prolonged period. For children younger than 6 years of age, the hallmarks of depression include poor appetite or failure to grow and gain weight appropriately, disturbance of sleep, hypoactivity, and indifference to the surroundings and to primary caretakers.[24] Treatment involves use of antidepressants in conjunction with psychotherapy to support the child and family, as well as child-life and recreational therapy. (See Chapter 25 for use of psychopharmacologic agents in children.)

Suicide Gestures and Attempts

Suicide is one of the leading causes of death among adolescents.[25,26] Although the incidence of completed suicide among children aged 6 to 12 years may be relatively low, suicidal threats and attempts by children in this age-group are not uncommon.[25] In most cases, children who have made a suicide gesture must remain in the hospital or another secure facility until a thorough evaluation and disposition are completed. This may occur via admission to the pediatric ward, in conjunction with crisis intervention services in the emergency department, or in some cases by transfer directly to a psychiatric facility.

During the assessment of a potentially suicidal child, one should take the following actions:

1. Gather details of the suicide attempt.
2. Assess the risk of an attempt—What did the child imagine would happen? What was the likelihood of rescue?
3. Determine the child's mind-set at the time of the attempt—Was there a clear precipitant? Was it an impulsive or a planned act?
4. Determine whether there is a history of suicide attempts.
5. Pursue the child's understanding of death and fantasy of what his or her death would elicit in the family or other significant person (such as a boyfriend or girlfriend).
6. Ask about the child's feelings of remorse about the attempt or regrets about having survived.
7. Assess whether the child expresses feelings of hopelessness, helplessness, or despair.
8. Determine whether the child used drugs or alcohol at the time of the attempt.
9. Determine whether the child is depressed, manic, or psychotic.
10. Determine whether the child identifies with someone who has committed suicide.
11. Assess the probability of physical or sexual abuse.
12. Conduct a family interview. Determine whether the parents are sad and frightened by the attempt or angry at the child for being manipulative.
13. Learn about therapeutic interventions that have been tried in the past. What is in place currently, and how good has compliance been with outpatient treatment in the past?

Family issues (including a family history of depression, whether a family is modeling suicide, intrafamilial tension, and real or imagined rejection of the suicidal child by the parents) should be assessed. If abuse is suspected, the appropriate child protective services agency must be contacted.

The consultant is initially asked to decide on the appropriate safety management for the suicidal child. This may include one or more of the following: one-to-one supervision, use of physical restraints, sedation, and the presence of or separation from the parents. Ultimately the consultant needs to determine whether the child or adolescent should be psychiatrically hospitalized or managed as an outpatient (while either living at home or in another setting). Criteria for psychiatric hospitalization include serious risk of death through suicide, little wish to be rescued, psychosis, identification with someone who has committed suicide, syntonic drug or alcohol abuse, intense feelings of hopelessness and helplessness, intense anger or severe depression, lack of support systems, history of inability to use help, and vulnerability to further losses.

Anorexia Nervosa

Anorexia nervosa (AN) is an illness characterized by significant weight loss or absence of appropriate weight gain for age and height, in the context of a fear of gaining weight and a distorted perception of the thin body as fat. Amenorrhea is also a symptom of AN in postmenarcheal females. The average age of onset is 17; some data supports bimodal peaks at 14 and 18 years of age.[20] The illness is predominantly seen in females but also occurs in males. Hospitalization of afflicted children is usually associated with severe weight loss, cardiovascular abnormalities, hypothermia, or electrolyte imbalance. The last-mentioned feature may reflect binging or purging. The goal of pediatric hospitalization is medical stabilization; nutritional assessment and treatment, psychological assessment of the child and family, and recommendations for appropriate levels of psychiatric intervention after medical stabilization.[27] The assessment as to whether or not medical stabilization must be followed by intensive day or inpatient psychiatric treatment includes determination of the adolescent's recognition that he or she has a problem with eating behavior and self image, the adolescent's motivation to participate in psychotherapy (e.g., is he or she in denial about the eating disorder and resistant to eating the adequate nutrition presented in the hospital diet), and the parents'

ability to support the adolescent and the need for psychotherapy (e.g., are they angry, intrusive, or controlling of the teen, or do they want to deny that the eating disorder is a problem?).

The consultant will be called on to make a recommendation about disposition. Can the adolescent safely live at home and attend outpatient treatment appointments (e.g., psychotherapy, nutrition, and pediatric), does the adolescent need a neutral place other than home to live for a while, or does the adolescent need to be transferred to a psychiatric hospital? If the adolescent is unable to consume adequate calories with support in the hospital, he or she will be unlikely to do so at home after discharge, just as he or she was unable before admission. Often the consultant, in conjunction with the social worker, spends a significant amount of time helping the parents accept the plan for psychotherapeutic treatment, especially if the team recommends that the adolescent not return home.

Somatoform Disorders

Some patients present to the pediatrician with intense somatic complaints, such as headaches, abdominal pain, constipation, dysmenorrhea, or fatigue. In general, when cases are referred for psychiatry consultation, the pediatrician suspects that the intensity or nature of the complaints are more likely to be an expression of emotional factors than medical conditions. Somatoform disorders, as described in DSM-IV refer to a clustering of physical symptoms suggestive of a medical condition, but the severity of the symptoms or the level of functional impairment are not fully explained by the medical condition.[20] Although the DSM-IV lists specific disorders, including somatization disorder, conversion disorder, pain disorder, hypochondriasis and body dysmorphic disorder, the criteria for these conditions were established for adults; children rarely meet full criteria for these specific diagnoses. Recurrent somatic complaints are common in the pediatric population, and are a frequent reason for psychiatric consultation. There may also be developmental considerations, with prepubertal children most often presenting with recurrent abdominal pain or headache; other pain and neurologic symptoms increase with age.[28]

The pediatrician's assessment that symptoms are emotional in origin is often at odds with the patient's and the parents' assessment. In psychosomatic illness, the child and family are highly invested in a medical cause to explain the somatic complaints and for seeking a medical treatment. They are not reassured by routine medical work-ups and they pressure the physician to continue to search for a medical cause. Although the families of somatizing children have been found to have higher rates of anxiety and depression, and to be more dysfunctional than other families,[28] they are typically resistant to psychiatric assessment. Parents may view any suggestion of the important role of psychological factors as an insult and an indication that the clinician does not believe the symptoms are real. These families prefer to have the child radiographed and endoscoped for abdominal pain, rather than to discuss stressors, such as the child's increasing difficulty at school, the death of a grandparent, or parental discord. Often the child and parents focus on borderline test findings and they pressure the physician to pursue these findings. They may connect a series of irrelevant bits of data to create a medical causal theory that is not supported by the pediatrician. Commonly the families seek multiple specialists in an attempt to find one who will support their medical theory. Unfortunately, if the parents search long enough, they will find either a specialist who will ignore the psychological factors and validate the parents' perspective or a more junior clinician who lacks the clinical experience to stop the rule-out approach. If the psychological issues are not attended to, the condition is likely to become chronic and result in significant morbidity.

The presenting somatic symptoms serve as a solution, albeit a maladaptive one, to an emotional dilemma. For example, it may be easier for a child to get his recently divorced mother to focus on his needs by vomiting and by complaining of relentless abdominal pain than by articulating his deep sadness at his father's absence. Moreover, it may be easier for the mother to champion the cause of discovering a medical cause for her child's vomiting than to support and acknowledge the child's level of distress about the divorce.

A helpful approach to psychosomatic conditions includes the following:

1. Watchful waiting: It is not necessary to make the whole diagnosis the first day, week, or month, despite the wishes of the family.
2. Judicious disregard: Use restraint in the pursuit of equivocal organic findings, yet ensure a complete and appropriate medical work-up.
3. Consideration of multiple diagnoses: It is not necessary to tie all of the symptoms to one disorder. (A child may have atypical asthma, a depressive disorder, and family discord.) Minimize the importance of a final diagnosis; instead, focus on reducing dysfunction.
4. Placing a diagnosis in context: Children often have shifting levels of functioning in different settings.

Therapeutic interventions for the somatizing patient include a medical-psychiatric team approach that emphasizes a consistent relationship between the clinicians, the child, and family. It is important to foster the continued presence of the pediatrician, because there may be a tendency for the pediatrician to withdraw after psychiatric referral has been made. If the family believes the presence of the psychiatrist leads to diminished access to the pediatrician, there may be escalating anxiety about physical symptoms, and it becomes difficult for the psychiatrist to maintain the critical alliance with the family. Pediatric reexamination without retesting helps calm the family's medical anxiety and reduces the likelihood of continued doctor shopping. Ongoing psychoeducation from team members can help the family reframe the medical symptoms and enhance communication with caregivers.

Often the child and family need different forms of psychotherapy to allow the child to let go of somatic symptoms, and to move on to a healthy role. The child's medical symptoms frequently serve to stabilize the family system; therefore family therapy may be required to change patterns of interactions. Couples therapy may also be used to help parents strengthen their adult relationship so the child's illness is not needed to hold the couple together or to distract from their discord. A child's individual therapy helps to build self-esteem, and allows the child to engage in developmentally appropriate activities that can increase his or her sense of agency or mastery, which leads to greater confidence and less need to rely on the sick role. Comorbid psychiatric disorders in the child or family members must also be identified and treated appropriately, with the use of pharmacologic agents as needed.

Psychiatric Factors Affecting a Medical Illness

Emotional factors affect all medical conditions, but in some children psychological issues are directly related to worsening of their medical illness and can lead to morbidity. Pediatricians rely on parental report in young children and self-report in older children to assess the need for intervention in many chronic conditions. When anxiety, dysphoria, emotional lability, or apathy is present, this increased distress often leads to more medical interventions. In a study of asthmatics, it was found that steroid prescription was correlated with the patient's expressed anxiety about an exacerbation and not with the degree of change on pulmonary function tests.[29] Anxiety and anger may aggravate inflammatory bowel syndromes and they routinely aggravate irritable bowel syndrome. Apathy or dysphoria in a patient with severe lung disease, as may be seen in a child with cystic fibrosis, can lead to less therapeutic coughing and to significant pulmonary compromise. Apathy as a result of frustration or helplessness in a child undergoing rehabilitation after a cerebrovascular accident (CVA) or car accident may prevent physical therapy from being optimal. Motivation is often a function of mood, and it is an essential feature of the sense of mastery and agency that we associate with striving toward maximal health. To help children be invested in their own best level of function, it is necessary to understand the emotional issues that impede the health-seeking process.

A helpful approach to understanding the psychiatric factors includes the following:

1. Ask the child what aspects of the illness and treatments are most difficult or scary for him or her.
2. Invite the child to describe his or her own treatment goals and any disappointments in reaching those goals.
3. Pursue the child's experience of how the illness and treatment affects his or her life outside the hospital.
4. Learn whether the child feels someone understands what it is like to be him or her.
5. Find out whether there is someone the child is particularly disappointed in for not understanding. Has the child felt deceived by anyone?
6. Determine whether the child knows someone with this condition, and how that person's condition has evolved and why.
7. Know the condition and its evolution.
8. Learn about what is the worst thing that could happen.

The goals of the physicians are sometimes at odds with the goals of the child. For example, a teenage girl, who after a CVA did not want to walk "like an old lady" with a cane, was sullen in rehabilitation because she did not want to give up her crutches. The many disappointments during hospitalization and the unexpected rehospitalizations in combination with the feeling that the patient's opinion was not sought or her or his best efforts still resulted in setbacks can lead to anger, frustration, mistrust, anxiety, or apathy.[30] Engaging the child in voicing his or her experience may be therapeutic in itself. There may be ways of altering the hospital protocols to suit the child or adapting the child's treatment program to accommodate home life priorities. The consultant is asked to assist the child during the hospital stay and to determine whether outpatient psychotherapy is warranted. How time is spent outside of the hospital and the content of the frustrations inform this decision. Psychopharmacologic interventions may also be helpful, depending on the symptoms and the psychiatric diagnosis.

Behavioral Difficulties Contributing to Hospitalization

Accidents and noncompliance are the two major categories of behavioral difficulties that lead to the hospitalization of children. Accidents are a leading cause of pediatric emergency department visits and childhood deaths. It is not uncommon to find multiple accident-related emergency department visits for the same child; therefore identifying the accident-prone child and gaining a better understanding of the causes of accidents may serve to prevent future and possibly more disabling injuries. Medical noncompliance is pervasive, but it runs along a spectrum from benign to potentially life-threatening. As a result, there are many cases of noncompliance that go undetected, such as an incomplete course of antibiotics for an ear infection; other cases of noncompliance can lead to death, such as a diabetic teen who skips his or her insulin and goes on a drinking binge.

Accidents

Accidents occur with all children, but they are more likely to occur in children who are reckless; active; impulsive; and afflicted with attention deficit hyperactivity disorder, fetal alcohol syndrome, or lead exposure or when supervision is inadequate or the two are combined. Adolescents tend to view themselves as invulnerable and therefore may be prone to greater risk-taking and to accidents. It is necessary to gather the following information about the child's behavior before the accident:

1. Has he had behavioral difficulty in school, at home, or with peers?
2. Has there been a change in the child's mood?
3. Is there evidence of a thought disorder?
4. Have there been problems leading to legal interventions?
5. Are these worrisome behaviors new or are they long-standing?

Supervision, particularly in younger children, plays a significant role in maintenance of child safety. When a child presents with an accidental injury, an assessment must be made as to whether the supervision has been adequate for the child's age; this usually involves an assessment of the parents or other caretakers. It is necessary to entertain the possibility that an accidental injury could be the result of abuse (see section on child abuse), a suicide gesture, or an act of self-destructiveness (see section on suicide). These causes should be part of the clinician's routine consideration; they should not be overlooked.

Noncompliance

Noncompliance may be secondary to an inadequate understanding of or a capacity to implement the intended medical regimen. Often noncompliance is not an active decision to defy treatment recommendations. Rather, noncompliance may result from the patient being overwhelmed by a medical regimen or being tired of the chronicity of one. Some children leave the hospital on numerous medications that are to be administered several times each day. It is crucial for the pediatrician to review the medications with the family before planned discharge. Simplification of medication regimens by as much as possible and having honest dialogues with parents and children about what is realistic at home is recommended. Research suggests that at-home medication compliance falls to approximately 50%.[31] Highlighting critical medications and the consequences of not taking them engages the child and family as educated collaborators in the child's health care.[32]

In contrast to the passive noncompliance just described, some children or parents actively disregard medical recommendations. There are many emotional issues that underlie such a course of action. Denial on the part of either the child or the parent may result in noncompliance. In this scenario, the child or caretaker has the conscious or unconscious notion that if the prescribed medication or prescribed restrictions are ignored, it is as if the illness does not exist. The clinician may hear from the child, "Taking my pills makes me feel like I am sick," or from the parent, "I cannot make myself bring him in for his doctor's appointments because sitting in the clinic reminds me he has a bad liver." Suppression of thoughts about illness is a healthy defense, which allows medically ill children and their families to cope with the stress of the illness, but denial when it leads to noncompliance is dangerous and warrants psychotherapeutic intervention.

Sometimes, noncompliance is an expression of anger, either the child's anger at the parent or the child or family's anger at the physician or at the illness itself. When the child is angry at the parents, noncompliance becomes a foolproof weapon guaranteed to elicit parental distress, which is then emotionally satisfying for the child. Psychologically absent in this schema is the child's awareness that he or she is actually harming himself or herself. The consultant can assist in altering the medical relationship, from a physician-to-parent-to-child relationship toward a more direct relationship between physician and child. By diminishing the parent's role in the communication of the health care regimen and of policing compliance, to the extent possible depending on the child's age, the pediatrician has the opportunity to build an alliance with the child that fosters a wish to please and thus to enhance compliance. Psychotherapy serves the function of allying with the healthy part of the child and helping the child or adolescent appreciate that this style of acting out anger and frustration with parents is self-injurious. Similarly, when the anger being acted out is against the illness or the physician, the psychotherapeutic goal is to ally with the healthy part of the child, helping the child articulate the frustration with words rather than by acting them out in a self-destructive way. The consultant is called on to assess what aspect of this goal can be achieved during the hospital stay and when outpatient psychotherapy is warranted. The noncompliant child may be resistant to the idea of outpatient psychotherapy. Hospitalization offers the consultant a valuable opportunity for alliance-building by letting the child experience how talking (therapy) can be helpful.

Behavioral Difficulties During Hospitalization

Some children are referred for consultation for the management of specific behavioral symptoms. Their symptoms may include excessive activity, agitation, verbal or physical threats to staff and other children, seizurelike episodes, and temper tantrums. Assessment should include medical, developmental, and social history from the child and family, a neurologic examination, nursing and child-life observations, and school reports, as needed.

Psychopharmacologic interventions may also be appropriate. The child with generalized anxiety or separation anxiety may benefit from a trial of a long-acting benzodiazepine[33] (e.g., clonazepam). Children with anxiety in association with particular procedures may benefit from premedication with shorter-acting benzodiazepines (e.g., lorazepam). Anticipatory anxiety can be managed with behavioral interventions (e.g., relaxation and visualization techniques) as well as pharmacologically.[34,35] When attention deficit hyperactivity disorder is diagnosed, the child may respond quite dramatically to the prescription of stimulants. Occasionally an underlying psychosis may be discerned, and the appropriate antipsychotic agent should be instituted. (See Chapter 25 for in-depth discussion of pediatric psychopharmacology.) Agitation associated with delirium may require the use of neuroleptics to maintain a child's safety and to help clear the delirium.

Behavioral plans, especially for younger children, may be instrumental in establishing good behavior. The guiding principle underlying behavioral plans is to identify the key behaviors that are most problematic and provide incentives for the child to behave in positive ways. In younger children, sticker charts for swallowing pills and allowing blood drawing without a temper tantrum are examples of common behavioral interventions. Younger children may receive stickers as the full reward, or after receiving a predetermined number of stickers, a child may earn a toy. Older children may work toward special privileges, such as a trip to the gift shop, time outside with the child-life specialist, or a favorite meal brought in from outside the hospital. Other incentives, such as tickets to a hockey game, may be provided by the family. In addition to behavioral plans, children benefit from having a schedule for the day. An unstructured day increases uncertainty, boredom, and anxiety. Scheduling activity times, meal times, rest times, and procedure times can be helpful in providing the child with an increased sense of control over the hospital milieu.

Parental interactions often play a major role in the child's behavior. Some behavioral outbursts may reflect the child's anxiety in response to the parent's escalating anxiety and inability to help the child feel more safe in the hospital setting. Some parents may find it difficult to set limits on the child, in light of the sadness the parent feels at the child's medical condition. The child's behavior may represent an unconscious need to reengage the parent in what had been the usual style of parenting. A parent's lack of limit-setting often feels to the child like emotional abandonment. In conjunction with the social worker doing family work or parent guidance, the consultant needs to help the parent feel competent to be an active parent again.

Children with behavioral difficulties invariably arouse negative feelings in the staff. There may be disagreements between staff members about how best to respond to particular behaviors, and the inconsistencies may foster further behavioral disturbances. Team meetings to develop a consistent plan and to facilitate good communication are essential. These team meetings are a good opportunity for the consultant to share his or her understanding of the psychological meaning of the behavior in a way that helps the staff feel more empathic with the child and the family.

Mental Status Assessments

Mental status examination of an adolescent is similar to the assessment of an adult, but the process is different for a younger child. Assessment at any age includes the child's current medical condition, including fever, infection, electrolyte imbalance, chronic and newly instituted medications, history of central nervous system (CNS) trauma, exposures, premorbid mood and behavior, and psychiatric history.

Adolescents should be oriented to person, place, and time. School-aged children should be oriented to person, place (a hospital, not a school or restaurant), and day versus night. Preschoolers should be able to identify family members, cartoon characters or other culturally appropriate characters, and types of animals.

Mood assessment for young children is made by history and observation because they are unable to provide accurate histories of mood across time. Older latency-aged children (10- to 12-year-olds) may be able to describe their mood of the moment accurately.

The normal adolescent's thought process has fully matured; therefore the presence of hallucinations, delusions, loosening of associations, or flight of ideas is abnormal. Logical, generally concrete thinking is typical of the latency-aged child. An isolated report of a hallucination or an individual distorted notion or delusion is of questionable diagnostic significance. Reports should be considered in connection with the full picture of the child's thinking and behavior. Are the thoughts

generally appropriate for age (e.g., do they occur in the context of nightmares) or is the child preoccupied with bizarre thoughts or does he or she exhibit bizarre behavior? Preschool thinking is characterized by an infusion of fantasy (e.g., imaginary friends). Abnormal preschool thinking is typified by a lack of relatedness, by a loss of previously achieved language milestones, or by unprovoked noises.

A change in mental status warrants neurologic assessment, including electroencephalogram and magnetic resonance imaging or computed tomography scan, metabolic and infectious assessment, toxicologic screening and consideration of environmental exposure, and interactions of (or reaction to) medications.

Child Abuse

Physical Abuse and Neglect

Physical abuse is defined as a child experiencing injury or risk of injury as a result of having been hit, kicked, shaken, thrown, burned, stabbed, or choked by a parent or parent-substitute. The incidence of child physical abuse has increased over the past decades, reaching levels of 5.7 per 1000 by 1993, with peak incidence in the 4- to 8-year-old range. Although gender does not predict the likelihood of abuse, there are specific risk factors for recurrent abuse. These include younger age of the child, the number of previous child protection services referrals, and caretaker characteristics (including emotional impairment), substance abuse, lack of social support, domestic violence, and a history of childhood abuse.[36]

Abuse must be suspected before it can be diagnosed. Certain types and locations of injuries are suspicious. Bruises that resemble finger or hand prints, and those that appear on body surfaces that normally do not bear the brunt of an accidental fall, such as welts on the back as opposed to anterior shin bruises, should raise suspicion. Multiple bruises in various stages of healing are suggestive of abuse that has been ongoing. Clinicians should be suspicious when bruises, broken bones, and accidents have occurred that are inconsistent with the caretaker's explanation, when the caretaker admits and then recants culpability, or admits having observed the abuse being perpetrated and then recants the story. The caretaker may blame the injury on the child, suggesting it was self-inflicted or blame a sibling for an injury that appears beyond the developmental capability of the child. There may have been an inexplicable delay in seeking medical attention, or the person bringing the child for medical assistance may be vague or report having not been with the child during the injury and not knowing how it happened.

Neglect, by comparison, is the absence of expectable parenting that results in the child being inadequately supervised, fed, clothed, cleaned, or emotionally attended to. These children may present with failure to thrive, the occurrence of preventable accidents, dermatologic conditions related to poor hygiene, lack of routine and specialized medical appointments, and school absences.

Abuse and neglect may occur in the setting of multigenerational inadequate parenting; substance abuse; or multiple family stressors, including domestic violence, a disrupted family unit, and cognitively limited or psychiatrically ill parents.[37] All physicians are mandated reporters of abuse. It is necessary to report a suspicion of abuse; it is not necessary to prove abuse to file with the appropriate state child welfare agency.

The child at risk should be kept in a safe facility until the child welfare agency has determined the safety of the child's disposition. A full physical examination should be performed and well documented, checking the whole child for evidence of bruising or injury in various stages of healing. This is important both to ensure the child's safety and because there may be subsequent legal proceedings. A radiologic bone series should be performed to look for evidence of old and new fractures. Retinal examination should be performed for evidence of traumatic shaking of a young child. Siblings of a child suspected of having been abused must be assessed immediately because they are also considered to be at high risk for abuse.

Sexual Abuse

Child sexual abuse is defined as exposure of a child to a sexual experience that is inappropriate for his or her emotional and developmental level and that is coercive in nature.[38] Studies have estimated the prevalence at approximately 15% for boys and as high as 38% for girls younger than the age of 18.[39] However, the incidence of sexual abuse is significantly underreported. The most common form of sexual abuse is father-daughter incest.[40] Incest is present when this sexual contact occurs between a child and a family member, including stepfamily members or members of a surrogate (foster) family. Sexual abuse tends to be so disturbing and so emotionally intense a topic that there is risk of medical professionals abandoning a logical approach to assessment.

There are three common presentations of sexual abuse in children: (1) presentation with an unmistakable traumatic injury or a sexually transmitted infection, (2) testimony that sexual abuse has occurred in the context of no physical evidence, and (3) presentation of a patient with physical or behavioral symptoms suggestive of sexual abuse but who has neither disclosed abuse nor implicated a perpetrator.[41]

In the first two presentations described, assessment and documentation of the sexual abuse and disclosure must be approached with the assumption that legal proceedings are likely to follow. In these cases, there is ample information to make mandated reporting of the suspicion of abuse a requirement. The fewest number of people should question the child to minimize further trauma to the child and to decrease distortions. Ideally a single interview of the child should be conducted by a mental health professional with expertise in child sexual abuse and the appropriate police agency representative. The child psychiatry consultant's role may be as the interviewer or as the supporter of the child on the pediatric unit, without being involved in the sexual abuse examination. In the third scenario, the child may present with medical symptoms, such as a urinary tract infection or vaginitis, or behavioral changes, such as sleep problems or depression.[38] These findings may arouse suspicion and should be followed up with a psychological assessment. A play therapy assessment of a preschooler may be helpful, looking for themes of abuse in the fantasy play. During the play, the young child may reveal new information about sexual experiences. In the latency-aged child, additional information may be gleaned from the child's drawings, especially self-portraits or pictures of the family. Children and teenagers should be invited to disclose sexual abuse to the consultant with questions such as, "Has anyone touched you in ways that made you feel uncomfortable or scared?" A follow-up question might be, "Would you tell me if they had?" and "Who could you tell, if someone was touching you or making you uncomfortable?" It is helpful to learn who a child feels he or she can talk to and to add new choices to the list, such as the pediatrician or school teacher as well as the consultant or another counselor. Even if a child is not yet ready to disclose, one hopes that it is therapeutic to assist a child in conceptualizing a plan for disclosing when he or she does feel ready.

In any case in which abuse is entertained, a family assessment is essential. There is no single personality profile of a sexual abuse perpetrator. Perpetrators may come from within the family or the community. The task of the psychiatric consultant is to explore sensitively the meaning of general symptoms that may be indicative of sexual abuse without suggesting that nonspecific symptoms are pathognomonic of sexual abuse.

Münchausen Syndrome by Proxy

Münchausen syndrome by proxy is a form of child abuse in which a parent, usually a mother, consciously distorts her description of her child's symptoms or does things to the child to fabricate a picture of medical illness and then seeks hospitalizations and medical interventions for the child. The parent may report periods of apnea or seizures at home that have not occurred, or may cause life-threatening illness by injecting the child with medication, blood, or feces to ensure that a medical work-up continues.

Some of the mothers with this syndrome have had medical training as nurses and they use their medical knowledge to create "illness" in their child. The mother is usually at the infant or young child's bedside. She tries to establish friendships with the nursing staff and is content as long as continued hospitalization and medical procedures are being scheduled and performed. She may become angry and agitated if she receives a report that her child is well and should be discharged home. Often she appears earnest and less anxious when serious diagnoses of the child are being

entertained. If discharged, she may return within hours or days to the emergency department with an escalation of symptoms. The psychological understanding of this syndrome is that the mother needs the child to be sick to maintain her role as a "nurturant" mother in the protected, supported environment of the pediatric ward. She perceives the nurses to be her friends and the male physicians as caretaking men in her life. She lacks the empathy to be troubled by the pain and suffering she is inflicting on her child.

Münchausen syndrome by proxy is a difficult diagnosis to make without observing the mother doing something to the child. It may be suspected when a child's medical condition does not follow the expected course and the symptoms are persistently inconsistent. The symptoms may be observed only by the mother or may occur in conjunction with the mother's presence, and may be consistent with an intentional action. Undertaking the investigation of this diagnosis, and seeking concrete evidence of risk to the child at the hands of a parent may require input from hospital legal counsel and administration.

It is crucial to protect the child's safety if this diagnosis is suspected. The reporters of this syndrome have described mortality rates and significant morbidity.[42,43] The hospital legal department and child protective services should be notified of this diagnosis to protect the best interest of the child. If the parent thinks that she is being suspected of having hurt her child she may become angry and leave against medical advice (sometimes going straight to another hospital under the same or an assumed name).

Living with Chronic Illness

The vast majority of children with chronic illnesses cope well. They are not defined by their illnesses but rather by their individual strengths, weaknesses, personalities, and age-appropriate developmental issues. However, children with chronic illnesses are more likely than their peers to have a psychiatric disorder.[6] There is no one personality that coincides with a particular illness, but each chronic illness, such as asthma, diabetes, rheumatoid arthritis, cystic fibrosis, and sickle cell anemia, presents with particular challenges. These challenges present in terms of coping with (1) the symptoms, such as pain or shortness of breath; (2) the timing of diagnosis, at birth, childhood, or adolescence; and (3) the requisite health care regimen, such as inhalers, intravenous antibiotics, or dietary restrictions. The meaning of the illness evolves according to relevant developmental issues throughout the child's life. The consultant's task is to understand the meaning of the illness to the individual child and family at this moment in development. The earlier section on development provides some general principles for understanding the effect of chronic illness throughout childhood, but the consultant must assess the unique experience of a particular child and family.[44–46]

The consultant needs to ask many questions to elucidate the child's subjective experience of living with the chronic illness. Diagnostic instruments used in physically healthy children may not be useful in children with chronic illnesses.[7] Some useful questions include what the worst or hardest thing is about the illness and if there is anything good about the illness. Similarly, what is the child's personal experience of the health care regimen? How has the child's experience of the disease changed as the child has grown older, or what events in the future are of concern? What are the child's peer relationships like, and how, if at all, does the illness affect these relationships? Who does the child tell about his or her illness, and when does the child do so in the course of the relationship? How does the child explain the illness to others, and how can he or she explain it to the consultant? What is the child's perception of the parental concerns about the illness? What are the areas of conflict between parent and child and between child and pediatrician or subspecialist?

Chronic illness requires adjustment on the part of the child, the family, and sometimes the school. The child's personal strengths, such as music, sports, or academics, are assets in maintaining self-esteem and building important peer supports. Some children enjoy peer group opportunities, such as specialized camps for children who share a particular illness. Temperament and interpersonal capacities are also factors in the ease of a child's adjustment. Parental attitude toward the illness is crucial in setting the stage for the child's attitude. Parental anxiety, anger, sadness, and guilt are likely to impede the child's adjustment.[46]

The extent to which an illness interferes with age-appropriate activities, especially school, is an important factor in adjustment. Multiple hospitalizations are associated with greater emotional morbidity than is seen in an individual hospital stay.[47] Structuring the admissions to provide the child with protected times and protected places for play and dialogue, appropriate to the child's age, decreases the stress of the hospital environment. In-hospital tutoring for prolonged hospital stays and continued contact with friends in person, by phone, or online, can assist the child's comfort in returning to school.

Grief Work in Life-Threatening Illness

A sense of vulnerability accompanies any hospitalization of a child, but children and families who face life-threatening illnesses must negotiate the most frightening and unsettling of emotions related to confronting the possibility of death. The capacity of the parents to bear the pain and to find the strength to reinvest in the life of the sick child is absolutely essential to the child's capacity to enjoy the life he or she has. The consultant can play an important role in supporting the child, the family, and the staff and can help optimize a shortened, compromised life. Children dying of cancer may experience significant suffering at the end of life, and require special attention to the treatment of fatigue, pain, and dyspnea.[48] In addition, seriously ill children should be assessed for evidence of depression, anxiety, or chronic pain. Pharmacologic agents, including benzodiazepines, antidepressants, stimulants, and narcotics, may be beneficial in the management of these children. Parents and siblings may also need to be referred for coping difficulties or treatment of depression and anxiety.

Helping the seriously ill child to communicate his or her many small preferences, from being called a nickname rather than a formal name to whether or not to wake him or her for optional events or social activities, can create a greater sense of agency and help stave off the destructive force of helplessness. Facilitating peer interactions in the hospital playroom for the child and encouraging both formal and informal support groups for children and their parents can be invaluable. Many parents and children feel that the enormity of the child's illness has so changed their lives that old friends feel inadequate. The worries of the well world can feel alienating and out of touch with the child and the family's new reality. This experience can be isolating. Sharing pleasures and frustrations with other families facing cancer, a terminal neurologic syndrome, or a metabolic disease can be an antidote to the isolation. Many family friendships that begin on the ward survive long after a child dies.

The consultant may assist the patient and the medical staff in the identification of short-term goals that modified treatment can permit, such as going home for a family celebration or attending a special sporting event. These events can bring great pleasure to the child and foster special memories for the family.

Support services for the family after the child dies are also important. A meeting with the pediatrician can be an opportunity to educate the parents about aspects of the child's illness or care, thus clearing up confusion, reducing unnecessary guilt, and acknowledging the parents' continued attachment to the physician. Some physicians may need support to follow through on these meetings, particularly if the physician feels inadequate in light of the child's death or imagines the parents will be angry (usually, rather than angry, parents are grateful). Grief after the death of a child is associated with higher rates of pathologic grief reactions, and parents may need additional support even through the course of uncomplicated bereavement.[49] One or several meetings with the pediatric social worker or child psychiatrist may help the family begin the process of grieving and help normalize the prolonged duration of the grief. Bereavement groups may be helpful in providing peer support for the enormous sadness associated with the loss of the child. Special attention should be paid to the needs of the surviving siblings because the parents may have difficulty being emotionally available to the children in the context of their own grief.

Initial Steps in the Consultation Process

The first step in any consultation is to fully understand the consultation question (e.g., Who initiated the consultation? What concerns underlie the question? What feedback does the consulting person need to be satisfied, and within what time frame?). Once the question is clarified, the consultant must gather the necessary history (including data provided by members of the medical team, the hospital record, and clinical interviews with the child and parents, as well as social agencies or nonparental caretakers when appropriate).

Some pediatricians are especially sensitive to psychological concerns and have known the patient and family for several years. In university-affiliated hospitals, the consultant often deals with less experienced house staff on monthly rotating schedules, and discussion with the referring physician is shifted toward teaching. A crucial function of ongoing consultation is the trusting relationship that should develop between pediatrician, ward personnel, and consultant. This trust creates an atmosphere in which the psychological needs of children are recognized, and the consultant's recommendations are carried out even when these take additional time and effort.

In the review of the medical record, it is especially important to note the observations of the nurses and child-life specialists. These individuals often have a wealth of information from sustained contact with the child and the family. They frequently have had considerable experience with other children of similar age and with the same diagnosis and thus have a sense of how this child is coping as compared with a relevant peer group. The nurse usually takes a self-care and daily habit history on admission that emphasizes the child's premorbid level of functioning. The nurse may also record the most careful observations of the child's level of anxiety, state of aggression, and temperamental characteristics.[50,51] The role of the child-life specialist, trained in development, is to help children cope with the stress of hospitalization by organizing individual and group play activities in the recreation room. The child life specialist often has the opportunity to observe children interacting with peers and using special hospital play materials.[52] The ward's staff input is a critical adjunct to the consultant's impression, which is based on one or two interviews. Many pediatric inpatient services have a social worker who reviews all or some of the admissions; this expanded social history may be helpful before the consultant meets the family and child.

Techniques of Child Psychiatric Consultation

The child and family should be prepared for the consultation. It is essential that the referring physician discuss the reasons for the referral with both the child and the parents so that the child feels more included and does not feel that information is being withheld. Parents of a preschool-aged and young school-aged child (younger than 8 years old) should be interviewed by the psychiatric consultant before the child is interviewed. The interview of the young child requires largely indirect means of expression of feelings and concerns via play rather than by direct questioning. In the initial interview, the psychiatrist needs to create as normal an environment as possible as he or she gets to know the child. The consultant's interactive style should be active, interested, and playful. The assessment room should contain some toys and not be the site of painful procedures. First, unstructured observation should be done and then a gross developmental assessment. In the child younger than 3 years of age, observations of the parent-child dyad are crucial. What is the eye contact like between parent and child? Does the parent respond to cues in the child and vice versa? Are the parent and child "in sync"? Does the child look to the parent for reassurance and comfort? What is the child's temperament like, and how does the parent handle frustration? How do the child and parent handle separation? How does the child respond to strangers? Stranger anxiety in the very young is expected, and the lack of any stranger anxiety may be a sign of attachment difficulties.

The 3- to 6-year-old child may still require that a parent be present throughout the interview. That request should be respected, although at some point in the interview an attempt should be made to have the parent leave the room. Developmental assessment, including language, social interaction, and gross and fine motor coordination, is a mandatory part of the interview. Drawings become a more important tool for some children to express troublesome thoughts and feelings. The psychiatrist should not expect to complete the evaluation in one visit. It may take several sessions, and the sessions may be shorter than the usual hour because of the child's fatigue or because other tests have been scheduled. The consultant may need to arrange visits to coincide with appropriate times for observing key behaviors, such as around meal times or dressing changes.

The latency-age child can be a more verbal participant in the interview. The child should be questioned about current and previous school attendance, school behavior, school performance, after-school activities, friends, health (including mental health) of family members, family problems, and interaction of family members in response to traumatic events. The mental status examination should initially focus on the manner of relating. The child may be active and verbal or shy and inhibited. The consultant's approach should be flexible depending on the child's way of relating. The active verbal child can be approached in the more traditional interview. The shy child may be engaged through drawings or games, such as checkers or video games. These activities can prove helpful in facilitating an alliance and in demonstrating organic deficits. The first several sessions may be necessary for the child to trust that the consultant will not be performing invasive or painful procedures. Many helpful observations of the child can occur in this initial phase, including assessment of pain, anorexia, and insomnia, assessment of coping strategies, and supportive comments about ways to deal with symptoms and difficult feelings.

Interviewing an adolescent can be most challenging with regard to building an alliance. Some adolescents flatly refuse to talk, and others substantially distort their psychosocial histories. Adolescents are often labile and experience emotions intensely. The consultant should not become discouraged by an adolescent's initial silence. This response may represent anxiety and vulnerability. The adolescent should be given a thorough explanation and reason for referral. The consultant should clarify the limits and expectations of the interview, as well as his or her knowledge of the adolescent's medical condition. The consultant can present himself or herself as a member of the medical treatment team with expertise in trying to understand what is most taxing about an illness or situation and working with the patient and the team to find the best approach for helping the patient.

Confidentiality should be addressed, and the interview should be conducted in a private setting. In general, the consultant should be patient and easygoing. It may be helpful to initiate the conversation with some safe topics, such as a sporting event, television show, or question about a photo or other belonging in the hospital room. The consultant should let the adolescent know the intended length of the visits, initially giving the adolescent some control over length and timing when possible. Over time, questions about body image, school, family relationships, friendship patterns, goals, and sexuality need to be addressed.

The role of the family interview as the initial interview for the assessment of a child is somewhat controversial. Many clinicians believe that a family evaluation is mandatory to understand the child,[53] but that the timing of the family assessment may vary. A family evaluation is necessary in certain disorders, specifically somatoform disorders, AN, school phobia, or with recurrent abdominal pain, in which family interaction may precipitate or maintain the symptoms. In the pediatric intensive care unit, we routinely prescribe family evaluation sessions for families with the following characteristics: when the response to the child's hospitalization is inappropriate (either excessive or severely constricted), when there is a history of psychiatric illness in family members, when there is a question of abuse or neglect, or when there is a question of whether the family is able to comprehend the clinical information adequately.[54]

For other families, the assessments are less urgent. Families of ill children need to express their feelings about hospitalization and to obtain emotional support. Siblings often have distorted concepts of the child's illness that need to be corrected. A carefully planned family meeting can begin to clarify distortions, reduce family turmoil, improve coping skills, and dispel conflict between family and staff. During the meeting, the ward staff or the psychiatrist should evaluate the family's psychological state, including an assessment of coping mechanisms, anxiety level, available support, and ability to comprehend information.

Working with Staff

Child psychiatric consultation almost always involves more than the patient and the referring physician. Parents are inherently a part of treatment as they give critical information and need to be actively involved in implementation of recommendations. During hospitalization, nurses may assume some parental roles while the ward is the child's temporary home. Child and family behaviors have an impact on other patients and staff, and are likely to evoke intense feelings. Because many pediatric units encourage parental visitation and rooming-in, the potential impact of a distraught or disturbed parent on the entire ward is substantial. Lastly, patients with chronic illness may return repeatedly to the same floor over a 5- to 10-year period. Thus many children become well known, and the depth of the staff's involvement grows over the years. Child psychiatric consultation includes an essential liaison role that is relevant to patient and family care, to interstaff tensions, and to individual staff stress.

Primary nursing encourages continuity of care as one or two nurses are assigned to the child during the hospitalization, often for repeated admissions. This practice is beneficial for the child's sense of trust, makes the nurse's role more personally satisfying, and can add a needed perspective if too many subspecialists forget the whole child's needs. Unavoidably, primary nurses become intensely involved in the child's personal and family life; thus they have critical information and share the stress of the child's illness. The child psychiatrist can provide suggestions and supervision for dealing with difficult families or crisis, review when psychiatric referral is indicated, and help in understanding the painful issues of chronic disease, suicide, and terminal illness.

For house staff, a basic stressor is being relatively inexperienced and yet forced to deal with complex medical and psychological circumstances. The source of stress is clearest in the intensive care unit, where frustration mounts rapidly as children do not respond to treatment or suffer life-long physical and neurologic damage. The consequences of multiple stresses (frustration with the patient's course, lack of sleep, and feeling incompetent) may lead to depression, substance abuse, or bitter tensions among house staff or nurses.

Part of the child psychiatrist's liaison function is to attend rounds, be aware of difficult clinical and family situations, get to know nurses and house staff through teaching and informal discussion concerning patients, and be aware of the early signs of behavior destructive to patient care and fellow staff. With sufficient credibility, the child psychiatric consultant can organize patient care, and family or interstaff meetings that have a beneficial impact on the unit's functioning, as well as relieve family or staff suffering.

Ethical Issues

The psychiatric consultant faces many challenging ethical issues in the hospital. The consultant may be involved in helping children and families come to terms with psychologically complex decisions, such as pursuing continued aggressive treatments or assenting to "do not resuscitate" orders. Staff and families need help assessing the extent to which a child at a particular developmental level can understand and be included in such decision-making.

Confidentiality is complex in the hospital setting. The consultant must be clear about whom he or she is consulting to and what the limits of confidentiality are. What cannot be kept confidential may be clear, such as suicidal ideation, but what can be confidential, such as a child's worry about a parent's sadness or a parent's trauma history, may be less apparent. The medical record is open to the full medical and support staff, and some personal information may be disclosed that is not relevant to the child's medical care.

Psychiatric consultation faces major barriers because of inadequate funding. Reimbursement guidelines do not recognize the time spent gathering data from many sources. The liaison role of the psychiatric consultant in assisting all the members of the medical team cope with the intense feelings elicited by working with seriously ill children and families in crisis goes unreimbursed if not supported financially by the hospital. As financial pressures on hospitals, especially teaching hospitals, increase, there is great risk of losing support for child psychiatry consultation.

Future Considerations

The long-term benefits of psychiatric intervention must be assessed through outcome studies examining the impact on quality of life, as well as impact on further use of health care dollars. The effect of liaison interventions on job satisfaction among physicians, nurses, social workers, and child-life specialists needs further assessment. As fewer and fewer professionals are asked to do more and more, often for lower salaries, hospitals must protect their most valuable assets—their human resources.

Professionals who work with children are called on to advocate for the special needs of the young because they are not yet able to do so for themselves. We need to be certain that our developmental expertise is heard in the debate about use of a finite health care budget. Interventions that improve the psychological well-being of children maximize their productivity long into the future, and interventions that support families strengthen the community. Health care is in a period of transition, and we must find the opportunities to effect positive change.

As managed care, critical pathways, and advances in care decrease lengths of stay, increasingly consultation work will bridge to or be centered in outpatient settings and schools.[55] Being accessible, responsive, and communicative with primary care pediatricians will continue to be essential in the future.

Efforts have resulted in closing some of the distance between pediatrics and child psychiatry. Some subspecialty clinics, including those treating cystic fibrosis, cancer, diabetes, and endocrine disorders, are more open to consultation at the time of diagnosis, at key points in the illness, and for noncompliance. For primary care settings, the Bureau of Child and Maternal Health of the Public Health Service and the American Academy of Pediatrics have collaborated on projects that emphasize the psychosocial needs of children. Bright Futures[56] integrates psychosocial issues into every recommended primary care visit. The *DSM—Primary Care*[57] bridges variations and problems common to pediatric practice with the DSM-IV. Symptom checklists, such as the Pediatric Symptom Checklist[58] are being used to screen for psychosocial dysfunction as part of ensuring comprehensive care and assessing mental health services. How these efforts to prevent, identify, diagnose, and treat child psychiatric disorders will fare under managed care, especially capitation, remains to be seen. In terms of clinical need, however, there is a clear role of child and adolescent consultation in inpatient and outpatient settings.

References

1. Stocking M, Rothney W, Grosser G, et al: Psychopathology in the pediatric hospital: implications for the pediatrician, *Am J Public Health* 62:551–556, 1972.
2. Burket RC, Hodgin JD: Pediatricians' perceptions of child psychiatry consultations, *Psychosomatics* 34:402–408, 1993.
3. Fritz GK, Bergman AS: Child psychiatrists seen through pediatricians' eyes: results of a national survey, *J Am Acad Child Psychiatry* 24:81–86, 1985.
4. Lloyd J, Jellinek MS, Little M, et al: Screening for psychosocial dysfunction in pediatric inpatients, *Clin Pediatr* 34:18–24, 1995.
5. Jellinek MS: Recognition and management of discord within house staff teams, *JAMA* 256:754–755, 1986.
6. Knapp P, Harris E: Consultation-liaison in child psychiatry: a review of the past ten years, *J Am Acad Child Adol Psychiatry* 37:139–146, 1998.
7. Jellinek MS: *Behavior problems of children and adolescence.* In Stern TA, Herman JB, Slavin PL, editors: *The Massachusetts General Hospital Guide to Primary Care Psychiatry, ed 2,* New York, 2004, McGraw-Hill.
8. Bowlby J: Separation anxiety, *Int J Psychoanal* 41:89–113, 1960.
9. Spitz RA: Hospitalism, *Psychoanal Study Child* 1:53–74, 1945.
10. Tronick E, Als H, Adamson L, et al: The infant's response to entrapment between contradictory messages in face to face interaction, *J Am Acad Child Psychiatry* 17:1–13, 1978.
11. Palmer SJ: Care of sick children by parents: a meaningful role, *J Adv Nurs* 18:185–191, 1993.
12. Prugh DG, Staub EM, Sands H, et al: A study of the emotional reactions of children and families to hospitalization and illness, *Am J Orthopsychiatry* 23:70–106, 1953.
13. Lewinsohn PM, Seeley JR, Hibbard J, et al: Cross-sectional and prospective relationships between physical morbidity and depression in older adolescents, *J Am Acad Child Adolesc Psychiatry* 35:1120–1129, 1996.
14. Freud A: The role of bodily illness in the child, *Psychoanal Study Child* 7:69–81, 1969.
15. Kazak AE, Barakat LP: Brief report: parenting stress and quality of life during treatment for childhood leukemia predicts child and parent adjustment after treatment ends, *J Pediatr Psychology* 22:749–58, 1997.
16. Sawyer MG, Steiner DL, Antoniou G, et al: Influence of parental and family adjustment on the later psychological adjustment of children treated for cancer, *J Am Acad Child Adolesc Psychiatry* 37:815–822, 1998.
17. Wright MC: Behavioral effects of hospitalization in children, *J Pediatr Child Health* 31:165–167, 1994.
18. Beresin EV, Jellinek MS, Herzog DB: The difficult parent: office assessment and management, *Curr Probl Pediatr* 20:620–633, 1990.
19. Sharpe D, Rossiter L: Siblings of children with a chronic illness: a meta-analysis. *J Pediatr Psychology* 27:699–710, 2002.
20. American Psychiatric Association: *Diagnostic and statistical manual of mental disorders,* ed 4 (DSM-IV), Washington, DC, 1994, American Psychiatric Association.
21. Birmaher B, Ryan ND, Williamson DE, et al: Child and adolescent depression: a review of the past 10 years: I. *J Am Acad Child Adol Psychiatry* 35:1427–1439, 1996.
22. Heilgenstein E, Jacobsen PB: Differentiating depression in medically ill children and adolescents, *J Am Acad Child Adolesc Psychiatry* 27:716–719, 1988.
23. Canning EH, Canning RD, Boyce WT: Depressive symptoms and adaptive style in children with cancer, *J Am Acad Child Adolesc Psychiatry* 31:1120–1124, 1992.
24. Kashani JG, Barbero GJ, Bolander FD: Depression in hospitalized pediatric patients, *J Am Acad Child Adolesc Psychiatry* 20:123–134, 1981.
25. Pfeffer CR: Suicide in mood disordered children and adolescents, *Child Adol Psychiatr Clin North Am* 11:639–647, 2002.
26. Catllozzi M, Pletcher JR, Schwarz DF: Prevention of suicide in adolescents, *Curr Opinion Pediatr* 13:417–422, 2001.
27. Anderson A, Bowers W, Evans K: *Inpatient treatment of anorexia nervosa.* In Garner DM, Garfinkel PE, editors: *Handbook of treatment for eating disorders,* New York, 1997, Guilford Press, pp 327–353.
28. Fritz GK, Fritsch S, Hagino O: Somatoform disorders in children and adolescents: a review of the past 10 years, *J Am Acad Child Adolesc Psychiatry* 36:1329–1338, 1997.
29. Hyland ME, Kenyon CA, Taylor M, et al: Steroid prescribing for asthmatics: relationship with Asthma Symptom Checklist and Living with Asthma Questionnaire, *Br J Clin Psychol* 32:505–511, 1993.
30. Bonn M: The effects of hospitalization on children: a review, *Curationis* 17:20–24, 1994.
31. Festa RS, Tamaroff MH, Chasalow F, et al: Therapeutic adherence to oral medication regimens by adolescents with cancer, *J Pediatr* 120:807–811, 1992.
32. Van Sciver M, D'Angelo E, Rapport L, Woolf A: Pediatric compliance and the roles of distinct treatment characteristics, treatment attitudes, and family stress: a preliminary report, *J Behav Pediatr* 16:350–358, 1995.
33. Biederman J: Clonazepam in the treatment of prepubertal children with panic-like symptoms, *J Clin Psychiatry* 48:38, 1987.
34. Lewis Claar R, Walker LS, Barnard JA: Children's knowledge, anticipatory anxiety, procedural distress, and recall of esophagogastroduodenoscopy, *J Pediatr Gastroent Nutrition* 34:68–72, 2002.
35. Zeltzer LK, Tsao JC, Stelling C, et al: A phase I study on the feasibility and acceptability of an acupuncture/

hypnosis intervention for chronic pediatric pain, *J Pain Sympt Management* 24:437–46, 2002.

36. Kaplan SJ, Pelcovitz D, Labruna V: Child and adolescent abuse and neglect research: a review of the past 10 years. I. physical and emotional abuse and neglect, *J Am Acad Child Adolesc Psychiatry* 38:1214–1222, 1999.

37. Merrick J, Browne KD: Child abuse and neglect: a public health concern, *Publ Health Reviews* 27:279–293, 1999.

38. Britton H, Hensen K: Sexual abuse, *Clin Obst Gynecol* 40:226–240, 1997.

39. Crewdson J: *By silence betrayed: sexual abuse of children in America*, Boston, 1988, Little, Brown.

40. Hilton MR: Victims and perpetrators of child sexual abuse, *Br J Psychiatry* 169:408–421, 1996.

41. Sugarman M: *Emergency ward evaluation and inpatient management of sexual abuse.* In Jellinek MS, Herzog DB, editors: *MGH psychiatric aspects of general hospital pediatrics*, Chicago, 1990, Year Book Medical Publishers.

42. Souid A, Keith D, Cunningham A: Munchausen syndrome by proxy, *Clin Pediatr* 37:497–503, 1998.

43. McClure RJ, Davis PM, Meadow SR, et al: Epidemiology of Munchausen syndrome by proxy, non-accidental poisoning, and non-accidental suffocation, *Arch Dis Childhood* 75:57–61, 1996.

44. Sawyer M, Antoniou G, Toogood I, et al: Childhood cancer: a 4-year prospective study of the psychological adjustment of children and parents, *J Pediatr Hem/Oncol* 22:214–20, 2000.

45. Meijer SA, Sinnema G, Bijstra JO, et al: Social functioning in children with a chronic illness, *J Child Psychol Psychiatry Allied Disciplines*, 41:309–317, 2000.

46. Hoekstra-Webbers J, Jaspers J, Kamps W, Klip E: Risk factors for psychological maladjustment of parents of children with cancer, *J Am Acad Child Adol Psychiatry* 38:1526–1535, 1999.

47. Geist RA: Consultation to a pediatric surgical ward: creating an empathic climate, *Am J Orthopsychiatry* 47:432–444, 1977.

48. Wolfe J, Grier HE, Klar N, et al: Symptoms and suffering at the end of life in children with cancer, *N Engl J Med* 342:326–333, 2000.

49. Goldman A: ABC of palliative care: special problems of children, *Br Med J* 316:49–52, 1998.

50. Graham P, Rutter M, George S: Temperamental characteristics as predictors of behavior disorders in children, *Am J Orthopsychiatry* 43:329–339, 1973.

51. Thomas A, Chess S: *Temperament and development*, New York, 1976, Brunner/Mazel.

52. American Academy of Pediatrics. Committee on Hospital Care. Child life services. *Pediatrics* 106:1156–1159, 2000.

53. Minuchin S: *The uses of an ecological framework in the treatment of a child.* In Anthony J, Koupernik C, editors: *The child in his family*, New York, 1970, John Wiley & Sons.

54. Herzog DB: *Psychiatrist in the pediatric intensive care setting.* In Manschreck TC, Murray GB, editors: *Psychiatric medicine update*, New York, 1984, Elsevier Biomedical Press.

55. Jellinek M: The present status of child psychiatry in pediatrics, *N Engl J Med* 306:1227–1230, 1982.

56. Green M, editor: *Bright futures: guidelines for health supervision of infants, children and adolescents*, Arlington, VA, 1994, National Center for Education in Maternal and Child Health.

57. American Psychiatric Association: *Diagnostic and Statistical Manual for Mental Disorders—Primary Care* (DSM-PC), Washington, DC, 1995, American Psychiatric Press.

58. Jellinek MS, Little M, Murphy JM, et al: The pediatric symptom checklist: support for a role in a managed care environment, *Arch Pediatr Adolesc Med* 149:740–746, 1995.

Chapter 25

Psychopharmacology for Children and Adolescents

Jefferson B. Prince, M.D.
Timothy E. Wilens, M.D.
Joseph Biederman, M.D.
Thomas J. Spenser, M.D.

Within medical settings use of psychopharmacologic agents should be tempered by knowledge of environmental and medical factors that can cause or exacerbate a child's condition, including the duration and severity of symptoms. Such psychiatric symptoms can emerge in children who face intense stress, loss of a caregiver, chronic illness, or a personal or family history of psychiatric disorders. Currently, a host of medications are being used and their benefits and short- and long-term risks are being investigated. The National Institute of Mental Health (NIMH) is actively assessing the risks and benefits of psychotropic medications in the pediatric population. (The institute recently held a conference, "Medication Safety Monitoring 2000: Developing Methodologies for Monitoring Long-Term Safety of Psychotropic Medications in Children," and it helps fund Research Units on Pediatric Psychopharmacology.[1] Likewise the Federal Drug Administration, through its Food and Drug Administration (FDA) Modernization Act, encourages the industry to monitor medication safety in children in exchange for extended patent exclusivity. Although the indications for the use of psychoactive compounds are modest, the appropriate use of these drugs within medical settings continues to increase. Despite increasing research, a gap remains between empirical support and clinical practice.[2] The following are general guidelines for the use of psychoactive medications in children and adolescents; they are consistent with the American Academy of Child and Adolescent Psychiatry's (AACAP) recent policy statement on prescribing psychotropic medications for children and adolescents (AACAP Policy Statement October 21, 2001).

1. The use of psychotropic medications should follow a careful evaluation of the child and the family, including psychiatric, medical, and social considerations. Consideration should be given to the child's psychiatric disorder and an exclusionary differential diagnosis should be considered, particularly in an acute medical setting. Children who manifest transient symptoms related to an adjustment to medical illnesses or to losses should be considered for nonpharmacologic treatment; pharmacologic care should be reserved for refractory cases.

2. Pharmacotherapy should be considered as part of a comprehensive treatment plan that includes individual and family psychotherapy, educational and behavioral interventions, and careful medical management; it should not be presented as an alternative to these other interventions. However, pharmacotherapy should be considered as an initial treatment when it is shown to be superior to other modalities.

3. If a patient has a psychiatric disorder that may respond to psychotropic medications, the clinician should decide which psychotropic medication to use, and take into consideration the age of the child and the severity and nature of the symptomatic picture. Diagnosis and target symptoms should be defined before initiating pharmacotherapy.

4. The family and the child should be familiarized with the risks and benefits of this intervention, the availability of alternative treatments, the possible adverse effects, the potential for interaction with other medications, the realization of possible unforeseeable adverse events, and the prognosis with and without treatment. Permission to use medications should be obtained from the custodial parent or the patient's legal guardian. Standard use of antipsychotics in children and adolescents who are in the custody of the state may require a legal hearing; however, antipsychotics can be used in these patients in emergency situations.

5. Ongoing pharmacologic assessment is necessary. When a medication is thought to be either ineffective or inappropriate to the current clinical situation, these agents should be tapered and discontinued under careful clinical observation. Appropriate alternative interventions should be reviewed with the family and then initiated.

6. Pediatricians, family practitioners, other medical staff, mental health professionals, and child psychiatrists should work collaboratively in the pharmacologic management of children and they should answer the family's questions.

In the following sections, salient information on common and severe psychiatric disorders in children and adolescents is reviewed, and current pharmacologic strategies and the use of medication in pediatric patients are described.

Clinical Management Issues

The use of psychotropic medications in pediatric patients raises a number of concerns. The first of these issues centers around the "off-label" use of medications. The FDA approves the use of medications in specified clinical situations. However, the FDA allows practitioners to use medications in clinical situations not included in the official labeling. That is, practitioners may use a medication for clinical situations other than the "approved" use or the use of medications in age-groups not formally studied. Often, medical advances are made with use of drugs in conditions that are not as yet included on the package insert.

A second issue centers around the concept of consent. Except in emergency situations, consent must be obtained from the custodial parent or legal guardian prior to use of any compounds in pediatric patients. This consent process involves a discussion of the diagnosis being treated, the prognosis with and without treatment, the potential risks and benefits of the proposed intervention, and a discussion of available treatment alternatives. The practitioner also needs to assess the reliability of the parents prior to the initiation of outpatient treatment, because it will be their responsibility to administer the drugs on an outpatient basis. If the parents cannot reliably administer the medication, then this type of intervention may be precluded.

A third issue involves developmental factors. Pharmacodynamic and pharmacokinetic factors may influence the safety, tolerability, and efficacy of medications in the pediatric population.[3] Pharmacodynamic factors, such as the ongoing development of neural networks, may affect response to medications. Similarly, pharmacokinetic factors may influence the absorption, distribution, metabolism, and excretion of medications. Pediatric patients often require higher doses of medication to achieve the same benefit, perhaps as a result of more extensive or rapid metabolism by the liver or increased excretion because of a higher glomerular filtration rate. Furthermore, the pharmacokinetics in children and adolescents may be different for short- and long-term exposures. Clinicians must keep these factors in mind as they monitor the use of medications in children and adolescents.

Medical Precautions

In the presence of active pediatric illness, special precautions apply when using psychotropic medications. For example, in the presence of a pre-existing cardiac disease that might impair cardiac conduction, tricyclic antidepressants (TCAs) and TCAs in combination with antipsychotics should be used cautiously. A cardiac evaluation might be necessary prior to the initiation of treatment in these patients. Recently the American Heart Association issued an official scientific statement on the cardiovascular monitoring of children and adolescents receiving psychotropic medications.[4] Clinicians are encouraged to refer to these recommendations to guide their selection and monitoring of psychotropic medications.

β-Blockers are contraindicated in patients with asthma, congestive heart failure (CHF), sinus bradycardia, first-degree atrioventricular block, and Wolff-Parkinson-White syndrome because they may cause severe bradycardia. β-Blockers should be used with caution in patients with diabetes and hyperthyroidism because they can mask the symptoms of hypoglycemic crisis and thyrotoxicosis. β-Blockers should not be used in conjunction with α-adrenergic medications because of concerns over heart block. TCAs and atypical antidepressants (e.g., bupropion) and antipsychotics have been reported to lower the seizure threshold. Although the Physicians Desk Reference[5] notes that stimulants are associated with seizures, clinical experience and recent investigations do not support this assertion. Furthermore, stimulants do not appear to exacerbate well-controlled epilepsy. Although recently published guidelines for the evaluation of attention deficit hyperactivity disorder (ADHD) do not recommend a baseline electroencephalogram (EEG) as part of the workup, recent data indicate that patients with ADHD and normal EEG results are at minimal risk of seizure. However, neurologically intact patients with ADHD, who had an epileptiform EEG, have an increased risk of seizure.[6] Antidepressants, antipsychotics, and antianxiety agents can produce central nervous system (CNS) depression and should be used with caution in patients with chronic respiratory disease.

Known drug interactions should also be considered. Psychostimulants generally do not have significant medication interactions except with the monoamine oxidase inhibitors (MAOIs), and many antidepressants, antipsychotics, and anticonvulsants can interact with a wide array of agents. Clinicians are encouraged to have ready access to databases that can provide up-to-date information about the metabolism and specific interactions of specific medications. For instance, antidepressants, antipsychotics (particularly those with strong anticholinergic properties), and antianxiety agents are contraindicated in patients with acute narrow-angle glaucoma and in untreated patients with open-angle glaucoma. The FDA has also issued warnings regarding liver toxicity secondary to magnesium pemoline and nefazodone. Psychotropic medications should be used with caution in the presence of renal or hepatic dysfunction. In these patients, psychotropic medications with specific metabolic pathways (i.e., renal or hepatic) should be selected or the dose decreased and closely monitored with serum levels.

Emergency Interventions: Treatment of Acute Agitation or Aggression

Typically, the request for the emergency use of psychotropic medication centers around the treatment of acutely assaultive, self-injurious, or "out-of-control" behaviors. These situations can arise in the context of psychosocial distress, acute psychopathology, drug intoxication or withdrawal states, and medical or neurologic disease. Acute psychopharmacologic interventions may be helpful in the initial management of the acutely disturbed patient.

This intervention should be based on diagnosis and conducted in concert with verbal and behavioral interventions aimed at addressing the crisis situation and its psychosocial impact. If reduced stimulation and general calming measures are ineffective, pharmacotherapy should be considered. Low doses of a short-acting benzodiazepine (e.g., lorazepam 0.5 to 1.0 mg.) or a sedating antihistamine (e.g., diphenhydramine 25 to 50 mg) can be used to reduce acute anxiety, agitation, and insomnia with few side effects. These agents can be administered orally, intravenously, or intramuscularly. Behavioral disinhibition can occur and should be monitored. In severe or agitated psychotic states, low doses of a sedating antipsychotic (e.g., chlorpromazine or thioridazine 25 to 50 mg; olanzapine 2.5 to 10.0 mg; or quetiapine 25 to 300 mg) may be very effective in reducing concomitant anxiety, agitation, or psychosis. For children with active hallucinations or severe disturbances of reality, a higher potency antipsychotic (e.g., risperidone at 0.25 to 4.0 mg orally) may be necessary. Often a combination of a benzodiazepine and an antipsychotic may be necessary for behavioral management. Resolution of the crisis should be followed by an ongoing psychiatric assessment to define an appropriate plan for follow-up.[7] Medications used for crisis management should not be continued indefinitely, unless they are indicated for the treatment of a coexisting psychiatric disorder.

Delirium

Delirium is a transient derangement of cerebral function with global impairment of cognition and attention accompanied frequently by disturbances of the sleep-wake cycle and changes in psychomotor activity. Delirium may be an early warning of a deteriorating medical condition, a toxic insult, or a brain injury, and it may be accompanied by self-injurious behaviors, such as pulling out IV lines. In adolescents, clinicians should consider substance intoxication and/or drug interactions (between prescribed medications and illicit substances, such as marijuana and TCAs) in the differential.[8]

Treatment is usually directed at both the cause and symptoms. Correction of metabolic abnormalities, removal of agents that may be exacerbating the symptoms, or treatment of the underlying injury or infection is generally followed by reversal in the delirium. After attempting to reorient and decrease the sensory input and contact with family, pharmacologic intervention may be necessary. Generally, antipsychotics are useful if hallucinations or delusions are present, whereas anxiolytics (i.e., benzodiazepines) help reduce anxiety and apprehension. As mentioned above, antihistamines (e.g., diphenhydramine 25 to 50 mg orally or intramuscularly every 6 to 8 hours) or benzodiazepines (e.g., lorazepam 0.5 to 1 mg orally, intramuscularly, sublingually, or intravenously every 4 to 6 hours) generally are considered to be the most benign choices for agitation and anxiety. In older children or adolescents who do not respond to these treatments or in those with psychosis, severe dyscontrol or agitation, haloperidol can be used with repeating the dose every 6 hours if needed. Psychotropic medications should be withdrawn with resolution of the delirium.

Childhood Anxiety Disorders

Children typically are anxious when receiving care in any medical setting. When the level of anxiety impairs the child (or practitioner) and is unremitting, a child should be assessed for an anxiety disorder. Anxiety problems may also be manifest in children as multiple somatic complaints, such as headaches, stomachaches, and nervous twitches of unknown physiologic nature. Often the child has a parent with an anxiety disorder. Childhood anxiety disorders are relatively common and tend to persist into adult life.[9,10] The three most common anxiety disorders in children seen in medical settings are separation anxiety, generalized anxiety disorder (GAD) of childhood, and acute stress disorder (ASD). Other anxiety disorders, such as posttraumatic stress disorder (PTSD), obsessive compulsive disorder (OCD), and/or tic disorders may be present in hospitalized children.

In separation anxiety, the predominant disturbance is a developmentally inappropriate excessive anxiety on separation from familial surroundings. It is called separation anxiety because it is assumed that the main disturbance is the child's inability to separate from the parent or from major attachment figures. When separation occurs or is anticipated, the child may experience severe anxiety to the point of panic. It may develop during the preschool age; however, it more commonly appears in older children.

GAD of childhood is common; it is more frequently seen in boys than in girls. Similar to GAD in the adult patient, the essential feature is excessive worry and fear that is not focused on a specific situation or object and not as a result of psychosocial stressors. Children may manifest an exaggerated or unrealistic response to the comments or criticisms of others. In addition, some children and adolescents experience panic attacks during hospitalization. The treatment of these juvenile anxiety disorders is similar to the treatment of adults; selective serotonin reuptake inhibitors (SSRIs), benzodiazepines, TCAs, or β-blockers, are efficacious.

ASD develops within 1 month of an acute traumatic event and is manifest by anxiety, dissociative symptoms, persistent re-experiencing of the trauma, and avoidance of stimuli that raise recollections of the trauma. This disorder is likely to be observed in pediatric patients or their parents after acute injuries. Recently, Winston et al. reported on the use of the Screening Tool for Early Predictors of PTSD (STEPP).[11] The STEPP is a 12-item questionnaire that obtains information from the child, the parents, and the medical record. A score of 4 or greater from the child or 3 or greater from the parent demonstrates sensitivity in predicting PTSD of 0.88 for children and 0.96 for parents. The STEPP's high sensitivity, brevity, and ease of scoring offers a quick way to identify children and families at high risk of developing PTSD in the acute care setting. The severity, duration, and proximity to the trauma are factors that influence the development of ASD. In addition to the nature (e.g., burns, self-injurious behaviors, or abuse) and extent of the injuries, preexisting psychiatric illness increases the risk of ASD. In patients with premorbid psychiatric illness, clinicians must carefully weigh risks and benefits of continuing previously prescribed psychotropic medications. In a number of patients, ASD may develop into PTSD. Effective management is organized around ensuring safety and reducing pain, anxiety, and fear. Recent investigations of children with burns suggest that aggressive management of pain with morphine may reduce and secondarily prevent PTSD.[12] Pediatric patients with PTSD are likely to have comorbidity with other psychiatric disorders and/or have a history of neglect or abuse.[13,14] Donnelly et al. recently reviewed the pharmacotherapy of pediatric PTSD.[15] Medications that enhance serotonergic neurotransmission, the selective serotonin-reuptake inhibitor (SSRIs), have been shown to be useful in reducing symptoms of anxiety, depressed mood, rage, and obsessional thinking in adults with PTSD.[15,16] In fact both sertraline and paroxetine are approved for treatment of PTSD in adults and are often used in pediatric patients. β-Blockers, in particular propranolol, have been studied as a means of reducing arousal symptoms of PTSD. Similarly, α-adrenergic agents, such as clonidine or guanfacine, may likewise reduce anxiety, hyperarousal, and impulsivity and improve attention.[15,16] In patients with dissociation, medications that enhance gamma aminobutyric acid (GABA), such as the benzodiazepines or gabapentin (Neurontin), may reduce the severity of anxiety. In patients with fear or terror, the short-term use of atypical antipsychotics in low doses may be useful. Long-term treatment of ASD/PTSD utilizes both pharmacologic and psychotherapeutic modalities.[17]

For anxiety disorders not co-occurring with depression, high-potency (e.g., alprazolam 0.25 to 1 mg three times per day or clonazepam 0.25 to 1 mg three times per day) or medium-potency (e.g., lorazepam 0.25 to 1 mg three times per day) benzodiazepines can be effective. In general, the clinical toxicity of benzodiazepines is low, but higher rates of disinhibition are observed in the pediatric population than in adults. The most commonly encountered short-term adverse effects of benzodiazepines are sedation, disinhibition, and depression. With the exception of the theoretical potential risk for tolerance and dependence that appears to be low in children, no known long-term adverse effects are associated with benzodiazepines. Adverse effects of withdrawal can occur, and benzodiazepines should be tapered slowly.

Long-acting benzodiazepines such as clonazepam may be preferable when long-term treatment with a benzodiazepine is warranted. For clonazepam, an initial dose of 0.25 to 0.5 mg can be given at bedtime. The dose can be increased by 0.5 mg every 5 to 7 days depending on the clinical response and the side effects. Typically, doses between 0.25 and 2.0 mg/day are effective. When utilizing high-potency benzodiazepines in pediatric patients, clinicians should monitor for signs of disinhibition, which may present as either excessively silly behavior or as agitation. As with other psychotropic medications, the daily dose should be slowly titrated to allow for use of the lowest effective dose. Potential benefits of the longer-acting compounds are single-daily dosage and a decreased risk of withdrawal symptoms upon discontinuation of treatment.

A short-acting compound such as lorazepam can be very effective in managing more acute situations (e.g., anxious or agitated reactions to psychosocial crises). As discussed, the dose should be titrated based on the individual's response. Doses of 0.5 to 1.0 mg of lorazepam given orally or sublingually are often effective. Use of short-acting benzodiazepines requires multiple daily dosage because of their short half-lives. Long-term use should be avoided whenever possible. Lorazepam may be administered intramuscularly in an emergency. Children who become disinhibited on high-potency benzodiazepines may respond more favorably to the mid- or low-potency agents, such as clorazepate or diazepam.

Buspirone is a novel nonbenzodiazepine anxiolytic without anticonvulsant, sedative, or muscle relaxant properties. Clinical experience with this drug suggests limited antianxiety efficacy that may be boosted by use of higher doses or by using it in combination with an SSRI. The effective daily dose is estimated to range from 0.3 to 0.6 mg/kg. It has also been suggested that buspirone may be effective in the treatment of aggressive behaviors in children with developmental disorders (e.g., pervasive developmental disorders).

Antidepressants may be helpful for children in whom anxiety does not respond to benzodiazepines when there is a risk of abuse of the medication or in cases where comorbidity, (e.g., depression or ADHD) is present. Many SSRIs used in doses similar to those incorporated in the treatment of adults have been shown to be helpful with the management of juvenile anxiety disorders. TCAs have also been useful for management of anxiety disorders; one controlled study with high-dose imipramine demonstrated efficacy under controlled conditions.[18]

Akathisia

Akathisia is a movement disorder associated with anxiety and an inability to sit still. The term is derived from Greek and it literally means 'not to sit.'[19] In children and adolescents it is most often seen as a side effect of either antipsychotics or antidepressants. Given the inability to sit still, akathisia may be confused with ADHD or agitation. Historically patients are free of this problem prior to starting an antidepressant or antipsychotic or reducing an anticholinergic medication. Treatment of akathisia involves reducing the dose of the precipitating medication to the lowest effective dose and then either using benzodiazepines (0.5 to 1 mg three times per day of lorazepam) or β-blockers. Although all β-blockers are likely to be effective, propranolol is typically used. Propranolol should be initiated at 10 mg two times per day and the dose increased every several days to good effect.

Of note, recent studies in adults demonstrate the efficacy of the potent selective β-1 blocking agent betaxolol in reducing akathisia. Betaxolol is a selective and potent β-1 blocker with a long half-life (allowing a dose once daily) with minimal medication interactions. Betaxolol is generally initiated at 5 mg and can be titrated as tolerated to doses between 10 to 20 mg/day.

Obsessive-Compulsive Disorder

OCD is the best studied of the juvenile anxiety conditions. OCD often develops early in life; nearly one-third of adults with obsessions report the onset of their symptoms before the age of 15 years, and cases of the disorder have been described as early as the age of 3. It is characterized by persistent ideas or impulses (obsessions) that are intrusive and senseless (e.g., thoughts of having caused violence, becoming contaminated, or severely doubting oneself) that may lead to persistent repetitive, purposeful behaviors (compulsions), (e.g., hand-washing, counting, checking, or touching in order to neutralize the obsessive worries).[20] Within the medical setting, this disorder is often associated with an exaggerated, persistent, and impairing obsession with an organ, disease process, or treatment. This disorder has been estimated to affect 1% to 2% of the adult population; it has been shown to be familial and associated with Tourette's syndrome (TS) and ADHD.

The drug treatment of OCD with serotonergic medications has been promising. Studies suggest that children with OCD respond in a similar fashion to these agents as their adult counterparts. Currently the SSRIs, (e.g., sertraline [Zoloft, initiated at 12.5 to 25 mg daily and titrated to 50 to 200 mg daily], fluvoxamine [Luvox, a more sedating drug that is initiated at 25 mg at bedtime and increased to 25 to 150 mg twice per day and fluoxetine [Prozac, initiated at 5 to 10 mg and increased to 60 mg/day]) are FDA-approved for OCD in the pediatric population.[21-25] In addition, the TCA, clomipramine (Anafranil), has been shown under controlled conditions to be useful for this chronic disorder. These studies suggest a clomipramine dosage of up to 250 mg/day, a fluoxetine dose of approximately 10 to 40 mg/day, and a sertraline dose of 50 to 200 mg/day, although anecdotal information indicates that some children may require higher dosages. Treatment with these agents should be initiated at a low dose (e.g., 25 mg/day of clomipramine) and increased slowly according to clinical response and side effects. In addition, the SSRIs paroxetine (Paxil), citalopram (Celexa), escitalopram (Lexapro), and the mixed agent venlafaxine (Effexor) may be useful in the management of OCD. Recently, interest has grown in a syndrome that resembles both OCD and tic disorders called pediatric autoimmune neuropsychiatric disorders associated with streptococcal infection (PANDAS). Investigators recently have studied plasma exchange, intravenous (IV) immunoglobulin, and penicillin to treat OCD/tics associated with PANDAS. Although many of these patients responded favorably to the treatments, the numbers studied remain small and the study designs were open.[26,27] These treatments appear effective only for those patients whose OCD/tics were associated with streptococcal infections.

Tic Disorders

The best known tic disorder is Torrete's Syndrome (TS), a childhood-onset neuropsychiatric disorder with an often life-long duration; it is manifest by multiple motor and phonic tics, and other behavioral and psychological symptoms. TS is commonly associated with OCD (in about 30% of cases) and ADHD (in about 50% of cases). It is noteworthy that in many cases it is not the tics but the comorbid disorders that are the major source of distress and disability. Much interest has been expressed in overlap of TS with ADHD. Some interesting associations include the findings that ADHD appears earlier in life than tics, and stimulants may exacerbate tics. For many patients with tics and ADHD, the symptoms of ADHD appear associated with the most severe impairment.

Several typical antipsychotics (e.g., haloperidol and pimozide) have been considered the drugs of choice in TS, however, antipsychotics have limited effects on the frequently associated comorbid disorders of ADHD and OCD, and they are associated with short-term (e.g., extrapyramidal side effects [EPS]) and long-term adverse effects (e.g., tardive dyskinesia [TD]). Recently,

pilot studies of the atypical antipsychotics, risperidone (Risperdal) and ziprasidone (Geodon), have been completed in the treatment of TS. These studies show that both ziprasidone (initially dosed at 20 mg/day and increased to a mean dose of approximately 60 mg per/day) and risperidone (titrated to a maximum dose of 0.06 mg/kg/day in one study and a maximum of 3 mg/day in another) were effective and generally well tolerated.[28–31] Both of these medications are potent blockers of D_2 and $5\text{-}HT_{2A}$ receptors, thereby reducing the theoretic risk of EPS and TD. Of note, dysphoria and depression are reported to occur in adolescents with TS who are treated with risperidone.[32] Clonidine has been shown to be highly effective in reducing the severity and frequency of tics and is considered a first-line drug for tic disorder and TS. Clonidine is usually begun at very low doses (i.e., 0.025 mg/day) to reduce the initial adverse effect of sedation and it is increased upward as necessary. Comparison between clonidine and risperidone and risperidone and pimozide demonstrated similar improvements in tic severity.[29,33] In addition, clonidine alone and in combination with methylphenidate was recently studied for effects on tics and ADHD.[34] Compared with placebo, clonidine and methylphenidate, clonidine alone, and methylphenidate alone were associated with reductions in tic severity. Although some patients experience an exacerbation of tics during treatment with stimulants (and it is still listed as a contraindication in the Physicians Desk Reference), many patients appear to benefit from treatment of their ADHD symptoms.

Recently, the TCAs have been found to be effective in some children with this disorder. There have been promising results in open and controlled investigations of TCAs (desipramine and nortriptyline) for ADHD and tic symptoms in juveniles with tic disorders and TS.[35] Given concerns over cardiac safety with the TCAs, atomoxetine (ATMX) may be an effective treatment for patients with ADHD and TS, although this remains to be formally studied. Additional recent reports indicate a variety of medications may prove useful in patients with TS with or without ADHD, including the selective type B, irreversible MAOI, L-deprenyl, the mixed $D_1/D_2/D_3$ dopamine agonist pergolide,[36,37] the hypotensive agent mecamylamine[38,39] and medications that enhance cholinergic neurotransmission (e.g., donepezil and nicotine).[40,41]

Cannabinoids have also been investigated as a potential treatment for TS, although this is not currently recommended.[42] Patients with comorbid OCD may need additional pharmacotherapy with serotonergic agents (e.g., clomipramine or the SSRIs).

Attention-Deficit Hyperactivity Disorder

ADHD is a common psychiatric condition shown to occur in 3% to 10% of school-age children.[43] ADHD is characterized by the classic triad of impaired attention, impulsivity, and excessive motor activity, although up to one third of children may only manifest the inattentive aspects of ADHD.[44] With developmental variations, ADHD affects children of all ages, as early as the age of 3, and it persists throughout adolescence and into adulthood about half of the time.[45] Within the medical setting, ADHD needs to be differentiated from environmental stimulation, iatrogenic causes (e.g., beta-agonists), or other psychiatric disorders, such as anxiety, depression, mania, or intoxication. Pharmacotherapy remains the cornerstone of ADHD treatment.[46–50]

For over 60 years stimulants have been used safely and effectively in the treatment of ADHD. Stimulants most commonly used are methylphenidate (MPH) (e.g., short-acting forms like Ritalin and Focalin and extended delivery forms such as Concerta, Ritalin-LA, Metadate-CD, and the older form of Ritalin-SR), dextroamphetamine (e.g., the short-acting form of Dexedrine tablets and the long-acting form in Dexedrine spansules) and a mixture of amphetamine salts (e.g., Adderall and an extended delivery form, Adderall-XR).

Stimulants have been shown to increase intrasynaptic concentrations of dopamine (DA) and norepinephrine (NE).[51,52] After oral administration, stimulants are rapidly absorbed and preferentially taken up into the CNS. Food has little impact on their absorption, but lowering the pH in the gastrointestinal (GI) tract may delay the C_{max} and T_{max} of the amphetamines and certain forms of extended delivery MPH. Stimulants bind poorly to plasma proteins. MPH is metabolized primarily by plasma-based esterases to ritalinic acid that is excreted in the urine. The amphetamines are 80% excreted in the urine unchanged, whereas 20% undergo hepatic metabolism. Acidification of the urine may enhance excretion of the amphetamines. Although the amphetamines are detected on routine urine drug screening, MPH is not usually detected.

As it was originally formulated in 1954, MPH was produced as an equal mixture of D, L-threo-MPH and D, L-erythro-MPH. Soon afterwards it was realized that the erythro form of MPH produced cardiovascular side effects, and thus MPH is now manufactured as an equal mixture of D, L-threo-MPH. Studies have indicated that the primarily active form of MPH is the D-threo isomer. Therefore the makers of Ritalin now produce the isomer or Ritalin called Focalin (D-threo-MPH or dex-MPH). Clinicians should note that in terms of potency that 10 mg of Ritalin is biologically equivalent to 5 mg of Focalin. Oral administration of immediate-release D, L-threo-MPH (available in generic MPH, Ritalin, Metadate ER, Methylin) results in a variable peak plasma concentration within 1 to 2 hours, with a half-life of 2 to 3 hours. Behavioral effects of immediate release MPH peak 1 to 2 hours after administration, and tend to dissipate within 3 to 5 hours. Although generic MPH has a similar pharmacokinetic profile to Ritalin, it is more rapidly absorbed and peaks sooner. Plasma levels of the sustained-release preparation of MPH (Ritalin-SR) peak in 1 to 4 hours, with a half-life of 2 to 6 hours. Clinicians observe variability in the absorption of the SR preparation and are using it less now that several alternative extended delivery systems are available. Peak behavioral effects of this preparation occur 2 hours after ingestion, and last up to 8 hours. Because of the wax-matrix preparation, absorption is clinically observed to be variable. Recently, several novel methods of delivering MPH and amphetamine have become available, all intended to extend the clinical effectiveness of the stimulants. Although these medications all deliver stimulant, their pharmacokinetic profiles differ. Concerta (Oros-methylphenidate) the first of these novel delivery systems, has been available since August 2000. Concerta uses the OROS technology to deliver a 50:50 racemic mixture of D, L-threo-MPH. An 18 mg caplet of Concerta delivers the equivalent of 15 mg of MPH (5 mg of

MPH three times per day) providing 12-hour coverage. Initially the 18-mg caplet provides 4 mg of MPH and delivers the additional MPH in an ascending profile over 12 hours.[53] The recommended dose of Concerta is between 18 to 54 mg/day, although a recent trial in adolescents studied doses up to 72 mg/day.[54] If Concerta is cut or crushed, its delivery system is compromised. Metadate-CD, available as a 20-mg capsule, which may be sprinkled, contains two types of beads containing D, L-threo-MPH.[55] Metadate-CD delivers 30% or 6 mg of D, L-threo-MPH initially and is designed for 8-hour coverage. Ritalin-LA, available in capsules of 20 mg, 30 mg, and 40 mg that may be sprinkled, delivers 50% of its D, L-threo-MPH initially and another bolus approximately 3 to 4 hours later, thereby providing around 8 hours of coverage. Recently, a MPH patch has shown encouraging results and may soon be available.

Dextroamphetamine achieves peak plasma levels 2 to 3 hours after oral administration, and it has a half-life of 4 to 6 hours.[51,56] Behavioral effects of dextroamphetamine peak 1 to 2 hours after administration and last 4 to 5 hours. For dextroamphetamine spansules, these values are somewhat longer. Adderall is a racemic mixture of D- and L-amphetamine. The two isomers have different pharmacodynamic properties, and some children with ADHD may have a preferential response to one isomer over the other. Recent data in children with ADHD suggest that, when compared with immediate-release Ritalin, peak behavioral effects of Adderall occur later and are more sustained.[57] Adderall-XR is a capsule that delivers two forms of mixed amphetamine salt in the form of beads. One type of bead releases its medication immediately, whereas another type of bead delays release by 4 hours. Studies of the pharmacokinetics of Adderall-XR show that a single dose of Adderall-XR 20 mg is bioequivalent to 10 mg of Adderall tablet dosed twice per day.

Pemoline is a CNS stimulant that is structurally different from both MPH and amphetamine and that seems to enhance central dopaminergic transmission. Pemoline reaches peak plasma levels 1 to 4 hours after ingestion and has a half-life of 7 to 8 hours in children and 11 to 13 hours in adults. A number of patients taking pemoline have developed significant hepatitis resulting in liver failure and in some cases death or need for liver transplant. Given concerns regarding potential hepatic toxicity, the FDA now recommends that patients taking pemoline have liver function tests assessed every 2 weeks. Although compliance with these recommendations has been scanty, pemoline has clinically been relegated to a third-line agent because of the availability of other long-acting stimulants and ATMX.

The AACAP has recently released guidelines on the use of stimulants in children, adolescents, and adults.[46] Short-acting stimulants are generally used for ADHD and are typically initiated at low doses (2.5 to 5 mg/day for children and adolescents, 5 to 10 mg/day for adults), given in the morning with food. Current treatment guidelines recommend starting with longer-acting preparations in most cases. Clinicians can initiate therapy at 18 mg of Concerta or 20 mg of Metadate-CD or Ritalin-LA for MPH products or 5 to 10 mg of Adderall-XR or Dexedrine spansules. Every few days the dose may be increased to optimize response. Although the PDR lists maximum dosages for amphetamine products at 40 mg/day and 60 mg/day for MPH, patients often benefit from suggested daily doses that range from 0.3 to 1.5 mg/kg/day for amphetamine products and from 0.5 to 2.0 mg/kg/day for MPH products. Frequently, patients benefit from adding immediate-release amphetamine or MPH in combination with longer-acting preparations in order to sculpt the dose to the patient's needs, although the efficacy of this practice has not been well studied.

Numerous short-term clinical trials (less than 12 weeks) show that approximately 70% of patients with ADHD respond to stimulants; a positive dose-response relationship is present for both the behavioral and cognitive effects of stimulants when used in children and adolescents with ADHD. Recently longer-term trials have demonstrated the tolerability and continued efficacy of stimulants in patients treated continuously over 2 years. Clinicians face a number of challenges when prescribing stimulants. Stimulants may decrease appetite in this patient population, so it often is useful to administer stimulants during or after meals. Food may even enhance their bioavailability. Stimulant-induced sleep disturbances are common and may diminish their effectiveness. Such disturbances may require alteration of the timing or amount of medication given or may require the administration of a sleep aid. Symptomatic treatment of ADHD-associated sleep disturbances include ensuring good sleep hygiene and use of clonidine (0.05 to 0.2 mg at bedtime), imipramine (25 to 100 mg at bedtime, which may be especially helpful if patient also suffers from enuresis), diphenhydramine (25 to 50 mg at bedtime, although its effectiveness is often short-lived), and trazodone (25 to 150 mg at bedtime, though one must monitor for priapism). Anecdotal reports describe the utility of melatonin in either oral or sublingual forms for ADHD-associated sleep disturbances in doses from 200 μg to 6 mg/day. Because melatonin is sold over the counter (OTC), patients may experience variability in the product. Irritability or dysphoria may occur 1 to 2 hours after administration of stimulants, which suggests an absorption peak phenomenon that may respond to lower and more frequent doses.

A majority of patients with ADHD experience at least one additional comorbid psychiatric disorder. ADHD is comorbid with oppositional defiant disorder (in up to 70%), conduct disorder (in approximately 25%), anxiety disorders (in approximately 40%), mood disorders (in approximately 33%), learning disorders (in approximately 40%), and substance use disorders.[58] These comorbid disorders may alter a stimulant's effectiveness. For instance, patients with ADHD and comorbid mood or anxiety disorders may respond differently to a stimulant, depending on the clinical state of their co-occurring disorders. In addition, stimulants may exacerbate tics, obsessions, or compulsions, although they are frequently used in patients with these conditions. Clinicians are often concerned about growth delays, tolerance, and abuse among stimulant-treated patients. Although short-term decreases in weight are often seen in children treated with stimulants, follow-up studies into adulthood have not demonstrated decreases in the ultimate height attained. Although tolerance to the effects of stimulants on ADHD symptoms has been debated, data from the NIMH Multimodal Treatment of ADHD demonstrated the persistence of stimulant medication effects. Dextroamphetamine, Adderall, and MPH are Schedule II medications that have the potential for abuse. Although the rates of substance abuse in patients with ADHD are increased, the use of stimulants does not appear to increase the risk of substance abuse; recent data suggest that successful stimulant treatment of children with ADHD may delay or decrease their risk of substance abuse in adolescence. Pemoline, a Schedule IV medication, has a low potential for abuse. Concerns remains regarding the addictive potential of stimulants. The design of the recently available extended delivery preparations makes misuse of stimulants more difficult. When administered orally in their intended dosages, stimulants do not appear to cause euphoria nor do they appear to be addictive. The order of addictive liability with available preparations from most to least addictive is amphetamine, MPH, then pemoline. Recent meta-analytic data show that in patients with ADHD treated for years with stimulants, the risk of substance abuse is cut in half compared with patients with ADHD who are not treated with stimulants.[59]

Stimulants can cause clinically significant anorexia, nausea, difficulty falling asleep, rebound phenomena, anxiety, nightmares, dizziness, irritability, dysphoria, and weight loss.[59] They also are associated with small increases in heart rate and blood pressure, which are usually not clinically significant. Occasionally, they may elicit a depressive reaction or psychosis. Stimulant use may exacerbate tics or TS. Although a physical withdrawal is not associated with stimulants, patients who have used high doses for a prolonged time may experience fatigue, hypersomnia, hyperphagia, dysphoria, and depression upon discontinuation. Given the abuse potential of these medications, it is important to inquire about concomitant use of drugs and alcohol. Other infrequent side effects include headaches, abdominal discomfort, lethargy, and fatigue. Mild increases in the baseline pulse and blood pressure (usually of little clinical significance) can also be observed, particularly in adults.

Stimulants can be safely administered with other medications, including antibiotics, anticonvulsants, dermatologic agents, antihistamines, and OTC preparations.[52] Interactions of stimulants with other prescription and nonprescription medications are generally mild and not a major source of concern. Concomitant use of sympathomimetic agents (e.g., pseudoephedrine) may potentiate the effects of both medications. Concurrent use of antihistamines may diminish the effects of stimulants. Although data on the co-administration of stimulants with TCAs suggest little interaction between these compounds, careful monitoring is warranted when prescribing stimulants with either TCAs or anticonvulsants. MPH taken along with ATMX is generally well tolerated. Co-administration of MAOIs with stimulants may result in a hypertensive crisis and be potentially life threatening.

Concerns have also centered on the effect of long-term administration of stimulants on growth. Whereas stimulants do not appear to significantly negatively impact growth for most patients, this issue has not been fully resolved. Although recent long-term trials with stimulants appear to alleviate concerns about growth, soon-to-be-published data from the Multimodal Treatment of ADHD (MTA) trial will add to the understanding of this complex issue. Current consensus is that stimulants may infrequently produce a small, negative (deficit) impact on growth velocity, however this delay may be related more to ADHD than its treatment.[60] If a decrease in growth rate occurs while a child is taking a stimulant, consideration should be given to either a medication "holiday" or alternative treatment options. Despite the vast literature and excellent safety of stimulants, studies indicate that approximately one third of children and adolescents with ADHD either do not respond or manifest intolerable adverse effects that necessitate alternative treatments. Fortunately, ATMX and other off-label treatments, including antidepressants and antihypertensives, are available.

ATMX is recently-approved non-stimulant agent for the treatment of ADHD. ATMX is a highly selective norepinephrine reuptake inhibitor (SNRI) that was initially studied as an antidepressant. Unlike the stimulants ATMX is not a Class II medication; therefore, clinicians can provide samples as well as prescribe refills. ATMX acts by blocking the norepinephrine reuptake pump on the presynaptic membrane, thus increasing the availability of intrasynaptic NE. ATMX is rapidly absorbed following oral administration and food does not appear to effect absorption, and C_{max} is 1 to 2 hours after the dose is administered.

In many patients ATMX can be initiated at 0.5 mg/kg/day (or at lower doses) and after a few days it can be increased to a target dose of 1.2 mg/kg/day; some patients may require a slower taper. Although ATMX was initially titrated up to 2 mg/kg/day in divided doses the current dosage guidelines recommend maximum dosage of 1.4 mg/kg/day in a single daily dose (usually after breakfast). Although the plasma half-life appears to be around 5 hours, the CNS effects appear to last over 24 hours. Therefore, most patients can be effectively covered by a single daily dose, although some patients may benefit from a twice-daily dose of medication.[61]

ATMX is associated with reduced appetite, dyspepsia, fatigue, and dizziness.[62] Extensive laboratory testing suggests the ATMX causes no organ toxicity and there were no discontinuations in the clinical trials as a result of abnormal laboratory tests. At this time, laboratory monitoring outside of routine medical care is not necessary. Similarly, the impact of ATMX on the cardiovascular system appears minimal. ATMX was associated with mean increases in heart rate of 6 beats per minute, and increases in systolic and diastolic blood pressure of 1.5 mm Hg. Extensive electrocardiogram (ECG) monitoring indicates that ATMX has no apparent effect on QTc intervals, and ECG monitoring outside of routine medical care does not appear necessary.

ATMX is metabolized primarily in the liver to 4-hydroxyatomoxetine by the cytochrome (CYP) P450 2D6 enzyme.[63,64] The minor metabolite of ATMX is desmethylatomoxetine that is primarily formed by CYP 2C19. In patients with compromised CYP 2D6 functioning, other enzymes were observed to be capable of forming 4-hydroxyatomoxetine. Although ATMX is primarily metabolized by 2D6, it does not appear to inhibit 2D6. ATMX is primarily excreted in the urine. Although patients identified as 'poor metabolizers' (i.e., low 2D6 activity) appear to generally tolerate ATMX, they seem to have more side effects, and a reduction in dose may be necessary. Therefore, in patients who are taking medications that are strong 2D6 inhibitors (e.g., fluoxetine, paroxetine, and quinidine), it may be necessary to reduce the dose of ATMX. Use of ATMX is contraindicated with MAOIs. ATMX has been co-administered with albuterol (600 μg intravenously) in patients with asthma. Mild elevations in heart rate and blood pressure with ATMX alone were observed. Similarly, in a small trial, ATMX was administered with MPH and appeared well tolerated, although co-administration of ATMX and the stimulants has not been fully studied.

Several controlled reports have shown that children and adolescents with ADHD may also respond favorably to bupropion hydrochloride (Wellbutrin), a unicyclic aminoketone with antidepressant properties.[65] Bupropion may be particularly helpful in children with ADHD with a prominent mood component.[66] When used in children, the risk factors and symptoms of an untreated seizure disorder should be reviewed carefully. Bupropion may cause irritability and agitation and has been reported to exacerbate tics. Treatment should be initiated at 37.5 mg/day of the IR or 100 mg SR and titrated gradually as indicated. Although dosage guidelines are not available for children, in one study, doses of 3 to 6 mg/day were utilized. As in adults, the medication should be given in divided doses and no single dose should exceed 150 mg. A recent open trial found the SR form of bupropion (mean dose 2.2 mg/kg in the morning and 1.7 mg/kg in the afternoon) helpful for reducing symptoms of depression and ADHD. Moreover, an additional method of delivering bupropion (Wellbutrin XL) is now available, which enables once-daily dosage for most patients.

Until recently the TCAs were considered the second line of medication for ADHD. Given concerns over cardiotoxicity and with the availability of ATMX, the role of TCAs has been curtailed. However, TCAs remain effective and will likely continue to have a role in the pharmacotherapy of patients with ADHD. Desipramine and nortriptyline are associated with somewhat lower risks of adverse effects (e.g., sedation, dry mouth, and impairment in cognition) than imipramine and other tertiary amine TCAs, and therefore may be better tolerated by patients.[67] Initial open trials were followed by controlled studies; they showed that TCAs were superior to placebo, although not superior to stimulants.[68] Possible advantages of TCAs over stimulants include a longer duration of action, the feasibility of a once-daily dosage without symptom rebound or insomnia, greater flexibility in dosage, the option of monitoring plasma drug levels, improved compliance, and a minimal risk of abuse or dependence.

Prior to treatment with a TCA, a baseline ECG should be obtained (as well as inquiry into any family history of early-onset or sudden cardiac arrhythmias).[4] Treatment with a TCA should be initiated with 10 mg or 25 mg depending on the size of the child (approximately 1 mg/kg) and increased slowly every 4 to 5 days by increments of 20% to 30%. For imipramine and desipramine, an upper dose limit of 5 mg/kg/day has been suggested for children, and for nortriptyline 2 mg/kg per day is suggested. When a daily dose of 2 to 3 mg/kg/day (or a lower effective dose for imipramine [IMI] and desipramine [DMI] or 1 mg/kg/day for nortriptyline [NT]) is reached, steady-state serum levels and an ECG should be obtained. A steady-state serum level obtained 10 to 14 hours after the last dose is usually achieved after at least 1 week on the same daily dose. Monitoring serum levels of TCAs is more helpful in avoiding toxicity than it is in determining optimal levels for response.

Common short-term adverse consequences of the TCAs include anticholinergic effects (e.g., dry mouth, blurred vision, and constipation). To date, no known deleterious effects have been associated with chronic administration of these drugs. The anticholinergic effects of TCAs limit salivary flow, so they may promote tooth decay in some children. Following the sudden death of a number of children receiving desipramine, concerns were raised regarding the possible cardiac toxicity of TCAs in children.[69] However, epidemiologic evaluation of the association between desipramine and sudden death in children has not supported a causal relationship.[70] TCAs predictably increase heart rate and are associated with conduction delays that generally affect the right bundle and thus require ECG monitoring.[71] However, these effects, when small, rarely seem to be pathophysiologically significant in noncardiac patients with normal baseline ECG readings. In children with documented congenital or acquired cardiac disease, pathologic rhythm disturbances (i.e., atrioventricular block, supraventricular tachycardia, ventricular tachycardia, and Wolff-Parkinson-White syndrome), family history of sudden cardiac death or cardiomyopathy, diastolic hypertension (>90 mm Hg), or when in doubt about the cardiovascular state of the patient, a complete (noninvasive) cardiac evaluation is indicated before initiating treatment with a TCA to help determine the risk-benefit ratio of such an intervention. A serious adverse event associated with use of TCAs is overdose either by the patient or by a sibling. Hence, parents should closely supervise the storage and administration of these medications.

Clonidine has achieved an increasing prominence in pediatric psychopharmacology because of its wide range of uses and relative safety.[72] Although clonidine ameliorates symptoms of ADHD,[73] its overall effect is less than the stimulants[74] and likely smaller than ATMX, TCAs, and bupropion. Clonidine appears particularly helpful in patients with ADHD and comorbid conduct or oppositional defiant disorder,[75,76] tic disorders,[77,78] and ADHD-associated sleep disturbances.[79,80] In addition, clonidine has been increasingly reported to be useful in developmentally disordered patients to control aggression to self and others.[81] Furthermore, clonidine appears to reduce anxiety and hypervigilance in traumatized children.[15]

Clonidine is an imidazoline derivative with alpha-adrenergic agonist properties; it has been primarily used in the treatment of hypertension.[82] At low doses, it appears to stimulate inhibitory, presynaptic autoreceptors in the CNS.[83] Clonidine is a relatively short-acting compound with a plasma half-life ranging from approximately 5.5 hours (children) to 8.5 hours (in adults). Usual daily dose ranges from 3 to 10 µg/kg given generally in divided doses, once per day, twice per day, or three times per day, and there is a transdermal preparation.[84] Therapy is usually initiated at the lowest manufactured dose of a half- or quarter-tablet of 0.1 mg depending on the size of the child (approximately 1 to 2 µg/kg) and increased depending on clinical response and adverse effects. Initial dosage can more easily be given in the evening hours or before bedtime because of sedation. The most common short-term adverse effect of clonidine is sedation, which tends to subside with continued treatment. It can also produce, in some cases, hypotension, dry mouth, vivid dreams, depression, and confusion. Except in overdose, clonidine is not known to be associated with long-term serious adverse effects. Because abrupt withdrawal of clonidine has been associated with rebound hypertension, slow tapering is advised.[85,86] In addition, extreme caution should be exercised with the co-administration of clonidine with β-blockers or calcium channel blockers as adverse reactions,

including complete heart block, have been reported.[87] After reports of several sudden deaths related to clonidine use, concerns about the safety of co-administration of clonidine with stimulants were raised.[88,89] However, these cases were thoroughly examined and no causative link between the combination and sudden death was found. For additional review of these issues, refer to Wilens et al.[90] Current guidelines are to monitor blood pressure when initiating and tapering clonidine, but ECG monitoring is not usually necessary.[4]

Recently the clonidine-like, more selective, α_2-adrenergic agonist compound guanfacine (Tenex) has been used as an alternative to clonidine for the same indications.[91,92] Possible advantages of guanfacine over clonidine include less sedation and a longer duration of action. Anecdotal information suggests that guanfacine may have less effectiveness in reducing the behavioral ramifications of ADHD (impulsivity, aggressiveness, and hyperactivity) but more usefulness in improving the cognitive deficits of ADHD. In open pilot trials, school-age children with ADHD and comorbid tic disorder, treated with guanfacine in doses ranging from 0.5 mg twice per day to 1.0 mg three times per day showed reduction in both tics and ADHD.[93] Recent controlled data demonstrated the benefit of guanfacine in reducing tic severity and ADHD symptomology.[94] In this study, guanfacine treatment was associated with minor, clinically insignificant decreases in blood pressure and pulse rate. The adverse effects of guanfacine include sedation, irritability, and depression. Recently, several cases of apparent guanfacine-induced mania have been reported, but the impact of guanfacine on mood disorders remains unclear.[95]

Mood Disorders

Depression

Children and adolescents may have various depressive disorders including major depression, dysthymia or mood disturbances associated with medical conditions, substance use/abuse, or as a result of psychosocial problems.[96] In the medical setting, clinicians are challenged to differentiate transient symptoms of depression from true depressive disorders. In the hospital setting, children and adolescents may experience depressive symptoms related to their illness or treatment. Children often manifest worry, hopelessness, and sadness as primary symptoms related to their own illness, whereas adolescents typically display anxiety, anger, or withdrawal. If the symptoms are episodic and associated with limited impairment, they are generally referred to as an adjustment disorder with depressed or anxious mood. These patients usually respond to reassurance, environmental intervention, or interpersonal or cognitive-behavioral psychotherapy. In the outpatient medical setting, children and adolescents with depression may present for evaluation of a variety of medical symptoms of unclear etiology. During routine examination these patients may present as sad, withdrawn, apathetic, anxious, angry, or irritable. Although an increasing number of families appear to be seeking care from primary care physicians for depression, recent data suggest that most family physicians and pediatricians believe they are inadequately trained in screening for, evaluating, and managing pediatric depression.[97,98]

Major depression increases in prevalence with age. Epidemiologic studies from community and clinical samples estimate the prevalence of major depressive disorder (MDD) as approximately 0.3% of preschoolers, 2% of children, and between 1.5% to 9% of adolescents.[99–107] By the end of adolescence, the cumulative incidence of MDD is estimated to be 20%.[102,105,106,108] Although the gender ratio appears equal in children, by the age of 14, girls appear twice as likely to experience depression as boys.[109] However, additional data suggest that boys and girls who have onset of depression during prepubescence experience similar symptoms, rates of recovery, relapse, and comorbidity.[110] Depressive disorders commonly co-occur with anxiety, ADHD, conduct, and substance use disorders in older children and adolescents.[111] The challenge to the clinician is to recognize the developmental progression of comorbidity. Children initially may be evaluated and treated for ADHD, only to develop depression several years later during their course of treatment for ADHD.

Pediatric depressive disorders are recognized with core symptoms similar to those found in adults, but with developmentally specific associated features including sudden-onset school difficulties, school refusal, irritability, sad faces, low energy, isolation, withdrawal, negativism, and aggression/prolonged irritability.[112,113] Diagnostic criteria for MDD include a 2-week period of symptoms that represent a change from previous functioning, with at least one of the symptoms being either depressed mood (which may manifest as irritability in pediatric patients) or loss of interest or pleasure. Other symptoms include decreased or increased appetite, weight loss (or, in children, failure to make expected weight gains), weight gain, insomnia or hypersomnia, psychomotor retardation or agitation, fatigue or loss of energy, feelings of worthlessness, inappropriate or excessive guilt (which may manifest in children as extreme sensitivity to rejection or requests), diminished ability to concentrate (which may manifest in children as indecisiveness), and recurrent thoughts of death or suicidal ideation, intent, or plan.[96] Assessing depression in preschoolers may require some adjustment from the *Diagnostic and Statistical Manual for Mental Disorders*, fourth edition (*DSM-IV*) and remains an area of active investigation.[114]

The duration of pediatric depression appears to be approximately 7 months, and in the course of a first episode, up to 40% appear to recover without specific treatment.[112,115] However, patients who do not recover are at high risk of chronic depression, and those who do recover have high rates of recurrence and dysthymia.[116,117] Evidence suggests that children of parents who suffered a depression, especially before the age of 30, have a significantly increased risk for recurrent bouts of depressions.[118,119] Mood disorders in children tend to be chronic compared with the more episodic nature typical of adult mood disorders. Furthermore, children and adolescents with depression have a higher rate of conversion to bipolar disorder. In follow-up, almost half of children who initially had single-episode, nonpsychotic MDD converted to bipolar disorder that lasts into their early twenties.[120,121] Similarly, up to 20% of adolescents who have MDD converted to bipolar disorder in follow-up.[122] Risk factors for switching from MDD to bipolar disorder include history of bipolar disorder in parents and grandparents and family history of antidepressant-induced mania. Other warning signs of conversion to mania include rapid onset of depression associated with psychosis, psychomotor retardation, and hypersomnia.[123] These patients may be at increased risk for self-injurious behaviors or suicide.

Suicidal ideation, threats, and behaviors are commonly seen among children and adolescents with psychiatric disorders. These behaviors are of great concern to clinicians who need to provide safety within the medical setting and to identify patients at increased risk of self-injurious behaviors. The American Academy of Pediatrics (AAP) and the AACAP recently published reviews and guidelines for the evaluation and management of suicidal behaviors in children and adolescents.[124,125] Suicide remains a leading cause of death in adolescents age 15 to 19 years because the numbers of adolescent suicides has increased dramatically in the past few decades. Overall, males are at increased risk compared with females; in particular boys with previous suicide attempts, a mood disorder (depression or bipolar), and associated substance abuse are at higher risk. Females at greatest risk have mood disorders (depression or bipolar) and a history of previous suicidal behaviors. After a suicide attempt, patients with a history of suicidal behaviors, who continue to think about suicide, who live alone and are agitated, who are irritable and have associated MDD, and who have bipolar disorder or substance abuse are at greatest risk. In addition to medical care, these patients require close monitoring, including possible restraint, seclusion, or observation by a sitter. Information needs to be obtained from outside sources (e.g., family, school, and therapist), and the patient must be evaluated for underlying psychiatric disorder(s) and treated appropriately. In outpatient settings, approximately half of children referred for depression are suicidal. For children in whom more malignant symptoms occur or in whom there is significant impairment or suicidality, the consideration of pharmacotherapy is necessary.

Similar to adults, children with subsyndromal depressive disorders, which are long-standing and often associated with anhedonia and negativity, may have dysthymic disorder. Dysthymia in children and adolescents is manifest by chronically depressed mood for at least 1 year, associated with change in appetite (too little or too much), sleep disturbance (insomnia or hypersomnia), low energy, easy fatigability, low self-esteem,

indecisiveness, poor concentration, and feelings of hopelessness.[20] Juveniles with dysthymia are often self-critical and feel easily criticized/rejected. Although dysthymic disorder is a major risk factor for future episodes of major depression,[126] juveniles with dysthymia have fewer melancholic symptoms and suicidality. In contrast to adults, children and adolescents must manifest their symptoms for at least 1 year rather than 2 years.[96]

Pharmacotherapy

Prescription of antidepressants for children and adolescents has increased dramatically over the past decade.[127–130] However, this increase must be put into context of the prevalence of pharmacologically responsive depression in this population.[131] Fortunately, research investigating the safety, tolerability, and efficacy of antidepressants in juveniles has expanded significantly. Initial studies of the pharmacotherapy of pediatric depression focused on the TCAs.[132] Despite solid methodology, through assessment, diagnosis, and treatment-controlled trials of TCAs in children and adolescents with depression have demonstrated minimal advantage of TCAs over placebo. Because pediatric depression appears refractory to treatment with TCAs, researchers are investigating the safety, tolerability, and efficacy of the SSRIs. Although these studies employ different methodologies, results are encouraging; currently the SSRIs appear to be the medications of choice for the treatment of pediatric depression and dysthymia.[107,133,134]

As a result of two large double-blind placebo-controlled trials demonstrating short-term safety, tolerability and efficacy of fluoxetine, the FDA recently approved fluoxetine to treat major depressive disorder in children and adolescents between the ages of 7 and 17.[135–137] In the first trial (single site NIMH-sponsored), 583 subjects with MDD were screened and 96 randomized to either placebo or fluoxetine (20 mg). Using the prime outcome measures of reduction on Childhood Depression Rating Scale (CDRS) scores, by week 5 fluoxetine separated from placebo. By the end of the study period, 56% (N = 27) of the fluoxetine-treated patients and 33% (N = 16) of the placebo-treated patients were rated as "much" or "very much" improved on the Clinical Global Impression (CGI) scale. Response rates were similar in adolescents and latency-aged children, as well as in males and females. Although patients responded well to the treatment, only 31% of the fluoxetine-treated patients achieved full remission, compared with 23% of placebo-treated patients. Lifetime comorbidities with anxiety disorders (N = 54, 55%), dysthymia (N = 34, 35%), ADHD (N = 29, 30%), and ODD (N = 29, 30%) were common in this sample. In the second trial (multisite, industry-sponsored), 420 pediatric subjects with MDD were screened and 219 randomized to either placebo (N = 110) or 20 mg of fluoxetine (N = 109). For most of the subjects, the current episode of MDD was. their index episode and the number of boys and girls experiencing the episode was equal. In this sample comorbidity with ADHD (N = 31, 14%), ODD (N = 34, 16%), CD (N = 4, 2%), and anxiety disorders (none reported, and baseline HAM-A scores in clinically insignificant range) appeared relatively low. Compared with patients randomized to placebo, patients treated with fluoxetine showed significant reductions in CDRS scores as early as week 1 of treatment that were maintained throughout the 9 weeks of the trial. Although significantly more fluoxetine-treated patients achieved remission (41.3% versus 19.8%; P < 0.05), based on the predefined definition of response (>30% reduction in CDRS scores) the percentage of patients responding to fluoxetine was not significantly different than placebo (65.1% versus 53.5%; P = .093). Compared with placebo, fluoxetine treatment was associated with significantly greater improvements in CGI-severity (52.3% vs. 36.8%; P = 0.028) scores. The most common side effect observed with fluoxetine treatment was headache, although difficulty paying attention and dizziness were commonly reported.

Results of large controlled trials of other SSRIs in the treatment of pediatric depression have recently been reported. Wagner et al. reported on pooled results of two 10-week (industry-sponsored multisite) double-blind placebo-controlled trials of sertraline (Zoloft) for pediatric depression.[138] In this protocol, 377 outpatients (177 children 6 to 11 years old and 189 adolescents 12 to 17 years old) were randomized to treatment with placebo or sertraline. Sertraline appears to have been started at 50 mg/day, although it could be titrated up to

200 mg/day as clinically indicated. Compared with placebo, sertraline treatment was associated with significant reductions in CDRS-R scores and improvements on CGIs (P < 0.05). Although generally well tolerated, sertraline treatment was associated with higher rates of diarrhea, vomiting, anorexia, and agitation. In an open trial of sertraline in depressed adolescents (N = 53), Ambrosini et al.[139] observed significant improvements in efficacy (measured using various rating scales) by ensuring adherence to the prescribed dose of sertraline between weeks 6 and 10. These results suggest that in clinical practice the acute phase of treatment for depression in adolescents needs to extend to at least 10 weeks. Wagner et al.[140] also reported on the efficacy of citalopram in the treatment of MDD in children and adolescents. In this trial, 174 pediatric patients (83 children 6 to 11 years old and 91 adolescents 12 to 17 years old) were randomized in a double-blind manner to treatment with either placebo or citalopram. Citalopram was initiated at 20 mg and increased to 40 mg after 4 weeks, if clinically indicated. In patients treated with citalopram significant reductions in mean CDRS-R scores were observed by week 1 (P < 0.02) and maintained thorough the end of the study (week 8, P < 0.04). By the end of the study period, significantly more patients treated with citalopram responded compared with placebo (36% vs. 24%; P < 0.05). Patients treated with citalopram more commonly reported nausea, influenza-like symptoms and rhinitis. Currently, a multisite controlled trial of escitalopram, the S-enantiomer of citalopram, is underway. Although well studied in pediatric anxiety disorders,[141] we are not aware of any controlled trials investigating the efficacy of fluvoxamine in the treatment of pediatric depression.

Earlier Keller et al.[142] reported the results of a trial comparing paroxetine, imipramine (Tofranil), and placebo in the treatment of adolescent depression. In this 8-week double-blind, placebo-controlled parallel design trial, 425 adolescents (ages 12 to 17 years old) were screened and 275 randomized (93 to paroxetine, 95 to imipramine, and 87 to placebo). Comorbidity with anxiety disorders (N = 73, 26.5%) and externalizing disorders (i.e., ADHD, ODD, and CD) (N = 71, 25.8%) commonly were observed in this cohort. Paroxetine was started at 20 mg/day, which could be titrated up to

30 mg at week 5 and to 40 mg at weeks 6 to 8. Imipramine was initiated at 50 mg and titrated up weekly to a target dose of 200 mg/day, which could be increased to 250 mg at week 5 or 300 mg during weeks 6 to 8 as clinically indicated. Although paroxetine was associated with significant improvements in CGI scores, it did not separate from imipramine or placebo on the total score of the primary outcome measure (Hamilton Rating Scale for Depression-17 item [HAM-D-17]). However, the HAM-D-17 is designed for adult patients and may not be the best way to measure change in adolescent depression. For this reason most current trials in pediatric depression use the CDRS-R to measure medication effect.[133] Nearly half of the paroxetine-treated patients were maintained on 20 mg/day. The most frequent side effects observed in the paroxetine-treated group included dry mouth, nausea, dizziness, insomnia, somnolence, and headache. Although 11 paroxetine-treated patients experienced serious adverse events, including emotional lability (N = 5), conduct problems or hostility (N = 2), worsening depression (N = 2), euphoria/expansive mood (N = 1), and headache during discontinuation (N = 1), investigators believe that only the discontinuation-related headache was directly related to paroxetine treatment.

On June 10, 2003 the British Medicines and Healthcare Products Regulatory Agency (MHRA) advised that paroxetine should not be used for the treatment of depression in patients younger than 18 years old. The MHRA's recommendation came after reviewing nine studies (three for depression) of paroxetine treatment in pediatric patients. In these studies the MHRA noted that 1.5 to 3.2 times as many patients on paroxetine as on placebo described severe mood swings, including suicidal ideation. Although the absolute rate of these behaviors was low, none of the self-injurious behaviors was life-threatening, and no patient completed suicide, the MHRA were concerned enough to say, ". . . the benefits of Seroxate (paroxetine) in children for the treatment of depressive illness do not outweigh the risks." The MHRA's full report and advice to prescribers is available online at www.medicines.mhra.gov.uk. Following the MHRA, the FDA recommended that paroxetine not be used to treat depression in patients younger than the age of 18. The FDA has dissuaded physicians from starting juvenile patients with depression on paroxetine, but advocated that patients currently receiving paroxetine be slowly tapered off the agent as treatment is completed. The issue of SSRIs causing suicidal behaviors is not new,[143] although a recent analysis of a large database (N = 48,277) of FDA reports failed to show any increase in suicide rates in patients treated with SSRIs.[144] Updated information on the FDA investigation is available online at www.fda.gov/cder/drug/infopage/paxil/paxilQ&A.html.

Several other antidepressants are used in juvenile depression. Venlafaxine (Effexor) possesses both SSRI and noradrenergic properties. Venlafaxine is effective in refractory adult depression and may be useful in the treatment of juvenile mood disorders and children with ADHD comorbid with their depression. The adverse effect profile of venlafaxine is similar to that of the SSRIs except for significant nausea, which can be reduced by using very low doses for the first 1 to 2 weeks. Venlafaxine did not show benefit over placebo in one published trial, although low doses (75 mg/day) were used.[145] Bupropion hydrochloride is a novel antidepressant with noradrenergic and dopaminergic properties. Bupropion may be helpful in children with prominent mood lability, dysthymia, and/or comorbid ADHD.[66] Similar to the management of ADHD (see above), bupropion should be started between 37.5 to 75 mg/day of the immediate-release preparation or 100 mg of the sustained-release preparation and titrated upward as necessary, eventually converting to the extended-release preparation for compliance and full-day coverage. The major side effects in children include insomnia, possible exacerbation of tics, and the theoretic risk of seizures with the short-acting preparation. Bupropion should not be used in patients with bulimia. No blood monitoring is required. Although open trials,[146] and a small case series[147] of nefazodone (Serzone) showed promise, results of a recent 15-site double-blind, placebo-controlled trial only approached statistical significance over placebo in adolescents with depression.[148] At this time, given concerns over hepatotoxicity and the availability of many alternative medications with demonstrated efficacy, the role of nefazodone in the treatment of pediatric depression appears limited. Results of a recent controlled trial of mirtazapine (Remeron) showed little difference in response between mirtazapine and placebo in a controlled study of juveniles with depression. Anecdotal reports and clinical experience suggest that mirtazapine may be helpful in patients with ADHD who benefit from treatment with a stimulant but who suffer insomnia and anorexia.

Pharmacokinetics of Antidepressants in Children and Adolescents

Although the main pharmacodynamic effect of the SSRIs is similar, they are structurally dissimilar to each other and vary in their pharmacokinetics and drug interactions. The SSRIs have been found to inhibit specific hepatic isoenzymes and thereby increase serum levels of other compounds. In the medical setting, treatment with antidepressants may produce clinically significant medication interactions. Parents and clinicians should be alerted to the concern that the SSRIs may interact with various antibiotics, especially the macrolide derivatives that are currently being used on pediatric patients. Clinicians need access to updated databases on medication interactions. An excellent current reference recently was published.[149]

Fluoxetine (Prozac) is a racemic mixture that is metabolized to its active metabolite, norfluoxetine. Both fluoxetine and norfluoxetine are substrates of CYP 2C9, 2C19, 3A4, and 2D6. Both fluoxetine and norfluoxetine are potent inhibitors of 2D6 and therefore may increase levels of medications that are metabolized through 2D6 (i.e., certain antidepressants, antipsychotics, analgesics, calcium channel blockers, β-blockers, dextromethorphan, and ATMX). Wilens et al.[150] recently reported on the pharmacokinetics of fluoxetine and its major metabolite, norfluoxetine, in 10 children (6 to 12 years old) and 11 adolescents (12 to 17 years old). In this open-label study patients received 20 mg/day of fluoxetine. Mean steady states of fluoxetine and norfluoxetine were achieved on average within 4 weeks, although high between-patient variability was observed. Furthermore, on average, children accumulated higher amounts of fluoxetine (2-fold) and norfluoxetine (1.7-fold) compared with adolescents. Accumulation of fluoxetine and norfluoxetine in adolescents was similar to profile for adult patients. Clinically, this implies that most children should be initiated at 10 mg/day of fluoxetine.

Sertraline (Zoloft) is produced as the S-enantiomer and metabolized to its active metabolite desmethylsertraline, both of which are substrates of 2B6, 2C9, 2C19, 2D6, and 3A4. Both sertraline and desmethylsertraline are modest inhibitors of 2C9, 2C19, and 3A4. Case reports have shown that sertraline increases concentrations of phenytoin, pimozide, warfarin, cyclosporine, and diazepam. Sertraline is known to inhibit glucuronidation, and it has been reported to cause toxic levels of lamotrigine. Levels of sertraline may be reduced by pain-inducers, such as carbamazepine and phenytoin.[149] Axelson et al. recently studied the pharmacokinetics of sertraline in adolescents.[151] They observed that the mean steady-state half-life of 50 mg/day of sertraline was significantly shorter than the single-dose half-life (15.3 ± 3.5 hours versus 26.7 ± 5.2 hours; $P < 0.001$) and the mean steady-state half-life of 100 to 150 mg/day of sertraline (20.4 ± 3.4 hours). These authors suggest that adolescent patients may need doses greater than 50 mg/day to achieve therapeutic response for depression. Similarly, Alderson et al. studied the pharmacokinetics of sertraline in 29 children (6 to 12 years old) and 32 adolescents (13 to 17 years old). These investigators found that during treatment with 200 mg/day of sertraline, the T_{max} (14.6 ± 16.1 vs. 10.8 ± 8 hours) and half-lives of sertraline (26.2 ± 8.4 versus 27.1 ± 8.2 hours) and its main metabolite desmethylsertraline (78.5 ± 50.6 versus 75.4 ± 37.1 hours) were similar in children and adolescents, respectively. These results also demonstrated that a single dose of 50 mg of sertraline and a steady-state dose of 200 mg/day of sertraline led to significantly increased C_{max} and the area under the curve in children, compared with adolescents or adults. However, when these pharmacokinetic parameters were normalized for body weight, no significant differences were observed. These results suggest linear pharmacokinetics of sertraline in pediatric patients across the dose range of 50 to 200 mg/day, and the authors conclude that sertraline can be safely used within the adult dosage schedule.

Paroxetine (Paxil) is an S-enantiomer that is a substrate of 2D6 and to a lesser degree 3A4. Paroxetine has no significant metabolites, is a potent inhibitor of 2B6 and 2D6, and is a mild inhibitor of 1A2, 2C9, 2C19, and 3A4. Co-administration of paroxetine with substrates of 2D6 (e.g., antidepressants, antipsychotics, analgesics, calcium channel blockers, β-blockers, antiarrhythmics), or 2B6 (e.g., bupropion, nicotine, sertraline, diazepam, tamoxifen) is likely to increase levels of the substrate.[149] Findling et al.[152] studied the pharmacokinetics of paroxetine in 30 children and adolescents with MDD. The mean steady-state half-life of paroxetine was 11.1 ± 5.2 hours, with tremendous interindividual variation. Urinary excretion of paroxetine correlated with cytochrome 2D6 activity. These authors conclude that paroxetine is metabolized more rapidly in pediatric patients than in adults.

Citalopram (Celexa), a racemic mixture of R and S-citalopram, is demethylated via 2C19, 2D6, and 3A4. It shows mild inhibition at 2D6, but in general has few medication interactions. Reis et al.[153], using data from two trials, studied the pharmacokinetics of citalopram in 44 patients younger than 21-years-old treated naturalistically with a mean dose of citalopram of 30 mg/day. As in adults, large interindividual variability in levels of serum citalopram (CIT) and its main metabolite desmethylcitalopram (DCIT) and didesmethylcitalopram (DDCIT) were observed in these adolescents. The mean serum half-life of CIT was 36 hours. These authors found the pharmacokinetics of citalopram were influenced by gender, smoking status, treatment with oral contraceptives, and menstrual period. The active enantiomer, S-citalopram has recently become available as Lexapro. Like citalopram, it has few medication interactions.

Fluvoxamine (Luvox) is a substrate of 2D6 and 1A2, which has no significant metabolites. It is described as a "pan-inhibitor" because it is a potent inhibitor of 2B6, 2C9, and 3A4 and a mild inhibitor of 2D6. When adding any medication to fluvoxamine clinicians are advised to be cautious.[149]

The profiles of the pK for novel antidepressants have been reported as well. Bupropion (Wellbutrin or Zyban) is mainly metabolized by 2B6 to its main metabolite hydroxybupropion. Bupropion acts as a modest inhibitor of 2D6. Although smoking does not affects the pK profile, co-administration with paroxetine, sertraline, or other 2B6 inhibitors may cause interactions. Stewart et al.[154] examined the single-dose pK profile of bupropion SR (150 mg) in 75 adolescents (13 to 18 years old). These investigators found no differences in pK profile between smokers and nonsmokers; however, girls in this sample were observed to have increased C_{max}, $t_{1/2}$, and area under the curve for both bupropion and hydroxybupropion.

Findling et al.[146] studied the PK profile of nefazodone in 28 patients (N = 15 children, 7 to 12 years old and N = 13 adolescents, 13 to 16 years old) treated for MDD. Nefazodone (NEF) is metabolized primarily by CYP 3A4 to at least three active metabolites: hydroxynefazodone (OH-NEF), triazoledione, and metachlorophenylpiperazine (mCPP). Formation of mCPP is dependent on CYP 2D6 activity. Although the PK profile showed a lot of variability, the C_{max} and AUC in children was observed to be greater than in adolescents and the serum half-life increased with increased dosage ($t_{1/2}$ 1.9 hours after first dose, 2.7 hours after 1 week, and 4.1 hours after 1 week on 100 mg twice per day). The PK profile for adolescents approximated that seen in adults. Substantial increases in concentration of mCPP were observed in the five patients (two children and three adolescents) determined to be poor metabolizers of CYP 2D6. A recent case series (two adults and one adolescent) described liver failure in three patients treated with NEF.[155] All patients developed jaundice and encephalopathy, and showed prominent necrosis in the centrolobular area. One patient recovered without transplantation, one died after transplantation, and one underwent successful transplantation. In response to these cases, the FDA added a black box warning to NEF's labeling. The FDA warning reports liver failure resulting in death or transplant in 1 per 250,000 to 300,000 patient years of NEF treatment (see www.fda.gov/medwatch/SAFETY/2002/ Serzone_deardoc.PDF). The FDA warning recommends not starting NEF in patients with active liver disease or elevated baseline serum transaminases. The FDA further advises that patients should be educated about signs of liver dysfunction, and NEF should be discontinued in patients who develop elevated serum AST or ALT levels.

Clinical Use of SSRIs

Given the likelihood of relatively similar efficacy, selection of an SSRI should take into consideration tolerability (e.g., side-effect profile), anticipated medication interactions, half-life (e.g., potential for bipolar switching), and adherence.[113] Whereas paroxetine, fluoxetine, citalopram, escitalopram, and sertraline may be associated with agitation and increased energy, fluvoxamine appears to be more sedating and can be useful in children with sleep difficulties associated with their mood symptoms. SSRIs should be initiated at low doses (e.g., 5 to 10 mg fluoxetine, 12.5 to 25 mg sertraline, 5 to 10 mg citalopram, 2.5 to 5 mg escitalopram, 5 to 10 mg paroxetine, 12.5 to 25 mg fluvoxamine, and 18.75 to 37.5 mg venlafaxine) and titrated upward slowly.[134] Like fluoxetine, sertraline, paroxetine, and citalopram, escitalopram is now available in an elixir form. Contrary to previously held beliefs, adolescents typically have the onset of depression prior to the onset of heavy tobacco use, which is associated with developing depressive symptoms.[156] Clinicians should consider directing adolescents with MDD and tobacco use to appropriate antismoking programs. Once positive antidepressant response is obtained, patients and their families often benefit from encouraging adherence to prevent relapse; however, the ideal length of treatment in pediatric patients remains understudied. After treatment is completed (typically 6 to 12 months after remission), the SSRIs should be slowly tapered, both to prevent a discontinuation syndrome and a recurrence of symptoms. Patients and their families need education regarding monitoring for future depressive episodes.

Side Effects and Complications

In general, SSRIs appear well tolerated and to have fewer side effects than the TCAs, especially in overdose. Common adverse effects of SSRIs include manic activation, agitation, gastrointestinal symptoms, irritability, insomnia, sexual side effects, and weight loss.[134,157] Whereas paroxetine, fluoxetine, citalopram, and sertraline may be associated with agitation and increased energy, fluvoxamine appears to manifest a relatively greater incidence of sedation and is useful in children with sleep difficulties associated with their mood symptoms. In approving fluoxetine for the treatment of juvenile depression and OCD, the FDA expressed concern that fluoxetine-treated patients may grow more slowly than patients treated with placebo (1.1 cm in height and 2 lbs in

weight) over a 19-week interval. Similarly, a small case series described slowing of growth during treatment with either fluoxetine (20 to 80 mg/day) or and 50 mg to 100 mg of fluvoxamine (50 to 100 mg/day) in four Middle Eastern patients with TS or OCD.[158] Although these agents have been used for almost 15 years in juveniles without detection of significant effects on growth, clinicians should consider alternative treatments if a patient's height/weight inexplicably decelerates. Given the lack of cardiovascular effects of SSRIs, vital sign and/or ECG monitoring does not appear necessary unless there is an additional medical concern.[4,159] Similarly, no specific blood monitoring appears necessary in children receiving SSRIs. Although it is not well studied, Walkup summarizes clinically relevant complications of SSRI pharmacotherapy in children and adolescents.[160] Activation, which is distinguished from a change in mood or impulse control and may be related to either akathisia, hyperactivity, or disinhibition, usually responds to lowering the dose. Signs of mania (which may include impulse dyscontrol, mood swings, grandiosity, hypersexuality, and aggression) may be observed and accompany bipolar switching. Treatment relies on pharmacologically addressing the mania. Celebration may occur in anxious children treated with SSRIs who experience relief of their anxiety, and they may seem impulsive or uninhibited. Developmental issues may be observed as patients' anxiety or depression lifts, after which additional comorbidities become evident (e.g., ADHD or Asperger's syndrome). Frontal lobe–type symptoms may appear and be manifest primarily by apathy. GI symptoms are very common, as noted above. Adolescents prescribed SSRIs may experience sexual side effects, although reports of these side effects are minimal in controlled studies in this population.

Like adults, children may experience a discontinuation syndrome either as they are tapered off SSRIs after treatment or if they miss their scheduled dose. Typically this syndrome occurs in patients who are taking SSRIs with shortened half-lives (e.g., paroxetine or venlafaxine), although it can occur with any antidepressant.[161] As in adults the discontinuation syndrome is typically characterized by physical symptoms (e.g., nausea, GI disturbance, diarrhea, dizziness, insomnia, lightheadedness, headache, shakiness, and sensations of mild electrical shock), cognitive symptoms (e.g., confusion, poor memory, cloudiness, and forgetfulness), and emotional symptoms (e.g., increased crying, mood lability, and anxiety).[162] Patients and parents should be educated about the discontinuation syndrome and steps taken to prevent its occurrence, including only using SSRIs when necessary, encouraging adherence, tapering SSRIs gradually, and ensuring that the manufacturer stays the same throughout treatment if patients are taking a generic preparation.[163] When patients experience a discontinuation syndrome, reintroducing the medication usually provides relief, although some patients may need to be switched to an SSRI with a longer half-life. A discontinuation syndrome has also been described as leading to a more complicated course of illness. Ali et al.[164] describe a review of the literature, noting that antidepressant withdrawal in general, and SSRI withdrawal in particular, appears to increase the risk of mania in adults with bipolar disorder. The authors postulate either noradrenergic hyperactivity or cholinergic overdrive as the possible underlying pathophysiology.

Bipolar Disorder

There is a growing awareness of the existence of a childhood symptom complex reminiscent of adult bipolar disorder.[165,166] The American Academy of Child and Adolescent Psychiatry (AACAP) and the NIMH have convened round-table meetings and the AACAP has issued practice parameters regarding the evaluation, diagnosis, management, and research into pediatric bipolar disorder.[167,168] It is common for many children and adolescents with bipolar disorder to seek medical attention in emergency departments or to develop severe, out-of-control symptoms during medical hospitalizations. Juveniles also may be referred to primary care physicians for unremitting temper tantrums. Prepubertal mania is usually comorbid with ADHD, and these patients typical presentation with extreme hyperactivity, impulsivity, and aggression.[169,170] In children, bipolar disorder commonly is manifest by an extremely irritable or explosive mood with associated poor psychosocial functioning that is often devastating to the

child and family. These children often overreact to the environment (mood reactivity). In milder conditions, additional symptoms consistent with mania include temper tantrums, unmodulated high energy, such as decreased sleep, over-talkativeness, racing thoughts, increased goal-directed activity (e.g., social, work, school, and sexual), and poor judgment, such as seeking out reckless activities. Although the juvenile symptom complex of mania should be differentiated from ADHD, conduct disorder, depression, trauma, substance use/abuse, and psychotic disorders, these disorders commonly co-occur with childhood mania.[171] The clinical course of juvenile mania is most frequently chronic and mixed with co-occurring manic and depressive features.[172–175]

There are no medications specifically approved to treat bipolar disorder in children younger than 12 years old. For bipolar patients between 12 and 17 years old, lithium is the only FDA-approved medication. However, investigators have noted that early-onset bipolar disorder appears less responsive to lithium.[176,177] Therefore, children and adolescents with bipolar disorder are often treated with combinations of lithium, anticonvulsants, and/or atypical antipsychotic mood stabilizers.[178,179] If is the patient does not respond to an adequate trial (in dose and time) of a single agent or cannot tolerate the medication, subsequent trials with alternative medication(s) are recommended. In manic or mixed presentations, with psychotic symptoms, additional antipsychotic treatment is recommended. In bipolar disorder with prominent symptoms of depression, combined treatment with a mood stabilizer and an antidepressant is indicated. One must be wary of the potential destabilizing effects of SSRIs in the treatment of bipolar depression in children and adolescents.[179] Recent data indicate that the management of bipolar disorder with or without comorbid disorders (depression, ADHD) may require an aggressive treatment approach that combines several therapeutic agents.

The use of lithium carbonate in mood disorders, particularly bipolar disorders and treatment-resistant unipolar depressions, appears useful; surprisingly, it has not been studied under controlled conditions. The usual starting dose of lithium ranges from 150 to 300 mg/day in divided doses, two or three times per day. Weller et al.[180]

published dosage guidelines for lithium in children 6 to 12 years old, suggesting initial total daily doses (administered three times per day) of 600 mg/day for patients weighing less than 25 kg, 900 mg for patients weighing 25 to 40 kg, 1200 mg/day for patients weighing 40 to 50 kg, and 1500 mg/day for patients weighing 50 to 60 kg. There is no known therapeutic serum lithium level in children. Based on the adult literature, serum levels of 0.8 to 1.5 mEq/L for acute episodes and levels of 0.4 to 0.8 mEq/L for maintenance therapy are suggested. Although lithium is commonly used in pediatric bipolar patients, only one prospective well-controlled study has been conducted. In this study Geller et al.[181] found treatment with lithium improved global assessment of functioning and reduced positive urine screens.

Common short-term adverse effects include GI symptoms (e.g., nausea and vomiting), renal symptoms (e.g., polyuria and polydipsia), and CNS symptoms (e.g., tremor, sleepiness, and memory impairment).[182] Short-term adverse effects associated with the use of lithium are generally dose-related. The incidence of toxicity increases directly with increased serum levels, and symptoms respond favorably to dose reduction. It is important to monitor a child's hydration status because lithium induces mild dehydration that, when more severe, may lead to toxic accumulation of lithium. Hence, it is prudent to consider withholding or reducing lithium doses in children who are dehydrated or who have experienced prolonged vomiting. The chronic administration of lithium may be associated with metabolic (substantial weight gain, decreased calcium metabolism), endocrine (decreased thyroid functioning), dermatologic (acne), cardiac, and possibly renal dysfunction. Thus, it is necessary that children be screened for renal function (blood urea nitrogen, creatinine), thyroid function (TSH), ECG, and calcium levels before lithium treatment is started and that these tests be repeated every 6 months. Females should undergo a pregnancy test and be educated about the dangers of lithium exposure during pregnancy. Particular caution should be exercised when lithium is used in patients with neurologic, renal, or cardiovascular disorders.

Alternative antimanic medications for children and adolescents include the anticonvulsants. Carbamazepine, approved for treatment of seizures

(e.g., psychomotor and grand mal) and trigeminal neuralgia, is structurally related to the TCAs. The plasma half-life after chronic administration is between 13 and 17 hours. The therapeutic plasma concentration is variably reported at 4 to 12 μg/ml and recommended daily doses in children range from 10 to 20 mg/kg administered twice per day. Because the relationship between dose and plasma level is variable and uncertain with marked interindividual variability, plasma level monitoring is recommended. Common short-term side effects include dizziness, drowsiness, nausea, vomiting, and blurred vision. Idiosyncratic reactions, such as bone marrow suppression, liver toxicity, and skin disorders (including Stevens-Johnson syndrome), have been reported but appear to be rare. However, given the seriousness of these reactions, careful monitoring of blood counts and liver and renal function is warranted initially and during treatment. Carbamazepine is not well studied in the treatment of pediatric mania; however, anecdotal reports and clinical experience support its consideration.[183,184] Although carbamazepine may be useful, worsening behavior during treatment has been reported.[185] Carbamazepine induces its own metabolism, which is usually complete after 3 to 5 weeks on the medication. Carbamazepine has many medication interactions,[149] induces the metabolism of substrates of 3A4 (e.g., haloperidol and phenytoin), and may reduce levels of valproic acid and increase lithium levels by reducing lithium clearance. Inhibitors of 3A4 (e.g., erythromycin) may increase levels of carbamazepine. Oxcarbazepine (Trileptal) appears to be increasingly considered because of fewer reports of medication interactions and adverse effects (e.g., less effect on bone marrow and skin). Although trials are ongoing, minimal data are currently available on oxcarbazepine's safety, tolerability, or efficacy in pediatric bipolar disorder. Clinicians who prescribe it should monitor for hyponatremia and be aware that it can induce the metabolism of ethinyl estradiol.

Valproic acid (VPA) is an anticonvulsant that is also FDA-approved for the acute and maintenance treatment of bipolar disorder in adults; therefore, it may be useful in the treatment of juvenile bipolar disorder. In a recent prospective 6- to 8-week randomized, open trial, Kowatch et al.[186] compared the efficacy of lithium, carbamazepine, and VPA in

42 children and adolescents with bipolar disorder I or II. Using improvements in scores on CGI and Young-Mania Rating Scale (>50% change from baseline), these investigators observed response rates of 38% with carbamazepine, 38% with lithium and 53% with VPA ($\chi2 = 0.85$, p = 0.60). In the initial open phase of another trial, Wagner et al.,[187] reported that 22 of 40 pediatric bipolar patients (55%) experienced more than 50% improvement in the Mania Rating Scale during open treatment with VPA in doses of 15 to 17 mg/kg/day.

VPA is primarily metabolized by the liver; it has a plasma half-life of 8 to 16 hours and a therapeutic plasma concentration of 50 to 100 μg/ml. Recommended initial daily doses are 15 mg/kg/day that are gradually increased to a maximum of 60 mg/kg/day, administered three times a day. Common short-term side effects include sedation, thinning of hair, anorexia, nausea, and vomiting. Idiosyncratic reactions, such as bone marrow suppression and liver toxicity, have been reported but appear to be rare. Asymptomatic elevations of SGOT usually resolve spontaneously. Although fatalities from hepatic dysfunction have been reported in children younger than 10 years old with monotherapy, these have occurred primarily in children younger than 2 years old. The risk of serious hepatic involvement is increased by concomitant use of other antiseizure medications and may be dose-related. Careful monitoring of blood counts and liver and renal function are warranted initially and during treatment. Hyperammonemia has been reported and based on clinical impression monitoring ammonia levels may be appropriate.

Increasingly the atypical antipsychotic medications, including clozapine (Clozaril), olanzapine (Zyprexa), quetiapine (Seroquel), risperidone (Risperdal), ziprasidone (Geodon), and aripiprazole (Abilify) are being used in the management of pediatric bipolar disorder. These medications differ from "typical" antipsychotics (e.g., chlorpromazine and haloperidol) in their receptor profile (D_2 blockade and that they affect multiple other receptors, including serotonin), reduced likelihood of causing EPS, reduced likelihood of causing hyperprolactinemia (the exception is risperidone), and a greater benefit on the negative symptoms of psychosis and on cognition.[188] Whenever these medications are used, patients and families should be informed about the potential for side effects including EPS, akathisia, neuroleptic malignant syndrome, and tardive dyskinesias/dystonias (TD). Although the risk of developing TD is lower with the atypical medications, the rate of occurrence is unknown. Patients treated with antipsychotic medications should be monitored with the Abnormal Involuntary Movement Scale (AIMS) exam regularly.

Olanzapine is currently FDA-approved for acute and maintenance treatment of bipolar disorder in adults.[189] Frazier et al.[190] openly treated 23 bipolar children (5 to 14 years old) with olanzapine for 8 weeks.[190] Of the 23 patients who completed this study, 61% responded (defined as >30% reduction in YMRS). Interestingly, these patients also experienced significant reductions in depressive symptomatology. The major side effects of olanzapine were sedation and weight gain (mean = 5 kg), although EPS were not observed. In some patients the weight gain outweighed clinical benefits and necessitated switching to an alternative treatment, although in some patients the weight gain remained stable. In adults on atypical antipsychotics, hyperglycemia, new-onset diabetes, and diabetic ketoacidosis (50% occurred in those without weight gain) have been observed during treatment.[191,192] Olanzapine is available in tablet and Zydis (melts on the tongue) forms. Olanzapine is typically initialed at 2.5 to 5.0 mg and can be titrated up to 20 mg. Olanzapine is metabolized, via glucuronidation (primary) and oxidation via CYP 1A2.[149] Grothe et al.[193] studied the pK of olanzapine in adolescents, observing a mean serum half-life of 37.2 ± 5.1 hours and that boys and smokers metabolize it more rapidly.

Risperidone also has been used to treat pediatric mania.[194] A retrospective chart review observed significant benefit of risperidone (mean dose of 1.7 ± 1.3 mg/day), on reducing manic and aggressive behaviors in 28 (N = 27 males, N = 25 bipolar type I) pediatric bipolar patients. Common side effects included weight gain, sedation, drooling, and elevation of prolactin. Although EPS was not observed, clinicians should be aware of this possibility and recognize it when it occurs. Like adults, children and adolescents with EPS can be treated with oral or IM diphenhydramine or benztropine. Although pK studies in children are lacking, data in adults indicates that risperidone reaches peak concentrations within 1 hour, is metabolized through CYP 2D6, and has a half-life of 3 hours in extensive metabolizers and 17 hours in poor metabolizers.[195] There are case reports of hepatotoxicity, tachycardia, increased QTc interval, and stroke (in elderly patients). Risperidone is available in tablet, liquid, or a dissolvable tablet. Risperidone is usually initiated at 0.25 mg once or twice per day and titrated up to 3 to 4 mg/day in most pediatric patients, although it appears to retain its atypical properties in doses up to 6 mg/day.

DelBello et al.[196] recently published results of an open trial that added quetiapine to VPA in the treatment of 30 adolescents with bipolar disorder.[196] In this trial, patients were treated openly with VPA (20 mg/kg) and then randomized to adjunct therapy with either placebo or quetiapine (titrated up to 450 mg/day). The group receiving the combination treatment showed significantly greater response rate (reductions in Y-MRS scores) compared with the VPA and placebo group. The patients receiving VPA and quetiapine experienced greater sedation and weight gain. The pK of quetiapine has not been formally studied in children and adolescents. Data from adult studies indicate that quetiapine is readily absorbed from the GI track and reaches peak concentrations 1.5 hours after ingestion. It is metabolized primarily in the liver by CYP 3A4 and does not appear impacted by gender, smoking, or race.[195] Occurrence of EPS appears low, but quetiapine can cause dizziness, sedation, and weight gain.

The atypical antipsychotic ziprasidone (Geodon) may also be used in the treatment of pediatric bipolar disorder. As of this writing, however, there are no reports on its safety, tolerability, or efficacy for bipolar disorder in this population. Ziprasidone may increase QTc intervals, and thus prior to use obtaining a baseline ECG, and family history of cardiac problems (especially early-onset arrhythmia) is wise. Although ziprasidone is primarily metabolized through aldehyde oxidase, it is also metabolized in part via CYP 3A4. Co-administration of ziprasidone with medications that may also lengthen QTc (e.g., thioridazine, pimozide, droperidol, and Class IA and III anti-arrhythmics) should be avoided. In children and adolescents ziprasidone is initiated at 10 to 20 mg per day or twice per day and can be increased upward to 40 to 60 mg twice

per day. Aripiprazole (Abilify) is the most recently available atypical agent. At present, no data exists on its safety, tolerability, or efficacy in pediatric patients with bipolar disorder. Aripiprazole appears to have mixed agonist/antagonist properties and is described as a "dopamine/serotonin stabilizer." Aripiprazole has a long half-life and does not appear to cause significant interactions with other medications that are metabolized through the CYP-450 system. Aripiprazole can cause dizziness. It is usually started at 2.5 to 5.0 mg/day and titrated to 10 to 15 mg/day (up to 30 mg/day in adult trials).

Additional treatments in pediatric bipolar disorder that are reasonable to consider, but have little data to support their use, include use of alternative anticonvulsants. Gabapentin (Neurontin) is approved as an adjunct therapy for seizures. It is not significantly metabolized in humans and has few medication interactions.[197] Trials with gabapentin for bipolar disorder in adults have been negative; however, it has shown benefit in reducing anxiety. Lamotrigine (Lamictal) is an anticonvulsant that was recently approved in the maintenance treatment of bipolar type I in adults. Lamotrigine's labeling contains a boxed warning that serious rashes, including Stevens-Johnson, occur in about 1% of patients younger than 16 years old. The risk for rash seems to increase if lamotrigine is increased too quickly, the initial dose is greater than recommended, or it is administered with VPA. Mandoki[198] reported on a case series of 10 pediatric bipolar patients treated with VPA (500 to 1500 mg/day) without adequate response. Lamotrigine (50 to 200 mg/day) was added to VPA, with significant improvement. Lamontrigine's role in treatment of pediatric bipolar disorder remains unclear.

Topiramate (Topamax) is an antiepileptic that has shown promise in treatment of bipolar disorder in adults.[199] In trials with epilepsy, topiramate was associated with weight loss; however, it also can cause word-finding difficulties, oligohidrosis, and renal stones.[197] Topiramate has a half-life of about 24 hours, is excreted unchanged in the urine, and inhibits carbonic anhydrase as well as CYP 2C19.

Investigations into the phenomenology, diagnosis, and pharmacotherapy of pediatric bipolar disorder are being pursued. Data upon which clinicians can make informed recommendations continue to expand. Current guidelines support using pharmacotherapy in the context of an overall treatment plan.

Developmental Disorders

This class of disorders includes mental retardation, pervasive developmental disorders (e.g., autism, Asperger's syndrome, pervasive developmental disorder NOS, and high-functioning autism), and specific developmental disorders, previously called "learning disabilities" (e.g., nonverbal learning disability).[200] It is estimated that at any given time approximately 1% to 3% of the population meet the diagnostic criteria for mental retardation (MR).[201,202] Children on "alien" medical units may manifest many behavior symptoms related to a novel environment coupled with their inability to tolerate change and anxiety related to pain and medical procedures.

Autism is a pervasive developmental disorder; symptoms develop before 30 months of age and involve disturbances in the rate of development and coordination of physical, social, and language skills, abnormal responses to sensory inputs (hyperactivity alternates with hyperreactivity), and disturbance in the capacity to relate appropriately to people, events, and objects.[200] Children who have relatively normal academic development but manifest more specific deficits in social interactions (social cues, few friends, oddities) may have Asperger's syndrome.[203] The specific developmental disorders represent a mixed group of cognitive dysfunctions in the context of an overall average or above-average intelligence quotient (IQ) and adequate educational opportunities.

Psychotropic agents, particularly antipsychotics, continue to be widely used and misused in the treatment of mentally retarded individuals, particularly when they are institutionalized. Although psychotropic medications can temporarily control behavioral and psychiatric complications in some children with developmental disorders, they do not affect the cardinal symptoms of the underlying disorder. In general, the treatment of specific developmental disorders is largely remedial and supportive. No medications are effective in altering the basic course of these disorders. If the child also meets diagnostic criteria for ADHD or a mood disorder, then the guidelines described for the treatment of these disorders are applicable. In fact, stimulants appear generally well tolerated and effective in reducing symptoms of hyperactivity/ impulsivity in patients with MR.[204]

Children with developmental disorders often have psychiatric disorders and behavioral problems that include hyperactive, aggressive, irritable, distractible, and self-abusive behaviors. They may also have prominent symptoms such as anxiety, obsessive behavior, and rigidity that may respond to pharmacologic treatment. Psychotropic medications are used in this population primarily for the treatment of anxiety, obsessive behavior, agitation, aggression, self-regulation, and self-injurious behaviors.

Atypical neuroleptic medications appear to improve target symptoms of aggression, irritability, and hyperactivity in patients with developmental disorders. In a 6-week multicenter double-blind placebo-controlled trial, Aman et al.[205] studied the effects of risperidone in a well-characterized group of 118 children with MR and disruptive behaviors. Dosage ranged from 0.02 to 0.06 mg/kg/day. Treatment with risperidone led to reduced aggression, irritability, and destructive behaviors. Common side effects included somnolence, headache, and weight gain (mean = 2.2 kg). McCracken et al.[206] conducted a multisite, randomized, double-blind trial of risperidone and placebo to treat irritable children and adolescents (N = 101, 5 to 17 years old) with autism and severe tantrums, aggression, and/or self-injurious behaviors. Significantly more patients (69%; 34/49) randomized to risperidone (dose range 0.5 to 3.5 mg/day) experienced meaningful reductions in irritability compared with patients treated with placebo (12%; 6/52; p < 0.001). Notably, many patients maintained these gains over the course of 6-month follow-up. Patients treated with risperidone gained an average of 2.7 kg and had more drooling, dizziness, fatigue, and drowsiness. Open trials with a variety of atypical antipsychotics, including olanzapine[207] and ziprasidone,[208] have similarly shown promise in modulating maladaptive behaviors in patients with developmental delay.

A number of alternative pharmacologic agents, in addition to antipsychotics, are being employed for complications or comorbidities of developmental disorders. Considering the relatively low toxicologic profile of these drugs compared with the antipsychotics, they are the preferred treatment for the management of these children. β-Blockers (e.g., propranolol) may improve modulation in patients with developmental disorder, and thus reduce agitation, aggression, and self-abusive behaviors.[209,210] Propranolol is usually given in divided doses throughout the day. Treatment is typically initiated at 10 mg twice per day and increased as clinically indicated. The dose range is 2 to 8 mg/kg/day. Short-term adverse effects of propranolol are usually not serious and generally abate upon decreasing or stopping the drug. Nausea, vomiting, constipation, and mild diarrhea have been reported. Psychiatric side effects appear to be relatively infrequent but can occur; symptoms include vivid dreams, depression, and hallucinations. Propranolol's capacity to induce β-adrenergic blockade can cause bradycardia, hypotension, and an increase in airway resistance. Thus, it is contraindicated in asthmatic and certain cardiac patients. Because abrupt cessation of this drug may be associated with rebound hypertension, a gradual taper is recommended. In a similar manner clonidine, lofexidine and buspirone have been used to diminish aggression in patients with developmental disorders.[211–214]

For children with prominent obsessive behavior, rigidity, or compulsive rituals, recent studies indicate that the SSRIs may be helpful. Often, the full antidepressant dosage (see below) is necessary; however, children should be started with the lowest possible dose to avoid adverse effects, for example, disinhibition or agitation. Controlled trials in adults with fluoxetine[215] and fluvoxamine[216] have show positive results. However, studies in children have been less robust. The long-acting benzodiazepines may also be useful as single or adjunct agents in children with prominent anxiety symptoms (e.g., difficulty when eating); although, a major adverse effect, disinhibition, may result in increased restlessness and more disturbed behavior. Antidepressant drugs and mood stabilizers may be effective in controlling affective disorders, and stimulants may improve symptoms of ADHD when these disorders coexist. Fenfluramine has been reported recently to have a beneficial effect in some children with autism; however, these results remain unsubstantiated in more controlled follow-up

investigations. In response to an initial positive report, great interest and study has focused on secretin.[217,218] However, of the 10 controlled studies that have been conducted, 8 demonstrated no benefit of secretin over placebo, regardless of the form of secretin (biologic versus synthetic),[219] following single dose,[220] or ongoing administration of secretin.[221] Despite mostly negative data for secretin, many parents elected to continue to use it. At this time, the role of secretin in the treatment appears limited at best.

Psychotic Disorders

The term *psychosis* is generally used to describe the abnormal behaviors of children with grossly impaired reality testing.[222] The diagnosis of psychosis requires the presence of either delusions, false implausible beliefs, or hallucinations, or false perceptions that may be visual, auditory, or tactile. Often, psychosis in children is seen with major depression, bipolar disorder, or severe dissociative states, such as PTSD. Psychotic disorders in children, as in adults, can be functional or organic. Functional psychotic syndromes include schizophrenia and related disorders and the psychotic forms of mood disorders. Organic psychosis can develop secondary to CNS lesions as a consequence of medical illness, trauma, or drug use. Children may manifest psychosis for a substantial amount of time without indicating its presence to parents or caregivers. Hence, all children with major mood disorders, or those who have manifest abnormal or bizarre behaviors should be queried for the presence of psychosis.

Currently the atypical antipsychotics, such as risperidone, olanzapine, quetiapine, ziprasidone, and aripiprazole, are first-line agents in the pharmacotherapy of psychosis in children and adolescents. Typically these medications are initiated at a low dose and gradually titrated up to achieve efficacy. Risperidone is started at 0.25 mg twice a day and can be increased every day or two with close observation.[223] In patients treated over the long term with risperidone, clinicians should monitor weight, vital signs, and laboratory results (e.g., triglyceride, cholesterol, and prolactin).[224,225] Olanzapine and quetiapine are generally more sedating and are initiated respectively at 2.5 to

5 mg/day and 25 to 50 mg/day.[226] Olanzapine has recently been investigated in two open studies in pediatric patients with schizophrenia.[227,228] Significant improvements were observed in children and adolescents; however, these patients experienced significant weight gain and sedation.

If trials with two or three atypical antipsychotics are ineffective, a trial with a typical agent (e.g., chlorpromazine or haloperidol) should be considered. The usual oral dosage of antipsychotics ranges between 3 and 6 mg/kg/day for the low-potency phenothiazines (e.g., chlorpromazine) and between 0.1 and 0.5 (up to 1.0) mg/kg/day for the high-potency antipsychotics (e.g., haloperidol). Antipsychotic medications have a relatively long half-life, and therefore they need not be administered more than twice daily.

Common short-term adverse effects of antipsychotics are drowsiness, increased appetite, and weight gain. Anticholinergic effects, such as dry mouth, nasal congestion, and blurred vision, are more commonly seen with the low-potency phenothiazines. Short-term adverse effects of antipsychotics are generally managed with adjustments of dose and timing of administration. Excessive sedation can be avoided by using less sedating agents and by prescribing most of the daily dose at night-time. Drowsiness should not be confused with impaired cognition; it can usually be corrected by adjusting the dose and the timing of administration. In fact, there is no evidence that antipsychotics adversely affect cognition when used in low doses. Anticholinergic adverse effects can be minimized by choosing a medium- or high-potency compound.

Extrapyramidal effects, such as acute dystonia, akathisia (motor restlessness), and parkinsonism (bradykinesia, tremor, and lack of facial expressions), are more commonly seen with the high-potency compounds (butyrophenones and thioxanthenes) and have been reported to occur in up to 75% of children receiving these agents. The extent to which antiparkinsonian agents (e.g., anticholinergic drugs, benztropine, trihexyphenidyl, antihistamines, and the antiviral agent amantidine) should be used prophylactically when antipsychotics are introduced is controversial. Whenever possible, antiparkinsonian agents should be used only when extrapyramidal symptoms emerge. Akathisia may be particularly problematic in young patients because of common under-recognition. When a child or adolescent starts on an antipsychotic and becomes acutely agitated with an associated inability to sit still and with aggressive outbursts, the possibility of akathisia should be considered. If suspected, the dose of the antipsychotic may need to be lowered. The centrally acting β-adrenergic antagonist propranolol often is very helpful in treating this adverse effect.

A benign withdrawal dyskinesia and a syndrome of deteriorating behavior have been associated with the abrupt cessation of these drugs. As in adults, the long-term administration of antipsychotic drugs may be associated with TD. Although children appear generally less vulnerable than adults to developing TD, there is an emerging consensus that this potentially worrisome adverse effect may affect children and adolescents in 10% to 15% of cases. Prevention (appropriate use for a clear indication, clear target symptoms, periodic drug discontinuation to assess the need for drug use) and early detection (with regular monitoring) are the only effective treatments for TD.

Little is known about the potentially lethal neuroleptic malignant syndrome (NMS) in juveniles; however, preliminary evidence indicates that its presentation is similar to that in adults. This syndrome may be difficult to distinguish from primary CNS pathology, concurrent infection, or other, more benign, side effects of antipsychotic treatment including EPS or anticholinergic toxicity. Treatment appears similar to those strategies used in adults.

In patients who do not respond to trials with either first-line atypical or typical antipsychotics or who experience significant dyskinesia from these medications, consideration should be given to a trial with clozapine (Clozaril).[229,230] In the United States and Europe, there has been a considerable experience with clozapine in adolescents. Established dose parameters are not yet available; however, in one open study of clozapine for schizophrenic youths, doses from 125 to 825 mg/day (mean = 375 mg/day) for up to 6 weeks were necessary for effectiveness. Although remarkably effective in chronic treatment-resistant schizophrenia and affective psychosis, there is a dose-related risk of seizures and an increased risk of leukopenia and agranulocytosis in adolescents that is similar to the risk in adults; it requires close monitoring.

Combined Agents

Increasingly, multiple agents have been utilized both in clinical practice and in research settings for the treatment of child and adolescent psychiatric disorders. This need has arisen out of an emerging awareness of the high rates of comorbidity described in clinical and epidemiologic studies of juvenile psychiatric disorders. Fluoxetine and MPH, for instance, have been described as useful in the management of children with depression and ADHD.[231] In addition, controlled investigations of single agents have produced inconclusive findings in many disorders. Enhanced response rates have been reported when traditional agents are combined. For example, improved anti-ADHD efficacy has been shown with the combination of stimulants and TCAs. Interest is growing in trials combining ATMX and stimulant pharmacotherapy for ADHD.

Previously the law of parsimony dictated a single cause for each symptom complex, which led to the use of large doses of individual agents for a given disorder often resulting in intolerable adverse effects. In contrast, the use of combined pharmacotherapy has permitted more targeted treatment and greater efficacy, often achieved with lower doses and fewer adverse effects.

References

1. Hoagwood K, Rupp A: *Mental health service needs, use, and costs for children and adolescents with mental disorders and their families: preliminary evidence.* In Services CCFMH, editor:, *Mental Health, United States, 1994* Washington, DC, 1994, U.S. Department of Health and Human Services, pp 52–64.
2. Jensen PS, Bhatara VS, Vitiello B, et al: Psychoactive medication prescribing practices for US children: gaps between research and clinical practice, *J Am Acad Child Adolesc Psychiatry* 38:557–565, 1999.
3. Popper C: *Psychiatric pharmacosciences of children and adolescents*, Washington, DC, 1987, American Psychiatric Press.
4. Gutgesell H, Atkins D, Barst R, et al: AHA scientific statement: cardiovascular monitoring of children and adolescents receiving psychotropic drugs, *J Am Acad Child Adolesc Psychiatry* 38:979–982, 1999.
5. *Physicians desk reference*. Montvale, NJ, Medical Economics Data Production Company, 1995.
6. Hemmer SA, Pasternak JF, Zecker SG, et al: Stimulant therapy and seizure risk in children with ADHD, *Pediatr Neurol* 24:99–102, 2001.
7. Steiner H, Saxena K, Chang K: Psychopharmacologic strategies for the treatment of aggression in juveniles, *CNS Spectr* 8:298–308, 2003.
8. Wilens T, Biederman J, Spencer T: Case study: adverse effects of smoking marijuana while receiving tricyclic antidepressants, *J Am Acad Child Adolesc Psychiatry* 36:45–48, 1997.
9. Bernstein G, Shaw K: AACAP official action-practice parameters for the assessment and treatment of anxiety disorders, *Am J Psychiatry* 32:1089–1098, 1993.
10. Bernstein G, Borchardt C, Perwein A: Anxiety disorders in children and adolescents: a review of the past 10 years, *J Am Acad Child Adolesc Psychiatry* 35:1110–1119, 1996.
11. Winston FK, Kassam-Adams N, Garcia-Espana F, et al: Screening for risk of persistent posttraumatic stress in injured children and their parents (comment), *JAMA* 290:643–649, 2003.
12. Saxe G, Stoddard F, Courtney D, et al: Relationship between acute morphine and the course of PTSD in children with burns, *J Am Acad Child Adolesc Psychiatry* 40:915–921, 2001.
13. Kessler R, Sonnega A, Bromet E, et al: Posttraumatic stress disorder in the national comorbidity survey, *Arch Gen Psychiatry* 52:1048–1060, 1995.
14. Famularo R: Psychiatric comorbidity in childhood posttraumatic stress disorder, *Child Abuse Negl* 20:953–961, 1996.
15. Donnelly CL: Pharmacologic treatment approaches for children and adolescents with posttraumatic stress disorder, *Child Adolesc Psychiatr Clin North Am* 12:251–269, 2003.
16. Donnelly CL, Amaya-Jackson L, March JS: Psychopharmacology of pediatric posttraumatic stress disorder, *J Child Adolesc Psychopharmacol* 9:203–220, 1999.
17. Pfefferbaum JD: Posttraumatic stress disorder in children: a review of the past 10 years, *J Am Acad Child Adolesc Psychiatry* 36:1503–1511, 1997.
18. Klein R, Koplewicz H, Kanner A: Imipramine treatment of children with separation anxiety disorder, *J Am Acad Child Adolesc Psychiatry* 31:21–28, 1992.
19. Sachdev P: *Akathisia and restless legs*, New York, 1995, Cambridge University Press.
20. American Psychiatric Association: *Diagnostic and statistical manual of mental disorders*, ed 4, Washington, DC, 1994, American Psychiatric Press.
21. Liebowitz MR, Turner SM, Piacentini J, et al: Fluoxetine in children and adolescents with OCD: a placebo-controlled trial, *J Am Acad Child Adolesc Psychiatry* 41:1431–1438, 2002.

22. Geller DA, Hoog SL, Heiligenstein JH, et al: Fluoxetine treatment for obsessive-compulsive disorder in children and adolescents: a placebo-controlled clinical trial(comment), *J Am Acad Child Adolesc Psychiatry* 40:773–779, 2001.

23. March J, Biederman J, Wolkow R, et al: Sertraline in children and adolescents with obsessive compulsive disorder: a multicenter double-blind placebo controlled study, *JAMA* 280:1752–1756, 1998.

24. Cook EH, Wagner KD, March JS, et al: Long-term sertraline treatment of children and adolescents with obsessive-compulsive disorder, *J Am Acad Child Adolesc Psychiatry* 40:1175–1181, 2001.

25. Riddle MA, Reeve EA, Yaryura-Tobias JA, et al: Fluvoxamine for children and adolescents with obsessive-compulsive disorder: a randomized, controlled, multicenter trial, *J Am Acad Child Adolesc Psychiatry* 40:222–229, 2001.

26. Garvey MA, Perlmutter SJ, Allen AJ et al: A pilot study of penicillin prophylaxis for neuropsychiatric exacerbations triggered by streptococcal infections, *Biol Psychiatry* 45:1564–1571, 1999.

27. Swedo SE, Leonard HL, Garvey M, et al: Pediatric autoimmune neuropsychiatric disorders associated with streptococcal infections: clinical description of the first 50 cases (comment) [erratum appears in *Am J Psychiatry* 1998 Apr;155(4):578]. *Am J Psychiatry* 155:264–271, 1998.

28. Sallee FR, Kurlan R, Goetz CG, et al: Ziprasidone treatment of children and adolescents with Tourette's syndrome: a pilot study, *J Am Acad Child Adolesc Psychiatry* 39:292–299, 2000.

29. Gaffney GR, Perry PJ, Lund BC, et al: Risperidone versus clonidine in the treatment of children and adolescents with Tourette's syndrome, *J Am Acad Child Adolesc Psychiatry* 41:330–336, 2002.

30. Dion Y, Annable L, Sandor P, et al: Risperidone in the treatment of Tourette's syndrome: a double-blind, placebo-controlled trial, *J Clin Psychopharmacol* 22:31–39, 2002.

31. Scahill L, Leckman JF, Schultz RT, et al: A placebo-controlled trial of risperidone in Tourette's syndrome, *Neurology* 60:1130–1135, 2003.

32. Margolese HC, Annable L, Dion Y: Depression and dysphoria in adult and adolescent patients with Tourette's disorder treated with risperidone, *J Clin Psychopharmacol* 63:1040–1044, 2002.

33. Bruggeman R, van der Linden C, Buitelaar JK, et al: Risperidone versus pimozide in Tourette's disorder: a comparative double-blind parallel-group study, *J Clin Psychiatry* 62:50–56, 2001.

34. Tourette's Syndrome Study G: Treatment of ADHD in children with tics: a randomized controlled trial (comment), *Neurology* 58:527–536, 2002.

35. Spencer T, Biederman J, Coffey B, et al: A double-blind comparison of desipramine and placebo in children and adolescents with chronic tic disorder and comorbid attention-deficit/hyperactivity disorder, *Arch Gen Psychiatry* 59:649–656, 2002.

36. Gilbert DL, Sethuraman G, Sine L, et al: Tourette's syndrome improvement with pergolide in a randomized, double-blind, crossover trial, *Neurology* 54:1310–1315, 2000.

37. Lipinski JF, Sallee FR, Jackson C, et al: Dopamine agonist treatment of Tourette disorder in children: results of an open-label trial of pergolide, *Mov Disord* 12:402–407, 1997.

38. Silver AA, Shytle RD, Sheehan KH, et al: Multicenter, double-blind, placebo-controlled study of mecamylamine monotherapy for Tourette's disorder, *J Am Acad Child Adolesc Psychiatry* 40:1103–1110, 2001.

39. Silver AA, Shytle RD, Sanberg PR: Mecamylamine in Tourette's syndrome: a two-year retrospective case study, *J Child Adolesc Psychopharmacol* 10:59–68, 2000.

40. Sanberg PR, Silver AA, Shytle RD, et al.: Nicotine for the treatment of Tourette's syndrome, *Pharmacol Ther* 74:21–25, 1997.

41. Hoopes SP: Donepezil for Tourette's disorder and ADHD, *J Clin Psychopharmacol* 19:381–382, 1999.

42. Muller-Vahl KR, Schneider U, Koblenz A, et al: Treatment of Tourette's syndrome with Delta 9-tetrahydrocannabinol (THC): a randomized crossover trial, *Pharmacopsychiatry* 35:57–61, 2002.

43. Pediatrics AAo, Committee on Quality Improvement SoA-DHD: Diagnosis and evaluation of the child with attention-deficit/hyperactivity disorder, *Pediatrics* 105:1158–1170, 2000.

44. Goldman L, Genel M, Bezman R, et al: Diagnosis and treatment of attention-deficit/hyperactivity disorder in children and adolescents, *JAMA* 279:1100–1107, 1998.

45. Wilens T, Biederman J, Spencer T: *Attention deficit hyperactivity disorder*. In Caskey CT, editor: *Annual Review of Medicine*, vol 53, 2002, pp 113–131.

46. Greenhill LL, Pliszka S, Dulcan MK, et al: Practice parameter for the use of stimulant medications in the treatment of children, adolescents, and adults, *J Am Acad Child Adolesc Psychiatry* 41:26S–49S, 2002.

47. Barkley R: *Attention-deficit/hyperactivity disorder: a handbook for diagnosis and treatment*, ed 2, New York, 1998, Guilford Press.

48. Barkley RA: International consensus statement on ADHD, *J Am Acad Child Adolesc Psychiatry* 41:1389, 2002.

49. American Academy of Pediatrics, Committee on Quality Improvement SoA-DHD: Clinical practice guideline: treatment of the school-aged child with attention-deficit/ hyperactivity disorder, *Pediatrics* 108:1033–1044, 2001.

50. Dulcan M: Practice parameters for the assessment and treatment of children, adolescents, and adults with attention-deficit/hyperactivity disorder, *J Am Acad Child Adolesc Psychiatry* 36:85S–121S, 1997.

51. Wilens T, Spencer T: *Pharmacology of amphetamines.* In Tarter R, Ammerman R, Ott P, editors: *Handbook of substance abuse: neurobehavioral pharmacology,* New York, 1998, Plenum Press, pp 501–513.

52. Wilens T, Spencer T: *The stimulants revisited.* In Stubbe C, editor: *Child and adolescent psychiatric clinics of north America,* vol 9, Philadelphia, 2000, WB Saunders, pp 573–603.

53. Wolraich M, Greenhill LL, Concerta Study Group: Randomized controlled trial of OROS Methylphenidate qd in children with attention deficit/hyperactivity disorder, *Pediatrics* 108:883–892, 2001.

54. Greenhill L: Efficacy and safety of OROS methylphenidate in adolescents with ADHD, American Academy of Child and Adolescent Psychiatry, San Francisco, 2002, Poster Presentation 4.

55. Greenhill LL, Findling RL, Swanson JM: A double-blind, placebo-controlled study of modified-release methylphenidate in children with attention-deficit/hyperactivity disorder, *Pediatrics* 109:E39, 2002.

56. Arnold LE: Methylphenidate vs. amphetamine: comparative review, *J Atten Disord* 3:200–211, 2000.

57. Pliszka SR, Browne RG, Olvera RL, et al: A double-blind, placebo-controlled study of Adderall and methylphenidate in the treatment of attention-deficit/hyperactivity disorder, *J Am Acad Child Adolesc Psychiatry* 39:619–626, 2000.

58. Biederman J, Newcorn J, Sprich S: Comorbidity of attention deficit hyperactivity disorder with conduct, depressive, anxiety, and other disorders, *Am J Psychiatry* 148:564–577, 1991.

59. Wilens T, Faraone S, Biederman J, et al: Does stimulant therapy of attention-deficit/hyperactivity disorder beget later substance abuse? A meta-analytic review of the literature, *Pediatrics* 111:179–185, 2003.

60. Spencer T, Biederman J, Harding M, et al.: Growth deficits in ADHD children revisited: evidence for disorder-associated growth delays? *J Am Acad Child Adolesc Psychiatry* 35:1460–1469, 1996.

61. Michelson D, Allen AJ, Busner J, et al: Once-daily atomoxetine treatment for children and adolescents with attention deficit hyperactivity disorder: a randomized, placebo-controlled study, *Am J Psychiatry* 159:1896–1901, 2002.

62. Michelson D, Faries D, Wernicke J, et al: Atomoxetine in the treatment of children and adolescents with attention-deficit/hyperactivity disorder: a randomized, placebo-controlled, dose-response study, *Pediatrics* 108:E83, 2001.

63. Ring BJ, Gillespie JS, Eckstein JA, et al: Identification of the human cytochromes P450 responsible for atomoxetine metabolism, *Drug Metab Dispos* 30:319–323, 2002.

64. Spencer T, Biederman J, Heiiigenstein J, et al: An open-label, dose-ranging study of atomoxetine in children with attention deficit hyperactivity disorder, *J Child Adolesc Psychopharmacol* 11:251–265, 2001.

65. Ascher JA, Cole JO, Colin J, et al: Bupropion: a review of its mechanism of antidepressant activity. *J Clin Psychiatry* 56:395–401, 1995.

66. Daviss WB, Bentivoglio P, Racusin R, et al: Bupropion SR in adolescents with combined attention-deficit/hyperactivity disorder and depression, *J Am Acad Child Adolesc Psychiatry* 40:307–314, 2001.

67. Wilens T, Biederman J, Baldessarini R, et al: Cardiovascular effects of therapeutic doses of tricyclic antidepressants in children and adolescents, *J Am Acad Child Adolesc Psychiatry* 35:1491–1501, 1996.

68. Biederman J, Baldessarini RJ, Wright V, et al: A double-blind placebo controlled study of desipramine in the treatment of ADD: I. efficacy, *J Am Acad Child Adolesc Psychiatry* 28:777–784, 1989.

69. Riddle MA, Nelson JC, Kleinman CS, et al: Sudden death in children receiving Norpramin: a review of three reported cases and commentary, *J Am Acad Child Adolesc Psychiatry* 30:104–108, 1991.

70. Biederman J, Thisted RA, Greenhill L, et al: Estimation of the association between desipramine and the risk for sudden death in 5- to 14- year old children, *J Clin Psychiatry* 56:87–93, 1995.

71. Daly J, Wilens T: The use of tricyclic antidepressants in children and adolescents, *Pedi Clin North Am*, 45:1123–1135, 1998.

72. Hunt R, Capper L, O'Connell P: Clonidine in child and adolescent psychiatry, *J Child Adolesc Psychopharmacol* 1:87–102, 1990.

73. Hunt RD, Inderaa RB, Cohen DJ: The therapeutic effect of clonidine and attention deficit disorder with hyperactivity: a comparison with placebo and methylphenidate, *Psychopharmacol Bull* 22:229–236, 1986.

74. Connor DF, Fletcher KE, Swanson JM: A meta-analysis of clonidine for symptoms of attention-deficit hyperactivity disorder, *J Am Acad Child Adolesc Psychiatry* 38:1551–1559, 1999.

75. Connor DF, Barkley RA, Davis HT: A pilot study of methylphenidate, clonidine, or the combination in ADHD comorbid with aggressive oppositional defiant or conduct disorder, *Clin Pediatr* 39:15–25, 2000.

76. Schvehla TJ, Mandoki MW, Sumner GS: Clonidine therapy for comorbid attention deficit hyperactivity disorder and conduct disorder: preliminary findings in a children's inpatient unit, *South Med J* 87:692–695, 1994.

77. Singer HV, Brown J, Quaskey S, et al: The treatment of attention-deficit hyperactivity disorder in Tourette's syndrome: a double-blind placebo controlled study with clonidine and desipramine, *Pediatrics* 95:74–81, 1995.

78. Steingard R, Biederman J, Spencer T, et al: Comparison of clonidine response in the treatment of attention deficit hyperactivity disorder with and without comorbid tic disorders, *J Am Acad Child Adolesc Psychiatry* 32:350–353, 1993.

79. Wilens TE, Biederman J, Spencer T: Clonidine for sleep disturbances associated with attention deficit

hyperactivity disorder, *J Am Acad Child Adolesc Psychiatry* 33:424–426, 1994.

80. Prince J, Wilens T, Biederman J, et al: Clonidine for sleep disturbances associated with attention-deficit hyperactivity disorder: a systematic chart review of 62 cases, *J Am Acad Child Adolesc Psychiatry* 35:599–605, 1996.

81. Fankhauser MP, Karumanchi VC, German ML, et al: A double-blind, placebo-controlled study of the efficacy of transdermal clonidine in autism, *J Clin Psychiatry* 53:77–82, 1992.

82. Roden DM, Nadeau JHJ, Primm RK: Electrophysiologic and hemodynamic effects of chronic oral therapy with the alpha₂-agonists clonidine and tiamenidine in hypertensive volunteers, *Clin Pharmacol Ther* 43:648–654, 1988.

83. Buccafusco JJ: Neuropharmacologic and behavioral actions of clonidine: interactions with central neurotransmitters, *Int Rev Neurobiol* 33:55–107, 1992.

84. Wilens T: *Straight talk about psychiatric medications for kids*, 1999 New York, 2002, Guilford Press.

85. Nami R, Bianchini C, Fiorella G, et al: Comparison of effects of guanfacine and clonidine on blood pressure, heart rate, urinary catecholamines, and cyclic nucleotides during and after administration to patients with mild to moderate hypertension, *J Cardiovasc Pharmacol* 5:546–551, 1983.

86. Leckman JF, Ort S, Caruso KA, et al: Rebound phenomena in Tourette's syndrome after abrupt withdrawal of clonidine: behavioral, cardiovascular, and neurochemical effects, *Arch Gen Psychiatry* 43:1168–1176, 1986.

87. Jaffe R, Livshits T, Bursztyn M: Adverse interaction between clonidine and verapamil, *Ann Pharmacother* 28:881–883, 1994.

88. Swanson J, Flockhart D, Udrea D, et al: Clonidine in the treatment of ADHD: Questions about safety and efficacy, *J Child Adolesc Psychopharmacol* 5:301–304, 1995.

89. Popper CW: Combining methylphenidate and clonidine: pharmacologic questions and news reports about sudden death, *J Child Adolesc Psychopharmacol* 5:157–166, 1995.

90. Wilens TE, Spencer TJ, Swanson JM, et al: Combining methylphenidate and clonidine: a clinically sound medication option, *J Am Acad Child Adolesc Psychiatry* 38:614–619; discussion 619–622, 1999.

91. Chappell PB, Riddle MA, Scahill L, et al: Guanfacine treatment of comorbid attention-deficit hyperactivity disorder and Tourette's syndrome: preliminary clinical experience, *J Am Acad Child Adolesc Psychiatry* 34:1140–1146, 1995.

92. Horrigan JP, Barnhill LJ: Guanfacine for treatment of attention-deficit hyperactivity disorder in boys, *J Child Adolesc Psychopharmacol* 5:215–223, 1995.

93. Scahill L: *Controlled clinical trial of guanfacine in ADHD youth with tic disorders*, Boca Raton, 2000, NCDEU.

94. Scahill L, Chappell PB, Kim YS, et al: A placebo-controlled study of guanfacine in the treatment of children with tic disorders and attention deficit hyperactivity disorder, *Am J Psychiatry* 158:1067–1074, 2001.

95. Horrigan JP, Barnhill LJ: Guanfacine and secondary mania in children, *J Affect Disord* 54:309–314, 1999.

96. American Psychiatric Association: *Diagnostic and statistical manual of mental disorders*, ed 4, Washington, DC, 1994, American Psychiatric Press.

97. Rushton JL, Clark SJ, Freed GL: Pediatrician and family physician prescription of selective serotonin reuptake inhibitors, *Pediatrics* 105:E82, 2000.

98. Rushton JL, Clark SJ, Freed GL: Primary care role in the management of childhood depression: a comparison of pediatricians and family physicians (comment), *Pediatrics* 105:957–962, 2000.

99. Fleming JE, Offord DR: Epidemiology of childhood depressive disorders: a critical review, *J Am Acad Child Adolesc Psychiatry* 29:571–580, 1990.

100. Kashani JH, Beck NC, Hoeper EW, et al: Psychiatric disorders in a community sample of adolescents. *Am J Psychiatry* 144:584–589, 1987.

101. Kashani J, Schmid LS: *Epidemiology and etiology of depressive disorders.* In Shafii M, Shafii S, editors: *Clinical guide to depression in children and adolescents*, Washington, DC, 1992, American Psychiatric Press, pp 43–64.

102. Lewinsohn P, Hops H, Roberts R, et al: Adolescent psychopathology: prevalence and incidence of depression and other DSM-III-R disorders in high school students, *J Abnorm Psychol* 102:133–144, 1993.

103. Rushton J, Forcier M, Schectman R: Epidemiology of depressive symptoms in the national longitudinal study of adolescent health, *J Am Acad Child Adolesc Psychiatry* 41:199–205, 2002.

104. Department of Health and Human Services: *Mental health: a report of the surgeon general*, Rockville, MD 1999, U.S. Public Health Service.

105. Birmaher B, Ryan ND, Williamson DE, et al: Childhood and adolescent depression: a review of the past 10 years, part I, *J Am Acad Child Adolesc Psychiatry* 35:1427–1439, 1996.

106. Birmaher B, Ryan ND, Williamson DE, et al: Childhood and adolescent depression: a review of the past 10 years: II. *J Am Acad Child Adolesc Psychiatry* 35:1575–1583, 1996.

107. Birmaher B, Brent DA, Benson RS: Summary of the practice parameters for the assessment and treatment of children and adolescents with depressive disorders. (comment), *J Am Acad Child Adolesc Psychiatry* 37:1234–1238, 1998.

108. Lewinsohn P, Clarke G, Seely J, et al: Major depression in community adolescents: age at onset, episode duration, and time to recurrence, *J Am Acad Child Adolesc Psychiatry* 33:809–818, 1994.

109. Wade T, Cairney J, Pevalin D: Emergence of gender differences in depression during adolescence: national panel results from three countries, *J Am Acad Child Adolesc Psychiatry* 41:190–198, 2002.

110. Kovacs M: Gender and the course of major depressive disorder through adolescence in clinically referred youngsters, *J Am Acad Child Adolesc Psychiatry* 40:1079–1085, 2001.

111. Biederman J, Faraone S, Mick E, et al: Psychiatric comorbidity among referred juveniles with major depression: Fact or artifact? *J Am Acad Child Adolesc Psychiatry* 34:579–590, 1995.

112. Kovacs M, Feinberg TL, Crouse-Novak MA, et al: Depressive disorders in childhood: a longitudinal prospective study of characteristics and recovery, *Arch Gen Psychiatry* 41:229–237, 1984.

113. Biederman J, Spencer T: Depressive disorders in childhood and adolescence: a clinical perspective, *J Child Adolesc Psychopharmacol* 9:233–237, 1999.

114. Luby JL, Heffelfinger AK, Mrakotsky C, et al: The clinical picture of depression in preschool children, *J Am Acad Child Adolesc Psychiatry* 42:340–348, 2003.

115. Kovacs M: Presentation and course of major depressive disorder during childhood and later years of the life span, *J Am Acad Child Adolesc Psychiatry* 35:705–715, 1996.

116. Kovacs M, Feinberg TL, Crouse-Novak M, et al: Depressive disorders in childhood: a longitudinal study of the risk for a subsequent major depression, *Arch Gen Psychiatry* 41:643–649, 1984.

117. Emslie G, Rush A, Weinberg W, et al: Recurrence of major depressive disorder in hospitalized children and adolescents, *J Am Acad Child Adolesc Psychiatry* 36:785–792, 1997.

118. Wickramaratne PJ, Greenwald S, Weissman MM: Psychiatric disorders in the relatives of probands with prepubertal-onset or adolescent-onset major depression, *J Am Acad Child Adolesc Psychiatry* 39: 1396–1405, 2000.

119. Wickramaratne PJ, Weissman MM: Onset of psychopathology in offspring by developmental phase and parental depression, *J Am Acad Child Adolesc Psychiatry* 37:933–942, 1998.

120. Geller B, Zimerman B, Williams M, et al: Adult psychosocial outcome of prepubertal major depressive disorder, *J Am Acad Child Adolesc Psychiatry* 40:673–677, 2001.

121. Geller B, Fox L, Clark K: Rate and predictors of prepubertal bipolarity during follow-up of 6- to 12-year-old depressed children, *J Am Acad Child Adolesc Psychiatry* 33:461–468, 1994.

122. Strober M, Carlson G: Predictors of bipolar illness in adolescents with major depression: a follow-up investigation, *J Adolesc Psychiatry* 10:299–319, 1982.

123. Bowden CL, Rhodes LJ: Mania in children and adolescents: recognition and treatment, *Psychiatric Ann* 26:S430–S434, 1996.

124. Gould MS, Greenberg T, Velting DM, et al: Youth suicide risk and preventive interventions: a review of the past 10 years *J Am Acad Child Adolesc Psychiatry* 42:386–405, 2003.

125. American Academy of Child and Adolescent Psychiatry: Practice parameter for the assessment and treatment of children and adolescents with suicidal behavior, *J Am Acad Child Adolesc Psychiatry* 40:24S–51S, 2001.

126. Kovacs M, Akiskal HS, Gatsonis C, et al: Childhood-onset dysthymic disorder: clinical features and prospective naturalistic outcome, *Arch Gen Psychiatry* 51:365–374, 1994.

127. Zito JM, Safer DJ: Services and prevention: pharmacoepidemiology of antidepressant use, *Biol Psychiatry* 49:1121–1127, 2001.

128. Zito JM, Safer DJ, dosReis S, et al: Trends in the prescribing of psychotropic medications to preschoolers, *JAMA* 283:1025–1030, 2000.

129. Zito JM, Safer DJ, dosReis S, et al: Rising prevalence of antidepressants among US youths, *Pediatrics* 109:721–727, 2002.

130. Zito JM, Safer DJ, dosReis S, et al Psychotropic practice patterns for youth: a 10-year perspective (comment), *Arch Pediatr Adolesc Med* 157:17–25, 2003.

131. Walkup J: Increasing use of psychotropic medications in children and adolescents: what does it mean? *J Child Adolesc Psychopharmacol* 13:1–3, 2003.

132. Geller B, Reising D, Leonard HL, et al: Critical review of tricyclic antidepressant use in children and adolescents, *J Am Acad Child Adolesc Psychiatry* 38:513–516, 1999.

133. Ryan ND: Medication treatment for depression in children and adolescents, *CNS Spectr* 8:283–287, 2003.

134. Bostic J, Wilens T, Spencer T, et al: Pharmacologic treatment of juvenile depression, *Child Adolesc Psychiatr Clin North Am* 6:175–191, 1999.

135. Anonymous: Prozac for pediatric use, *FDA Consumer* 37:3, 2003.

136. Emslie GJ, Rush AJ, Weinberg WA, et al: A double-blind, randomized, placebo-controlled trial of fluoxetine in children and adolescents with depression, *Arch Gen Psychiatry* 54:1031–1037, 1997.

137. Emslie GJ, Heiligenstein JH, Wagner KD et al: Fluoxetine for acute treatment of depression in children and adolescents: a placebo-controlled, randomized clinical trial, *J Am Acad Child Adolesc Psychiatry* 41:1205–1215, 2002.

138. Wagner KD, Ambrosini P, Rynn M et al: Efficacy of sertraline in the treatment of children and adolescents with major depressive disorder: two randomized controlled trials, *JAMA* 290:1033–1041, 2003.

139. Ambrosini PJ, Wagner KD, Biederman J, et al: Multicenter open-label sertraline study in adolescent outpatients with major depression, *J Am Acad Child Adolesc Psychiatry* 38:566–572, 1999.

140. Wagner KD, Robb AS, Findling R, et al: *Citalopram treatment of pediatric depression: results of a placebo-*

controlled trial, American College of Neuropsychopharmacology. Waikoloa, Hawaii, 2001.

141. Cheer SM, Figgitt DP: Fluvoxamine: a review of its therapeutic potential in the management of anxiety disorders in children and adolescents [erratum appears in *Paediatr Drugs* 3(11):801, 2001], *Paediatric Drugs* 3:763–781, 2001.

142. Keller MB, Ryan ND, Strober M, et al: Efficacy of paroxetine in the treatment of adolescent major depression: a randomized, controlled trial, *J Am Acad Child Adolesc Psychiatry* 40:762–772, 2001.

143. Teicher MH, Glod C, Cole JO: Emergence of intense suicidal preoccupation during fluoxetine treatment (comment), *Am J Psychiatry* 147:207–210, 1990.

144. Khan A, Khan S, Kolts R, et al: Suicide rates in clinical trials of SSRIs, other antidepressants, and placebo: analysis of FDA reports, *Am J Psychiatry* 160:790–792, 2003.

145. Mandoki MW, Tapia MR, Tapia MA, et al: Venlafaxine in the treatment of children and adolescents with major depression, *Psychopharmacol Bull* 33:149–154, 1997.

146. Findling RL, Preskorn SH, Marcus RN, et al: Nefazodone pharmacokinetics in depressed children and adolescents, *J Am Acad Child Adolesc Psychiatry* 39:1008–1016, 2000.

147. Wilens T, Spencer T, Biederman J, et al: Case study: nefazodone for juvenile mood disorders, *J Am Acad Child Adolesc Psychiatry* 36:481–485, 1997.

148. Emslie G: *A double-blind placebo controlled study of nefazodone in depressed children and adolescents,* New Drug Clinical Evaluation Unit, Boca Raton, Fla, 2002.

149. Cozza KL, Armstrong SC, Oesterheld JR: *Concise guide to drug interaction principles for medical practice*, Washington, DC, 2003, American Psychiatric Press.

150. Wilens TE, Cohen L, Biederman J, et al: Fluoxetine pharmacokinetics in pediatric patients, *J Clin Psychopharmacol* 22:568–575, 2002.

151. Axelson DA, Perel JM, Birmaher B, et al: Sertraline pharmacokinetics and dynamics in adolescents, *J Am Acad Child Adolesc Psychiatry* 41:1037–1044, 2002.

152. Findling RL, Reed MD, Myers C, et al: Paroxetine pharmacokinetics in depressed children and adolescents, *J Am Acad Child Adolesc Psychiatry* 38:952–959, 1999.

153. Reis M, Olsson G, Carlsson B, et al: Serum levels of citalopram and its main metabolites in adolescent patients treated in a naturalistic clinical setting, *J Clin Psychopharmacol* 22:406–413, 2002.

154. Stewart JJ, Berkel HJ, Parish RC, et al: Single-dose pharmacokinetics of bupropion in adolescents: effects of smoking status and gender, *J Clin Psychopharmacol* 41:770–778, 2001.

155. Aranda-Michel J, Koehler A, Bejarano PA, et al: Nefazodone-induced liver failure: report of three cases, *Ann Intern Med* 130:285–288, 1999.

156. Goodman E, Capitman J: Depressive symptoms and cigarette smoking among teens, *Pediatrics* 106: 748–755, 2000.

157. Masand PS, Gupta S: Long-term side effects of newer-generation antidepressants: SSRIS, venlafaxine, nefazodone, bupropion, and mirtazapine, *Ann Clin Psychiatry* 14:175–182, 2002.

158. Weintrob N, Cohen D, Klipper-Aurbach Y, et al: Decreased growth during therapy with selective serotonin reuptake inhibitors, *Arch Pediatr Adolesc Med* 156:696–701, 2002.

159. Wilens TE, Biederman J, March JS, et al: Absence of cardiovascular adverse effects of sertraline in children and adolescents, *J Am Acad Child Adolesc Psychiatry* 38:573–577, 1999.

160. Walkup J, Labellarte M: Complications of SSRI treatment, *J Child Adolesc Psychopharmacol* 11:1–4, 2001.

161. Rosenbaum JF, Fava M, Hoog SL, et al: Selective serotonin reuptake inhibitor discontinuation syndrome: a randomized clinical trial (comment), *Biol Psychiatry* 44:77–87, 1998.

162. Zajecka J, Tracy KA, Mitchell S: Discontinuation symptoms after treatment with serotonin reuptake inhibitors: a literature review, *J Clin Psychiatry* 58:291–297, 1997.

163. Sher L: Prevention of the serotonin reuptake inhibitor discontinuation syndrome, *Med Hypotheses* 59: 92–94, 2002.

164. Ali S, Milev R: Switch to mania upon discontinuation of antidepressants in patients with mood disorders: a review of the literature, *Can J Psychiatry* 48:258–264, 2003.

165. Geller B, Luby J: Child and adolescent bipolar disorder: a review of the past 10 years, *J Am Acad Child Adolesc Psychiatry* 36:1168–1176, 1997.

166. Biederman J: Developmental subtypes of juvenile bipolar disorder, *Harv Rev Psychiatry* 3:227–230, 1995.

167. McClellan J, Werry J, Ayres W, et al: Practice parameters for the assessment and treatment of children and adolescents with bipolar disorder.

168. Biederman J, Birmaher B, Carlson GA, et al: National Institute of Mental Health Research Roundtable on Prepubertal Bipolar Disorder, *J Am Acad Child Adolesc Psychiatry* 40:871–878, 2001.

169. Wozniak J, Biederman J, Kiely K, et al: Mania-like symptoms suggestive of childhood-onset bipolar disorder in clinically referred children, *J Am Acad Child Adolesc Psychiatry* 34:867–876, 1995.

170. Biederman J: Resolved: mania is mistaken for ADHD in prepubertal children, *J Am Acad Child Adolesc Psychiatry* 37:1091–1096, discussion 1096–1099, 1998.

171. Spencer TJ, Biederman J, Wozniak J, et al: Parsing pediatric bipolar disorder from its associated comorbidity with the disruptive behavior disorders, *Biol Psychiatry* 49:1062–1070, 2001.

172. Geller B, Sun K, Zimerman B, et al: Complex and rapid-cycling in bipolar children and adolescents: a preliminary study. *J Affect Disord* 34:259–268, 1995.

173. Geller B, Zimerman B, Williams M, et al: Diagnostic characteristics of 93 cases of a prepubertal and early adolescent bipolar disorder phenotype by gender, puberty and comorbid attention deficit hyperactivity disorder, *J Child Adolesc Psychopharmacol* 10:157–164, 2000.

174. Biederman J, Mick E, Faraone SV,: Pediatric mania: a developmental subtype of bipolar disorder? (comment), *Biol Psychiatry* 48:458–466, 2000.

175. Strober M, Schmidt-Lackner S, Freeman R, et al: Recovery and relapse in adolescents with bipolar affective illness: a five-year naturalistic, prospective follow-up, *J Am Acad Child Adolesc Psychiatry* 34:724–731, 1995.

176. Strober M, Morrell W, Lampert C, et al: Relapse following discontinuation of lithium maintenance therapy in adolescents with bipolar I illness: a naturalistic study, *Am J Psychiatry* 147:457–461, 1990.

177. Schurhoff F, Bellivier F, Jouvent R, et al: Early and late onset bipolar disorders: two different forms of manic-depressive illness? *J Affect Disord* 58:215–221, 2000.

178. Biederman J, Mick E, Bostic J, et al: The naturalistic course of pharmacologic treatment of children with manic like symptoms: a systematic chart review, *J Clin Psychiatry* 59:628–637, 1998.

179. Biederman J, Mick E, Spencer TJ, et al: Therapeutic dilemmas in the pharmacotherapy of bipolar depression in the young, *J Child Adolesc Psychopharmacol* 10:185–192, 2000.

180. Weller EB, Weller RA, Fristad MA: Lithium dosage guide for prepubertal children: a preliminary report, *J Am Acad Child Adolesc Psychiatry* 25:92–95, 1986.

181. Geller B, Cooper T, Sun K, et al: Double blind and placebo controlled study of lithium for adolescent bipolar disorders with secondary substance dependency, *J Am Acad Child Adolesc Psychiatry* 37:171–178, 1998.

182. Alessi N, Naylor MW, Ghaziuddin M, et al: Update on lithium carbonate therapy in children and adolescents, *J Am Acad Child Adolesc Psychiatry* 33:291–304, 1994.

183. Woolston J: Case study: carbamazepine treatment of juvenile-onset bipolar disorder, *J Am Acad Child Adolesc Psychiatry* 38:335–338, 1999.

184. Wozniak J, Biederman J, Richards JA: Diagnostic and therapeutic dilemmas in the management of pediatric-onset bipolar disorder, *J Clin Psychiatry* 62:10–15, 2001.

185. Pleak RR, Birmaher B, Gavrilescu A, et al: Mania and neuropsychiatric excitation following carbamazepine, *J Am Acad Child Adolesc Psychiatry* 27:500–503, 1988.

186. Kowatch RA, Suppes T, Carmody TJ, et al: Effect size of lithium, divalproex sodium, and carbamazepine in children and adolescents with bipolar disorder, *J Am Acad Child Adolesc Psychiatry* 39:713–720, 2000.

187. Wagner KD, Weller EB, Carlson GA et al: An open-label trial of divalproex in children and adolescents with bipolar disorder, *J Am Acad Child Adolesc Psychiatry* 41:1224–1230, 2002.

188. Stahl S: What makes an antipsychotic atypical? *J Clin Psychiatry* 59:402–404, 1998.

189. Tohen M, Jacobs TG, Grundy SL, et al: Efficacy of olanzapine in acute bipolar mania: a double-blind, placebo- controlled study: The Olanzipine HGGW Study Group, *Arch Gen Psychiatry* 57:841–849, 2000.

190. Frazier JA, Biederman J, Tohen M, et al: A prospective open-label treatment trial of olanzapine monotherapy in children and adolescents with bipolar disorder, *J Child Adolesc Psychopharmacol* 11:239–250, 2001.

191. Lindenmayer JP, Nathan AM, Smith RC: Hyperglycemia associated with the use of atypical antipsychotics, *J Clin Psychiatry* 62:30–38, 2001.

192. Jin H, Meyer JM, Jeste DV: Phenomenology of and risk factors for new-onset diabetes mellitus an diabetic ketoacidosis associated with atypical antipsychotics: an analysis of 45 published cases, *Ann Clin Psychiatry* 14:59–64, 2002.

193. Grothe DR, Calis KA, Jacobsen L, et al: Olanzapine pharmacokinetics in pediatric and adolescent inpatients with childhood-onset schizophrenia, *J Clin Psychopharmacol* 20:220–225, 2000.

194. Frazier JA, Meyer MC, Biederman J, et al: Risperidone treatment for juvenile bipolar disorder: a retrospective chart review, *J Am Acad Child Adolesc Psychiatry* 38:960–965, 1999.

195. Green WH: *Child & adolescent clinical psychopharmacology*, Philadelphia, 2001, Lippincott Williams & Wilkins, 2001.

196. Delbello MP, Schwiers ML, Rosenberg HL, et al: A double-blind, randomized, placebo-controlled study of quetiapine as adjunctive treatment for adolescent mania, *J Am Acad Child Adolesc Psychiatry* 41:1216–1223, 2002.

197. Wang PW, Ketter TA: Pharmacokinetics of mood stabilizers and new anticonvulsants, *Psychopharmacol Bull* 36:44–66, 2002.

198. Mandoki M: Lamontrigine/valproate in treatment resistant bipolar disorder in children and adolescents, *Biol Psychiatry* 41:93S–94S, 1997.

199. Roy Chengappa KN, Levine J, Rathore D, et al: Long-term effects of topiramate on bipolar mood instability, weight change and glycemic control: a case-series, *Eur Psychiatry* 16:186–190, 2001.

200. Tanguay PE: Pervasive developmental disorders: a 10-year review, *J Am Acad Child Adolesc Psychiatry* 39:1079–1095, 2000.

201. State M, King B, Dykens E: Mental retardation: a review of the past 10 years: II. *J Am Acad Child Adolesc Psychiatry* 36:1664–1671, 1997.

202. King BH, State MW, Shah B, et al: Mental retardation: a review of the past 10 years: I. *J Am Acad Child Adolesc Psychiatry* 36:1656–1663, 1997.

203. Volkmar FR, Klin A, Schultz RT, et al: Asperger's disorder, *Am J Psychiatry* 157:262–267, 2000.

204. Pearson DA, Santos CW, Roache JD, et al: Treatment effects of methylphenidate on behavioral adjustment in children with mental retardation and ADHD, *J Am Acad Child Adolesc Psychiatry* 42:209–216, 2003.

205. Aman MG, De Smedt G, Derivan A, et al: Double-blind, placebo-controlled study of risperidone for the treatment of disruptive behaviors in children with sub-average intelligence, *Am J Psychiatry* 159:1337–1346, 2002.

206. McCracken JT, McGough J, Shah B, et al: Risperidone in children with autism and serious behavioral problems (comment), *N Engl J Med* 347:314–21, 2002.

207. Malone RP, Cater J, Sheikh RM, et al: Olanzapine versus haloperidol in children with autistic disorder: an open pilot study, *J Am Acad Child Adolesc Psychiatry* 40:887–894, 2001.

208. McDougle CJ, Kem DL, Posey DJ: Case series: use of ziprasidone for maladaptive symptoms in youths with autism, *J Am Acad Child Adolesc Psychiatry* 41:921–927, 2002.

209. Ratey JJ, Mikkelsen E, Sorgi P, et al: Autism: the treatment of aggressive behaviors, *J Clin Psychopharmacol* 7:35–41, 1987.

210. Ratey JJ, Bemporad J, Sorgi P, et al: Open trial effects of beta-blockers on speech and social behaviors in 8 autistic adults, *J Autism Dev Disord* 17:439–446, 1987.

211. Ratey JJ, Sovner R, Mikkelsen E, et al: Buspirone therapy for maladaptive behavior and anxiety in developmentally disabled persons, *J Clin Psychiatry* 50:382–384, 1989.

212. Niederhofer H, Staffen W, Mair A: Lofexidine in hyperactive and impulsive children with autistic disorder, *J Am Acad Child Adolesc Psychiatry* 41:1396–1397, 2002.

213. Jaselskis CA, Cook EH, Jr, Fletcher KE, et al: Clonidine treatment of hyperactive and impulsive children with autistic disorder, *J Clin Psychopharmacol* 12:322–327, 1992.

214. Fankhauser MP, Karumanchi VC, German ML, et al: A double-blind, placebo-controlled study of the efficacy of transdermal clonidine in autism, *J Clin Psychiatry*. 53:77–82, 1992.

215. Buchsbaum MS, Hollander E, Haznedar MM, et al: Effect of fluoxetine on regional cerebral metabolism in autistic spectrum disorders: a pilot study, *Int J Neuropsychopharmacol* 4:119–125, 2001.

216. McDougle CJ, Naylor ST, Cohen DJ, et al: A double-blind, placebo-controlled study of fluvoxamine in adults with autistic disorder (comment), *Arch Gen Psychiatry* 53:1001–1008, 1996.

217. Horvath K: Secretin treatment for autism (comment), *New Engl J Med* 342:1216, discussion 1218, 2000.

218. Horvath K, Stefanatos G, Sokolski KN, et al: Improved social and language skills after secretin administration in patients with autistic spectrum disorders, *Assoc Acad Minority Physicians* 9:9–15, 1998.

219. Unis AS, Munson JA, Rogers SJ, et al: A randomized, double-blind, placebo-controlled trial of porcine versus synthetic secretin for reducing symptoms of autism (comment), *J Am Acad Child Adolesc Psychiatry* 41:1315–1321, 2002.

220. Sandler AD, Sutton KA, DeWeese J, et al: Lack of benefit of a single dose of synthetic human secretin in the treatment of autism and pervasive developmental disorder (comment), *New Engl J Med* 341:1801–6, 1999.

221. Sponheim E, Oftedal G, Helverschou SB: Multiple doses of secretin in the treatment of autism: a controlled study, *Acta Paediatr* 91:540–5, 2002.

222. McClellan J, Werry J: Practice parameters for the assessment and treatment of children and adolescents with schizophrenia, *J Am Acad Child Adolesc Psychiatry* 33:616–635, 1994.

223. Armenteros JL, Whitaker AH, Welikson M, et al: Risperidone in adolescents with schizophrenia: an open pilot study *J Am Acad Child Adolesc Psychiatry* 36:694–700, 1997.

224. Martin A, L'Ecuyer S: Triglyceride, cholesterol and weight changes among risperidone-treated youths: a retrospective study, *Eur Child Adolesc Psychiatry* 11:129–133, 2002.

225. Martin A, Landau J, Leebens P, et al: Risperidone-associated weight gain in children and adolescents: a retrospective chart review, *J Child Adolesc Psychopharmacol* 10:259–268, 2000.

226. Bryden KE, Carrey NJ, Kutcher SP: Update and recommendations for the use of antipsychotics in early-onset psychoses, *J Child Adolesc Psychopharmacol* 11:113–130, 2001.

227. Findling RL, McNamara NK, Youngstrom EA, et al: A prospective, open-label trial of olanzapine in adolescents with schizophrenia, *J Am Acad Child Adolesc Psychiatry* 42:170–175, 2003.

228. Sholevar EH, Baron DA, Hardie TL: Treatment of childhood-onset schizophrenia with olanzapine, *J Child Adolesc Psychopharmacol* 10:69–78, 2000.

229. Remschmidt H, Schulz E, Martin M: An open trial of clozapine in thirty-six adolescents with schizophrenia, *J Child Adolesc Psychopharmacol* 4:31–41, 1994.

230. Kumra S, Frazier JA, Jacobsen LK, et al: Childhood-onset schizophrenia: a double-blind clozapine trial, *Arch Gen Psychiatry* 53(12): 1090–1097, 1996.

231. Gammon GD, Brown TE: Fluoxetine and methylphenidate in combination for treatment of attention deficit disorder and comorbid depressive disorder, *J Child Adolesc Psychopharmacol* 3:1–10, 1993.

Chapter 26
Care of the Geriatric Patient

M. Cornelia Cremens, M.D., M.P.H.

Consultation with Geriatric Patients

The patient population in the United States over the age of 65 is increasing at an alarming rate; this trend reflects improvements in health, nutrition, and medical care for the elderly. The impact of medical and psychiatric illness in this population is growing due to comorbidity and the effects of drug-drug interactions. Unfortunately, elderly individuals are more susceptible to disease and the side effects of drugs, both prescribed and over-the-counter.

Roughly 40% to 60% of those hospitalized with medical and surgical illnesses are over the age of 65; this places them at greater risk for functional decline.[1] In addition, a reduction in hepatic, renal, and gastric function further impairs the elderly patient's ability to metabolize drugs and degrade medications.[2] Psychiatric consultation with this group of patients is ever more necessary; it provides complicated challenges and rewards.

Depression

Mood disorders associated with later life are a major public health problem. Depression is prevalent, unrelenting, immobilizing, and frequently fatal, especially in those with comorbid medical illness.[3,4] In the United States, depression in the elderly is accompanied by higher rates of suicide than any other condition. Moreover, rates of suicide are higher in later life than they are in any

other age-group.[5] Certainly, the use and abuse of alcohol increases the risk of suicide in all groups; in the elderly its impact is dramatic.[6] Many variables (e.g., in mental, physical, and social realms) are correlated with completed suicide in older adults, but case control studies indicate that affective disorders are a powerful independent risk factor for suicide.[6] Physical illness and functional impairment also increase the risk, but their influence appears to be mediated by depression.

Approximately 50% of those with neurologic diseases, cardiac diseases, and cancers have depressive symptoms. Major depression following stroke is also common; it occurs in one quarter to one half of all post-stroke patients. The prevalence of major depression in Alzheimer's disease (AD) is approximately 10%, and with Parkinson's disease (PD) it is approximately 20%.[7] Longitudinal data on depression in AD and PD suggest that depressive symptoms in these conditions decrease over time.[7] In short, the elderly are at greater risk for depression due to the prevalence of these illnesses and their downstream sequelae.

Despite the fact that depression is a mood disorder comprised by far-ranging symptoms involving disordered sleep, diminished interests, guilt and ruminations, decreased energy or fatigue, impaired concentration, disturbed appetite, and suicidal thoughts or attempts, somatic complaints, rather than depressed mood, are often the reason for referral in the elderly and the medically ill.[8] These physical complaints lie on a continuum and can mimic medical problems (e.g., chest pain, headache, joint pain, nausea, dizziness, and weakness). Teasing out the symptoms of medical or surgical problems from the symptoms of depression can be a daunting task in the hospitalized patient. Physicians often misdiagnose or undertreat depression in the medically ill due to an overlap of these symptoms. At the same time, substantial progress has been made in the treatment of elderly individuals with mood disorders, especially major depression.[9] Once the diagnosis has been established, prescription of an appropriate medication is part of the art of geriatric psychiatry. Since the list of prescribed medications is long for those with numerous medical problems, knowledge of how the addition of an antidepressant may alter the metabolism and therapeutic drug levels of the various medications is crucial. One needs to review the side effects of the antidepressant and then tailor its use to treat the patient's symptoms. For example, if a depressed patient is sleeping poorly and losing weight, one should select a sedating medication that is associated with weight gain. Moreover, since depression can complicate recovery from the medical or surgical problems, treatment must be swift and aggressive. Often, stimulants are used alone or in conjunction with a traditional antidepressant, such as a selective serotonin-reuptake inhibitor (SSRI).[10] Consideration of electroconvulsive-therapy (ECT) if a patient is not responsive to medications should be discussed with patients and their family members (Table 26-1).[11]

Table 26-1. Treatments Recommended for Depression in the Elderly

Drugs	Dose Range (mg/d)	Comments
Tricyclic Antidepressants		
Nortriptyline	10–150	Mildly anticholinergic
Desipramine	10–250	Reliable blood levels, minimal orthostasis
Monoamine Oxidase Inhibitors		
Tranylcypromine	10–30	Orthostasis (may be delayed), pedal edema, weakly anticholinergic, dietary restrictions
Stimulants		
Dextroamphetamine	2.5–40	
Methylphenidate	2.5–60	Agitation, mild tachycardia
Selective Serotonin-Reuptake Inhibitors		
Fluoxetine	5–60	
Sertraline	25–200	
Paroxetine	5–40	
Fluvoxamine	25–300	
Citalopram	10–40	
Escitalopram	2.5–20	Akathisia, headache, agitation, GI complaints, diarrhea/constipation
Serotonin/Norepinephrine-Reuptake Inhibitors (SNRI)		
Venlafaxine	25–300	Increased systolic blood pressure (SBP), confusion, lightheadedness
Alpha-2 Antagonist/Selective Serotonin		
Mirtazapine	15–45	Sedation, weight gain
Atypical Antidepressants		
Trazodone	25–250	Sedation, orthostasis, incontinence, hallucinations, priapism
Nefazodone	50–600	Pedal edema, rash
Bupropion	75–450	Seizures, less mania/cycling headache, nausea

Bipolar Disorder

Patients with bipolar disorder over the age of 65 years do not always develop their affective illness early in life.[12] Many elderly patients have the onset of their illness in middle age or later and often have etiologically related comorbid neurologic insults.[13] Those patients with comorbid neurologic diseases have a significantly later age of onset of their affective illness and are less likely to have a family history of affective illness. Snowdon[14] reported that 25% of patients whose mania arose after the age of 50 had a history of

neurologic disease and had significantly fewer genetic (familial) risk factors.[14] A number of biologic risk factors have been identified for bipolar mood disorders in the elderly, including genetic factors and medical illnesses, particularly vascular conditions.[15] Moreover, the differential diagnosis of secondary mania warrants special consideration.[16] Many of those with dementia or delirium present with mania secondary to their underlying illness. Although the treatment of secondary affective symptoms is similar to those of primary affective illness, an accurate diagnosis is important (Table 26-2).

Table 26-2. Antipsychotics Commonly Used in the Elderly

Agent/dose (mg)	Sedation	Anticholinergic	Extrapyramidal	Comments
Low Potency				
Thioridazine (Mellaril)	High	High	Low	Significant hypotension
10–50				
Intermediate Potency				
Perphenazine (Trilafon)	Medium	Medium	Medium	
0.5–5				
High Potency				
Haloperidol (Haldol)	Low	Low	High	
0.25–2				
Thiothixene (Navane)	Low	Low	High	
0.5–4				
Fluphenazine (Prolixin)	Low	Low	High	
0.5–2				
Atypical Antipsychotics				
Clozapine (Clozaril)	High	High	Very low	White blood cell (WBC) check each week
2.5–100				Excessive drooling Hypotension
Risperidone (Risperdal)	Low	Low	Low	More EPS than initially reported
0.25–3				
Olanzapine (Zyprexa)	Moderate	Medium	Low	
2.5–10.0				
Quetiapine (Seroquel)	High	Low	Low	
12.5–200				
Ziprasidone (Geodon)	Moderate	Low	Low	
Aripiprazole (Abilify)	Low	Low	Moderate	
15–30				

Dementia

The prevalence of dementia increases as age advances; 3% to 12% of patients over the age of 65 and 25% to 46% of those over the age of 85 have dementia.[17] Age is the most robust risk factor for dementia. AD, the most common form of dementia, affects 5% to 8% of individuals over the age of 65 years, 15% to 20% of individuals over the age of 75 years, and 25% to 50% of individuals over the age of 85 years.

Dementia is an acquired syndrome that consists primarily of a decline in memory, as well as at least one other area of cognition (e.g., language or visuospatial or executive function), that is sufficient to interfere with social or occupational functioning.[18] It is characterized by a decline in intellectual functioning that can be severe enough to make the patient unable to perform activities of daily living. Typically, the deterioration of intellectual functioning occurs over months to years. The diagnosis is often overlooked or goes undiagnosed until it is moderately or severely disabling. The prevalence of dementia and cognitive impairment is higher in women; of note, women have higher rates of AD, whereas men have higher rates of vascular dementia.

Numeric rating scales can quantify the severity of AD (0 to 5) throughout its course until the final stage of the illness. The decline is gradual but steady, over the course of 8 to 10 years. The use of rating scales can facilitate evaluation of patients with dementia, but their results need to be placed in the context of what may be a brief evaluation. Although the Mini-Mental-State Examination does not provide an in-depth assessment, its brevity is an advantage.[19]

Mild cognitive impairment describes the functional and cognitive abilities of those who function between what is considered to be normal aging and what is classified as very mild AD.[20] Those with mild cognitive impairment should be seen in follow-up, as different individuals develop dementia at different rates. As will be mentioned later in the discussion on delirium, a patient with mild dementia is at greater risk for developing delirium during a hospitalization; such a complication can lead to serious behavioral problems.[21]

The major causes of dementia include AD, vascular dementia, Lewy body disease (LBD), trauma to the central nervous system (CNS), PD, Creutzfeldt-Jakob disease, Huntington's disease, Pick's disease, and infection with the human immunodeficiency virus (HIV).[22] Potentially reversible causes of symptoms that are suggestive of dementia include thyroid dysfunction, deficiencies of vitamins (such as B_{12} and folate), infections, metabolic abnormalities, and normal pressure hydrocephalus (NPH).

Of these causes, AD is the most common; vascular dementia is second, but it often coexists with AD and is a difficult diagnosis to discern. Vascular dementia presents with a step-wise decline in function that is usually not global. It is common in patients with a history of coronary artery disease (CAD) and multiple ischemic events or strokes; about 8% of patients who suffer strokes develop dementia.[20] LBD has often been confused with AD. However, it usually presents with a Parkinsonian gait, visual hallucinations, fluctuations in cognitive problems, and at times a transient loss of consciousness. Recognizing LBD is important, as afflicted patients are exquisitely sensitive to the adverse side effects of psychiatric medications.

Treatment of dementia is controversial. Cummings[23] outlined the multiple uses of cholinesterase inhibitors in patients with a variety of dementias, not just those ascribed to AD. The use of cholinesterase inhibitors to reduce the behavioral symptoms and to improve the function of activities of daily living leads to dramatic impact on quality of life. Currently, several cholinesterase inhibitors are available, including donepezil, rivastigmine, galantamine, and the soon-to-be-released memantine.[23–27] Donepezil has been the most widely used due to its once-daily dosing; however, all are effective, albeit limited, with regard to reduction of cognitive decline. Side effects are minimal within all of these medications,[28] but in any given patient one medication may be better tolerated than another. Donepezil, rivastigmine, and galantamine have a cholinomimetic mechanism of action, while memantine has an antiglutaminergic mechanism. Memantine is indicated for moderate to severe AD. The goal of treatment is to reduce the rate of decline; unfortunately, they are not able to affect the ultimate prognosis.[27]

Delirium

Delirium, a syndrome with a prodromal phase, an abrupt onset, a rapid fluctuating course, disorientation, decreased attention, altered arousal, psychomotor abnormalities, a disturbed sleep-wake cycle, impaired memory, disorganized thinking, disordered speech, hallucinations (usually visual), delusions (persecutory), and altered perceptions, often goes misdiagnosed or undertreated due to the overlap of symptoms with medical illnesses and the erroneous assumption that confusion is secondary to aging. The elderly are more vulnerable to delirium because of the numbers of medical problems encountered, changes in brain function, brain disorders (such as dementia), reduced hepatic metabolism of medications, and multisensory dysfunction. Elderly patients are at the highest risk for delirium, as are those with brain damage (including dementia and strokes), cardiac surgery, burns, substance withdrawal, and autoimmune diseases.[29–32] The morbidity and mortality in the elderly with delirium are high; 15% to 26% will die, often as a result of the problem responsible for the delirium.[32]

Performing a comprehensive medical evaluation (e.g., with assessment of oxygenation and infections [urinary tract infection is common in elderly]), examination of the patient (including careful neurological assessment, even if it has been done by another physician), use of medications, and review of medication compliance, are keys to uncovering the etiology of the delirium and directing appropriate management. Medications with anticholinergic effects are often responsible for cognitive dysfunction and should be avoided. Diphenhydramine, a medication commonly given to patients for sleep, can be dangerous for an elderly patient due to its strong anticholinergic properties.

Neurologic abnormalities of delirium include dysphagia, constructional apraxia, dysnomic aphasia, motor abnormalities, and an abnormal EEG. Emotional disturbances can be prominent with intense anger or fear, mania, irritability, depression, euphoria, sadness, rage, apathy, anxiety, and panic.[32] Hyperactive, hypoactive, or mixed clinical subtypes of delirium are widely accepted; the hyperactive type is the more frequently reported.[33] Motor subtypes are perplexing in that patients who are more agitated are more often diagnosed, while those with hypoactive or mixed states may be at greater risk from delirium but go undiagnosed.[34] Although there is no significant difference in terms of etiology or outcome profile between clinical subtypes, the variety of presentations of delirium confuses the diagnosis, hence the discrepancy among criteria for delirium used by neurologists and psychiatrists. Symptoms of delirium can develop over hours to days and rarely weeks. Delirium tends to have an abrupt onset of symptoms, while dementia develops more slowly. Each is a neuropsychiatric state of altered and fluctuating consciousness that develops from a generalized cerebral impairment or dysfunction related to an illness, intoxication with a substance, or withdrawal from a substance.

Numerous conditions cause delirium; implicated are medical or surgical illness and adverse effects of pharmacologic agents. Reversible causes of delirium require accurate diagnosis and treatment because of the danger of permanent brain damage (e.g., from Wernicke's encephalopathy, hypoxia, hypoglycemia, hypertensive encephalopathy, intracerebral hemorrhage, meningitis or encephalitis, and poisoning).[35]

Patients with dementia may exhibit paranoia, irrational suspiciousness, or mistrust of those caring for them, even when they are close family members. Delusions are common with dementia, and they often present as fixed, false ideas or beliefs despite evidence to the contrary. For example, a person may complain that someone has stolen something from them or poisoned their food, or that someone who is deceased has come to see them. Hallucinations are usually visual in nature, ranging from a dream-like state to terrifying but realistic visions.

Management and treatment of delirium are multifaceted. Identification and diagnosis is key since the treatment is predicated on the underlying cause.[36–40] Contributing factors should be eliminated and the environment structured to avoid clinical deterioration.[35]

Low doses of antipsychotics, either typical or atypical, are generally adequate to treat delirium in the elderly; one should increase the dose slowly, so as not to overshoot the target dose. Table 26-2 lists the types and doses of antipsychotics frequently used in the elderly. Whenever possible, family or a familiar person should stay with the patient to reorient them; this may prevent the need for medications or restraints. However in patients with significant delirium, both restraint and medication may be indicated. Restraints may be required as a reminder not to get out of bed without supervision, as falls and subsequent hip fractures may result. Hip fractures are associated with delirium and lead to a bleak prognosis for the elderly; they may never return to independent functioning after a hip fracture.[41] On the other hand, the risks associated with restraints are also greater among the elderly; if possible, other means to prevent falls should be considered. Prolonged memory impairment in patients who have been delirious can persist in 50% of patients and become permanent.[42] Nursing home patients and patients with dementia are also at greater risk of delirium due to their impaired status.

When patients are agitated and do not cooperate with care or are unable to take oral medications, then intravenous (IV) haloperidol is often used to sedate and reduce the symptoms of psychosis when delirious.[43,44] Elderly patients are initially started on lower doses (e.g., 0.5 to 2.0 mg of haloperidol IV). To adequately treat the delirium, the appropriate dose should be titrated.[42] Haloperidol IV can cause cardiac problems with QTc widening and torsades de pointes, but with the multiple medical causes for delirium, the etiology of polymorphic ventricular tachycardia is often difficult to determine.[45]

Atypical antipsychotics have been successful in the treatment of delirium and agitation in elderly and in those who are critically ill.[46,47] Again, doses must be titrated slowly to minimize adverse side effects. Patients are maintained on the optimal dose until their symptoms resolve. Symptoms of delirium in the elderly can last up to 6 to 12 months, and it may be necessary to discharge patients home on antipsychotic medications. Patients with underlying dementia are clearly at greater risk for delirium; the impact of cholinesterase inhibitors have been studied in this population.[23,48]

Psychosis

Criteria for the diagnosis of psychosis include one or more of the following: delusions, hallucinations, disorganized speech, or disorganized or catatonic behavior.

Psychosis in dementia is often manifested by one of three general categories (i.e., delusions, hallucinations, and misconceptions). Delusions often include the themes of stolen items, infidelity, imposters, disorientation, a lack of familiarity with ordinary items, and fear of being alone or abandoned. Hallucinations may relate to sensory losses and to the usual sensory domains (i.e., visual, auditory, and tactile). Frequent misconceptions include the misperceptions of objects, not recognizing oneself, and believing that television scenes are real here-and-now events. The risk of delirium and the psychotic symptoms that accompany that diagnosis increases with age. Psychosis is most commonly associated with schizophrenia and delusional disorders, but in the elderly it is more common for delirium and psychosis to be associated with dementia and to have behavioral complications that accompany these diagnoses.

Further complications from treatment of psychosis are the side effects associated with medications. In the elderly these side effects are often dramatic and may lead to iatrogenic complications. Drugs that induce anticholinergic, orthostatic, sedative, and extrapyramidal symptoms are relatively commonplace.[39] The elderly are more susceptible to tardive dyskinesia than are other populations. The older antipsychotic medications have more adverse side effects, and higher potency agents are more useful than lower potency agents. Atypical antipsychotics are most useful in the elderly because of their sedative properties and their lack of extrapyramidal side effects (EPS) when used in lower doses.[44,45] These atypical antipsychotics have more beneficial side effects, such as sedation of the agitated patient, a calming effect in anxious patients, and an ability to reduce aggression in dementia.[7,49] In certain instances, when agitation is the primary symptom without psychosis, other medications to reduce anger, such as SSRIs, or other antidepressants that may cause sedation are beneficial and have a more calming effect.[7,50] Dose equivalents of the atypical antipsychotics have been problematic, but a recent report by Woods[49] using 100 mg/day of chlorpromazine as the standard, compared the following doses: 2 mg/day for risperidone, 5 mg/day for olanzapine, 75 mg/day for quetiapine, 60 mg/day for ziprasidone, and 7.5 mg/day for aripiprazole, and outlined a more useful schedule. The caveat to begin low and titrate up slowly remains the gold standard; adding more medication is less harmful than giving a large bolus of a drug with a long half-life.

Substance Abuse and Withdrawal

Alcoholism is common, often not reported by patients, and overlooked in the elderly.[51,52] Alcohol-related problems in the elderly are a growing public health concern. A life-long pattern of drinking every day, even though only small amounts, is problematic. The National Institute on Alcohol Abuse deems one drink (12 oz beer, 1.5 oz spirits, or 5 oz wine) per day to be the maximum intake considered to be moderate alcohol use for men and women 65 years of age or older.[53,54] The prevalence of alcoholism in the elderly is about 10% to 18% and is the second most frequent reason for admission to an inpatient psychiatric facility.[54] As with those in the general population, the risk of suicide in the elderly who abuse alcohol is staggering and is second only to major depression.[55]

Older alcoholics often decline treatment due to perceived negative stigma and significant denial of the problem.[53] Screening tools have not been of significant benefit, but as in all aspects of geriatric care, use of the team approach to diagnosis and treatment is essential.[56] Alcohol withdrawal is characterized by two or more of the following symptoms: autonomic hyperactivity; tremor; insomnia; nausea or vomiting; transient visual, tactile, or auditory hallucinations or illusions; psychomotor agitation; anxiety; or tonic-clonic seizures.[51] With the loss of lean body mass due to aging, the volume of alcohol distribution is reduced, which results in an increased peak ethanol concentration after any amount of alcohol is consumed.[2]

Comorbid illnesses, both psychiatric and medical, confound accurate diagnosis of both alcoholism and medical presentations.[52] Patients seen in consultation often are admitted for infection, trauma, cardiac disease, gastrointestinal disorders, renal diseases, and pulmonary conditions. Treatment of withdrawal in the elderly is more complex and requires close monitoring. Shorter-acting benzodiazepines are the medications of choice, and one should begin with low doses and increase them slowly, so as to avoid oversedation (Table 26-3). In some older patients, larger doses and longer-acting benzodiazepines are indicated, especially with those who have a history of seizures or delirium tremens (DTs). Often in chronic alcoholics with history of DTs or seizures, the gold standard remains chlordiazepoxide because of its long-acting metabolites that provide a slow taper and reduce the risk of seizures. Most important, aggressive treatment of symptoms limits the possibility of complications due to withdrawal or the development of DTs.

Table 26-3. Benzodiazepines

Medications	Equivalent Dose (mg)	Onset of Action	Active Metabolites	Method of Metabolism
Short-acting				
Midazolam	Not PO	Fast	Yes	Hydroxylation
Triazolam	0.25	Intermediate	No	Hydroxylation
Intermediate				
Alprazolam	0.5	Intermediate	Yes	Hydroxylation
Lorazepam	1.0	Intermediate	No	Glucuronidation
Oxazepam	15.0	Slow	No	Glucuronidation
Temazepam	15.0	Slow	No	Glucuronidation
Prolonged				
Diazepam	5.0	Fast	Yes	n-Demethylation
Clonazepam	0.25	Slow	No	Hydroxylation
Clorazepate	7.5	Fast	Yes	Hydroxylation
Chlordiazepoxide	10.0	Intermediate	Yes	n-Demethylation
Flurazepam	15.0	Fast	Yes	Hydroxylation

Anxiety

Anxiety disorders have not been as widely studied in the context of depression and dementia.[57,58] Aartjan et al.[57] noted that loss of control and vulnerability to stress were the strongest risk factors for anxiety. Both of these risk factors were common to elderly hospitalized patients. In the general hospital, the treatment for anxiety involves use of benzodiazepines (see Table 26-3); however, since some older patients may have a paradoxical reaction to benzodiazepines, they should be used cautiously (observe for exacerbation of other problems, such as sleep apnea). Other agents (including selected antidepressants, such as trazodone and mirtazapine) can be used as well.

Elder Abuse

Each year thousands of elderly are abused, neglected, and exploited by family members, caregivers, and others. Many of the victims are frail and vulnerable; they are unable to help themselves and they depend on those who abuse them to assist them with their basic needs. The psychiatric consultation service often identifies these issues that may result in noncompliance with medications or with medical care. These issues may have contributed to the hospital admission and to ongoing medical or psychiatric problems.[57] All 50 states have reporting systems and toll-free hotlines to report concerns anonymously. Adult protective services (APS) agencies investigate the reports of suspected elder abuse and determine if abuse or neglect exists. Types of abuse are physical, sexual, psychological, financial, exploitative, and negligent. More than one-half million cases were reported to the APS in 1996 during a national incidence study done through the Administration on Aging. The cohort at greatest risk were those 80 years of age and older. In 90% of the cases the perpetrator was a family member; in two thirds they were either adult children or spouses.[59]

The warning signs of abuse are subtle, and the patient may not be willing to cooperate or agree to go forward with an investigation. Family or caregivers may be overwhelmed, depressed, or physically unable to continue to care for the elderly

patient; the APS can guide them to appropriate services.

Families and Caregivers

Dementia often causes tremendous suffering for patients, their families, and society. Patients are forced to become more dependent and to lose their independence in basic caring for themelves; this complicates other comorbid conditions. Family members or caregivers can develop anxiety and depression and become isolated due to the increased time spent caring for the elderly patient. While caring for a patient it is important to watch out for those caring for the patient.[60]

References

1. Francis J, Martin D, Kapoor WN: Prognosis after hospital discharge of older medical patients with delirium, *J Am Geriatr Soc* 40:601–606, 1992.
2. Cremens MC: *Polypharmacy in the elderly*. In: Ghaemi SN, *Polypharmacy in psychiatry*. New York, 2002, Marcel Dekker.
3. Callahan CM, Hendrie HC, Nienaber NA, et al: Suicidal ideation among older primary care patients, *J Am Geriatr Soc* 44:1205–1209, 1996.
4. Callahan CM, Hui SL, Nienaber NA, et al: Longitudinal study of depression and health services use among elderly primary care patients. *J Am Geriatr Soc* 42:833–838, 1994.
5. Waern M, Rubenowitz E, Runeson B, et al: Burden of illness and suicide in elderly people: case-control study. *BMJ* 324:1355, 2002.
6. Szanto K, Mulsant BH, Houck P, et al: Occurrence and course of suicidality during short-term treatment of late-life depression, *Arch Gen Psychiatry* 60:610–617, 2003.
7. Lyketsos CG, Sheppard JM, Steele CD, et al: Randomized, placebo-controlled, double-blind clinical trial of sertraline in the treatment of depression complicating Alzheimer's disease: initial results from the depression in Alzheimer's disease study. *Am J Psychiatry* 157:1686–1689, 2000.
8. Koenig HG, George LK: Depression and physical disability outcomes in depressed medically ill hospitalized older adults. *Am J Geriatr Psychiatry* 6:230–247, 1998.
9. Lebowitz BD, Pearson JL, Schneider LS, et al: Diagnosis and treatment of depression in late life: consensus statement update, *JAMA* 278:1186–1190, 1997.
10. Masand PS, Tesar GE: Use of stimulants in the medically ill, *Psychiatr Clin North Am* 19: 515–547, 1996.

11. Rasmussen KG, Rummans TA, Richardson JW: Electroconvulsive therapy in the medically ill, *Psychiatr Clin North Am* 25:177–193, 2002.

12. Shulman K, Post F: Bipolar affective disorder in old age. *Br J Psychiatry* 136:26–32, 1980.

13. Stone K: Mania in the elderly. *Br J Psychiatry* 155:220–224, 1989.

14. Snowdon J: A retrospective case-note study of bipolar disorder in old age. *Br J Psychiatry* 158:485–490, 1991.

15. Cummings JL: Cholinesterase inhibitors: a new class of psychotropic compounds, *Am J Psychiatry* 157:4–15, 2000.

16. Krauthammer C, Klerman GL: Secondary mania. *Arch Gen Psychiatry* 35:133–1339, 1978.

17. Cremens MC, Okereke OI: *Alzheimer's disease and dementia.* In: Carlson KJ, Eisentstat SA. *Primary care of women, ed 2*, St Louis, 2002, Mosby, p. 214–219.

18. American Psychiatric Association Task Force on DSM-IV: *Diagnostic and statistical manual of mental disorders, ed 4 (DSM IV-tr)*, Washington, DC, 2000, American Psychiatric Association.

19. Folstein MF, Folstein SE, McHugh PR: Mini-Mental State: a practical method for grading the cognitive state of patients for the clinician. *J Psychiatr Res* 12:189–198, 1975.

20. Petersen RC, Stevens JC, Ganguli M, et al: Practice parameter: early detection of dementia—mild cognitive impairment (an evidence-based review): report of the quality standards subcommittee of the American Academy of Neurology. *Neurology* 56:1133–1142, 2001.

21. O'Hara R, Mumenthaler MS, Davies H, et al: Cognitive status and behavioral problems in older hospitalized patients, *Ann Gen Hosp Psychiatry* 1:1–8, 2002.

22. Geldmacher DS, Whitehouse PJ: Evalution of dementia. *N Engl J Med* 335:330–336, 1996.

23. Cummings JL: Use of cholinesterase inhibitors in clinical practice: evidence-based recommendations, *Am J Geriatr Psychiatry* 11:131–145, 2003.

24. Feldman H, Gauthier S, Hecker J, et al: Efficacy of donepezil on maintenance of activities of daily living in patients with moderate to sever Alzheimer's disease and the effect of caregiver burden, *Am J Geriatr Soc* 51:737–744, 2003.

25. Farlow M, Potkin S, Koumarasa B: Analysis of outcome in retrieved dropout patients in a rivastigmine vs placebo, 26-week, Alzheimer disease trial, *Arch Neurol* 60: 843–848, 2003.

26. Erkinjuntti T, Kurz A, Gauthier S, et al: Efficacy of galantamine in probable vascular dementia and Alzheimer's disease combined with cerebrovascular disease: a randomised trial. *Lancet* 359:1283–1290, 2002.

27. Reisberg B, Doody R, Stoffler A, et al: Memantine in moderate-to-severe Alzheimer's disease, *N Engl J Med* 348:1333–1341, 2003.

28. Devanand D, Marder K, Michaels K, et al: A randomized, placebo-controlled dose-comparison trial of haloperidol for psychosis and disruptive behaviors in Alzheimer's disease. *Am J Psychiatry* 155:1512–1520, 1998.

29. Franco K, Litaker D, Locala J, et al: The cost of delirium in the surgical patient, *Psychosomatics* 42: 68–73, 2001.

30. Lindesay J, Rockwood K, MacDonald A, editors: *Delirium in old age*, Oxford, UK, 2002.

31. McNicoll L, Pisani MA, Zhang Y, et al: Delirium in the intensive care unit: occurrence and clinical course in older patients, *J Am Geriatr Soc* 51:591–598, 2003.

32. Lipowski ZJ: Delirium in the elderly patient, *N Engl J Med* 320:578–582 1989.

33. Camus V, Gonthier R, Dubos G, et al: Etiologic outcomes in hypoactive and hyperactive subtypes of delirium. *J Geriatr Psych Neurol* 13:38–42, 2000.

34. Meagher DJ, Trzepacz PT: Motoric subtypes of delirium. *Semin Clin Neuropsychiatry* 5:76–85, 2000.

35. Cassem NH, Murray GB: *Delirious patients.* In Cassem NH, Stern TA, Rosenbaum JF, Jellinek MS, editors: *Massachusetts General Hospital handbook of general hospital psychiatry, ed 4*, St. Louis, 1997, Mosby.

36. Cremens MC, Gottlieb GL: *Acute confusional state: delirium, encephalopathy.* In Sirven JI, Malamut BL, editors: *Clinical neurology of the older adult*, Philadelphia, 2002, Lippincott Williams & Wilkins, pp. 65–75.

37. Trzepacz PT: Is there a final common neural pathway in delirium? *Semin Clin Neuropsychiatry* 5:132–148, 2000.

38. Trzepacz PT: Delirium: Advances in diagnosis, pathophysiology, and treatment, *Psychiatr Clin North Am* 19: 429–448, 1996.

39. Tune LE: Serum anticholinergic activity levels and delirium in the elderly, *Semin Clin Neuropsychiatry* 5:149–53, 2000.

40. Levkoff SE, Evans DA, Liptzin B, et al: Delirium: the occurrence and persistence of symptoms among elderly hospitalized patients, *Arch Intern Med* 152:334–340 1992.

41. Marcantonio ER, Flacker JM, Michaels M, et al: Delirium is independently associated with poor functional recovery after hip fracture, *J Am Geriatr Soc* 48: 618–624, 2000.

42. Inouye SK: Delirium in hospitalized older patients: recognition and risk factors, *J Geriatr Psych Neurol* 11:118–125, 1998.

43. Tesar GE, Stern TA: Rapid tranquilization of the agitated intensive care unit patient, *J Intensive Care Med* 3:195–201,1988.

44. Stern TA: Continuous infusion of haloperidol in agitated, critically ill patients, *Crit Care Medicine* 22:378–379, 1994.

45. Hunt N, Stern TA: The association between intravenous haloperidol and torsades de pointes: three

cases and a literature review, *Psychosomatics* 36:541–549, 1995.

46. Schwartz TL, Masand PS: The role of atypical antipsychotics in the treatment of delirium, *Psychosomatics* 43:171–174, 2002.

47. Brietbart W, Tremblay A, Gibson C: An open trial of olanzapine for the treatment of delirium in hospitalized cancer patients, *Psychosomatics* 43:175–182, 2002.

48. Wengel SP, Burke WJ, Roccaforte WH: Donepezil for postoperative delirium associated with Alzheimer's disease, *J Am Geriatr Soc* 47:379–380, 1999.

49. Woods SW: Chlorpromazine equivalent doses for the newer atypical antipsychotics, *J Clin Psychiatry.* 64:663–667, 2003.

50. Fava M, Rosenbaum JF: Anger attacks in patients with depression, *J Clin Psychiatry* 60 Suppl 15:21–24, 1999.

51. American Medical Association, Council on Scientific Affairs: alcoholism in the elderly, *JAMA* 275:797–801, 1996.

52. O'Connor PG, Schottenfeld RS: Patients with alcohol problems, *N Engl J Med* 338:592–602, 1998.

53. Blow FC, Barry KL: Older patients with at risk and problem drinking patterns: new developments and brief interventions, *J Geriatr Psychiatry Neurol* 13:134–140, 2000.

54. Moss RH, Mortens MA, Brennan PL: Patterns of diagnosis and treatment among late-middle-aged and older substance abuse patients, *J Stud Alcohol* 54:479–487, 1993.

55. Waern M: Alcohol dependence and misuse in elderly suicides, *Alcohol* 38:249–254, 2003.

56. Fink A, Tsai MC, Hays RD, et al: Comparing the alcohol-related problems survey (ARPS) to traditional alcohol screening measures in elderly outpatients, *Arch Gerontol Geriatr* 34:55–78, 2002.

57. Aartjan TF, Beekman, E deB, Anton JLM, et al: Anxiety and depression in later life: co-occurrence and communality of risk factors, *Am J Psychiatry* 157:89–95, 2000.

58. Porter VR, Buxton WG, Fairbanks LA, et al: Frequency and characteristics of anxiety among patients with Alzheimer's disease and related dementias, *J Neuropsychiatry Clin Neurosci,* 15:180–186, 2003.

59. Kahan FS, Paris BE: Why elder abuse continues to elude the health care system, *Mt Sinai J Med,* 70:62–68, 2003.

60. Brodaty H, Green A, Koschera A: Meta-analysis of psychosocial interventions for caregivers of people with dementia, *J Am Geriatr Soc,* 51:657–664, 2003.

Chapter 27

Patients with Neurologic Conditions I. Seizure Disorders (Including Nonepileptic Seizures), Cerebrovascular Disease, and Traumatic Brain Injury

Jeff C. Huffman, M.D.
Felicia A. Smith, M.D.
Theodore A. Stern, M.D.

The structure and function of the central nervous system (CNS) is altered by many neurologic disorders. Because the CNS controls affect, behavior, and cognition, neurologic disorders can lead to neuropsychiatric symptoms that resemble those found in primary psychiatric conditions. Because of this, the general hospital psychiatrist is frequently called upon to assess patients with neurologic disorders. Often such patients appear to have "classic" psychiatric symptoms, but an underlying neurologic disease may impact diagnosis and treatment.

In this chapter, we will review the psychiatric management of patients with neurologic illnesses that are frequently associated with neuropsychiatric phenomena. We will discuss seizure disorders and will describe the diagnosis and management of nonepileptic seizures (also known as *pseudoseizures*). Furthermore, we will outline important considerations in the treatment of neuropsychiatric symptoms in patients with cerebrovascular disease and traumatic brain injury. Chapter 28 will discuss the management of neuropsychiatric conditions associated with movement disorders, demyelinating disease, and CNS neoplasm or infection.

The Management of Psychiatric Symptoms in Patients with Seizure Disorders

Approximately half of all patients with seizure disorders have comorbid psychiatric syndromes[1]; therefore, the general hospital psychiatrist should have a working knowledge of seizure disorders and the neuropsychiatric syndromes that are commonly associated with these disorders. Patients with seizures may have psychiatric symptoms that occur during a seizure (*ictal* symptoms), immediately before or after a seizure (*perictal* symptoms), or between seizures (*interictal* symptoms).

It may be useful to begin with some definitions. A *seizure*, as defined by Schwartz and Marsh,[2] is an abnormal paroxysmal discharge of cerebral neurons sufficient to cause clinically detectable events that are apparent to the patient or to an observer. Seizures can be *partial* (focal) or *generalized*; partial seizures are localized in one area of the brain, while generalized seizures result in abnormal electrical activity throughout the cortex. Patients with a chronic course of repeated, unprovoked seizures are said to have *epilepsy*.

Generalized seizures are also subclassified into a number of subtypes.[3,4] *Tonic-clonic* (grand mal) seizures are the most common form of generalized seizure. These seizures are characterized by a sudden loss of consciousness, followed by a brief tonic phase with contraction of skeletal muscles and an upward deviation of the eyes. A more prolonged clonic phase follows; this stage is characterized by rhythmic, symmetric jerking of the extremities. *Absence* (petit mal) seizures are characterized by brief (usually 5 to 10 seconds) lapses in consciousness and by motionless staring; these occur primarily in children and are rare after puberty. *Myoclonic* seizures are characterized by brief and sudden muscle jerks that may occur unilaterally or bilaterally; these are more commonly seen in children but they may also occur in adults. Finally, *atonic* seizures ("drop attacks") are characterized by sudden loss of muscle tone in the neck, upper extremities, or lower extremities.

Partial seizures may be classified as *simple partial seizures* when consciousness is unaffected or as *complex partial seizures* when consciousness is altered. Partial seizures may secondarily progress to become generalized seizures. An aura prior to a generalized seizure (e.g., an unusual sensation prior to the onset of a convulsive seizure) is essentially a partial seizure that secondarily generalizes. Complex partial seizures (CPS) deserve special mention. Complex partial seizures are the most common type of seizure in adults[4] and are commonly associated with neuropsychiatric phenomena (especially when the seizures have a temporal lobe focus; in this case the syndrome is often called temporal lobe epilepsy [TLE]).

CPS may involve unusual sensations and abnormalities of affect, behavior, and cognition. CPS may include hallucinations of any sensory modality; they can be olfactory (usually an unpleasant smell), gustatory (metallic or other tastes), auditory, visual, or tactile in nature. The most common affective symptoms are fear or anxiety, although depression may also occur. Such affective symptoms usually have a sudden onset and offset.

Behavior during CPS may also be abnormal; automatisms are common and may include oral or buccal movements (such as lip smacking or chewing), picking behaviors, or prolonged staring. Cognitive symptoms associated with CPS include déjà vu, jamais vu, macropsia, micropsia, and dissociative or "out of body" experiences. Patients with neuropsychiatric symptoms secondary to CPS often appear to have a primary psychiatric disorder. This is because CPS cause symptoms that overlap with primary psychiatric disorders, because CPS are generally not associated with "classic" tonic-clonic seizure activity, and because the interictal (and even ictal) scalp electroencephalogram (EEG) may appear normal in CPS. Therefore, the general hospital psychiatrist is frequently called upon to evaluate patients with CPS for affective symptoms, psychosis, or pseudoseizures.

In the following discussion, we outline the phenomenology and treatment of neuropsychiatric symptoms among patients with seizure disorders. We discuss ictal, peri-ictal, and interictal neuropsychiatric symptoms and delineate how these symptoms differ from those seen in patients without seizure disorders. In addition, we discuss practical approaches to treatment.

Ictal Neuropsychiatric Phenomena

Ictal psychiatric symptoms are generally associated with partial seizures, although they can also occur with generalized seizures.[1] Anxiety, fear, and psychosis are the most common psychiatric symptoms experienced during a seizure. Anxiety or fear is a component of the aura in one third of patients with partial seizures[5]; the anxiety is intense, and it may last throughout the course of the seizure. It may be most common in patients with right temporal foci.[6]

Such symptoms may resemble those of panic attacks, with autonomic symptoms, nausea, and depersonalization, and be accompanied by anxiety. The clinical situation may be further confused by the fact that patients with epilepsy have high rates (approximately 20%) of comorbid panic attacks[7]; therefore, patients with epilepsy may have both ictal anxiety and interictal panic attacks that can be difficult to distinguish. When the symptoms occur in concert with automatisms or hallucinations during an episode, or with confusion or severe lethargy after the event, this suggests that the anxiety is ictal in nature.

Ictal psychosis is also common in patients with partial seizures. Ictal psychotic symptoms are most often associated with temporal lobe foci, but nearly one third of patients with ictal psychosis have nontemporal lobe foci.[8] Hallucinations during a seizure are much more likely to be olfactory or gustatory in nature; auditory hallucinations (common in primary psychotic disorders) are less common. Paranoia is uncommon and is usually short-lived. In contrast to patients with primary psychosis, consciousness is usually impaired during ictal psychosis, and affected patients are usually amnestic for the episode.[9]

Ictal depression is uncommon, occurring as part of the aura in approximately 1% of epilepsy patients.[10] Such depressive symptoms, as with other ictal symptoms, appear abruptly and without obvious psychosocial precipitants. While depressive symptoms often disappear abruptly, some authors have noted that ictal depressed mood may extend beyond other ictal or postictal symptoms.[10,11]

Ictal aggression has been reported, but it appears to be exceedingly rare (less than 0.5% of patients in one large series[12]). Furthermore, such aggressive symptoms are poorly directed and do not involve significant interactive behavior; stereotyped shouting and pushing are among the most common aggressive symptoms. Patients rarely perform intricate, directed acts of violence during a seizure.

Distinguishing whether anxiety, depression, or other psychiatric symptoms are ictal events or part of a primary psychiatric condition may be difficult. Table 27-1 describes some distinguishing characteristics between ictal and nonictal symptoms. In general, ictal symptoms are more often abrupt in their onset and offset, occur in concert with other stereotyped manifestations of seizures (e.g., automatisms and jerking), and are frequently short-lived, usually lasting less than 3 minutes.[1] Furthermore, ictal symptoms are usually stereotyped; that is, a patient will not experience fear with one seizure and depressive symptoms with another—the pattern of symptoms will generally be the same.

In most cases, these factors should help the clinician to distinguish ictal psychiatric symptoms from primary psychiatric phenomena. However, complicating factors may be present, and partial status epilepticus may result in prolonged ictal psychiatric symptoms. Therefore, the EEG remains the gold standard for determining whether symptoms are ictal.

Treatment of ictal psychiatric symptoms relies upon a careful evaluation. Because primary

Table 27-1. Differences Between Ictal and Nonictal Neuropsychiatric Symptoms

Appearance of Symptoms	Length of Symptoms	Associated Symptoms	Psychotic Symptoms	Consciousness During Event	Recall for Event	EEG During Episodes	EEG Between Episodes	Postevent Prolactin Level
Ictal Symptoms								
Sudden onset and offset	Usually <3 minutes	Stereotyped ictal symptoms: rhythmic blinking, abnormal movements, unusual sensations, automatisms	Usually olfactory, gustatory, or tactile hallucinations	May be altered	Frequently none or limited	Almost always abnormal	Frequently normal	Often elevated
Nonictal Symptoms								
More often gradual in nature	Usually 20–30 minutes (panic attack); usually days-weeks (depression, psychosis)	Absence of blinking, jerking, automatisms	Usually auditory hallucinations; paranoia common	Generally intact	Usually intact	Usually normal	Normal	Normal

psychiatric symptoms and ictal psychiatric symptoms are similar, and because they may be comorbid, careful clinical evaluation, EEG monitoring, and, when indicated, other diagnostic procedures (e.g., determination of prolactin levels) should be performed to distinguish these phenomena because the treatment differs considerably. Once symptoms have been identified as ictal, treatment of the associated psychiatric symptoms requires treatment of the seizure with anticonvulsants. Treatment of ictal psychosis with antipsychotics or ictal anxiety with nonanticonvulsant anxiolytics is generally not indicated. Nonpharmacologic strategies, including close observation and measures to reduce the risk of falls or other injury, are crucial for patients whose seizure disorders remain active.

Peri-ictal Neuropsychiatric Phenomena

The majority of peri-ictal neuropsychiatric disturbances are postictal; they usually occur several hours after a seizure. Preictal symptoms can occur and include psychosis, mood changes, or aggression in the days, hours, or minutes prior to a seizure. These symptoms tend to increase until the onset of ictus[13] and, depending on the time course and nature of the symptoms, may be conceptualized as prodromes separate from the ictus or as ictal events (i.e., as a partial seizure).

Postictal symptoms are relatively common. Approximately 8% to 10% of patients with seizures have postictal psychiatric disturbances.[14] These psychiatric symptoms may occur in the context of a postictal delirium or in the setting of clear consciousness. In general, postictal symptoms remit spontaneously and are often short-lived; in one study, symptoms lasted approximately 72 hours.[15] However, such symptoms may persist for days or even weeks, and patients with well-defined, prolonged postictal neuropsychiatric syndromes may be more likely to develop persistent interictal symptoms.

Postictal psychosis is the most common postictal neuropsychiatric symptom, generally appearing after a nonpsychotic postictal period of hours to days. It most commonly presents in patients with CPS that become secondarily generalized,[9] especially in those with temporal lobe or bilateral foci. Psychotic symptoms vary widely, and affective symptoms (depressive or manic) may also be present. Symptoms can include paranoid or grandiose delusions and hallucinations in a variety of sensory modalities; Schneiderian first-rank symptoms of schizophrenia are rare.[15] Symptoms tend to resolve spontaneously, but recur on average two to three times per year.[16] In a minority of patients, such symptoms become chronic.

Postictal depression is also associated with CPS, but is less common than is postictal psychosis.[17] Patients with postictal depression may have flattened affect and anhedonia more often than sadness, and postictal depression is commonly associated with delirium and other postictal cognitive disturbances.[18] Kanner et al.[17] found that symptoms last an average of 24 hours, although symptoms may be more prolonged.[11] In most cases, postictal depressive symptoms do not just represent a reactive response to the stress of having a seizure.

Other postictal symptoms are less common. Acute postictal anxiety is relatively infrequent and is usually associated with postictal depression.[17] Postictal mania and hypomania occur infrequently. Postictal aggression can also occur; it is generally associated with delirium, psychotic symptoms, or abnormal mood states.

The management of patients with postictal neuropsychiatric symptoms has a number of tenets. First, enhanced treatment of the seizure disorder is crucial; patients whose seizure disorders are poorly controlled appear to have a greater tendency toward postictal affective and psychotic symptoms. In addition to anticonvulsants for seizure prophylaxis, other psychotropic medication may be indicated, especially if symptoms are prolonged, present a risk to the patient or to others, or adversely effect the patient's ability to receive appropriate treatment. Such situations occur most commonly with psychosis; low doses of antipsychotics can reduce agitation and diminish psychotic symptoms. If such symptoms are limited to the postictal period, these medications can be discontinued once symptoms resolve, as the best prophylaxis against recurrence of psychosis is treatment with anticonvulsants to avoid seizures. Antidepressants are uncommonly indicated for depressive symptoms limited to the postictal period.

In addition to medications, behavioral treatments can be instituted to facilitate coping and to maintain the patient's safety. Such interventions could include the use of restraints or sitters, frequent reorientation, or the presence of familiar family members. Finally, it is important to know the patient's postictal pattern of symptoms to prepare caregivers and family members for what lies ahead. Seizures and their neuropsychiatric sequelae are commonly stereotyped; that is, patients tend to have the same postictal symptomatology from seizure to seizure. If a patient is known to become psychotic or dangerous after a seizure, the treatment team can be prepared with antipsychotic treatments or other safety-enhancing measures.

Interictal (Chronic) Neuropsychiatric Phenomena

Psychiatric syndromes are also common in the period between seizures; patients with seizure disorders have chronic psychiatric disorders at substantially higher rates than do those in the general population. Depression, anxiety, and psychosis are all common, with depressive disorders being the most prevalent. In contrast, interictal hypomanic or manic symptoms are uncommon.

Interictal depression is common and can be disabling. Rates of depression and suicide among patients with epilepsy are four to five times greater than those in the general population,[1,19,20] and up to 80% of patients with epilepsy report having some feelings of depression.[21,22] A constellation of biological and psychosocial factors likely coalesce to result in these elevated rates of depression, but risk factors for depression that are specific to seizure disorders include poor seizure control and CPS,[23,24] especially with left-sided temporal lobe seizure foci. In fact, suicide may be 25 times more likely among patients with TLE than among those in the general population.[25]

Furthermore, this relationship between depression and seizures may be bidirectional. History of depression has been associated with the onset of seizures, as a history of depression increases (by threefold) the risk of developing a seizure disorder.[18,26] Some have hypothesized that depression and epilepsy share neurotransmitter abnormalities (e.g., reduced noradrenergic, dopaminergic, and serotonergic activity), and that these shared abnormalities may explain the link between the two conditions.

The symptoms of interictal depression are often distinctive. Atypical features are common,[21] and many patients have depressive symptoms that are more consistent with dysthymia than with major depression. Furthermore, these dysthymic symptoms are often interrupted by symptom-free periods that can last for hours or days.[27] Blumer et al.[28] have described a clinical syndrome called *interictal dysphoric disorder*; this syndrome is characterized by interictal dysthymic symptoms with intermittent irritability, impulsivity, anxiety, and somatic symptoms.

Interictal anxiety disorders vary in frequency. Anxiety symptoms are more common in patients with epilepsy than those in the general population, and, of the anxiety disorders, panic disorder appears to be the most common. Interictal panic disorder is present in approximately 20% of patients with epilepsy,[7] with symptoms that differentiate the panic attacks from the feelings of panic that occur during a seizure. Other anxiety disorders, such as generalized anxiety disorder (GAD) or obsessive-compulsive disorder (OCD), are less common.[1]

Interictal psychosis can be intermittent (with brief, recurrent episodes), but more commonly it is continuous and chronic. Psychotic symptoms are approximately 10 times more likely to occur in patients with epilepsy.[29] Psychosis is more common in patients with CPS (especially those with TLE), and in those with multiple seizure types, a poor response to treatment, or a history of status epilepticus.[30] Clinically, interictal psychotic symptoms most often consist of paranoid delusions with associated visual or auditory hallucinations. Affective blunting, a lack of motivation, and catatonia are also common.[30] Compared to patients with primary schizophrenia, patients with interictal psychosis have a greater preservation of affect and more visual hallucinations.

Finally, some evidence supports an interictal personality change among patients with TLE. The TLE personality syndrome, described primarily by Gastaut et al.[29] and by Geshwind,[31] has features that include moral rigidity, hyperreligiosity, hypergraphia, hyposexuality, and hyperviscosity. However, this concept remains controversial, with other authors[32] refuting the existence of such a syndrome.

The management of interictal psychiatric phenomena is similar to the treatment of primary psychiatric disorders. However, there are a number of special considerations in this population. Given that most interictal psychiatric symptoms are more common when seizures are poorly controlled, effective treatment with anticonvulsants is of vital importance. Treatment of psychiatric symptoms associated with epilepsy should also include behavioral and educational interventions that reduce the risk related to their seizure disorder (e.g., having family ensure that depressed patients take their anticonvulsants or keeping manic or psychotic patients from driving when this is unsafe).

Treatment of psychiatric symptoms with psychotropics is frequently indicated, but the effects of these agents on the seizure threshold should be considered. Treatment of epileptic patients with antidepressants has been controversial, given the propensity of some antidepressants to increase the risk of seizure. However, the risk of seizure with most antidepressant agents is quite small when these agents are used at standard doses.[33] Citalopram,[34] sertraline,[33,34] venlafaxine,[18] and tricyclic antidepressants (TCAs)[28] have all been used successfully in patients with epilepsy without significantly exacerbating the underlying seizure disorder.

Given their relative safety with regard to seizure exacerbation and their overall safety and tolerability, selective serotonin-reuptake inhibitors (SSRIs) should be considered first-line treatment for patients with interictal depression. In general, starting with a low dose and increasing the dosage gradually should minimize the risk of seizure in these patients. In general, bupropion and maprotiline should be avoided, as these agents are more strongly associated with the development of seizures. Among the TCAs, clomipramine may be associated with a greater risk of seizure and should probably be avoided as well.[35] Monoamine oxidase inhibitors (MAOIs) have not been associated with an elevated risk of seizure, though they have not been studied in patients with seizure disorders. Finally, electroconvulsive therapy (ECT) can be used in patients with epilepsy and severe depression[36]; ECT appears to increase the seizure threshold,[37] and it has been used safely in patients with epilepsy.[38]

Patients with anxiety disorders can be treated with antidepressants or with benzodiazepines; buspirone, sometimes used for the treatment of GAD, can lower seizure threshold and should generally be avoided in this population.[39] Interictal psychosis can be treated with antipsychotics. It appears that all antipsychotics may modestly lower the seizure threshold; however, low-potency antipsychotics, such as chlorpromazine, may have greater effects on the seizure threshold than higher-potency agents.[40,41] Furthermore, clozapine has been associated with an elevated seizure risk and, in general, should be avoided. Therefore, atypical antipsychotics, such as risperidone, or high-potency typical antipsychotics should be used when needed. Again, titrating the dosage slowly and using the lowest effective dose should minimize the risk of seizure in this population.

In sum, virtually any psychiatric symptom can occur with any type of seizure at any time before, during, or after the seizure. However, anxiety is most common during a seizure, psychosis is most common postictally, and depression is the most common chronic symptom between seizures. Virtually all symptoms are more common in patients with CPS than with other types of seizure disorders. Treatment of ictal phenomena involves treatment of the seizure, while postictal and interictal phenomena may require the use of antipsychotics, anxiolytics, or antidepressants for optimal symptomatic relief. Careful attention to the patient's safety is always an important consideration (whether from seizure or suicidality), and a knowledge of the patient's pattern of symptoms associated with their seizures helps caregivers and family members prepare for sequelae.

Nonepileptic Seizures

Patients who appear to be having epileptic seizures may, in fact, be having abnormal movements as the result of another medical or neurologic problem, or, most often, as a consequence of psychological factors (e.g., a conversion reaction). These events, called nonepileptic seizures (NES) pose a common and important problem. Patients with NES have convulsive events more frequently and are more significantly disabled by their events than are those with true seizure disorders.[42] Even after a diagnosis of NES has been made, affected patients continue to be disabled by recurrent convulsive events.[43]

The general hospital psychiatrist is frequently called upon to assess patients suspected of having NES. Knowledge of the epidemiology, differential diagnosis, clinical features, and relevant diagnostic studies that may suggest the presence of NES can significantly aid diagnosis during these assessments.

Once the diagnosis of NES is suspected, it is just as important for the general hospital psychiatrist to be able to discuss the diagnosis of NES with the patient in a way that is validating, reassuring, and supportive.

NES are common. They are seen in approximately 10% of outpatients with intractable seizure disorders; this rate climbs to approximately 20% in patients with intractable seizures who are referred to epilepsy monitoring units.[44,45] About three quarters of individuals with NES are women, and they most often present between the ages of 15 and 35.[43] Sexual abuse is common among patients with NES; it occurs in at least 25% of those with the condition.[46,47] Further complicating the picture is the fact that patients with NES often have true seizure disorders as well, with roughly 25% of patients with NES also having true seizures.[48]

NES are associated with general medical conditions, deceptive acts, and unconscious productions of symptoms that appear to be epileptic seizures. Table 27-2 displays a number of conditions that can be mistaken for epilepsy. Of these conditions, unconscious, psychologically mediated convulsive activity (essentially, conversion seizures) are the most common[44] and we will focus on this etiology of NES. Other causes of functional somatic symptoms, such as factitious disorder and malingering, are more extensively covered in Chapter 19.

Clinical Considerations

In this section, we discuss methods for making a clinical diagnosis of NES. For the purposes of this discussion, we assume that medical and neurologic causes of NES have been ruled out, and that the etiology of the NES is psychogenic (i.e., conversion disorder).

With regard to making a clinical diagnosis of psychogenic NES, certain clinical features of the convulsive event are suggestive of NES. However, it should be noted that all of the features that suggest NES (discussed later) can also occur in true seizure disorders, and, therefore, a single clinical feature taken in isolation should not be used to confirm a diagnosis of NES. However, careful observation during the convulsive event (and during the preictal and postictal periods) can be very useful in the diagnostic assessment. Most NES simulate generalized tonic-clinic (GTC) seizures. The more features that deviate from the usual characteristics of a GTC seizure, the more likely that the event is, in fact, an NES. Therefore, it is useful to know the usual characteristics of GTC seizures.

GTC seizures usually are sudden in onset; though there may be an aura prior to the seizure, there is usually a sudden loss of consciousness, followed by a brief tonic period of less than 30 seconds. A more prolonged period of convulsive, clonic activity follows. This activity is characterized by bilateral, symmetric, and rhythmic jerking of the upper and lower extremities; trunk activity and pelvic thrusting are uncommon. Loss of continence, tongue-biting, and other injuries may occur. The patient remains unconscious and unresponsive throughout the event and is amnestic for the episode. After the event, the patient may be confused, drowsy, or complain of headache; the patient is rarely completely lucid in the immediate postictal period. Most GTC seizures are quite brief, lasting less than 3 minutes, and have a stereotyped pattern in a given individual.

Table 27-3 lists the clinical features that suggest NES. The gradual onset of seizure, responsiveness during the seizure, pelvic thrusting, asymmetric clonic activity, and lucidity immediately after the event are indicative that the event may not be

Table 27-2. Differential Diagnosis of Nonepileptic Events

General Medical Conditions
Transient ischemic attack (TIA)
Complicated migraine
Syncope
Hypoglycemia
Parasomnia (e.g., REM behavior disorder or night terrors)
Narcolepsy
Myoclonus (from metabolic disturbance)

Psychiatric Causes
Conversion disorder
Somatization disorder
Dissociative disorder
Panic disorder (simulating partial seizures)

Volitional Deception
Factitious disorder (goal is to maintain the sick role)
Malingering (goal is to obtain secondary gain, e.g., disability income)

Table 27-3. Features that Suggest Nonepileptic (Conversion) Seizures

Historical Features

History of sexual abuse

History of other unexplained neurologic symptoms occurring during stress

Seizures despite multiple adequate trials of anticonvulsants at therapeutic levels

Features of Event

Events occur with suggestion/provocation

Gradual onset and offset of symptoms

Responsiveness during event

Weeping, speaking, or yelling during event

Asymmetric clonic activity

Head bobbing or pelvic thrusting

Rapid kicking or thrashing

Prolonged duration of symptoms (>3 minutes)

No EEG abnormalities during event

Postevent Features

Lucid during immediate postictal period

Able to recall event

Lack of incontinence, tongue biting, or physical injury despite numerous events

Postictal prolactin is normal

Neuropsychological testing suggestive of conversion symptoms

---

epileptic in nature. It should be emphasized again that certain types of seizure are manifest by symptoms that appear to suggest NES. Simple partial seizures may have asymmetric jerking with preserved consciousness. CPS can manifest with only behavioral or psychiatric symptoms. Frontal lobe seizures may cause pelvic thrusting. Automatisms during partial seizures may result in acts that appear volitional. However, combinations of atypical features suggest that NES are the more likely diagnosis.

A number of diagnostic procedures can be performed to aid in the diagnosis of NES. The two most useful of these may be video-EEG monitoring and so-called *provocative testing*. The use of video-EEG monitoring allows one to correlate EEG changes (or the lack thereof) during a convulsive event. If a patient has one of his or her typical events and the EEG remains normal, this strongly suggests NES, especially when there are other clinical features that are inconsistent with epilepsy. However, it should be noted that both complex and simple partial seizures may result in normal EEGs in 10% to 40% of cases.[44,49] The EEG capture of multiple events

reduces the likelihood of such false-negative EEG findings.

In addition to using video-EEG monitoring, suggestion or provocative stimuli may be used to provoke a seizure-like event during EEG monitoring. Provocative stimuli have included injection of normal saline or placement of a tuning fork on the head after a suggestion has been given that the procedure will likely cause a seizure. It is crucial that EEG monitoring be done during these procedures, as true epileptic seizures can also be more frequent during periods of stress, and because patients may have both epileptic and nonepileptic events. There has been much discussion about the ethics of deception under these circumstances; researchers have found that such provocative testing can be frequently approached honestly with the patient with high rates of suggestibility and little adverse effect on the patient-physician alliance.[50,51]

In addition, a number of other ancillary studies can be used when considering a diagnosis of NES. The measurement of prolactin levels has been used to aid NES diagnosis, as prolactin levels typically rise during seizures, possibly due to disruption of hypothalamic inhibition of prolactin release during a seizure. This rise is maximal within the first 30 minutes after a seizure. However, in more than 10% of patients with GTC seizures, in 30% of patients with temporal lobe seizures, and in 60% of patients with frontal lobe seizures, prolactin is not elevated.[52] Cragar et al.,[52] in their review of the literature, found that a rise in prolactin is suggestive of epilepsy, but that a failure of prolactin to rise is less predictive of NES. Other diagnostic laboratory values, such as creatine phosphokinase (CPK), may be even less sensitive and specific, especially when taken in isolation.

Neuropsychological testing can be a useful adjunct to a clinical and laboratory evaluation. Such testing can provide information about comorbid psychiatric diagnoses, personality styles, and tendency toward conversion reactions. However, such testing cannot definitively make or exclude a diagnosis of NES, and there is significant overlap of results between those patients with NES and in those with epilepsy.[53]

In short, making a definitive diagnosis of NES can be difficult. There are characteristic features of epidemiology, clinical events, laboratory values, and EEG monitoring that may suggest NES, but for each individual thought to have NES, there are others in whom true epilepsy can result in a "diagnosis" of NES. However, a thorough evaluation using each of these domains—with EEG-video monitoring being perhaps the best diagnostic test— can help the psychiatrist determine whether NES is more or less likely.

It is important to allow for the possibility that one's diagnosis of NES may be incorrect. Patients with NES typically have symptoms that are quite convincing for epileptic seizures; conversely, patients diagnosed with conversion symptoms are found to have an organic syndrome related to the "conversion" symptom roughly 20% of the time.[54] This should not prevent the clinician from moving forward based on his or her clinical findings, but should simply serve as a reminder to maintain an open mind about the diagnosis.

General medical providers often feel that once the diagnosis of NES has been made, treatment is over. However, fortunately *and* unfortunately, treatment is truly just beginning. After the diagnosis is made, patients with NES continue to have frequent and disabling NES events; only about 30% will stop having convulsive events.[43,55] However, early diagnosis is associated with better outcome,[55] and, therefore, presenting the diagnosis and a treatment plan in a way that is acceptable to the patient is critical.

Table 27-4 lists the important features of NES diagnosis and the treatment plan for patients with the disorder. In general, the tenets of revealing the diagnosis are similar to those outlined for conversion disorder by Barsky et al. in Chapter 19. First of all, the diagnosis should be framed in a positive way: it is tremendously reassuring that these events are not due to abnormal electrical discharges in the brain, and that there is no need to take anticonvulsant medications and deal with their side effects.

If a patient feels as if he or she is being told that there is nothing wrong, it can be useful to emphasize that, while there is not a *structural* or *electrical* abnormality present, it is clear that there is an abnormality of *function* of their nervous system that will require integrated treatment. Furthermore, the physician should make it clear that he or she understands that these events are

Table 27-4. Guidelines for Presenting a Diagnosis of NES and Developing a Treatment Plan

Presentation of the Diagnosis

1. Frame diagnosis in a positive way: symptoms are not due to abnormal electrical activity, and risks of anticonvulsants need not be undertaken.
2. Explain that symptoms are likely due to a problem with the *function* of the nervous system, rather than electrical or structural abnormalities.
3. Explain that these symptoms are common and are likely to improve gradually over time. Give specific suggestions regarding how they will improve (e.g., episodes become less prolonged, then become less frequent, then have fewer symptoms during each episode, and so forth).
4. Acknowledge the disability that such symptoms have caused and the importance of developing a treatment plan that will improve the function of the nervous system and reduce disability.
5. Introduce the idea that anxiety, stress, and mood significantly affect the frequency and severity of these events, and that reduction of these symptoms is crucial in the patient's treatment.
6. Describe a treatment plan that includes integrated, consistent treatment from psychiatry, neurology, and a primary care physician.

Treatment Plan

1. The treatment plan should include as much psychiatric care as the patient will allow. Weekly psychotherapy to assess unconscious motivation, to allow psychoeducation, and to provide support is ideal.
2. Psychotropic medications should be used to treat comorbid psychiatric symptoms (e.g., major depression).
3. Regular follow-up from other caregivers is a key component of the treatment plan. Appointments should be scheduled at regular intervals, whether or not the patient is symptomatic, and patients should receive positive reinforcement (and not a decrease in frequency of follow-up) when symptoms subside.
4. Physical examinations should be done regularly, but diagnostic studies should be avoided unless clearly indicated.
5. Despite the diagnosis of NES, all caregivers should remain vigilant for the possibility that an organic diagnosis has been missed, or that NES and epilepsy are both present.

having a significant impact on the patient's life and obviously require ongoing efforts to reduce their negative impact.

Next, the impact of mood, anxiety, and stress on these symptoms should be described, and the physician should tell the patient that reduction of these symptoms is absolutely imperative to help the patient improve his or her function and quality of life. However, rather than simply making a referral to a psychiatrist, the physician should also emphasize that the patient will continue to see his or her neurologist or primary care physician on a regular basis as a crucial part of the treatment. The regularity of this follow-up is important—the patient should have an appointment with the caregiver whether or not he or she is having active symptoms, thus disconnecting the link between symptoms and medical attention.

Finally, suggesting to the patient that his or her symptoms are likely to gradually improve over time can be helpful. As with the management of patients with pain, the goal of treatment should be to optimize function and quality of life rather than to focus on the total absence of symptoms.

Cerebrovascular Disease

Given that cerebrovascular accidents (CVAs) result in brain areas with reduced or absent function, it is not surprising that abnormalities of affect, behavior, and cognition are common after a CVA. This section discusses the prevalence, diagnosis, and management of patients with psychiatric symptoms after CVAs.

Approximately 3 million stroke survivors are alive at any given time[56]; more than half of them suffer from significant poststroke neuropsychiatric sequelae.[57] Such neuropsychiatric sequelae of strokes have been recognized for decades. More than 50 years ago, both Kraeplin[58] and Bleuler[59] noted an association between cerebrovascular disease and depressive illness, and Ironside,[60] in 1956, was the first to describe pathologic crying and laughing associated with cerebral infarction; this has become a well-described poststroke syndrome, termed pseudobulbar affect. Despite the high incidence of these disorders and their frequent description in the literature, acute emotional and behavioral sequelae of stroke go largely unrecognized and untreated.[61]

Neuropsychiatric syndromes caused by stroke can be conceptualized based on lesion location. While our understanding of brain circuitry has become much more sophisticated than prior models

that postulated that certain cortical lobes performed specific cognitive functions, it remains true that lesions in specific cortical areas are more likely to cause characteristic cognitive and neuropsychiatric deficits. For example, strokes in the left frontal lobe are more likely to result in a nonfluent aphasia, while strokes affecting the right parietal lobe most frequently cause anosognosia, an unawareness of illness or of neurologic deficits. Table 27-5 provides a list of some correlations between neuropsychiatric deficits and lesion locations.

Table 27-5. Correlations Between Cortical Lesion Location and Neuropsychiatric Symptoms

Cortical Area	Potential Neuropsychiatric Symptoms
Frontal Lobes	
Orbitofrontal region	Disinhibition, personality change, irritability
Dorsolateral region	Executive dysfunction: poor planning, organizing, and sequencing
Medial region	Apathy, abulia
Left frontal lobe	Nonfluent (Broca's) aphasia, poststroke depression (possibly)
Right frontal lobe	Motor dysprosody
Temporal Lobes	
Either side	Hallucinations (olfactory, gustatory, tactile, visual, or auditory), episodic fear, or mood changes
Left temporal lobe	Short-term memory impairment (verbal, written stimuli), fluent (Wernicke's) aphasia (left temporoparietal region)
Right temporal lobe	Short-term memory impairment (nonverbal stimuli; e.g., music), sensory dysprosody (right temporoparietal region)
Left parietal lobe	Gerstmann's syndrome (finger agnosia, right/left disorientation, acalculia, agraphia)
Right parietal lobe	Anosognosia, constructional apraxia, prosopagnosia, hemineglect
Occipital lobes	Anton's syndrome (cortical blindness with unawareness of visual disturbance)

Neuropsychiatric syndromes caused by strokes can also be discussed with regard to symptomatology. The following section discusses poststroke depression, mania, psychosis, anxiety, and other common neuropsychiatric sequelae of stroke.

Poststroke depression

Poststroke depression (PSD) is the prototypical acute psychiatric manifestation of stroke. It is common; approximately 20% of patients meet criteria for major depression in the poststroke period, and another 20% meet criteria for minor depression.[62–64] Untreated, episodes of poststroke major depression last approximately 9 months, with a minority of patients remaining depressed for several years.[65,66] Risk factors for PSD include a history of depression, prestroke functional impairment, living alone, poststroke social isolation, and possibly female gender.[67]

There has been controversy regarding the correlation between location of stroke and the likelihood of developing PSD. Early study of the topic found that PSD seemed to be more prevalent when the stroke occurred in the left cerebral cortex.[68,69] Further study found higher rates of PSD in two specific regions of the left hemisphere—the left frontal lobe and the basal ganglia.[63,70,71] Furthermore, such studies found increasing rates of depression with increased proximity of the lesion to the left frontal pole. In contrast, a number of other studies have found no such correlation between lesion location and PSD; most striking among these was a recent meta-analysis of 143 studies by Carson et al.[72] that found no correlation between lesion location and the risk of PSD.

PSD has significant long-term negative effects on social functioning, motor abilities, and quality of life.[73–75] The negative effect of depression on functional impairment continues well beyond the period of mood symptoms.[76] Such extended functional disability may be due to poor initial rehabilitation efforts by patients with PSD, limiting the recovery of strength and mobility.

Diagnosis of PSD is straightforward in many cases, though certain situations can make diagnosis quite challenging. A number of nondepressive neurologic stroke sequelae can appear similar to symptoms of depression. Patients with expres-

sive aprosodias have monotonous speech that may make them appear sad or withdrawn, and their affect may appear blunted. The presence of anosognosia (neurologically mediated unawareness of illness usually associated with right parietal lesions) may look like denial associated with depression, and this symptom can itself lead to frustration and to anger when others insist that the patient has a problem that he or she simply cannot recognize. Finally, aphasias can make the diagnosis of depression—or any diagnosis—more difficult because of the difficulty communicating with such patients. By being aware of these potential neurologic sequelae, and by carefully using DSM-IV[77] criteria to determine the presence of depressed mood, anhedonia, and neurovegetative symptoms, in most cases the psychiatrist can accurately determine the presence or absence of PSD.

Despite the significant consequences of PSD, it is often undertreated, both because of underdiagnosis[61] and the fear of intolerable side effects from antidepressant medications. However, early and effective treatment of depression is perhaps even more crucial in this patient population than it is in other populations, given the need for full mobilization for occupational and physical therapy and other functional retraining early in the course of recovery.

A number of placebo-controlled trials have demonstrated that antidepressants are effective in the treatment of PSD. SSRIs[78,79] and nortriptyline[80] have been shown to relieve symptoms of PSD; another study of nortriptyline found that treatment of depression resulted in improved cognitive outcome.[81] A recent study by Robinson et al.[82] found that nortriptyline was more effective than either fluoxetine or placebo in treating PSD and improving functional outcomes.

Studies of PSD have found disruptions of both noradrenergic and serotonergic pathways[78]; therefore, newer antidepressants with effects on both norepinephrine and serotonin, such as mirtazapine and venlafaxine, may also be effective in the treatment of PSD. However, there have been no clinical trials using these medications to treat PSD. Psychostimulants have also been used in the treatment of PSD. Retrospective studies using psychostimulants (methylphenidate and dextroamphetamine) to treat PSD found these medications to be effective, with response rates of 47% to 80%.[83,84] Response to psychostimulants was rapid (usually within 48 hours), and adverse events were rare. However, unlike SSRIs and TCAs, psychostimulants have not been studied under placebo-controlled, double-blind conditions for the treatment of PSD.

ECT also appears to be an effective treatment for PSD, with high rates of response and low rates of medical complications.[85] ECT is more extensively discussed in Chapter 10. In addition to these somatic treatments of PSD, group and family psychotherapy have also been reported to safely and effectively treat PSD.[86,87] Individual psychotherapy, a safe and effective treatment for depression, has not yet been evaluated for patients with PSD.

For most patients with mild to moderate PSD, SSRIs are probably the treatments of choice, given their proven efficacy, their favorable side effect profile, and their cardiovascular safety. However, TCAs, despite higher rates of side effects than SSRIs, might also be considered first-line agents for PSD because of their potentially superior efficacy. For more severe depression that impairs decision-making capacity, nutritional intake, or ability to participate in rehabilitation, psychostimulants should be strongly considered; methylphenidate or dextroamphetamine can be started at 2.5 to 5 mg in the morning, and a protocol for dosing and patient monitoring can be followed (Table 27-6). ECT can also be considered in patients with incapacitating depression.

Other Poststroke Psychiatric Phenomena

Other psychiatric syndromes than can occur in the poststroke period include anxiety, mania, and psychosis. Poststroke anxiety is common, and usually occurs in concert with PSD. Approximately one fourth of patients meet criteria for GAD (except for duration criteria) in the acute poststroke period; at least three fourths of these patients with poststroke GAD symptoms have comorbid depression.[88,89] Poststroke anxiety has a negative impact on the functional recovery of stroke victims and has been associated with impairment in activities of daily living (ADL) up to 3 years after the event.[89] The functional impairment of PSD and poststroke GAD appear to be additive, as patients with both GAD and PSD have greater ADL-impairment at follow-up than those with isolated PSD.[90]

Poststroke mania occurs in less than 1% of patients.[3] Symptoms of poststroke mania are identical to those of primary mania, with flight of ideas, pressured speech, a decreased need for sleep, grandiosity, and associated psychotic symptoms. Lesions in the right orbitofrontal cortex and thalamus appear to be most often associated with poststroke mania.[91–93] Poststroke psychosis is also uncommon, occurring at a rate of approximately 1% to 2%.[94] Such patients most often have right temporoparietal lesions and a high rate of associated seizures.[94,95] This suggests that temporal lobe damage that leads to complex partial seizures and

Table 27-6. Guidelines for the Use of Psychostimulants to Treat Depression

1. Consider possible (relative) contraindications to psychostimulant use:
   (a) history of ventricular arrhythmia
   (b) recent myocardial infarction
   (c) congestive heart failure with reduced ejection fraction
   (d) poorly controlled hypertension
   (e) tachycardia
   (f) concurrent treatment with MAOIs
2. Initiate treatment with morning dose of 5 mg of methylphenidate or dextroamphetamine (2.5 mg in frail elderly or medically tenuous patients)
3. Check vital signs and response to treatment in 2–4 hours (the period of peak effect)
4. If the initial dose is well-tolerated and effective throughout the day, continue with single daily morning dose.
5. If the initial dose is well-tolerated and effective for several hours, with a loss of effect in the afternoon, give the same dose twice per day (in the morning and the early afternoon)
6. If the initial dose is well-tolerated but is without significant clinical effect, increase dose by 5 mg per day until a clinical response is achieved, intolerable side effects arise, or 20 mg dose is ineffective (i.e., a failed trial).
7. Continue treatment throughout the hospitalization; stimulants can usually be discontinued at discharge.

to associated psychosis may account for symptoms in a significant percentage of these patients.

Finally, there are two other clinical neuropsychiatric syndromes that are common in the poststroke period. The first is termed *catastrophic reaction*, a collection of symptoms involving patient desperation and frustration. Such symptoms include anxiety, aggression, refusal of reassurance and treatment, and compensatory boasting. This syndrome is relatively common; rates of poststroke catastrophic reaction are 3% to 20%.[96,97] Catastrophic reactions are strongly associated with PSD, with roughly three quarters of patients with catastrophic reaction having PSD.[97] Catastrophic reactions are also associated with a personal and family history of psychiatric disorders.[96]

Catastrophic reactions also appear to be associated with anterior subcortical lesions and with left cortical lesions.[96–98] Given the strong association of catastrophic reactions and depression, some feel that such a reaction is a behavioral symptom of depression (provoked by anterior subcortical damage) rather than a discrete syndrome. Others feel that catastrophic reactions result from damage to left hemispheric areas involved in the regulation of emotions related to social communication.[97]

The second of these clinical syndromes is *pseudobulbar affect*, also termed pseudobulbar palsy. This syndrome is present to some degree in approximately 15% of poststroke patients.[99,100] The syndrome consists of frequent and easily provoked spells of laughing or crying. It is usually seen in a mild form, with brief fits of crying or laughing with appropriate changes in mood, but in more serious cases it may involve frequent and spontaneous fits of laughing and crying inappropriate to the context.

Treatment of these poststroke phenomena generally parallels the treatment of primary psychiatric syndromes. Poststroke anxiety can be treated like any primary anxiety syndrome. SSRIs are effective in the treatment of a variety of anxiety disorders including GAD, and, given that most patients with poststroke anxiety have comorbid PSD, these agents are often the treatments of choice. Benzodiazepines can also be given for isolated anxiety, but they can lead to ataxia, sedation, and paradoxical disinhibition, and therefore must be used with caution in this population. Furthermore, these agents do not treat comorbid depression.

Treatment of poststroke mania follows the same rules as does the treatment of primary mania: mood stabilizers and adjunctive antipsychotic medications or benzodiazepines are used to control symptoms. Treatment studies of poststroke mania have found lithium, valproic acid, carbamazepine, neuroleptics, and clonidine to be efficacious, though none of these treatments has been examined in placebo-controlled, double-blind trials for this condition.[101,102] Poststroke psychosis can be treated symptomatically with antipsychotics. However, anticonvulsants (especially valproic acid and carbamazepine) should be used when psychotic symptoms are the result of complex partial seizures, as psychotic symptoms should improve with better seizure control.

Finally, pseudobulbar affect and catastrophic reaction may respond well to antidepressants. Two studies of pseudobulbar affect found significant improvement using nortriptyline[103] and citalopram.[104] Symptoms of catastrophic reaction may also improve with antidepressant treatment of comorbid PSD.

In short, psychiatric symptoms after stroke are common and have a significant impact on the long-term outcome of poststroke patients. Awareness of neurologic symptoms that may mimic psychiatric illness (e.g., anosognosia) and careful diagnostic interview can allow accurate diagnosis and prompt treatment. In general, psychiatric symptoms secondary to stroke are treated in the same way as are non–stroke-related psychiatric syndromes with similar symptoms.

The Management of Patients with Traumatic Brain Injury

Traumatic brain injury (TBI) is a leading cause of death and disability in the United States; nearly 1.6 million head injuries occur every year.[105,106] Of these, approximately 250,000 result in hospital admission,[105,106] while between 50,000 and 60,000 result in death.[105–107] Permanent neuropsychiatric disabilities affect an estimated 70,000 to 90,000 patients who suffer a TBI.[105,106,108] Of this group, psychosocial and psychological impairments lead to substantial disability and cause significant stress to their families.[108] The consulting psychiatrist plays an important role in the evaluation and treatment of these patients. In this section, the epidemiology and pathophysiology of TBI will first be addressed. This will be followed by a discussion of clinical features and treatment of the cognitive, behavioral, and affective aspects of TBI.

Epidemiology

Disorders that result from TBI are more common than any other neurologic disease except for headache.[108] Motor vehicle accidents cause approximately half of TBIs, while falls, assaults, and recreational accidents make up the majority of other causes.[108] Men from 15 to 24 years old are at highest risk; alcohol has been shown to be a contributing factor in 40% to 56% of cases.[105,108] Average length of stay in the hospital is roughly 6.7 days for moderate TBI and 17.5 days for more severe TBI.[106] It should be noted, however, that even more mild TBIs (without an associated hospital stay) may result in neuropsychiatric sequelae.

Pathophysiology

TBI may be divided into primary and secondary brain injury. Primary injury, in turn, consists of focal and diffuse lesions. Focal TBI generally results from a blow to the head that produces cerebral contusions or hematomas. The location, size, and progression of the injury determine resultant morbidity and mortality.[105] Most injuries occur in the polar temporal lobes and on the inferior surface of the frontal lobes as a result of contact with the bony prominences along the base of the skull.[108,109] Epidural hematomas, subdural hematomas, and cerebral contusions are all types of focal lesions. All are diagnosed by computed tomography (CT) scan or magnetic resonance imaging (MRI) of the brain. An epidural hematoma is usually caused by head trauma that is associated with a lateral skull fracture and with tearing of the middle meningeal artery and vein and, therefore, is most often located in the temporal or temporoparietal region.[105,110] There is often loss of consciousness followed by a period of lucency, and then neurologic deterioration. Prompt surgical evacuation of the hematoma is essential. Subdural hematoma is more common than is epidural hematoma, and it generally results from

tearing of a bridging vein between the cortex and a venous sinus. Much of the force of an impact is often transmitted to the brain, and the underlying brain injury actually determines the outcome in approximately 80% of cases.[105] Treatment also involves surgical evacuation. Finally, traumatic cerebral contusion is often associated with an initial bout of unconsciousness, generally followed by recovery. Edema may cause fluctuations in the level of consciousness, seizures, or focal neurologic signs.[110] Surgery is rarely undertaken for cerebral contusions.

Diffuse lesions, or *diffuse axonal injury*, are caused by shearing forces to axons that traverse large areas of the brainstem. Mechanical or chemical damage to white matter axons occurs during injuries associated with acceleration or deceleration.[111,112] The sites most prone to such injury are the reticular formation, basal ganglia, superior cerebellar peduncles, limbic fornices, hypothalamus, and corpus callosum.[108] Patients who suffer diffuse axonal injury have high rates of morbidity and mortality. The diagnosis may be made by use of diffusion-weighted MRI. Deficits in arousal, attention, and cognition (i.e., processing speed) often result from diffuse axonal injury.

Whereas primary brain injury (focal and diffuse) results from mechanical injury at the time of the trauma, secondary brain injury is caused by the physiologic responses to the initial injury. This may include hypoxia, hypotension, infection, cerebral edema, increased intracranial pressure, and neurotoxicity from release of biochemical substances. While a full discussion of each of these is beyond the scope of this chapter, each must be considered when evaluating the status of a brain-injured individual in the acute care setting.

Clinical Presentation

TBI is often divided into three categories according to its severity; however, there is no definitive breakdown of specific types of sequelae that may be affiliated with each. While more severe injuries are often thought to have more severe consequences, there are certainly instances of significant morbidity even with mild TBI. The severity of the injury is classified by the Glasgow Coma Scale (GCS; Table 27-7). Mild head injury correlates

Table 27-7. Glasgow Coma Scale

Eye Opening

Spontaneous	4
To voice	3
To painful stimulus	2
None	1

Verbal Response

Oriented	5
Confused	4
Inappropriate words	3
Unintelligible sounds	2
None	1

Motor Response

Follows commands	6
Localizes pain	5
Withdraws from pain	4
Flexor response	3
Extensor response	2
None	1

with a GCS score of 13 to 15, moderate injury with a GCS score of 9 to 12, and severe head injury corresponds to a GCS score of less than 8.

Other factors that may increase morbidity include: lower IQ, a concomitant substance abuse disorder, older age, and a history of previous brain injury.[108] Moreover, the DSM-IV[77]suggests the following criteria to establish the severity of injury significant enough to cause postconcussional disorder, a diagnosis under research (two of the following): (1) a period of unconsciousness lasting more than 5 minutes; (2) a period of posttraumatic amnesia that lasts more than 12 hours after the closed head injury; or (3) new seizures (or a marked worsening of a preexisting seizure disorder) that occurs within the first 6 months after the closed head injury. Diagnostic criteria for this disorder will also likely include cognitive disturbances and three or more of the following[75]:

1. Fatigue
2. Disordered sleep
3. Headache
4. Vertigo or dizziness
5. Irritability or aggressivity
6. Anxiety, depression, or affective lability
7. Changes in personality
8. Apathy or lack of spontaneity

These features are representative of the three major categories of neuropsychiatric sequelae that

may be seen with TBI: cognitive impairment, changes in personality, and Axis I psychiatric disorders (e.g., mood, anxiety, and psychotic disorders). Each of these is outlined briefly.

Cognitive Impairment

Cognitive difficulties in acute care settings may be due to delirium or posttraumatic amnesia.[112] Delirium is generally caused by the trauma itself; however, one should also consider other potential causes (e.g., infection of use or withdrawal from medications; see Chapter 12 for a full discussion of delirium). As recovery progresses, more subtle cognitive deficits and intellectual impairment may develop. Such manifestations include diminished concentration, memory problems, perseveration, poor planning, dyspraxia, poor attention, distractibility, impaired abstraction and calculation, language difficulties, and impaired executive functioning.[108,109] Children often manifest behavioral and learning problems. Neurocognitive testing is essential to further specify and quantify deficits. Moreover, neuropsychological testing is invaluable in designing an individualized rehabilitation program to meet the specific needs of each patient.

Personality Changes

Personality change due to TBI is a DSM-IV[77] diagnosis that is characterized by a persistent personality disturbance that represents a change from the individual's prior personality. It results as a direct consequence of the injury and is not better explained by delirium, dementia, or another Axis I disorder. The disturbance must also cause clinically significant distress or impairment in occupational or social functioning.[77] *Frontal lobe syndrome* and *organic personality syndrome* are terms that are often used to describe these personality changes.[113] Personality changes and behavioral manifestations often include labile affect, disinhibition, poor social judgment, apathy, lewdness, loss of social graces, perseveration, aggressive behavior, paranoia, and inattention to personal hygiene. In a 30-year follow-up study of patients with TBI, Koponen et al.[114] found that 23% of adult patients manifested an Axis II diagnosis. Children have also been shown to suffer from personality changes, with labile subtypes being the most common (49%), followed by disinhibited (38%) and aggressive (38%) subtypes.[113] These percentages support the idea that mixed types (i.e., two or more types together) are common. When evaluating personality changes, it is particularly important to note that the patient may have little insight into the change. It is therefore helpful to include family members in the evaluation and planning of treatment. Families may need significant support to cope with these changes present in their loved ones.

Mood and Anxiety Disorders

Patients with TBI are at risk for developing both depression and mania. Depression occurs in 12% to 44% of those with mild TBI, while rates of depression associated with more severe injuries are higher.[115–118] While results are inconsistent, a higher rate of depression is found in head-injured patients than in the general population. Prominent signs and symptoms include fatigue, distractibility, anger, irritability, and rumination.[115] Since there may be significant overlap with cognitive impairment and personality changes, diagnosis must be made with care. Neuropsychological testing may be helpful in these individuals. Major depression is associated with poor outcome across multiple domains[116]; this makes its early diagnosis and treatment particularly important. Finally, there is an increased risk of suicide after TBI; up to 15% of individuals make a suicide attempt in the 5 years after TBI.[108] This may be due to a combination of depression and disinhibition associated with frontal lobe injury.[108]

Mania has also been shown to occur more often after TBI than it does in the general population.[118] Predisposing factors may include a family history of affective illness, right temporal lobe lesions, and right orbitofrontal cortex injuries; unfortunately, consensus is lacking.[108,118] Furthermore, seizures seem to be more common in this group[118]; this makes the EEG an important diagnostic tool following TBI. For this reason, anticonvulsant medications are the preferred mood stabilizers after TBI (see treatment section).

Regarding anxiety disorders after TBI, GAD and posttraumatic stress disorder (PTSD) appear to be the most common.[118–120] OCD, specific phobias, and panic disorder have also been reported.[117,121] GAD is a comorbid condition with depression in approximately 11% of patients.[108] There is some

evidence that early intervention with cognitive-behavioral therapy (CBT) for acute stress disorder may prevent PTSD following mild TBI.[119] Other investigators have shown a relationship between impaired memory of the traumatic event and lower rates of PTSD,[120] however more research is needed in this area.

Psychosis

Psychosis as a consequence of TBI is thought to be relatively rare. While some authors doubt that a correlation exists,[118] others argue that psychosis may appear immediately after brain injury or years later (with rates between 3.4% and 8.9%).[108,122] Frontal and temporal lobe injuries are associated with psychosis, as are posttraumatic seizures.[122] Cognitive impairment and behavioral changes (already described) may mimic the symptoms of schizophrenia. Since individuals with schizophrenia have also been found to have a higher incidence of brain injury than those in the general population,[122] it may be true that head injury predisposes these individuals to schizophrenia. Alternatively, it may be that individuals who are already predisposed to schizophrenia have a higher incidence of brain injury for other reasons. More research is needed in this area.

Treatment

Treatment of neuropsychiatric sequelae of TBI is best accomplished with a comprehensive, multidisciplinary, rehabilitative approach. This may include psychiatric, neurologic, psychological, behavioral, occupational, and vocational evaluations.[109] Specific brain-injury centers are best equipped to undertake this; however, not all communities have such resources. Psychiatric evaluation and consultation generally focus on several areas of intervention: pharmacologic, behavioral, cognitive, and social (family support). These are discussed in the following section.

Pharmacology

Psychopharmacologic care following TBI is symptom based. The presence of mood disorders, anxiety, psychosis, aggression, or seizures are general indications for pharmacologic management. Since brain-injured patients may respond differently to certain medications, there are several guidelines that should be considered. Brain-injured patients may be more sensitive to the side effects of medications and require lower doses. The principle of "start low, and go slow" is helpful in this regard. However, there is also a danger of inadequate medication trials if therapeutic doses are not achieved or if medications are not given sufficient time to work. Slow titration as tolerated by side effects and an adequate duration of trials should be the goal.

The treatment of depression and anxiety in patients with TBI should follow the same principles as those followed for the treatment of depression and anxiety in the general population. However, medications with a high potential to cause sedation, anticholinergic side effects, and hypotension must be used with great care. For this reason, TCAs are not first-line agents. TCAs and bupropion lower the seizure threshold, which is problematic given the already higher incidence of seizure in these patients. SSRIs are in general well tolerated. Psychostimulants may be employed for depression and concentration difficulty, although paradoxical dysphoria, agitation, and paranoia may be seen in the brain-injured patient.[108] ECT remains a good option and is often underutilized. Care should be taken to assess memory and cognitive dysfunction before undergoing ECT, given potential side effects of this treatment.

Mania should be treated using standard agents. However, neurotoxicity from lithium may develop at higher rates in patients with TBI[108]; anticonvulsant mood-stabilizers, such as valproic acid or carbamazepine, may be preferable. For those patients with comorbid seizures, anticonvulsants are the treatment of choice.

Neuroleptics are used to treat psychosis and may be beneficial for aggression as well. Brain-injured patients are at increased risk for dystonias, akathisias, and Parkinsonian side effects[109]; therefore, typical agents should be used with care. Moreover, anticholinergics and antipsychotics that lower the seizure threshold, such as clozapine, need to be monitored carefully. Finally, benzodiazepines and barbiturates should be used sparingly in patients with TBI due to their potential for causing paradoxical disinhibition. If rapid sedation is desired in an agitated patient, low doses may be used with caution.

Behavioral, Cognitive, and Social Interventions

Behavioral treatments may be helpful for management of maladaptive social behaviors (including aggression) and personality disorders. Specific cognitive rehabilitation programs may be helpful, depending on individual deficits. These deficits are best assessed by administration of neuropsychiatric testing. Teaching about stress management and coping skills may also be particularly useful. Finally, social interventions, including family education and supportive therapy, may prove useful given the sense of loss and distress often felt by family members and by loved ones.

Conclusion

TBI is an important cause of neuropsychiatric disability in the United States. A thorough assessment of mood, anxiety, personality change, and cognition should be a routine part of postinjury screening. The consulting psychiatrist plays an important role in the evaluation and treatment of these patients. Prompt diagnosis and treatment, as well as appropriate referral using a multidisciplinary approach, greatly benefits patients and their families.

References

1. Marsh L, Rao V: Psychiatric complications in patients with epilepsy: a review, *Epilepsy Res* 49(1):11–33, 2002.
2. Schwartz JM, Marsh L: The psychiatric perspectives of epilepsy, *Psychosomatics* 41(1):31–38, 2000.
3. Commission on Classification and Terminology of the International League Against Epilepsy: Proposal for revised classification of epilepsies and epileptic syndromes, *Epilepsia* 30(4):389–399, 1989.
4. Khoshbin S: *Seizure disorders*. In Stern TA, Herman JB, editors: *Psychiatry update and board preparation, ed 2*, New York, 2004, McGraw-Hill.
5. Engel J: *Seizures and epilepsy*, Philadelphia, 1989, F.A. Davis.
6. Hermann BP, Seidenberg M, Haltiner A et al: Mood state in unilateral temporal lobe epilepsy, *Biol Psychiatry* 30:1205–1218, 1991.

7. Pariente PD, Lepine LP, Lellouch J: Lifetime history of panic attacks and epilepsy: an association from a general population survey (letter), *J Clin Psychiatry* 52:88–89, 1991.

8. Williamson PD, Spencer SS: Clinical and EEG features of complex partial seizures of extratemporal origin, *Epilepsia* 27(suppl 2):S46–S63, 1986.

9. Sachdev P: Schizophrenia-like psychosis and epilepsy: the status of the association, *Am J Psychiatry* 155(3): 325–336, 1998.

10. Williams D: The structure of emotions reflected in epileptic experiences, *Brain* 79:29–67, 1956.

11. Robertson M: *Mood disorders associated with epilepsy.* In McConnell HW and Snyder PJ, editors: *Psychiatric comorbidity in epilepsy: basic mechanisms, diagnosis, and treatment*, Washington, DC, 1998, American Psychiatric Press.

12. Delgado-Escueta AV, Mattson RH, King L et al: The nature of aggression during epileptic seizures, *N Eng J Med* 305:711–716, 1981.

13. Fenwick P: The basis of behavioral treatments in seizure control, *Epilepsia* 36:S46–S50, 1995.

14. Lancman M: Psychosis and peri-ictal confusional states, *Neurology* 53(5 suppl 2):S33–38, 1999.

15. Kanner AM, Stagno S, Kotagal P et al: Postictal psychiatric events during prolonged video-electroencephalographic monitoring studies, *Arch Neurol* 53(3):258–263, 1996.

16. Lancman ME, Craven WJ, Asconape JJ et al: Clinical management of recurrent postictal psychosis, *J Epilepsy* 7:47–51, 1994.

17. Kanner AM, Soto A, Kanner-Gross HR: There is more to epilepsy than seziures: a reassessment of the postictal period, *Neurology* 54:7(suppl 3):A352, 2000.

18. Kanner AM, Balabanov A: Depression and epilepsy: how closely related are they? *Neurology* 58:S27–S39, 2002.

19. Standage K, Fenton G: Psychiatric symptom profiles of patients with epilepsy: a controlled investigation, *Psychol Med* 5:152–160, 1975.

20. Barraclough B: The suicide rate of epilepsy, *Acta Psychiatr Scand* 76:339–345, 87.

21. Mendez MF, Cummings JL, Benson DF et al: Depression in epilepsy: significance and phenomenology, *Arch Neurol* 43:766–770, 1986

22. Robertson M, Trimble M, Townsend H: Phenomenology of depression in epilepsy, *Epilepsia* 28:364–372, 1987.

23. Currie S, Heathfield K, Henson R: Clinical course and prognosis of temporal lobe epilepsy: a survey of 666 patients, *Brain* 94:173–190, 1971.

24. Blumer D, Zielinski J: Pharmacologic treatment of psychiatric disorders associated with epilepsy, *J Epilepsy* 1:135–150, 1988.

25. Harris EC, Barraclough B: Suicide as an outcome for mental disorders: a meta-analysis, *Br J Psychiatry* 170:205–228, 1997.

26. Forsgren L, Nystrom L: An incident case referent study of epileptic seizures in adults, *Epilepsy* 6:66–81, 1990.

27. Kanner AM, Barry J: Is the psychopathology of epilepsy different from that of non-epileptic patients? *Epilepsy Behav* 2:170–186, 2001.

28. Blumer D, Montouris G, Hermann B: Psychiatric morbidity in seizure patients on a neurodiagnostic monitoring unit, *J Neuropsychiatry Clin Neurosci* 7:445–456, 1995.

29. Gastaut H, Roger J, Lesevre N: Differenciation psycholoique des epileptiques en fonction des formes electrocliniques de leur maladie, *Rev Psychol Appl* 3:237–249, 1953.

30. Slater E, Beard AW, Glithero E: The schizophrenia-like psychoses of epilepsy, i–v, *Br J Psychiatry* 109:95–150, 1963.

31. Geshwind N: Behavioral changes in temporal lobe epilepsy, *Psychol Med* 9:217–219, 1979.

32. Devinsky O, Najjar S: Evidence against the existence of a temporal lobe epilepsy personality syndrome, *Neurology* 53(suppl 2):S13–S25, 1999.

33. Kanner AM, Kozak AM, Frey M: The use of sertraline in patients with epilepsy: is it safe? *Epilepsy Behav* 1:100–105, 2000.

34. Hovorka J, Herman E, Nemcová I: Treatment of interictal depression with citalopram in patients with epilepsy, *Epilepsy Behav* 1:444–447, 2000.

35. Rosenstein DL, Nelson JC, Jacobs SC: Seizures associated with antidepressants: a review, *J Clin Psychiatry* 54:289–299, 1993.

36. Post R, Putnam F, Uhde T et al: *Electroconvulsive therapy as an anticonvulsant: implications for its mechanisms of action in affective illness.* In Malitz S, Sackeim H, editors: *Electroconvulsive therapy: clinical and basic research issues*, New York, 1986, New York Academy of Sciences.

37. Sackeim HA: The anticonvulsant hypothesis of the mechanisms of action of ECT: current status, *ECT* 15:5–26, 1999.

38. Fink M, Kellner C, Sackheim HA: Intractable seizures, status epilepticus and ECT, *J ECT* 15:282–284, 1999.

39. McConnell H, Duncan D: *Treatment of psychiatric comorbidity in epilepsy.* In McConnell HW and Snyder PJ, editors: *Psychiatric comorbidity in epilepsy: basic mechanisms, diagnosis, and treatment*, Washington, DC, 1998, American Psychiatric Press.

40. Arana GW, Rosenbaum JF: *Handbook of psychiatric drug therapy*, Philadelphia, 2000, Lippincott Williams and Wilkins.

41. Pisani F, Oteri G, Costa C et al: Effects of psychotropic drugs on seizure threshold, *Drug Saf* 25(2):91–110, 2002.

42. Barry E, Krumholz A, Bergey GK et al: Nonepileptic posttraumatic seizures. *Epilepsia* 39(4):427–431, 1998.

43. Krumholz A, Niedermeyer E: Psychogenic seizures: a clinical study with follow-up data, *Neurology* 33(4):498–502, 1983.

44. Krumholz A: Nonepileptic seizures: diagnosis and management, *Neurology* 53(5 suppl 2):S76–83, 1999.

45. Kuyk J, Leijten F, Meinardi H et al: The diagnosis of psychogenic nonepileptic seizures: a review, *Seizure* 6(4):243–253, 1997.

46. Alper K, Devinsky O, Perrine K et al: Nonepileptic seizures and childhood sexual and physical abuse, *Neurology* 43(10):1950–1953, 1993.

47. Bowman ES, Markand ON: Psychodynamics and psychiatric diagnoses of pseudoseizure subjects, *Am J Psychiatry* 153(1):57–63, 1996.

48. Devinsky O, Thacker K: Nonepileptic seizures, *Neurol Clin* 13(2):299–319, 1995.

49. Bare MA, Burnstine TH, Fisher RS et al: Electroencephalographic changes during simple partial seizures, *Epilepsia* 35(4):715–720, 1994.

50. Devinsky O, Fisher R: Ethical use of placebos and provocative testing in diagnosing nonepileptic seizures, *Neurology* 47(4):866–870, 1996.

51. McGonigal A, Oto M, Russell A et al: Outpatient video EEG recording in the diagnosis of non-epileptic seizures: a randomised controlled trial of simple suggestion techniques, *J Neurol Neurosurg Psychiatry* 72:549–551, 2002.

52. Cragar DE, Berry DT, Fakhoury TA et al: A review of diagnostic techniques in the differential diagnosis of epileptic and nonepileptic seziures, *Neuropsychol Rev* 13(1):31–64, 2002.

53. Henrichs TF, Tucker DM, Farha J et al: MMPI indices in the identification of patients evidencing pseudoseizures, *Epilepsia* 29(2):184–187, 1988.

54. Lazare A: Conversion symptoms, *N Engl J Med* 305:745–748, 1981.

55. Walczak TS, Papacostas S, Williams DT et al: Outcome after diagnosis of psychogenic nonepileptic seizures, *Epilepsia* 36:1131–1137, 1995.

56. American Heart Association: *1989 stroke facts*, Dallas Meeting, 1989.

57. Robinson RG, Starkstein SE: *Neuropsychiatric aspects of cerebrovascular disorders.* In Hales RE, Yudofsky SC, editors: *The American Psychiatric Press textbook of neuropsychiatry*, Washington DC, 1997, American Psychiatric Press.

58. Kraeplin E: *Manic depressive insanity and paranoia*, Edinburgh, Scotland, 1921, E and S Livingstone.

59. Bleuler EP: *Textbook of psychiatry*, New York, 1924, Macmillian.

60. Ironside R: Disorders of laughter due to brain lesions, *Brain* 79:589–609, 1956.

61. Schubert DS, Burns R, Paras W, et al: Increase in medical hospital length of stay by depression in stroke and amputation patients: a pilot study, *Psychother Psychosom* 57:61–66, 1992.

62. Astrom M, Adolfsson R, Asplund K: Major depression in stroke patients: a three-year longitudinal study, *Stroke* 24:976–982, 1993.

63. Eastwood MR, Rifat SL, Hobbs, et al: Mood disorder following cerebrovascular accident, *Br J Psychiatry* 154:195–200, 1989.

64. Robinson RG, Bolduc PL, Price TC: Two-year longitudinal study of poststroke mood disorders: diagnosis and outcome at one and two years, *Stroke* 18:837–843, 1987.

65. Morris PLP, Robinson RG, Raphael B: Prevalence and outcome of poststroke depression in hospitalized patients, *Intl J Psychiatric Med* 20:327–342, 1990.

66. Astrom M, Olsson T, Asplund K: Different linkage of depression to hypercortisolism early vs. late after stroke: a 3-year longitudinal study, *Stroke* 24:52–57, 1993.

67. Ouimet MA, Primeau F, Cole MG: Psychosocial risk factors in poststroke depression: a systematic review, *Can J Psychiatry* 46(9):819–828, 2001.

68. Starkstein SE, Robinson RG, Price TC: Comparison of cortical and subcortical lesions in the production of poststroke depression matched for size and location of lesions, *Arch Gen Psychiatry* 45:247–252, 1988

69. Starkstein SE, Robinson RG, Price TR: Comparison of cortical and subcortical lesions in the production of poststroke mood disorders, *Brain* 110:1045–1059, 1987.

70. Robinson RG, Kubos KL, Starr LB, et al: Mood disorders in stroke patients: importance of location of lesion, *Brain* 107:81–93, 1984.

71. Morris PL, Robinson RG, Raphael B: Lesion location and depression in hospitalized stroke patients: evidence supporting a specific relationship in the left hemisphere, *Neuropsychiatry Neuropsychol Behav Neurol.* 3:75–82, 1992.

72. Carson AJ, MacHale S, Allen K, et al: Depression after stroke and lesion location: a systematic review, *Lancet* 356:122–126, 2000.

73. King RB: Quality of life after stroke, *Stroke* 27(9):1467–1472, 1996.

74. Clark MS, Smith DS: The effects of depression and abnormal illness behaviour on outcome following rehabilitation from stroke, *Clin Rehabil* 12(1):73–80, 1998.

75. Schubert DS, Taylor C, Lee S, et al: Physical consequences of depression in the stroke patient, *Gen Hosp Psychiatry* 14(1):69–76, 1992.

76. Parikh RM, Robinson RG, Lipsey JR, et al: The impact of post-stroke depression on recovery of activities of daily living over two year follow-up, *Arch Neurol* 47(7):785–789, 1990.

77. American Psychiatric Association: *Diagnostic and statistical manual of mental disorders, ed 4,* Washington, DC, 1994, American Psychiatric Press.

78. Andersen G, Vestergaard K, Lauritzen L: Effective treatment of poststroke depression with the selective serotonin reuptake inhibitor citalopram, *Stroke* 25:1099–1104, 1994.

79. Wiart L, Petit H, Joseph PA, et al: Fluoxetine in early poststroke depression: a double-blind placebo-controlled study, *Stroke* 31(8):1829–1832, 2000.

80. Lipsey JR, Robinson RG, Pearlson GD, et al: Nortriptyline treatment of poststroke depression: a double-blind study, *Lancet* 1:297–300, 1984.

81. Kimura M, Robinson RG, Kosier JT: Treatment of cognitive impairment after poststroke depression: a double-blind treatment trial, *Stroke* 31(7):1482–1486, 2000.

82. Robinson RG, Schultz SK, Castillo C et al: Nortriptyline vs. fluoxetine in the treatment of depression and in short-term recovery after stroke: a placebo-controlled, double-blind study, *Am J Psychiatry* 157(3):351–359, 2000.

83. Masand P, Murray GB, Pickett P: Psychostimulants in poststroke depression, *J Neuropsychiatry Clin Neurosci* 3(1):23–27, 1991.

84. Lingam VR, Lazarus LW, Groves L, et al: Methylphenidate in treating poststroke depression, *J Clin Psychiatry* 49(4):151–153, 1988.

85. Currier MR, Murray GR, Welch CC: Electroconvulsive therapy for poststroke depressed geriatric patients, *J Neuropsychiatry Clin Neurosci* 4(2):140–144, 1992.

86. Oradei DM, Waite NS: Group psychotherapy with stroke patients during the immediate recovery phase, *Am J Orthopsychiatry* 44:386–395, 1974.

87. Watziawick P, Coyne JC: Depression following stroke: brief, problem-focused family treatment, *Family Process* 19:13–18 1980.

88. Castillo CS, Schultz SK, Robinson RG: Clinical correlates of early-onset and late-onset poststroke generalized anxiety, *Am J Psychiatry* 152:1174–1179, 1995.

89. Astrom M: Generalized anxiety disorder in stroke patients: a three-year longitudinal study, *Stroke* 27:270–275, 1996.

90. Starkstein SE, Robinson RG, Price TC: Comparison of cortical and subcortical lesions in the production of post-stroke depression matched for size and location of lesions, *Arch Gen Psychiatry* 45.247–252, 1988.

91. Robinson RG, Boston JD, Starkstein SE et al: Comparison of mania with depression following brain injury: causal factors, *Am J Psychiatry* 145:172–178, 1988.

92. Cummings JL, Mendez MF: Secondary mania with focal cerebrovascular lesion, *Am J Psychiatry* 141:1084–1087, 1984.

93. Starkstein SE, Mayberg HS, Berthier ML et al: Secondary mania: neuroradiological and metabolic findings, *Ann Neurol* 27:652–659, 1990.

94. Rabins PV, Starkstein SE, Robinson RG: Risk factors for developing atypical (schizophreniform) psychosis following stroke, *J Neuropsychiatry Clin Neurosci* 3:6–9, 1991.

95. Levine DN, Finklestein S: Delayed psychosis after right temporoparietal stroke or trauma: relation to epilepsy, *Neurology* 32:267–272, 1982.

96. Starkstein SE, Fedoroff JP, Price TR et al: Catastrophic reaction after cerebrovascular lesions: frequency, correlates, and validation of a scale, *J Neurol Neurosurg Psychiatry* 5:189–194, 1993.

97. Carota A, Rossetti AO, Karapanayiotides T, et al: Catastrophic reaction in acute stroke: a reflex behavior in aphasic patients, *Neurology* 57:1902–1905, 2001.

98. Morrison JH, Molliver ME, Grzanna R: Noradrenergic innvervation of the cerebral cortex: widespread effects of local cortical lesions, *Science* 205:313–316, 1979.

99. Andersen G: Treatment of uncontrolled crying after stroke, *Drug Ther* 6:105–111, 1999.

100. Morris PLP, Robinson RG, Raphael B: Emotional lability after stroke, *Aust NZ J Psychiatry* 27:601–605, 1993.

101. Starkstein SE, Ferderoff JP, Berthier ML et al: Manic depressive and pure manic states after brain lesions, *Biol Psychiatry* 29:149–158, 1991.

102. Bakchine S, Lacomblez L, Benoit N et al: Manic-like state after orbitofrontal and right temporoparietal injury: efficacy of clonidine, *Neurology* 39:778–781, 1989.

103. Robinson RG, Parikh RM, Lipsey JR et al: Pathological laughing and crying following stroke: validation of measurement scale and double-blind treatment study, *Am J Psychiatry* 150:286–293, 1993.

104. Andersen G, Vestergaard K, Riis J: Citalopram for poststroke pathological crying, *Lancet* 342:837–839, 1993.

105. Marik PE, Varon J, Trask T: Management of head trauma, *Chest* 122(2):699–711, 2002.

106. McGarry LJ, Thompson D, Millham FH et al: Outcomes and costs of acute treatment of traumatic brain injury, *J Trauma* 53(6):1152–1159, 2002.

107. Adekoya N, Thurman DJ, White DD et al: Surveillance for traumatic brain injury deaths: United States, 1989–1998, *MMWR Surveill Summ* 51(10):1–14, 2002.

108. Silver JM, Hales RE, Yudofsky SC: *Neuropsychiatric aspects of traumatic brain injury.* In Yudofsky SC, Hales RE, editors: *Neuropsychiatry and Clincial Neurosciences, ed 4,* Washington, DC, 2002, American Psychiatric Publishing.

109. Sanders KM, Smith FA: *Approach to the patient following closed head injury.* In Stern TA, Herman JB, Slavin PL, editors: *MGH guide to psychiatry in primary care, ed 2,* New York, 2004, McGraw-Hill Professional.

110. Simon RP, Aminoff MJ, Greenberg DA: *Clinical Neurology, ed 4,* Stamford, CT, 1999, Appleton & Lange, 1–49, 309–327.

111. Onaya M: Neuropathological investigation of cerebral white matter lesions caused by closed head injury, *Neuropathology* 22(4):243–251, 2002.

112. Capruso DX, Levin HS. *Neuropsychiatric aspects of head trauma.* In Sadock BJ, Sadock VA, editors: *Kaplan & Sadock's comprehensive textbook of psychiatry, ed 6,* Philadelphia, 2000, Lippincott Williams & Wilkins.

113. Max JE, Robertson BA, Lansing AE: The phenomenology of personality change due to traumatic brain injury in children and adolescents, *J Neuropsychiatry Clin Neurosci* 13(2):161–170, 2001.

114. Koponen S, Taiminen T, Portin R, et al: Axis I and II psychiatric disorders after traumatic brain injury: a 30-year follow-up study, *Am J Psychiatry* 159(8):1315–1321, 2002.
115. Seel RT, Kreutzer JS, Rosenthal M, et al: Depression after traumatic brain injury: a National Institute on Disability and Rehabilitation Research Model Systems multicenter investigation, *Arch Phys Med Rehabil* 84(2):177–184, 2003.
116. Rapoport MJ, McCullagh S, Streiner D, et al: The clinical significance of major depression following mild traumatic brain injury, *Psychosomatics* 44(1):31–37, 2003.
117. Deb S, Lyons I, Koutzoukis C, et al: Rate of psychiatric illness one year after traumatic brain injury, *Am J Psychiatry* 156(3):374–378, 1999.
118. van Reekum R, Cohen T, Wong J: Can traumatic brain injury cause psychiatric disorders? *J Neuropsychiatry Clin Neurosci* 12(3):316–327, 2000.
119. Bryant RA, Moulds M, Guthrie R, et al: Treating acute stress disorder following mild traumatic brain injury, *Am J Psychiatry* 160(3):585–587, 2003.
120. Klein E, Caspi Y, Gil S: The relation between memory of the traumatic event and PTSD: evidence from studies of traumatic brain injury, *Can J Psychiatry* 48(1):28–33, 2003.
121. Stengler-Wenzke K, Muller U: Fluoxetine for OCD after brain injury, *Am J Psychiatry* 159(5):872, 2002.
122. Fujii DE, Ahmed I: Risk factors in psychosis secondary to traumatic brain injury, *J Neuropsychiatry Clin Neurosci* 13(1):61–69, 2001.

Chapter 28
Patients with Neurologic Conditions
II. Movement Disorders, Multiple Sclerosis, and Other Neurologic Conditions

Joshua L. Roffman, M.D.
Karsten Kueppenbender, M.D.
Felicia A. Smith, M.D.
Jeff C. Huffman, M.D.
Theodore A. Stern, M.D.

Chapter 27 discussed the epidemiology, diagnosis, and management of neuropsychiatric symptoms associated with seizures, strokes, and traumatic brain injuries (TBI). In this chapter, we extend such discussion to other neurologic conditions. We discuss neuropsychiatric symptoms associated with movement disorders, multiple sclerosis, connective tissue diseases, brain neoplasms, and central nervous system (CNS) infections; as in the last chapter, the focus will be on phenomenology, diagnosis, and the practical management of patients with such symptoms.

Movement Disorders

Movement disorders are characterized by abnormalities in the extrapyramidal motor system that result in progressively impaired regulation of voluntary motor activity in the setting of normal strength. Depending on the particular illness, as well as on the stage of the disease, a patient can exhibit hyperkinetic, involuntary movement or hypokinetic, impoverished motor activity. These clinical features reflect dysfunction or degeneration of subcortical gray matter structures, known as the *basal ganglia*. Three movement disorders discussed in the following sections—Parkinson's disease, Huntington's disease, and Wilson's disease—are associated with particularly high psychiatric comorbidity, ranging from mood and thought disorders to dementia. These disorders pose a particular diagnostic challenge for psychiatrists, for in each case, behavioral symptoms can reflect the primary pathophysiology of the disease, psychological reactions to debilitating illness, or both. Treatment can be equally challenging, for although medications used to treat the underlying neurologic process can also induce psychiatric symptoms, certain treatments directed at psychiatric symptoms can worsen the movement disorder.

Parkinson's Disease

Parkinson's disease (PD), a neurodegenerative disorder characterized by the clinical triad of resting tremor, rigidity, and bradykinesia/akinesia, affects up to 2.5% of the geriatric population, although its onset in young adults has also been reported.[1]

The pathophysiology of PD likely reflects both genetic and environmental influences; it involves loss of dopamine neurons in the midbrain substantia nigra, with subsequent downstream effects in striatal, frontal, and cingulate regions and disruption of cortical-basal ganglia-thalamic circuitry. Postmortem examination can reveal the presence of Lewy bodies as well as the degeneration of noradrenergic neurons in the locus ceruleus, cholinergic neurons in the nucleus basalis, and serotonergic neurons in the dorsal raphe nucleus.[2] Anti-parkinsonian medications potentiate dopamine transmission as well as modulate the dopamine-acetylcholine balance in the basal ganglia. The mainstay of treatment is the dopamine precursor levodopa, usually given with carbidopa (which inhibits peripheral metabolism of dopamine). Other useful agents include dopamine agonists (e.g., bromocriptine, pergolide, pramipexole, and ropinirole), inhibitors of dopamine metabolism (e.g., monoamine oxidase B inhibitors, such as deprenyl and selegiline, and the catecholamine transferase inhibitor tolcapone), anticholinergics (e.g., trihexyphenidyl and benztropine), and amantadine.

Psychiatric disturbances in PD are common and multifactorial. These complications, which encompass dysregulated mood, psychosis, and cognitive impairment, can be primary to the underlying neurodegenerative process or secondary to its pharmacologic treatment; in some cases, they may be engendered or exacerbated by the psychological stress of experiencing a severe, progressive illness. The following sections will discuss the more common psychiatric sequelae of PD and review approaches to management, bearing in mind that in most cases, well controlled clinical trials establishing safety and efficacy have yet to be conducted.

Depression in Parkinson's Disease (PD)

The reported occurrence of depression in PD ranges widely, possibly due to variations among diagnostic instruments and disease-defining criteria, but in many studies (as reviewed by Burn[3]) it approaches 50%. Indeed, early PD is often mistaken for depression, given the sizable overlap in clinical phenomenology between the two disorders. Features common to both disorders are summarized in Table 28-1. According to the Global

Table 28-1. Symptoms Common to Parkinson's Disease and Major Depression

Motor
Bradykinesia/psychomotor retardation
Masked facies/restricted affect
Stooped posture

Cognitive
Impaired memory
Impaired concentration
Indecisiveness

Vegetative
Decreased energy
Fatigue
Impaired sleep
Appetite changes

Somatic
Physical complaints

Damier P: *The role of dopamine, serotonin, and noradrenaline in Parkinson's disease.* In Wolters ECH, Scheltens PH, Berendse HW, editors: *Mental dysfunction in Parkinson's disease II*, Utrecht, 1999, Academic Pharmaceutical Productions.

Parkinson's Disease Survey conducted by the World Health Organization in 1999,[4] even among patients with established diagnoses of PD, depression was recognized by clinicians in only 1% of cases. The same study indicated that among all measured factors, including severity of motor disability, depression accounted for the greatest impairment in quality of life.[4]

Given the mixture of potential neurobiologic, pharmacologic, and psychosocial substrates that could account for mood disorders in patients with known PD, careful consideration should be given to differential diagnosis. Depressive features thought to be related to the underlying neuropathology of PD have been well characterized and likely reflect altered monoamine transmission in the brain regions described earlier. In contrast to primary major depressive disorder, patients with parkinsonian depression primarily exhibit anhedonia, anxiety, and sleep disturbance, with far less prominent guilt, irritation, and psychotic features. Although suicide attempts are rare, suicidal ideation is common.[5,6] Alterations in mood can parallel the "on-off" phenomenon related to abrupt changes in motor activation[7]; depression associated with the "off" period can be reversed with acute administration of levodopa.[8] However, the degree of depression does not usually correlate with either severity of motor symptoms or the duration of PD.[3] Caregivers should also bear in mind the possibility that depressive symptoms in PD might alternatively reflect dysthymia, adjustment disorder, or (rarely) bipolar disorder.[9]

Few controlled studies have examined the safety and efficacy of antidepressant medications in patients with PD and depression. Several reports suggest some benefit from use of dopamine agonists, although it is unclear whether improvement in depressive symptoms merely reflects improved motor performance.[10,11] Recently the D_2 and D_3 receptor agonist pramipexole, which appears to provide significant antidepressant effect when used as an adjuvant in refractory major depressive disorder (MDD),[12] has also shown some promise in treating depression among patients with PD.[13] Selegiline, a selective type B monoamine oxidase inhibitor (MAOI) originally developed as an antidepressant, has been used to slow the progression of motor decline in PD. Limited studies have not consistently demonstrated an antidepressant effect for selegiline in PD.[14,15] The most widely used treatments for depression in PD are tricyclic antidepressants (TCAs) and selective serotonin-reuptake inhibitors (SSRIs). A single double-blind study indicated a greater effect of nortriptyline (up to 150 mg per day) than placebo in improving depressive symptoms in PD patients[16]; similar results have been obtained with imipramine and desipramine in smaller studies.[17,18] Given their particular efficacy in improving sleep as well as their mild anticholinergic action, TCAs can be especially useful in the PD population; at the same time, though, elderly PD patients are at greater risk for TCA-induced adverse effects, including delirium, cardiac arrhythmias, orthostatic hypotension, and urinary retention.[3] Several SSRIs, which exhibit an improved safety profile compared to TCAs, ameliorated depression among PD patients in open-label trials and case reports (see Poewe and Seppi[6] for a review); however, to date neither placebo-controlled trials nor comparison studies with TCAs have been reported in PD. There are also conflicting reports about SSRI-induced exacerbations of motor symptoms in PD.[6] Caution must also be exercised when prescribing both an MAOI and an SSRI or (especially) a TCA, given the risk of serotonin syndrome.[19] Efficacy of newer antidepressants in PD (including norepinephrine- and combined serotonin/norepinephrine-reuptake inhibitors) is plausible but remains to be studied.[6]

Although again not supported by well-controlled studies, electroconvulsive therapy (ECT) appears to be effective in improving depression among PD patients. One retrospective study described a similar benefit of ECT among 25 patients with parkinsonism and 25 age- and gender-matched patients without neurologic comorbidity.[20] Two studies have also indicated a transient improvement in motor symptoms among PD patients receiving ECT for depression.[20,21] However, the same studies also report that PD patients can demonstrate an increased vulnerability to ECT-related mental status changes, including delirium. There is some preliminary evidence that transcranial magnetic stimulation may improve both the depressive and motor symptoms in PD, putatively via effects on brain monoamine levels.[22,23]

Psychosis in PD

Psychotic features are also common and multifactorial in PD patients, occurring in as many as 20% to 30% of cases.[24,25] Especially prominent in patients with dementia, psychotic symptoms are often manifest initially as illusions or as "friendly" visual hallucinations (e.g., beloved relatives or animals). With time, hallucinations progress to include frightening or threatening images (e.g., insects or snakes) and paranoid delusions, often involving persecution or spousal infidelity.[24–26] As in depressive syndromes among patients with PD, consideration should be given to several potential etiologies. Psychotic features were recognized as part of the natural course of PD in up to 10% of patients before the advent of antiparkinson medication,[25] potentially related to altered subcortical dopamine transmission and to diffuse Lewy body pathology.[27] Both dopamimetic and anticholinergic medications given to alleviate motor symptoms can induce psychosis in PD. Dopaminergic agents can provoke a subacute psychotic disorder (perhaps akin to the putative role of dopamine in primary psychoses); there is no apparent relationship between dose, duration, or plasma levels of dopamimetic drugs and the incidence or severity of psychosis.[28,29] Anticholinergic agents can induce a toxic delirium with associated autonomic dysfunction (e.g., sweating, tachycardia, mydriasis, and priapism). Other factors predisposing PD patients to psychosis include cognitive deterioration, preexisting psychiatric diseases, infection or other medical illness, and dehydration.[25] Of note, virtually all PD patients eventually exhibit cognitive impairment,[30] and at the time of autopsy, up to 75% of PD brains exhibit pathologic evidence of Alzheimer's disease.[31]

Optimal management of psychosis in PD is highly dependent on consideration of differential diagnosis, as detailed in Table 28-2. Once other causes of mental status alteration have been ruled out, the next step is to reduce or eliminate anti-PD medications in order of the most psychotogenic and least antiparkinsonian agents first (i.e., anticholinergic and other agents) followed by dopamine antagonists, and finally levodopa/carbidopa. Nighttime psychosis can be alleviated by reduction or discontinuation of bedtime medications.[24] Finally, treatment with antipsychotics can be attempted. The best-studied antipsychotic for use in PD is clozapine, an atypical antipsychotic associated with virtually no extrapyramidal symptoms.[32,33] Poewe and Seppi[6] reviewed several case reports with a total of 432 patients receiving clozapine for psychotic symptoms in PD and found

significant benefit in approximately 85% of patients; similar results were obtained in two recent placebo-controlled trials, which also yielded no evidence of motor decline attributable to clozapine.[32,34] In most cases, the dose of clozapine used (e.g., 50 mg) was much lower than the dose typically used in schizophrenia. The use of clozapine is associated with life-threatening agranulocytosis in 1% to 2% of cases, necessitating weekly white blood cell count monitoring; no leukopenia-related deaths have been reported in PD patients.[6] A randomized, controlled study that assessed the use of the atypical antipsychotic olanzapine in PD patients with psychosis was stopped prematurely due to exacerbation of motor symptoms in the olanzapine group[35]; although no improvement in psychosis was observed in this study, several open-label and case studies have documented amelioration of psychotic symptoms with olanzapine.[36,37] Preliminary reports on the atypical antipsychotic quetiapine have suggested efficacy in treating psychosis but contradictory data regarding worsening of motor symptoms.[6] With regard to risperidone and the typical antipsychotics, given their propensity toward inducing extrapyramidal and parkinsonian symptoms in patients with primary psychosis, these medications should only be used as a last resort in PD.

Table 28-2. Stepwise Management of Psychosis in Parkinson's Disease

I. Consider etiologies unrelated to PD or anti-PD medications and treat accordingly

Medications: antihistamines, anticholinergics, benzodiazepines, antispasmodics, narcotics, and corticosteroids
Metabolic, electrolyte, or fluid-related abnormalities
Infection
Alcohol, benzodiazepine, or opiate withdrawal; Wernicke's encephalopathy
Hypoxia
Stroke or intracranial hemorrhage
Hypertensive encephalopathy
Seizure

II. Reduce anti-PD medications

Reduce or discontinue anticholinergic medications, amantadine, or MAOIs; then
Reduce or discontinue dopamine agonists; then
Reduce levodopa

III. Consider a trial of antipsychotics

Treatment of choice: clozapine
Next line: quetiapine, olanzapine
Last resort: risperidone, low-potency typical antipsychotics

From Cantello R, Gill M, Riccio A et al: Mood changes associated with "end-of-dose deterioration" in Parkinson's disease, *J Neurol Neurosurg Psychiatr* 49:1182–1190, 1986 and Kuzuhara S: Drug-induced psychotic symptoms in Parkinson's disease. problems, management and dilemma, *J Neurol* 248(suppl 3):III 28–31, 2001.

Other Neuropsychiatric Aspects of PD

Patients with PD suffer from a variety of other neuropsychiatric problems, including dementia, behavioral disorders, sleep pathology, and anxiety. As previously mentioned, there is significant clinical and neuropathologic overlap between PD and Alzheimer's disease, although it remains to be determined whether one or several concurrent etiologies are at work.[30,31] Whether as a function of age or primary disease progression, the frequency of dementia and cognitive impairment increases with PD duration.[38] PD patients, especially men, can exhibit a marked increase in libido and hypersexual behavior as a result of levodopa treatment.[39] Excessive daytime sleepiness, sleep attacks, and parasomnias also occur with increased frequency in PD patients; these symptoms can be treated effectively with sleep hygiene, intermittent use of nonbenzodiazepine hypnotics, and occasionally with a reduction in dopamimetics.[40] Finally, especially in PD patients with coexisting depression, anxiety disorders can significantly detract from quality of life[41]; although no randomized studies have been conducted to assess pharmacologic intervention, citalopram has demonstrated good anxiolytic effect in an open-label study of depressed PD patients.[42]

Huntington's Disease

An autosomal dominant disorder occurring with a frequency of 4 to 8 per 100,000, Huntington's disease (HD) is characterized by progressive choreiform movements, dementia, and neuropsychiatric symptoms. The usual course involves initial presentation in the fourth and fifth decades of life, with gradual deterioration and death occurring within 10 to 15 years.[43,44] Although expression of neurologic and psychiatric symptoms is variable, the underlying disease process reflects a single mutation on chromosome 4p16.3.[45] Expansion of CAG repeats beyond the usual number (wild type, approximately <37) and results in an elongated huntingtin protein, which (due to a variety of putative mechanisms) induces neuronal death.[46] The neuronal population most severely affected includes GABAergic medium spiny striatal neurons, causing decreased inhibitory

output to the substantia nigra and globus pallidus; some cortical neurons in layers III and VI also appear to be directly affected.[47–49] Accordingly, disruptions in dorsolateral prefrontal-subcortical, orbitofrontal, and medial prefrontal-thalamic circuitry may underlie respective alterations in executive function, mood, and response inhibition.[50]

In his description of the disorder, Huntington himself noted a "tendency to insanity and suicide."[51] Indeed, HD appears to incorporate a spectrum of psychopathology, including mood, anxiety, and psychotic symptoms. Notably, suicide risk in HD is as high as 12.7%.[52] In a prospective study of 52 HD patients, Paulsen and co-workers[50] described neuropsychiatric symptoms in 98% of subjects, with dysphoria, agitation, and irritability occurring most frequently (65% to 69%); 52% exhibited anxiety symptoms, while 13% demonstrated hallucinations or delusions. Symptoms did not correlate with dementia or chorea-scale ratings or with disease duration. Of 102 HD patients evaluated by Dewhurst and associates,[53] 42 exhibited depressive symptoms, and 50% were described as delusional (12 with hallucinations). Another large study indicated the presence of major depressive disorder in 28 of 88 HD patients, with bipolar disorder diagnosed in an additional 8 cases.[54] Although in the latter study the onset of affective symptoms preceded chorea and dementia by an average of 5.1 years, De Marchi and Mennella[55] similarly concluded that psychotic symptoms often emerged significantly earlier than motor dysfunction in HD. These studies, as well as others which described clustering of psychiatric symptoms in specific HD families, suggested that affective and psychotic symptoms in HD may be primary expressions of the disease process.[55] As always, though, medical causes of new-onset psychiatric symptoms in HD patients should first be ruled out; particular consideration should be given to alcohol withdrawal, as ethanol abuse has been reported in up to 24% of men with HD.[56]

As in PD, there are few well-controlled trials that establish the efficacy of treatment strategies for psychiatric problems in HD. The observations of Rosenblatt and LeRoi[57] suggested that SSRIs are well-tolerated in HD patients with depression and perhaps are safer than TCAs, given the vulnerability of HD patients to anticholinergic delirium, sedation, and falls. They also report that SSRIs are useful in managing the irritability, aggression, apathy, and obsessiveness often seen in HD.[57] ECT can be useful in treating severe or psychotic depression in HD, although again the risk of ECT-induced delirium must be weighed.[58] For treatment of psychotic symptoms in early HD, small doses of high-potency neuroleptics (e.g., haloperidol) should be considered; these medications are also useful for management of chorea and motor tics. However, in more advanced HD, when parkinsonism and dystonia are more likely to occur, atypical antipsychotics (e.g., quetiapine and clozapine) are preferable.[57,59]

Wilson's Disease

Wilson's disease (WD) is a rare, autosomal recessive disorder of copper metabolism with an incidence of 12 to 30 per 1 million.[60] Mutations on chromosome 13q14 result in altered function of apoceruloplasmin, a copper-transporting protein[61]; subsequent toxic accumulations of copper in the liver, brain, and other organs lead to progressive hepatic and neuropsychiatric dysfunction. Onset usually occurs in the first four decades of life, with a mean onset at age 17.[62] Low serum ceruloplasmin and high urinary copper levels are diagnostic; associated neuroimaging findings include increased signal in the putamen on T2-weighted magnetic resonance imaging (MRI),[63] reduced striatal glucose metabolism,[64] and reduced N-acetylaspartate levels in the globus pallidus.[65]

Initial clinical presentation can be divided among predominantly hepatic, neurologic, or psychiatric symptoms with roughly equal frequency. Liver-related presentations include hepatitis and cirrhosis, whereas neurologic presentations most commonly involve dysdiadochokinesia and dysarthria[66]; tremor, spasticity, rigidity, or chorea in the absence of sensory changes can also occur. Psychiatric symptoms are varied, but personality change and incongruous behavior are the most frequently described.[67] A prospective study of major depression in WD indicated an incidence of 27%,[66] although it remains unclear whether this reflects primarily a reactive or biologic process. Psychotic symptoms are seen infrequently, but catatonia can occur in 8% of patients with other neurologic manifestations of WD.[68] Kayser-Fleischer rings, which reflect copper deposition in the corneal limbus, occur much more frequently with neuropsychiatric than with hepatic presentations.[66]

Given the clinical heterogeneity with which WD can present, a high degree of clinical suspicion is important in making the diagnosis and therefore in establishing treatment. Moreover, treatment with copper-chelating and depleting agents (e.g., penicillamine and zinc) is only effective during the first few years of illness, so early intervention is essential.[62] Improvement in psychiatric symptoms has been less well studied than neurologic recovery, but incongruous behavior and psychosis appear to respond better than irritability and depression.[69] There have been no controlled evaluations of adjunctive psychotropic medications in WD, although there are reports of increased sensitivity to neuroleptic-induced extrapyramidal symptoms.[70]

Multiple Sclerosis

Multiple sclerosis (MS) is a chronic disorder of white matter in the brain and spinal cord, characterized pathologically by inflammatory demyelination of axonal sheaths and by gliosis. The illness is disseminated in space and time (i.e., it affects different locations within the CNS and is manifest by separate symptomatic attacks). Neurologic dysfunction frequently involves changes in vision (e.g., blurred vision, alteration of color perception, and diplopia), spastic paresis, hypoesthesia and paresthesia, ataxia, and bladder or bowel dysfunction.

Epidemiology

MS affects approximately 250,000 to 350,000 people in the United States. The disease usually becomes manifest between the ages 18 and 50. Most cases (80%) are of the relapsing-remitting type; episodes of dysfunction last for several weeks and they are followed by substantial or complete improvement. Some patients remain well for decades. The prevalence of the relapsing-remitting type of MS is roughly twice as high in women as in men. Primary progressive MS, which is characterized by a steady neurologic decline, more often affects men.[71]

Etiology

The pathogenesis of MS remains enigmatic. Its inflammatory white matter changes are thought to be immune-mediated. The absolute risk of disease for a first-degree relative of an MS patient is less than 5%, but is still approximately 20 to 40 times higher than the rate in the general population. Several linkage studies have shown an association between major histocompatibility complex (MHC) alleles and other genes related to the immune system. Infectious agents and other environmental factors may also contribute; however, no causal link has yet been established.[71]

Psychiatric Changes

Cognition. Cognitive changes occur in 45% to 60% of patients with MS.[72–75] The impairment is often not readily apparent; it is frequently missed by bedside cognitive screening, such as with the Mini-Mental State Examination (MMSE).[76] Systematic psychological testing has shown impaired memory function within the first 5 years of diagnosis in at least half of afflicted patients.[74,77] In most studies, cognitive decline was not significantly correlated with physical impairment or depressed mood, and there has been no association with the duration of disease (but see McIntosh-Michaelis et al.[73]). Dramatic worsening of cognitive function that occurs during an acute episode may remit completely over several months, as described in a case series by Franklin et al.[78]

Mood and Behavior. MS greatly increases the risk for affective illness. The lifetime prevalence of a major depressive episode for patients with MS is roughly 50%.[79–82] Several studies describe a higher incidence of depression in MS patients compared to those with other chronic neurologic disorders[83,84]; patients with prominent plaque formation in the cerebrum were more likely to be depressed than were patients with solely spinal involvement and comparative physical disability.[82] Fatigue is also a problem for 80% to 97% of MS patients.[85] The risk of bipolar disorder is 2 to 13 times higher for MS patients than for those in the general population.[80,86]

Pathologic laughing and crying, a neurological phenomenon that occurs in the absence of subjective emotional lability, has been reported in 10% to 20% of patients with MS.[87–89] Population studies in Denmark and Canada showed a 2- and 7.5-fold increase of suicide risk, respectively, for patients with MS compared to the general population. The Danish investigators found that suicide was most likely during the first 5 years after diagnosis was made.[90,91]

Psychosis. Patients with MS do not typically have psychotic symptoms. Rarely, however, MS may initially manifest as a psychotic break, as described by Matthews.[92] An MRI study of psychotic MS patients reported more extensive lesions in the temporal horns compared to other MS patients.[93]

Sexual Dysfunction. Up to 70% of MS patients experience sexual dysfunction.[94] Both genders experience decreased libido, orgasmic dysfunction, and decreased genital sensation. The incidence of these symptoms may be higher in men, who also describe difficulty with erection and ejaculatory dysfunction.[95] Women report decreased vaginal lubrication and decreased vaginal sensation.[96] Sexual dysfunction is a common contributor to marital problems for MS patients.

Iatrogenic Neuropsychiatric Changes. Corticosteroids, which are used in high doses to treat MS exacerbations, are known to induce insomnia, irritability, mood lability, and maniform psychosis.[97] Minden et al.[98] described a higher incidence of steroid-associated mania or hypomania in MS patients with a history of depression.

Concerns that interferon beta may induce or exacerbate depression were raised after the first controlled clinical trial of interferon beta-1b and follow-up data reported one completed suicide and four suicide attempts in the active treatment group.[99,100] This association, however, was not replicated in subsequent trials of interferon beta-1a and 1b.[101,102] Prospective studies of MS patients during interferon-beta therapy suggest that patients with a recent depressive episode may experience a recurrence of their symptoms after initiation of interferon treatment; a family history of affective disorder by itself was not an independent risk factor for depression during interferon treatment.[103,104]

Treatment. Neuropsychiatric changes associated with MS are primarily treated in the same way as are neuropsychiatric changes in other types of psychiatric patients.

Depression, which is the strongest predictor of poor quality of life in MS patients,[105] responds well to treatment with SSRIs and psycho-therapy. Supportive psychotherapy, and therapies focused on developing problem-solving skills, are more effective than are insight-oriented approaches.[104,106,107]

Fatigue may be improved by aerobic exercise, timed rest periods, improved sleep, and avoidance of heat. Often patients with MS-associated fatigue require pharmacologic treatment. Amantadine (100 to 200 mg/day) and modafinil (200 to 400 mg/day) have both been effective in controlled trials. If fatigue recurs despite continuing treatment with amantadine, drug holidays may restore its efficacy.[107–109]

Patients with a history of steroid-induced mania may be treated prophylactically with lithium or with low-dose chlorpromazine (100 to 200 mg/day) prior to, and during, the treatment with steroids to prevent the recurrence of a manic episode.[110,111] Pathologic laughing and crying have also been shown to improve with low-dose amitriptyline (25 to 75 mg/day).[112]

Few studies have addressed the treatment of sexual dysfunction. Foley et al.[113] reported a successful pilot study involving couples counseling. Male patients with MS who have erectile dysfunction may benefit from sildenafil, 50 to 100 mg, administered 1 hour prior to intercourse. Because sildenafil can enhance the effect of nitrates, which produce severe hypotension, this combination should be avoided.[114] Often it is appropriate to refer patients with sexual dysfunction to a urologist or gynecologist with expertise in this area.

Cognitive dysfunction can be treated with rehabilitation, which focuses on retraining and the development of compensatory strategies.[115] An open-label pilot study to treat cognitive impairment in patients with MS with donepezil showed improvement of memory, attention, and executive functioning.[116] However, to date no controlled study of the pharmacologic treatment of cognitive dysfunction in MS has been reported.

Connective Tissue Diseases

Connective tissue diseases (also known as collagen vascular diseases) are characterized by inflammation, small vessel damage, and serosal surface inflammation and cause a constellation of symptoms ranging from arthritis to severe, multisystem illness. Although the etiology of many connective tissue diseases is unknown, autoimmune processes have been implicated in most cases. Neuropsychiatric presentations of connective tissue disease are variable and again can reflect the primary disease process, psychological stress related to the illness, or side effects of medications. The following sections will discuss neuropsychiatric manifestations and treatment approaches for common connective tissue diseases including systemic lupus erythematosus, rheumatoid arthritis, Sjögren's syndrome, and other rheumatologic disorders.

Systemic Lupus Erythematosus

Systemic lupus erythematosus (SLE) is an autoimmune disease with multiorgan involvement primarily affecting adult women, in particular African-American women in their third through fifth decades of life.[117] Non-CNS manifestations of the disease are varied and include malar or discoid rash, arthritis, proteinuria, hematologic disorders, photosensitivity, oral ulcers, and serositis. The diagnosis is made by satisfying minimal criteria as established by the American Rheumatological Association,[118] as well as by the presence of serum autoantibodies including antinuclear antibodies (ANA), as well as anti-DNA, anti-Smith, and anti-RNP antibodies.

Neuropsychiatric manifestations of SLE occur in approximately 50% of patients[119] and can be divided into focal and nonfocal signs (see Table 28-3). Not surprising, whereas focal signs have been correlated with macroscopic CNS pathology at autopsy (including infarction, hemorrhage, and thrombosis), patients with nonfocal signs exhibit more subtle findings, such as encephalomalacia, arteriolar infarction, and fatty infiltration.[120] Clinically, though, there is inconsistent evidence to support a relationship between emergence of neuropsychiatric symptoms and changes in biologic markers. In general, CNS symptoms do not correlate with increases in autoantibody titers,[121]

Table 28-3. Presenting Features in Systemic Lupus Erythematosus

Non-CNS	CNS	
	Focal	Nonfocal
Malar rash	Seizure (generalized, partial)	Headache
Discoid rash	Hemiplegia	Delirium
Photosensitivity	Cranial neuropathy	Psychosis
Oral ulcers	Transverse myelitis	Mood disorders
Arthritis	Peripheral neuropathy	Cognitive dysfunction
Serositis (pleuritis, pericarditis)	Abnormal movements	
Renal disorder (proteinuria, casts)		
Hematologic disorder (hemolytic anemia, leukopenia, lymphopenia, thrombocytopenia)		

although in cases of severe depression or psychosis, elevations in anti-RNP can be seen.[122,123] Although many patients with CNS manifestations exhibit cerebrospinal fluid (CSF) abnormalities (e.g., elevated protein, immunoglobulin G [IgG], and immunoglobulin M [IgM]),[124,125] and most demonstrate electroencephalographic (EEG) abnormalities (e.g., diffuse slowing),[126] neither test appears to be sensitive or specific. MRI studies can be useful, but abnormal findings often do not correlate with clinical changes.[127]

Psychiatric symptoms in SLE are varied and occur with an unpredictable course. They can reflect primary effects of SLE, secondary metabolic abnormalities, side effects of treatment (steroid treatment or withdrawal in particular), or psychological reactions to illness.[119] Depressed mood can occur in 41% to 70% of patients,[128] although the exact prevalence is difficult to determine due to a lack of standardized diagnostic criteria; other mood-related symptoms can include lability, irritability, and anger.[127] Although the prevalence of psychotic symptoms was initially reported at greater than 50%,[129] many of these patients may have in fact exhibited delirium; a more recent study employing a more standardized diagnosis indicated an incidence of 5%.[130] Cognitive impairment, with specific impairment in concentration and attention, occurs quite frequently, perhaps in as many as two thirds of SLE patients.[131]

Because psychiatric symptoms related to SLE are so heterogeneous, the general hospital psychiatrist will often face the problem of deciding whether these symptoms are due to SLE itself or to some other primary etiology (including a psychiatric one). It is therefore important to consider the timing of symptom emergence in relation to medication changes and new physical examination or laboratory findings. If an SLE flare is detected in concert with psychiatric symptoms, a combination of immunosuppressant and adjunctive psychotropic medication should be initiated, again with the caveat that corticosteroids may induce or worsen depression, psychosis, or delirium. Lithium has been used prophylactically to prevent manic and psychotic symptoms in patients receiving corticosteroid treatment for other disorders.[132]

Rheumatoid Arthritis

Rheumatoid arthritis (RA) is a common and debilitating disease of unknown etiology that causes symmetric inflammation of the joint synovium. First symptoms usually occur in the hands, with sparing of the distal interphalangeal joints; morning stiffness is common. Extraarticular manifestations occur in more than three fourths of patients and can involve the heart (e.g., pericarditis, cardiomyopathy, and valvular lesions), lungs (e.g., pleurisy, fibrosis, and pneumoconiosis), eyes (e.g., scleritis and iridocyclitis), and peripheral nervous system. Rheumatoid factor is a sensitive although nonspecific diagnostic test.

Although there is a high (40% to 50%) prevalence of depressive symptoms in RA, it is unclear whether these reflect the underlying disorder or a secondary psychological reaction to the disease[133]; treatment should include both analgesics and adjunctive antidepressants or psychotherapy.[119] Of particular concern, though, is the potential for psychiatric complications related to RA treatment. The rare ability of salicylates to cause delirium and psychosis has been known since 1965.[134] Nonsteroidal antiinflammatory drugs (NSAIDs) have been reported to cause paranoia, depression, hallucinations, and delirium,[135] and can also increase plasma lithium levels by decreasing its renal clearance.[119] Finally, as mentioned previously, the use of corticosteroids has been associated with manic and psychotic symptoms as well as delirium.

Sjögren's Syndrome

Sjögren's syndrome, a chronic inflammatory disorder characterized most commonly by keratoconjunctivitis sicca (dry eyes), xerostomia (dry mouth), and xerosis (dry skin), can also induce peripheral neuropathy and both focal and nonfocal CNS manifestations. Psychiatric symptoms have been reported with varying frequency and often include affective disturbance (e.g., depression or hypomania) and personality changes (e.g., hypochondriasis).[136] In addition, patients with Sjögren's syndrome appear vulnerable to cognitive dysfunction ranging from mild problems with attention and concentration to severe dementia.[136] Treatment of Sjögren's symptoms, both glandular and extraglandular, is generally supportive, with use of steroids and other immunosuppressants reserved for severe, systemic cases.[137] Caution should be exercised when using anticholinergic medications as these can exacerbate glandular symptoms.

Other Connective Tissue Diseases

Several other connective tissue diseases are sometimes associated with neuropsychiatric sequelae, but these phenomena have not been extensively described. End-stage scleroderma can cause delirium as a consequence of renal or hepatic failure.[138] Fibromyalgia has been associated with sleep disturbance, hypochondriasis, and depression.[139] Finally, vasculitides (e.g., temporal arteritis) can cause transient blindness, cerebral ischemia, delirium, and stroke.[140]

Brain Tumors

Brain tumors may originate in the CNS, where they are derived from neuroepithelium, glia, or meninges (a *primary brain tumor*), or may be metastases from tumors in another locations in the body (a *secondary brain tumor*).

Epidemiology

Each year, roughly 16,500 patients in the United States are diagnosed with a primary brain tumor. In addition, approximately 120,000 individuals experience morbidity resulting from brain metastases of a systemic neoplasm. In adults, more than one half of the primary brain tumors are gliomas (i.e., tumors derived from the interstitial tissue of the nervous system). High-grade tumors, predominantly glioblastoma multiforme, constitute up to 80% of the gliomas. Unfortunately, the prognosis associated with glioblastomas remains poor; even with treatment, few patients survive longer than one year. Meningioma, a slow-growing tumor of the meninges, is the second most common CNS tumor; it accounts for about 20% of cases. Unlike glioblastomas, meningiomas can be cured with surgery or controlled by use of radiation. Although primary CNS lymphomas represent only 1% of adult brain tumors, their incidence has tripled during the past 20 years. Advances in high-dose chemotherapy, with or without radiation therapy, have increased the median survival of patients with these tumors to at least 40 months. In children, the two most common brain tumors are low-grade astrocytic or glial tumors and medulloblastomas. Meningiomas in children occur infrequently.[141–143]

Neuropsychiatric Changes Associated with Brain Tumors

All brain tumors can produce changes in affect, behavior, cognition, and perception. Upon initial presentation, mental status changes are most often seen in those with lymphoma (61%) and high-grade gliomas (40% to 60%) and less frequently seen with meningiomas (21%).[141] Most of these mental status changes are typically associated with infiltration of the tumor into the frontal and temporal lobes, and rarely with occipital and parietal tumors.

Mood

Alterations in mood lead to anxiety, depression, fatigue, irritability, anger, and full-blown mania, especially with lesions of the ventral frontal and temporoparietal cortices.[144–146] Symptoms inconsistently correlate with lesion size and location. Prospective studies have shown both higher rates of depression with left-sided tumors[147] and no effect based upon hemisphere involvement.[148] One crucial distinction to make is between depression and abulia. *Abulia* or *akinetic mutism* (manifest by reduced spontaneity of speech, motion, and goal-directed behavior and by the absence of despair, sadness, or crying) is distinct from depression.[149] Tumors that cause abulia most frequently invade and affect the frontal lobes. Caplan and Ahmed[150] described bedside testing suggestive of abulia. This involves asking a patient to give lists of common objects, such as animals, fruits, or vegetables. The abulic patient will often produce only two or three items. Another strategy is to ask the patient to count out loud from 1 to 20 and then backward from 20 to 1. Abulic patients often stop in the middle of the task, and then will either lose interest in the task, or take significantly longer than the normal (10 to 20 seconds) to complete the task. Patients with depression may also fail to pay full attention to these tasks, but with prodding their behavior changes. Delirious patients may be unable to respond appropriately; in contrast to abulic patients, they often exhibit other cognitive deficits such as disorientation. Fluctuations in performance over time, a hallmark of delirium, is not anticipated in abulic patients, whose lack of persistence and effort is more stable.

Psychosis

Perceptual disturbances are caused by mass lesions that impinge directly on the auditory, visual, tactile, or olfactory pathways (located in the temporal and

occipital cortices), the brainstem, and the base of the frontal lobes. Less frequently, brain tumors cause hallucinations indirectly through increased intracranial pressure. Paranoid ideation and other delusions are also associated with lesions of the temporal lobes.[144,145]

Cognition

When cognitive testing is performed on patients with frontal and temporal lobe tumors, measurement of memory, attention, language, and executive functions shows significant impairment in at least one area of function in most patients assessed immediately after the diagnosis. Verbal fluency and learning is most often impaired in patients with left-sided tumors.[147,151] Tucha et al.[152] found only a weak correlation between self-reports of cognitive dysfunction (of 139 brain tumor patients) and formal neuropsychological assessment.

Iatrogenic Neuropsychiatric Changes

Neuropsychiatric changes are commonly caused by cancer treatments. Dexamethasone, which frequently relieves headaches and improves cognitive function by reducing brain edema, is known to induce insomnia, irritability, mood lability, and maniform psychosis.[153] Whole brain irradiation may cause sudden, transient cognitive changes. In addition, a delayed-onset subcortical dementia, thought to be related to delayed white matter necrosis, has been reported between 6 months and 20 years after radiotherapy.[154,155] Memory impairment also occurs more frequently in patients who receive high doses of radiation and in patients older than 60 years of age.[156,157] Combined radiotherapy and chemotherapy increase the risk of neurotoxicity. Reports of cognitive dysfunction in adults with primary brain tumors treated exclusively with chemotherapy are few and far between. Recent long-term follow-up studies of patients with primary CNS lymphoma suggested that chemotherapy alone does not contribute to cognitive impairment.[158,159]

Tumor resection or *debulking* often produces neuropsychiatric improvement, once the postsurgical edema has resolved; however, it carries the risk of creating lesions in functional brain areas. Careful preoperative mapping of target regions with the help of conventional and functional MRI reduces the morbidity surrounding eloquent brain areas.[160]

Treatment

The consulting psychiatrist may be called to help with the treatment of mood and behavior symptoms in patients with brain tumors. Such symptoms may be sequelae of tumor invasion into the patient's brain, of tumor-related brain edema, or of neurotoxic side effects of treatments. In addition, the psychiatrist can help the patient and family members to cope with and adapt to a devastating illness.

Psychopharmacologic Interventions

Clinical depression is best treated with SSRIs, such as citalopram, sertraline, paroxetine, or fluoxetine. Use of TCAs and bupropion may lower the seizure threshold and thus should be avoided (unless the patient has a therapeutic level of an anticonvulsant medication). Abulia and apathetic depression respond best to psychostimulants.[161] Methylphenidate or dextroamphetamine are usually given in the morning and around lunch time. Administration later in the day may cause insomnia.

Anxiety, especially surrounding the initial diagnosis and before procedures or imaging studies, responds well to low doses of benzodiazepines (such as lorazepam or oxazepam), given two to four times per day. Acute psychosis, due to the tumor, postoperative delirium, or use of steroids, is treated best with high-potency neuroleptics (e.g., haloperidol), given intravenously, intramuscularly, or by mouth. Chlorpromazine and clozapine may lower the seizure threshold and create anticholinergic symptoms and are best avoided. Mania after initiation of dexamethasone treatment is often short-lived and quickly controlled with neuroleptics. If prolonged treatment with steroids is necessary and is accompanied by intolerable mood swings, lithium or valproic acid can help stabilize the patient. These medications can also be prescribed prophylactically to patients with a history of bipolar disorder, or with a previous episode of steroid-induced mania, prior to a future course of dexamethasone.[110,162]

Psychosocial Interventions

Supportive psychotherapy (conducted individually or in a group) may be helpful to both the patient and his or her family. Patients struggle with vulnerability and mortality; they wonder "Why me?" According to Elvin Semrad, the ideal talking therapies help patients acknowledge, bear, and place in perspective their emotional pain (cited by Rogers and Mendoza).[162] Patients may redefine the meaning and priorities of their life and ponder their legacy left behind. A patient with young children may want to make a recording or leave a picture album or a letter, which can be addressed to his or her children for when they are older. Family members often struggle with the patient's decline in function and behavior that may be induced by the tumor. Studies have repeatedly shown that caregivers tend to give lower estimates of patient quality of life and hope than do patients themselves.[163,164] Cognitive rehabilitation, originally developed for patients with traumatic brain injuries, can help to improve function and dysphoric mood in patients with brain tumors.[165]

CNS Infections

Infections of the CNS must be considered in the differential diagnosis of both acute and chronic neuropsychiatric symptoms. Manifestations of CNS infections may involve the entire gamut of neuropsychiatric disorders, including delirium, psychosis, mania, depression, dementia, catatonia, behavioral changes, agitation, or anxiety.[166–168] The consequence of missing a CNS infection may contribute to increased morbidity and a devastating outcome for the patient. The general hospital psychiatrist plays an important role in ensuring that such diagnoses are considered and evaluated. The following section will first describe the signs and symptoms that should prompt a more thorough medical evaluation in this regard. This will be followed by a discussion of specific types of CNS infection most likely to be seen by the psychiatric consultant. These include meningitis and encephalitis due to bacteria, viruses, and parasites.

Table 28-4. Factors Suggestive of Medical Illness

Sudden onset of symptoms
Absence of prior psychiatric history
Vital sign abnormalities
Disorientation
Younger or older age (younger than 12 or older than 40)
Immunocompromised host
Concurrent physical symptoms
Focal neurologic signs
Nonauditory hallucinations

From Reeves RR, Pendarvis EJ, Kimble R: Unrecognized medical emergencies admitted to psychiatric units, *Am J Emerg Med* 18(4):390–393, 2000.

Since CNS infections may present with such a wide array of neuropsychiatric symptoms, the diagnosis may not be readily apparent. However, certain clues suggest that neuropsychiatric symptoms are due to a medical illness rather than a primary psychiatric disease (Table 28-4).

Moreover, the presence of fever, nuchal rigidity, headache, visual changes, or focal neurologic signs puts CNS infection atop the list of possible etiologies. Work-up may then include serum laboratory tests, CSF analysis, CT scan or MRI scans of the head, and an EEG. These will be discussed in more detail below with each of the specific types of infection.

Bacterial Meningitis

Bacterial meningitis often presents with a constellation of signs and symptoms including fever, headache, lethargy, confusion, vomiting, irritability, and a stiff neck.[170,171] Focal neurologic abnormalities and seizures may also be seen. Early diagnosis

greatly improves outcome. Although a complete discussion of etiologic agents is beyond the scope of this chapter, the most common pathogens include *Neisseira meningitides, Streptococcus pneumoniae*, and *Haemophilus influenzae*. The propensity of infection with specific pathogens varies according to age of the patient and with the following factors: neurosurgical procedure, immunocompromised state, alcoholism, systemic illness, cancer, and head trauma.[171,172] Bacteria may enter the subarachnoid space via hematogenous spread, which generally begins in the nasopharynx. Alternatively, bacteria may invade the meninges directly through structural defects. Because of the diffuse nature of bacterial involvement, confusion and altered sensorium are typical manifestations. Focal findings often suggest a localized cerebritis or abscess.[171]

Bacterial meningitis is diagnosed by lumbar puncture, which should be performed at the earliest suspicion, given high rates of mortality. Table 28-5 illustrates typical CSF findings for different types of CNS infections. CSF should also be sent for culture to identify specific organisms involved. Other diagnostic measures include a complete blood count (CBC), which may show leukocytosis or leukopenia. An EEG is most commonly marked by generalized slowing. Brain imaging is most helpful in instances where an abscess or focal disease is suspected.

Intravenous (IV) antibiotics are the mainstay of treatment for bacterial meningitis. Although specific agents will not be discussed here, the standard practice involves starting broad coverage and then narrowing the range once an etiologic agent is discovered. Corticosteroids may also be used for patients with cerebral edema or with high levels of bacteria in the CSF.[172] Neuropsychiatric side effects of steroid treatment may complicate the situation.

Table 28-5. Typical CSF Findings with CNS Infections

	Cell Type Predominance	Glucose	Protein (mg/dl)
Bacterial meningitis	Polymorphonuclear cells	Low	>150
Viral meningitis	Lymphocytes	Normal	<100
Tuberculous meningitis	Lymphocytes	Low	>150
Syphilitic meningitis	Lymphocytes	Low	<100
Herpes simplex encephalitis	Lymphocytes	Normal	<100

From Andreoli TE, Bennett JC, Carpenter CC et al: *Cecil essentials of medicine, ed 4,* Philadelphia: W.B. Saunders Company, 1997 and Sagar SM, McGuire D: *Infectious diseases.* In Samuels MA, editor: *Manual of neurologic therapeutics, ed 6,* Philadelphia, 1999, Lippincott Williams & Wilkins.

Despite intervention, bacterial meningitis may be fatal in an estimated 20% to 30% of cases.[170,171]

Viral Meningitis

Viral meningitis is commonly referred to as *aseptic meningitis* because of characteristic aseptic CSF. Diagnosis is made by lumbar puncture (see Table 28-5), and care must be taken to exclude fungal or mycobacterial etiologies since these may take days or weeks to grow in culture medium. Viruses generally infect the subarachnoid space and leptomeninges with rare involvement of the brain parenchyma.[172,173] Clinical features most commonly include a triad of fever, meningismus, and vomiting. Irritability, clouding of consciousness, and lethargy are less frequent.[173] Focal neurologic signs, seizures, or more severe presentation suggest encephalitis.

Viral meningitis is most often caused by the Enterovirus family; however, the most common single causal agent is mumps.[170] It often affects young adults in the late summer or early fall. Herpes viruses and human immunodeficiency virus (HIV) infection may also produce viral meningitis and is discussed separately. The course of aseptic meningitis is usually benign and treatment involves supportive measures. Fatalities are extremely rare, as are long-term sequelae. However, at least one study suggests that viral meningitis in adults may result in underdiagnosed mild cognitive impairment, especially in areas of nonverbal learning and cognitive speed.[173] Neuropsychological testing may prove to be beneficial in this regard.

Herpes Simplex Virus Encephalitis

Herpes simplex virus (HSV) is the most frequent and potentially dangerous cause of sporadic and focal encephalitis in the United States. Mortality rates are estimated at 10% to 40% with similar rates of significant sequelae.[170,172] HSV typically invades the inferior frontal and anterior temporal lobes via cell-to-cell spread along branches of the trigeminal nerve.[170,174] Due to its predisposition for these locations, typical presentations include behavioral disturbances, personality changes, aphasia, memory loss, and dementia. Fever and headache are also frequently present.

Definitive diagnosis of HSV encephalitis may be difficult as brain biopsy is the gold standard, and CSF often does not reveal virus. However, brain imaging by CT or MRI may demonstrate inflammation and edema in characteristic temporal and frontal areas. An EEG with periodic sharp waves in the temporal regions should also raise suspicion. In cases in which there is a high index of suspicion, treatment with acyclovir is started empirically, as delay increases the risk of mortality.

Tuberculous Meningitis

Tuberculous meningitis is important to consider in patients who present with confusion, especially in those with a history of pulmonary tuberculosis, alcohol abuse, homelessness, HIV infection, or chronic steroid treatment.[171] It is caused by a rupture of latent parameningeal tubercles, which remain dormant in the subarachnoid space from earlier exposure. Tuberculous meningitis is characteristically subacute with symptoms generally present for up to 4 weeks at the time of presentation. Clinically, one sees headache, fever, meningismus, and delirium most frequently. Papilledema and ocular palsies are also notable. CSF usually reveals low glucose and mononuclear predominance (see Table 28-5). Acid-fast smears may be initially negative, though they are an aid in early diagnosis when positive. Definitive diagnosis may be delayed given that *Mycobacterium tuberculosis* may take up to four weeks to be cultured, and only 50% to 65% of patients have a positive purified protein derivative (PPD) skin test or chest x-ray evidence of prior exposure to tuberculosis.[172,173] Treatment is therefore initiated with antituberculous medications when the level of suspicion is high while awaiting culture results. Once a diagnosis is established, treatment continues for 4 to 10 months. Recurrences may occur due to poor compliance. Even with treatment, mortality is significant, at about 30%.[171]

Syphilitic Meningitis

The incidence of syphilis increased significantly in the 1980s.[172] Neurosyphilis occurs when *Treponema pallidum* invades the CNS and is reactivated up to years later. Since neurologic symptoms rarely appear until at least the secondary stage of the disease, earlier detection of syphilis infection is essential to prevent long-term sequelae. The serologic test for syphilis (STS) or Venereal Disease Research Laboratory (VDRL) test is used for large screening programs, but the fluorescent treponemal antibody (FTA-ABS) is much more sensitive and should be used when suspicion is high. There are several categories of neurosyphilis that occur when *T. pallidum* enters the CNS (including meningeal and parenchymal). Patients may exhibit confabulation, dysarthria, impaired judgment, and psychosis.[168] *General paresis* refers to dementia associated with parenchymal neurosyphilis; it had been a common cause of admission to psychiatric facilities. *Tabes dorsalis*, also of the parenchymatous type, results from chronic infection, and it causes a progressive sensory neuropathy. Other complications of neurosyphilis include communicating hydrocephalus, lightning pains (associated with tabes dorsalis), Charcot joints, parenchymal or meningeal gummas, and spinal pachymeningitis.[172] Treatment is with penicillin; however, once later stages of neurosyphilis are reached, full recovery is not expected.

Lyme Meningitis

Lyme disease is caused by *Borrelia burgdorferi,* a spirochete transmitted by ticks primarily on the Atlantic coast of the United States and in parts of the West and Midwest, as well as parts of western Europe. Lyme is the major vector-borne infection in the United States, and in endemic areas (as above), the attack rate may be as high as 2% to 3%.[175] Initial presentation is marked by *erythema migrans*, an expanding skin lesion at the location of the tick bite. Due to a typical central clear region, the lesion has been called the *bull's eye* lesion.[175] If untreated, Lyme disease may progress to a subacute or chronic meningitis marked by lymphocytic predominance in the CSF. Serologic tests are generally positive for Lyme as well; however, during late neurologic disease CSF serology may be negative. Of particular note, patients with Lyme disease may have a false-positive test for syphilis (and vice versa) because of cross reactivity.[172]

Particular neuropsychiatric sequelae from Lyme disease have been noted to include paranoia, dementia, psychosis, mania, panic attacks, depression, anorexia, obsessive-compulsive disorder, and cognitive impairment.[176,177] Depression has been reported to be as high as 26% to 66%.[176] Other studies suggest that impairment in verbal memory is significant.[177] However, more recent studies suggest that long-term sequelae may not be as common as initially suspected, and that the psychiatric sequelae (listed previously) may not be caused by Lyme disease in a majority of patients.[178,179] Nevertheless, prompt diagnosis and treatment with doxycycline is important to prevent long-term complications that may occur.

Parasitic Meningitis

Parasitic infections are an important cause of meningitis, especially in immunocompromised hosts and in certain areas of the world. While the scope of such organisms is too large to discuss fully in this chapter, one organism is of particular note due to increasing reemergence in the United States and other developed areas of the world.

Neurocysticercosis is caused when the larval form of *Taenia solium* (pork tapeworm) infects the CNS. The parasite is typically ingested from undercooked pork, and later eggs from the tapeworm residing in the human gut make their way to the CNS. While autoinfection is possible, more commonly eggs are passed on by fecal-oral transmission by food handlers and such. Cysticercosis is endemic in rural Latin America, Asia, and Africa, and immigration has recently caused a reemergence of the disease in the United States (California, Texas, and the Southwest United States are particularly affected).[179-181]

Neurocysticercosis may present in a number of ways depending on the part of the CNS involved. The main clinical manifestations are seizures, headache, and focal neurologic deficit. Hydrocephalus may contribute to acute presentations of psychosis and delirium. A more chronic picture of depression and dementia is also seen.[179,181] Definitive diagnosis is by brain biopsy; however, CT or MRI often shows the characteristic cysts. Treatment for neurocysticercosis depends on clinical presentation. Anticonvulsants are the mainstay for seizures. Steroids may be used for edema, whereas shunting is used to manage hydrocephalus. Standard antidepressants and neuroleptic medications are used for psychiatric manifestations. Anthelmintic medications are standard as well, however, no controlled trial has established definitive doses or durations of treatment.[181]

Human Immunodeficiency Virus Infection

CNS infections related to HIV may result from meningitis due to HIV itself, or from superimposed infections due to an immunocompromised state. Moreover, the differential diagnosis of neuropsychiatric disturbance in patients with HIV infection or AIDS may result from a variety of factors. These include primary psychiatric illness, primary effects of HIV infection of the CNS, opportunistic infections, and side effects of medications used to treat HIV-related illnesses.[182] Because HIV infection is described in detail elsewhere in this book, only a short overview is provided here.

In brief, of the two categories of CNS infection seen with HIV infection (meningitis due to the HIV itself and CNS opportunistic infections), meningitis usually runs a more benign course. HIV meningitis is marked by a syndrome of fever, headache, acute confusional state, meningeal irritation, and cranial nerve palsies (especially cranial nerve VII).[171] This often occurs at the time of HIV seroconversion as a complication of the flu-like illness experienced by approximately one third of HIV-infected people.[182] Symptoms generally resolve spontaneously. The CSF reveals mononuclear plcocytosis. Meningitis, encephalitis, and abscesses caused by opportunistic infections are generally more serious, and they signify worsening of the immune status. Others include cryptococcal meningitis, HSV encephalitis, varicella-zoster encephalitis, cytomegalovirus encephalitis, and cerebral toxoplasmosis. Each of these must be excluded since treatments vary depending on the pathogen. In general, organic causes of psychiatric symptoms should be at the top of the list of possible causes in people with HIV infection or AIDS, especially at later stages of the illness.

Conclusion

Infections of the CNS may cause both acute and chronic neuropsychiatric symptomatology. Presentation may be quite varied; it includes delirium, psychosis, dementia, depression, behavioral changes, and mania, among others. The general hospital psychiatrist plays an important role in safeguarding patients from medical diagnoses that may be missed due to psychiatric manifestations. This introduction to the more commonly seen CNS infections and their neuropsychiatric sequelae should provide a starting point for such consultations and evaluations.

References

1. Cummings JL: Understanding Parkinson's disease, *JAMA* 281:376–378, 1999.
2. Jellinger JA: *Neuropathological correlates of mental dysfunction in Parkinson's disease: an update*. In Wolters ECH, Scheltens PH, Berendse HW, editors: *Mental dysfunction in Parkinson's disease*, Utrecht, Netherlands, 1999, Academic Pharmaceutical Productions.
3. Burn DJ: Beyond the iron mask: towards better recognition and treatment of depression associated with Parkinson's disease, *Mov Disord* 17:445–454, 2002.
4. Damier P: *The role of dopamine, serotonin, and noradrenaline in Parkinson's disease*. In Wolters ECH, Scheltens PH, Berendse HW, editors: *Mental dysfunction in Parkinson's disease II*, Utrecht, Netherlands, 1999, Academic Pharmaceutical Productions.
5. Yamamoto M: Depression in Parkinson's disease: its prevalence, diagnosis, and neurochemical background, *J Neurol* 248 (suppl 3):III 5–7, 2001.
6. Poewe W, Seppi K: Treatment options for depression and psychosis in Parkinson's disease, *J Neurol* 248 (suppl 3):III 12–21, 2001.
7. Cantello R, Gill M, Riccio A et al: Mood changes associated with "end-of-dose deterioration" in Parkinson's disease, *J Neurol Neurosurg Psychiatr* 49:1182–1190, 1986.
8. Nissenbaum H, Quinn NP, Brown RG, et al: Mood swings associated with the "on-off" phenomenon in Parkinson's disease, *Psychol Med* 17:899–904, 1987.
9. Marsh L: Neuropsychiatric aspects of Parkinson's disease, *Psychosomatics* 41:15–23, 2000.
10. Bennet J Jr, Piercey MF: Pramipexole: a new dopamine agonist for the treatment of Parkinson's disease, *J Neurol Sci* 163:25–31,1999.
11. Jouvent R, Abensour P, Bonnet AM, et al: Anti-Parkinson and antidepressant effects of high doses of bromocriptine, an independent comparison, *J Affect Disord* 5:141–145, 1983.
12. Lattanzi L, Dell'Ossa L, Cassano P, et al: Pramipexole in treatment-resistant depression: a 16 week naturalistic study, *Bipolar Disord* 4:307–314, 2002.
13. Reichmann H, Brecht HM, Kraus PH, et al: Pramipexole in Parkinson's disease: results of a treatment observation, *Nervenarzt* 73:745–750, 2002.

14. Knoll J: Pharmacology of selegiline ((-) deprenyl) new aspect, *Acta Neurol Scand* 80(suppl 126):83–91, 1989.
15. Tom T, Cummings JL: Depression in Parkinson's disease: pharmacological characteristics and treatment, *Drugs Age* 12:55–77, 1998.
16. Anderson J, Aabro E, Gulmann N et al: Antidepressive treatment in Parkinson's disease: a controlled trial of the effect of nortriptyline in patients with Parkinson's disease treated with L-DOPA, *Acta Neurol Scand* 62:210–219, 1980.
17. Strang RR: Imipramine in treatment of Parkinson's disease: a double-blind study, *Br Med J* 2:33–34, 1965.
18. Laitinen L: Desipramine in treatment of Parkinson's disease: a placebo-controlled study, *Acta Neurol Scand* 45:109–113, 1969.
19. Richard IH, Kurlan R, Tanner C, et al: Serotonin syndrome and the combined use of eldepryl and an antidepressant in Parkinson's disease, *Neurology* 48: 1070–1077, 1997.
20. Moellentine C, Rummans T, Ahlskog JE, et al: Effectiveness of ECT in patients with Parkinsonism, *J Neuropsychiatry Clin Neurosci* 10:187–193, 1998.
21. Douyon R, Serby M, Klutchko B, et al: ECT and Parkinson's disease revisited: a "naturalistic" study, *Am J Psychiatry* 146:1451–1455, 1989.
22. Mally J, Stone TW: Therapeutic and "dose-dependent" effect of repetitive microelectroshock induced by transcranial magnetic stimulation in Parkinson's disease, *J Neurosci Res* 57:935–940, 1999.
23. Mally J, Stone TW: Improvement in Parkinsonian symptoms after repetitive transcranial magnetic stimulation, *J Neurol Sci* 162:179–184, 1999.
24. Kuzuhara S: Drug-induced psychotic symptoms in Parkinson's disease: problems, management and dilemma, *J Neurol* 248(suppl 3):III 28–31, 2001.
25. Wolters E CH: Intrinsic and extrinsic psychosis in Parkinson's disease, *J Neurol* 248(suppl 3):III 22–27, 2001.
26. Marsh L: Psychosis in Parkinson's disease (abstract), American Association of Geriatric Psychiatry 16th Annual Meeting, 2003, Honolulu[AU10].
27. Mjønes H: Paralysis agitans: a clinical and genetic study, *Acta Psychiatr Scand*[AU11] S54, 1949.
28. Aarsland D, Larsen JP, Cummings JL, et al: Prevalence and clinical correlates of psychotic symptoms in Parkinson's disease, *Arch Neurol* 56:595–601, 1999.
29. Goetz CG, Pappert EJ, Blasucci EJ, et al: Intravenous levodopa in hallucinating Parkinson's disease patients: high-dose challenge does not precipitate hallucinations, *Neurology* 50:515–517, 1998.
30. Mortimer JA, Sun SP, Kuskowski MA, et al: *Cognitive and affective disorders in Parkinson's disease*. In Franks AJ, Ironside JW, Mindham RHS, et al, editors: *Function and dysfunction in the basal ganglia*, Manchester, 1990, Manchester University Press.
31. Boller F, Mizutani T, Roessmann U, et al: Parkinson's disease, dementia and Alzheimer's disease: clinico-pathological correlations, *Ann Neurol* 7:329–335, 1980.
32. Kane J, Honigfeld G, Singer J, et al: Clozapine for the treatment-resistant schizophrenic: a double-blind comparison with chlorpromazine, *Arch Gen Psychiatry* 45:789–796, 1988.
33. The French Clozapine Parkinson Study Group: Clozapine in drug-induced psychosis in Parkinson's disease: The French Clozapine Parkinson Study Group, *Lancet* 353:2041–2042, 1999.
34. The Parkinson Study Group: Low-dose clozapine for the treatment of drug-induced psychosis in Parkinson's disease. The Parkinson study group, *N Engl J Med* 340:757–763, 1999.
35. Goetz CG, Blasucci LM, Leurgans S, et al: Olanzapine and clozapine: comparative effects on motor function in hallucinating PD patients, *Neurology* 55:789–794, 2000.
36. Aarsland D, Larsen JP, Lim NG, et al: Olanzapine for psychosis in Parkinson's disease with and without dementia, *J Neuropsychiatry Clin Neurosci* 11:392–394, 1999.
37. Wolters EC, Jansen EN, Tuynman QH, et al: Olanzapine in the treatment of dopaminomimetic psychosis in patients with Parkinson's disease, *Neurology* 47:1085–1087, 1996.
38. Mindham RH, Biggins CA, Boyd JL, et al: A controlled study of dementia in Parkinson's disease over 54 months, *Adv Neurol* 60:470–474, 1993.
39. Brown B, Brown GM, Kofman O, et al: Sexual function and affect in Parkinsonian men treated with L-dopa, *Am J Psychiatry*, 135:1552–1555, 1978.
40. Larsen JP, Tandberg E: Sleep disorders in patients with Parkinson's disease: epidemiology and management, *CNS Drugs* 15:267–275, 2001.
41. Menza MA, Robertson-Hoffman DE, Bonapace AS: Parkinson's disease and anxiety: comorbidity with depression, *Biol Psychiatry* 33:465–470, 1993.
42. Menza MA, Marin H, Kaufman K, et al: Citalopram treatment of depression in Parkinson's disease: the impact on anxiety, disability, and cognition, *Neuropsychiatry Clin Neurosci*, 2003, in press.
43. Harper PS: The epidemiology of Huntington's disease, *Hum Genet* 89:365–376, 1992.
44. Folstein SE: *Huntington's disease: a disorder of families*, Baltimore, 1989, Johns Hopkins University Press.
45. Gusella JF, Wexler NS, Conneally PM, et al: A polymorphic DNA marker genetically linked to Huntington's disease, *Nature* 306:234–238, 1983.
46. Huntington's Disease Collaborative Research Group: A novel gene containing a trinucleotide repeat that is expanded and unstable on Huntington's disease chromosomes, *Cell* 72:971–983, 1993.
47. Glass M, Dragunow M, Faull RLM: The pattern of neurodegeneration in Huntington's disease: a comparative study of cannabinoid, dopamine, adenosine, and GABA$_A$ receptor alterations in the human basal ganglia

in Huntington's disease, *Neuroscience* 97:505–519, 2000.

48. Reddy PH, Williams M, Tagle DA: Recent advances in understanding the pathogenesis of Huntington's disease, *Trends Neurosci* 22:248–255, 2001.

49. Ho LW, Carmichael J, Swartz J et al: The molecular biology of Huntington's disease, *Psychol Med* 31:3–14, 2001.

50. Paulsen JS, Ready RE, Hamilton JM, et al: Neuropsychiatric aspects of Huntington's disease, *J Neurol Neurosurg Psychiatry* 71:310–314, 2001.

51. Huntington G: On Chorea, *Med Surg Rep Philadelphia* 26:317–321, 1872.

52. Schoenfeld M, Myers RH, Cupples LE, et al: Increased rate of suicide among patients with Huntington's disease, *J Neurol Neurosurg Psychiatry* 47:1283–1287, 1984.

53. Dewhurst K, Oliver J, Trick KLK, et al: Neuropsychiatric aspects of Huntington's disease. *Confin Neurol* 31:258–268, 1969.

54. Folstein S, Abbott MH, Chase GA, et al: The association of affective disorder with Huntington's disease in a case series and in families, *Psychol Med* 13:537–542, 1983.

55. De Marchi N, Mennella R: Huntington's disease and its association with psychopathology, *Harvard Rev Psychiatry* 7:278–289, 2000.

56. King M: Alcohol abuse in Huntington's disease, *Psychol Med* 15:815–819, 1996.

57. Rosenblatt A, LeRoi I: Neuropsychiatry of Huntington's disease and other basal ganglia disorders, *Psychosomatics* 41:24–30, 2000.

58. Ranen NG, Peyser KR, Folstein SE: ECT as a treatment for depression in Huntington's disease, *J Neuropsychiatry* 6:154–158, 1994.

59. Bonucelli U, Ceravolo R, Maremmani C, et al: Clozapine in Huntington's chorea, *Neurology* 44:821–823, 1994.

60. Hoogenraad TU, Houwen RHJ: *Prevalence and genetics*. In Hoogenraad TU, editor: *Wilson's disease*, London, 1996, WB Saunders.

61. Frydman M: Genetic aspects of Wilson's disease, *J Gastroenterol Hepatol* 5:483–490, 1990.

62. ANPA Committee on Research et al: Neuropsychiatric correlates and treatment of lenticulostriatal disorders, *J Neuropsychiatry Clin Neurosci* 10:249–266, 1998.

63. Starosta-Rubenstein S, Young AB, Kluin K, et al: Clinical assessment of 31 patients with Wilson's disease: correlations with structural changes on magnetic resonance imaging, *Arch Neurol* 44:365–370, 1987.

64. Kuwert T, Hefter H, Scholz D, et al: Regional cerebral glucose consumption measured by positron emission tomography in patients with Wilson's disease, *Eur J Nucl Med* 19:96–101, 1992.

65. van Den Huevel AG, Van der Grond J, Van Rooij LG, et al: Differentiation between portal-systemic encephalopathy and neurodegenerative disorders in patients with Wilson's disease: H-1 MR spectroscopy, *Radiology* 203:539–543, 1997.

66. Oder W, Grimm G, Kollegger H, et al: Neurological and neuropsychiatric spectrum of Wilson's disease: a prospective study of 45 cases, *J Neurol* 238:281–287, 1991.

67. Akil M, Schwartz JA, Dutchak D, et al: The psychiatric presentations of Wilson's disease, *J Neuropsychiatry Clin Neurosci* 3:377–382, 1991.

68. Brewer GJ, Yuzbasiyan-Gurkan V: Wilson's disease, *Medicine (Baltimore)* 71:139–164, 1992.

69. Dening TR, Berrios GE: Wilson's disease: a longitudinal study of psychiatric symptoms, *Biol Psychiatry* 28:255–265, 1990.

70. Hoogenraad TU: *Wilson's disease*, London, 1996, WB Saunders.

71. Noseworthy JH, Lucchinetti C, Rodriguez M, et al: Multiple sclerosis, *N Engl J Med* 343:938–952, 2000.

72. Ivnik RJ: Neuropsychological test performance as a function of the duration of MS-related symptomatology. *J Clin Psychiatry* 39:304–312, 1978.

73. McIntosh-Michaelis SA, Roberts MH, Wilkinson SM, et al: The prevalence of cognitive impairment in a community survey of multiple sclerosis, *Br J Clin Psychol* 30:333–348, 1991.

74. Peyser JM, Edwards KR, Poser CM, et al: Cognitive function in patients with multiple sclerosis. *Arch Neurol* 37:577–579, 1980.

75. Rao SM, Leo GJ, Bernardin L, et al: Cognitive dysfunction in multiple sclerosis: I. frequency, patterns, and prediction. *Neurology* 41:685–691, 1991.

76. Folstein MF, Folstein SE, McHugh PR: "Mini Mental State": a practical method for grading the cognitive state of patients for the clinician, *J Psychiatr Res* 12:189–198, 1975

77. Truelle JL, Palisson E, Le Gall D, et al: Troubles intellectuels et thymique dans la sclérose en plaques, *Rev Neurol* 143:595–601, 1987.

78. Franklin GM, Nelson LM, Filley CM, et al: Cognitive loss in multiple sclerosis, case reports and review of the literature, *Arch Neurol* 46:162–167, 1989.

79. Sadovnick AD, Remick RA, Allen J, et al: Depression and multiple sclerosis, *Neurology* 46:628–32, 1996.

80. Joffe RT, Lippert GP, Gray TA, et al: Mood disorder and multiple sclerosis, *Arch Neurol* 44:376–378, 1987.

81. Minden SL, Schiffer RB: Affective disorders in multiple sclerosis: review and recommendations for clinical research, *Arch Neurol* 47:98–104, 1990.

82. Rabins PV, Brooks BR, O'Donnell P, et al: Structural brain correlates of emotional disorders in multiple sclerosis, *Brain* 109:585–597, 1986.

83. Schubert DS, Foliart RH: Increased depression in multiple sclerosis patients. A meta-analysis, *Psychosomatics* 34:124–130, 1993.

84. Schiffer RB, Babigian HM: Behavioral disorders in multiple sclerosis, temporal lobe epilepsy, and amyotrophic

lateral sclerosis: an epidemiologic study, *Arch Neurol* 41:1067–1069, 1984.

85. Krupp LB: *Mechanisms, measurement, and management of fatigue in multiple sclerosis.* In Thompson AJ, Polman C, Reinhard H, editors: *Multiple sclerosis: clinical challenges and controversies,* London, 1997, Martin Dunitz.

86. Schiffer RB, Wineman NM, Weitkamp LR: Association between bipolar affective disorder and multiple sclerosis, *Am J Psychiatry* 143:94–95, 1986.

87. Langworthy OR, Kolb LC, Androp S: Disturbances of behavior in patients with disseminated sclerosis, *Am J Psychiatry* 98:243–249, 1941.

88. Pratt RTC: An investigation of psychiatric aspects of disseminated sclerosis, *J Neurol Neurosurg Psychiatry* 14:326–336, 1951.

89. Surridge D: An investigation into some psychiatric aspects of multiple sclerosis, *Br J Psychiatry* 115:749–764, 1969.

90. Sadovnick AD, Eisen K, Ebers GC, et al: Cause of death in patients attending multiple sclerosis clinics, *Neurology* 41:1193–1196, 1991.

91. Stenager EN, Stenager E, Koch-Henriksen N, et al: Suicide and multiple sclerosis: an epidemiological investigation, *J Neurol Neurosurg Psychiatry* 55:542–545, 1992.

92. Matthews WB: Multiple sclerosis presenting with acute remitting psychiatric symptoms, *J Neurol Neurosurg Psychiatry* 42:859–863, 1979.

93. Feinstein A, du Boulay G, Ron MA: Psychotic illness in multiple sclerosis: a clinical and magnetic resonance imaging study, *Br J Psychiatry* 161:680–685, 1992.

94. Minderhoud JM, Leemhuis JG, Kremer J, et al: Sexual disturbances arising from multiple sclerosis, *Acta Neurol Scand* 70:299–306, 1984.

95. Mattson D, Petrie M, Srivastava DK, et al: Multiple sclerosis: sexual dysfunction and its response to medications, *Arch Neurol* 52:862–868, 1995.

96. Hulter BM, Lundberg PO: Sexual function in women with advanced multiple sclerosis, *J Neurol Neurosurg Psychiatry* 59:83–86, 1995.

97. Kershner P, Wang-Cheng R: Psychiatric side effects of steroid therapy, *Psychosomatics* 30:135–139, 1989.

98. Minden SL, Orav J, Schildkraut JJ: Hypomanic reactions to ACTH and prednisone treatment for multiple sclerosis, *Neurology* 38:1631–1634, 1988.

99. IFNB Multiple Sclerosis Study Group: Interferon beta-1b is effective in relapsing-remitting multiple sclerosis, *Neurology* 43:655–661, 1993.

100. Klapper JA: Interferon beta treatment of multiple sclerosis, *Neurology* 44:188; author reply 188–190, 1994.

101. PRISMS Study Group: Randomised double-blind placebo-controlled study of interferon β-1a in relapsing/remitting multiple sclerosis, *Lancet* 352:1498–1504, 1998.

102. European Study Group on interferon beta-1b in secondary progressive MS: Placebo-controlled multicentre randomised trial of interferon beta-1b in treatment of secondary progressive multiple sclerosis, *Lancet* 352:1491–1497, 1998.

103. Mohr DC, Likosky W, Dwyer P, et al: Course of depression during the initiation of interferon beta-1a treatment for multiple sclerosis, *Arch Neurol* 56:1263–1265, 1999.

104. Feinstein A, O'Connor P, Feinstein K: Multiple sclerosis, interferon beta-1b and depression a prospective investigation, *J Neurol* 249:815–820, 2002.

105. Fruehwald S, Loeffler-Stastka H, Eher R, et al: Depression and quality of life in multiple sclerosis, *Acta Neurol Scand* 104:257–261, 2001.

106. Mohr DC, Goodkin DE: Treatment of depression in multiple sclerosis: review and meta-analysis, *Clin Psychol Sci Pract* 6:1–9, 1999.

107. Krupp LB, Rizvi SA: Symptomatic therapy for underrecognized manifestations of multiple sclerosis, *Neurology* 58:S32–39, 2002.

108. Rammohan KW, Rosenberg JH, Lynn DJ, et al: Efficacy and safety of modafinil (Provigil®) for the treatment of fatigue in multiple sclerosis: a two center phase 2 study, *J Neuro Neurosurg Psychiatry* 72:179–183, 2002.

109. Krupp LB, Coyle PK, Doscher C, et al: Fatigue therapy in multiple sclerosis: results of a double-blind, randomized, parallel trial of amantadine, pemoline, and placebo, *Neurology* 45:1956–1961, 1995.

110. Falk WE, Mahnke MW, Poskanzer DC: Lithium prophylaxis of corticotropin-induced psychosis, *JAMA* 241:1011–1012, 1979.

111. Bloch M, Gur E, Shalev A: Chlorpromazine prophylaxis of steroid-induced psychosis, *Gen Hosp Psychiatry* 16:42–44, 1994.

112. Schiffer RB, Herndon RM, Rudick RA: Treatment of pathologic laughing and weeping with amitriptyline, *N Engl J Med* 312:1480–1482, 1985.

113. Foley FW, LaRocca NG, Sanders AS, et al: Rehabilitation of intimacy and sexual dysfunction in couples with multiple sclerosis, *Mult Scler* 7:417–21, 2001.

114. Fernández O: Mechanisms and current treatment of urogenital dysfunction in multiple sclerosis, *J Neurol* 249:1–8, 2002.

115. Prosiegel M, Michael C: Neuropsychology and multiple sclerosis: diagnostic and rehabilitative approaches, *J Neurol Sci* 115(suppl):S51–54, 1993.

116. Greene YM, Tariot PN, Wishart H, et al: A 12-week, open trial of donepezil hydrochloride in patients with multiple sclerosis and associated cognitive impairments, *J Clin Psychopharmacol* 20:350–356, 2000.

117. Fessel WJ: Systemic lupus erythematosus in the community, *Arch Intern Med* 134:1027–1035, 1974.

118. Hochberg MC: Updating the American College of Rheumatology revised criteria for the classification of systemic lupus erythematosus, *Arthritis Rheum* 40:1725, 1997.

119. Morgan MG: Connective tissue disorders. In Stoudemire A, Fogel BS, Greenberg DB, editors:

Psychiatric care of the medical patient, New York, 2000, Oxford University Press.

120. O'Connor JF, Musher DM: Central nervous system involvement in systemic lupus erythematosus, *Arch Neurol* 14:157–164, 1966.

121. Hay EM, Isenberg DA: Autoantibodies in central nervous system lupus, *Br J Rheumatol* 32:329–332, 1993.

122. Schneebaum AB, Singleton JD, West SG, et al: Association of psychiatric manifestations with antibodies to ribosomal P proteins in systemic lupus erythematosus, *Am J Med* 90:54–62, 1991.

123. Kozora E, Thompson LL, West SG, et al: Analysis of cognitive and psychological deficits in systemic lupus erythematosus patients with and without overt central nervous system disease, *Arthritis Rheum* 39:2035, 1996.

124. Winfield JB, Shaw M, Silverman LM, et al: Intrathecal IgG synthesis and blood-brain barrier impairment in patients with systemic lupus erythematosus and central nervous system dysfunction, *Am J Med* 74:837–844, 1983.

125. Ernerudh J, Olsson T, Lindstrom F, et al: Cerebrospinal fluid immunoglobulin abnormalities in systemic lupus erythematosus, *J Neurol Neurosurg Psychiatry* 48:807–813, 1985.

126. Bresnihan B: Systemic lupus erythematosus, *Br J Hosp Med* 22:16–25, 1979.

127. Calabrese LV, Stern TA: Neuropsychiatric manifestations of systemic lupus erythematosus, *Psychosomatics* 36:344–359, 1995.

128. Liang MH, Rogers M, Larson M, et al: The psychosocial impact of systemic lupus erythematosus and rheumatoid arthritis, *Arthritis Rheum* 27:13–19, 1984.

129. O'Connor JF: Psychoses associated with systemic lupus erythematosus, *Ann Intern Med* 51:526–536, 1959.

130. Brey RL, Holliday SL, Saklad AR, et al: Neuropsychiatric syndromes in lupus: prevalence using standardized definitions, *Neurology* 58:1214–1220, 2002.

131. Carbotte RM, Denburg SD, Denburg JA: Prevalence of cognitive impairment in systemic lupus erythematosus, *J Nerv Ment Dis* 174:347–364, 1986.

132. Falk WK: *Steroid psychosis: diagnosis and treatment.* In Manschreck TC, editor: *Psychiatric medicine update*, New York, 1981, Elsevier.

133. Silverman AJ: *Rheumatoid arthritis.* In Kaplan HI, Sadock BJ, editors: *Comprehensive textbook of psychiatry*, Baltimore, Williams & Wilkins, 1985.

134. Greer HD, Ward HP, Corbin KB: Chronic salicylate intoxication in adults, *JAMA* 193:555–558, 1965.

135. Browning CH: Nonsteroidal anti-inflammatory drugs and severe psychiatric side effects, *Int J Psychiatry Med* 26:25–34,1996.

136. Malinow KL, Molina R, Gordon B, et al: Neuropsychiatric dysfunction in primary Sjogren's syndrome, *Ann Intern Med* 103:344–349, 1985.

137. Fox RI, Tornwall J, Maruyama T, et al: Evolving concepts of diagnosis, pathogenesis, and therapy of Sjogren's syndrome, *Curr Opin Rheumatol* 10:446–456, 1998.

138. Ochtill HN, Amberson J: Acute cerebral symptomatology, a rare presentation of scleromyxedema, *J Clin Psychiatry* 39:471–475, 1978.

139. Epstein SA, Kay G, Clauw D, et al: Psychiatric disorders in patients with fibromyalgia: a multicenter investigation, *Psychosomatics* 40:57–63, 1999.

140. Cochran JW, Fox JH, Kelly MP: Reversible mental symptoms in temporal arteritis, *J Nerv Ment Dis* 166:446–447, 1978.

141. DeAngelis LM: Brain tumors, *N Engl J Med* 344:114–123, 2001.

142. Yung WKA, Janus T: *Primary neurological tumors.* In Goetz CG, Pappert EJ, editors: *Textbook of clinical neurology*, Philadelphia, 1999, WB Saunders.

143. Das A, Hochberg FH: *Metastatic neoplasms and paraneoplastic syndromes.* In Goetz CG, Pappert EJ, editors: *Textbook of clinical neurology*, Philadelphia, 1999, Saunders.

144. Weitzner MA: Psychosocial and neuropsychiatric aspects of patients with primary brain tumors, *Cancer Invest* 17:285–291, 1999.

145. Filley CM, Kleinschmidt-DeMasters BK: Neurobehavioral presentation of brain neoplasms, *West J Med* 163:19–25, 1995.

146. Avery TL: Seven cases of frontal tumor with psychiatric presentation, *Br J Psychiatry* 119:19–23, 1971.

147. Hahn CA, Dunn RH, Logue PE, et al: Prospective study of neuropsychologic testing and quality-of-life assessment of adults with primary malignant brain tumors, *Int J Radiat Oncoly Biol Phys* 55:992–999, 2003.

148. Irle E, Peper M, Wowra B, et al: Mood changes after surgery for tumors of the cerebral cortex, *Arch Neurol* 51:164–174, 1994.

149. Fisher CM: Honored guest presentation: abulia minor versus agitated behavior, *Clin Neurosurg* 31:9–31, 1983.

150. Caplan LR, Ahmed I: Depression and neurological disease, *Gen Hosp Psychiatry* 14:177–185, 1992.

151. Scheibel RS, Meyers CA, Levin VA: Cognitive dysfunction following surgery for intracerebral glioma: influence of histopathology, lesion location and treatment, *J Neuro-oncology* 30:61–69, 1996.

152. Tucha O, Smely C, Preier M, et al: Cognitive deficits before treatment among patients with brain tumors, *Neurosurgery* 47:324–333, 2000.

153. Kershner P, Wang-Cheng R: Psychiatric side-effects of steroid therapy, *Psychosomatics* 30:135–139, 1989.

154. Armstrong CL, Hunter JV, Ledakis GE et al.: Late cognitive and radiographic changes related to radiotherapy: initial prospective findings, *Neurology* 59:40–48, 2002.

155. Hochberg FH, Slotnick B: Neuropsychologic impairment in astrocytoma survivors, *Neurology* 30:172–177, 1980.

156. Abrey LE, DeAngelis LM, Yahalom J: Long-term survival in primary CNS lymphoma, *J Clin Oncol* 1998:859–863, 1998.

157. Klein M, Heimans JJ, Aaronson NK, et al: Effect of radiotherapy and other treatment-related factors on mid-term to long-term cognitive sequelae in low-grade gliomas: a comparative study, *Lancet* 360:1361–1368, 2002.

158. Guha-Thakurta N, Damek D, Pollack C, et al: Intravenous methotrexate as initial treatment for primary central nervous system lymphoma: response to therapy and quality of life of patients, *J Neurooncol* 43:259–268, 1999.

159. Fliesbach K, Urbach H, Helmstaedter C, et al: Cognitive performance and magnetic resonance imaging findings after high-dose systemic and intraventricular chemotherapy for primary central nervous system lymphoma, *Arch Neurol* 60:563–568, 2003.

160. Wilkinson ID, Romanowski CA, Jellinek DA, et al: Motor functional MRI for pre-operative and intraoperative neurosurgical guidance, *Br J Radiol* 76:98–103, 2003.

161. Meyers CA, Weitzner MA, Valentine AD, et al: Methylphenidate therapy improves cognition, mood, and function of brain tumor patients, *J Clin Oncol* 16:2522–2527, 1998.

162. Rogers MP, Mendoza AY: *Psychiatric aspects of brain tumors*, In Black PM, Loeffler JS, editors: *Cancer of the nervous system*, Cambridge: Blackwell Science, Inc.; 1997:310–334.

163. Salander P, Bergenheim T, Henrikson R: The creation of protection and hope in patients with malignant brain tumours, *Soc Sci Med* 42:985–996, 1996.

164. Sneeuw KC, Aaronson NK, Osoba D, et al: The use of significant others as proxy raters of the quality of life of patients with brain cancer, *Med Care* 35:490–506, 1997.

165. Sherer M, Meyers CA, Bergloff P: Efficacy of postacute brain injury rehabilitation for patients with primary malignant brain tumors, *Cancer* 80:250–257, 1997.

166. Talbot-Stern JK, Green T, Royle TJ: Psychiatric manifestations of systemic illness, *Emerg Med Clin North Am* 18(2):199–209, 2000.

167. Szokol JW, Vender JS: Anxiety, delirium, and pain in the intensive care unit, *Crit Care Clin* 17(4):821–842, 2001.

168. Ross GW, Bowen JD: The diagnosis and differential diagnosis of dementia, *Med Clin North Am* 86(3):455–476, 2002.

169. Reeves RR, Pendarvis EJ, Kimble R: Unrecognized medical emergencies admitted to psychiatric units, *Am J Emerg Med* 18(4):390–393, 2000.

170. Andreoli TE, Bennett JC, Carpenter CC et al: *Cecil essentials of medicine, ed 4*, Philadelphia: W.B. Saunders Company, 1997.

171. Simon RP, Aminoff MJ, Greenberg DA: *Clinical neurology, ed 4*, Stamford, Conn., 1999, Appleton and Lange.

172. Sagar SM, McGuire D: *Infectious diseases*, In Samuels MA, editor: *Manual of neurologic therapeutics, ed 6*, Philadelphia, 1999, Lippincott Williams & Wilkins.

173. Sittinger H, Muller M, Schweizer I, et al: Mild cognitive impairment after viral meningitis in adults, *J Neurol* 249(5):554–560, 2002.

174. Chu K, Kang DW, Lee JJ, et al: Atypical brainstem encephalitis caused by herpes simplex virus 2, *Arch Neurol* 59(3):460–463, 2002.

175. Coyle PK, Schutzer SE: Neurologic aspects of Lyme disease, *Med Clin North Am* 86(2):261–84, 2002.

176. Fallon BA, Nields JA: Lyme disease: a neuropsychiatric illness, *Am J Psychiatry* 151(11):1571–1583, 1994.

177. Shadick NA, Phillips CB, Logigian EL, et al: The long-term clinical outcomes of Lyme disease. A population-based retrospective cohort study, *Ann Intern Med* 121(8):560–567, 1994.

178. Seltzer EG, Gerber MA, Cartter ML, et al: Long-term outcomes of persons with Lyme disease, *JAMA* 283(5):609–616, 2000.

179. Schneider RK, Robinson MJ, Levenson JL: Psychiatric presentations of non-HIV infectious diseases: neurocysticercosis, Lyme disease, and pediatric autoimmune neuropsychiatric disorder associated with streptococcal infection, *Psychiatr Clin North Am* 25(1):1–16, 2002.

180. Garcia HH, Del Brutto OH: Taenia solium cysticercosis, *Infect Dis Clin North Am* 14(1):97–119, 2000.

181. Carpio A: Neurocysticercosis: an update, *Lancet Infect Dis* 2(12):751–62, 2002.

182. Querques J, Worth JL: *HIV infection and AIDS*. In Stern TA, Herman JB, editors: *Massachusetts General Hospital Psychiatry Update and Board Review, ed 2*, New York, 2004, McGraw-Hill Professional.

Chapter 29
Aggressive and Impulsive Patients

Kathy M. Sanders, M.D.

Patients who display aggressive and impulsive behavior frequently come to the attention of the consultation psychiatrist.[1] Because aggression and violence are complex behaviors that occur both inside and outside the medical setting, a systematic approach is useful for the management of patients with these behaviors and the support of staff who care for them. Care of the violent or impulsive patient poses a serious challenge to the psychiatrist, who needs to both rapidly and accurately assess the cause of aggression while initiating treatment. In the medical setting aggressive behavior can be associated with delirium, dementia, and other organic medical conditions; these must be evaluated prior to considering whether the behavior is the consequence of antisocial personality disorder or other types of character pathology.[2] Additionally, there is debate as to whether individuals with mental illness are at greater risk for violence than the general population. Current data suggest that people who suffer from mental illness commit violent acts more often than individuals without psychiatric diagnosis.[3–5] The psychiatrist must have a frame of reference to adequately assess for the risk of violence as well as the skills to manage it.[6]

Because of the complex nature of aggressive and impulsive behavior, this chapter focuses on the differential diagnosis of aggressive acts as it pertains to the medical setting and discusses the range of disorders associated with impulsivity. An exhaustive review of aggression and violence

within society and its larger economic and sociocultural impact is beyond the scope of this chapter.[7,8] Although workplace violence has a significant impact on the medical and hospital environment, it is not be discussed here.[9,10] In an era of growing sensitivity to the ongoing effects of terrorism and the residual psychological and behavioral effects on tortured patients, psychiatrists must be able to recognize the complex biopsychosocial context of each patient with such a history who displays aggression or impulsive behavior.[11] Traumatic brain injury, which leads to impulsive and aggressive behavior, may be the first evidence of a patient's trauma history.[12]

Neurobiology

Violent acts and aggression have biologic, environmental, and psychological determinants.[4,13] While there has never been an identifiable "aggression center" in the brains of humans, many animal studies have implicated several brain regions that may be involved in the hierarchical control of this complicated set of behaviors. Some of these areas are excitatory in nature, while others are inhibitory.[13,14–17] The hypothalamus regulates neuroendocrine responses through output to the pituitary gland and the autonomic nervous system. Within the hypothalamus, the anterior, lateral, ventromedial, and dorsomedial nuclei often are described as areas crucial to

501

animal aggression; they are considered to be involved in the control of aggression in humans. The limbic system (which includes the amygdala, hippocampus, septum, cingulate, and fornix), has regulatory control of aggressive behaviors in humans and animals. The prefrontal cortex modulates input from both the limbic system and the hypothalamus; it may have a role in the social context and judgmental aspects of aggression.[18] Damage to the frontal lobe from many causes (including violent trauma and closed head injury [CHI]) results in increased impulsivity behavior and less executive control of emotional reactivity. Anoxic injury to the brain also results in similar impairment.

Low central serotonin (5-HT) function has been correlated with impulsive aggression. Violent patients have been found to have a low turnover of 5-HT, as measured by its major metabolite 5-hydroxyindoleacetic acid (5-HIAA) in the cerebrospinal fluid (CSF). Acetylcholine in the limbic system stimulates aggression in animals; cholinergic pesticides have been cited as provoking violence in humans. Gamma aminobutyric acid (GABA) is thought to have inhibitory effects on aggression in both humans and animals. Norepinephrine may enhance some types of aggression in animals and could play a role in impulsivity and episodic violence in humans. Dopamine increases aggressive behavior in animal models, but its effect in humans is less clear due to its psychotomimetic effects.[19-21]

In considering the genetics of aggressive and impulsive behavior, there has been no specific chromosomal abnormality yet associated with an increased risk for aggression; however, polymorphisms of tryptophan hydroxylase may be correlated with impulsive aggression. The relationship between the syndrome involving XYY and impulsivity is questionable, and the relationship remains inconclusive. Hormonal influences of androgens often are cited as a major factor in aggressive behavior because they may play an organizational role in the development of these behaviors. Some attribute a lower threshold for violence in women to lower levels of estrogen and progesterone during the menstrual cycle. More recently, lower cholesterol levels in patients with personality disorders have been associated with aggressive and impulsive behavior.[22,23]

Differential Diagnosis

The multiaxial *Diagnostic and Statistical Manual of Mental Disorders*, fourth edition *(DSM-IV)*[24] diagnostic system has five domains that may help categorize aggressive or violent behaviors. It is important to make an accurate diagnosis because the acute and chronic management of aggressive behaviors hinges on the diagnosis. The diagnosis of underlying psychiatric disorders associated with aggression rests on initial consideration of its organic causes. These may include intoxication or withdrawal from substances of abuse (e.g., alcohol, cocaine, opiates, and sedative-hypnotics). Once it is determined that these factors are not involved, then a psychiatric differential should be created; conditions ranging from major mental illness to personality disorders, interpersonal situations that alter coping mechanisms, such as being a victim or witness of violence, and family and job stress should be considered.

Medical Causes

When considering the differential diagnosis of violent and impulsive behavior, the psychiatrist should first assume that a medical condition or substance abuse problem is the root of the behavior before considering psychiatric illnesses.

A variety of primary central nervous system (CNS) disorders can generate aggressive and violent behavior; particular attention should be paid to seizure disorders. Seizure-related aggression involves ictal aggression (typically nonpurposeful, stereotyped behavior during the seizure), postictal aggression (secondary to confusion or agitation), and interictal aggression (may result from subthreshold electrical brain activity) that elicits violence.

Other medical causes include dementias of any etiology, delirium from a host of underlying medical conditions, traumatic brain injury, and hormonal and metabolic abnormalities. For a more exhaustive differential of the underlying medical causes of delirium and dementias, see Table 29-1 and Chapters 12 and 13.

Violence is more prevalent in patients with alcohol abuse and dependence than in those without a substance abuse diagnosis. In an acutely intoxi-

Table 29-1. Differential Diagnosis of Psychosis and Agitation

General Category	Cause/Diagnosis
Organic mental disorders	Aphasia
	Catatonia
	Delirium
	Dementia
	Frontal lobe syndrome
	Organic hallucinosis
	Organic delusional disorder
	Organic mood disorder (secondary mania)
	Seizure disorders
Drugs	Substance abuse (e.g., cocaine and opiates)
	Steroids
	Procarbazine HCl
	Antibiotics
	Anticholinergics
Drug withdrawal	Alcohol and sedative-hypnotics (barbiturates and benzodiazepines)
	Clonidine
	Opiates
Psychotic disorders	Schizophrenia
	Delusional disorder
	Psychotic disorders NOS
	Brief reactive psychosis
	Schizoaffective
	Shared paranoid disorder (*folie a deux*)
Mood disorders	Manic-depressive disorder
	Major depression with psychotic/agitated features
	Catatonia
Anxiety/fear	Anxiety disorders
	Acute reaction to stress
Discomfort	Pain
	Hypoxia
	Akathisia
Personality disorder	Antisocial
	Borderline
	Paranoid
	Schizotypal
Disorders of infancy, childhood, or adolescence	Autism
	Mental retardation
	ADHD
	Conduct disorder

cated state, patients may be disinhibited and therefore at greater risk for violence. During the withdrawal state, delirium and/or agitation may also precipitate violence. Chronic alcohol abuse that causes brain damage or dementia may lead to aggressive behaviors that persist beyond the state of acute intoxication or withdrawal. Acute intoxication or withdrawal from psychostimulants (e.g., cocaine and amphetamine) can lead to agitation, paranoia, psychosis, and violence. Hallucinogens (e.g., phencyclidine and lysergic acid diethylamide [LSD]) may precipitate psychosis and violence. Sedative-hypnotics (e.g., barbiturates or benzodiazepines) can result in disinhibition, and withdrawal from these agents may cause delirium. States of opiate intoxication and withdrawal, as well as behaviors required to obtain these drugs, may also increase the risk for violence.

Other prescription medications (e.g., anticholinergics and steroids) and over-the-counter preparations may induce aggression. In the fitness subculture, the use of various herbal and nutritional supplements and the abuse of hormone therapies may result in an altered mental status that could be manifest as violence, aggression, and impulsivity.

In evaluating and determining the likelihood of organic and medical factors that play a role in an aggressive or impulsive episode, one should take a history, obtain corroborating information from family or friends, perform pertinent laboratory studies, and conduct a physical examination that will narrow the differential diagnosis. For example:

Mr. A, a 37-year-old with chronic alcohol abuse, was brought by police to the emergency department (ED) after getting into an argument with staff at a local shelter. The argument escalated in an uncharacteristic manner for Mr. A; he pulled a knife on a staff member but was subdued before being able to use it. During examination in the ED, he was uncooperative at triage; he shouted expletives at nursing and security staff. He was thought to be acutely intoxicated until his vital signs were checked; both his temperature and blood pressure were elevated. After laboratory studies were drawn for alcohol levels and for evidence of substances of abuse, Mr. A's treating doctors were surprised to find that the blood alcohol level was negligible. He was treated for alcohol withdrawal with rapid abatement of obstreperous behavior.

Ms. B, a 45-year-old woman with chronic mental illness returned to the ED for the third time in a week. Each time, she was evaluated for a decompensation of her chronic schizoaffective illness. After a dose of her usual neuroleptic, she became calm and capable of returning to her group home. The day she came back to the ED, her case manager had found her roaming the streets of her neighborhood and picking fights with neighbors and strangers. Although she readily backed down before actually becoming violent, her persistent and impulsive flares of temper required containment and further evaluation. This time, more extensive laboratory studies showed a sodium blood level of 115 mEq/L. She was admitted to the medical service for management of her hyponatremia and probable syndrome if inappropriate antidiuretic hormone (SIADH) secretion.

Ms. C, a young woman, was brought to the ED by her family when she started to aggressively shove her mother without provocation. Ms. C had been invited to a family dinner in honor of her recent job change. She was extremely irritable and accused her family of being part of a plot to prevent her from being successful in her new job. When they tried to dissuade her from her thinking, she became belligerent, aggressive, and threatening. The family brought her to the ED, worried she was emotionally unbalanced. At triage, she was fully alert but visibly shaking and irritated by any questions or delay in the process. She admitted to intentionally taking extra isoniazid tablets (which had been prescribed for a positive purified protein derivative [PPD] skin test during a pre-employment medical screening) in an overdose attempt while overwhelmed by concerns about her new job. Although she took fewer than 10 tablets, the psychiatrist recommended medical management before further psychiatric evaluation. Within minutes of her arrival in the ED, she had a grand mal seizure.

Psychiatric Causes

Violent and impulsive behaviors are nonspecific symptoms that may be part of most major mental illnesses at some time in the course of the illness. When considering whether a psychiatric illness is causative of violent behavior, it is important to distinguish among major mental illnesses on Axis I, personality disorders on Axis II, and organic causes on Axis III.

Schizophrenia/Psychosis Not Otherwise Specified (NOS)

The prevalence for violent behavior in individuals with schizophrenia is similar to that for those with major depression and bipolar disorder; however, it is five times higher than individuals with

no Axis I diagnosis. Individuals who are paranoid with delusions of persecution may act violently toward a perceived threat. Command hallucinations, associated with violent content toward oneself or others, dramatically increase the potential for violence in individuals with schizophrenia. Disorganized thought and behavior may also lead to violence.

Affective Illness

Unipolar depression may be accompanied by an increase in hostility and by anger attacks (nearly half of the time) that can lead to violent behavior.[25] Depression with psychotic features may further increase the chances of violence. Bipolar patients with a manic, hypomanic, or mixed presentation often display irritability, anger outbursts, omnipotence, and paranoia, which may lead to impulsive aggression.

Impulsive disorders as classified by the *DSM-IV* are a "residual" diagnostic category.[26] Diagnoses in this category include kleptomania, pyromania, pathologic gambling, trichotillo-mania, intermittent explosive disorder, and impulse-control disorder NOS (not otherwise specified).[27,28] Each of these conditions involves a drive or a temptation to perform an act that is harmful to the person or to others or the failure to resist an impulse. Other associated features are the experience of increasing tension (of dysphoria or arousal) before committing the act, which is followed by a release of tension, a sense of gratification, or a sense of pleasure and relief during and after the act. There also may be a sense of guilt, regret, or self-reproach following the behavior.

Controversy exists concerning whether these conditions are distinct diagnoses or variants of another Axis I disorder. In some ways, they are similar to obsessive-compulsive disorder (OCD), substance dependence, mood disorders, eating disorders, paraphilias, and mental disorders due to a general medical condition because similar treatments work for each of these disorders.[29,30] Patients diagnosed with impulse-control disorders have an increased risk of being diagnosed with substance abuse disorders, OCD and other anxiety disorders, eating disorders, and mood disorders. Moreover, there is an increased incidence of substance abuse disorders and mood disorders in family members of those with impulse-control disorders. Theories place impulse-control disorders on a spectrum of affective disorders, as a variant of OCD, or as a blend of mood, impulse, and compulsive disorders. Historically these disorders were thought to result from psychodynamic conflicts; however, more biologic hypotheses have been explored recently since improvement of impulsive symptoms has been accompanied by use of the serotonergic antidepressants.[31]

Intermittent explosive disorder is a diagnosis that characterizes individuals who have episodes of dyscontrol, assaultive acts, and extreme aggression that is out of proportion to the precipitating event and is not explained by another Axis I or Axis II disorder. It is considered very rare and mostly a diagnosis of exclusion.[31,32] Intermittent explosive disorder and personality change resulting from a general medical condition, aggressive type, are the current diagnoses available to patients with episodic violent behavior. Most violent behavior can be accounted for by a variety of psychiatric and medical conditions. The most common diagnosis associated with violence is personality change resulting from a general medical condition (e.g., seizures, head trauma, neurological abnormality, dementia, or delirium), aggressive or disinhibited type. Personality disorders of the borderline or antisocial type must also be ruled out. Psychosis from schizophrenia or a manic episode may cause episodic violence. Aggressive outbursts while intoxicated or while withdrawing from a substance of abuse would rule out the diagnosis of intermittent explosive disorder. Psychopharmacology is commonly employed in the chronic management of this disorder. Anticonvulsants, lithium, β-blockers, anxiolytics, neuroleptics, antidepressants (both serotonergic and polycyclic agents), and psychostimulants are used with varying success. The acute management of aggressive and violent behavior may involve the use of physical restraints and the rapid use of parenteral neuroleptics and benzodiazepines. Long-term outpatient management of intermittent explosive disorder requires attention to the therapeutic alliance between the clinician and the patient.

Impulse control disorder NOS is a category of disorders that do not meet diagnostic criteria for any of the previously discussed impulse-control disorders or for another mental disorder involving impulse control. Included in this category are diagnoses, such as pathologic spending, pathologic shopping, repetitive self-mutilation, compulsive sexual behavior, and compulsive face picking. Most of the literature on this diagnostic category focuses on repetitive self-mutilation. It is more common in women than in men. However, it is considered endemic in male prisons. Two thirds of self-mutilators have a history of sexual and physical abuse during childhood. The disorder starts in adolescence and is characterized by severe psychosocial morbidity.[26]

Attention deficit disorder with (ADHD) or without (ADD) hyperactivity begins in childhood and can persist into adulthood. The impulsivity, inattentiveness, and behavioral problems that accompany this condition may lead to aggressive acts. Other childhood developmental disorders and learning disorders may have concomitant aggressive and impulsive behaviors, including self-mutilation.

Diagnoses on Axis II

Antisocial personality disorder is frequently associated with violent and impulsive behavior and criminality. Further complicating this is the fact that sociopathic individuals frequently have co-morbid substance abuse. Patients with borderline personality disorder may display aggression toward themselves and/or others as part of their impulsive behaviors. Individuals with a paranoid personality disorder react to perceived threats with violent reactions toward that perceived threat. Those with mental retardation and other developmental disorders have poor impulse control; depending on the underlying causes (e.g., head trauma) of retardation, these states may lead to violence.[33–35]

Diagnoses on Axes IV and V

Environmental precipitants are as important as underlying psychiatric or medical diagnoses when determining a patient's level of dangerousness. The parameters on Axis IV (e.g., occupational, social relationship, educational, housing, economic, and legal problems) can lead to aggression and violence. A patient's current level of functioning (as measured on Axis V) will aid the clinician in predicting the threat of violence in a particular patient. The more stressors one has on Axis IV and the lower the level of functioning on Axis V, the higher the possibility for violence in those prone to act in a violent manner.

Assessment of the Violent Patient

General Considerations

To ensure safety of the patient and those around him or her, the evaluator must act swiftly to provide an accurate diagnosis and acute management.[37] Under more emergent conditions, the "ABCs" of emergency evaluation of aggressive and impulsive behavior are (1) safety, (2) diagnosis, and (3) management.[6] Safety is the first priority in the assessment of the violent patient. Control of the patient and of the environment must be obtained to prevent harm to the staff and to the individual being assessed. Without proper safety mechanisms, adequate evaluation is impossible. Diagnosis of underlying psychopathology, substance abuse, and/or medical conditions guides specific treatment. If there is no condition amenable to medical or psychiatric interventions, then one must consider that the legal authorities may more suitably manage the patient's behavior. Management, in the form of chemical sedation, with neuroleptics and/or benzodiazepines, and seclusion and restraint, may be required to allow the evaluator to perform a safe and accurate assessment.[36,37]

Interview of the Potentially Violent Patient

Before the examiner can interview the potentially violent patient, a safe environment must be secured. All potentially dangerous materials should be removed from the patient and from the interview room. Objects that can be used as weapons (e.g., pens, needles, and phones) should be scrutinized prior to and during the interview. The interview room should allow for possible escape and should be highly visible. The ideal room for such an interview should contain an

emergency call button; the room should not be able to be locked from within. The consultant should pay careful attention to the patient's behavior for signs of imminent danger. Escalating behaviors may include: (1) verbal threats and/or gestures; (2) rapid movements, agitation, pacing, knocking over furniture, and/or slamming doors; and (3) invasion of personal space, clenching of the jaw, or signs of muscular tension. At this time, the examiner's interventions are designed to direct the patient to regain the locus of control. If the examiner's attempts to redirect the patient fail to decrease the patient's level of agitation and increase his or her level of self-control, then tranquilization and emergency restraints may be necessary to regain control and to ensure safety.

History

The medical history must be obtained in the initial phases of the interview process to ascertain and to treat any potentially life-threatening medical causes for the patient's agitation or aggressive behavior. The mnemonic, WWHHHHIMPS, can be used to quickly rule-out life-threatening causes (Table 29-2).

Other pertinent history includes a search for previous head trauma, neurologic or seizure disorders (e.g., febrile childhood seizures), and previous psychiatric illness and substance abuse that may increase the patient's risk for aggressivity and guide treatment.

Table 29-2. WWHHHHIMPS, A Mnemonic for Life-Threatening Causes of Delirium

Withdrawal (e.g., from barbiturates)
Wernicke's encephalopathy
Hypoxia and *Hypoperfusion* of the brain
Hypertensive crisis
Hypoglycemia
Hyper/hypothermia
Intracranial bleed/mass
Meningitis/encephalitis
Poisoning
Status epilepticus

Adapted from Wise MG: *Delirium.* In Yudofsky SC, Hales RE, editors: *Textbook of neuropsychiatry and clinical neurosciences,* Washington, DC, 2002, American Psychiatric Publishing.

Assessment for violence is one of the most difficult tasks for the medical and psychiatric professional. The best indicator of future violence remains a history of violence. Therefore, seeking a history of previous violence in a patient is an integral part of the interview. Given the nature of violent perpetrators, it is difficult to elicit an accurate account. The best approach is indirect questioning of violent behaviors (Table 29-3).

Examination of the Violent Patient

The mental status examination of the potentially violent patient begins like a standard examination. However, as has been previously emphasized, careful consideration must be given to safety. If at any time during the exam, the examiner feels unsafe, the interview should cease until proper measures can be put in place to ensure safety. The initial assessment should focus on elements of the mental status (e.g., the sensorium, disordered thought, mood and affect, cognition, agitation, hallucinations, and evidence of intoxication by drugs

Table 29-3. Assessment of Violence

1. Determine the specifics of past violence.
   a. At what age did violent acts begin?
   b. How frequently did those acts occur?
   c. What was the most recent act?
   d. How severe were the actions?
   e. Has there been a recurring pattern of escalation preceding violence?
   f. Have there been common precipitants surrounding the acts?
   g. Have any violent actions resulted in legal recourse or incarceration?
   h. Has there been a history of recklessness, suicidal ideations, arrests, or impulsivity?
   i. Does the patient have a family history of violence, abuse, or gang involvement?
2. Ask screening questions.
   a. Do you ever think of harming anyone else?
   b. Have you ever seriously injured another human being? (Tell me about the most violent thing that you have ever done.)
3. Ask about prior evaluations and treatments related to violent behavior, including medical workups, diagnostic tests, and old records.
4. Collect information from as many ancillary sources as possible, including family members, victims, court records, medical records, and previous treaters.

or alcohol). Mental status abnormalities or symptoms (as listed above) can increase the likelihood of aggressive action and alert the physician to medical conditions that require further workup or immediate treatment. For example, affective disorders, either mania or depression, may impair a patient's judgment and lead to violence. The impulsivity accompanied by mania can lead to irrational thoughts and aggression. The hopelessness of a depressed individual, combined with psychotic thoughts, may lead a person to attempt suicide or murder. Thought disorders, psychosis with paranoid features, and command hallucinations make for a situation that can produce dangerous and difficult-to-predict behavior. Just as in the evaluation of the suicidal patient, patients with violent thoughts toward others must be assessed in terms of their specific plan, the lethality of their plan, and the possibility that the plan can actually be carried out. Determination of the relative risk of violence in this manner helps one develop a disposition plan (e.g., inpatient versus outpatient management). Documentation of agitation through standardized rating scales, such as the Overt Agitation Severity Scale (OASS), is useful in anticipating escalating behaviors and determining when to intervene.[1]

Physical examination is targeted to find medical causes of violence and is guided by findings in the history. Because violence is more likely in a patient with an organic brain syndrome or acute intoxication, one should focus on elements of the examination that will help to identify these diagnoses. Based on physical findings and the patient's medical history, appropriate diagnostic tests should be performed. These include but are neither mandatory nor limited to: (1) routine chemistry tests, blood counts, and tests of serum and/or urine toxicology; (2) an organic workup for dementia; (3) neuroimaging, electroencephalogram (EEG), and other radiological tests as indicated; and (4) neuropsychological and cognitive testing.

Approach to the Treatment of the Violent Patient

Management of the aggressive patient can be divided into acute management and chronic management. There are no medications that specifically target aggressive behavior; the psychiatrist must apply general principles to guide treatment. One should attempt to optimize treatment of the underlying psychiatric illness if present; if that fails, it is best to use the most benign treatments in an empirical and systematic way. Target symptoms should be well defined and monitored in response to specific interventions. Efficacy should be defined by parameters that can be observed and measured. The symptom checklist in the OASS is useful for documenting progress in the management of agitation and aggressive behaviors. In the acute setting the goal in treatment of the violent patient should be to reduce the risk of harm to both the staff and the patient and to facilitate the diagnostic process. Medications that can be delivered intramuscularly and that have a rapid onset and a favorable side-effect profile should be first-line treatments. Once the patient is calm and a more thorough assessment is achieved, the psychiatrist can decide between outpatient management or hospitalization (voluntary versus involuntary).

Benzodiazepines are rapid, safe, and easily administered first-line drugs for moderate to severe agitation and for cases in which the potential for escalating behavioral dyscontrol exists. The caveat concerning use of benzodiazepines is the paradoxic reaction seen in certain character-disordered patients or the worsening of symptoms in the elderly. When these medications are given in the intramuscular or oral form, they are effective sedatives in the acute care setting. Alprazolam acts rapidly, but it can only be administered orally. Its initial dose is usually 0.5 mg, and acutely the dose should not in general exceed 4 mg/day. Diazepam (with an initial dose of 5 mg) has a rapid onset of action and can be administered intramuscularly, orally, or intravenously. It has a long half-life (30 to 100 hours), and therefore it should be used cautiously in elderly patients who will not metabolize it efficiently. Lorazepam may be given sublingually, orally, intramuscularly, or intravenously. The usual starting dose is 1 mg; its moderate half-life (10 to 20 hours) makes it an ideal medication for initial treatment. Because it has no active metabolites there is little risk of accumulation if the patient requires more than one dose to manage and maintain behavioral calm. In addition, lorazepam is metabolized by both the liver and kidneys, which makes it easier to use in medically ill patients with organ system failure.[38]

Mr. D, a 54-year-old married executive, was seen in the cardiac care unit (CCU) because he was unable to remain in bed and cooperate with the nursing staff. He had been admitted earlier that day from the ED, where he was diagnosed with an acute myocardial infarction (MI) and was given intravenous tissue plasminogen activator (TPA). Upon arrival in the CCU, he was distractible; he made frequent attempts to get out of bed and pace. He could be redirected only briefly before resuming efforts to get out of bed. Prior to the consultant arriving in the CCU, Mr. D was given diazepam and morphine for sedation to allow a computed topography (CT) scan of the head to be completed. The neuroimaging study revealed a midline intraventricular bleed presumably associated with the anticoagulant treatment initiated in the ED. Although initially seen as a type A personality with restlessness in a structured and controlled environment, his agitated and impulsive behavior stemmed from central nervous system irritability due to the presence of blood in his ventricles. Ongoing management with a high-potency neuroleptic was begun as further use of benzodiazepines and opiates altered his mental status.

Antipsychotics, particularly high-potency agents, are often effective in reducing agitation and violence in both the psychotic and nonpsychotic patients. Haloperidol, a high-potency neuroleptic, is frequently used in this setting because of its favorable side-effect profile and overall cardiopulmonary safety. It may be given orally, intramuscularly, or intravenously, and is usually effective when one or two 5-mg doses are administered intramuscularly or intravenously. Given intravenously, it is less likely to precipitate extrapyramidal side effects; however, regardless of route, one must attend to the risk of torsades de pointes. Virtually any neuroleptic may diminish aggressivity, but careful consideration should be given to the potency, history of response, side-effect profile of the particular medication, and the psychiatric and medical history of the patient. Atypical antipsychotics (e.g., clozapine, olanzapine, ziprasidone, and risperidone) have been used more in recent years.[39–41] Currently, ziprasidone is the only atypical neuroleptic that is available in a parenteral form. Intramuscular olanzapine has been Food and Drug Administration (FDA)-approved but has not yet been released.[42] In general atypical neuroleptics are better tolerated with than conventional agents; they have fewer extrapyramidal side effects and are associated with better long-term compliance.[43–45]

Mr. E, a 32-year-old single Russian immigrant, was forcibly brought to the ED after calling 911 and seeking "help" by provocatively expressing passive suicidal ideation. He was intoxicated with alcohol, agitated, and angry, which made staff unable to reason with him. He was placed in four-point restraints and a psychiatry consult was called to assess his mental status and risk for suicide. His agitation was intense as was his anger toward the police and their treatment of him. He would not engage in a meaningful exchange without the use of medications. After haloperidol (5 mg intramuscularly) was administered, he became more cooperative and could be examined. It became apparent that his right arm hurt. He described how he was forcibly removed from his apartment and taken down four flights of stairs. Once adequately calm and in control, his restraints were removed for an x-ray examination of his swollen elbow, which revealed a fractured elbow that was then placed into a cast. His rage and anger returned, and he demanded to be released from the hospital.

The long-term management of the violent patient poses a complex challenge for the treating psychiatrist. First, one should maximize appropriate treatment of any underlying psychiatric disorder, using both psychotherapy and pharmacotherapy. Selective serotonin-reuptake inhibitors (SSRIs) have been used with some efficacy in patients with personality disorders, dementia, and mental retardation. One should be cautious when using any antidepressant in patients with bipolar disorder because this may exacerbate, rather than lessen, certain symptoms.[46] Lithium has been used to reduce aggression in patients with mental retardation, conduct disorder, and antisocial personality disorder and in prison inmates; the target lithium level should be between 0.6 and 0.9 mEq/L. Anticonvulsants (e.g., carbamazepine, valproic acid, and phenytoin) have been used with some success in reducing impulsive aggression. Gabapentin also has significant mood-stabilizing benefits that may be used in the management of aggression in a wide range of patients. Gabapentin has also been used for patients with substantial anxiety and character pathology. Benzodiazepines may be used in chronic, as well as acute, settings. Buspirone, a $5-HT_{1A}$ partial agonist, is a nonbenzodiazepine anxiolytic that has been used as an adjunct treatment for agitation and aggression.[47] β-Adrenergic blockers have been used in high doses to treat aggression; their effects may not be seen for several months. All patients should be started at a low dose and then titrated to effect and tolerance. Propranolol may be gradually

increased up to 1 g/day; it has been used successfully in patients with dementia and organic brain disorders.[48] Nadolol (40 to 120 mg/day) and metoprolol (200 to 300 mg/day) may also be used in patients who are chronically aggressive. Psychostimulants may be effective in reducing impulsive aggression in children with ADD/ADHD and in adults with residual ADHD. Bupropion and desipramine are other medications have been efficacious in adults with residual ADHD.

The long-term use of atypical neuroleptics in the management of aggression may provide good behavioral control while addressing the underlying psychotic and affective components of aggression. Clozapine, risperidone, olanzapine, ziprasidone, and aripiprazole broaden the options for the treatment of psychosis.[49,50] Their relatively benign side-effect profile allows for compliance, and their ability to enhance mood increase the options for the types of patients that can be treated for aggressive and impulsive behaviors.

Psychotherapeutic approaches (e.g., behavioral techniques, cognitive-behavioral therapy, and group and family therapy) have also been used to treat aggression and violence.[51] Such techniques (e.g., limit setting, contingent reinforcement, distraction and redirection, relaxation, and biofeedback) have been utilized in the ongoing inpatient and outpatient management of aggressive and impulsive patients with mixed success. The combination of medication and psychotherapy is still the best approach to the chronic management of aggression and violence.

References

1. Hales RE, Silver JM, Yudofsky SC, et al: *Aggression and agitation*. In Wise MG, Rundell JR, editors: *Textbook of consultation-liaison psychiatry: psychiatry in the medically ill*, Washington, DC, 2002, American Psychiatric Publishing.
2. Wise MG: *Delirium*. In Yudofsky SC, Hales RE, editors: *Textbook of neuropsychiatry and clinical neurosciences*, Washington, DC, 2002, American Psychiatric Publishing.
3. Monahan J: Mental disorder and violent behavior: perceptions and evidence, *Am Psychol* 47(4):511–521, 1992.
4. Renfrew JW: *Aggression and its causes: a biopsychosocial approach*, New York, 1997, Oxford University Press.
5. Crowner ML: *Understanding and treating violent psychiatric patients*, Washington, DC, 2000, American Psychiatric Publishing.

6. Sanders KM: *Approach to the violent patient.* In Stern TA, Herman JB, Slavin PL, editors: *The MGH guide to psychiatry in primary care*, New York, 1998, McGraw-Hill.

7. Beck JC: Legal and ethical duties of the clinician treating a patient who is liable to be impulsively violent, *Behav Sci Law* 16(3):375–389, 1998.

8. Blue HC, Griffith EE: Sociocultural and therapeutic perspectives on violence, *Psychiatr Clin North Am* 18(3):571–87, 1995.

9. Fleming P, Harvery HD: Strategy development in dealing with violence against employees in the workplace, *J R Soc Health* 122(4):226–232, 2002.

10. Viitasara E, Menckel E: Developing a framework for identifying individual and organizational risk factors for the prevention of violence in the health-care sector, *Work* 19(2):117–23, 2002.

11. Pferrerbaum B, North CS, Flynn BW, et al: The emotional impact of injury following an international terrorist incident, *Public Health Rev* 29(2–4):271–280, 2001.

12. Smith F, Sanders K: *The patient following closed head injury.* In Stern TA, Herman JB, Slavin PL, editors: *The MGH guide to primary care psychiatry, ed 2*, New York, 2004, McGraw-Hill.

13. Kavoussi R, Armstead P, Coccaro E: The neurobiology of impulsive aggression, *Psychiatr Clin North Am* 20(2):395–403, 1997.

14. Garza-Trevino ES: Neurobiological factors in aggressive behavior, *Hosp Comm Psychiatry* 45(7):690–699, 1994.

15. Volavka J: *Neurobiology of violence*, Washington DC, 2002, American Psychiatric Publishing.

16. Stein DJ, Hollander E, Liebowitz MR: Neurobiology of impulsivity and the impulse control disorders, *J Neuropsychiatr Clin Neurosci* 5(1):9–17, 1993.

17. Oquendo MA, Mann JJ: The biology of impulsivity and suicidality, *Psychiatr Clin North Am* 23(1):11–25, 2000.

18. Best M, Williams JM, Coccaro EF: Evidence for a dysfunctional prefrontal circuit in patients with an impulsive aggressive disorder, *Proc Natl Acad Sci* 99(12):8448–8453, 2002.

19. Miczek KA, Fish EW, DeBold JF, DeAlmeida RM: Social and neural determinants of aggressive behavior: pharmacotherapeutic targets at serotonin, dopamine and gamma-aminobutyric acid system, *Psychopharmacology* 163(3–4):434–458, 2002.

20. Coccaro EF: Impulsive aggression and central serotonergic system function in humans: an example of a dimensional brain-behavior relationship, *Int Clin Psychopharmacol* 7(1):3–12, 1992.

21. Schmahl CG, McGlashan TH, Bremner JD: Neurobiological correlates of borderline personality disorder, *Psychopharmacol Bull* 36(2):69–87, 2002.

22. Buydens-Branchey L, Branchey M, Hudson J, Fergeson P: Low HDL cholesterol, aggression and altered central serotonergic activity, *Psychiatry Res* 93(2):93–102, 2000.

23. New AS, Sevin EM, Mitropoulou V, et al: Serum cholesterol and impulsivity in personality disorders, *Psychiatry Res* 85(2):145–150, 1999.

24. American Psychiatric Association: *Diagnostic and statistical manual of mental disorders*, ed 4, Washington, DC, 1994, American Psychiatric Press.

25. Fava M, Buolo RD, Wright EC, et al: Fenfluramine challenge in unipolar depression with and without anger attacks, *Psychiatry Res* 94(1):9–18, 2000.

26. Wise MG, Tierney JG: *Impulse-control disorders not elsewhere classified.* In Hales RE, Yudofsky SG, editors: *Textbook of clinical psychiatry*, ed 4, Arlington, Va, 2003, American Psychiatric Publishing.

27. DeCaria CM, Hollander E, Grossman R, et al: Diagnosis, neurobiology, and treatment of pathological gambling. *J Clin Psychiatry* 57(suppl. 8):80–84, 1996.

28. Burt VE: *Impulse-control disorders not elsewhere classified.* In Sadock BJ, Sadock Va, editors: *Kaplan and Sadock's comprehensive textbook of psychiatry,* ed 7, Baltimore, 1999, Lippincott Williams and Wilkins.

29. McElroy SL, Hudson JI, Pope HG Jr, et al: The DSM-III-R Impulse Control Disorder not elsewhere classified: clinical characteristics and relationship to other psychiatric disorders, *Am J Psychiatry* 149(3):318–327, 1992.

30. McElroy SL, Pope HG Jr, Keck PE Jr, et al: Are impulse-control disorders related to bipolar disorder? *Comp Psychiatry* 37(4):229–240, 1996.

31. Coccaro EF, Kavoussi RJ, Berman ME, Lish JD: Intermittent explosive disorder-revised: development, reliability, and validity of research criteria, *Comp Psychiatry* 39(6): 368–376, 1998.

32. McElroy SL, Soutullo CA, Beckman DA, et al: DSM-IV intermittent explosive disorder: a report of 27 cases, *J Clin Psychiatry* 59(4):203–210, 1998.

33. Stein DJ, Hollander E, Cohen L, et al: Neuropsychiatric impairment in impulsive personality disorders, *Psychiatry Res* 48(3):257–266, 1993.

34. Hollander E: Managing aggressive behavior in patients with obsessive-compulsive disorder and borderline personality disorder, *J Clin Psychiatry* 60(suppl 15):38–44, 1999.

35. Goodman M, New A: Impulsive aggression in borderline personality disorder, *Curr Psychiatry Rep* 2(1):56–61, 2000.

36. Blumenreich P, Lippmann S, Bacani-Oropilla T: Violent patients. Are you prepared to deal with them? *Postgrad Med* 90(2):201–206, 1991.

37. Lande RG: The dangerous patient, *J Fam Pract* 29(1):74–78, 1989.

38. Lavine R: Psychopharmacological treatment of aggression and violence in the substance abusing population, *J Psychoactive Drugs* 29(4):321–329, 1997.

39. Fava M: Psychopharmacologic treatment of pathologic aggression, *Psychiatr Clin North Am* 20(2):427–451, 1997.

40. Spivak B, Mester R, Wittenberg N, et al: Reduction of aggressiveness and impulsiveness during clozapine

treatment in chronic neuroleptic-resistant schizophrenic patients, *Clin Neuropharmacol* 20(5):442–446, 1997.

41. Schwartz TL, Masand PS: The role of atypical antipsychotics in the treatment of delirium, *Psychosomatics* 43(3):171–174, 2002.

42. Currier GW, Buckley PF, Daniel DG, Glick RL: Intramuscular atypical antipsychotics: their promise and practice, *Psych Issues Emerg Care Settings* Fall: 3–18, 2002.

43. Keck PE, McElroy SL, Arnold LM: Ziprasidone: a new atypical antipsychotic, *Expert Opin Pharmacother* 2(6):1033–1042, 2001.

44. Brook S, Lucey JV, Gunn KP: Intramuscular ziprasidone compared with intramuscular haloperidol in the treatment of acute psychosis, *J Clin Psychiatry* 61(12):933–941, 2000.

45. Daniel DG, Potkin SG, Reeves KR, et al: Intramuscular ziprasidone 20 mg is effective in reducing acute agitation associated with psychosis: a double-blind, randomized trial, *Psychopharmacology* 155(2): 128–134, 2001.

46. Coccaro EF, Kavoussi RJ: Fluoxetine and impulsive aggressive behavior in personality-disordered subjects, *Arch Gen Psychiatry* 54(12):1081–1088, 1997.

47. Ratey JJ, Leveroni CL, Miller AC, et al: Low-dose buspirone to treat agitation and maladaptive behavior in brain-injured patients: two case reports, *J Clin Psychopharmacol* 12(5):362–364, 1992.

48. Greendyke RM, Kanter DR, Schuster DB, et al: Propranolol treatment of assaultive patients with organic brain disease: a double-blind crossover, placebo-controlled study, *J Nerv Ment Dis* 174(5):290–294, 1986.

49. McGavin JK, Goa KL: Aripiprazole, *CNS Drugs* 16(11):779–786, 2002.

50. Kelleher JP, Centorrino F, Albert MJ, Baldessarini RJ: Advances in atypical antipsychotics for the treatment of schizophrenia: new formulations and new agents, *CNS Drugs* 16(4):249–261, 2002.

51. Alpert JE, Spellman MK: Psychotherapeutic approaches to aggressive and violent patients, *Psychiatr Clin North Am* 20(2): 453–472, 1997.

Chapter 30

Catatonia, Neuroleptic Malignant Syndrome, and Serotonin Syndrome

Gregory L. Fricchione, M.D.
Jeff C. Huffman, M.D.
Theodore A. Stern, M.D.
George Bush, M.D.

The syndromes described in this chapter each involve a complex interaction of motor, behavioral, and systemic manifestations that are derived from unclear mechanisms. What *is* clear is that neurotransmitters, such as dopamine (DA), gamma aminobutyric acid (GABA), and glutamate (GLU) are of major importance in catatonia and neuroleptic malignant syndrome (NMS), while serotonin (5-hydroxytryptamine [5-HT]) is a key to the serotonin syndrome (SS). Many now believe that NMS represents a catatonic state secondary to use of DA-blocking medications. These syndromes have symptoms and treatments that overlap.

As psychopharmacologic armamentarium grows and as drugs with potent effects on modulation of monoamines proliferate, the diagnosis and management of these complex disorders becomes even more important. In this chapter NMS is treated as a drug-induced case of malignant catatonia, a condition with multiple etiologies. SS is viewed as a separate and hyperserotonergic condition.

How can we approach such vexing clinical syndromes? Use of vignettes should help to clarify issues of diagnosis and treatment.

Case 1: Catatonia

A 42-year-old man with a long history of complex partial seizures and a history of a left temporal lobectomy had intermittent seizures despite use of phenytoin and other antiepileptics. After admission to the hospital following a seizure, he became catatonic and withdrawn. After administration of intravenous (IV) lorazepam he became alert, agitated, and aggressive; moreover, he was paranoid, and reported nihilistic and religious delusions. After several more doses of lorazepam, a higher dose of phenytoin, and a dose of an atypical antipsychotic (risperidone), his psychosis gradually dissipated. At that point he was able to state that he felt alone and dissociated, and he was unsure as to whether he even existed. "I feel separated from the human race, like I am on another planet," he said.

Definition

The catatonic syndrome comprises a constellation of motor and behavioral signs and symptoms that often occurs in relation to neuromedical insults. Structural brain disease, intrinsic brain disorders (e.g., epilepsy, toxic-metabolic derangements, infectious diseases), a variety of systemic disorders that affect the brain, and idiopathic psychiatric disorders (such as affective and schizophrenic psychoses) have each been associated with catatonia.[1-3] First defined in 1847 by Karl Kahlbaum, who published a monograph that described 21 patients with a severe psychiatric disorder, the condition was called "catatonia."[4] It was among the first studies in the area of mental illness to use the symptom-based approach of Sydenham to diagnose disorders without a known etiopathogenesis.[1]

Kahlbaum believed that patients with catatonia passed through several phases of illness: a short stage of immobility (with waxy flexibility and posturing), a second stage of stupor or melancholy, a third stage of mania (with pressured speech, hyperactivity, and hyperthymic behavior), and finally, after repeated cycles of stupor and excitement, a stage of dementia.[4]

Kraepelin,[5] who was influenced by Kahlbaum, included catatonia in the group of deteriorating psychotic disorders named "dementia praecox." Bleuler[6] adopted Kraepelin's view that catatonia was subsumed under severe idiopathic deteriorating psychoses, which he renamed "the schizophrenias."

Kraepelin and Bleuler both recognized that catatonic symptoms could emerge as part of a mood disorder (either mania or depression). It also was well known that catatonia developed secondary to neurologic, toxic-metabolic, and infectious etiologies. These states were considered phenomenologically indistinguishable from primary psychogenic catatonias. Nevertheless, catatonia was strongly linked with schizophrenia until the 1990s, thanks in large part to the work of Fink and Taylor,[7] the *Diagnostic and Statistical Manual of Mental Disorders*, fourth edition (*DSM-IV*), which includes new criteria for mood disorders with catatonic features and for the catatonic type of schizophrenia.[8] Catatonia, whether a consequence of medical illness, major depression, mania, a mixed affective disorder, or schizophrenia, is diagnosed when the clinical picture includes at least two of the following:

1. Motoric immobility, as evidenced by catalepsy (including waxy flexibility) or stupor
2. Excessive motor activity that is apparently purposeless and not influenced by external stimuli
3. Extreme mutism or negativism that is characterized by an apparently motiveless resistance to all instructions or by maintenance of a rigid posture against attempts to be moved
4. Peculiarities of voluntary movement, such as the voluntary assumption of inappropriate or bizarre postures, stereotyped movements, prominent mannerisms, or grimacing)
5. Echolalia or echopraxia

Signs and symptoms of the catatonic syndrome are outlined in Table 30-1. A key is to differentiate catatonia from other syndromes with similar manifestations and with different etiologies (Table 30-2).[9-32] One should question whether catatonia is the result of a neurologic disorder, a toxic state, a metabolic derangement, or an idiopathic psychiatric disorder.

Unfortunately, no specific test can make the diagnosis of catatonia. However, some studies help hone in on the diagnosis and the etiology. These tests include the electroencephalogram (EEG), neuroimaging, optokinetic and caloric testing, and amobarbital "narcoanalysis."[33] A personal and family history of psychiatric illness is important although not diagnostic.

The specific number and nature of signs and symptoms required to make a diagnosis of catatonia remains controversial. Lohr and Wiesniski[10] proposed that one or more cardinal features (including catalepsy, positivism [such as seen in automatic obedience], and negativism), and two of the other features should be present to diagnose catatonia. Rosebush and colleagues[15] suggested that catatonia was present when three cardinal features (e.g., immobility, mutism, and withdrawal [with refusal to eat or drink]) or when two cardinal features and two secondary characteristics were present.

Taylor[1] contended that even one cardinal characteristic has as much clinical significance (for diagnosis and treatment) as the presence of seven or eight characteristics. The evidence does not support a relationship among the number of catatonic features, the diagnosis, and response to treatment. Fink and Taylor[7] later argued that a minimum of two classic symptoms was sufficient to diagnose the syndrome, and more recently, Bush et al.[34] developed a rating scale and guidelines for the diagnosis of catatonia. They found that two or more signs identified all of their patients with catatonia (Table 30-3; see also Table 30-1). Their

Table 30-1. Modified Bush-Francis Catatonia Rating Scale

Catatonia can be diagnosed by the presence of 2 or more of the first 14 signs listed below.

1. Excitement	Extreme hyperactivity, and constant motor unrest, which is apparently nonpurposeful. Not to be attributed to akathisia or goal-directed agitation.
2. Immobility/stupor	Extreme hypoactivity, immobility, and minimal response to stimuli.
3. Mutism	Verbal unresponsiveness or minimal responsiveness.
4. Staring	Fixed gaze, little or no visual scanning of environment, and decreased blinking.
5. Posturing/catalepsy	Spontaneous maintenance of posture(s), including mundane (e.g., sitting/standing for long periods without reacting).
6. Grimacing	Maintenance of odd facial expressions.
7. Echopraxia/echolalia	Mimicking of an examiner's movements/speech.
8. Stereotypy	Repetitive, non–goal-directed motor activity (e.g., finger-play, or repeatedly touching, patting, or rubbing oneself); the act is not inherently abnormal but is repeated frequently.
9. Mannerisms	Odd, purposeful movements (e.g., hopping or walking on tiptoe, saluting those passing by, or exaggerating caricatures of mundane movements); the act itself is inherently abnormal.
10. Verbigeration	Repetition of phrases (like a scratched record).
11. Rigidity	Maintenance of a rigid position despite efforts to be moved; exclude if cogwheeling or tremor present.
12. Negativism	Apparently motiveless resistance to instructions or attempts to move/examine the patient. Contrary behavior; one does the exact opposite of the instruction.
13. Waxy flexibility	During reposturing of the patient, the patient offers initial resistance before allowing repositioning, similar to that of a bending candle.
14. Withdrawal	Refusal to eat, drink, or make eye contact.
15. Impulsivity	Sudden inappropriate behaviors (e.g., running down a hallway, screaming, or taking off clothes) without provocation. Afterward, gives no or only facile explanations.
16. Automatic obedience	Exaggerated cooperation with the examiner's request or spontaneous continuation of the movement requested.
17. *Mitgehen*	"Anglepoise lamp" arm raising in response to light pressure of finger, despite instructions to the contrary.
18. *Gegenhalten*	Resistance to passive movement that is proportional to strength of the stimulus; appears automatic rather than willful.
19. Ambitendency	The appearance of being "stuck" in indecisive, hesitant movement.
20. Grasp reflex	Per neurologic examination.
21. Perseveration	Repeatedly returns to the same topic or persistence with movement.
22. Combativeness	Usually aggressive in an undirected manner, with no or only facile, explanation afterward.
23. Autonomic abnormality	Abnormal temperature, blood pressure, pulse, or respiratory rate, and diaphoresis.

Modified from the Bush-Francis Catatonia Rating Scale (BFCRS).[34] The full 23-item BFCRS measures the severity of 23 signs on a 0–3 continuum for each sign. The first 14 signs combine to form the Bush-Francis Catatonia Screening Instrument (BFCSI). The BFCSI measures only the presence or absence of the first 14 signs, and it is used for case detection. Item definitions on the two scales are the same.

method is consistent with the *DSM-IV* criteria for catatonia.

Subtypes of Catatonia

When encountering the catatonic patient, the clinician must be aware that subtypes of catatonia have been described. Catatonic withdrawal is characterized by psychomotor hypoactivity, whereas catatonic excitement is characterized by psychomotor hyperactivity. These presentations may alternate during the course of a catatonic episode. Kraepelin identified a "periodic" catatonia with an onset in adolescence characterized by intermittent excited states, followed by catatonic stuporous stages and a remitting and relapsing course.[35] This disorder was further elaborated upon by Gjessing[36] in 1932 and by Stauder[37] in 1934, who described lethal catatonia that was distinguished by the rapid onset of a manic delirium, high temperatures, catatonic stupor, and a mortality rate of greater than 50%. In 1986, Mann et al.[38] reviewed the world's literature on lethal catatonia, dating back to the

Table 30-2. Potential Etiologies of the Catatonic Syndrome

Primary Psychiatric
Acute psychoses[11]
Conversion disorder[12]
Dissociative disorders[13]
Mood disorders[1]
Obsessive-compulsive disorder[14]
Personality disorders[15]
Schizophrenia[1]
Secondary Neuromedical
Cerebrovascular
   Arterial aneurysms[1]
   Arteriovenous malformations[1]
   Arterial and venous thrombosis[11,16]
   Bilateral parietal infarcts
   Temporal lobe infarct
   Subarachnoid hemorrhage[16]
   Subdural hematoma[16]
   Third ventricle hemorrhage
   Hemorrhagic infarcts
Other Central Nervous System Causes
Akinetic mutism[17]
Alcoholic degeneration and Wernicke's encephalopathy[13]
Cerebellar degeneration[18]
Cerebral anoxia[11]
Cerebromacular degeneration[13]
Closed head trauma[11, 13]
Frontal lobe atrophy[16]
Hydrocephalus[16]
Lesions of thalamus and globus pallidus[19]
Narcolepsy[16]
Parkinsonism[15]
Postencephalitic states[11]
Seizure disorders[11, 13]*
Surgical interventions[11, 16]
Tuberous sclerosis[13]
Neoplasm
Angioma[11]
Frontal lobe tumors[13]
Gliomas[11]
Langerhans' carcinoma[1]
Paraneoplastic encephalopathy[20]
Periventricular diffuse pinealoma[11]
Poisoning
Coal gas[16]
Organic fluorides[13]
Tetraethyl lead poisoning[11]
Infections
Acquired immunodeficiency syndrome[21]
Bacterial meningoencephalitis[22]
Bacterial sepsis[11]

General paresis[11]
Malaria[11]
Mononucleosis[11]
Subacute sclerosing panencephalitis[11]
Tertiary syphilis[17]
Tuberculosis[16]
Typhoid fever[11]
Viral encephalitides (especially herpes)[1, 13]
Viral hepatitis[11]
Metabolic and Other Medical Causes
Acute intermittent porphyria[1, 13]*
Addison's disease[11]
Cushing's disease[11]
Diabetic ketoacidosis[13]
Glomerulonephritis[13]
Hepatic dysfunction[1, 13]
Hereditary copronphyria[16]
Homocystinuria[1, 13]
Hyperparathyroidism[1]
Idiopathic hyperadrenergic state[23]
Multiple sclerosis[18]
Pellagra[13]
Idiopathic[16]
Peripuerperal[24]
Systemic lupus erythematosus[11]*
Thrombocytopenic purpura
Uremia[1, 11]
Drug Related
Neuroleptics (typical and atypical) clozapine[25]
   and risperidone[26]* (all neuroleptics have
   been associated)
Non-neuroleptic
   Alcohol
   Anticonvulsants (tricyclics, monoamine oxidase
      inhibitors, and others)[27,28]
   Anticonvulsants (e.g., carbamazepine,
      primidone)[15, 27]
   Aspirin[16]
   Disulfiram[16]*
   Metoclopramide[27]
   Dopamine depleters (e.g., tetrabenazine)[28]
   Dopamine withdrawal (e.g., levadopa)[28]
   Hallucinogens (e.g., mescaline, phencyclidine*, and
      lysergic acid diethylamide)[29]
   Lithium carbonate[27]
   Morphine[16]
   Sedative-hypnotic withdrawal[11]
   Steroids[26]*
Stimulants (e.g., amphetamines, methylphenidate, and
   possibly cocaine)[16,30,31]

*Signifies most common medical conditions associated with catatonic disorder from literature review done by Carroll BT, Anfinson TJ, Kennedy JC, et al. Catatonic disorder due to general medical conditions. *J Neuropsychiatry Clin Neurosci* 6:122–133, 1994.
Modified from Philbrick KL, Rummans TA. Malignant catatonia. *J Neuropsychiatry Clin Neurosci* 6:1–13, 1994.

Table 30-3. Standardized Examination for Catatonia

The method described here is used to complete the 23-item Bush-Francis Catatonia Rating Scale (BFCRS) and the 14-item Bush-Francis Catatonia Screening Instrument (BFCSI). Item definitions on the two scales are the same. The BFCSI measures only the presence or absence of the first 14 signs.

Ratings are based solely on observed behaviors during the examination, with the exception of completing the items for "withdrawal" and "autonomic abnormality," which may be based on directly observed behavior or chart documentation.

As a general rule, only items that are clearly present should be rated. If the examiner is uncertain as to the presence of an item, rate the item as "0."

Procedure

1. Observe the patient while trying to engage in a conversation.
2. The examiner should scratch his or her head in an exaggerated manner.
3. The arm should be examined for cogwheeling. Attempt to rep--osture and instruct the patient to "keep your arm loose." Move the arm with alternating lighter and heavier force.
4. Ask the patient to extend his or her arm. Place one finger beneath his or her hand and try to raise it slowly after stating, "Do *not* let me raise your arm."
5. Extend the hand stating, "Do *not* shake my hand."
6. Reach into your pocket and state, "Stick out your tongue. I want to stick a pin in it."
7. Check for grasp reflex.
8. Check the chart for reports from the previous 24-hour period. Check for oral intake, vital signs, and any incidents.
9. Observe the patient indirectly, at least for a brief period each day, regarding:
   Activity level
   Abnormal movements
   Abnormal speech
   Echopraxia
   Rigidity
   Negativism
   Waxy flexibility
   Gegenhalten
   Mitgehen
   Ambitendency
   Automatic obedience
   Grasp reflex

preneuroleptic era. Cases from the preneuroleptic era classically began with a period of intense motor excitement, which lasted uninterrupted for an average of 8 days. These patients often acted in a bizarre and violent fashion, refused to eat, and displayed intermittent mutism, posturing, catalepsy, and rigidity that alternated with their excitement. They manifested thought disorders with disorganized incoherent speech and experienced delusions and hallucinations. During the hyperactive stage their fever rose rapidly, and they were diaphoretic and tachycardic. This stage would be followed by exhaustion, characterized by stupor and high body temperatures.

Terminal rigidity and posturing were noted in Stauder's series of 27 cases,[37] although others reported cases of flaccidity.[38] Some cases in the preneuroleptic era were characterized by catatonic stupor and rigidity in the absence of an early excitement phase. Preneuroleptic era lethal catatonia was fatal in more than three out of four cases.

For Kraepelin, lethal catatonia was a syndrome with various neuromedical and psychiatric etiologies; the review by Mann and co-workers[38] of 292 cases since 1960 supports this concept. Most of the patients in this series received neuroleptics at some point during their treatment. Of those, 60% died. The "classic" hyperactive form of catatonia was found in 69% of the cases. Patients either presented with catatonic excitement or it developed early on; stupor typically followed. High fever, altered consciousness, autonomic instability, anorexia, electrolyte imbalance, cyanosis, and associated catatonic signs (e.g., posturing, stereotypies, and mutism) were present from the early stages.

More recent literature indicates that 31% of patients with catatonia present with stupor. Stupor and fever emerge only after neuroleptics are begun. Once stupor and rigidity emerge, patients with catatonic stupor act in a fashion similar to those with NMS, which also has a substantial mortality rate.[39] Indeed, the symptoms of predominantly stuporous patients with catatonia were clinically indistinguishable from those with NMS.

Philbrick and Rummans[40] reviewed this "lethal" form of catatonia. They suggested using the term "malignant catatonia" (since not all cases are lethal) to describe cases marked by autonomic instability or hyperthermia, in contradistinction to cases of "simple, nonmalignant catatonia." The causes of malignant catatonia are the same as those of simple catatonia. "Pernicious catatonia" is another term that has been used to describe this catatonic variant.[41]

Consideration of neuroleptics as potential causative agents is important because NMS is currently considered by many as a severe form of neuroleptic-induced catatonia. NMS is a syndrome of autonomic dysfunction with tachycardia and elevated blood pressure, fever, rigidity, mutism, and stupor, associated with the use of neuroleptics. In 1985 Fricchione[42] suggested that NMS is to lethal catatonia what neuroleptic-induced catatonia is to simple catatonia. Moreover, if neuroleptic-induced catatonia is a form of catatonia, then NMS is a form of malignant catatonia with a similar pathophysiology.[42] Goforth and Carroll[43] also noted the overlap of catatonia and NMS. All 27 of their cases of NMS met the *DSM-IV* diagnostic criteria for catatonia; 24 met stricter research criteria. The authors concluded that the two syndromes were identical, with NMS presenting as a more severe and iatrogenic variant of malignant catatonia. Fink[44] also arrived at this conclusion (Table 30-4).

NMS and lethal catatonia appear to be part of a single syndrome, with minor differences in their presentations (i.e., there is a behavioral prodrome and hyperthermia in the prestuporous stage of lethal catatonia, as opposed to its occurrence in the stage with stupor and rigidity in NMS). Indeed, although early reports suggested that the level of creatine phosphokinase (CPK) is increased in NMS and not

in primary lethal catatonia, a survey of 13 cases of primary malignant catatonia revealed that CPK levels were elevated in all nine of the cases in which they were tested.[40]

In 1991 Rosebush and Mazurek[45] found decreased levels of serum iron in NMS and suggested a role for lowered iron stores in the reduction of dopamine (DA) receptor function. Supporting the hypothesis of NMS as a severe variant of catatonia, Carroll and Goforth[46] reported a similar decrease of serum iron in 3 of 12 cases of catatonia, with NMS developing in 2 of the 3 cases. The third was without neuroleptic exposure and did not progress to NMS.[46] Lee[47] prospectively studied 50 patients with catatonia; serum iron was measured in 39 of the episodes. The low serum iron level found in 14 (44%) cases was associated with lethal catatonia and with a poorer response to benzodiazepines. In seven episodes of lethal catatonia, a low level of serum iron was detected. Neuroleptics were used in 5 cases and all 5 progressed to NMS.

Providing further support for the relationship between primary "psychogenic" catatonias and neuroleptic-induced catatonias, White and Robins[48] reported 5 consecutive cases of NMS that were each preceded by a catatonic state; none had received prior neuroleptics and none had a prior psychiatric history. White[49] concluded that NMS and lethal catatonia are not separate disorders. Mann and Caroff[50] also viewed NMS as "a neuroleptic-induced iatrogenic form of organic lethal catatonia."

Table 30-4. Catatonia and NMS: Associated Features

	NMS	Catatonia
Clinical Signs		
Hyperthermia	Yes	Often
Motor Rigidity	Yes	Yes
Mutism	Yes	Yes
Negativism	Often	Yes
Altered Consciousness	Yes	Yes
Stupor or Coma	Yes	Yes
Autonomic Dysfunction	Yes	Often
Tachypnea	Yes	Often
Tachycardia	Yes	Often
Abnormal BP	Yes	Yes
Diaphoresis	Yes	Yes
Laboratory Results		
CPK elevated	Yes	Often
Serum iron reduced	Yes	Probable
Leucocytosis	Yes	Often

NMS = neuroleptic malignant syndrome; CPK = creatine phosphokinase; BP = blood pressure.

Case 2: Neuroleptic Malignant Syndrome

A 56-year-old woman with a history of bipolar disorder was admitted to the hospital after arguing with her husband; she became agitated and combative and required haloperidol (5 mg IM) on two occasions in the emergency room. Psychiatric history was notable for depression, suicidal ideation, and auditory hallucinations as a teenager that required electroconvulsive therapy (ECT) and long-term treatment with perphenazine, lithium, and imipramine. Soon after her admission she became psychomotorically withdrawn, hypokinetic, mute, and rigid. Her temperature reached 101.6 °F and her CPK level was elevated (2260). An EEG revealed generalized slowing. A diagnosis of NMS was made and her medications were discontinued. Her catatonic symptoms responded to lorazepam (2 mg IV × 2). Divalproex sodium and olanzapine were started two weeks after the resolution of her NMS.

Evaluation

A neuromedical workup is essential to identify an etiology of catatonia, especially when the patient's history is complicated (See Table 30-2). Treatment of a specific etiology can be life-saving. An EEG also can facilitate an accurate diagnosis. In one series, 4 out of 10 patients with "idiopathic" catatonia actually had epilepsy.[24] An EEG read as normal might be consistent with primary catatonia, although psychiatric patients may have nonspecific, diffuse changes on the EEG. Neuroimaging, especially magnetic resonance imaging (MRI) of the brain, should be obtained. Again, a negative result does not rule out a neuromedical etiology because toxic, metabolic, and infectious etiologies may exist that would not be identified by MRI. CPK levels are often elevated in malignant catatonia.

In catatonic stupor, a skillful amobarbital interview may relieve the syndrome long enough to gather data from the patient. When brain function changes after administration of a sedative (i.e., a barbiturate or benzodiazepine) or a stimulant (i.e., amphetamine or methamphetamine), there is often a temporary recovery from stupor, mutism, or excitement. Such relief can be diagnostically helpful as patients with catatonia associated with psychiatric illness often respond to an amobarbital interview. The procedure involves the slow administration of an IV barbiturate, accompanied by an interview.[11,13] In one study, only 50% of psychiatric patients with catatonic mutism responded to an amobarbital interview.[51] Benzodiazepines given intravenously are a reliable alternative to barbiturates. They often lyse the catatonic episode completely. Benzodiazepines also may relieve secondary catatonias, such as those secondary to neuroleptics and to complex partial seizures.

Plum and Posner[33] pointed out that those with idiopathic catatonia, as opposed to catatonia associated with structural neurologic disease, have normal optokinetic responses, normal pupillary responses, and normal ocular nystagmus on cold caloric tests. Patients with hysterical stupor, when turned on their sides, will elicit a downward gaze, as if due to gravity.[50]

Management and Treatment

Whatever its etiology, catatonia is accompanied by significant morbidity and mortality from systemic complications. In addition many of the physical illnesses responsible for catatonia can be hazardous (Table 30-5). Thus, timely diagnosis and treatment are essential. If a neurologic or medical condition is found, then treatment for that specific illness is indicated. Occasionally psychiatric therapies will be used to treat catatonia as a behavioral manifestation of a medical illness. For example, ECT has been used to treat lupus patients with catatonia.[53]

Table 30-5. Some Medical Complications Associated with Catatonia

Simple Nonmalignant Catatonia
Aspiration
Burns
Cachexia
Dehydration and its sequelae
Pneumonia
Pulmonary emboli
Thrombophlebitis
Urinary incontinence
Urinary retention and its sequelae

Malignant Catatonia
Acute renal failure
Adult respiratory distress syndrome
Cardiac arrest
Cheyne-Stokes respirations
Death
Dysphagia due to muscle spasm
Disseminated intravascular coagulation
Electrocardiographic abnormalities
Gait abnormalities
Gastrointestinal bleeding
Hepatocellular damage
Hypoglycemia (sudden and profound)
Intestinal pseudo-obstruction
Laryngospasm
Myocardial infarction
Myocardial stunning
Necrotizing enterocolitis
Respiratory arrest
Rhabdomyolysis and sequelae
Seizures
Sepsis
Unresponsiveness to pain

Modified from Philbrick KL, Rummans TA: Malignant catatonia, *J Neuropsychiatry Clin Neurosci* 6:1–13, 1994.

Response to treatment is usually good for individuals with acute primary catatonia; 67% are improved by time of discharge.[54] Patients with manic features respond particularly well. Rates of long-term recovery range from 33% to 75%.[1] ECT remains the most effective treatment for catatonia.[28] Fatality rates of 50% or more were the rule prior to the introduction of ECT.[55] Two or three ECT treatments are usually sufficient to lyse the catatonic state, though a course of four to six treatments is usually given to prevent relapse. Nevertheless, patients' families are often reluctant to agree to ECT because of the stigma associated with it and the fear of side effects.

IV amobarbital is rapidly successful in some patients with catatonic stupor.[56] However, these effects tend to be short-lived. Repeated IV doses lead to oversedation; amobarbital administered orally does not appear to prolong its benefits.

Neuroleptics have been used frequently to treat catatonia. In addition to the variable response of catatonia to these drugs, neuroleptics may complicate matters; their use also has precipitated catatonic reactions and NMS.[39] At times higher doses of antipsychotics are used to treat psychosis and agitation, but it may worsen catatonia. Moreover, among the 292 patients with malignant catatonia reviewed by Mann et al.,[38] 78% of those treated with a neuroleptic alone died, compared with an overall mortality rate of 60%. In 18 cases (reviewed by Philbrick and Rummans[40]), only one patient received a neuroleptic alone—this patient also died. Therefore, neuroleptics may be contraindicated during an acute episode of malignant catatonic stupor.[38,40]

In 1983, Lew and Tollefson[57] reported on the usefulness of IV diazepam; in the same year, Fricchione et al.[58] reported on the benefit of lorazepam given intravenously to patients in neuroleptic-induced catatonic states (including NMS) and suggested its use in primary psychiatric catatonia. McEvoy and Lohr[59] had already and successfully administered diazepam intravenously to two catatonic patients whose conditions had not improved with haloperidol regimens (that had been initiated after the onset of catatonia). Rosebush et al.[60] diagnosed catatonia 15 times in 12 patients during a 1-year period. Lorazepam (1 to 2 mg oral, IM, or IV) was administered to each patient. Of these patients, 80% had a complete and dramatic response within 2 hours of lorazepam treatment; one showed a partial response, and two

showed no response. Side effects were uncommon. Catatonia related to a central nervous system abnormality was evident in 8 of 12 responders, which suggested that a beneficial response to lorazepam was not limited to patients with psychogenic catatonia.

Bush et al.[61] studied the use of lorazepam and ECT in the treatment of catatonia. Twenty-eight prospectively identified patients entered their open-trial protocol (including use of parenteral lorazepam, oral lorazepam [1 to 2 mg orally 2 to 3 times a day], or both for 3 to 5 days, with referral for ECT if lorazepam failed). Of 21 (76%) patients who received a complete trial of lorazepam (11 received an initial 2-mg IV challenge), 16 had their catatonic signs resolve. All four patients referred for ECT (after failing lorazepam therapy) responded promptly. Bush et al.[61] specifically suggested a trial of lorazepam (2 mg IM or IV) with monitoring of respiratory status. Sometimes higher doses were required. With a drug distribution that is less rapid and less extensive, a relatively high plasma level can be maintained, thus prolonging the clinical benefit of IV lorazepam.[2] Given intramuscularly in the deltoids, lorazepam is more reliably absorbed than other IM benzodiazepines.[2] A switch to regular doses of lorazepam or diazepam maintains the therapeutic effect. Lorazepam given orally or via nasogastric tube in a daily dose of 6 mg to 20 mg also has been used effectively. Diazepam (10 to 50 mg/day) or clonazepam (1 to 5 mg/day) also has been used successfully, as has midazolam.[2] If lorazepam is unsuccessful within 5 days, ECT should be considered.[2]

In a study of lorazepam treatment for NMS, rigidity and fever abated in 24 to 48 hours, whereas secondary features of NMS dissipated within 64 hours (without adverse effects).[62] If lorazepam does not briskly reverse the lethal catatonia, the clinician should not wait for 5 days to begin ECT. Mann et al.[63] found that in one series of cases lethal catatonia where ECT was used, 40 of 41 patients survived. In another series,[63] although 16 out of 19 patients who had received ECT within 5 days of symptom onset survived, none of the 14 patients who had received ECT after 5 days after symptom did.

Philbrick and Rummans[40] reviewed 18 cases of lethal catatonia; 11 out of 13 patients treated with ECT survived, whereas only 1 out of 5 not treated with ECT died. In terms of NMS, 39 reported cases of ECT treatment have been reported; 34 of them improved. The message is clear—when a patient presents with malignant catatonia of any type, ECT should be used expeditiously. Although an initial trial of lorazepam, a dopaminergic agent, or both is reasonable for malignant catatonia, ECT should be instituted early (i.e., within 5 days) if a medication trial is unsuccessful. Muscle relaxants, calcium channel-blockers, carbamazepine, anticholinergics, lithium, thyroid medication, and corticosteroids have each had anecdotal success in catatonia.[40] Adrenocorticotropic hormone and corticosteroids also have been reported to work in cases of lethal catatonia.[38] Dopaminergic agents, bromocriptine, and amantadine have been used successfully in NMS.[64] In a retrospective review of 734 cases, Sakkas et al.[65] concluded that these agents and the muscle relaxant dantrolene led to improvement; bromocriptine and dantrolene also were associated with a significant reduction in the mortality rate. However, in a prospective study of 20 patients, Rosebush et al.[66] found that bromocriptine and dantrolene were not efficacious. Another DA agonist, lisuride, has been used intravenously with success in four patients with NMS, three of whom had failed to respond to other dopaminergic agents.[67]

In 1985, when it was suggested that psychogenic catatonia and neuroleptic-induced catatonia (including NMS) shared a common pathophysiology, use of specific dopaminergic or GABAergic drugs in psychogenic catatonia untreated by neuroleptic medication also was suggested.[42] Accordingly, it is of interest that 2.5 mg of oral bromocriptine twice a day was used successfully in a 16-year-old girl with catatonia that preceded neuroleptic exposure,[68] and that Rogers[69] used L-dopa to treat a patient with a 50-year history of severe catatonic schizophrenia (off neuroleptics for 5 years) with improvement in catatonic akinesia and without worsening of positive symptoms. Neppe[70] also successfully used L-dopa to treat catatonic stupor. Dopaminergic agents may also be helpful in catatonia and NMS. Table 30-6 outlines recommendations for the treatment of catatonia, lethal catatonia, and NMS, and Table 30-7 reviews management principles.

Rechallenging a patient who has had NMS with an antipsychotic is controversial. Most investigators suggest that antipsychotics should not be given until at least 2 weeks after an episode of NMS has resolved and that rechallenge should be with a neuroleptic of a lower potency.

Table 30-6. Treatment of Catatonia

Simple catatonia (including neuroleptic-induced catatonia)

↓

Lorazepam (or another benzodiazepine) (if still catatonic)

↓

Dopamine agonist (if still catatonic)

↓

ECT

Lethal catatonia (including NMS)

↓

Lorazepam (or another benzodiazepine)
  and/or
Dopamine agonist ± dantrolene (if still catatonic)

↓

ECT (should be instituted prior to day 5 of syndrome)

Modified from Fricchione G, Bush G, Fozdur M, et al. The recognition and treatment of the catatonic syndrome, *J Intensive Care Med* 12:135–147, 1997.
ECT = electroconvulsive therapy; NMS = neuroleptic malignant syndrome.

Neuropathophysiology

What type of neuropathophysiology involving DA and GABA neurons in mesostriatal, mesolimbic, and hypothalamic systems can lead to the similar symptomatology seen in neuroleptic catatonia (including NMS) and psychogenic catatonia?[42] In the mesostriatal and mesocorticolimbic systems, the

Table 30-7. Principles of Management of Catatonia

1. Early recognition is important; once catatonia has been diagnosed, the patient must be closely observed and vitals signs taken frequently.
2. Supportive care is essential. Such care involves hydration, nutrition, mobilization, anticoagulation (to prevent thrombophlebitis), and precautions against aspiration.
3. Discontinue antipsychotics or other drugs, such as metoclopramide, which can cause or worsen catatonia.
4. Restart recently withdrawn dopamine agonists, especially in patients with parkinsonism.
5. Institute supportive measures (e.g., a cooling blanket if hyperthermia is present or parenteral fluids and antihypertensives or pressors if autonomic instability emerge and if malignant catatonia is suspected.
6. Maintain a high index of suspicion for the development of medical complications and for new medical problems.

Modified from Philbrick KL, Rummans TA: Malignant catatonia, *J Neuropsychiatry Clin Neurosci* 6:1–13, 1994.

long feedback loops from DA neurons are regulated by GABA pathways. Given its extensive projections on both limbic and motor structures, the nucleus accumbens may be a hub for the linkage between motivation and movement.[71] By extrapolating from animal evidence (i.e., $GABA_A$ antagonists lead to catalepsy and $GABA_A$ agonists protect against catalepsy), and from the hypothesis that neuroleptic-induced catatonia may result from reduced DA and $GABA_A$ activity in the mesostriatum, it has been proposed that primary psychogenic catatonia results from a similar destabilization.[42] $GABA_A$ agonists could be restorative by inhibiting the pars reticulata's inhibitory $GABA_B$ neurons, resulting in disinhibition of the neighboring pars compacta's DA cells with a resultant striatal DA agonism.[42]

ECT may be effective in catatonia on the basis of this GABA-DA interaction. Sackeim et al.[72] proposed that the neural state following ECT is produced by increased GABA transmission. They cited animal studies in which the concentration of GABA in the striatum became elevated following ECT. Some investigators have believed that ECT may increase the sensitivity of postsynaptic DA receptors to available DA.

Kish et al.[73] described the neuropathophysiologic findings in three patients who died of fatal hyperthermia from catatonia and NMS. They found reduced concentrations of norepinephrine in the hypothalamus of all three patients and speculated that this depletion was a product of hyperthermia and hypothalamic stress. They also found evidence, however, of a reduced level of the DA metabolite homovanillic acid (HVA) in the striatum of one patient, the lack of an elevated HVA:DA ratio in another, and a reduced striatal level of HVA in the third (although that patient had been receiving a monoamine oxidase inhibitor [MAOI] that that could have affected these results). They postulated that the DA system had a reduced ability to respond to stress, to neuroleptic-induced hypodopaminergic postsynaptic activity, or to both. These findings are supported by the work of Nisijima and Ishiguro,[74] who found significantly lower levels of HVA in the cerebrospinal fluid of eight patients with NMS during the active phase of the illness and after recovery, suggesting that a decrease in DA metabolism may have made the patients prone to NMS. In line with the impression that NMS represents a severe form of

catatonia, Northoff et al.[75] reported findings in 18 neuroleptically naïve, acutely catatonic patients. They found that higher plasma HVA concentrations were present in patients who responded to lorazepam than in those who did not respond to lorazepam. The latter patients also scored significantly higher on scales of extrapyramidal symptoms. NMS has been postulated to be secondary to DA blockade in the mesostriatum (which is responsible for the motor disorder), the mesolimbic system (which is responsible for the mutism), and the preoptic anterior hypothalamus (which is responsible for the hyperthermia).[76]

In rats, the application of the DA agonist apomorphine to the prefrontal cortex will increase the ability of haloperidol to produce catalepsy.[77] This finding suggests that if stress dramatically increases DA activity in the mesocorticolimbic system, it will result in catatonic withdrawal and catalepsy via feedback to the ventral tegmental and nigral DA areas. Animal evidence suggests that prefrontal cortical DA synthesis and metabolism are accelerated by stress, which suggests an increase in impulse flow in dopaminergic neurons that project to the prefrontal cortex. These increases in DA synthesis and metabolism are antagonized by diazepam.[78] Also, electroconvulsive stimulation causes a rapid rise in diazepam binding site density in the rat cerebral cortex; when applied for a long time, it potentiates the effects of diazepam and upregulates benzodiazepine receptors in the rat's frontal cortex.[79] Sequential or concurrent lorazepam and ECT have been used successfully to treat catatonia, perhaps because of this synergism.[80]

Some researchers[1] have concluded that the catatonic syndrome is primarily a frontal lobe disorder, whereas some have cited evidence that it is primarily a disorder of the basal ganglia.[69] We have proposed that the catatonic syndrome is actually a disorder of basal ganglia-thalamo (limbic) cortical circuits.[2,81] In particular, the "orbitofrontal," the "dorsolateral prefrontal," the "anterior cingulate-medial orbitofrontal," and the "motor" circuits would be major candidates for involvement. Each circuit has cortical/limbic, striatal, pallidal/nigral, and thalamic nodal points with the loops closed by thalamocortical connections. Any neuromedical or psychiatric disturbance strong enough to disrupt the GABA-DA balance in the mesostriatal-mesocorticolimbic medial fore-brain bundle DA tracts, with terminal fields in the nucleus accumbens, the anterior cingulate, and the prefrontal cortex system, will potentially set off a catatonic response. Using functional magnetic resonance imaging (MRI) and magnetoencephalography, Northoff and co-workers[82] recently presented findings that indicate primary psychogenic catatonia involves reduced activity in the medial orbitofrontal cortex during negative emotional stimulation; this suggests that psychogenic catatonia initiates there.[82] Insofar as disorders of the basal ganglia, cerebellum, and brainstem also will disturb this circuitry, they will also have the potential to cause catatonia. Hypodopaminergia in the tuberoinfundibular DA system and in the mesolimbic or mesostriatal DA system may precipitate NMS (with hyperthermia and reactive hyperadrenalism).[40]

The restitutive hypothesis of DA receptor activity may offer an explanation for the relationship of catatonia, lethal catatonia, and NMS.[42,83] It assumes that the dopaminergic system is involved in protecting against the emergence of psychotic symptoms through physiologic downregulation of DA receptors in the face of psychological or biologic events that would tend to destabilize the system.[56] The dopaminergic system then may stabilize mental homeostasis by spontaneous down- regulation of its own function.[42] In some patients, this downregulation is sufficient to maintain a nonpsychotic state. However, the biologic or psychological stresses may be so severe that down-regulation is not adequate to prevent psychosis. In some patients, treatment with neuroleptics will help in remission of symptoms by producing a further decrease in DA activity. Still others, however, will not benefit from neuroleptic treatment. Indeed, the further decrease in DA activity by DA blockade may lead to neuroleptic-induced catatonia.

The hyperdopaminergic mesolimbic system may attempt restoration of homeostasis (i.e., down-regulation of DA receptors, or a restitutive hypothesis). As Friedhoff pointed out, an adjustment will likely affect other brain systems.[83] The systems likely to be adjusted rapidly are the mesostriatal system (with GABAergic feedback from the nucleus accumbens through the globus pallidus to the pars reticulata of the substantia nigra), and the

hypothalamic DA system (which may have cell bodies in the substantia nigra). They too may then downregulate. If these areas become hypodopaminergic to a relatively large degree, psychosis may continue, and then lethal catatonia may ensue. Use of cataleptogenic neuroleptics could hasten the catatonia through DA blockade and decreased GABA in the ventral tegmentum and the substantia nigra.[84]

An animal model of catatonia bears this out. Stevens et al.[85] instilled bicuculline, a $GABA_A$ antagonist, into the ventral tegmentum of cats; slinking, hiding, looking fearful, staring, sniffing, and taking a catatonic stance were noted. Waxy flexibility of the limbs developed and animals stood still and stared for extended periods.[85] When bicuculline was given in the ventral tegmentum after systemic haloperidol, marked dystonic postures were produced. Picrotoxin, an antagonist at the chloride channel of the benzodiazepine-$GABA_A$ recognition site, was administered in the ventral tegmentum area as well. Smaller doses induced fear and staring, whereas larger doses produced prolonged severe dystonia, especially following haloperidol. Microinjection of the $GABA_A$ agonist muscimol into the ventral tegmentum area of the rat caused a dose-dependent motor activation. This response was antagonized by administration of bicuculline or by haloperidol administration.[86] Neuroleptics reduce the conditioned avoidance response, which is thought to be secondary to decreased DA activity in the nucleus accumbens and the striatum. Stress has been shown to increase medial prefrontal cortical DA release, which in turn is thought to reduce DA activity in subcortical DA terminal fields in the mesolimbic and mesostriatal systems.[77,87] Friedhoff et al.[88] were able to show that rats undergoing twice-daily tail-shock stress for 8 days displayed conditioned avoidance response inhibition, along with a reduction in nucleus accumbens DA use. The findings provided support for a restitutive hypothesis involving an endogenous DA-dependent system that mimicked the effects of neuroleptics in the context of repeated stress-induced medial prefrontal cortical hyperdopaminergia. When such a system down-regulates too much because of neurologic or medical insult, primary psychiatric dysfunction, neuroleptic medication, or a combination or all three, catatonic stupor may occur. These state changes may be tied to a genetic trait vulnerability for acute NMS, perhaps having to do with defective calcium regulation that leads to a dysregulated hyperactive sympathetic nervous system response in the presence of severe psychic stress and neuroleptic-induced hypodopaminergia.[89]

Recently a "universal field hypothesis of catatonia and NMS" has been proposed.[90] It speculates that some type of neurochemical predisposition, be it low activity at the D_2 or $GABA_A$ receptor for which most evidence exists, N-methyl-D-aspartate (NMDA) receptor dysregulation, or even high $5\text{-}HT_{1A}$ receptor activity can modulate the circuits involved in catatonia and NMS and lower the threshold for the syndrome. In any event the DA and $GABA_A$ disturbances in the basal ganglia thalamo-cortical circuits appear to be the primary physiologic derangements. It is of interest that the potential secondary disturbance of $5\text{-}HT_{1A}$ in catatonia becomes the primary component of SS (discussed next).

Summary

Catatonia is a fascinating condition that graphically links emotion and behavior, motivation, and movement. Given the morbidity and mortality associated with catatonia, concerted efforts at supportive care are essential. When catatonia is of the malignant variety, treatment should take place in the intensive care unit (ICU). All potential offending agents, especially neuroleptics and DA blockers (e.g., metoclopramide) should be discontinued. If antiparkinsonian dopaminergic agents have recently been discontinued or tapered, they should be reinstituted. Lorazepam (or another benzodiazepine) should be used in an effort to lyse catatonia, be it simple or malignant. ECT should be considered early because it is the definitive treatment of catatonia, especially in malignant instances of the syndrome; it can be life-saving.

If the condition is not life-threatening and if ECT is not available, DA agonists or dantrolene may be added to supportive measures. If the condition is life-threatening and if ECT is not available, transfer to a facility where ECT is performed is appropriate. By examining the nature of basal ganglia thalamo-limbic-cortical loops, we can hypothesize why such a wide array of neuromedical and psychiatric etiologies can present with the catatonic syndrome and why the discussed treatments may be therapeutic.

Case 3: Serotonin Syndrome

A 69-year-old woman with a history of depression partially responsive to paroxetine (40 mg/day) had her dose increased (to 60 mg/day); 2 weeks later buspirone was added (5 mg tid) along with trazodone 100 mg for sleep. She became confused, diaphoretic, febrile (to 101.2 °F), hyperreflexic, and mildly rigid and was admitted to the hospital. Paroxetine and buspirone were discontinued; over the next 2 days her condition improved (with acetaminophen and supportive care).

Definition

Serotonin is a neurotransmitter involved in many psychiatric disorders. With this in mind many pharmacologic agents have been designed that affect central serotonergic tone. As serotonin increases it is known to have certain nervous system effects and toxicity, when available in excess. Heightened clinical awareness is necessary to prevent, recognize, and intervene when a toxic syndrome secondary to serotonin excess emerges. SS, as it is called, most commonly occurs as a result of an interaction between serotonergic agents and MAOIs. Signs of SS include mental status changes (e.g., confusion, anxiety, irritability, euphoria, and dysphoria), gastrointestinal symptoms (e.g, nausea, vomiting, diarrhea, and incontinence), behavioral manifestations (e.g., restlessness and agitation), neurologic findings (e.g., ataxia or incoordination, tremor, myoclonus, hyperreflexia, ankle clonus, and muscle rigidity), and autonomic nervous system abnormalities (e.g., hypertension, hypotension, tachycardia, diaphoresis, shivering, sialorrhea, mydriasis, tachypnea, and hyperthermia).[91,92]

There is no formal consensus regarding the diagnostic criteria for SS. Based on his review of 38 cases, Sternbach[93] proposed the first operational definition of the syndrome in humans. Diagnosis requires the following three criteria:

1. An increase in or addition of a serotonergic agent to an established medication regimen, in addition to least three of the following features:

mental status changes, agitation, myoclonus, hyperreflexia, diaphoresis, shivering, tremor, diarrhea, and incoordination

2. Other etiologies need to be ruled out
3. A neuroleptic must not have been started or increased in dosage prior to the onset of the signs and symptoms listed previously

Based on a review of other diagnostic criteria, Keck and Arnold[91] recently modified Sternbach's criteria to include mental status changes, agitation, restlessness, myoclonus, hyperreflexia, diaphoresis, tremor, shivering, incoordination, autonomic nervous system dysfunction, hyperthermia, and muscle rigidity.

Epidemiology

The incidence of SS is unknown. There are no data to suggest that sex or gender differences confer any particular vulnerability to the syndrome. Given the overlap of symptoms with NMS, SS is often mistaken for it and thus may be underreported. The existence of the syndrome in varying degrees also may confound its recognition. SS most often occurs in individuals being treated with psychotropics for a psychiatric disorder. Most often this involves some combination of a selective serotonin-reuptake inhibitor (SSRI), an MAOI, an antiparkinsonian agent, and lithium. At the outset, patients will develop a peripheral tremor, confusion, and ataxia, which is followed by systemic signs (e.g., hyperreflexia, diaphoresis, shivering, and agitation). If the condition becomes more severe, fever, myoclonic jerking, and diarrhea may develop. The syndrome can last from hours to days after the offending agents have been stopped and supportive treatment has been initiated.

Pathophysiology

From both animal and human studies, the role 5-HT has been implicated in the pathogenesis of SS. The 5-HT$_{1A}$ receptor in particular appears to be overactive in this condition, which has led some to use 5-HT$_{1A}$ antagonists in the management of the SS. The animal model of SS seems to be associated with receptors in the lower brainstem and spinal cord. Ascending serotonergic projections are likely to play a role, particularly in hyperthermia, mental status, and autonomic changes. The roles of catecholamines and 5-HT$_2$ and 5-HT$_3$ receptor interactions are unclear.

Evaluation

As with NMS, taking a detailed history is crucial. Use of two or more psychotropics confers a greater risk of developing SS. Obtaining a history of neuroleptic use and of psychosis can be especially important since NMS shares many clinical features with SS (Table 30-8).

A temporal relationship between the start of pharmacotherapy and the development of the syndrome exists. Laboratory abnormalities are mostly nonspecific or are secondary to the medical complications of the syndrome. A complete laboratory evaluation is nevertheless essential to rule out other etiologies for the signs and symptoms that are shared with SS. Leukocytosis, rhabdomyolysis, and liver function test abnormalities have all been reported in SS along with hyponatremia, hypomagnesemia, and hypocalcemia. These latter disturbances are thought to be related to fluid and electrolyte abnormalities. Disseminated intravascular coagulation (DIC) also has been reported in SS. Acute renal failure secondary to myoglobinuria can occur and it has been associated with fatalities, as has DIC.

It is interesting to note that certain secreting tumors like carcinoid and oat cell carcinoma have been associated with SS. X-ray examinations and imaging of the abdomen and lung may sometimes be helpful in working up SS. An EEG and neuroimaging often are useful in uncovering a seizure disorder or another neurologic condition as well.

The most common drug interactions associated with SS include MAOI-SSRI, MAOI–tricyclic antidepressants, and MAOI-venlafaxine combinations. In general when an SSRI is used in combination with an MAOI, an SS is more likely to occur. Drugs associated with SS are included in Table 30-9.

Overdoses of MAOIs also have caused SS. Because of the potential problems of using an MAOI and any medicine with serotonergic

Table 30-8. Comparison of Serotonin Syndrome (SS) with Neuroleptic Malignant Syndrome (NMS)

Feature	SS	NMS
Temperature	Hyperthermia variable	Hyperthermia
Mental status	Anxiety	Coma
	Coma	Confusion
	Confusion	Delirium
	Delirium	Stupor
	Euphoria	
	Irritability	
	Stupor	
Neurological	Ankle clonus	Hyperreflexia (uncommon)
	Hyperreflexia,	Muscle rigidity
	Incoordination	Tremor
	Muscle rigidity variable	
	Myoclonus	
	Tremor	
Behavioral	Agitation	Agitation
	Restlessness	Restlessness
Autonomic	Diaphoresis	Diaphoresis
	Hypertension/hypotension	Hypertension/hypotension
	Incontinence	Incontinence
	Mydriasis	Mydriasis
	Shivering	Sialorrhea
	Sialorrhea	Tachycardia
	Tachycardia	Tachypnea
	Tachypnea	
Gastrointestinal	Diarrhea	
	Nausea	
	Vomiting	
Laboratory	Elevated (uncommon)	Elevated (common)
	CPK	CPK
	WBC	WBC
	LFTs	LFTs

CPK = creatine kinase; WBC = white blood cell count; LFTs = liver function tests.
Modified from Keck PE, Arnold LM: The serotonin syndrome, *Psychiat Ann* 30: 333–343, 2000, p 339.

properties, caution on the part of the prescribing physician is required. With this in mind, it is good to be reminded that a 2-week wash-out interval following discontinuation of an MAOI is required before starting any serotonergic medications. In the case of fluoxetine discontinuation, there should be a minimum 5-week wash-out period before an MAOI is initiated.

Treatment

No prospective studies have looked at treatment of SS. Recommendations for treatment are based solely on anecdotes. SS is often self-limited, and removal of the offending agents will frequently result in resolution of symptoms within 24 hours. Therefore, the initial step in managing SS is to discontinue the suspected offending agent or agents. The next step is to provide supportive measures to prevent potential medical complications. These supportive measures include the use of antipyretics and cooling blankets to reduce hyperthermia, monitoring, and support of the respiratory and cardiovascular systems, IV hydration to prevent renal failure, use of clonazepam for myoclonic jerking, use of anticonvulsants if seizures arise, and use of hypertensive agents (such as nifedipine) for significantly elevated blood pressures. The syndrome rarely leads to

Table 30-9. Central Nervous System Serotonergic Agents

Enhanced serotonin synthesis
   L-tryptophan
Increased serotonin release
   Cocaine
   Amphetamines
   Fenfluramine
   Dextromethorphan
   Meperidine
   Methylene dioxymethamphetamine
   Sibutramine
Serotonin agonists
   Buspirone
   Dihydroergotamine (DHE)
   Lithium
   Meta-chlorophenylpiperazine (mCPP)
   Sumatriptan
   Trazodone
Inhibited serotonin catabolism
   Isocarboxazid
   Moclobemide
   Phenelzine
   Selegiline
   Tranylcypromine
Inhibited serotonin reuptake
   Amitriptyline
   Bromocriptine
   Clomipramine
   Desipramine
   Dextromethorphan
   Fenfluramine
   Fluoxetine
   Fluvoxamine
   Imipramine
   Meperidine
   Mirtazapine
   Nefazodone
   Nortriptyline
   Paroxetine
   Pethidine
   Sertraline
   Tramadol
   Trazodone
   Venlafaxine

Modified with permission from: Keck PE, Arnold LM: The serotonin syndrome, *Psychiat Ann* 30:333–343, 2000, p 336.

respiratory failure. When it does, it usually is because of aspiration, and artificial ventilation may be required.

Specific 5-HT receptor antagonism has occasionally been advocated for the treatment or prevention of the symptoms associated with SS. Cyproheptadine (4 to 24 mg/day) has been used. Mirtazapine, a 5-HT_3 and 5-HT_2 antagonist and ketanserin a 5-HT_2 antagonist, and propranolol, which has 5-HT_{1A} receptor-blocking properties, have all been used in a small number of cases. Benzodiazepines also have been reported to help.

Summary

The SS occurs infrequently as a toxic state secondary to serotonin excess produced by high doses or combinations of serotonergic medications. It usually begins soon after the addition of a serotonin agent or an increase in the dose of one. This syndrome is often mild and goes unrecognized; it also is self-limiting. Symptoms often disappear soon after the offending agents are discontinued. Supportive measures are required in more severe cases, which often come to the attention of physicians. Nonspecific serotonin receptor antagonists may be helpful in the treatment of the SS. Prevention, early recognition, and intervention will benefit from a heightened clinical awareness of medications that can cause serotonin excess.

References

1. Taylor MA: Catatonia: a review of a behavioral neurologic syndrome, *Neuropsychiatry Neuropsychol Behav Neurol* 3:48–72, 1990.
2. Fink M, Bush G, Francis A: Catatonia: a treatable disorder, occasionally recognized, *Direct Psychiatry* 13:1–7, 1993.
3. Fricchione G, Bush G, Fozdar M, et al: Recognition and treatment of the catatonic syndrome, *J Intensive Care Med* 12:135–147, 1997.
4. Kahlbaum K: *Catatonia*. Levy Y, and Priden T, translators; Baltimore: Johns Hopkins University Press, 1973.
5. Kraepelin E: *Dementia praecox and paraphrenia*. Barclay RM, translator; Robertson CM, editor, Huntington, NY, 1971, RE Krieger Publishing (facsimile edition).
6. Bleuler E: *Dementia praecox and the group of schizophrenia*. J. Zinkin J, translator; New York, 1950, International University Press.
7. Fink M, Taylor MA: Catatonia: a separate category in DSM IV? *Integrative Psychiatry* 7:2–5, 1991.
8. American Psychiatric Association: *Diagnostic and statistical manual of mental disorders, ed 4*, Washington, DC, 1994, American Psychiatric Press.
9. Philbrick KL, Rummans TA: Malignant catatonia, *J Neuropsychiatry Clin Neurosci* 6:1–13, 1994.

10. Lohr JB, Wisniewski AA: *Catatonia.* In Lohr JB, Wisniewski AA, editors: *The Neuropsychiatric basis of movement disorders,* Baltimore, 1987, Guilford Press, 201–117.

11. Mann SC, Caroff SN, Bleir HR, et al: Lethal catatonia, *Am J Psychiatry* 143:1374–1381, 1986.

12. Dabholkar PD: Use of ECT in hysterical catatonia: a case report and discussion, *Br J Psychiatry* 153:246–247, 1988.

13. Gelenberg AJ: The catatonic syndrome, *Lancet* 1:1339–1341, 1976.

14. Hermesh H, Hoffnung RA, Aizenberg D, et al: Catatonic signs in severe obsessive compulsive disorder, *J Clin Psychiatry* 50:303–305, 1989.

15. Rosebush PI, Hildebrand AM, Furlong BG, et al: Catatonic syndrome in a general psychiatric inpatient population: frequency, clinical presentation, and response to lorazepam, *J Clin Psychiatry* 51:357–362, 1990.

16. Barnes MP, Saunders M, Walls TJ, et al: The syndrome of Karl Ludwig Kahlbaum, *J Neurol Neurosurg Psychiatry* 49:991–996, 1986.

17. Altshuler LL, Cummings JL, Miles MJ: Mutism: review, differential diagnosis and report of 22 cases, *Am J Psychiatry* 143:1409–1414, 1986.

18. Clothier JL, Pazzaglia P, Freeman TW: Valuation and treatment of catatonia (letter), *Am J Psychiatry* 146:553–554, 1989.

19. Goeke JE, Hagan DS, Goelzer SL, et al: Lethal catatonia complicated by the development of neuroleptic malignant syndrome in a middle-aged female, *Crit Care Med* 19:1445–1448, 1991.

20. Tandon R, Walden M, Falcon S: Catatonia as a manifestation of paraneoplastic encephalopathy, *J Clin Psychiatry* 49:121–122, 1998.

21. Synder S, Prenzlauer S, Maruyama N, et al: Catatonia in patient with AIDS-related dementia (letter), *J Clin Psychiatry* 53:414, 1992.

22. Orlando RM, Daghestahi AN: A case of catatonia induced by bacterial meningoencephalitis, *J Clin Psychiatry* 48:489–490, 1987.

23. Wheeler AH, Ziegler MG, Insel PA, et al: Episodic catatonia, hypertension, and tachycardia: elevated plasma catecholamines, *Neurology* 35:1053–1055, 1985.

24. Korkina MV, Tsivl'ko MA, Kareva MA, et al: Features of catatono-oneiroid paroxysms of schizophrenia manifesting in the puerperal period, *ZH Nevropatol Psikhiatr* 83:1702–1707, 1983.

25. Miller DD, Sharafuddin MJA, Kathol RG: A case of clozapine-induced neuroleptic malignant syndrome, *J Clin Psychiatry* 52:99–101, 1991.

26. Najara JE, Enikeer IE: Risperidone and neuroleptic malignant syndrome: a case report, *J Clin Psychiatry* 56:534–535, 1995.

27. Kellam AMP: The (frequently) neuroleptic (potentially) malignant syndrome, *Br J Psychiatry* 157:169–173, 1990.

28. Kellam AMP: The neuroleptic malignant syndrome, so-called: a survey of the world literature, *Br J Psychiatry* 150:752–759, 1987.

29. Behan WMH, Bekheit AMO, More IAR: The muscle findings in the neuroleptic malignant syndrome associated with lysergic acid diethylamide, *J Neurol Neurosurg Psychiatry* 54:741–743, 1991.

30. Wetli CV, Fishbain DA: Cocaine-induced psychosis and sudden death in recreational cocaine users, *J Foren Sci* 30:873–880, 1985.

31. Kosten TR, Kleber HD: Sudden death in cocaine abusers: relation to neuroleptic malignant syndrome (letter), *Lancet* 1:1198–1199, 1987.

32. Carroll BT, Anfinson TJ, Kennedy JC, et al: Catatonic disorder due to general medical conditions, *J Neuropsychiatry Clin Neurosci* 6:122–133, 1994.

33. Plum F, Posner J: *Diagnosis of stupor and coma.* In *Contemporary neurology series, ed 3,* Philadelphia, PA, 1980, FA Davis, pp 308–311.

34. Bush G, Fink M, Petrides G, et al: Catatonia I. Rating scale and standardized examination, *Acta Psychiatr Scand* 93:129–136, 1996.

35. Kraepelin E: *Psychiatrie,* vol. 3, ed 8, Leipzig, Germany, Johann Ambrosius Barth, 1913, p 806.

36. Gjessing R: Contributions to the understanding of the pathophysiology of catatonic stupors, *Arch Gen Psychiatry* 96:379–392, 1932.

37. Stauder KH. Die toldliche katatinie, *Arch Psychiatry Nervenkr* 102:614–634, 1934.

38. Mann SC, Caroff SN, Bleier HR, et al: Lethal catatonia, *Am J Psychiatry* 143:1374–1381, 1986.

39. Caroff S: The neuroleptic malignant syndrome, *J Clin Psychiatry* 41:79–83, 1980.

40. Philbrick KL, Rummans TA: Malignant catatonia, *J Neuropsychiatry Clin Neurosci* 6:1–13, 1994.

41. Kalinowsky LB: Lethal catatonia and neuroleptic malignant syndrome, *Am J Psychiatry* 144:1106–1107, 1987.

42. Fricchione GL: Neuroleptic catatonia and its relationship to psychogenic catatonia, *Biol Psychiatry* 20:304–313, 1985.

43. Goforth HW, Carroll BT: The overlap of neuroleptic malignant syndrome (NMS) and catatonic diagnoses, *J Neuropsychiatry Clin Neurosci* 7:402, 1995.

44. Fink M: Neuroleptic malignant syndrome and catatonia: one entity or two? *Biol Psychiatry* 39:1–4, 1996.

45. Rosebush PI, Mazurek MF: Serum iron and neuroleptic malignant syndrome, *Lancet* 338:149–151, 1991.

46. Carroll BT, Goforth HW: Serum iron in catatonia, *Biol Psychiatry* 38:776–777, 1995.

47. Lee JW: Serum iron in catatonia and neuroleptic malignant syndrome, *Biol Psychiatry* 44:499–507, 1998.

48. White DA, Robins AH: Catatonia: harbinger of the neuroleptic malignant syndrome, *Br J Psychiatry* 158:419–421, 1991.

49. White DA: Catatonia and the neuroleptic malignant syndrome: a single entity? *Br J Psychiatry* 161:558–560, 1992.

50. Mann SC, Caroff SN: *Lethal catatonia and the neuroleptic malignant syndrome.* In Stefanis CN, Soldatos CR,

Rambazilas AD, editors: *Psychiatry: a world perspective*, vol. 3, Amsterdam, 1990, Elsevier Science, 287–292.

51. McCall WV, Shelp FE, McDonal WM: Controlled investigation of the amobarbital interview for catatonic mutism, *Am J Psychiatry* 149:202–206, 1992.

52. Henry JA, Woodruff GHA: A diagnostic sign in states of apparent unconsciousness, *Lancet* 2:920–921, 1978.

53. Guze SB: The occurrence of psychiatric illness in systemic lupus erythematosus, *Am J Psychiatry* 123:1562–1570, 1967.

54. Altshuler LL, Cummings JL, Miles MJ: Mutism: review, differential diagnosis and report of 22 cases, *Am J Psychiatry* 143:1409–1414, 1986.

55. Fink M: *Catatonia*. In Trimble M, Cummings J, editors: *Contemporary behavioral neurology*, Oxford, 1997, Butterworth/Heinemann, pp 289–308.

56. Dysken MW, Kooser JA, Haraszti JS, Davis JM: Clinical usefulness of sodium amobarbital interviewing, *Arch Gen Psychiatry* 36:789–794, 1979.

57. Lew TY, Tollefson G: Chlorpromazine-induced neuroleptic malignant syndrome and its response to diazepam, *Biol Psychiatry* 18:1441–1446, 1983.

58. Fricchione GL, Cassem NH, Hooberman D, Hobson D: Intravenous lorazepam in neuroleptic induced catatonia, *J Clin Psychopharmacol* 3:338–342, 1983.

59. McEvoy JP, Lohr JB: Diazepam for catatonia, *Am J Psychiatry* 141:284–285, 1984.

60. Rosebush PI, Hildebrand Am, Furlong BG, Mazurek MF: Catatonic syndrome in a general psychiatric inpatient population: frequency, clinical presentation, and response to lorazepam, *J Clin Psychiatry* 51:357–362, 1990.

61. Bush G, Fink M, Petrides G, et al: Catatonia: II. Treatment with lorazepam and electroconvulsive therapy, *Acta Psychiatr Scand* 93:137–143, 1996.

62. Francis A, Chandragiri S, Rizvi S: Lorazepam therapy of the neuroleptic malignant syndrome. Presented at the Annual Meeting of the American Psychiatric Association; May 30-June 4, 1998; Toronto, Ontario, Canada.

63. Mann SC, Caroff SN, Bleier HR, et al: Electroconvulsive therapy of the lethal catatonia syndrome, *Convulsive Therapy* 6:239–247, 1990.

64. Caroff SN, Mann SC: Neuroleptic malignant syndrome, *Med Clin North Am* 77:185–202, 1993.

65. Sakkas P, Davis JM, Hua J, et al: Pharmacotherapy of neuroleptic malignant syndrome, *Psychiat Ann* 21: 157–164, 1991.

66. Rosebush PI, Stewart T, Mazurek MF: The treatment of neuroleptic malignant syndrome: are dantrolene and bromocriptine useful adjuncts to supportive care? *Br J Psychiatry* 159:709–712, 1991.

67. Sczesni B, Bittkau S, von Baumgarten F, et al: Intravenous lisuride in the treatment of the neuroleptic malignant syndrome, *J Clin Psychopharmacol* 11: 185–188, 1991.

68. Mahmood T: Bromocriptine in catatonic stupor, *Br J Psychiatry* 158:437–438, 1991.

69. Rogers D: Catatonia: a contemporary approach, *J Neuropsychiatry Clni Neurosci* 3:334–340, 1991.

70. Neppe VM: Management of catatonic stupor with L-dopa, *Clin Neuropharmacol* 11:90–91, 1988.

71. Jones DL, Mogenson GJ: Nucleus accumbens to the globus pallidus GABA projection subserving ambulatory activity, *Am J Physiol* 238:R63–R69, 1980.

72. Sackeim HA, Decina P, Prohovnik I, et al: Anticonvulsant and antidepressant properties of electroconvulsive therapy: a proposed mechanism of action, *Biol Psychiatry* 18:1301–1310, 1983.

73. Kish SJ, Kilnert R, Miriauf M, et al: Brain neurotransmitter changes in three patients who had a fatal hyperthermia syndrome, *Am J Psychiatry* 147:1358–1363, 1990.

74. Nisijima K, Ishiguro T: Neuroleptic malignant syndrome: a study of CSF monoamine metabolism, *Biol Psychiatry* 27:280–288, 1990.

75. Northoff G, Wenke J, Demisch L, et al: Catatonia: short-term response to lorazepam and dopaminergic metabolism, *Psychopharmacology* 122:182–186, 1995.

76. Mann SC, Caroff SN, Lazarus A: Pathogenesis of neuroleptic malignant syndrome, *Psychiat Ann* 23: 175–180, 1991.

77. Busber M, Schmidt WJ: Injection of apomorphine into the medial prefrontal cortex of the rat increases haloperidol-induced catalepsy, *Biol Psychiatry* 36:64–67, 1994.

78. Reinhard JF, Bannon MJ, Roth RH: Acceleration by stress of dopamine synthesis and metabolism in prefrontal cortex: antagonism by diazepam, *Naunyn-Schmiedeberg's Archive Pharmacologia* 318:374–377, 1982.

79. Gulati A, Srimal RC, Shawan BN: Up-regulation of brain benzodiazepine receptors by electroconvulsive shocks, *Pharmacology Research Communications* 18: 581–589, 1986.

80. Petrides G, Divadeenam KM, Bush G, Francis A: Synergism of lorazepam and electroconvulsive therapy in the treatment of catatonia, *Biol Psychiatry* 42:375–381, 1997.

81. Alexander GE, Crutcher MD, DeLong MR: Basal ganglia-thalamo-cortical circuits: parallel substrates for motor, oculomotor, "prefrontal" and "limbic" functions, *Prog Brain Res* 85:119–146, 1990.

82. Northoff G, Bogerts B, Leseunges A, et al: Alternations in orbitofrontal activity in catatonia: a combined FMRI/MEG study. Presented at the XI World Congress of Psychiatry meeting; August 6–11, 1999; Hamburg, Germany.

83. Friedhoff AJ: A strategy for developing novel drugs for the treatment of schizophrenia, *Schizophr Bull* 9: 555–562, 1983.

84. Kim JS, Hassler R: Effects of acute haloperidol on the gamma aminobutyric acid system in rat striatum and substantia nigra, *Brain Res* 88:150–153, 1975.

85. Stevens J, Wilson K, Foote W: GABA blockade, dopamine and schizophrenia: experimental studies in the cat, *Psychopharmacologia (Berl)* 39:105–119, 1974.

86. Kalivas PW, Duffy P, Eberhardt H: Modulation of A10 dopamine neurons by gamma-a aminobutyric acid agonists, *J Pharmacol Exp Ther* 253:858–866, 1990.

87. Jaskiw GE, Weinberger DR, Crawley JN: Microinjection of apomorphine into the prefrontal cortex of the rat reduces dopamine metabolite concentration in the microdialystate from the caudate nucleus, *Biol Psychiatry* 29:703–706, 1991.

88. Friedhoff AJ, Carr KD, Uysal S, Schweitzer J: Repeated inescapable stress produces a neuroleptic like effect on the conditioned avoidance response, *Neuropsychopharmacology* 13:129–138, 1995.

89. Gurrera R: The role of calcium and peripheral catecholamines in the pathophysiology of neuroleptic malignant syndrome, *Psychiatric Annals* 30:356–362, 2000.

90. Carroll BT: The universal field hypothesis of catatonia and neuroleptic malignant syndrome, *CNS Spectrums* 5:26–33, 2000.

91. Keck PE, Arnold LM: The serotonin syndrome, *Psychiat Ann* 30:333–343, 2000.

92. Reddick B, Stern TA: *Catatonia, neuroleptic malignant syndrome, and serotonin syndrome*. In Stern TA, Herman JB, editors: *Psychiatry. update and board preparation, ed 2*, New York, 2004, McGraw Hill, pp 219–226.

93. Sternbach H: The serotonin syndrome, *Am J Psychiatry* 148:705–713, 1991.

Chapter 31
Patients with Disordered Sleep

Patrick Smallwood, M.D.
Theodore A. Stern, M.D.

Scholars have long sought the cause and nature of sleep and sleep disorders, yet theories have far exceeded clear facts. Plato, for example, believed that sleep was caused by vapors arising from the stomach and condensing in the head, while Hippocrates believed that sleep was the result of blood and its warmth retreating into the body. Sixteenth- and seventeenth-century scholars debated whether sleep was induced by oxygen deprivation, accumulated toxins, or the daily thickening of blood that impaired spirits from entering the nerves.[1] Despite these age-old theories, only in recent years have the mysteries of sleep been slowly unraveled. Indeed, we now know that sleep is an active biochemical process complete with various physiologic markers, stages, and patterns that, like vital signs, provide a basic indication of overall well being. This chapter examines the biologic and psychiatric aspects of normal and disordered sleep, followed by a brief discussion of the diagnosis and treatment of common sleep disorders.

Sleep Stages and Normal Sleep

Aserinsky and Kleitman (1953) were the first to investigate eye movements during sleep. Kleitman postulated that depth of sleep could be assessed through eye motility, and both he and Aserinsky began testing this hypothesis through direct observation of eye movements of infants during sleep.[2] They noted slow rolling eye movements during the early stages of sleep that disappeared as sleep

progressed, and they saw periods of rapid eye movements associated with irregular breathing and increased heart rate.[2,3] They coined the terms *non-rapid eye movements* (NREM) to indicate the slow rolling rhythmic eye movements and *rapid eye movements* (REM) to indicate the fast erratic eye movements. In 1957 Kleitman and Dement discovered that REM and NREM sleep occurred cyclically throughout the night and named this overall NREM-REM pattern *sleep architecture*.[2,3]

Polysomnography

Polysomnography is the gold standard method for the evaluation of disordered sleep. It involves the simultaneous recording of multiple physiologic variables in a standardized fashion known as the *polysomnogram* (PSG).[4] The parameters recorded by the PSG include, but are not limited to, the following:

Electroencephalogram (EEG): A recording of the electrical activity of cortical neurons via scalp electrodes that are placed in standardized positions according to the International 10–20 System.

Electro-oculogram (EOG): A recording of eye movements.

Electrocardiogram (ECG): A recording of heart rhythm.

Electromyogram (EMG): A recording of the activity of the left and right tibialis anterior muscles and the submental (chin) muscles.

Respiratory efforts: A recording of nasal and oral airflow by means of nasal thermistors, and thoracoabdominal movements by means of strain gauges.

Pulse oximetry: A recording of oxygen saturation in the blood.

Snore monitor: A detection and recording of snoring by means of a microphone placed on the lateral aspect of the neck.

Through the use of the PSG, wakefulness, sleep onset, NREM sleep, and REM sleep can be identified and studied.

The *waking state* is defined by polysomnography in the following manner: (1) the EEG reveals an 8 to 14 hertz (Hz) wave pattern known as *alpha waves*, (2) the EMG reveals muscle tone and activity, and (3) the EOG demonstrates variable eye movements, including blinking.[2] In the normal subject, *sleep onset* follows the transition from wake to NREM stage 1 sleep.[2,5–8] Being a highly subjective state, sleep onset is not reliably obtained by asking the individual and must therefore be determined by specific polysomnographic criteria, which include (1) a decrease in alpha activity and the emergence of relatively low-voltage mixed-frequency (RLVMF) activity and (2) slow rolling eye movements on the EOG.[5] The EMG usually, but not always, registers a modest decrease in muscle activity. Some patients do not perceive themselves as asleep and may engage in *automatic behavior*, a phenomenon in which very complex cognitive and behavioral tasks are performed outside awareness.[5,9]

Sleep is normally entered through *NREM sleep*. NREM is divided into four stages; each one is identified by specific criteria on the PSG.[2,5]

Stage 1: Alpha waves, present during the waking state, comprise less than 50% of an *epoch* (a 30-second interval on the PSG). RLVMF waves emerge, with the most prominent ones being *theta waves* (4 to 7 Hz).

Stage 2: Theta activity continues. During this stage, two new wave types emerge: *sleep spindles* (rhythmic 12 to 14 Hz waves lasting 0.5 seconds or more) and *K-complexes* (high amplitude negative waves followed by a positive deflection, lasting 0.5 seconds or more).

Stage 3: During this stage, *delta waves* (high amplitude, slow frequency 0.5 to 2.0 Hz waves) occur. Delta waves occupy at least 20%, but not more than 50%, of an epoch. The EMG begins to show less muscle activity.

Stage 4: Almost identical to stage 3, except delta waves now occupy greater than 50% of an epoch.

Stage 3 and 4 NREM sleep is also known as *delta* or *slow wave sleep*. The distinction between stage 3 and 4 NREM sleep, while scientifically intriguing, has no known clinical significance at this time.

REM sleep, also known as *paradoxical sleep* due to its similarity to wakefulness and NREM sleep, is defined by three principle features. First, the EEG demonstrates RLVMF wave patterns that are virtually indistinguishable from those of NREM stage 1. Second, the EMG reveals an absence of, or a marked decrease in, muscle activity. Finally, conjugate rapid eye movements become evident on the EOG.[4]

Sleep Cycle and Architecture

NREM and REM sleep do not occur randomly throughout the night; instead, they alternate in a rhythmic fashion known as the *NREM-REM cycle*.[2,5,6] In healthy individuals, this cycle begins with NREM stage 1 and progresses to NREM stages 2, 3, 4, 3, 2, and then REM. This pattern generally repeats itself every 90 to 120 minutes throughout the night. NREM stages 3 and 4 are most prominent in the first half of the night; they diminish during the latter half of the night. REM sleep, however, is less prominent in the first half of the night, and it increases as the night progresses. *Sleep latency* typically lasts 10 to 20 minutes; it is the time from "lights out" to the first NREM stage 1. The time (which is usually 90 to 100 minutes) from sleep onset to the first REM is known as *REM latency*. *Sleep efficiency* is the actual amount of sleep/total time in bed times 100. The average amount of sleep a night for adults is between 6 and 9 hours.

The distributions of sleep stages across an average night are as follows:

Time awake after sleep onset: less than 5%
NREM stage: 2% to 5%
NREM stage 2: 45% to 55%
NREM stages 3 and 4: 13% to 23%
REM sleep: 20% to 25%

Although sleep architecture is influenced by a host of variables, the amount of wakefulness is influenced by an internal biologic cycle known as the *circadian rhythm*.[1,10] This rhythm or "biologic clock" is an endogenous rhythm of bodily functions that is influenced by environmental cues, or *zeitgebers*, the main one of which is daylight. The cycle is unique to each individual, averaging 25 hours for most individuals, but possibly 50 hours for others. Sleep disorders related to the circadian rhythm emerge when an individual's circadian rhythm clashes with environmental and societal expectations.

Sleep Across the Life Span

Sleep and sleep quality changes across the lifespan. Infants spend about two thirds of the day sleeping, whereas in adulthood, this amount decreases to less than one third. As a result of degenerative changes in the central nervous system (CNS), sleep architecture becomes altered as people age. These changes include increases in sleep latency, nocturnal awakenings, and time spent in NREM stage 1 sleep, and decreases in delta sleep, REM sleep, REM latency, and overall sleep efficiency.[11–13]

Neuroanatomic Basis for Sleep

Although the actual neuroanatomic basis for the sleep-wake cycle remains uncertain, current research reveals that specific regions of the brain are critical for wakefulness and for sleep. These neuronal systems are located in the brainstem, hypothalamus, and basal forebrain, and they project diffusely throughout the neocortex.[14–16] Any disruption of these regions invariably leads to alterations in the sleep-wake cycle and gives rise to sleep disorders. Wakefulness is maintained by tonic activity in the ascending reticular activating system (ARAS) and is strongly influenced by sensory stimuli, the most powerful of which are sound and pain. Sleep develops when there is decreased activity in the ARAS and activation of a hypnagogic sleep system located predominately in the dorsal raphe nucleus. Although no specific neural generator for REM sleep has been identified, REM sleep is known to be an active process involving both the nucleus ceruleus and the gigantocellular tegmental field.

Sleep Disorders

Although several classification systems for sleep disorders exist, the *Diagnostic and Statistical Manual of Mental Disorders*, fourth edition, text revision (*DSM-IV-TR*)[17] and the International Classification of Sleep Disorders (ICSD)[18] systems are the most widely used. The ICSD systems offers a comprehensive nosology of sleep disorders and is the official classification recognized by the American Sleep Disorder Association (ASDA), and the *DSM-IV-TR* is complaint-based; as such, it is perhaps the simplest and easiest to understand. The *DSM-IV-TR* divides sleep disorders into primary and secondary sleep disorders based on presumed etiology. Primary sleep disorders are the most common and are therefore emphasized.

Primary Sleep Disorder

The *DSM-IV-TR* subdivides primary sleep disorders into dyssomnias and parasomnias, based on whether the problem involves the quality of sleep itself or a behavioral and physiologic event that occurs during sleep or sleep transitions.

Dyssomnias

Dyssomnias are primary sleep disorders that result in complaints of either too little sleep (insomnia) or too much sleep (hypersomnia). Included in the dyssomnias are primary insomnias, primary hypersomnias, narcolepsy, breathing-related sleep disorders, circadian rhythm disorders, and dyssomnias not otherwise specified.

Primary Insomnia.   *Primary insomnia* is the classic form of insomnia in which patients complain of deficient, inadequate, or unrefreshing sleep; malaise; and fatigue. Sufferers often experience overarousal and anxiety at bedtime and have decreased daytime functioning with mild to moderate impairment in concentration and psychomotor functioning.[19] To diagnose this disorder, there must be objective daytime sleepiness and/or subjective feelings of not being well rested, as well as an absence of psychiatric or medical conditions that better account for the symptoms. Objective findings include prolonged sleep latency (an inability to fall asleep in less than 30 minutes) and shallow or fragmented sleep as evidenced by multiple arousals on a PSG.

Sleep-state misperception, also known as *subjective insomnia* and *nonrestorative sleep*, is a primary insomnia in which sufferers complain of inadequate and/or poor sleep, but objective findings on the PSG are lacking. Invariably, patients with sleep-state misperception underestimate total sleep time and efficiency and overestimate sleep latency. *Idiopathic insomnia* is chronic primary insomnia that is present from childhood and is most likely the result of an innate process.

Primary insomnias are perhaps the hardest sleep disorders to treat; treatment involves the selection of a specific modality based on the cause. Nonpharmacologic techniques, such as application of good sleep hygiene, the relaxation response, or meditation should be attempted before any pharmacologic interventions. Table 31-1 provides a guideline for proper sleep hygiene. Sleep restriction therapy, a specific method of graded matching of time spent in bed to actual sleep, is useful for more persistent and severe cases, but it often requires consultation with sleep disorders specialist. Other behavioral techniques can be learned through self-help tapes or manuals or

Table 31-1. Basic Sleep Hygiene

Limit in-bed time to the amount present before the sleep
  disturbance
Lie down only when sleepy, and sleep only as much as
  necessary to feel refreshed
Use the bed for sleep only
Maintain comfortable sleeping conditions and avoid
  excessive warmth and cold
Wake up at a regular time each day
Avoid daytime naps
Exercise regularly, but early in the day
Limit sedatives
Avoid alcohol, tobacco, and caffeine near bedtime
Eat at regular times daily and avoid large meals near
  bedtime
Eat a light snack, if hungry, near bedtime
Practice evening relaxation routines, such as progressive
  muscle relaxation, meditation, or taking a very hot,
  20-minute, body temperature-raising bath near bedtime

from consultation with mental health clinicians. If behavioral techniques are unsuccessful, brief intermittent use of sedative-hypnotics may be appropriate. The long-term use of benzodiazepines, although controversial, is common in practice and may be appropriate for those patients with insomnia secondary to an anxiety disorder. Benzodiazepines should either be used cautiously or avoided in patients with a history of alcohol or substance abuse, a personality disorder, or a sleep-related breathing disorder. To avoid dose escalation with these agents, prescriptions should be carefully monitored when used for more than 4 weeks. Newer nonbenzodiazepine agents, such as zolpidem and zaleplon, are often preferred. Melatonin remains incompletely studied; some authors suggest that 2 mg at bedtime may be effective. Sedating antihistamines can be used as alternatives to benzodiazepines; however, they may cause delirium in the elderly or in those with a compromised CNS. Chloral hydrate, short-acting barbiturates, and ethchlorvynol are less effective and more toxic than other agents; they should be used rarely, if ever, and then only under closely monitored conditions.

Primary Hypersomnia.   The hallmark of *primary hypersomnia* is the complaint of somnolence and excessive daytime sleep. Other complaints include difficulty waking, sleep drunkenness, headache, intellectual dysfunction, and Raynaud's phenomenon. Like primary insomnia, primary hypersomnia is not the direct result of an underlying medical or psychiatric conditions; it is confirmed by objective PSG findings. *Recurrent hypersomnia*, also known as *Kleine-Levin syndrome*, is a rare, often self-limiting condition that primarily affects adolescent males. Symptoms include hypersomnia, hyperphagia, and hypersexuality. While the exact cause is unknown, it often follows an acute viral infection. Treatment includes the use of psychostimulants, selective serotonin-reuptake inhibitors (SSRIs), and monamine oxidase inhibitors (MAOIs).

Narcolepsy.   *Narcolepsy* is a primary hypersomnia associated with a classic tetrad of symptoms:

1. *Sleep attacks*: Irresistible and brief sleep episodes with sleep-onset REM periods (SOREMPs) that occur several times a day, often at inappropriate times.

2. *Cataplexy*: Sudden and brief bilateral loss of motor tone without impairment of consciousness, triggered by strong emotions, such as laughter, anger, or surprise.
3. *Sleep paralysis*: Brief episodes of muscular paralysis associated with the transitions of sleep onset or awakening.
4. *Hypnagogic* or *hypnopompic hallucinations*: Vivid visual and auditory phenomena that are associated with the transitions to sleep onset or awakening.

Narcolepsy occurs in approximately 0.07% of the general population; it typically arises in the second decade of life. Symptoms usually begin with sleep and are associated with excessive sleepiness. Current research suggests that genetics play a role in this disorder because a strong association exists between narcolepsy and the human leukocyte antigens HLA-DR2 and DQwl phenotypes. The probability of developing narcolepsy is 40 times greater if an immediate family member suffers from it.[20–22] While the exact abnormality of narcolepsy is unknown, leading theories implicate a mutation in the gene that codes for the production of the neurotransmitter *hypocretin*.[23]

Treatment for narcolepsy is aimed at reducing both daytime sleepiness and cataplexy. Daytime sleepiness is effectively treated with psychostimulants, particularly methylphenidate (Ritalin), dextroamphetamine (Dexedrine), and to a lesser extent, pemoline (Cylert).[24,25] Modafinil (Provigil), a new central adrenergic stimulant, is gaining popularity because it promotes wakefulness, has minimal side effects, and a low potential for abuse.[26–29] Antidepressants, due to their ability to suppress REM sleep, particularly the tricyclic antidepressants (TCAs), are the treatment of choice for cataplexy, sleep paralysis, and hypnagogic hallucinations. Prophylactic naps, when feasible, can reduce the total daily dose of stimulants required.

Breathing-Related Sleep Disorders. *Breathing-related sleep disorders*, particularly sleep apnea syndromes, are the most commonly encountered hypersomnias. The essential feature of these disorders is disrupted sleep due to repeated apnea and oxygen desaturation. Prior to a discussion of breathing-related sleep disorders, several terms must be defined. *Apnea* is defined as the cessation

of nasobuccal airflow longer than 10 seconds. The type of apnea that a person experiences during sleep is based on its proposed cause and the presence or absence of respiratory effort during the event. *Central apneas* are identified by the cessation of airflow with no attempt to initiate thoracoabdominal respiratory effort. The etiology of the central apnea, while debated, is felt to lie in abnormal CNS processes. *Obstructive apneas*, on the other hand, are identified by the cessation of airflow as a result of a collapse in the upper airway. Unlike central apneas, obstructive apneas demonstrate continued or even increased respiratory effort. These obstruction can be so complete and the effort so powerful that the chest and abdomen can move in opposite directions, which is a phenomenon known as *paradoxical breathing*. *Mixed apneas*, the most common type of apneas encountered, are events in which a central apnea is followed by an obstructive apnea. An *hypopnea* is simply a reduction, rather than cessation, of nasobuccal airflow or thoracoabdominal movements during sleep. To be a clinically significant, an hypopnea must result in at least a 4% decrease in the oxygen saturation and/or be associated with an arousal pattern on the EEG. The *apnea index* (AI) is the number of clinically significant apneas per hour of sleep, and the *hypopnea index* (HI) is the number of clinically significant hypopneas per hour of sleep. The *respiratory disturbance index* (RDI),[30] also known as *apnea-hypopnea* index (AHI), is the sum of the AI and the HI. An AI of greater than 5, HI of greater than 5, or an RDI of greater than 10 is considered pathologic and warrants treatment.[30]

Of all the sleep apnea spectrum disorders and disorders of excessive daytime sleepiness (EDS), obstructive sleep apnea syndrome (OSA) is the most common, accounting for 40% to 50% of all patients seen in sleep disorder centers.[2,31,32] The estimated prevalence of OSA is 1% to 4% of the U.S. adult male population, with the prevalence increasing to 8.5% of men between the ages of 40 to 65 years.[3,10,21,30–33] Women account for 12% to 35% of OSA patients, with the majority of them being postmenopausal, suggesting that female hormones may be somewhat protective against OSA.[17] The most significant risk factors for OSA are as follows: male, 40 to 65 years old, obese, smoker, user/abuser of alcohol, and poor physical health.[31–33] The principle defect is repetitive occlusion of the upper airway at the level of the pharynx (which results from an abnormal decrease in oropharyngeal musculature tone), excessive tissue mass in the pharynx and tongue, malposition of the jaw or tongue, or a narrow airway. Nocturnal symptoms include snoring, choking, enuresis, reflux, hypoxemia, hypercapnia, and cardiac dysrhythmias; daytime symptoms include headaches, hypersomnolence, automatic behavior, neuropsychiatric abnormalities, and hypertension.[34–36]

The treatment of OSA involves identification and correction of the underlying etiology. Patients should be encouraged to lose weight and avoid alcohol and sedatives, which prolong apneas by increasing vagal tone, relaxing muscles, and preventing arousal for breathing. Because apneas are affected by gravity, positional therapy can be utilized in mild to moderate OSA. No medication has been shown to be clearly beneficial in the treatment of OSA, although pharmacologic agents, such as protriptyline, fluoxetine, and medroxyprogesterone have been used in the treatment of OSA.[10,11,17,37] Oral appliances aimed at altering the position of structures of the upper airway to create a larger airway or to prevent further collapse are indicated for those patients with primary snoring, mild OSA, or moderate to severe OSA (who are intolerant of or refuse either continuous positive airway pressure [CPAP] or surgical interventions).[10,38,39] Uvulopalatopharyngoplasty (UPPP) is an option selected by some patients. Mainly used to prevent snoring, UPPP aims to increase the volume of the oropharynx by removing the tonsils, adenoids, posterior soft palate, and redundant tissue on the sides of the pharynx by means of primary or laser-assisted surgery.[5,17] The overall success rate for UPPP, as measured by at least a 50% reduction in apnea index, is only 40% to 50%; moreover, there is often a gradual return of apneas to pretreatment levels.[3,5,17] Until very recently, tracheostomy was considered the treatment of choice for severe OSA. First-line therapy now includes nasal continuous positive airway pressure (nCPAP) and bilevel positive airway pressure (BiPAP), both of which work by providing an air pressure "splint" to the upper airway. For patients who receive no treatment and who have an apnea index of greater than 20, the probability of a cumulative 8-year survival is reported at

63% ± 17%. With the use of nCPAP, regardless of the initial apnea index, the probability of a cumulative 8-year survival rises to 100%.[40]

Circadian Rhythm Sleep Disorders

Circadian rhythm sleep disorders emerge when societal expectations conflict with an individual's endogenous sleep-wake cycle. Although patients suffering from these disorders may complain of insomnia, hypersomnia, sleepiness, and fatigue, the timing of sleep—not its quality and architecture—is adversely affected. The most frequently encountered circadian rhythm disorders include jet lag syndrome, shift-work sleep disorder, delayed sleep phase disorder, advanced sleep phase disorder, and non-24 hour day (or hypernyctohemeral) syndrome. *Jet lag* occurs when an individual rapidly crosses several time zones, often from western to eastern time zones, which results in an advancement in the sleep-wake cycle and leaves the individual feeling tired earlier in the evening.[41] *Shift-work sleep disorder* occurs when the circadian rhythm conflicts with a work schedule that does not coincide with a conventional day-night cycle.[42] *Delayed sleep phase disorder* occurs in individuals whose circadian rhythm is set for a later time than the conventional sleep-wake cycle.[43] Considered "night owls," these individuals are most alert in the evening and at night, and become sleepy several hours after the conventional bedtime. If left undisturbed, they can sleep 7 to 8 hours, with problems arising when they are required to adhere to conventional daytime schedules. *Advanced sleep phase disorder* occurs in individuals whose circadian rhythm is set for an earlier time than the conventional sleep-wake cycle.[44] Considered "larks," these individuals (who are frequently elderly) are most alert in the earlier morning and they become sleepy several hours earlier than the conventional bedtime. While sleeping for 7 to 8 hours, they may awaken at 2 to 3 AM, complaining of an inability to stay asleep all night. The *non-24-hour day* (or "*hypernyctohemeral*") *syndrome* is a phenomenon seen most commonly in individuals who are totally blind and who are unable to perceive visual *zeitgebers*. These patients, who function on a natural circadian rhythm of 24.5 to 25.0 hours, go to sleep and wake up about 45 minutes later each day.[45] As opposed to individuals who follow a conventional sleep-wake schedule, their sleep-wake cycle will literally go "around the clock" in approximately a 3-week period.

The diagnosis of circadian rhythm disorders is based primarily on the history, which can be obtained through a detailed sleep-wake diary maintained for several weeks. Because most circadian rhythm disorders are self-limited and resolve as the individual adjusts to the new sleep-wake schedule, aggressive treatment is unnecessary. Common treatment options include gradually delaying sleep until they achieve a new schedule, or receive light therapy or melatonin.

Dyssomnias Not Otherwise Specified. *Periodic limb movement disorder* (PLMD), sometimes called *nocturnal myoclonus*, is a common dyssomnia that affects up to 40% of people older than 65 years of age and 11% of sleep disorder clinic patients who complain of insomnia.[46–48] PLMD manifests as brief (0.5 to 5.0 seconds), stereotypic, and involuntary contractions of the lower limbs (frequently the dorsiflexors of the foot and flexors of the lower legs), at intervals of 20 to 40 seconds. Contractions appear more commonly during NREM stages 1 and 2: although patients are unaware of them, the EEG demonstrates nocturnal arousals and actual awakenings. Sleep is often unrefreshing, with hypersomnia being the most common complaint. Diagnosis is made by overnight polysomnography and is confirmed when the *myoclonus index* (number of leg jerks per hour of sleep accompanied by arousals) reaches five or more. While the pathogenesis of PLMD is unknown, a variety of medical conditions (e.g., renal failure, diabetes, chronic anemia, peripheral nerve injuries, and even uncomplicated pregnancy) and medications (e.g., antidepressants, neuroleptics, lithium, diuretics, and narcotics [especially with narcotic withdrawal]) are associated with it. Treatment is symptomatic and includes use of dopamine agonists (e.g., levodopa), dopaminergic facilitating agents (e.g., selegiline), and benzodiazepines (particularly clonazepam).[49]

A disorder closely related to PLMD is the *restless leg syndrome* (RLS). RLS is characterized by intense aching or crawling sensations inside the legs and calves that occur while sitting or lying; it causes an irresistible urge to move or rub the legs. Symptoms arise mainly at bedtime and are partially relieved by movement, which unfortunately interrupts sleep initiation because the patient frequently paces. Like PLMD, RLS is associated with various medical problems, especially renal failure, diabetes, iron-deficiency anemia, and peripheral nerve injury, as well as with use of medications, particularly SSRIs. Symptomatic relief may be provided by medications, such as L-dopa and clonazepam.[50]

Parasomnias

Parasomnias are a group of primary sleep disorders in which abnormal behaviors or physiologic events arise during specific sleeps stages or during the transitions between wakefulness and sleep. These events are often bizarre; however, they rarely are a cause for great concern for the patient or the physician. Different from dyssomnias, children are more commonly affected by parasomnias than are adults. Sleepwalking disorder, sleep terror disorder, nightmare disorder, REM behavior disorder, and sleep-related seizures are the more clinically significant parasomnias, and therefore will be the primary focus of this discussion.

Non-Rapid Eye Movement Sleep Disorders. The hallmarks of this group of parasomnias are its occurrence primarily during delta sleep, and amnesia for the specific events carried out during sleep. The most commonly encountered NREM sleep disorders are sleepwalking disorder and night terrors. With s*leepwalking disorder* or "somnambulism," the patient experiences episodic motor behaviors while emerging from delta sleep, most often during the first third of the night. While the behaviors are often simple (e.g., walking, sitting up in bed, or picking at bed sheets), more complex and serious behaviors can occur (e.g., running, eating, driving, or committing murder).[51] Patients are frequently unresponsive to efforts to wake them, confused and disoriented when actually awakened, and amnestic to the sleep-related event the next day. Sleepwalking is not uncommon in childhood; it is rare in adulthood, a fact that should prompt a search for a possible underlying medical, neurologic, or pharmacologic etiology. No definitive treatment for sleepwalking exists, but some patients respond to low-dose benzodiazepines or sedating antidepressants. Adjunctive therapies include reassurance, hypnosis, and provision of a safe sleep environment, as patients have been known to trip or to fall out of open windows.

Like sleepwalking disorder, *sleep terror disorder*, also known as *night terrors, pavor nocturnus*, or *incubus*, occurs during partial arousal from delta sleep, usually during the first third of the night. As in sleepwalking disorder, patients are difficult to awaken, they lack dream recall, and they are amnestic for the episodes. Caretakers are often bothered more by this disorder than are patients. Symptoms include repeated awakenings from sleep followed by intense fear, screaming, flailing, and autonomic hyperarousal (e.g., tachycardia, tachypnea, and mydriasis).[52] In adults, this disorder is associated with posttraumatic stress disorder (PTSD), generalized anxiety disorder, and borderline personality disorder. Treatment includes use of low-dose benzodiazepines, which suppress delta sleep. Adjunctive therapies include psychotherapy and stress reduction techniques.

REM Sleep Disorders. The hallmarks of this group of parasomnias are occurrence in REM sleep, dreaming, and awareness of the specific events. The most commonly encountered REM sleep disorders are nightmare disorder and REM behavior disorder. The essential feature of *nightmare disorder* is repeated episodes of terrifying dreams that awaken the patient. In contrast to patients with sleep terror disorder, patients with nightmare disorder often have vivid recall of the events, are atonic while experiencing them, demonstrate no autonomic arousal, and experience the events in the latter half of the night when REM sleep is longest and most dense. The specific etiology for nightmares is often underlying emotional stress, and treatment is aimed at stress reduction; however, it may include psychotherapy, rehearsal instructions, and reassurance.

REM behavior disorder (RBD) is perhaps the most dramatic of all the parasomnias. As in sleepwalking disorder, patients with RBD may exhibit simple to quite complex behaviors while asleep, including jumping out of bed, walking, running, or singing.[53] In contrast to sleepwalking disorder, RBD, like all REM sleep disorders, occurs later in the night when REM is longest and it is accompanied by vivid dream recall. Unlike other REM sleep disorders, however, patients with RBD lack the muscle atonia that normally accompanies REM

sleep, resulting in patients literally acting out dream content.[54] The disorder is idiopathic in more than half of the cases, but it may be due to underlying organic processes, such Parkinson's disease, vascular and Alzheimer's dementia, multiple system atrophy, focal brain stem lesions, and alcoholism. It is more common in the elderly, and it affects males nine times more frequently than females. Low-dose clonazepam, which suppresses REM density and length, has an 80% to 90% success rate. Other treatment options, if clonazepam is ineffective, include levodopa-carbidopa, clonidine, or carbamazepine.

Diffuse Sleep Disorders. The key feature of this group of parasomnias is that the event can arise during any phase of sleep. The most clinically relevant disorder in this group is *sleep-related seizures*. Sleep-related seizures are quite rare and are often confused with parasomnias, such as sleep terror disorder, REM sleep behavior disorder, sleepwalking disorder, enuresis, or nocturnal panic attacks.[55] Seizures occur predominately during the first 2 hours of sleep and most often during light NREM sleep or in transitional states to and from REM sleep. Seizure type may be either generalized or partial, with temporal and frontal lobe seizures being the most commonly encountered variety of partial seizures.[56] The chief complaint is often nonspecific and may include disturbed sleep, torn-up bed linens, confusion, or muscle soreness. Some patients may be unaware that they suffer from sleep-related seizures until someone observes a convulsion. The treatment for sleep-related seizures, as with most forms of seizures, is anticonvulsants.

Secondary Sleep Disorders

Secondary sleep disorders are disorders in which the disturbance of sleep is the presenting problem, but the cause is another underlying problem. As such, secondary sleep disorders frequently masquerade as primary sleep disorders; they require skill and vigilance on the part of psychiatrists and primary care physicians to ensure proper treatment for the principal disorder. The *DSM-IV-TR* subdivides secondary sleep disorders into those related to another mental disorder, those related to a general medical condition, and those related to use of substances.

Sleep Disorders Related to Another Mental Disorder

Sleep disturbance is such a common feature of psychiatric illness that it is often the first neurovegetative symptom about which psychiatrists inquire. In patients with known psychiatric illness, however, care must be taken to avoid attribution of a sleep disturbance solely to the mental disorder because psychiatric patients also suffer from primary sleep disorders and comorbid medical problems with associated disturbances of sleep. If a primary sleep disorder is not present and the complaint of sleep disturbance is not the only predominant complaint but is also temporally related to a mental disorder, then a sleep disorder related to another mental illness can be diagnosed. While patients may complain of either hypersomnia or insomnia, insomnia is the most common sleep-related complaint resulting from psychiatric disorders. Because the mental disorder is the cause of the sleep disturbance, treatment consists of treating the primary psychiatric condition.

Mood Disorders. Sleep abnormalities occur in up to 60% of outpatients and 90% of inpatients with depression. Consequently, more is known about sleep disturbances in depressed patients than in any other psychiatric illness. Most individuals who suffer from depression complain of initial, middle, and terminal insomnia and early morning awakening. Hypersomnia and neurovegetative reversal, however, tends to occur in atypical depression. Objective findings on the PSG include (1) prolonged sleep latency, (2) decreased delta sleep, (3) decreased REM latency, (4) increased duration and density of the first REM period, and (5) early morning awakening. Evidence suggests that these abnormalities may persist after remission and that they precede the onset of another episode. In addition, some studies suggest that decreased REM latency or decreased delta sleep may predict relapse in depressed patients.[57] Sleep disturbance in bipolar illness depends on which phase of the illness the patient is experiencing. During a depressed phase, for example, bipolar patients experience hypersomnia and an increased percentage of REM sleep, while during a manic episode they experience insomnia and a decreased percentage of REM sleep. Unlike other patients with insomnia, however, patients with mania rarely complain of their inability to sleep.

Psychotic Disorders. The most common sleep abnormalities in patients with psychotic disorders are difficulties with sleep initiation and maintenance, which become apparent during the acute phase of these illnesses. Patients with psychosis, like those with depression, also experience decreased REM latency, total sleep time, sleep efficiency, and delta sleep. Because many of the medications used for treating psychosis can cause similar disruptions in sleep architecture, medication side effects must be ruled out. Current evidence suggests, however, that many of these sleep abnormalities, particularly delta sleep deficits, are the function of a psychotic disorder rather than the result of medication use.[58]

Anxiety Disorders. Although anxiety disorders are perhaps the most common cause of insomnia, their exact effect on sleep architecture is tenuous. As a general rule, patients with anxiety disorders frequently complain of disturbed sleep and have poor sleep efficiency.[59] Patients suffering from panic disorder can experience attacks during sleep, usually during the transition from NREM stage 2 sleep and early delta sleep.[60,61] Patients with obsessive-compulsive disorder (OCD) report difficulties with the initiation and maintenance of sleep, which is often a result of presleep anxiety and bedtime rituals prior to sleep onset. Of all the anxiety disorders, PTSD is the best studied. Sleep findings in patients with PTSD include easy arousability, nightmares, night terrors, and increased sleep-related movements.[62] In addition, total sleep time is often reduced due to recurrent awakenings and impaired sleep maintenance.[59,62] Patients suffering from generalized anxiety have difficulty falling asleep, and may awaken with anxious ruminations throughout the night.

Sleep Disorders Related to a General Medical Condition

Because pain, discomfort, and unremitting symptoms can interfere with sleep continuity, sleep complaints are common in a host of medical conditions. To diagnose a sleep disorder related to a general medical condition, the history and physical examination must demonstrate a solid connection between the sleep disorder and the underlying medical problem; in addition, the sleep disturbance must be severe enough to warrant independent clinical attention. While the most frequent sleep complaint is insomnia, general medical conditions can produce sleep disturbances that mimic any sleep disorder. The list of medical conditions that result in a sleep disorder is quite lengthy and this section will highlight the more common ones. As with all secondary sleep disorders, the definitive treatment rests on treatment of the underlying medical condition.

Patients who suffering from pain syndromes often complain of symptoms that worsen at bedtime. Consequently, these patients frequently have disrupted sleep patterns, insomnia, early morning awakening, and daytime fatigue.[63–65] Polysomnographic features include increased NREM stage 1 sleep, decreased delta sleep, an increased number of arousals, and an alpha pattern known as *alpha-delta sleep anomaly*. (This anomaly can also be seen in sleep-deprived individuals and in individuals in whom deep pain has been induced.)[64,66,67] Adequate pain control can substantially improve sleep for these individuals. Sedating antidepressants or benzodiazepines, while they do not directly treat the pain, can help with sleep initiation and maintenance.

Patients who suffer from respiratory conditions, such as asthma and chronic obstructive pulmonary disease, often complain of frequent nocturnal awakening, light sleep, terminal insomnia, and daytime hypersomnia. Many of these symptoms are attributable to an inability to enter or to maintain REM sleep due to decreases in ventilatory drive, which cause hypoxia and hypoxemia that signals the patient to awaken. In such cases, supplemental oxygen may improve the quality of sleep. Other polysomnographic features are identical to those found in patients with OSA, as many patients with primary respiratory disorders also suffer from comorbid breathing-related sleep disorders.

While sleep complaints are common in other chronic medical problems, they are less well investigated. Patients with angina and cardiac arrhythmias may experience exacerbations of their symptoms during sleep, most often during REM sleep. Patients in congestive heart failure often suffer orthopnea, paroxysmal nocturnal dyspnea, and nocturia, which may be confused with primary sleep disorders, such as breathing-related sleep disorder, sleep terror disorder, nocturnal panic disorder, and sleep-related seizures.[68]

A discussion of sleep disorders associated with medical conditions would be incomplete without mention of paroxysmal nocturnal hemoglobinuria (PNH), even though it is not a true sleep disorder. A rare condition, PNH is an acquired hemolytic anemia exacerbated by sleep. Sufferers complain of rust-colored morning urine that is the result of hemolysis.[69] Patients often have chronic PNH without it effecting their life span. Death most often results from thrombosis or various cytopenias. Treatment includes blood transfusions, immunosuppressive therapies, or a bone marrow transplant.

Substance-Induced Sleep Disorder

Substances, whether prescribed or illicit, can have profound effects on sleep. These effects may arise during regular use, acute ingestion, or withdrawal and can masquerade as any primary sleep disorder. As a general rule, if the substance is a CNS depressant, intoxication will result in sedation and withdrawal will result in insomnia. Similarly, if the substance is a CNS stimulant, intoxication will result in insomnia and withdrawal will result in sedation. Diagnosis of these disorders can only be made if the sleep disturbance is severe enough to warrant independent clinical attention, it is caused by the direct physiological effects of a substance, if it developed during or within a month of intoxication or withdrawal from the substance, and if it is not the result of a mental disorder or delirium. Once a substance-related sleep disorder is suspected, a thorough substance abuse history must be obtained to recognize the offending substance. Treatment consists of judicious discontinuation of the substance, management of any acute withdrawal, and treatment of any underlying comorbid psychiatric problems that initiated or contributed to the substance abuse in the first place.

Alcohol is perhaps the most commonly used sleep aid, but its soporific value is limited by significant side effects, including dependence, addiction, and withdrawal. Its effects on sleep are well documented and are dependent on the pattern of use and the state of intoxication or withdrawal. During acute intoxication, alcohol alters sleep architecture by decreasing sleep latency, increasing delta sleep, and decreasing REM sleep. During acute withdrawal, however, its effects on sleep architecture are reversed; initial insomnia, decreased delta sleep, short REM latency, an increased percentage of REM sleep, decreased total sleep time, and decreased sleep efficiency all develop. Each of these features may be a contributing factor for alcohol relapse in dependent patients.[70–72] For recovering alcoholics, insomnia, poor sleep continuity, and decreased delta sleep may persist for several years after detoxification.[70,71] The definitive treatment for alcohol-related sleep complaints is detoxification and abstinence, in addition to treatment of comorbid psychiatric conditions. Benzodiazepines, hypnotics, and sedating antidepressants should, in general, be avoided due to cross-tolerance, risk of alcohol relapse, and synergistic sedative effects that may lead to CNS depression should the patient relapse.

The effects of nonalcoholic substances on sleep are not as well established as are the effects of alcohol. In general, intoxication with either amphetamine or cocaine prolongs sleep latency, decreases the amount of REM sleep, disrupts sleep continuity, and shortens total sleep time. During the first week of withdrawal from these substances, patients often experience hypersomnia (a "crash") and excessive REM sleep, followed perhaps by several days of insomnia.[73] Sedative-hypnotics, particularly benzodiazepines, shorten sleep latency, increase delta sleep, and decrease REM sleep. Caution must be taken when prescribing benzodiazepines, particularly those with a short half-life, as one or two days of withdrawal-based insomnia can occur after just a few days of benzodiazepine administration.[74] Opiates are known to increase sleep and to reduce REM sleep, with rebound insomnia occurring upon their discontinuation. Finally, SSRIs can produce arousal and insomnia in some patients, and sedation in others. The effects of SSRIs on sleep architecture include decreased REM sleep and decreased delta sleep. They may also aggravate sleepwalking and REM sleep behavior disorder, and they may induce REM during NREM sleep.[75]

Approach to the Patient with Disordered Sleep

Once a sleep complaint has reached clinical attention, it is important to conduct a careful evaluation to correctly assess, diagnose, and treat any potential sleep disorder. Because this process can be complex and time-consuming, the special skills of a board-certified sleep specialist might be required. The following discussion is based on the general approach that many sleep specialists recommend for proper diagnosis and management of sleep complaints and disorders.

The initial step in the diagnostic process is to obtain a detailed sleep history, either through direct inquiry of the patient and his or her bed partner or by means of a sleep questionnaire. Table 31-2 provides a list of specific areas that should be addressed.[76] In addition to a detailed sleep history, patients are encouraged to keep a 2-week sleep diary that details the time and amount of sleep, the number and length of any naps, the number of awakenings, wake-up times, any medications taken, and subjective mood during the day. For patients in whom hypersomnia is the major complaint, an Epworth Sleepiness Scale (ESS)—a simple, self-administered questionnaire that requires patients to rate their degree of sleepiness

Table 31-2. Sleep History

Times of retiring and arising? Note any variations between weekdays and weekends.

Note changes in sleep-wake schedule.

Subjective quality of sleep?

Amount of sleep needed to feel ideally alert and energetic during daily functioning? Note any drugs needed.

Frequency with which ideal amount of sleep is achieved compared to the average amount of sleep obtained? Note any disagreement between patient and bed-partner about time spent asleep.

Sleep habits and requirement in childhood and other major periods of life? Note subjective quality of sleep and attitudes toward sleep during those periods.

Difficulties with sleep initiation, maintenance, or early termination? Note daytime symptoms and effect on daily functioning.

Problems with daytime sleepiness? Note if the problem is worsening. Note any snoring, intermittent snoring with gagging, episodes of muscle weakness with laughter, leg jerking in sleep, or other troublesome events during sleep.

Drugs and alcohol before 6 PM; after 6 PM?

General emotional and physical problems? Note treatment modalities.

Sleep hygiene?

Modified from: Roffward H, Erman M: Evaluation and diagnosis of the sleep disorders: implications for psychiatry and other clinical specialties. In: Hales RE, Frances AJ, eds: *Psychiatry update: American Psychiatric Association annual review*, vol 4, Washington, DC, 1985, American Psychiatric Press 1985, pp 204–328.

Table 31-3. The Epworth sleepiness scale. (From Johns MW: A new method for measuring daytime sleepiness: the Epworth sleepiness scale, *Sleep* 14(6):540–545, 1991.)

How likely are you to doze off or fall asleep in the following situations, in contrast to feeling just tired? This refers to your usual way of life in recent times. Even if you have not done some of these things recently try to work out how they would have affected you. Use the following scale to choose the most appropriate number for each situation:

0 = no chance of dozing
1 = slight chance of dozing
2 = moderate chance of dozing
3 = high chance of dozing

SITUATIONS

Situation	
Sitting and reading	_____
Watching TV	_____
Sitting inactive in a public place (e.g. a theater or a meeting)	_____
As a passenger in a car for an hour without a break	_____
Lying down to rest in the afternoon when circumstances permit	_____
Sitting and talking to someone	_____
Sitting quietly after a lunch without alcohol	_____
In a car, while stopped for a few minutes in traffic	_____
Total	_____

in a variety of routine situations,)—is often given. A total score of 10 or more on the ESS significantly distinguishes normal patients from patients with various hypersomnias, including obstructive sleep apnea, narcolepsy, and idiopathic hypersomnia (Table 31-3).[77] Once the sleep history and screening examinations have been completed, a medical history (including past medical history, current medications, alcohol and drug history, family history, and psychiatric history) is undertaken.

After a comprehensive history has been completed, and if clinically indicated, the patient receives a detailed physical examination. For patients suffering from hypersomnia, this examination focuses on the distribution of obesity, the respiratory system, the cardiovascular system, and the oronasomaxillofacial region

(with careful attention to the tongue, tonsils, uvula, and pharynx).[12,13,78,79] If indicated, laboratory examinations including a complete blood cell (CBC) count, blood gas analysis, pulmonary function tests, an ECG, thyroid function tests, serum iron analysis, and electrolyte count are ordered. Cephalometric x-rays of the skull and neck may be obtained to evaluate for skeletal discrepancies if craniofacial malformations are suspected as a possible etiology for any breathing-related sleep disorder.[10,12,13,78,79] Polysomnography completes the evaluation and often confirms the diagnosis.

Once a diagnosis has been confirmed, patients are offered appropriate treatment. Table 31-4 summarizes nonpharmacologic and pharmacologic treatments for the most commonly encountered primary sleep disorders.

Table 31-4. Treatment Options for Frequently Encountered Primary Sleep Disorders

Primary Sleep Disorder	Nonpharmacologic Treatment	Pharmacologic Treatment
Dyssomnias		
Primary insomnia	Sleep hygiene Stimulus control Sleep restriction Biofeedback Relaxation training Paradoxical intention Cognitive therapy Psychotherapy	**Benzodiazepines** Triazolam 0.125 to 0.25 mg/hs Temazepam 15 to 30 mg/hs Oxazepam 15 to 30 mg/hs Lorazepam 1 to 2 mg/hs Diazepam 2.5 to 10 mg/hs Clonazepam 0.5 to 2 mg/hs **Imidazopyridines** Zolpidem 10 to 20 mg/hs **Pyrazolopyrimidines** Zaleplon 10 to 20 mg/hs **Antihistamines** Diphenhydramine 25 to 50 mg/hs **Sedating antidepressants** Amitriptyline 10 to 75 mg/hs Imipramine 25 to 100 mg/hs Doxepin 10 to 75 mg/hs Trazodone 25 to 100 mg/hs
Primary hypersomnia	Regular bedtime Avoid daytime naps	**Amphetamines** Dextroamphetamine 5 to 60 mg/day Methamphetamine 5 to 40 mg/day Methylphenidate 5 to 80 mg/day **Nonamphetamines** Pemoline 18.75 to 112.5 mg/day Modafinil 200 to 400 mg/day
Narcolepsy	Regular bedtime Daytime naps	**Amphetamines** Dextroamphetamine 5 to 60 mg/day Methamphetamine 5 to 40 mg/day Methylphenidate 5 to 80 mg/day **Nonamphetamines** Pemoline 18.75 to 112.5 mg/day Modafinil 200 to 400 mg/day **Tricyclic Antidepressants** Imipramine 25 to 100 mg/day Desipramine 25 to 100 mg/day
Breathing-related sleep disorders	Weight loss Avoidance of sedating substances Positional therapy UPPP Tracheostomy CPAP/BiPAP	Protriptyline 5 to 20 mg/day Fluoxetine 20 to 40 mg/day
PLMD and RLS	None	**Dopaminergic agents** Carbidopa/levodopa 12.5/50 mg/hs Pergolide 0.05 to 1 mg/hs Pramipexole 0.125 to 1.0 mg/hs **Benzodiazepines** Clonazepam 0.5 to 2 mg/hs **Opioids** Codeine 15 to 30 mg/hs Oxycodone 5 to 10 mg/hs

Continued

Table 31-4. Treatment Options for Frequently Encountered Primary Sleep Disorders—*Cont'd*

Primary Sleep Disorder	Nonpharmacologic Treatment	Pharmacologic Treatment
		Others
		Gabapentin 100 to 800 mg/hs
Parasomnias		
Sleepwalking disorder	Reassurance	Diazepam 2.5 to 10 mg
	Maintenance of safe environment	Clonazepam 0.5 to 2.0 mg
	Psychotherapy	
	Hypnosis	
Sleep terror disorder	Reassurance	Diazepam 2.5 to 5 mg/hs
	Stress reduction	Clonazepam 0.5 to 2.0 mg/hs
Nightmare disorder	Reassurance	None
	Stress reduction	
	Psychotherapy	
	Desensitization	
	Rehearsal therapy	
REM behavior disorder	Reassurance	Clonazepam 0.5 to 2.0 mg/hs
	Maintenance of safe environment	

BiPAP = bilevel positive airway pressure; CPAP = continuous positive airway pressure; PLMD = periodic limb movement disorder; RLS = restless leg disorder; UPPP = Uvulopalatopharyngoplasty.

References

1. Chokroverty S: *An overview of sleep.* In Chokroverty S, editor: *Sleep disorders medicine: basic science, technical considerations, and clinical aspects*, Boston, 1994, Butterworth-Heinemann, pp 7–16.
2. Bootzin RR, Lahmeyer H, Lillie JK, editors: *Integrated approach to sleep management*, Belle Mead, NJ, 1994, Cahners Healthcare Communications.
3. Carskadon MA, Roth T: *Normal sleep and its variations.* In Kryger MH, Roth T, Dement WC, editors: *Principles and practice of sleep medicine, ed 2*, Philadelphia, 1994, WB Saunders Company, pp 3–15.
4. Sheldon SH, Spire JP, Levy H: *Introduction to polysomnography.* In Sheldon SH, Spire JP, Levy H, editor: *Pediatric sleep medicine*, Philadelphia, WB Saunders Company, 1992, pp 167–177.
5. Sheldon SH, Spire JP, Levy H: *Normal sleep in children and young adults.* In Sheldon SH, Spire JP, Levy H, editor: *Pediatric sleep medicine*, Philadelphia, 1992, WB Saunders Company, pp 14–27.
6. Carskadon MA, Roth T: *Normal human sleep: an overview.* In Kryger MH, Roth T, Dement WC, editors: *Principles and practice of sleep medicine, ed 2*, Philadelphia, 1994, WB Saunders Company, pp 16–25.
7. Mahowald MW, Schenck CH: Dissociated states of wakefulness and sleep, *Neurology* 42(S6):44S–51S, 1992.
8. Mahowald MW, Schenck CH: Status dissociatus: a perspective on states of being, *Sleep* 14(1):69–79, 1991.
9. Aldrich MS: *Cardinal manifestations of sleep disorders.* In Kryger MH, Roth T, Dement WC, editors: *Principles and practice of sleep medicine, ed 2*, Philadelphia, 1994, WB Saunders Company,, pp 418–434.
10. Mendelson WB: Circadian rhythms and sleep. In Human sleep. *Research and clinical care*, New York, Plenum Medical, 1987:295–314.
11. Hauri J, Orr WC: *Sleep disorders, ed 2*, Kalamazoo, Mich, 1982, The Upjohn Co.
12. Mendelson WB: An introduction to sleep studies. In *Human sleep: research and clinical care*, New York, 1987, Plenum Medical, pp 3–31.
13. Williams RL, Gokcebay N, Hirshkowitz M, Moore CA: *Ontogeny of sleep.* In Cooper R, editor: *Sleep*, London, 1994, Chapman and Hall Medical, pp 60–75.
14. Culebras A: Update on disorders of sleep and the sleep-wake cycle, *Psychiatric Clin North America* 15(2):467–489, 1992.
15. Siegel JM: Mechanisms of sleep control, *J Clin Neurophysiol* 7:49–65, 1990.
16. Vertes RP: Brainstem control of the events of REM sleep, *Prog Neurobiol* 22:241–88, 1984.
17. American Psychiatric Association: *Diagnostic and statistical manual of mental disorders, ed 4*, text revision, Washington, DC, 2000, American Psychiatric Association.
18. Diagnostic Classification Steering Committee (Thorpy MJ, chairman): *ICSD—International classification of sleep disorders: diagnostic and coding manual,*

Rochester, Minn, 1990, American Sleep Disorders Association.

19. Weilburg, JB, Richter JM: *Approach to patients with disordered sleep*. In Stern TA, Herman JB, Slavin PL, editors: *MGH guide to psychiatry in primary care*, New York, 1998, McGraw-Hill, pp 67–77.

20. Mignot E, Wang C, Rattazzi C, et al: Genetic linkage of autosomal recessive canine narcolepsy with a mu immunoglobulin heavy-chain switch-like segment, *Proc Natl Acad Sci U S A* 88:3475–3478, 1991.

21. Honda Y, Juji T, Matsuki K, et al: HLA-DR2 and Dw2 in narcolepsy and in other disorders of excessive somnolence without cataplexy, *Sleep* 9:133–142, 1986.

22. Rosenthal L, Roehrs TA, Hayashi H, et al: HLA DR2 in narcolepsy with sleep-onset REM periods but not cataplexy, *Biol Psychiatry* 30:830–836, 1991.

23. Krahn LE, Black JL, Silber MH: Narcolepsy: new understanding of irresistible sleep, *Mayo Clin Proc* 76(2):185–194, 2001.

24. Mitler MM, Hajdukovic R, Erman MK: Treatment of narcolepsy with methamphetamine, *Sleep* 16:306–317, 1993.

25. Mitler M, Hajdukovic R: Relative efficacy of drugs for the treatment of sleepiness in narcolepsy, *Sleep* 14:218–220, 1991.

26. Laffont F, Mayer G, Minz M: Modafinil in diurnal sleepiness: a study of 123 patients, *Sleep* 17(suppl. 8):S113–S115, 1994.

27. Billiard M, Besset A, Montplaisir J: Modafinil: a double-blind multicentric study, *Sleep* 17(suppl 8):S107–S112, 1994.

28. Warot D, Corruble E, Payan C, et al: Subjective effects of modafinil, a new central adrenergic stimulant in healthy volunteers: a comparison with amphetamine, caffeine and placebo, *Eur Psychiatry* 8:201–208, 1993.

29. Lyons TJ, French J: Modafinil: the unique properties of a new stimulant, *Aviat Space Environ Med* 62:432–435, 1991.

30. Smallwood P: Obstructive sleep apnea revisited, *Med Psychiatry* 1:42–52, 1998.

31. Lugaresi E, Coccagna G, Cirignotta F: *Snoring and its clinical implications*. In Guilleminault C, Dement WC, editors: *Sleep apnea syndromes*, New York, 1978, Alan R. Liss, Inc, pp 13–21.

32. Partinen M, Telakivi T: Epidemiology of obstructive sleep apnea syndrome, *Sleep* 15:S1–S4, 1992.

33. Partinen M: *Epidemiology of sleep disorders*. In Kryger MH, Roth T, Dement WC, editors: *Principles and practice of sleep medicine, ed 2*, Philadelphia, 1994, WB Saunders, pp 437–453.

34. Shepard JW Jr: Hypertension, cardiac arrhythmias, myocardial infarction, and stroke in relation to obstructive sleep apnea, *Clin Chest Med* 13:437–458, 1992.

35. Aldrich MS, Chauncey JB: Are morning headaches part of obstructive sleep apnea syndrome? *Arch Intern Med* 150:1265–1267, 1990.

36. Roehrs T, Conway W, Wittig R, et al: Sleep-wake complaints in patients with sleep-related respiratory disturbances, *Am Rev Respir Dis* 132:520–523, 1990.

37. Hanzel Da, Proia NG, Hudgel DW: Response of obstructive sleep apnea to fluoxetine and protriptyline, *Chest* 100:416–421, 1991.

38. Schmidt-Nowara W, Lowe A, Wiegand L, et al: Oral appliances for the treatment of snoring and obstructive sleep apnea: a review, *Sleep* 18(6):501–510, 1995.

39. Standards of Practice Committee, American Sleep Disorders Association. Practice parameters for the treatment of snoring and obstructive sleep apnea with oral appliances, *Sleep* 18(6):511–513, 1995.

40. Sullivan CE, Grunstein RR: *Continuous positive airway pressure in sleep-disordered breathing*. In Kryger MH, Roth T, Dement WC, editors: *Principles and practice of sleep medicine, ed 2*, Philadelphia, 1994, WB Saunders, pp 694–706.

41. Moore-Ede MC: Jet lag, shift work, and maladaption, *News Physiol Sci* 1:156–160, 1986.

42. Akerstedt T: *Shift work and sleep disturbances*. In Peter JH, Penzel T, Podszus T, et al, editors: *Sleep and Health Risk*, New York, 1991, Springer-Verlag, pp 265–278

43. Vignau J, Dahlitz M, Arendt J, et al: *Biological rhythms and sleep disorders in man*: the delayed sleep phase syndrome. In Wettering L, editor: *Light and biological rhythms in man*, Stockholm, 1993, Pergamon Press, pp 261–271.

44. Richardson GS: Circadian rhythms and aging, *Biol Aging* 13:275–305, 1990.

45. Kamgar-Parsi B, Wehr TA, Gillin JC: Successful treatment of human non-24 hour sleep-wake syndrome, *Sleep* 6:257–264, 1983.

46. Ancoli-Israel S, Kripke DF, Klauber MR, et al: Periodic limb movements in sleep in community-dwelling elderly, *Sleep* 14:496–500, 1991.

47. Coleman R, Bliwise DL, Sajben N, et al: *Epidemiology of periodic movements during sleep*. In Guilleminault C, Lugaresi E, editors: *Sleep/wake disorders: natural history, epidemiology, and long-term evolution*, New York, 1983, Raven Press, pp 217–229.

48. Ancoli-Israel S, Kripke DF, Mason W, et al: Sleep apnea and periodic movements in an aging sample, *J Gerontol* 40:419–425, 1985.

49. Mitler MM, Browman CP, Menn SJ, et al: Nocturnal myoclonus: treatment efficacy of clonazepam and temazepam, *Sleep* 9:385–392, 1986.

50. Trenkwalder C, Walter AS, Hening W: Periodic limb movements and restless leg syndrome, *Neurol Clin* 14(3):629–650, 1996.

51. Luchins D, Sherwood PM, Gillin JC, et al: Filicide during psychotropic-induced somnambulism: a case report, *Am J Psychiatry* 135:1404–1405, 1978.

52. Kales JD, Kales A, Soldatos CR, et al: Night terrors, *Arch Gen Psychiatry* 37:1413–1417, 1980.

53. Schenk C, Bundlie S, Ettinger M, et al: Chronic behavioral disorders of human REM sleep: a new category of parasomnia, *Sleep* 9:293–308, 1986.

54. Schenk CH, Bundlie SR, Patterson AL, Mahowald MW: Rapid eye movement sleep behavior disorder, *JAMA* 257:1786–1789, 1987.

55. Culebras A: Neuroanatomic and neurologic correlates of sleep disturbances, *Neurology* 42(suppl 6):19–27, 1992.

56. Shouse MN, Martins da Silva A, Sammaritano M: Circadian rhythm, sleep and epilepsy, *J Clin Neurophysiol* 13:32–50, 1995.

57. Giles DE, Jarrett RB, Roffwarg HP: Reduced REM latency: a predictor of recurrence in depression, *Neuropsychopharmacology* 1:33–39, 1988.

58. Keshavan, MS, Matcheri S, Reynolds CF III, et al: Delta sleep deficits in schizophrenia: evidence from automated analyses of sleep data, *Arch Gen Psychiatry* 55:443–448, 1998.

59. Uhde TH: *The anxiety disorders*. In Kryger MH, Roth T, Dement WC, editors: *principles and practice of sleep medicine, 2 ed*, Philadelphia, 1994, WB Saunders, pp 871–898.

60. Mellman TA, Uhde TW: Electroencephalographic sleep in panic disorder, *Arch Gen Psychiatry* 46:178–184, 1989.

61. Hauri PJ, Friedman M, Ravaris CL: Sleep in patients with spontaneous panic attacks, *Sleep* 12:323–337, 1989.

62. Mellman TA, Kulick-Bell R, Ashlock LE, Nolan B: Sleep events among veterans with combat-related posttraumatic stress disorder, *Am J Psychiatry* 152:110–115, 1995.

63. Korszun A: Sleep and circadian rhythm disorders in fibromyalgia, *Current Rheumatol Rep* 2(2):124–130, 2000.

64. Harding SM: Sleep in fibromyalgia patients: subjective and objective findings, *Am J Med Sci* 315(6):367–376, 1998.

65. Weintraub JR: Cluster headaches and sleep disorders, *Current Pain & Headache Reports* 7(2):150–156, 2003.

66. Saskin P, Moldofsky H, Lue FA: Sleep and posttraumatic rheumatic pain modulation disorder (fibrositis syndrome), *Psychosom Med* 48:319–323, 1986.

67. Manu P, Lane TJ, Matthews DA, et al: Alpha-delta sleep in patients with a chief complaint of chronic fatigue, *South Med J* 87:465–470, 1994.

68. Bradley TD: Sleep disturbances in respiratory and cardiovascular disease, *J Psychosom Res* 37(suppl) 1:13–17, 1993.

69. Johnson RJ. Hillmen P: Paroxysmal nocturnal haemoglobinuria: nature's gene therapy, *Mol Path* 55(3):145–152, 2002.

70. Brower KJ: Alcohol's effects on sleep in alcoholics, *Alcohol Research & Health: J Natl Inst Alcohol Abuse & Alcoholism* 25(2):110–125, 2001.

71. Landolt HP, Gillin JC: Sleep abnormalities during abstinence in alcohol-dependent patients: aetiology and management, *CNS Drugs* 15(5):413–425, 2001.

72. Gillin JC, Smith TL, Irwin M, et al: Increased pressure for REM sleep at admission to an alcohol treatment program predicts relapse at 3 months post-discharge in primary, nondepressed alcoholic patients, *Arch Gen Psychiatry* 50:1–9, 1994.

73. Watson R, Bakos L, Compton P, et al: Cocaine use and withdrawal: the effect on sleep and mood, *J Drug Alcohol Abuse* 18:21–28, 1992.

74. Gillin JC, Spinweber CL, Johnson LC: Rebound insomnia: a critical review, *J Clin Psychopharmacol* 9:161–172, 1989.

75. Sharpley AL, Cowen PJ: Effect of pharmacologic treatments on the sleep of depressed patients, *Biol Psychiatry*. 37(2):85–98, 1995.

76. Roffward H, Erman M: *Evaluation and diagnosis of the sleep disorders: implications for psychiatry and other clinical specialties*. In: Hales RE, Frances AJ, editors: *Psychiatry update: American Psychiatric Association annual review*, 4 vol, Washington, DC, 1985, American Psychiatric Press, pp 204–328.

77. Johns MW: A new method for measuring daytime sleepiness: the Epworth sleepiness scale, *Sleep* 14(6):540–545, 1991.

78. Guilleminault C: Obstructive sleep apneas, the clinical syndrome and historical perspective, *Med Clin North America* 69(6):1187–1203, 1985.

79. Guilleminault C: *Clinical features and evaluation of obstructive sleep apnea*. In: Kryger MH, Roth T, Dement WC, editors: *Principles and practice of sleep medicine, ed 2*, Philadelphia, 1994, WB Saunders, pp 667–678.

Chapter 32

The Psychiatric Management of Patients with Cardiac Disease

Jeff C. Huffman, M.D.
Theodore A. Stern, M.D.
James L. Januzzi, M.D.

Caring for cardiac patients can present a host of dilemmas for the general hospital psychiatrist. Patients with psychiatric conditions may present with cardiac symptoms, psychotropic agents can result in electrocardiographic abnormalities, and psychiatric manifestations may result from cardiac conditions. Moreover, patients with cardiac conditions can present with psychiatric symptoms, and cardiac drugs can result in psychiatric and neuropsychiatric symptoms. Since the overlap between psychiatry and cardiology is so great, knowledge of how one can manage specific problems can be of tremendous benefit. For instance, knowing how to deal with chest pain in the face of a psychiatric syndrome, an electrocardiographic complication from a psychotropic agent, or delirium due to invasive technology or cerebral hypoperfusion can facilitate comprehensive and compassionate care.

This chapter will focus on three main psychiatric syndromes related to the cardiac patient: anxiety, depression, and delirium. For each of these syndromes, we will consider epidemiology, clinical manifestations, differential diagnosis, psychopharmacologic approaches, and practical management strategies for patients with cardiac disease in the general hospital. Additional information on the interface between psychiatric and cardiac care will also be provided in other chapters.

Anxiety in the Cardiac Patient

Anxiety and the heart have long been linked. In 1836, Williams[1] published a text called *Practical Observations on Nervous and Sympathetic Palpitations of the Heart*. In 1871, Da Costa[2] described *irritable heart*, a condition in which chest discomfort was caused by emotional upset. Osler[3] (in 1882) discussed the difficulty of differentiating cardiac and noncardiac etiologies of chest pain and described a subset of patients with atypical chest pain and nervousness. Since then, numerous authors have linked anxiety and chest pain and have described such symptoms using terms that have included Da Costa syndrome, soldier's heart, neurocirculatory asthenia, and effort syndrome. For years, it has been suggested that anxiety and worry might cause heart conditions; more recent work has shown that both acute and chronic anxiety (as measured, for example, on the Cornell Medical Index[4]) are associated with sudden cardiac death (SCD) and coronary artery disease (CAD).[5,6]

The assessment of anxiety in the cardiac patient in the general hospital is often complex. First of all, it may be difficult to ascertain whether the patient is experiencing distress as a result of a myocardial event, an acute confusional state, or a primary anxiety condition or as a complex interaction between these factors. Furthermore, there are many potential causes of anxiety for the cardiac patient, from an adjustment reaction to a serious cardiac event to the anxiogenic effects of cardiac medications administered to treat such events. Among hospitalized inpatients, the threshold for treatment of anxiety tends to be lower than it is in the outpatient setting, as the elevations in catecholamine levels and vital signs associated with mild to moderate anxiety may have profound cardiovascular effects in the patient who is post-myocardial infarction (MI), post-coronary artery bypass grafting (CABG), or in congestive heart failure (CHF).

Epidemiology

Anxiety Among Cardiac Patients

Patients who have an acute coronary syndrome or undergo CABG are commonly anxious. Cardiac patients who are more critically ill (e.g., those on intraaortic balloon pumps [IABPs]) also experience significant anxiety; the presence of technology (e.g., automatic implanted cardiac defibrillators [AICDs]) can increase such symptoms further. Furthermore, those patients who are initially identified as "cardiac" patients—including those who present with chest pain but who have no known cardiac cause for their symptoms—may also have severe anxiety. Such anxiety may be both the cause of their chest pain and the result of being told that the cause for their symptoms is unknown.

Approximately 50% of patients with an acute coronary syndrome experience abnormal anxiety,[7] and 25% are at least as anxious as the average inpatient on a psychiatric unit.[8] These symptoms peak in the first two hospital days, then slowly drop over the next few days[8,9]; however, those with elevated levels of anxiety while in the hospital continue to be anxious 1 year later.[10] In addition, up to 40% of post-CABG patients have clinically significant anxiety[11]; such symptoms are generally greatest prior to CABG,[12] but they can persist throughout the hospitalization.

Cardiac patients with invasive technology may also experience panic and fear associated with these devices. Approximately 10% to 15% of outpatients with pacemakers and AICDs have elevated levels of anxiety.[13,14] Not surprisingly, patients whose AICDs discharged frequently (10 or more shocks received) are significantly more anxious; over one half of such patients had abnormal anxiety in one study.[14]

In addition to high levels of free-floating anxiety, cardiac patients also experience elevated rates of formal anxiety disorders. Approximately 20% of all patients who present to emergency departments with chest pain meet criteria for panic disorder (PD).[15] Patients who present to outpatient cardiology clinics for evaluation of their chest pain have rates of PD that are even higher. However, not all patients with PD are free of cardiac disease; in fact, patients with CAD appear to have PD at approximately four times the rate of the general population.[15] Patients with comorbid CAD and PD can be among the most difficult for the general hospital psychiatrist, as the cause of chest pain, palpitations, and other symptoms is often unclear.

Cardiac patients who experience events as traumatic during their hospitalization may exhibit symptoms of posttraumatic stress disorder (PTSD). Recent studies have found that 8% to 16% of patients who have an MI develop symptoms of PTSD[16–18]; such PTSD symptoms also arise at a similar rate among patients who undergo CABG.[18,19] Studies of intensive care patients with burn injuries and acute respiratory distress syndrome (ARDS)[20,21] suggest that PTSD may be even more prevalent among cardiac patients in intensive care units (ICUs). Finally, generalized anxiety disorder (GAD), though not formally studied in cardiac patients, appears to be common among patients with CAD. As noted above, anxiety is prevalent 1 year after MI, and this may correlate with elevated rates of GAD.

Association Between Anxiety and Cardiac Illness

Epidemiologic studies suggest that cardiac illness may lead to increased anxiety and that anxiety may also exacerbate cardiac illness. Acute and chronic emotional stress has been linked to the development of ventricular arrhythmias[22] and to the exacerbation of silent myocardial ischemia.[23]

A number of studies have also found a correlation between anxiety and SCD. The Normative Aging Study,[24] an epidemiologic study of 2280 men, found that those with two or more anxiety symptoms on the Cornell Medical Index[4] had a fourfold greater risk of SCD than those without anxiety symptoms. Further, prospective epidemiologic studies[25,26] of phobic anxiety have found a significantly increased rate of SCD.

One anxiety disorder in particular, PD, has been associated with a number of cardiovascular illnesses, (e.g., episodic and baseline hypertension,[27,28] small-vessel cardiac ischemia,[29] and the development of idiopathic cardiomyopathy[30,31]); idiopathic cardiomyopathy has been hypothesized to result from elevated catecholamine levels that cause a dilated cardiomyopathy.[32] Furthermore, a large community survey of over 5000 patients found that, controlling for demographic factors, patients with PD had more than four times the risk of MI than those without PD.[33] Small longitudinal studies have suggested that PD may be associated with a greater overall cardiovascular mortality than those without PD; this effect appears to be largest in men.[34,35] It is important to note that these links are at the level of association; it is not yet clear that PD *causes* these cardiovascular conditions; rather, patients with PD have them more frequently.

In the post-MI setting, anxiety may be associated with worse in-hospital and longitudinal outcome. Moser and Dracup[36] found that patients with post-MI anxiety were nearly five times more likely to have in-hospital ischemic or arrhythmic complications than those who did not. Frasure-Smith, Lespérance, and Talajic[37] found that patients with elevated levels of anxiety immediately post-MI were more than twice as likely to have recurrent cardiac events over the next year. However, three other studies[38–40] found that post-MI anxiety did not predict cardiac morbidity over the following year. One of these studies[38] did find that anxiety predicted poor quality of life, greater recurrent chest pain, more use of primary care services, and reduced adherence with medical recommendations. Despite these different findings, the studies were largely similar, using similar inclusion and exclusion criteria, standard instruments, and comparable numbers of patients.

Anxiety among patients undergoing CABG appears to have a similar effect. Two studies found that pre-CABG anxiety predicted poor psychosocial adjustment and quality of life both before and after surgery.[41,42] These studies are consistent with the literature on psychiatric outpatients with PD and GAD; investigators have found that these anxiety disorders were associated with a lower quality of life as well as increases in functional morbidity and the use of primary care services.[43–45]

In sum, cardiac patients have high rates of situational anxiety and of formal anxiety disorders (such as PD, GAD, and PTSD). Such anxiety has been associated with elevated rates of myocardial ischemia, SCD, and other cardiac diseases, and, in the post-MI setting, may be associated with worse in-hospital and longitudinal cardiac outcomes. Furthermore, in addition to suboptimal medical outcomes, anxiety among cardiac patients in the general hospital is also associated with poor psychosocial outcomes.

Differential Diagnosis of Anxiety in the Cardiac Patient

Anxiety in the general hospital is often a primary psychiatric problem caused by stressful medical events. However, anxiety in the cardiac patient can also be caused by a number of general medical conditions and medications commonly associated with cardiac care (Table 32-1).

Not uncommonly, cardiac events cause anxiety. Myocardial ischemia, arrhythmias, and CHF

Table 32-1. Selected General Medical Causes of Anxiety Among Cardiac Patients in the General Hospital

Cardiac Events
Myocardial ischemia
Atrial and ventricular arrhythmias
Congestive heart failure

Other Medical Conditions
Pulmonary embolism
Asthma/chronic obstructive pulmonary disease (COPD) exacerbation
Hyperthyroidism
Hypoglycemia

Medications
Sympathomimetics
Thyroid hormone
Bronchodilators
Stimulants

Illicit Substances
Cocaine or amphetamine intoxication
D-Lysergic acid diethylamide (LSD) or phencyclidine (PCP) intoxication
Alcohol or benzodiazepine withdrawal

can each cause anxiety due to the sympathetic discharge associated with these conditions *and* because of what they may represent to the patient (e.g., the fear of dying, the worsening of medical illness, or the loss of role identity). Other general medical conditions may cause or exacerbate anxiety in the cardiac patient; important among these is pulmonary embolism in the sedentary cardiac patient. Anxiety may also be a side effect of medications administered to cardiac patients and can result from substance intoxication or withdrawal (e.g., cocaine intoxication or alcohol withdrawal). Finally, impaired sleep in the coronary care unit (as the result of an unfamiliar setting, frequent nursing interventions, and significant noise) can lead to or exacerbate anxiety.

The general hospital psychiatrist should consider general medical causes of anxiety when evaluating cardiac patients; this is especially true when the anxiety has developed during an uneventful hospitalization, when the patient has no history of anxiety, or when anxiety persists despite appropriate treatment.

Psychopharmacologic Issues in the Anxious Cardiac Patient

Agents used in the treatment of anxiety in the general hospital patient include benzodiazepines, antidepressants, and antipsychotics. Benzodiazepines are the most frequently used medications for the treatment of anxiety in cardiac patients. These medications rapidly relieve anxiety and appear to have a number of beneficial cardiovascular effects.

Benzodiazepines. Among patients with myocardial ischemia or infarction, benzodiazepines reduce catecholamine levels[46,47] and decrease coronary vascular resistance.[48] Although β-blockers, now commonly prescribed to cardiac patients, have similar effects, anxious patients tend to have elevations in vital signs, catecholamines, and coronary pressures as the result of their anxiety, despite the use of β-blockers; benzodiazepines can effectively treat these abnormalities. Furthermore, there is some suggestion that benzodiazepines may inhibit platelet aggregation[49] and raise the ventricular fibrillation (VF) threshold.[50,51] Furthermore, benzodiazepines are generally well tolerated by the general hospital population; low rates of hypotension, virtually no anticholinergic effects, and very low

rates of respiratory compromise develop when standard doses of benzodiazepines are used.[52] Benzodiazepines also appear to be safe even in seriously ill patients. A naturalistic study of 173 seriously ill medical inpatients (25% of whom died while in the hospital) who received IV diazepam for a variety of indications found that rates of any adverse effect from the benzodiazepine were low (3.5%).[53] Although clinicians may be concerned about the development of benzodiazepine dependence, when these agents are used in the acute care setting, at adequate doses, and for appropriate indications, the risk of dependence is minimal.[54]

Studies of benzodiazepines in cardiac patients have found that these agents effectively reduce anxiety and may have beneficial effects on cardiovascular outcome in selected cardiac populations. For example, patients with cocaine-induced chest pain are effectively treated with benzodiazepines; a recent study of patients who presented to an emergency department (ED) with chest pain after cocaine use found that the use of IV lorazepam in combination with nitroglycerin (NTG) was safe and more efficacious in relieving cocaine-associated chest pain than was the use of NTG alone.[55] In addition, benzodiazepines may have beneficial effects in patients with more conventional causes of acute myocardial ischemia. A report by Wheatley[56] combined the results of three studies using benzodiazepines in post-MI patients; Wheatley found that the addition of benzodiazepines to standard cardiac medications led to significantly lower rates of reinfarction over the study period. It should be noted that the patients in these studies, however, were not taking β-blockers.

In short, benzodiazepines are rapidly effective in the treatment of anxiety in the cardiac patient. They are well tolerated and are associated with low rates of adverse effects and minimal risk of dependence when used in acute care settings. Benzodiazepines have favorable effects on catecholamines and coronary pressures and may have favorable effects on cardiac outcome when administered in the post-MI period. One important caveat for the use of benzodiazepines is that they can exacerbate confusion and paradoxically worsen agitation in patients with delirium or dementia; therefore, other agents (e.g., antipsychotics) may be more appropriate for the treatment of anxiety, fear, and distress in the delirious or demented cardiac patient.

Antidepressants.   Antidepressants can also be used in the treatment of anxiety in the general hospital. However, these agents often take several weeks to work and are best used to treat Axis I anxiety disorders, such as PD, GAD, or PTSD. For acutely anxious cardiac patients in the general hospital, when antidepressants are prescribed, it is often wise to coadminister benzodiazepines to acutely reduce anxiety during a vulnerable cardiovascular state. Among the antidepressants, selective serotonin-reuptake inhibitors (SSRIs) are generally the agents of choice for cardiac patients, as tricyclic antidepressants (TCAs) can cause orthostasis, tachycardia (due to anticholinergic effects), and arrhythmias. The SADHART trial by Glassman et al.[57] established that the SSRI sertraline appears to be safe when administered one month after MI, with no adverse effects on cardiac function; smaller studies[58,59] and our own clinical experience have found that sertraline and other SSRIs may be used safely in the days and weeks post-MI. Antidepressants will be discussed more extensively in the section on depression.

Antipsychotics.   Antipsychotics can also be used for the treatment of heightened anxiety in the general hospital. Though there has been little study of the use of antipsychotics for anxiolysis, the consultation-liaison service at MGH has long used antipsychotics when fear impairs reason in general hospital patients; both typical and atypical antipsychotics appear effective for this indication. Atypical antipsychotics, especially quetiapine,[60] but also olanzapine and risperidone, are also being used more frequently in the treatment of acute anxiety. Though this off-label use of antipsychotics has not been extensively investigated, these antipsychotics do appear to effectively reduce anxiety in cardiac (and other) patients in the general hospital. These agents have the additional beneficial effects of symptomatically treating comorbid delirium, and they do not cause the paradoxical disinhibition that is sometimes associated with benzodiazepines. Antipsychotics, however, can cause orthostasis and anticholinergic effects (associated with low-potency typical agents and, to a lesser degree, some atypical agents), and may be associated with prolongation of the corrected QT (QTc) interval. Antipsychotics will be discussed more extensively in the section on delirium.

Other Agents.   Anticonvulsants, such as valproate and gabapentin, have been used in the acute treatment of anxiety. These agents are associated with essentially no risk of physiologic dependence, and they do not cause orthostasis or anticholinergic effects. Like antipsychotics, their efficacy in the treatment of acute anxiety in hospitalized cardiac patients has not been examined. They may be especially effective in patients with anxiety and comorbid neuropathic pain.

Approach to the Anxious Cardiac Patient

The psychiatric consultant is frequently called to cardiac floors to assess and treat anxiety. A careful, stepwise approach to these consultations can ensure an accurate diagnosis and appropriate treatment.

1. *Consider a broad differential diagnosis for the patient's distress.* A primary role of the general hospital psychiatrist is to accurately characterize a patient's distress as anxiety, denial, depression, delirium, or as another psychiatric phenomenon. When one is consulted for "anxiety," it is easy to be biased toward making a diagnosis of anxiety. However, patients who appear anxious and tremulous may in fact be disoriented, paranoid, and frightened—that is, delirious. Therefore, the consultant should be careful in the interview to assess affect, behavior, and cognition.

If the patient's primary psychiatric symptom appears to be anxiety, the consultant should then consider the potential contribution of medications or medical symptoms to this anxiety. As noted earlier, there is a long list of conditions that can cause or exacerbate anxiety, and the consultant should carefully consider these and recommend appropriate diagnostic studies if appropriate. It may be especially useful to note correlations between anxiety levels and the initiation or discontinuation of potentially offending medications or substances. For example, the development of anxiety, tremulousness, insomnia, and fluctuations in vital signs 24 to 48 hours after admission might suggest alcohol withdrawal, even in a patient who denies alcohol use.

2. *Evaluate sources of anxiety, and assess how the patient has dealt with difficult situations in the past.* A careful psychiatric interview of the anxious patient will help to determine what factors are

causing his or her anxiety. Is the preoperative CABG patient anxious because a relative died during cardiac surgery years ago? Is the post-MI mother of three worried because she is afraid that no one will be able to care for her children if she dies from cardiac disease? Is the patient with an AICD fearful that his defibrillator will painfully discharge again? By determining the sources of anxiety, the consultant will be able to address these anxieties through education, reassurance, medication, or brief psychotherapy. Often, many of these worries (e.g., worries about being able to sleep in the hospital and worries that family members have not been contacted) can be directly addressed. Furthermore, knowledge of the factors that contribute to anxiety may allow the consultant to estimate the duration of such symptoms; for example, a patient who reports that he will be "just so relieved" once the surgery to place his AICD has been performed is likely to have a relatively short course of anxiety, while the patient with chronic, uncontrollable worries is likely to have anxiety throughout the hospitalization.

A related task is to determine the patient's coping style and coping strengths. How does he or she manage anxiety outside of the hospital? How has he or she managed difficult situations in the past? The consultant can use this information to ally with the patient's strengths and to determine the best approach to the patient's anxieties. Patients who identify themselves as "survivors," or as people who persevere and succeed despite difficult obstacles, often take quite well to a consultant who also identifies this quality in them.

Another question for patients regards stimulation and control. Some cardiac patients crave control and wish to know every detail of their care; they feel anxious when they do not feel that they have comprehensive information about their illness and when they are not part of all treatment decisions. In contrast, other patients find such information and the "pressure" to make decisions overstimulating, and feel less anxious when told only the general details of their condition.

3. *Recommend appropriate behavioral and therapeutic interventions.* Having learned about the patient's sources of anxiety, coping strengths, and preferences regarding control, the consultant is in an excellent position to design a treatment plan that reduces a patient's anxiety. For example,

if a patient reports that the hospitalization is overwhelming, the treatment team can be encouraged to limit detailed information and to provide reassurance to the patient that they see this condition frequently (if true) and that they plan to provide excellent care to the patient. On the other hand, for the patient whose anxiety increases with lack of perceived control, the treatment team can be encouraged to provide the patient with detailed information and written materials. The patient should also be included in treatment decisions; inclusion in even small decisions (e.g., the best time for dressing changes) can allay anxiety and allow the patient to feel in control.

In other cases, worried cardiac patients simply need to express their anxieties to someone. If the consultant, treating physician, and nursing staff can set aside short periods to reflectively listen to the patient's fears, this investment of time often results in significantly less anxiety, greater compliance with treatment, and less chaos for patient and staff alike. If the patient seems to have an insatiable desire to discuss his or her fears, staff can be taught to consistently set aside time to listen to the patient while setting limits on his or her time; for example, a nurse may tell the patient that she will sit with him or her for 5 minutes at the beginning, middle, and end of the shift to talk about his or her worries. If the patient attempts to engage the nurse in further conversation about this topic, the nurse can calmly refer the patient to their future appointment.

4. *Intelligently use psychiatric medications for specific target symptoms.* Benzodiazepines are often the agents of choice for the anxious cardiac patient. If the anxi-ety appears to be short-term or situation-specific (e.g., whenever a procedure is performed), a short-acting benzodiazepine can be used on an as-needed basis, (e.g., lorazepam 0.5 to 1.0 mg as needed for acute anxiety). However, for most patients, longer-acting benzodiazepines given on a standing basis provide the smoothest and most consistent reduction of anxiety. Most anxious cardiac patients can be started on clonazepam 0.5 mg at night or twice per day; doses can be adjusted upward if this dose is well-tolerated and anxiety persists. In general, these agents can be discontinued upon discharge from the hospital if they were only used on a short-term basis.

Benzodiazepines may not be the agents of choice for patients with acute or chronic organic brain syndromes (e.g., delirium, dementia, or traumatic brain injury), in those with tenuous respiratory function (including obstructive sleep apnea), or in those with a history of substance dependence. In these patients, antipsychotics are often useful, alleviating agitation and confusion in delirious patients while also reducing anxiety. We often start with doses of quetiapine at 12.5 to 25.0 mg at night or twice per day, or olanzapine at 2.5 to 5.0 mg at night or twice per day.

Anticonvulsants may be useful when a patient has anxiety that is comorbid with neuropathic pain or with a chronic brain disturbance, such as a dementia or head injury. Antidepressants may be useful in the treatment of Axis I anxiety disorders and when depression is comorbid with anxiety; we generally coadminister a benzodiazepine to reduce initial anxiety associated with initiation of antidepressants.

5. *Return frequently to see the patient.* Anxious patients generally are relieved to see a familiar face, especially one that has attempted to understand and address their anxiety. Such frequent follow-up, therapeutic in itself, allows for careful monitoring of behavioral and pharmacologic interventions.

Case 1

Mr. A, a 53-year-old executive without a psychiatric history, was admitted for CABG after cardiac catheterization revealed three-vessel cardiac disease. He initially had an uneventful perioperative course. However, on the day after his operation, psychiatry was consulted to assess his capacity to leave the hospital against medical advice.

On interview, Mr. A was alert, oriented, lucid, and initially quite angry. He reported that, "I have no assurance that I'm getting the right care; the doctors and nurses come in and out of my room and bark orders to one another but they don't include me at all. They haven't even listened to the fact that I always take my sleeping pill at 9 PM every night instead of 11 PM like they give it to me. I'm fed up." By the end of his tirade, Mr. A's anger had changed to fear and anxiety.

The consultant told Mr. A that he would bring his concerns to the team. The consultant was able to meet with members of the treatment team and encouraged them to provide as much information as possible about his care, and to allow him to mandate his treatment when possible (e.g., getting his sleeping pill at 9 PM). The consultant, nurse, and Mr. A then met together to allow Mr. A to express his concerns, and

for the nurse and consultant to outline how things would change so that he could have more information and more control. Mr. A was agreeable to this plan and also agreed to clonazepam 0.5 mg twice per day to reduce his anxiety.

The consultant checked back frequently with Mr. A to assess his response to this treatment plan. Small changes in the plan were instituted at his request, and his anxiety steadily decreased. He was discharged to cardiac rehabilitation, and thanked the nursing staff for their "compassionate care."

Depression in the Cardiac Patient

The link between depression and cardiac disease has been scrutinized over the last several years in the wake of studies that have found that patients with depression may have a greater risk of developing cardiovascular disease.[61] Especially provocative has been research by Frasure-Smith, Lespérance, and Talajic[62,63] that suggests that depressive symptoms immediately post-MI are associated with greater cardiac mortality 6 and 18 months later. Such findings have renewed interest in the treatment of post-MI depression and led to questions about the safety and efficacy of antidepressants in the post-MI period. In addition, patients undergoing cardiac surgery are more likely to have adverse medical outcomes if they are depressed before surgery.[64] These findings have underscored the importance of the general hospital psychiatrist's role in identifying depressed cardiac patients and considering appropriate treatments.

Epidemiology

Depression Among Cardiac Patients

Depression is common among patients with CAD, with prevalence rates of major depression hovering around 20%.[65–67] This rate of depression is greater than that in the general population. Such elevated rates of depression are also present among cardiac patients in the general hospital: 15% to 30% of post-MI patients have major depression, and 65% manifest at least minor depression.[68,69] Moreover, a study by Baker et al.[70] found that more than 30% of pre-CABG patients were depressed.

With regard to depression, post-MI patients have been the most extensively studied cardiac population. Despite the high prevalence of depression, only 10% of post-MI depressed patients are recognized as such.[1,71] Several factors likely account for these low rates of recognition. The pattern of depression (with hostility, listlessness, and withdrawal being more common than sad mood) is often somewhat atypical[72]; furthermore, depression is often seen as a normal consequence of a serious medical event, such as MI. Finally, most patients with uncomplicated MI have brief inpatient stays, and it may be difficult to assess a patient's mood or to obtain psychiatric consultation during this limited time frame.

Strik, Honig, and Maes[68] in a review of post-MI depression, delineated a number of putative risk factors for the development of post-MI depression. These risk factors included smoking, hypertension, female gender, social isolation, medical complications during acute hospitalization, a history of depression, and first-time prescription of benzodiazepines (suggesting potential comorbidity between anxiety and depression).

The course of post-MI depression remains somewhat unclear. It appears that depression is most likely to develop immediately post-MI; furthermore, the development of depression in the first 6 months after MI is also common, with the incidence declining sharply thereafter. Post-MI depression is frequently persistent; Travella and associates[73] reported that the average length of a depressive episode after MI is 4 to 5 months. Frasure-Smith et al.[74] found that more than half of patients with post-MI depression remained depressed after 1 year. Even more strikingly, Lespérance, Frasure-Smith, and Talajic[75] found that only 26% of the patients who were depressed immediately post-MI were alive and known to be depression-free at follow-up.

Other cardiac patients may also have elevated rates of depression. Shapiro, Levin, and Oz[76] followed 30 recipients of left ventricular assist devices (LVADs) and found that 17% became depressed in the postoperative period. Candidates for cardiac transplantation have elevated rates of anxiety and depression[77]; depressive symptoms can persist for years after transplantation.[78] Dew et al.[79] found that one quarter of transplant recipients developed major depressive disorder (MDD) in the 3 years posttransplantation.

In short, depression is common among cardiac patients, and it has been best studied in those with recent MI. Post-MI depression is highly prevalent, poorly recognized, and frequently persistent. Further characterization of depression in other populations of cardiac patients should help to facilitate diagnosis and treatment of this mood disorder.

Depression and Cardiac Outcome

A number of longitudinal studies have examined the hypothesis that patients with depression are at greater risk for the development of cardiac disease. Several studies have found that patients with depressive symptoms are 1.5 to 3.5 times more likely to have an MI than are those without such symptoms.[80–85] Patients with full-blown MDD appear to have an even greater risk (4.5 times greater than nondepressed patients) of suffering an MI.[83] Another study of patients with asymptomatic CAD (noted on coronary angiography) found that 18% were depressed, a rate of depression that is more than threefold greater than in the general population.[84] In addition, the Johns Hopkins Precursor Study[80] found that, in a 40-year follow-up of male physicians, depression was associated with a strongly significant twofold risk of developing heart disease.

A recent meta-analysis examined these and other studies to determine the role of depression as a predictor of CAD.[86] The author identified 11 relevant articles and found that these longitudinal studies revealed an elevated risk for the development of CAD among patients with depression, with more severe depression correlating with higher risk of CAD development. He concluded that depression predicts the development of CAD among initially healthy persons.

In addition to predicting the development of CAD in healthy people, depression has also been associated with significantly higher rates of cardiac death and overall mortality among patients with established CAD. In the specific population of post-MI patients, numerous studies have examined the relationship between post-MI depressive symptoms and cardiac mortality; the majority of these studies,[40,62,63,87,88] though not all,[38,39] have found that depressive symptoms after MI predict cardiac mortality 6 to 18 months later. These effects on mortality appear to be largely independent of the severity of cardiac disease, demographic variables, medications, or other confounding factors. The best known of these studies (by Frasure-Smith, Lespérance, and Talajic[62,63]) found that depressive symptoms immediately post-MI were associated with a four- to sixfold augmentation of risk of cardiac mortality 6 and 18 months post-MI. Bush, Ziegelstein, and Tayback[87] found that even minimal depressive symptoms were associated with an elevated risk of cardiac mortality, though more severe depressive symptoms more strongly predicted cardiac mortality.

Depressive symptoms also appear to predict cardiac morbidity and mortality in other cardiac populations as well. At least three studies have found that pre-CABG depressive symptoms have been associated with an increase in cardiac morbidity at 6 or 12 month follow-up.[64,70,89] Among patients undergoing cardiac transplantation, persistent depression was associated with increased rates of incident CAD.[79] Furthermore, a recent study by Zipfel et al.[90] found that preoperative depressive symptoms predicted mortality in cardiac transplant recipients.

The mechanisms by which depression may contribute to increased cardiac morbidity and mortality have not yet been clearly outlined. This increased morbidity may be attributable to increased catecholamine levels. Depressed patients have increases in baseline levels of circulating catecholamines and exaggerated rises in catecholamine levels during stress[91]; elevated catecholamine levels can result in increased myocardial oxygen demand and elevations in blood pressure and heart rate. Furthermore, elevated catecholamine levels have been associated with infarct initiation, infarct extension, and the development of ventricular fibrillation in patients with myocardial ischemia.[92,93]

The association between depression and cardiac morbidity may be mediated by changes in autonomic nervous system tone, which may be manifested as decreased heart rate variability (HRV) or as abnormalities in baroreflex sensitivity. HRV is a measure of autonomic regulation of cardiac activity, and decreased HRV has been established as an independent risk factor for the development of SCD. Both depressed psychiatric outpatients and patients with post-MI depression have been found to have decreased HRV,[94,95] and depressed patients with CAD have been shown to have elevated rates of ventricular arrhythmias.[96] Therefore, depressed patients with CAD may have decreased HRV, leading to increased susceptibility to ventricular arrhythmias and SCD; this may explain increases in cardiac morbidity and mortality. A third possible mechanism concerns platelet aggregation; depressed patients with CAD appear to have increased platelet aggregation,[65,97] and this could increase vulnerability to myocardial ischemia.

A last potential "mechanism" by which depression may be linked to poor cardiac outcomes is poor compliance with medical recommendations. Depressed patients appear to have decreased adherence to medication regimens,[98] and depressed cardiac patients less frequently attend cardiac rehabilitation programs.[99] Furthermore, patients who are depressed after MI are less adherent to recommendations about diet, exercise, and smoking cessation.[100,101]

The link between depression in cardiac patients and increased cardiac morbidity is likely mediated by multiple factors. One crucial question that remains unanswered is whether treatment of depression among cardiac patients improves cardiac prognosis.

Differential Diagnosis of Depression in the Cardiac Patient

As with anxiety in the cardiac patient, there are a number of medical conditions and medications that can cause or exacerbate depressive symptomatology. Table 32-2 lists a number of these medical influences on mood. Conditions associated with depressed mood that are common in the cardiac patient include hypothyroidism (both idiopathic and secondary to amiodarone, which is increasingly prescribed to cardiac patients), Cushing's disease (idiopathic or cushingoid symptoms secondary to steroid administration), neoplasm (especially pancreatic), vitamin B_{12} and folate deficiency, and depression associated with vascular dementia.

A number of medications sometimes used in cardiac populations have been associated with

Table 32-2. Selected General Medical Causes of Depression Among Cardiac Patients in the General Hospital

Medical Conditions
Hypothyroidism (idiopathic or
    amiodarone-induced)
Cushing's disease
Vitamin B_{12} or folate deficiency
Neoplasm (especially pancreatic, lung, or central nervous
    system tumors)
Vascular dementia
Movement disorders (e.g., Parkinson's disease or
    Huntington's disease)

Medications
Methyldopa
Reserpine
Steroids
Interferon

Illicit Substances
Chronic alcohol or benzodiazepine abuse
Cocaine or amphetamine withdrawal

depression. Steroids, methyldopa, and reserpine have each been linked with increased rates of depression. Substances can also influence mood; chronic alcohol use and withdrawal from cocaine or amphetamines commonly lead to depression. β-Blockers have long been associated with depression; however, a recent reexamination of the literature suggests a minimal association between β-blockers and depression.[102]

Because depression can have significant effects on cardiac and psychosocial outcome in cardiac patients, and because these conditions are often reversible or treatable, the general hospital psychiatrist should consider these in all depressed cardiac patients.

Psychopharmacologic Issues in the Depressed Cardiac Patient

Antidepressants are effective in the treatment of depression. However, older antidepressants (i.e., TCAs and monoamine oxidase inhibitors [MAOIs]) have effects that make their use in cardiac patients difficult. TCAs have anticholinergic effects (including tachycardia) and they can cause orthostasis; these effects make their use questionable in patients with significant cardiac disease. Even more concerning is the propensity of TCAs to prolong cardiac conduction and to have a proarrhythmic effect in some patients as a result of their quinidine-like properties.[103,104] A recent study, controlling for medical and demographic factors, found that depressed patients on TCAs had more than a twofold risk of MI, while SSRIs did not enhance risk of MI.[105] For these reasons, the use of TCAs is generally avoided among patients with cardiac conduction disease,[106] and in the 2- to 3-month period after MI;[104,107] unfortunately, this peri-MI period appears to be the time when post-MI depression is both most prevalent and most dangerous.

Newer antidepressants (such as SSRIs, bupropion, and mirtazapine) do not appear to have the negative cardiovascular effects of TCAs. They are generally not associated with significant anticholinergic effects or orthostasis, and they do not appear to result in adverse effects on cardiac conduction. These properties make SSRIs and other new agents a more logical choice for most patients with cardiac disease. This recommendation is supported by a study (by Roose et al.[108]) that compared paroxetine and nortriptyline in depressed patients with ischemic heart disease. The two agents were equally efficacious, but the TCA was associated with a significantly higher rate of serious adverse cardiac events.

One cardiac population in whom the cardiac safety of SSRIs has been scrutinized is the post-MI population. Though a small study of fluoxetine found this agent to be safe in a post-MI population,[109] the most extensive study has been on the SSRI sertraline. The preliminary SADHAT trial by Shapiro et al.[59] found that the open-label administration of sertraline to 26 post-MI patients was associated with clinical improvement of depression and resulted in no significant changes in heart rate, blood pressure, cardiac conduction, left ventricular ejection fraction, or coagulation measures. This study paved the way for the more extensive multicenter SADHART trial by Glassman et al.[57] This study used a double-blind placebo-controlled design to administer sertraline or placebo to 369 post-MI patients. The investigators found that, compared to placebo, sertraline significantly improved depressive symptoms and was not associated with changes in ejection fraction, cardiac conduction, or adverse cardiac events. Two important limitations of this study were that patients did not begin treatment until an average of 34 days after their MI, and that the patients were followed for only 24 weeks.

Therefore, it appears that sertraline (and probably other SSRIs) is safe and effective in the treatment of post-MI depression in the first 24 weeks of treatment when administered to patients approximately 1 month after MI. Our clinical experience with SSRI administration in cardiac patients has also found SSRIs to be safe, and we have safely prescribed SSRIs in post-MI patients earlier than 1 month after the MI when indicated by the severity of depression or the follow-up circumstances.

Though other new non-SSRI antidepressants appear to have properties that would render them safe in cardiac populations, these agents have been less extensively studied. Bupropion, at therapeutic doses, does not have adverse effects on blood pressure, heart rate, or other cardiovascular parameters.[110] Furthermore, a study of bupropion in depressed patients with CAD found that this agent had a favorable cardiovascular side effect profile in this specific population.[111] While bupropion overdose can cause hypertension and tachycardia,[112] it generally does not lead to adverse cardiovascular events[113,114]; however, some studies of bupropion overdose have noted cardiovascular effects, including tachycardia, hypertension, wide-complex tachycardia, and cardiac arrest.[115] Therefore, bupropion should be used cautiously in depressed cardiac patients with a history of overdose or significant impulsivity. The use of bupropion in the cardiac patient is made more appealing by its ability to aid smoking cessation.[116,117] Bupropion (at 300 mg per day) has been found to be effective for this indication, and therefore cardiac patients who are depressed and who continue to smoke might be excellent candidates for bupropion therapy.

Mirtazapine is another new antidepressant that has a favorable cardiovascular side effect profile. It has not been formally studied among cardiac patients, although a large-scale study is planned.[118] However, it has few effects on cardiac conduction or vital signs, even in overdose,[119] and is otherwise well-tolerated. One potential drawback of the use of mirtazapine in cardiac patients is its propensity to cause weight gain in some patients as the result of its interaction with histamine receptors.

Psychostimulants have also been shown to be rapidly acting, efficacious antidepressants in medically hospitalized patients.[120,121] Though they may elevate blood pressure or heart rate, stimulants may be indicated in cardiac patients whose depression requires rapid treatment (e.g., depression that is severe, is negatively affecting rehabilitation due to anergia or minimal oral intake, or is affecting the patient's capacity to make medical decisions). Stimulants are relatively contraindicated in patients with a history of ventricular tachycardia, recent MI, CHF, uncontrolled hypertension or tachycardia, or those who are concurrently taking MAOIs. However, in many cardiac patients, psychostimulants can be safely used with slow dosage titration, beginning with 2.5 to 5.0 mg in the morning, and increasing up to 20 mg per day.

Approach to the Management of the Depressed Cardiac Patient

The approach to the depressed cardiac patient is in many ways similar to the approach to the anxious cardiac patient. The consultant must first confirm that depression is the primary psychiatric symptom and evaluate for comorbid psychiatric conditions. Furthermore, the psychiatrist must consider the presence of medical conditions or medications that can cause or exacerbate mood symptoms. Once these steps have been completed, an approach to treatment involves an identification of the patient's coping strengths and support network; it may also involve the weighing of the risks and benefits of antidepressant treatment. Below we outline the approach to the depressed cardiac patient:

1. *Consider appropriate psychiatric and medical differential diagnoses.* As with consultations on cardiac floors for "anxiety," we also find that consultations for "depression" often reveal that a patient's distress is caused by another psychiatric syndrome. Commonly, disordered sleep, inability to engage with caregivers, and social withdrawal may result from a hypoactive delirium rather than from depression, and therefore cognitive status must be addressed. Furthermore, anxiety is often prominent in cardiac patients, and the patient's distress may be more accurately assessed and treated as anxiety.

The consultant should also note the course of depressive symptoms to see if the onset or worsening of such symptoms correlated with the administration of a new medication or new physical symptoms, or if there are other indications that a physical disorder might be implicated in the evolution of the depressive symptoms. The general hospital psychiatrist should also order laboratory tests and other studies as indicated (e.g., vitamin B_{12} and folate in an elderly patient with poor nutrition; thyroid function tests in a patient with recent cold intolerance, weight gain, loss of appetite, and thinning of hair; or toxicologic screening tests when clinical suspicion of substance use arises).

2. *Attempt to identify the patient's coping style and the triggers for depressive symptoms.* Determining the external factors that exacerbate depressive symptoms may help the consultant to reduce the patient's stressors. Is the patient feeling more depressed because he must face his mortality? Does he feel that his children will not respect him? Is he stuck in the hospital and unable to attend an important family function? The consultant can use this information to utilize solutions that are psychotherapeutic in nature (e.g., discussing mortality and life goals) or more concrete (e.g., having family members call the patient to let him know he is missed and important to them). Identification of the patient's coping strengths—especially, how the patient has previously managed difficult situations—will inform the treatment team's approach to the patient.

3. *Make use of existing social supports or help develop a network.* Social support has been associated with superior medical outcomes in depressed patients after MI[122]; therefore, if such social support does not exist, the consultant can work with the treatment team to consider options to improve the patient's support system. Such options could include participation in cardiac rehabilitation, having visiting nurses, joining a support group, or beginning psychotherapeutic treatment for depressive symptoms (cognitive-behavioral therapy [CBT] has been found to be effective in the treatment of post-MI depression,[123] and it carries no concern of drug-drug interactions). Such interventions should not be limited to post-MI patients; all cardiac patients can benefit from increased social support, and by creating a more coherent system of support

for a cardiac patient, the chances of recovery improve.

4. *Carefully consider the use of antidepressant medication.* SSRIs, bupropion, and mirtazapine appear to be both safe and effective for patients with CAD, with few cardiovascular side effects. Therefore, in most cardiac patients who meet criteria for MDD, these antidepressants can be administered at standard doses. The SSRIs sertraline, citalopram, and escitalopram have the additional advantage of having few drug-drug interactions and little interaction with the cytochrome p450 system; therefore, we use these agents more frequently in cardiac patients on multiple medications. Bupropion also has few drug-drug interactions and may be the agent of choice in patients with comorbid MDD and a desire to stop smoking.

The risks and benefits of antidepressant medications should be more carefully considered in patients with recent MI, and probably by extension, all patients with severe cardiac disease, a history of ventricular arrhythmia, or recent cardiac surgery. For most patients who are immediately post-MI or post-CABG, we typically do not prescribe antidepressants for the onset of depressive symptoms within days after MI, both because such patients have not yet met criteria for MDD and because there are not extensive data establishing the safety of these agents in the post-MI or postcardiac surgery period. For most patients who become depressed post-MI, a reasonable and conservative approach is to have the patient follow up with a psychiatrist (or primary care physician) within 2 to 3 weeks; then, if the patient remains depressed, one can start sertraline or another antidepressant.

There are certain factors that may cause a clinician to lead toward the earlier prescription of antidepressants. These include:

Depression with suicidal ideation
Severe depression that inhibits participation in rehabilitation or self-care
The development of depressive symptoms during hospitalization in a patient with a history of severe depression
An inability or unwillingness to follow-up in the next 2 to 3 weeks (We often see patients who wish only to see their primary care physicians, and then only every 2 to 3 months. These

patients are quite compliant with their medication regimen and would therefore take an antidepressant if prescribed on discharge, but would be unlikely to return to see their physician in the next 6 weeks)

When one or more of these factors is present, we frequently initiate antidepressant therapy in the hospital in coordination with cardiology. As noted previously, when anxiety is present comorbidly, it is best to use benzodiazepines when beginning an antidepressant, as most antidepressants can cause initial anxiety or insomnia in the first few days of use.

Case 2

Mr. B, a 52-year-old gentleman with a history of MDD, was admitted to the hospital with chest pain. His electrocardiogram showed ST-segment depression in the anterolateral leads, his cardiac enzymes were elevated, and he ruled in for an MI by cardiac enzymes. Though he had not been depressed in the year prior to admission, he developed depressive symptoms in the days after his MI; psychiatric consultation was obtained.

On interview, Mr. B was dysphoric but alert, oriented, and able to actively engage in conversation with the interviewer. He reported depressed mood, anhedonia, and low energy, along with disturbed concentration and appetite; he denied significant anxiety. He denied feeling suicidal or being unable to care for himself. Mr. B reported one episode of relatively mild MDD 3 years ago that was well-treated with citalopram (20 mg per day, for 1 year); he had also had several episodes of "feeling low" for 3 to 5 days that spontaneously resolved. He appeared to be invested in getting better, he had a strong social support network, and he planned to follow up with his cardiologist shortly after his hospitalization.

Given Mr. B's relatively mild current depressive symptoms, his history of having only one mild episode of MDD, and his ability and willingness to follow up with his cardiologist, the consultant decided to defer antidepressant treatment while Mr. B was in the hospital. The consultant contacted Mr. B's cardiologist and they agreed that citalopram should be started (given Mr. B's history of good response to this medication) if he continued to be depressed upon returning for his follow-up appointment in 2 weeks.

Mr. B had an uneventful medical course and was discharged 3 days after his MI. He followed up in 2 weeks with his cardiologist; he remained depressed and was started on citalopram. He tolerated the citalopram (20 mg per day) well, and his depressive symptoms sub-sided over the next 8 weeks.

Delirium in Cardiac Patients

Patients with cardiac disease have long been found to have a propensity for delirium. In an era when open-heart surgery was common, the incidence of postcardiotomy delirium was found to be 32%.[124] Despite advances in the treatment of cardiac illness and the utilization of noninvasive procedures to open coronary arteries and replace abnormal valves, general hospital patients with cardiac disease continue to suffer delirium at high rates. High rates of comorbid medical illness, complex medication regimens, and central nervous system (CNS) hypoperfusion due to poor cardiac output all contribute to elevated rates of delirium among cardiac patients. The general hospital psychiatrist should be aware of the special issues in the diagnosis and management of delirium in cardiac patients.

Epidemiology

Delirium and Cardiac Disease

Delirium is more generally reviewed elsewhere in this handbook; this section focuses more specifically on delirium in patients with cardiac illness.

Among cardiac patients in the general hospital, rates of delirium are high. A study of patients suffering acute MI found that approximately 20% suffered delirium during the hospitalization.[125] Though estimates vary widely, postoperative delirium affects about 20% to 25% of the patients undergoing cardiac surgery.[126–128] Furthermore, two studies of patients receiving IABP therapy found that 34% of such patients were delirious.[129,130]

Reports of risk factors for the development of delirium in cardiac patients have varied, but it appears that increased age, preoperative cognitive impairment, and the use of anticholinergic drugs have been significantly associated with the development of postoperative delirium.[131,132] Other potential risk factors for delirium among patients undergoing cardiac surgery have been history of stroke,[126,133] low postoperative cardiac output,[133] MI prior to surgery,[127] low albumin,[134] and hypotension requiring high-dose ionotropic support.[135]

Factors related to the hospital setting may also increase the risk of delirium. Sleep deprivation as the result of light, noise, and an unfamiliar setting can predispose patients to delirium. Furthermore, discomfort (resulting from a prolonged need to remain supine, from IV catheters, or from multiple painful procedures) may be treated with narcotics or benzodiazepines which can then induce delirium.

In short, rates of delirium are high among patients with cardiovascular disease. Acute MI, cardiac surgery, and cardiac failure requiring IABP support are each associated with high rates of delirium, and a number of risk factors for delirium have been established in the cardiac population.

Delirium and Medical Outcome

To our knowledge, there have been no studies that have looked at the outcome of delirium specifically in cardiac patients. However, a number of studies have examined the effects of delirium on the medical outcome of general hospital patients. Studies of ICU patients have found that delirium significantly increases length of stay in the ICU,[136–138] overall length of hospitalization,[136,137] and amount of time on a ventilator[138]; one such study found that when other factors (such as severity of illness, age, gender, race, and days of benzodiazepine and narcotic drug administration) were controlled, delirium was the strongest independent determinant of hospital length of stay.[136]

In addition to increased length of stay in the ICU and in the hospital, delirium can significantly affect other important outcome measures. Delirium has been associated (independently of disease severity, age, and other medical and demographic factors) with significantly greater rates of functional decline during hospitalization, increased rates of admission to long-term care after admission, and reduced ability to perform activities of daily living (ADLs) compared to patients without delirium.[139–142]

Finally, and perhaps most importantly, delirium appears to be independently associated with increased mortality. Delirium is associated with high rates of in-hospital mortality.[142,143] Furthermore, prospective studies have found that delirium predicts mortality at 1,[144] 2,[139] and 3[145] years after discharge in elderly patients; in some of these studies, these effects of delirium on lifespan are

independent of medical comorbidity, functional status, and baseline cognitive status.

In short, delirium is common among cardiac patients in the general hospital, including post-MI patients, patients undergoing cardiac surgery, and severely ill patients on IABP therapy. Risk factors for delirium in cardiac patients appear to include age, baseline dementia, administration of anticholinergic medications, and hypotension. While the effects of delirium on outcome have not been studied specifically in cardiac patients, in the general medical population, delirium has been associated with increased length of stay, worsened functional outcome, and elevated in-hospital and long-term outcome. Still needed are studies that examine the effects of delirium treatment on long-term outcome.

Differential Diagnosis of Delirium in the Cardiac Patient

A wide variety of medical conditions and medications can cause or exacerbate delirium, and it is helpful for the psychiatrist to use mnemonics (such as VINDICTIVE MAD[146] cited by Cassem et al. in Chapter 12) to allow for a systematic approach to delirium. In the cardiac patient, there are a number of specific causes that should be carefully considered in all delirious patients (Table 32-3). CNS hypoperfusion is a common mechanism of delirium in the cardiac population; this can result from poor cardiac output due to CHF or myocardial ischemia, from comorbid carotid disease, from CNS bleeding (in the setting of anticoagulation), or from relative hypotension.

The phenomenon of relative hypotension deserves special mention. Patients with baseline uncontrolled hypertension who are admitted with myocardial ischemia or another cardiac event are often placed on one or more antihypertensives, and blood pressure is run "low," with systolic blood pressure typically between 100 and 120 mm Hg. In such patients, who may have significant baseline hypertension that is untreated or who are noncompliant with antihypertensives, hypertension may lead to stiffening of cerebral vessels with impaired ability to autoregulate. When these patients are presented with significantly lower "normal" blood pressures, cerebral

Table 32-3. Selected Causes of Delirium Among Cardiac Patients in the General Hospital

Central Nervous System Hypoperfusion
Myocardial infarction/ischemia
Cerebrovascular accident (ischemic or hemorrhagic)
Hypovolemia (due to dehydration or bleeding)
Relative hypotension

Other General Medical Conditions
Electrolyte abnormalities (especially sodium with diuretic
     administration)
Thyroid abnormalities
Hypertensive encephalopathy
Hypoxia (during pulmonary edema)
Infections (e.g., pneumonia, urinary tract infections)
Alcohol withdrawal

Medication-Related Causes
Digoxin toxicity
Narcotic analgesics
Benzodiazepines
Anticholinergic medications
H_2-Blockers

hypoperfusion and ischemia may result, leading to delirium.

Other common causes of delirium in the cardiac patient include hypoxia during CHF, hypertensive encephalopathy, electrolyte abnormalities (e.g., hyponatremia in the context of diuretic therapy), and medication effects (e.g., digoxin toxicity). The general hospital psychiatrist should rule out each of these potential etiologies of delirium in the cardiac patient.

Psychopharmacologic Issues in the Delirious Cardiac Patient

As noted in the APA Practice Guideline for the Treatment of Patients with Delirium,[147] the use of medications is an important component of a multipronged approach to the psychiatric management and treatment of delirium; such an approach also includes monitoring and ensuring safety, educating the patient and family regarding the illness, and utilizing environmental and supportive interventions (e.g., placing the patient near the nursing station and frequently reorienting the patient).

In general, psychotropic agents are used for the supportive treatment of delirium. They can reduce agitation and psychotic symptoms and may help to normalize the sleep-wake cycle. They usually are not the primary treatment or antidote for delirium (i.e., determining and specifically treating the etiology of the delirium), but they can reduce the risk of patient harm and alleviate patient distress until the etiology is identified and effectively treated.

Antipsychotics are the symptomatic treatment of choice for most delirious patients. These agents effectively reduce agitation and provide sedation for the delirious patient; moreover, they are generally quite safe. The greatest experience has been with haloperidol. This agent can be given orally or intramuscularly, but the IV form is both more rapidly acting and much less associated with the development of extrapyramidal symptoms (EPS); prospective study[148] and clinical experience have found the rate of EPS with IV haloperidol to be minimal. Haloperidol generally has no significant effects on heart rate, blood pressure, or respiratory status, and it has essentially no anticholinergic effects.

Haloperidol has, however, been associated with the development of torsades de pointes (TDP), a malignant polymorphic ventricular arrhythmia that can occur with medications that lengthen the cardiac QTc interval. More than two dozen cases of TDP have been reported with haloperidol,[149–151] and rates of TDP from haloperidol in the treatment of delirious patients have ranged from 0.36% to 3.5%.[149,152] TDP appears more common at high doses (>35 mg per day) of haloperidol, though it has also occurred at low doses as well.[149] Because hypokalemia and hypomagnesemia have been associated with the development of TDP, it is recommended that patients receiving IV haloperidol have these electrolytes monitored and repleted as needed. IV droperidol has also been used effectively in the treatment of delirium, though concerns about its propensity to cause TDP have significantly reduced its availability and use.

More recently, atypical antipsychotics, especially risperidone[153,154] and olanzapine[155] have been used in the treatment of delirium. These agents are also well-tolerated; risperidone and quetiapine can cause orthostatic hypotension and olanzapine has mild anticholinergic effects, but in general, these agents have little effect on heart rate, blood pressure, or respiratory status and can be safely used in cardiac patients.

There has been limited study of the use of atypical antipsychotics in delirium. In the two largest retrospective case series[153,154] describing the use of risperidone in the treatment of delirium from a variety of causes, 15 of 18 patients clinically improved with the use of risperidone, which was well-tolerated in these subjects. The largest study of olanzapine was a prospective open trial in hospitalized cancer patients with delirium by Breitbart, Tremblay, and Gibson;[155] the authors found that olan-zapine was well tolerated and led to complete resolution of delirium in 76% of cases. Finally a retrospective study by Schwartz and Masand[156] found that 10 of 11 patients receiving quetiapine for delirium showed substantial improvement of their symptoms; furthermore, the rate of peak improvement was similar to that seen in patients treated with haloperidol. There has been no study that has examined the efficacy or tolerability of atypical antipsychotics in the specific population of cardiac patients.

There have been concerns about the potential for atypical antipsychotics to cause QTc prolongation (potentially predisposing to TDP), especially in patients with cardiac disease. To address this, a study of the effects of a number of antipsychotics on the QTc of 154 subjects was undertaken.[157] In the study, six antipsychotics (thioridiazine, haloperidol, ziprasidone, risperidone, quetiapine, and olanzapine) were orally administered to the highest dose tolerated. Thioridazine (the antipsychotic most associated with TDP with oral administration[158]) and ziprasidone were associated with the greatest QT prolongation, while olanzapine and haloperidol had the least. It is difficult to extrapolate the results of this study to delirious cardiac patients, however, as the subjects were largely healthy young men without comorbid medical illness.

Treatment of cardiac patients with delirium with benzodiazepine monotherapy is generally contraindicated, as these agents can worsen confusion or cause paradoxical disinhibition, especially in elderly, demented, or brain-injured patients. However, benzodiazepines are the treatment of choice in delirium secondary to alcohol or benzodiazepine withdrawal and in delirious patients unable to tolerate high doses of antipsychotics (or who have significant cardiovascular side effects such as hypotension). Benzodiazepines may be used in combination with antipsychotics in the symptomatic treatment of delirium.

Other agents may be used to treat certain delirious states in cardiac patients. For example, physostigmine can be used to treat delirium from anticholinergic toxicity,[159] naloxone can use used to treat delirium due to opioid intoxication, and IV thiamine can be administered to those with Wernicke's encephalopathy.

The Practical Management of the Delirious Cardiac Patient

As with other conditions involving cardiac patients, the management of delirium involves careful diagnosis and the consideration of comorbid conditions. Once diagnosis and etiology have been established, the general hospital psychiatrist can then utilize optimal behavioral and nonpharmacologic strategies and intelligently use psychotropic agents that reduce medical risk while effectively decreasing symptoms:

1. *Make an informed diagnosis of delirium and carefully consider potential etiologies.* Delirium is characterized by an acute onset, disorientation, poor attention, fluctuation of levels of consciousness, and alterations in sleep-wake cycle. Psychotic symptoms, anxiety, worry, and reports of depressed mood may or may not be present. A careful review of the chart and cognitive evaluation (that considers orientation, attention, and executive function) can allow the consultant to use these factors to distinguish delirium from other psychiatric illnesses. Once a diagnosis has been made, the psychiatrist should work to consider all possible causes of delirium. The cause of delirium is frequently multifactorial; therefore, the identification of one potential contributing factor of delirium should not preclude the search for further potential abnormalities leading to an acute confusional state. The consultant should pay special attention to the initiation and termination of medications and their relationship to the onset of delirium; a careful review of nursing medication sheets often reveals a wealth of valuable information that can "crack the case" in a delirium of unknown etiology.

2. *Aggressively treat all potential etiologies of delirium.* Treating the core etiology of delirium is the

only way to definitively reverse delirium; all other behavioral and pharmacologic remedies are symptomatic treatments that reduce risk and increase comfort until the primary etiologies of the delirium resolve. Therefore, treatment of urinary tract infections, vitamin B_{12} deficiency, mild metabolic abnormalities, and other "small" contributing factors to delirium is absolutely crucial.

3. *Use nonpharmacologic strategies to minimize confusion and ensure safety.* Having the patient situated near the nursing station or in other areas where the patient can be frequently monitored can reduce the risk of falls, wandering, or other dangerous actions. The use of Posey vests, sitters, or locked restraints may be required when a delirious patient's inability to safely navigate places him or her at risk; in almost all cases, medication should be given in combination with physical restraint to reduce discomfort and risk of harm while in restraints. Having reassuring family members or friends at the bedside can mitigate paranoia and agitation, while in some cases visitors that overstimulate the patient may worsen symptoms. The consultant can recommend that the team either encourage or dissuade interaction with certain visitors based on the response of the patient's symptoms to the visitors.

4. *Use antipsychotic medications to reduce agitation and psychotic symptoms, and to regulate the sleep-wake cycle.* IV haloperidol is often the drug of choice for agitated, paranoid, or hyperactive patients with delirium. As noted earlier, this agent is associated with low rates of EPS, and it has little effect on heart rate or blood pressure. It is rapidly effective in the IV form. Cardiac patients may be at increased risk for TDP, and therefore, risk factors for this arrhythmia (e.g., prolonged QTc interval and electrolyte abnormalities) must be considered before its use. The protocol used at the MGH (Table 32-4) for the use of IV haloperidol considers these risk factors for TDP and uses a progressive dosing schedule. An initial dose (from 0.5 to 10.0 mg based on the age and size of patient and the extent of agitation) is selected and administered to the patient. If the patient is not calm within 20 to 30 minutes, the dose is doubled, and continues to be doubled every 20 to 30 minutes until the patient is calm. This effective dose is then used when and if the patient again becomes agitated. Though most patients require standard doses of haloperidol (2 to 10 mg), some patients have

required (and safely received) thousands of milligrams for agitation.[160]

If an agitated, delirious patient is or becomes unable to receive IV haloperidol (e.g., due to QTc prolongation), there are a number of other options. Sublingual olanzapine wafers are also fast-acting and effective in the treatment of delirium. Mildly agitated patients willing to take oral medications can be given oral atypical antipsychotics, such as risperidone, olanzapine, or quetiapine. Finally, patients whose agitation requires rapidly acting IV medication and who cannot receive IV antipsychotics may be given narcotics (e.g., morphine) or benzodiazepines (e.g., lorazepam) parenterally when immediate sedation is required; though these agents may worsen confusion, they are effective in the short-term when sedation is urgently needed.

Table 32-4. Massachusetts General Hospital Protocol for IV Haloperidol in Agitated Delirious Patients

---

Check pre-haloperidol QTc interval
If QTc > 450 ms, proceed with care
If QTc > 500 ms, consider other options

Check potassium and magnesium, and correct abnormalities
Aim for potassium > 4 mEq/L, magnesium >2 mEq/L

Give dose of haloperidol (0.5–10 mg) based on level of agitation, and patient's age and size
Goal is to have patient calm and awake
Haloperidol precipitates with phenytoin and heparin; flush line before giving haloperidol if these agents have been used in the same intravenous tubing
Wait 20–30 minutes. If patient remains agitated, double dose.
Continue to double dose every 30 minutes until patient calm

Follow QTc interval to ensure that QTc is not prolonging
If QTc increases by 25% or becomes >500, consider alternative treatments

Once effective dose has been determined, use that dose for future episodes of agitation
Depending on likely course of delirium, may schedule haloperidol or give on as-needed basis
For example, may divide previous effective dose over next 24 hours, giving q 6 hours.
Or may simply give effective dose as needed for agitation
Consider small dose at night to regulate sleep-wake cycle in all delirious patients

---

IV benzodiazepines are also the agents of choice in delirium tremens caused by benzodiazepine or alcohol withdrawal.

Once the agitated delirious patient has been safely and adequately sedated, there is often a question of whether to schedule antipsychotic medication or to use it on an as-needed basis for agitation. Such a decision may depend on the likely duration of the delirium, if this can be determined. For example, if the delirium is secondary to CNS hypoperfusion in a patient with low cardiac output on an IABP, such delirium may well be prolonged, and scheduling of an antipsychotic would be reasonable. In contrast, delirium in an elderly cardiac patient resulting from narcotic administration may be short-lived once the narcotic has been eliminated, and standing antipsychotics may not be needed. In most cases of delirium, we have found that it is often reasonable to schedule a low dose of IV haloperidol or an oral atypical antipsychotic at bedtime to help regulate the sleep-wake cycle, which is often seriously perturbed in delirious patients. We have found that, by ensuring adequate sleep at appropriate hours, delirious cardiac patients have the best possible chance to recover.

Case 3

Mr. C, a 64-year-old man with three-vessel CAD and no significant psychiatric history, was admitted for CABG. Though he was alert, oriented, pleasant, and cooperative prior to his surgery, on postoperative day 2, he became angry and threatening, reporting that the nurses were the "minions of the devil" and that he needed to leave the hospital immediately; notes revealed that he had not slept for 24 hours. Psychiatry was urgently consulted for "psychosis and capacity to leave against medical advice."

The psychiatrist found Mr. C sitting on his bed, wearing only his pajama tops. He angrily reported that the nursing staff was stealing money from him and that they had injected "poisons" into him. He was disoriented to time and place, and he was unable to attend to conversation for more than a few seconds. He had pulled off his telemetry leads and not allowed the nurses to check his vital signs. The psychiatrist was able to get Mr. C to agree to stay for the moment, and, after confirming a normal postoperative QTc interval and normal electrolyte levels, he got Mr. C to accept an injection of 3 mg of IV haloperidol. After 20 minutes, the patient became sedated, and he fell asleep after 45 minutes.

When Mr. C's leads were reattached, and vital signs checked, he was noted to have new-onset atrial fibrillation with a rate of 119. His heart rate was slowed with the use of b-blockers, and he returned to normal sinus rhythm within 12 hours. He received two further doses of IV haloperidol, and 25 mg of quetiapine each night. His delirium slowly resolved over the next 6 days, coinciding with resolution of his atrial fibrillation and with treatment of a urinary tract infection, and the quetiapine was discontinued on his discharge to a cardiac rehabilitation facility.

References

1. Williams JC: *Practical observations on nervous and sympathetic palpitations of the heart*, London, 1936, Longman Rees Orme Browne.
2. Da Costa JM: On irritable heart, *Am J Med Sci* 61:17–52, 1871.
3. Osler W: *The principles and practice of medicine*, Edinburgh, 1882, J Pentland Young.
4. Abramson JH, Terespolsky L, Brook JG: Cornell Medical Index as a health measure in epidemiological studies, a test of the validity of a health questionnaire, *Br J Prev Soc Med* 19(3):103–110, 1965.
5. Kawachi I, Colditz GA, Acherio A, et al: Prospective study of phobic anxiety and risk of coronary heart disease in men, *Circulation* 89:1992–1997, 1994.
6. Dimsdale JE: Emotional causes of sudden death, *Am J Psychiatry* 134(12):1361–1366, 1977.
7. Cassem NH, Hackett TP: Psychiatric consultation in a coronary care unit, *Ann Intern Med* 75:9–14, 1971.
8. Crowe JM, Runions J, Ebbesen LS, et al: Anxiety and depression after myocardial infarction, *Heart Lung* 25:98–107, 1996.
9. Philip AE, Cay EL, Vetter NJ, et al: Short-term fluctuations in anxiety in patients with myocardial infarction, *J Psychosom Res* 23:277–280, 1979.
10. Billing E, Lindell B, Sederholm M, et al: Denial, anxiety, and depression following myocardial infarction, *Psychosomatics* 21:639–645, 1980.
11. Hallas CN, Thortnon EW, Fabri BM, et al: Predicting blood pressure reactivity and heart rate variability from mood state following coronary artery bypass surgery, *Int J Psychophysiol* 47(1):43–55, 2003.
12. Koivula M, Tarkka MT, Tarkka M, et al: Fear and anxiety in patients at different time-points in the coronary artery bypass process, *Int J Nurs Stud* 39(8):811–822, 2002.
13. Duru F, Buchi S, Klaghofer R, et al: How different from pacemaker patients are recipients of implantable cardioverter-defibrillators with respect to psychosocial adaptation, affective disorders, and quality of life? *Heart* 85(4):375–379, 2001.

14. Herrmann C, von zur Muhen F, Schaumann A, et al: Standardized assessment of psychological well-being and quality-of-life in patients with implanted defibrillators, *Pacing Clin Electrophysiol* 20(1 Pt 1):95–103, 1997.

15. Huffman JC, Pollack MH: Predicting panic disorder among patients with chest pain: an analysis of the literature, *Psychosomatics* 44(3): 222–236, 2003.

16. Ginzburg K, Solomon Z, Bleich A: Repressive coping style, acute stress disorder, and posttraumatic stress disorder after myocardial infarction, *Psychosom Med* 64(5):748–757, 2002.

17. Shemesh E, Rudnick A, Kaluski E, et al: A prospective study of posttraumatic stress symptoms and nonadherence in survivors of myocardial infarction, *Gen Hosp Psychiatry* 23(4):215–222, 2001.

18. Doerfler LA, Pbert L, DeCosimo D: Symptoms of posttraumatic stress disorder following myocardial infarction and coronary artery bypass surgery, *Gen Hosp Psychiatry* 16(3):193–199, 1994.

19. Stoll C, Schelling G, Goetz AE, et al: Health-related quality of life and post-traumatic stress disorder in patients after cardiac surgery and intensive care treatment, *J Thorac Cardiovasc Surg* 120:505–512, 2000.

20. Ehde DM, Patterson DR, Wiechman SA, et al: Post-traumatic stress symptoms and distress following acute burn injury, *Burns* 25(7):587–592, 1999.

21. Schelling G, Stoll C, Haller M, et al: Health-related quality of life and posttraumatic stress disorder in survivors of the acute respiratory distress syndrome, *Crit Care Med* 26(4):651–659, 1998.

22. Reich P, DeSilva RA, Lown B, et al: Acute psychological disturbances preceding life-threatening ventricular arrhythmias, *JAMA* 246(3):233–235, 1981.

23. Freeman LJ, Nixon PG, Sallabank P, et al: Psychological stress and silent myocardial ischemia, *Am Heart J* 114(3):477–482, 1987.

24. Kawachi I, Sparrow D, Vokonas PS, et al: Symptoms of anxiety and risk of coronary heart disease: the Normative Aging Study, *Circulation* 90:2225–2229, 1994.

25. Haines AP, Imeson JD, Meade TW: Phobic anxiety and ischaemic heart disease, *Br Med J* 295:297–299, 1987.

26. Myerberg RJ, Kessler KM, Castellanos A: Sudden cardiac death: epidemiology, transient risk, and intervention assessment, *Ann Intern Med* 119:1187–1197, 1993.

27. Katon W, Vitaliano PP, Russo J, et al: Panic disorder: epidemiology in primary care, *J Fam Prac* 23:233–239, 1986.

28. Balon R, Ortiz A, Pohl R, et al: Heart rate and blood pressure during placebo-associated panic attacks, *Psychosom Med* 50:434–438, 1988.

29. Roy-Byrne PP, Schmidt P, Cannon RO, et al: Microvascular angina and panic disorder, *Int J Psychiatry Med* 19:315–325, 1989.

30. Kahn JP, Drusin RE, Klein DF: Idiopathic cardiomyopathy and panic disorder: clinical association in cardiac transplant candidates, *Am J Psychiatry* 144:1327–1330, 1987.

31. Kahn JP, Gorman JM, King DL, et al: Cardiac left ventricular hypertrophy and chamber dilatation in panic disorder patients: implications for idiopathic dilated cardiomyopathy, *Psychiatry Res* 32:55–61, 1990.

32. Gillette PC, Smith RT, Garson A, et al: Chronic supraventricular tachycardia: a curable cause of congestive cardiomyopathy, *JAMA* 253:391–392, 1985.

33. Coryell W, Noyes R, House JD: Mortality among outpatients with anxiety disorders, *Am J Psychiatry* 143:508–510, 1986.

34. Coryell W, Noyes R, Clancy J: Excess mortality in panic disorder: a comparison with primary unipolar depression, *Arch Gen Psychiatry* 139:701–703, 1982.

35. Weissman MM, Markowitz JS, Ouellette MD, et al: Panic disorder and cardiovascular/cerebrovascular problems: results from a community survey, *Am J Psychiatry* 147:1504–1508, 1990.

36. Moser DK, Dracup K: Is anxiety early after myocardial infarction associated with subsequent ischemic and arrhythmic events? *Psychosom Med* 58:395–401, 1996.

37. Frasure-Smith N, Lespérance F, Talajic M: The impact of negative emotions on prognosis following myocardial infarction: is it more than depression? *Health Psychol* 14:388–398, 1995.

38. Mayou RA, Gill D, Thompson DR, et al: Depression and anxiety as predictors of outcome after myocardial infarction, *Psychosom Med* 62:212–219, 2000.

39. Lane D, Carroll D, Ring C, et al: Mortality and quality of life 12 months after myocardial infarction: effects of depression and anxiety, *Psychosom Med* 63(2):221–230, 2001.

40. Ahern DK, Gorkin L, Anderson JL, et al: Biobehavioral variables and mortality or cardiac arrest in the Cardiac Arrhythmia Pilot Study (CAPS), *Am J Cardiol* 66(1):59–62, 1990.

41. Underwood MJ, Firmin RK, Jehu D: Aspects of psychological and social morbidity in patients awaiting coronary artery bypass grafting, *Br Heart J* 69(5):382–384, 1993.

42. Duits AA, Boeke S, Taams MA, et al: Prediction of quality of life after coronary artery bypass graft surgery: a review and evaluation of multiple, recent studies, *Psychosom Med* 59(3):257–268, 1997.

43. Jones GN, Ames SC, Jeffries SK, et al: Utilization of medical services and quality of life among low-income patients with generalized anxiety disorder attending primary care clinics, *Int J Psychiatry Med* 31(2):183–198, 2001.

44. Eaton WW, Kessler LG, editors: *Epidemiologic field methods in psychiatry: the NIMH epidemiologic catchment Area Program.* Orlando, Fla, 1985, Academic Press.

45. Simon GE, Von Korff M: Somatization and psychiatric disorder in the Epidemiologic Catchment Area study, *Am J Psychiatry* 148:1494–1500, 1991.

46. Dixon RA, Edwards IR, Pilcher J: Diazepam in immediate post-myocardial infarct period: a double blind trial, *Br Heart J* 43(5):535–540, 1980.

47. Melsom M, Andreassen H, Melsom T, et al: Diazepam in acute myocardial infarction: clinical effects and effects on catecholamines, free fatty acids, and cortisol, *Br Heart J* 38:804–810, 1976.

48. Nitenberg A, Marty J, Blanchet F, et al: Effects of flunitrazepam on left ventricular pressure, coronary haemodynamics and myocardial metabolism in patients with coronary artery disease, *Br J Anaesth* 55(12): 1179–1184, 1983.

49. Kornecki E, Ehrlich YH, Lenox RH: Platelet-activating factor-induced aggregation of human platelets specifically inhibited by triazolobenzodiazepines, *Science* 225:1454–1456, 1986.

50. Van Loon GR: Ventricular arrhythmias treated by diazepam, *Can Med Assoc J* 98(16):785–787, 1968.

51. Muenster JJ, Rosenberg MS, Carleton RA, et al. Comparison between diazepam and sodium thiopental during DC countershock, *JAMA* 199:758–760, 1967.

52. Roche Laboratories: *Valium*. In Sifton D, editor: *Physicians' desk reference*, Montvale, NJ, 2000, Medical Economics Company.

53. Greenblatt DJ, Koch-Weser J: Adverse reactions to intravenous diazepam: a report from the Boston Collaborative Drug Surveillance Program, *Am J Med Sci* 266(4):261–266, 1973.

54. Tesar GE, Rosenbaum JF: *The anxious patient*. In: Hyman SE, Tesar GE, editors. *Manual of psychiatric emergencies, ed 3*, Boston: 1994, Little, Brown, and Company, pp 129–142.

55. Honderick T, Williams D, Seaberg D, et al: A prospective, randomized, controlled trial of benzodiazepines and nitroglycerine or nitroglycerine alone in the treatment of cocaine-associated acute coronary syndromes, *Am J Emerg Med* 21(1):39–42, 2003.

56. Wheatley D: Anxiolytic drug use in cardiovascular disease: an overview, *Psychopharmacol Bull* 20(4): 649–659, 1984.

57. Glassman AH, O'Connor CM, Califf R, et al: Sertraline treatment of major depression in patients with acute MI or unstable angina, *JAMA* 288:701–709, 2002.

58. Strik JJ, Honig A, Lousberg R, et al: Efficacy and safety of fluoxetine in the treatment of patients with major depression after first myocardial infarction: findings from a double-blind, placebo-controlled trial, *Psychosom Med* 62(6):783–789, 2000.

59. Shapiro PA, Lespérance F, Frasure-Smith N, et al: An open-label preliminary trial of sertraline for treatment of major depression after acute myocardial infarction (the SADHAT Trial), Sertraline Anti-Depressant Heart Attack Trial, *Am Heart J* 137(6):1100–1106, 1999.

60. Adityanjee, Schulz SC: Clinical use of quetiapine in disease states other than schizophrenia, *J Clin Psychiatry* 63 (suppl) 13:32–38, 2002.

61. Rabins PV, Harvis K, Koven S: High fatality rates of late-life depression associated with cardiovascular disease, *J Affect Disord* 9:165–167, 1985.

62. Frasure-Smith N, Lespérance F, Talajic M: Depression following myocardial infarction: impact on 6-month survival, *JAMA* 270:1819–1825, 1993.

63. Frasure-Smith N, Lespérance F, Talajic M: Depression and 18-month prognosis after myocardial infarction, *Circulation* 91:999–1005, 1995.

64. Burg MM, Benedetto MC, Rosenberg R, et al: Presurgical depression predicts medical morbidity 6 months after coronary artery bypass graft surgery, *Psychosom Med* 65(1):111–118, 2003.

65. Musselman DL, Evans DL, Nemeroff CB: The relationship of depression to cardiovascular disease: epidemiology, biology, and treatment, *Arch Gen Psychiatry* 55:580–592, 1998.

66. Carney RM, Rich MW, Freeland KE, et al: Major depressive disorder predicts cardiac events in patients with coronary artery disease, *Psychosom Med* 50: 627–633, 1988.

67. Gonzalez MB, Snyderman TB, Colket JT, et al: Depression in patients with coronary artery disease, *Depression* 4:57–62, 1996.

68. Strik JJ, Honig A, Maes M: Depression and myocardial infarction: relationship between heart and mind, *Progr Neuropsychopharmacol Biol Psychiatry* 25(4):879–892, 2001.

69. Januzzi JL, Stern TA, Pasternak RC, et al: The influence of anxiety and depression on outcomes of patients with coronary artery disease, *Arch Intern Med* 160(13):1913–1921, 2000.

70. Baker RA, Andrew MJ, Schrader G, et al: Preoperative depression and mortality in coronary artery bypass surgery: preliminary findings, *ANZ J Surg* 71(3):139–142, 2001.

71. Freedland KE, Lustman PJ, Carney RM, et al: Underdiagnosis of depression in patients with coronary artery disease: the role of nonspecific symptoms, *Int J Psychiatry Med* 22(3):221–229, 1992.

72. Honig A, Lousberg R, Wojciechowski FL, et al: Depression following a first heart infarct: similarities with and differences from 'ordinary' depression [article in Dutch], *Ned Tijdschr Geneeskd* 141(4):196–199, 1997.

73. Travella JI, Forrester AW, Schultz SK, et al: Depression following myocardial infarction: a one year longitudinal study, *Int J Psychiatry Med* 24(4):357–369, 1994.

74. Frasure-Smith N, Lespérance F, Gravel G, et al: Social support, depression, and mortality during the first year after myocardial infarction, *Circulation* 101(16):1919–1924, 2000.

75. Lespérance F, Frasure-Smith N, Talajic M: Major depression before and after myocardial infarction: its nature and consequences, *Psychosom Med* 58(2):99–110, 1996.

76. Shapiro PA, Levin HR, Oz MC: Left ventricular assist devices. Psychosocial burden and implications for

heart transplant programs, *Gen Hosp Psychiatry* 18(6 suppl):30S–35S, 1996.

77. Kuhn WF, Myers B, Brennan AF, et al: Psychopathology in heart transplant candidates, *J Heart Transplant* 7(3):223–236, 1988.

78. Bunzel B, Laederach-Hofmann K, Grimm M: Survival, clinical data and quality of life 10 years after heart transplantation: a prospective study [article in German], *Z Kardiol* 91(4):319–327, 2002.

79. Dew MA, Kormos RL, Roth LH, et al: Early posttransplant medical compliance and mental health predict physical morbidity and mortality one to three years after heart transplantation, *J Heart Lung Transplant* 18(6):549–562, 1999.

80. Ford DE, Mead LA, Chang PF, et al: Depression is a risk factor for coronary artery disease in men: the Precursors Study, *Arch Intern Med* 158:1422–1426, 1998.

81. Anda R, Williamson D, Jones D, et al: Depressed affect, hopelessness, and the risk of ischemic heart disease in a cohort of U.S. adults, *Epidemiology* 4:285–294, 1993.

82. Zyzanski SJ, Jenkins CD, Ryan TJ, et al: Psychological correlates of coronary angiographic findings, *Arch Intern Med* 136:1234–1237, 1976.

83. Aromaa A, Raitasalo R, Reunanen A, et al: Depression and cardiovascular diseases, *Acta Psychiatr Scand Suppl* 377:77–82, 1994.

84. Pratt LA, Ford DE, Crum RM, et al: Depression, psychotropic medication, and risk of myocardial infarction, *Circulation* 94:3123–3129, 1996.

85. Barefoot JC, Schroll M: Symptoms of depression, acute myocardial infarction and total mortality in a community sample, *Circulation* 93:1976–1980, 1996.

86. Rugulies R: Depression as a predictor for coronary heart disease, *Am J Prev Med* 23(1):51–61, 2002.

87. Bush DE, Ziegelstein RC, Tayback M: Even minimal symptoms of depression increase mortality risk after acute myocardial infarction, *Am J Cardiol* 88:337–341, 2001.

88. Ladwig KH, Kieser M, Konig J, et al: Affective disorders and survival after acute myocardial infarction. results from the post-infarction late potential study, *Eur Heart J* 12:959–964, 1991.

89. Connerney I, Shapiro PA, McLaughlin JS, et al: Relation between depression after coronary artery bypass surgery and 12-month outcome: a prospective study, *Lancet* 358:1766–1771, 2001.

90. Zipfel S, Schneider A, Wild B, et al: Effect of depressive symptoms on survival after heart transplantation, *Psychosom Med* 64(5):740–747, 2002.

91. Krantz D, Helmers K, Bairey CN, et al: Cardiovascular reactivity and mental stress-induced myocardial ischemia in patients with coronary artery disease, *Psychosom Med* 53:1–12, 1991.

92. Dixon RA, Edwards IR, Pilcher J: Diazepam in immediate post-myocardial infarct period: a double blind trial, *Br Heart J* 43(5):535–540, 1980.

93. Jewitt DE, Mercer CJ, Reid D, et al: Free noradrenaline and adrenaline excretion in relation to the development of cardiac arrhythmias and heart-failure in patients with acute myocardial infarction, *Lancet* 1:635–641, 1969. .

94. Gorman JM, Sloan RP: Heart rate variability in depressive and anxiety disorders, *Am Heart J* 140 (4 suppl):77–83, 2000.

95. Carney RM, Blumenthal JA, Stein PK, et al: Depression, heart rate variability, and acute myocardial infarction, *Circulation* 104(17):2024–2028, 2001.

96. Follick MJ, Ahern DK, Gorkin L, et al: Relation of psychosocial and stress reactivity variables to ventricular arrhythmias in the Cardiac Arrhythmia Pilot Study, *Am J Cardiol* 66:63–67, 1990.

97. Levine SP, Towell BL, Saurez AM: Platelet activation and secretion associated with emotional stress, *Circulation* 71:1129–1134, 1995.

98. Carney RM, Freedland KE, Rich MW, et al: Depression as a risk factor for cardiac events in established coronary heart disease: a review of possible mechanisms, *Ann Behav Med* 17:142–149, 1995.

99. Lane D, Carroll D, Ring C, et al: Predictors of attendance at cardiac rehabilitation after myocardial infarction, *J Psychosom Res* 51(3):497–501, 2001.

100. Welin C, Lappas G, Wilhelmsen L: Independent importance of psychosocial factors for prognosis after myocardial infarction, *J Intern Med* 247:629–639, 2000.

101. Sykes DH, Hanley M, Boyle DM, et al: Socioeconomic status, social environment, depression and postdischarge adjustment of the cardiac patient, *J Psychosom Res* 46:83–98, 1999.

102. Ko DT, Hebert PR, Coffey CS, et al: Beta-blocker therapy and symptoms of depression, fatigue, and sexual dysfunction, *JAMA* 288(3):351–357, 2002.

103. Sheline YI, Freedland KE, Carney RM: How safe are serotonin reuptake inhibitors for depression in patients with coronary heart disease? *Am J Med* 102:54–59, 1997.

104. Warrington SJ, Padgham C, Lader M: The cardiovascular effects of antidepressants, *Psychol Med Monogr Suppl* 16:1–40, 1989.

105. Cohen HW, Gibson G, Alderman MH: Excess risk of myocardial infarction in patients treated with antidepressant medications: association with use of tricyclic agents, *Am J Med* 108(1):2–8, 2000.

106. Arana GW, Rosenbaum JF: *Handbook of psychiatric Drug Therapy, ed 4*, Philadelphia, 2000, Lippincott Williams and Wilkins.

107. Stern TA: The management of depression and anxiety following myocardial infarction, *Mt Sinai J Med* 52:623–633, 1985.

108. Roose SP, Laghrissi-Thode F, Kennedy JS, et al: Comparison of paroxetine and nortriptyline in depressed patients with ischemic heart disease, *JAMA* 279(4):287–291, 1998.

109. Strik JJ, Honig A, Lousberg R, et al: Efficacy and safety of fluoxetine in the treatment of patients with major depression after first myocardial infarction: findings from a double-blind, placebo-controlled trial, *Psychosom Med* 62(6):783–789, 2000.

110. Kiev A, Masco HL, Wenger TL, et al: The cardiovascular effects of bupropion and nortriptyline in depressed outpatients, *Ann Clin Psychiatry* 6(2):107–115, 1994.

111. Roose SP, Dalack GW, Glassman AH, et al: Cardiovascular effects of bupropion in depressed patients with heart disease, *Am J Psychiatry* 148(4):512–516, 1991.

112. Balit CR, Lynch CN, Isbister GK: Bupropion poisoning: a case series, *Med J Aust* 178(2):61–63, 2003.

113. Wenger TL, Stern WC: The cardiovascular profile of bupropion, *J Clin Psychiatry* 44(5 Pt 2):176–182, 1983.

114. Paoloni R, Szekely I: Sustained-release bupropion overdose: a new entity for Australian emergency departments, *Emerg Med (Fremantle)* 14(1):109–112, 2002.

115. Tracey JA, Cassidy N, Casey PB, et al: Bupropion (Zyban) toxicity, *Ir Med J* 95(1):23–24, 2002.

116. Jorenby DE, Leischow SJ, Nides MA, et al: A controlled trial of sustained-release bupropion, a nicotine patch, or both for smoking cessation, *N Engl J Med* 340(9):685–691, 1999.

117. Ahluwalia JS, Harris KJ, Catley D, et al: Sustained-release bupropion for smoking cessation in African Americans: a randomized controlled trial, *JAMA* 288(4):468–474, 2002.

118. van den Brink RH, van Melle JP, Honig A, et al: Treatment of depression after myocardial infarction and the effects on cardiac prognosis and quality of life: rationale and outline of the Myocardial Infarction and Depression-Intervention Trial (MIND-IT), *Am Heart J* 144(2):219–225, 2002.

119. Velazquez C, Carlson A, Stokes KA, et al: Relative safety of mirtazapine overdose, *Vet Hum Toxicol* 43(6):342–344, 2001.

120. Masand P, Pickett P, Murray GB: Psychostimulants for secondary depression in medical illness, *Psychosomatics* 32(2):203–208, 1991.

121. Woods SW, Tesar GE, Murray GB, et al: Psychostimulant treatment of depressive disorders secondary to medical illness, *J Clin Psychiatry* 47(1):12–15, 1986.

122. Frasure-Smith N, Lespérance F, Gravel G, et al: Social support, depression, and mortality during the first year after myocardial infarction, *Circulation* 101(16):1919–1924, 2000.

123. Carney RM, Freedland KE, Stein PK, et al: Change in heart rate and heart rate variability during treatment for depression in patients with coronary heart disease, *Psychosom Med* 62(5):639–647, 2000.

124. Smith LW, Dimsdale JE: Postcardiotomy delirium: conclusions after 25 years? *Am J Psychiatry* 146(4):452–458, 1989.

125. Kagoshima M, Miyashita Y, Takei K, et al: Acute myocardial infarction in elderly patients: medical and social problems [article in Japanese], *J Cardiol* 35(4):267–275, 2000.

126. van der Mast RC, Roest FH: Delirium after cardiac surgery: a critical review, *J Psychosom Res* 1996; 41(1):13–30, 1996.

127. Eriksson M, Samuelsson E, Gustafson Y, et al: Delirium after coronary bypass surgery evaluated by the organic brain syndrome protocol, *Scand Cardiovasc J* 36(4):250–255, 2002.

128. Kornfeld DS, Heller SS, Frank KA, et al. Delirium after coronary artery bypass surgery, *J Thorac Cardiovasc Surg* 76(1):93–96, 1978.

129. Sanders KM, Stern TA, O'Gara PT, et al: Delirium during intra-aortic balloon pump therapy. incidence and management, *Psychosomatics* 33(1):35–44, 1992.

130. Sanders KM, Stern TA, O'Gara PT, et al: Medical and neuropsychiatric complications associated with the use of the intra-aortic balloon pump, *J Intensive Care Med* 7:154–164, 1992.

131. Dyer CB, Ashton CM, Teasdale TA: Postoperative delirium: a review of 80 primary-data-collection studies, *Arch Intern Med* 155(5):461–465, 1995.

132. Rolfson DB, McElhaney JE, Rockwood K, et al: Incidence and risk factors for delirium and other adverse outcomes in older adults after coronary artery bypass graft surgery, *Can J Cardiol* 15(7):771–776, 1999.

133. Litaker D, Locala J, Franco K, et al: Preoperative risk factors for postoperative delirium, *Gen Hosp Psychiatry* 23(2):84–89, 2001.

134. van der Mast RC, van den Broek WW, Fekkes D, et al: Incidence of and preoperative predictors for delirium after cardiac surgery, *J Psychosom Res* 46(5):479–483, 1999.

135. Gokgoz L, Gunaydin S, Sinci V, et al: Psychiatric complications of cardiac surgery postoperative delirium syndrome, *Scand Cardiovasc J* 31(4):217–222, 1997.

136. Ely EW, Gautam S, Margolin R, et al: The impact of delirium in the intensive care unit on hospital length of stay, *Intensive Care Med* 27(12):1892–1900, 2001

137. Aldemir M, Ozen S, Kara IH, et al: Predisposing factors for delirium in the surgical intensive care unit, *Crit Care* 5(5):265–270, 2001.

138. Granberg Axell AI, Malmros CW, Bergbom IL, et al: Intensive care unit syndrome/delirium is associated with anemia, drug therapy and duration of ventilation treatment, *Acta Anaesthesiol Scand* 46(6):726–731, 2002.

139. Dolan MM, Hawkes WG, Zimmerman SI, et al: Delirium on hospital admission in aged hip fracture patients: prediction of mortality and 2-year functional outcomes. *J Gerontol A Biol Sci Med Sci* 55(9):M527–534, 2000.

140. Inouye SK, Rushing JT, Foreman MD, et al: Does delirium contribute to poor hospital outcomes? A three-site epidemiologic study, *J Gen Intern Med* 13(4):234–242, 1998.

141. O'Keeffe S, Lavan J: The prognostic significance of delirium in older hospital patients, *J Am Geriatr Soc* 45(2):174–178, 1997.

142. Rabins PV, Folstein MF: Delirium and dementia: diagnostic criteria and fatality rates, *Br J Psychiatry* 140:149–153, 1982.

143. Cameron DJ, Thomas RI, Mulvihill M, et al: Delirium: a test of the Diagnostic and Statistical Manual III criteria on medical inpatients, *J Am Geriatr Soc* 35:1007–1010, 1987.

144. McCusker J, Cole M, Abrahamowicz M, et al: Delirium predicts 12-month mortality, *Arch Intern Med* 162(4):457–463, 2002.

145. Curyto KJ, Johnson J, TenHave T, et al: Survival of hospitalized elderly patients with delirium: a prospective study. *Am J Geriatr Psychiatry* 9(2):141–147, 2001.

146. Ludwig AM: *Principles of clinical psychiatry*, New York, 1980, The Free Press.

147. American Psychiatric Association: Practice guideline for the treatment of patients with delirium, *Am J Psychiatry* 156(suppl 5):1–20, 1999.

148. Menza MA, Murray GB, Holmes VF, et al: Controlled study of extrapyramidal reactions in the management of delirious, medically ill patients: intravenous haloperidol versus intravenous haloperidol plus benzodiazepines, *Heart Lung* 17(3):238–244, 1988.

149. Sharma ND, Rosman HS, Padhi ID, et al: Torsades de pointes associated with intravenous haloperidol in critically ill patients, *Am J Cardiol* 81(2):238–240, 1998.

150. Metzger E, Friedman R: Prolongation of the corrected QT and torsades de pointes cardiac arrhythmia associated with intravenous haloperidol in the medically ill, *J Clin Psychopharmacol* 13:128–132, 1993.

151. Hunt N, Stern TA: The association between intravenous haloperidol and torsades de pointes: three cases and a literature review, *Psychosomatics* 36:541–549, 1995.

152. Wilt JL, Minnema AM, Johnson RF, et al: Torsades de pointes associated with the use of intravenous haloperidol, *Ann Intern Med* 119:391–394, 1993.

153. Sipahimalani A, Rime RM, Masand PS: Treatment of delirium with risperidone, *Int J Geriatr Psychopharmacol* 1:24–26, 1997.

154. Furmaga KM, DeLeon OA, Sinha SB, et al: Psychosis in medical conditions: response to risperidone, *Gen Hosp Psychiatry* 19(3):223–228, 1997.

155. Breitbart W, Tremblay A, Gibson C: An open trial of olanzapine for the treatment of delirium in hospitalized cancer patients, *Psychosomatics* 43(3):175–182, 2002.

156. Schwartz TL, Masand PS: Treatment of delirium with quetiapine, *J Clin Psychiatry (Primary Care Companion)* 2:10–12, 2000.

157. Food and Drug Administration, Center for Drug Evaluation and Research Psychopharmacological Drugs Advisory Committee. Meeting Transcript (for the approval of Zeldox [ziprasidone]), July 19, 2000. (Available at: http://www.fda.gov/ohrms/docket/ac/00/transcripts/ 3619t1a.pdf, 3619t1b.pdf, and 3619t1c.pdf).

158. Mehtonen OP, Aranko K, Malkonen L, et al: A survey of sudden death associated with the use of antipsychotic or antidepressant drugs: 49 cases in Finland, *Acta Psychiatr Scand* 84:58–64, 1991.

159. Greene LT: Physostigmine treatment of anticholinergic-drug depression in postoperative patients, *Anesth Analg* 50:222–226, 1971.

160. Sanders KM, Murray GB, Cassem NH: High-dose intravenous haloperidol for agitated delirium in a cardiac patient on intra-aortic balloon pump, *J Clin Psychopharmacol* 11(2):146–147, 1991.

Chapter 33

Patients with Cancer and the Evolution of the Role of Psychiatry in Oncology

Donna B. Greenberg, M.D.
Halyna Vitagliano, M.D.
William F. Pirl, M.D.
Annah N. Abrams, M.D.
Anna C. Muriel, M.D.
Paula K. Rauch, M.D.

In *Case Histories of Psychosomatic Medicine*, written in 1952 by the staff of the Massachusetts General Hospital (MGH) Psychiatric Service,[1] Harley Shands presented a 41-year-old married woman whose breast cancer was misdiagnosed as it progressed during her first pregnancy. Just after the delivery of a daughter, she was told she had cancer and would require a radical mastectomy. A painful clavicle metastasis 2 months later led to removal of both ovaries. She did well for a year until back pain developed. Despite testosterone treatment, she continued to worsen. Three years after diagnosis, she was receiving radiation treatment for sudden-onset diabetes insipidus and palsy of the right sixth nerve.

At the time of oophorectomy, she wept bitterly, and psychiatry was consulted. After two visits in the hospital by Shands, she agreed to review some of her life experiences in a psychiatric setting. She had been in the Women's Army Corps in World War II and had an episode of prolonged crying during her service. When the cancer was diagnosed, she became preoccupied with being injured, spoiled, and dirty. Over the first few months, she improved emotionally, and psychiatric visits became landmarks in her course; however, she worsened later as the cancer progressed. She continued to see Shands several times each week over 18 months.

Shands[1] remarked on the power of a steady, dependable, nonrejecting psychiatrist offering emotional support. He commented on the patient's idealization of physicians and the difficult medical assignment of staying with a patient who was deteriorating. The psychiatrist's ability to understand the emotional impact and fantasy associated with the cancer made it easier to answer questions and to decide how much to tell the patient and what to avoid. Child Psychiatry felt it was important for the mother to establish a relationship with the infant daughter before the patient died. Ruth Abrams, the social worker who worked with the patient, described the efforts made to help the patient's husband accept the fact that his wife would likely die.

Patients preferred to assign responsibility for the cancer than to see the cause as mysterious.[2] Abrams and Finesinger,[3] in 1953, reported that half of 60 cancer patients believed that the cancer was their fault; 26 thought it was due to an injury inflicted by someone else.

Abrams[4] emphasized the loneliness of cancer and the humiliation of long illness. The first lesson, she wrote later, describing 25 years of work with cancer patients, was: "Listen to the patient; she will tell you how much, how little and with whom she wishes to discuss her fears or anxieties . . . Let her make the choices that she . . . can tolerate . . . Let her manage the course of her life and herself to the best of her ability." (p. xvi)

Early Psychosomatic Medicine

The psychiatrist's ability to work together with practitioners of medicine, surgery, and other specialties to help the patient with a condition like cancer was the essence of psychosomatic medicine for Stanley Cobb,[5] who in 1952 was the Chairman of the MGH Psychiatry Service. Cobb's discussion of emotions included the role of the visceral brain, hereditary predisposition, corticosteroids, conditioning, and phobias. He believed that psychotherapy was best taught by individual supervision of clinical work in detailed discussion with an instructor. The work required an appreciation of unconscious processes, particularly the dynamics of the doctor–patient relationship.

Three components of the doctor–patient relationship were described by Avery Weisman[6] in 1950 and published in the Case Histories. These were what the patient brought spontaneously to the relationship; how the doctor managed the relationship; and how both doctor and patient also brought a transference relationship, the repetitive reenactment of certain unresolved conflicts with important real or fantasied figures in their own life. The doctor could judiciously choose interview topics in order to increase the patient's capacity to feel equal with the physician. An objective, yet sympathetic attitude with a warm, human interest was suggested. The doctor–patient relationship could be satisfactory without persuasion, flattery, or reassurance. The patient should feel that he or she is the center of the interview with ample time to tell his or her story.

Weisman and Thomas Hackett collaborated from 1956 on several studies[7–9] that led to Weisman's explication of the existential core of psychoanalysis,[10] the fuller description of denial in the face of cancer, and the principles that became the basis of his own approach to psychotherapy for cancer patients.

The Existential Core of Psychoanalysis

Weisman noted that we are inevitably immersed in our own existence.[10] In other words, each person has a "highly personal, private, idiosyncratic attitude" toward the dilemma of his or her own life and death.[11] (p. xv) Moreover, existential events are the basic unit of reality sense and organic memory.[10]

Responsibility

For an autonomous man, according to Weisman,[10] responsibility is that "quality of reality sense that allows [him or her] to choose, control, and consummate intended acts with a high level of self-esteem." (p. 174) The autonomous man has a "strong sense of reality for himself and for the world he helps to create . . . At the heart of responsibility is the capacity to respond and to bring about responses, and the ability to choose and to carry out one form of conduct instead of another." (p. 174) Responsibility is a response to a variety of directives and prohibitions connected to the cultural standards for what is expected of us.[11] Although psychoanalysis recognizes and studies unconscious forces, it does not advocate surrender to those forces. Responsibility remains.

Sickness

In Weisman's view,[10] sickness is the opposite pole of responsibility. The state of being sick has an impersonal dimension of disease, an interpersonal dimension of crisis, and an intrapersonal dimension of conflict. On the crisis dimension, the sick person's aim is to meet the challenge of a decisive moment. From the perspective of conflict, the patient wishes that his or her sense of autonomous responsibility be restored, so that the patient can once more achieve a measure of cause and control over what the patient does and what his or her ego ideal requires.

Conflict

From Weisman's perspective, the individual comes to terms with sickness and mortality through the same psychic mechanisms that govern other conflicts. Within the person who struggles with conflict is a "feeling of being hopelessly suspended between antithetical affects, paradoxical ideas, and incompatible alternatives"[10] (p. 207). Resolution exacts pain, fear, guilt, or some other emotional penalty.[10]

Although he acknowledged that we do not know how conflict is relieved and hopeful enthusiasm for living is restored, "neither relief from painful emotion nor resolution of conflict comes without prolonged antecedent oscillation between one form of polarized experience and another. Successfully or not, people try to solve problems of all kinds, as well as conflict, by trial-and-error performance of whatever alternative acts may be suggested by different polarities."[10] (p. 219) This understanding of the dynamic process by which humans resolve conflict was the basis for Weisman's later work on "middle knowledge" and on coping strategies.

Paradox

Psychiatrists are trained to recognize persons in conflict by paying attention to "laboring affect and inappropriate emotion" as clues to underlying meaning. The therapist may spontaneously express the taboo feeling or deliberately evoke antithetical affect in order to diagnose the conflict. Asking a patient about his feelings may modify those feelings and insisting that he feel any particular affect may suppress or bring about its antithesis, particularly when there is conflict. This technique may relieve symptoms, suppress another affect, or bring out a more appropriate but unacknowledged attitude to a specific event.[10]

The physician's impartial involvement sometimes relieves conflict because it is antithetical to what the distressed patient expects. The psychiatrist does not prod, praise, get angry, criticize, or rebuke; so the patient has the comfort to confront the latent side of a conflict or the intensity of the conflict decreases.[10]

Weisman focused on paradoxes or conflicts of meaning as a reliable way to detect nearby conflict.[10] Confrontation of incompatible ideas is a key feature of psychotherapy, a valuable and familiar psychotherapeutic technique in the office. Patients can at least recognize paradoxical ideas. When confronted with inconsistencies, they can at least make an effort to understand.[10] When the

apparent inconsistency is understood, a curious sense of validity develops.[11]

The *primary paradox* is that a dying man believes in the fact of his own death but hopes that he is an exception.[12]

Eros and Agape[10]

A person's ability to move beyond this paradox is related to his or her ability to tolerate anxiety about dissolution at the same time as he or she sustains an ego ideal and an authentic self. Sickness can deprive a person of the sense of autonomous responsibility and the sense that the person can strive toward his or her ego ideal. For Weisman, the opposite of annihilation anxiety is *Eros*, "that form of love that idealizes both the object loved and the process of loving, concordant with the ego ideal, responsive and responsible in the loftiest sense." (p. 233) *Eros* is a "process of seeking perfect love through the love of perfection." *Agape* is "the antithesis of hopeless abandonment and the antithesis of dread generated by primary anxiety. It is a love that reaches down to the bereft and undeserving regardless [of merit], . . acceptance of another person on existential terms."[10] (pp. 233–236) *Eros* and *agape*, both idealized versions of reality sense and responsibility, "attest to the meaning of belief itself and urge us to believe in limitless human potential and a world that cares rather than the opposite: unreality, anonymity, and meaningless existence (p. 234)."

"At the very least," Weisman said, "fear of imminent annihilation can prompt hopeful anticipation of a pervasive love that outlasts fears, withstands despair, forgives wrongdoing, and counters every other alienating force."[10] (p. 234) ". . . To believe that whatever happens has significance is the antithesis of meaningless existence[10] (p. 235)."

"If a person facing nothing but death can retain a sense of awe for the inner affinity of existence, and for his own significance, the inevitability of extinction can become a necessary harmonic among the antitheses of life" (p. 236), and hope is sustained.[10]

The existential core of psychoanalysis is whatever nucleus of *meaning* and *being there* can confront both life and death.[10] It requires a reality sense, responsibility, and meaning.

Psychological Autopsy

Hackett and Weisman[9] in 1961 noted that some patients believed that death offered a promise of resolution and relief. These patients looked to death with "yearning, acceptance, serenity, and a measure of impatience, without dejection and with only a minimum of denial." Concepts of neurosis, psychosis, and character disorders did not seem to describe the psyche of medical and surgical patients facing death. They set about studying man facing the human predicament.

To study dying patients, Weisman adapted a technique used retrospectively to evaluate suicide. In the Los Angeles County coroner's office, to clarify whether the case was a suicide or not, the staff of the Suicide Prevention Center did a psychological autopsy to examine the intentions, attitude, and ambivalence of the person who had died in an accident. Weisman[13] adapted this technique to assess the psychological events that preceded the death of a medical patient with the idea that the psychological autopsy would be a forum for the nonorganic factors in patients on or near the threshold of death. The major purpose was to develop a uniform method by which trained and compassionate observers could systematically assess patients. The core staff, including psychiatrists, psychologists, a social worker, and a nurse-clinician, spoke to the patient for days or weeks and reviewed the history and chart. Multidisciplinary assessments included interviews with primary staff and significant others, as well as psychological testing during the hospitalization. Bedside observations, clinical constructions, organic diagnoses, physical and physiologic principles, postmortem information, social network, personal behaviors, relationships, and socioeconomic status were recorded. This study of more than 100 patients was an effort to say to the resurrected person, "If we had met before death, how could I have been of any help?"

Psychotherapeutic Interview

Out of this work came a psychotherapeutic interview to assess the patient with cancer. Weisman[13] noted that the interview is an instrument of assessment that requires constant monitoring and adjustment. How the interviewer tolerates the threat of death, for instance, may affect the answers. to questions. The goal of the interview is existential contact acquired with tact but persistence, sitting down with eye contact to reduce disparity between the patient and interviewer. Questions asked of the cancer patient were:

1. How did you happen to see the doctor and come to the hospital at this time?
2. Who suggested that you come? How undecided were you?
3. In your opinion, what might have brought on this condition? What did you think when it first developed?
4. Right now, what bothers you most of all? How does this condition make a difference in the people you're closest to? What have you said to them if anything?
5. As a rule whom do you depend on most? like to be with? trust?
6. What do you usually do when you're feeling down? angry? afraid? What happens when you don't get your own way?
7. When someone you really cared about went away, say, in the past-for any reason-how did you feel? What could make you feel like that again now?
8. As you look back over the past few years, what are some things you really feel good about? What about the things that didn't turn out well, disappointed you, caused some heartache or regrets? Whose fault was it? If you had it to do over, what would you do differently?
9. What would you see yourself doing, say, a year from now? What could interfere, if anything?
10. Tell me at this very moment, what do you think about your entire situation?[13] (pp. 59–60)

From these questions, the interviewer could assess key elements: the personal past, present plight, anticipated future, regrets, salient concerns, problem areas, physical symptoms, disabilities, coping strategies, and psychosocial vulnerability. The Profile of Mood States (POMS)[14] and thematic apperception test (TAT)[15] were also sources of data[13] (p. 54).

Appropriate Death and Life

Weisman[13] used what he learned from the psychological autopsy to understand how the death might have been made more acceptable or appropriate. These objectives outlined the death we would choose if we had a choice, as well as a way of living as long as possible, and striving for the highest aspirations of mankind. He defined as feasible:

1. Adequate medical care, alleviation of pain and suffering, full use of technical resources, prolongation of life, but not prolongation of dying when recovery is wholly out of the question.
2. Informed consent or, even better, informed collaboration between doctor and patient.
3. Encouragement of conscious, competent control, helping the patient to use available, practical, and appropriate coping strategies.
4. Maintenance of behavior on as high a level as seems consistent with physical and psychological limitations.
5. Preservation and, if necessary, enhancement of self-esteem, which is an essential ingredient of a dignified death.
6. Support of the significant key others, a gesture that helps them to help the patient.
7. Gradual relinquishment of control to those who have shown themselves to be trustworthy and acceptance of counter-control.
8. Safe conduct in sustaining life until it ceases.
9. Honest communication, designed to support acceptance, reduce bitterness, and replace denial with courage to confront what cannot be changed[13] (pp. 188–189).

This description of "purposeful death" includes "a measure of fulfillment, quiescence, resolution, and even traces of personal development."[12] (p. 33) It serves as a guide to significant survival with a measure of competence and pride.[12]

Participatory Interview and Consultation

Given the primary paradox and "our uncertainty about how this world can be separated from our own sense of self"[12] (p. 14), Weisman took on the question of how ordinary people adapt to the personal reality of their own death. He and

Hackett interviewed 350 patients with cancer, myocardial infarction, and old age between 1962 and 1965. They adapted the psychotherapeutic consultation that had emphasized the patient as a unique and responsible individual to a participatory interview in which the personal dimensions of illness could be elicited.[7,8] The psychiatrist was an active participant who then formulated the salient problems as succinctly as possible and implemented recommendations during continued patient care. The psychiatrist encounters the patient at a moment of high vulnerability, a moment when relationships to the world are in critical transition. Weisman's style was impersonal as he asked factual information, but he became more humane and interpersonal as he asked about the patient's relationships.[12]

Denial and Middle Knowledge

Weisman did not see denial as an "independent, unambiguous, self-contained mental mechanism"[12] (p. xiv). He viewed it as an interpersonal rather than an intrapersonal phenomenon like repression. Denial, he noted, can bend reality to conform to an inner wish or fantasy in order to maintain a relationship. Even when organic meaning is negated by repression, "objective meaning survives till another time, on another occasion in relation to another person when there is a more favorable attitude toward an unwelcome reality."[10] (pp. 238–239)

Patients tend to deny their knowledge of fatal illness to different people at different times, perhaps in order to preserve a relationship.[13] Tactful discussion of mortality between a patient and caretakers allows them to be responsive to each other as long as possible.[12] Weisman noted "somewhere between open acknowledgment of death and its utter repudiation is an area of uncertain certainty called 'middle knowledge'"[12] (p. 65). It occurs particularly at serious transition points. This concept of middle knowledge captures the observation that patients often seemed to know and want to know about the gravity of illness, yet often talked as if they did not know and did not want to be reminded.[12] Patients may deny facts, inferences, or extinction.[12] However, "denial is almost impossible to maintain; inner perceptions force themselves on the most reluctant patient"[12] (p. 133). The balance between denial and acceptance changes during a fatal illness[12] (p. 112).

Hope

Hope, a sense of reality for future events, comes from a desirable self-image and a belief in the personal ability to exert a degree of influence on the world.[12] It further comes from self-acceptance and the conviction that a person may do something worth doing.[12] That sense of purpose adds value to life regardless of the time frame. "Hope has a way of outlasting the facts of illness."[12] (p. 133) Authentic hope and acceptance of death naturally accompany each other. Respect for the person who must die sustains authentic hope. "The will to live is an expression of hope coupled with a sense of effort"[12] (p. 27).

Coping and Vulnerability

Faced with the conflict between sickness and responsibility, cancer patients by trial and error seek a way forward. Coping is a complicated mixture of cognitive appraisal and reappraisal, "first responses and corrected responses over a long time continuum"[16] (pp. 264–267). Weisman[13] compiled a list of coping strategies, systematized responses to the question, "What did you do about it?" Patients tried to find more information, share their concern, laugh it off, forget or wait and see, distract themselves, confront or negotiate a plan based on present understanding, make virtue out of necessity, submit to the inevitable, act out, consider alternatives, drain off tension, avoid, blame, comply, or blame themselves.[17] (pp. 29–30) Since they were interested in the factors that got in the way of coping, they developed an Index of Vulnerability. Vulnerability had 13 dimensions: the worst points were described by hopelessness, perturbation, frustration, despondence, helplessness, anxiety, exhaustion, worthlessness and self-rebuke, no self-esteem, painful isolation/abandonment, denial/avoidance, truculence/resentment, repudiation of significant key others compared to mutuality, and closed time perspective.[17] Weisman later defined vulnerability as the disposition to

behave or to conduct oneself at less than full efficiency.[16]

Newly Diagnosed Cancer Patients

Weisman, with J. William Worden,[18] went on to study the ways in which newly diagnosed cancer patients (with Hodgkin's disease, or cancers of breast, colon, or lung) coped or failed to cope with different psychosocial problems at various stages of illness. With semistructured interviews and special inventories of coping strategies, vulnerability, and predominant concerns, they made serial prospective assessments, something that they could not have done using the retrospective view of the psychological autopsy. Patients were also given the Minnesota Multiphasic Personality Inventory (MMPI), TAT, and POMS. Over 4 to 6 weeks, each of the 163 patients had five evaluations followed by less frequent visits over 18 months.

The Existential Plight (First 100 Days) Versus Syndromes of Anxiety/Depression

In their study, Weisman and Worden[18] identified the existential plight, a previously unrecognized psychosocial phase that developed shortly after diagnosis and initial treatment of cancer. The peak of distress varied from a day or two to 2 to 3 months after diagnosis, but the intense distress abated over the first 100 days. "Cancer patients usually came to terms with the facts and circumstances of their illness"[18] (p. 11).

These patients, faced with a threat to life, differed from most psychiatric patients. Patients with the hopelessness of clinical depression were usually more hopeless than dying patients. Depressed patients saw no end to their suffering, whether or not they had cancer.[12]

Death and fear were not inseparable.[12] Panic attacks or fear of dying that came with the feeling of impending doom occurred throughout life and were not particularly more frequent in dying patients. They were associated with derealization, emptiness, and loneliness. Fear of death, Weisman thought, reflected man's helplessness and was associated with obsessive worry.

High Risk for Distress at Diagnosis[17]

Weisman and Worden[18] found that patients with high levels of emotional distress tended to use more submissive and suppressive tactics, whereas patients with low levels of emotional distress confronted problems directly, shared concerns, and (within realistic limits) did something about them. The group with high emotional distress was more pessimistic and regretful and had more marital problems and alcohol abuse. They were more apt to have a history of psychiatric treatment or suicidal ideation. On the MMPI, they had lower ego strength and more anxiety. Socioeconomic status was lower. They were less apt to go to church and more apt to have an advanced stage of cancer and more physical symptoms. They expected little support from family and saw the doctor as less helpful. They had more concerns of all types, poorer problem resolution, and were more apt to feel like giving up. Weisman and Worden[18] suggested that a screening instrument and a concise interview would be helpful to identify patients at high risk for social vulnerability and ineffective coping.

Psychotherapy for Vulnerable Cancer Patients at Diagnosis

Between 1977 and 1980 Weisman and Worden, along with Harry Sobel, went on to validate the Index of Vulnerability as a screening instrument for high emotional distress and to develop a psychosocial intervention.[19] The index included dimensions of hopelessness, turmoil, frustration, depression, powerlessness, anxiety, exhaustion, worthlessness, abandonment, denial, truculence (distrust of caregivers), repudiation of significant key others, and a closed time perspective.

The researchers had learned that high-risk patients were unable to generate a number of alternate coping strategies. These patients tended to overuse strategies that were ineffective for finding relief and resolution; therefore, Weisman, Worden, and Sobel[19] designed the psychosocial intervention to lower levels of distress, to correct deficits in coping, to reclaim personal control, and to improve morale and self-esteem.

Patients were approached by a social worker, who asked about current concerns (from an inventory of 36 concerns). They interviewed 381 patients with cancers of the breast, colon, or lung; melanoma; or Hodgkin's Disease. They found 125 (33%) were at high risk, and 59 of these were randomized to one of two interventions.

Newly diagnosed and distressed patients were encouraged to examine their plight in relation to cancer (their current concerns); to articulate their understanding of what might interfere with good coping; and, by looking beyond, to use options that were feasible in order to find satisfactory solutions. It was the staff's view that change was possible, and that patients could be helped to take steps on their own behalf as problems were revised into manageable proportions. The therapist functioned best "as an ally, guide, preceptor, or instructor, depending on the format of the intervention"[19] (p. 22). They focused on coping and adaptation rather than on psychopathology and conveyed an expectation of positive change, a sense that options and alternatives were seldom completely exhausted, a flexibility to change strategies and to see that the nature of perceived problems changed, and resourcefulness in seeking additional information and support. They used two different four-session interventions over 6 weeks and made assessments at 2, 4, 6, and 12 months.

Two Psychotherapy Interventions at Diagnosis. One intervention was similar to the model used in brief liaison consultations. The main focus was "How is this illness now affecting you and the people who are important in your life?" The therapist facilitated identification of problems, encouraged expression of affect associated with these problems, and explored with the patient various ways to solve problems. They emphasized clarification, cooling off, confrontation, and collaboration. Clarification included focusing on the problems, setting priorities, making clear what the patient was doing or not doing about a problem, and exploring strategies that might be more effective. They heard and sanctioned feelings, including those that had otherwise not been shared; and they encouraged confrontation and active strategies. Sometimes role-playing and rehearsal were used. The therapist's role as an ally and the suggestion of resources in the hospital or community modeled collaboration. The staff saw short-term consultation therapy as an opportunity to get at sources of preexisting conflict that were aggravated in the setting of cancer and an opportunity "to reinforce the reality of personal choice, control, or competence in the 'here and now' encounter."[19]

The second intervention was a short-term, structured, problem-oriented approach (i.e., a cognitive modality). Patients were taught how to recognize, confront, and solve commonly encountered cancer problems. They were taught a specific step-by-step approach to problem-solving that was practiced with the therapist. These general methods were applied to personal problems related to the cancer. To strengthen the coping process, patients were taught progressive body relaxation to relieve anxiety. A series of drawings facilitated problem-solving. A series of paired cards illustrating a cancer-relevant task and resolution was shown to the patient. The pictures facilitated the patient discussion of alternate solutions. The therapist could suggest possible alternatives or ask, "What do you think other people might do in a similar situation?" Handouts and homework reinforced relaxation and step-wise problem-solving. This intervention was more structured, and talking about personal concerns was discouraged; both interventions had similar objectives.

Those cancer patients who were screened, noted to be at high-risk for distress, and had either intervention, were noted to be less distressed at follow-up than the control group of high-risk patients. The intervention reduced feelings of frustration, depression, anxiety, apathy, truculence, and repudiation. While distress was reduced, denial was also reduced. Patients did not change their sense of hopelessness about the illness or their perspective of limited time. Those who refused the intervention had more denial of the diagnosis and its implications. Patients who were least helped were more depressed and pessimistic and tended to externalize their locus of control and to have higher vulnerability scores. The psychosocial interventions developed in this project put into play the principles that Weisman had defined to help patients face life-threatening illness. He and his colleagues succeeded in showing that a psychosocial intervention could prevent distress in newly diagnosed patients with cancer who were at high risk for distress. When Weisman wrote about how he helped patients, he purposely avoided writing a manual. He believed that "most practice is a mixture of improvisation, hypothesis, and deviation from . . . baseline procedures"[11] (p. 94). The goal of treatment was

collaboration with and comprehension of another.[11] Empathy, in this setting, was respect for another's irrationality and an authentic desire to see the world through another's eyes.[11]

Specifically, with the tasks of counter-coping, the strategic techniques of the caregiver were spelled out by Weisman:

1. Clarification and control
   Examine the problem forthrightly.
   Provide only reliable and accurate information.
   Redefine and reduce problems to manageable size.
   Consider feasibility and probable consequence of any action.
2. Collaboration
   Share concern without sharing distress.
   Refer certain problems to the respected judgment of another.
   Veto or prevent hasty, ill-considered actions.
   Suggest various directions and proposals that reflect your understanding.
3. Directed relief
   Encourage expression of pent-up feelings.
   Permit temporary avoidance, distraction, and respite.
   Look at familiar strategies that worked in the past.
   Allow yourself to express doubt, misgivings, or confusion.
4. Cooling off
   Modulate and mollify tendencies to emotional extremes.
   Encourage self-esteem and self-confidence.
   Emphasize rational, practical, prudent actions.
   At times be content to share silence and adopt a constructive resignation[11] (p. 93).

Weisman believed that patients come to psychotherapy when they are demoralized, and autonomy has failed.[11] Although psychotherapy can never cure, it can "mitigate misery and maybe help establish a stronger sense of morale," such that a patient can "take a place again . . . with confidence and competence, willing even to assume responsibility for being a part of the world"[11] (p. 98). For Weisman, "courage and morale are inseparable; each strengthens the other"[20] (p. xiv). Coping is a way of negotiating a series of obstacles, some of which are due to self-deception. The idealized goal in coping is to be at one's best. This is a "product of cultivating versatility, open-mindedness, skepticism and resiliency, and still being able to imagine whether being at one's best is really feasible"[11] (p. 138). At the same time, each of us must accept fallibility without condemning ourselves for not reaching perfection.[11]

Weisman[10,13,17,19] clarified the existential core of psychoanalysis, a method that explored motives, conflicts, and deceptions in the human psyche; he looked retrospectively via psychological autopsy at the ways patients confronted death, and then prospectively as patients tried to adapt to knowledge of newly diagnosed cancer. He further developed a strategy to facilitate meaning, morale, and the ability to negotiate with mortality.

More Recent Psychosocial Interventions

Weisman's study[19] move foreshadowed major studies of preventive psychosocial interventions for cancer patients. Fawzy et al.[21] described a 6-week structured group intervention for patients with melanoma (stage I and II); it included health education, stress management, coping skills, and supportive group psychotherapy. They were taught simple relaxation exercises: progressive muscle relaxation, guided imagery or self-hypnosis, as well as problem solving and coping methods. The interaction of the patients within the group provided a source of emotional support. The group that had the 6-week treatment had a survival benefit at 5 to 6 years, but this comparative benefit was not as evident in the tenth year.[22–24]

Spiegel[25–27] and others[28] more recently developed a supportive-expressive group therapy for women with metastatic breast cancer. In two randomized multisite studies, the benefit of this therapy for survival has not been found, but the ability of this intervention to reduce distress, to offer patients social support and safe conduct, and to increase their ability to confront difficult challenges has been documented.

Even more recently, Chochinov[29] focused on conserving dignity at the end of life by asking patients what they felt was most important and what they wanted their loved ones to remember. A life manuscript was returned to the patient and in many cases passed on to survivors. Informed by the work of Victor Frankl,[30] Greenstein and Breitbart[31] reported on a group intervention for patients with advanced cancer that focused on a sense of meaning. Meaning and faith, scored as subscales of a measure of spiritual well-being, were negatively correlated to depression, hopelessness, suicidal ideation, and a desire for hastened death.[32]

Combinations of interventions[33] augment patients' coping skills. Teaching about relaxation, one component of some combination regimens, was beneficial for cancer patients.[34,35] A variety of educational interventions that were tailored to disease type and phase, stress management, cognitive therapy, and behavioral training improved coping and decreased distress with treatment.[34]

Medical and Psychiatric Diagnosis

Hackett and Cassem, as they led the Psychiatric Consultation Service, reemphasized the medical model and the role of the psychiatric consultant as a physician. Their teaching was guided by clinical experience.[36] For Cassem,[36] "clinical work boiled down to diagnosis and treatment" (p. 35). Medical diagnosis has pragmatic value if it clarifies the course of illness and the benefits of treatment. The prompt diagnosis owed to cancer patients leads to a protocol of recommended medical treatment. By 1980, psychiatric diagnosis was further systematized in the *Diagnostic and Statistical Manual, Third Edition (DSM-III)*, and specific psychotropic medications became more widely used. A specific psychiatric diagnosis had implications for relief of suffering, for treatment, and for prognosis. The consulting psychiatrist integrated medical and psychiatric diagnosis, knowledge of the natural course of disease, and the complications of medical treatment, as well as a psychopharmacologic and psychological formulation.

Optimum Care Committee

Cassem's approach to the dying patient has been articulated in his words in Chapter 23. To assess hopelessly ill patients at the end of life, the MGH established the Optimum Care Committee in 1973 to advise the physicians of record about difficult cases.[37] Since its inception, Cassem has led this committee and operationalized the formal assessment of the patient. Most common reasons for consultation[38] by the Optimum Care Committee have been: (1) prior conflict within the family of an incompetent patient; (2) families who were asked for a do-not-resuscitate order when a clear medical plan was not offered; (3) physician hesitancy to proceed with futile treatment; (4) physician confusion about legal or ethical issues, and (5) concerns about stopping nutrition.

The assessment has included careful specialty evaluation of what is best care. "The criterion that determines every aspect of the therapeutic regimen is the overall welfare of the patient. . . . The therapeutic plan must be clearly detailed to the other members of the care team so that all understand and are united about their caring efforts and responsibilities."[37] The most knowledgeable consultant spelled out the medical realities and the uncertainties about benefit and prognosis. "Everyone, physicians and family alike, wants to know what the most knowledgeable physician thinks."[38] Furthermore, the therapeutic plan and the rationale are documented in the chart. The medical data are then explicit and juxtaposed to the wishes of the patient, the psychiatric assessment of the patient, and the dynamics of the family. This multidisciplinary assessment holds as an ideal the optimum standard of care. The patient may or may not choose to receive it.

By analogy, the psychiatric consultant's optimum assessment of the cancer patient throughout his or her course requires an understanding of the physical disease, treatment plan, treatment complications, and the uncertainty of prognosis. The modern day patient consents to treatment. The patient faces the crisis with the psychological advantages and limitations that Weisman outlined for the ordinary man who faces sickness. The patient copes with the crisis by getting medical help. The crisis dimension of sickness is interpersonal,[11] and depends on the relationship to the physician and medical system. The consulting psychiatrist should understand the technical aspect of the patient's medical predicament with a clearer judgment and with more training than the patient. Some decisions and behaviors are more urgent than others. Clarification of what needs to be decided rapidly and what does not is a service to the patient. In addition, the psychiatrist brings to the fore an understanding of intrapersonal conflict, the existential plight, and psychiatric diagnosis. Contributions of character

and neuropsychiatric consequences of treatment, for instance, sleep disorder with estrogen deficiency or fatigue with brain radiation, can also be clarified. Table 33-1 lists common concerns of patients with specific tumors.

Axes I, II, and III Diagnoses

The psychiatric consultant evaluates in particular anxiety, depression, and disturbances of cognition. The anxiety and distress associated with the existential plight describes the human normative, emotional adjustment to the news of a life-threatening illness like cancer. Those most vulnerable to distress are those with the most severe physical disease, the least social support, and the greatest predisposition to anxiety and depressive disorders.[39] In Weisman's terms, those vulnerable to Axis I diagnoses would be those who feel hopeless, despondent, helpless, anxious, and exhausted, as well as those who feel worthless and have low self-esteem and those with a perspective that time is short. Some who are vulnerable have a history of psychiatric treatment. Those with maladaptive coping skills, the truculent and resentful, who repudiate key others and who have the least amount of ego strength might be the same individuals who are diagnosed with a personality disorder (an Axis II disorder).

The patient is entitled to an accurate diagnosis of serious and treatable psychiatric syndromes. Among cancer patients, these conditions occur more often in those with a lifetime history of anxiety or mood disorders that predate cancer.[40,41] The challenge is to recognize the platonic ideal of the syndrome amidst the existential plight and the somatic complications of cancer.

Anxiety Syndromes. Claustrophobia becomes clinically important when a magnetic resonance imaging (MRI) scan is required for careful physical evaluation or when a patient is trapped in bed by orthopedic repair of a leg with osteogenic sarcoma. Needle phobia can be treated with rapid desensitization.[42]

The roller coaster of life-threatening experiences and uncertainty in cancer treatment parallels the unpredictable aversive stimuli that provoke conditioned helplessness and depression.[43] Patients with ovarian cancer anticipate the report of the CA125,

Table 33-1. Concerns of Patients with Specific Tumors

Prostate Cancer
Significance of serum prostate specific antigen (PSA) test results: anxiety
Once diagnosed, the initial choices of watchful waiting, surgery, or radiation treatment
Side effects of surgery or radiation: incontinence or erectile dysfunction
Sexual function and dysfunction
Androgen blockade and its effects on fatigue and loss of sexual interest

Breast Cancer
Body image related to mastectomy and/or to reconstruction
Adjuvant chemotherapy and its side effects: alopecia, weight gain, fatigue, and impaired concentration
Menopausal symptoms: insomnia, sexual dysfunction, and hot flashes related to adjuvant treatment, antiestrogens or
    aromatase inhibitors
The question of prophylactic mastectomy
Sexuality and fertility (or infertility)

Colon Cancer
Adjustment to surgery and/or an ostomy
Body image and sexual function
Bowel dysfunction

Lung Cancer
Physical limitations of reduced lung capacity
Post-thoracotomy neuralgia
Cough
Guilt about nicotine addiction, past and present

Ovarian Cancer
Anxiety about the tumor marker CA125
Sexual dysfunction and infertility
Pain and recurrent bowel obstruction

Pancreatic Cancer
Maintenance of adequate nutrition
Poor appetite
Bowel function (and the need for pancreatic enzymes and laxatives)
Pain
Diabetes
Depressed mood

Head and Neck Cancer
Facial deformity
Dry mouth
Poor nutrition
A weak voice and difficulty with communication
Post-treatment hypothyroidism
Alcohol and nicotine dependency

Lymphoma
Corticosteroid-induced mood changes
The need for recurrent chemotherapy and its effects

Hodgkin's Disease
Post-treatment hypothyroidism
Fatigue

Osteosarcoma
Amputation/prosthesis vs. bone graft
Impaired mobility
Post-thoracotomy neuralgia

and their mood rises and falls with the results of the tumor marker and reports of progressive disease.[44] Most patients are alert to physical symptoms after treatment, and they worry that those symptoms signify recurrent disease. A visit to the doctor is reassuring for most, but some people are unreassurable and are preoccupied with fear. Every symptom signifies a cancer recurrence. Over the course of cancer treatment, chronic recurrent anxiety may be indistinguishable from clinical depression. Since both syndromes improve with use of antidepressants, antidepressant medications are preferable to the long-term use of benzodiazepines.

When patients vomit as part of treatment, they can develop conditioned anxiety to the smells and sights associated with treatment and then anticipatory anxiety with insomnia, nausea, and aversion to treatment. Hypnosis, cognitive-behavioral therapy (CBT), and use of antianxiety agents, like alprazolam or lorazepam, can reduce the phobic response and the anticipatory nausea and vomiting that occurs during and after chemotherapy.[45]

If patients receive the best antiemetic drugs with treatment, the chances of developing conditioned associations are reduced; however, patients may still vomit after doxorubicin, cisplatin, or carboplatin, even with a 5-hydroxytryptamine-3 receptor antagonist and dexamethasone.[46] Some patients still develop anticipatory anxiety for treatment, and they avoid the hospital or its smells long afterward. Those who have developed conditioned responses tend to be younger, to have had more emetic treatments, and to have trait anxiety.[47]

Cancer treatment can be traumatic. Pitman et al.[48] have shown that women with breast cancer have a physiologic response to the personal narrative of the two most stressful experiences in their cancer story 2 years after the onset of cancer. Leukemia survivors who developed anticipatory nausea with treatment are more apt to become nauseated at reminders of treatment years later.[49] Numbness and tingling of peripheral neuropathy can be a physical reminder of treatment and trigger the intrusive thoughts and avoidant behaviors of post-traumatic stress disorder (PTSD).[50] The symptoms of PTSD are often associated with comorbid depression.[48] Antidepressants are useful in the setting of hypochondriasis and chronic anxiety.

Panic disorder and other anxiety disorders occur among cancer patients at about the same rate as are seen in the general population[51]; however, in patients with cancer, a pulmonary embolism should always be in the differential diagnosis of a panic attack.

Major Depressive Disorder. Major depressive disorder (MDD) in a patient with cancer is more common when a history of depressive disorder is present.[40] Overall, MDD in a patient with cancer is at least as common as is depression in those with other medical illness.[52] However, patients have difficulty distinguishing between the existential plight associated with a cancer diagnosis and its treatment, and a depressive disorder that might benefit from use of medication. Patients take pride in their responsibility to cope. They are loathe to tell their oncologists that they are depressed lest their physicians think less of them, and oncologists tend to note anxiety and crying but often do not learn about the suicidal thoughts of their patients.[53]

Case 1

Ms. A, a 42-year-old woman with a small breast tumor that was diagnosed on her first screening mammogram, talked during her first visit about her can-do perspective and the conflicts and challenges she faced as a working mother. It was not until the second visit that she acknowledged her symptoms of persistent sadness, a feeling that her absence made no difference to her 6-year-old son, and the comments from her college friends about how depressed she seemed. Persistent morbid thoughts, morning anxiety, panic attacks, and suicidal thoughts are clues to the syndrome, which is treatable with antidepressant medication.

A variety of screening tests for depression have been advocated to improve case-finding and to begin the conversation about feelings in the oncology setting.[54] The National Comprehensive Cancer Network guidelines describe a method of asking about distress, assessing concerns, and initiating consultations with social workers, psychologists, psychiatrists, and pastoral counselors. They illustrate how a member of one discipline, like a pastor, can call upon a psychiatrist if a depressive symptom, like inordinate guilt, raises the specter of mood disorder; or a psychiatrist may suggest consultation with a member of the clergy for concerns about reconciliation with tradition.[55]

FATIGUE. Fatigue is a symptom of major depressive disorder, often characterized by dread of getting out of bed to face the day, trouble getting going, broken sleep, a sense that everything is effortful, rejection sensitivity, and phobic inhibition. By comparison, chemotherapy causes a loss of stamina that is worse mid-chemotherapy cycle when blood counts are low. A cumulative loss of stamina develops with repeated cycles of treatment. Recovery takes many months. Localized radiation treatment for breast cancer and prostate cancer cause a gradual increase in fatigue beginning at about 17 fractions (3.5 weeks).[56,57] It is associated with a tendency to sleep for more hours. Radiation treatments that involve more volume, particularly to viscera, cause more fatigue.

In addition to the use of effective treatments for depression and anxiety, strategies to reduce fatigue are crucial; these include reduction of sedative medications, improvement in physical conditioning, adjustment of antihypertensive medications, and treatment of anemia and hypothyroidism. From the perspective of psychotherapy, patients are often advised in the tradition of Janet to manage their energy budget[58]: to set priorities, delegate, consider what brings pleasure, and to allow caregivers flexibility.[59] Smart use of energy is related to the give and take of good collaboration. Stimulants may be used strategically to increase alertness.

Patients with breast cancer often develop insomnia, dysphoria, and nighttime hot flashes that are associated with menopause. Adjuvant chemotherapy suppresses ovarian function, and antiestrogen treatment is a mainstay of antitumor treatment for estrogen receptor–positive breast cancers. Mood symptoms are noted in 15% of those taking tamoxifen or an aromatase inhibitor like anastrazole.[60] The contribution of the menopausal syndrome can be clarified.[61] Of note, antidepressants, like venlafaxine and paroxetine, have been shown to reduce hot flashes associated with tamoxifen and may improve mood in a timely fashion.[62,63] Androgen blockade in men with prostate cancer also causes hot flashes that may improve with antidepressant medications.

DRUGS LINKED TO DEPRESSION. The anticancer agents most likely to cause clinical depression are interferon and corticosteroids. Interferon treatment causes depression, insomnia, anxiety, cognitive impairment, and, more rarely, hypomania.[64]

Paroxetine given 1 month in advance has reduced the incidence of depression during the first month of high-dose treatment of advanced melanoma, thus showing in a controlled trial that serotonin reuptake-inhibitors can treat the interferon-related depression.[65] Interferon itself can suppress some of the P-450 enzymes that metabolize antidepressants. The associated autoimmune thyroiditis[66] that can cause hypothyroidism may complicate treatment; therefore, thyroid function should be monitored.

Corticosteroids are used in a one-time 10 mg dexamethasone dose to prevent vomiting associated with chemotherapy, 5 days of 100 mg prednisone for lymphoma treatment, or 4 mg of dexamethasone every 6 hours to suppress brain swelling with radiation. Patients may become agitated and hypomanic with use of steroids and then become depressed when taken off of treatment. The gravity of the response is generally dose-related, but the psychiatric effects of each cycle of treatment can vary. Neuroleptics and mood stabilizers are useful for treatment of steroid-induced side effects.

Procarbazine, asparaginase, vincristine, and vinblastine are also anticancer agents that have been less often associated with depression. (Table 33-2)

TREATMENT. Treatment of MDD in cancer patients should involve the best psychopharmacologic and psychotherapy strategies available. The first-line medications have the fewest side effects and may facilitate sleep or reduce pain or hot flashes.[67]

Cognitive Impairment. Some chemotherapy drugs can cause confusional states during treatment and leukoencephalopathy later.[68] In most cancer protocols, the doses and timing have been adjusted to minimize these adverse effects. However, sometimes patients with vulnerable brains or delayed metabolism of drugs (e.g., methotrexate, carmustine, cisplatin, levamisole, fludarabine, thiotepa, ifosfamide, cytarabine, and fluorouracil) may be prone to confusion. Immunosuppressive drugs (e.g., cyclosporine, tacrolimus, or the antifungal drug amphotericin B) have also been implicated (Table 33-2).

Patients who receive adjuvant chemotherapy for breast cancer often complain about troubles with working memory and concentration ability.[69] Although they refer to "chemo brain," the subjective complaints often do not match neuropsychiatric

Table 33-2. Neuropsychiatric Side Effects of Cancer Drugs[87]

Drug	Side Effect
HORMONES	
Antiestrogens	
Tamoxifen, toremifene	Hot flashes, insomnia, and mood disturbance
Anastrozole, letrozole, vorozole, exemestane	Hot flashes, fatigue, and mood disturbance
Leuprolide, goserelin	Hot flashes, fatigue, and mood disturbance
Androgen blockade	
Leuprolide	Hot flashes, fatigue, and mood disturbance
Flutamide, bicalutamide, nilutamide	Hot flashes, fatigue, and mood disturbance
Glucocorticoids	Dose-related, variable psychiatric side effects (including insomnia, hyperactivity, hyperphagia, depression, hypomania, irritability, and psychosis); often easily treated by antipsychotics; lithium, valproate, lamotrigine, or mifepristone also used
BIOLOGICS	
Interferon-alpha	Depression, cognitive impairment, hypomania, psychosis, fatigue, and malaise
	Mood responsive to antidepressants, hypnotics, antipsychotics, stimulants, and antianxiety agents
	Associated with autoimmune thyroiditis, check thyroid function
	May inhibit metabolism of some antidepressants by P-450 isoenzymes
	Interferon-beta has less neurotoxicity
Interleukin-2	Delirium, flu-like syndrome, dose-dependent neurotoxicity, and hypothyroidism
CHEMOTHERAPY	
Vincristine, vinblastine, vinorelbine	Seizures, hyponatremia, depression, fatigue, rarely autonomic neuropathy, and postural hypotension with vincristine; less common with vinblastine and vinorelbine
Procarbazine	Mild reversible delirium or depression
	Weak MAOI
	Antidepressant use must consider timing of procarbazine or risk serious interaction
	Disulfiram-like effect; avoid alcohol
Asparaginase	Depression, lethargy, and delirium
Cytarabine	Somnolence and rarely, delirium 2–5 days into treatment, cerebellar syndrome, and rare leukoencephalopathy
Fludarabine	Rare somnolence, delirium, and rare progressive leukoencephalopathy
5-Fluorouracil (5-FU)	Fatigue, rare seizure or confusion
	Cerebellar syndrome
	Rare deficiency of enzyme that metabolizes drug-dihydropyrimidine dehydrogenase (DPD)
Capecitabine	Less neurotoxicity than 5-FU
Methotrexate	Dose- and route-related risk of delirium,
	Rare progressive leukoencephalopathy after intrathecal treatment
	Worse neurotoxicity when combined with radiation
	Folinic acid rescue, alkalinization if high serum level suspected

Continued

Table 33-2. Neuropsychiatric Side Effects of Cancer Drugs[87]—cont'd

Drug	Side Effect
Gemcitabine	Fatigue, flu-like syndrome, and rare autonomic neuropathy
Etoposide	Postural hypotension and rare disorientation
Thalidomide	Drowsiness and somnolence (which improves over 2–3 weeks)
Carmustine	Delirium (only at high dose), and rare leukoencephalopathy
Thiotepa	Rare leukoencephalopathy
Ifosfamide	Transient delirium, lethargy, seizures, and drunkenness Cerebellar signs (which improves within days of treatment) Hyponatremia Leukoencephalopathy
Cisplatin	Rare reversible posterior leukoencephalopathy; parietal, occipital, and frontal changes with cortical blindness Peripheral neuropathy, poor proprioception, rarely autonomic signs Hypomagnesemia (secondary to renal wasting) Vitamin E 300 mg and amifostine may limit peripheral toxicity Hearing decreased due to sensorineural hearing loss
Carboplatin	Neurotoxicity (only at high doses)
Oxaliplatin	Acute dysesthesias of hands, feet, perioral region, jaw tightness, and pharyngo/laryngo-dysesthesias
Paclitaxel	Sensory peripheral neuropathy (not worse with continued treatment) Rarely seizures and transient encephalopathy, and motor neuropathy Given with steroids
Docetaxel	Signs and symptoms like paclitaxel, but less neurotoxic
IMMUNOSUPPRESSIVES	
Cyclosporine and tacrolimus	Delirium (dose-related); leukoencephalopathy Tremor and headache Serum level available
ANTIINFECTIVES	
Amphotericin B	Delirium and leukoencephalopathy

deficits. At the very least, the combination of fatigue, catabolic effects of treatment, and hormonal change are associated with a sense of impairment that seems to improve gradually.

Radiation treatment to the whole brain can cause leukoencephalopathy or radiation necrosis.[70] Neurobehavioral effects of leukoencephalopathy occur in up to one fourth acutely, and the sequelae are a consideration in cancer survivors. The latest techniques for treatment of metastases target specific areas in an effort to reduce the necessity of whole-brain radiation, but whole-brain radiation is used prophylactically in small cell lung cancer and commonly in non–small cell lung cancer. In survivors of tumors that required radiation over the neck or pituitary gland, hypothyroidism may cause cognitive impairment or depressive symptoms later. Oxygen treatment at night or all day may improve the cognition of lung cancer survivors who are chronically hypoxic.

Cancer itself causes cognitive impairment in patients with primary brain tumors or brain metastases. Metastatic brain tumors are common complications of breast cancer, lung cancer, and melanoma. They also occur less commonly in sarcoma as well as renal, colorectal, thyroid, pancreatic, ovarian, uterine, prostate, testicular, and bladder cancers. In patients with small cell lung cancer, brain metastases are anticipated and whole-brain radiation is prescribed prophylactically.[71] Isolated brain metastases from non–small cell lung cancer may be treated surgically, and modern radiation techniques target small areas of the brain. Carcinomatous meningitis or leptomeningeal disease is a consideration when brain images do not show metastases, but cranial nerve signs, headache, ataxia, or seizures are present. This can occur with non-Hodgkin's lymphoma, leukemia, melanoma, or adenocarcinoma of the lung, breast, or gastrointestinal system.

Hypercalcemia in patients with lung cancer or bone metastases can cause cognitive impairment or delirium, as can the hyperviscosity syndrome in myeloma or lymphoma patients, and hyponatremia in patients with the cancer-related syndrome of inappropriate antidiuretic hormone (SIADH) secretion. Hypercalcemia can be treated with diphosphonates, hydration, and diuresis, while hyponatremia responds to fluid restriction. Hyperviscosity syndrome results from paraproteins that impair blood circulation in the brain. A serum viscosity level above 4.0 centipoise (1.56 to 1.68 cp) has been associated with symptoms.[72,73] The clinical signs are bleeding, visual signs and symptoms, and delirium. Cushing's syndrome with delirium and psychosis may be a presenting syndrome of adrenocortical carcinoma or lung cancer with the paraneoplastic production of adrenocorticotropic hormone (ACTH).

Autoimmune paraneoplastic encephalopathy is a rare complication associated with antineuronal antibodies.[74] Limbic encephalopathy is a specific autoimmune encephalopathy that presents with memory difficulties, anxiety, depression, and seizures. These paraneoplastic syndromes are most likely in the context of small cell carcinoma of the lung, but they also occur with non–small cell lung cancer; Hodgkin's disease; and breast, ovarian, stomach, uterine, renal, testicular, thyroid, and colon cancers.[75]

Opiates and benzodiazepines are the most common medications associated with acute cognitive impairment in the setting of cancer treatment. Patients with structural brain disease, vascular problems, and kidney or liver impairment, as well as the elderly, are more prone to delirium.

Patients with primary brain tumors, particularly low-grade tumors, present the problems of both cancer diagnosis and chronic brain injury.

Case 2

> Mr. B., a 40-year-old obsessive engineer with a history of temporal lobe epilepsy in college learned after several years that his seizures may be due to mesial fibrosis. When a biopsy was ultimately recommended, the diagnosis was a low-grade astrocytoma in the hippocampus. In addition to worry about tumor progression, he had to cope with frustration at delayed and inadequate diagnosis, current memory deficits, and grief over his loss of function.

A lesion in the limbic system affects the hardwiring of motivation, attention, emotion, and memory. As Murray described in Chapter 3, the hippocampus has an important role in memory and a role in a person knowing his or her place in the world. Temporal lobe epilepsy can be associated with psychological symptoms, such as memory dysfunction, anxiety, hypergraphia, and interpersonal viscosity. For such an afflicted patient, neuropsychiatric consultation and testing may be critically important to define the specific loss. Once the neurologic basis of specific difficulties has been clarified, cognitive rehabilitation can facilitate compensatory strategies. Multimodal interventions for attention, memory, word retrieval, and problem-solving may be appropriate.[76] Loved ones can understand more clearly the basis of necessary limitations, and the patient can acknowledge his deficits and make required adjustments. Psychotropic medications can serve as adjuncts to anticonvulsants and anticancer treatment.

Children and Cancer

For many years all children hospitalized with cancer at MGH have been seen by a child psychiatrist. The most common diagnoses are leukemia, lymphoma, brain tumors, osteogenic sarcoma, Ewing's sarcoma, and Wilms' tumor. Fortunately, childhood cancers are now more commonly considered a serious chronic illness than a uniformly terminal illness. A child psychiatrist works side-by-side in the outpatient setting with the pediatric hematology-oncology team to treat the emotional needs of the child in age-appropriate ways during active treatment and thereafter. With consideration of the child's stage of development, the psychiatrist can judge what the child will understand and what the child will want and need to know.

Common domains for consultation with children with cancer include anticipatory anxiety, sleep disturbances, behavioral problems, and mood changes. Despite advances in antiemetic medication, anticipatory anxiety still affects many children. Children may feel nauseated or vomit upon approaching the hospital, clinic, or phlebotomist. Behavioral modification, visualization and relaxation techniques, and medication help to diminish apprehension. Sleep disturbances may be related to a child's worries about the illness or to medications like steroids. Child psychiatry is also consulted for behavior problems in younger children who become more aggressive or difficult to manage. The emphasis in treatment of depression or withdrawal is placed on the child's ability to experience joy. Overall, children tend to be resilient. Although children and their parents are very distressed at the time of diagnosis, the prevalence of psychological problems among survivors of childhood cancer is similar to that in the community.[77]

Genetic Testing

Genetic testing for cancer susceptibility has become a clinical service in many cancer centers and hospitals. Testing for genes associated with breast, ovarian, and colon cancer is available in clinical practice and in research protocols for these and other cancers. People who present for genetic testing usually have a family history of cancer or have cancer themselves. Such testing is done to help them make medical decisions for their own care or to facilitate decision-making for family members. Although many people who present for genetic testing are distressed, so far it does not appear that positive results for cancer susceptibility increase suicidal thoughts or actions to the degree seen with screening for Huntington's disease. Not surprisingly, pretest anxiety and depression decrease in individuals who test negative for cancer and persist or increase in individuals who test positive. Psychological distress may also be unrelated to the testing experience, but related to concurrent life stressors or to preexisting psychopathology like character disorders or paranoid delusions. Common themes of testing-related distress include grief, either over self-loss or family; complex decision-making and risk analysis; adherence to medical treatment; management of anxiety and depression; and, if tests are negative, survival guilt. Genetic information once revealed can reverberate in the family constellation with the personal and interpersonal issues that already exist. The psychiatrist's role is to help the patient to understand and live with the concept of risk as well as to understand the emotional consequences for others in the family.[78,79]

Parenting and Cancer

One of the most deeply felt concerns of parents with cancer is how their illness will affect their children. The National Cancer Institute estimates that one fourth of adults with cancer have children under the age of 18 years living at home with them,[80] and up to one third of women with breast cancer are parents.[81] Studies of grieving children note their vulnerability during the terminal phases of a parent's illness,[82] as well as the longitudinal process of coping with the death of a parent.[83] In 1997 Paula Rauch[84] developed a program of consultation for parents with cancer; its goal was to help them to communicate with their children and to plan for care of the children during the illness. Bringing to parents the expert knowledge of a child psychiatrist, she asked about the ages, sensitivities, and psychiatric history of their children, so that advice could be tailored to the individual needs and developmental capacity of each child. She and Anna Muriel reviewed the impact that illness had on these children and the benefits of helping parents to communicate effectively.[85]

For patients who are parents, their role as parents may be central to their identity. Consultation that does not take parenting into consideration misses a critical part of their life. Adult psychiatrists can enhance their confidence about their ability to address parenting issues by reviewing and keeping in mind developmental principles in order to know how children at different ages understand illness and death. Guiding principles include maximizing childrens' support systems, maintaining their routines, facilitating parent-child communication about the illness, and preserving quality family time and connection with the ill parent.[84]

Summary

Cobb and Shands wrote about the contribution of the psychiatrist to care of the cancer patient when the psychiatrist made a relationship that was steadfast even as the patient deteriorated. The psychiatrist brought to the patient an expert ability to understand who the patient is, fantasies, transference, hopes, and fears. Weisman[10,12] described the patient's oscillation between denial and acknowledgment of mortality, the use of paradox to understand and to relieve the patient's conflicts, and the psychic mechanisms that facilitate hope and morale in the setting of progressive disease.

In the first encounters, the psychiatrist hears the patient's concerns as well as the patient's story and existential predicament. As the psychiatrist sits with the patient in the here and now, the psychiatrist tries to understand the patient in front of him or her, who the patient was before the diagnosis, and the nature of the patient's existential predicament. In the participatory interview, the physician conveys respect as he or she explores the patient's capacity to cope. The patient regains a sense of responsibility and control as he or she appraises and reappraises what choices to make. Trust between the physician and patient requires mutual respect; hope and trust are sturdy enough to withstand truth.[20] Weisman[20] found that resiliency and courage are there to be developed and that confidence in the patient transmits respect. He believed that suffering was intensified by a lack of meaning, and that meaning is an antidote to annihilation anxiety. The patient's hope is not directly related to the facts of illness. It is related to the patient's desirable self-image, to an ego ideal, and the conviction that he or she can have an influence on the world. As the patient copes, he or she may strive to be his or her optimal self, but the patient is forced to accommodate as well to his or her failings, losses, and need for help. If the patient trusts the psychiatrist, failings and losses will be revealed. The psychiatrist's capacity to hear out the patient in a nonjudgmental way without condescension allows the patient to express doubts and weaknesses, to accept who he or she is and why the patient sees things as he or she does. The physician's "being there" is testimony that the patient is not abandoned.

When Cassem et al. (Chapter 23) explore a patient's spiritual history for an agnostic in relation to meaning, or for a believer in relation to God, they are exploring the patient's personal understanding of what matters and what can be forgiven. The taking of the spiritual history allows the patient to glimpse forgiveness and healing (agape). The very nature of the interaction between the therapist and the patient in both settings facilitates the patient's acceptance of who he or she is and what the patient has to say—the authentic self. The patient tolerates the lapse from an ego ideal with the possibility that he or she is neither judged nor abandoned.

The consulting psychiatrist also brings to the patient medical understanding of cancer. The psychiatrist ought to understand the medical imperative and the medical choices that apply to the individual case better than the patient. The diagnosis, treatment, and prognostic decisions are complex as set forth by medical experts,[86] but the psychiatrist hears them as a colleague. When the patient's judgment is clouded by anxiety, shock, and denial, good coping mandates collaboration with experts who can clarify the priorities. As the psychiatrist gets to know the patient's idiosyncratic thinking and adds appropriate psychopharmacologic treatment, the psychiatrist has to maintain a focus on the priority of the anticancer treatment necessary to keep the patient alive. Which choices clearly jeopardize life? Decisions about initial cancer treatment in breast cancer and prostate cancer, in particular, are complex. The challenge is to provide clarification. To Weisman, clarification meant focusing on problems, setting priorities, making clear what the patient is doing and not doing about a problem, and exploring strategies. This technique allows patients to make the decisions most critical and most important to them. Meanwhile, the consulting psychiatrist, in collaboration with the oncology staff, sorts through the differential diagnoses as new psychological symptoms develop and as the medical condition and treatment progress.

Now in the twenty-first century, the tools to diagnose and to treat breast cancer have improved, but some 41-year-old women still die of progressive disease. The young woman treated by Shands in 1952 should still have the relationship with an expert listener, now skilled at consideration of the existential plight and facilitation of coping strategies, but she may also receive the diagnosis of recurrent MDD and antidepressant treatment.

The hormonal influence on emotions noted by Cobb in 1952 can be clarified, so that she understands the source of sudden menopausal symptoms postoophorectomy and the irritability associated with testosterone treatment. She and her husband would have the opportunity to consider her role as a parent to her toddler daughter. The genetic contribution to her early breast cancer and its relevance to her daughter might also be clarified.

For the many patients who tackle oncology treatments and survive, the path to optimal treatment and optimal negotiation with mortality can be charted by the goals that Weisman defined as appropriate: the treatment we would choose if we had a choice. These include the opportunity for excellent medical care and alleviation of pain and suffering with full use of technical resources available, including those of modern psychiatry. As an informed, consenting collaborator with the doctor, the patient is encouraged to use feasible and practical coping strategies that offer the possibility for as high a level of behavior as is consistent with his physical and psychosocial limitations. This strategy allows for further enhancement of self-esteem. The work includes an education about how to support significant key others and how to allow help or relinquish control to those who have shown themselves trustworthy. The goal of honest communication is to support acceptance, to reduce bitterness, and to replace denial with the courage to confront what cannot be changed.

References

1. Shands HC: *The emotional significance of cancer.* In Staff of Psychiatric Service, MGH, editors. Miles HHW, Cobb S, Shands HC. *Case histories of psychosomatic medicine*, New York, 1952, WW Norton, 236–248.
2. Shands H, Finesinger JE, Cobb S, et al: Psychological mechanisms in patients with cancer, *Cancer* 4: 1159–1170, 1951.
3. Abrams RD, Finesinger JE: Guilt reactions in patients with cancer, *Cancer*, 6:474–482, 1953.
4. Abrams RD: *Not alone with cancer*, Springfield, Ill., 1974, Charles C Thomas.
5. Cobb S: *Some principles and applications of psychosomatic medicine.* Staff of Psychiatric Service, MGH, editors. Miles HHW, Cobb S, Shands HC. *Case histories of psychosomatic medicine,* New York, 1952, WW Norton, 3–21.
6. Weisman AD: The doctor-patient relationship: its role in therapy, *Am Pract Digest Treatment* 1:1144, 1950.
7. Reprinted in Staff of Psychiatric Service, MGH, editors. Miles HHW, Cobb S, Shands HC: *Case histories of psychosomatic medicine*, New York, 1952, WW Norton, 22–40.
8. Hackett T, Weisman AD: Psychiatric management of operative syndromes: I. the therapeutic consultation and the effect of noninterpretive intervention, *Psychosom Med* 122:267–282, 1960.
9. Hackett TP, Weisman AD: Psychiatric management of operative syndromes: II. psychodynamic factors in formulation and management, *Psychosom Med* 22:356–372, 1960.
10. Weisman AD, Hackett TP: Predilection to death, *Psychosom Med* 23:232–255, 1961.
11. Weisman AD: *The existential core of psychoanalysis: reality sense and responsibility*, Boston, 1965, Little, Brown & Company.
12. Weisman AD: *The coping capacity. on the nature of being mortal*, New York, 1984, Human Sciences Press.
13. Weisman AD: *On denying and dying*, New York, 1972, NY Behavioral Publications.
14. Weisman AD: *The realization of death: a guide for the psychological autopsy.* New York, 1974, Jason Aronson.
15. McNair D, Lorr M, Dropplemann L: *Manual for profile of mood states*, San Diego, 1971, Educational and Industrial Testing Service.
16. Murray HA and the staff of the Harvard psychological clinic: *Thematic apperception test manual*, Cambridge, Mass., 1943, Harvard University Press.
17. Weisman AD: *Coping with illness.* In Hackett T, Cassem NH, editors: *Massachusetts General Hospital handbook of general hospital psychiatry*, St. Louis, 1978, Mosby, 264–275.
18. *Coping and vulnerability in cancer patients report of results.* National Cancer Institute Grant # R18-CA-14104, Project Omega, 1976
19. Weisman AD, Worden JW: The existential plight in cancer: significance of the first 100 days, *Int J Psychiatry Med* 7:1–15, 1976.
20. Weisman AD, Worden JW, Sobel HJ: *Psychosocial screening and intervention with cancer patients*, Project Omega. NCI grant 19797 (1977–1980) 1980.
21. Weisman AD: *The vulnerable self: conquering the ultimate questions*, New York, 1993, Plenum Press.
22. Fawzy FI, Cousins N, Fawzy N, et al: A structured psychiatric intervention for cancer patients: I. changes over time in methods of coping and affective disturbance, *Arch Gen Psychiatry* 47:720–725, 1990.
23. Fawzy FI, Fawzy NW, Hyun CS, et al: Malignant melanoma: effects of an early structured psychiatric intervention, coping, and affective state on recurrence and survival six years later, *Arch Gen Psychiatry* 50:681–689, 1993.
24. Fawzy FI, Kemeny ME, Fawzy N, et al: A structured psychiatric intervention for cancer patients: II. changes over time in immunological measures, *Arch Gen Psychiatry* 47:729–735, 1990.

24. Fawzy FI, Canada AL, Fawzy NW: Effects of a brief, structured psychiatric intervention on survival and recurrence at 10-year follow-up, *Arch Gen Psychiatry* 60:100–103, 2003.

25. Kogon MM, Biswas A, Pearl D, et al: Effects of medical and psychotherapeutic treatment on the survival of women with metastatic breast carcinoma, *Cancer* 28:225–230, 1997.

26. Spiegel D: Mind matters: group therapy and survival in breast cancer, *N Engl J Med* 345:1767–1768, 2001.

27. Classen PJ, Butler LD, Koopman C, et al: Supportive-expressive group therapy and distress in patients with metastatic breast cancer: a randomized clinical intervention trial, *Arch Gen Psychiatry* 58:494–501, 2001.

28. Goodwin PJ, Leszcz M, Ennis M, et al: The effect of group psychosocial support on survival in metastatic breast cancer, *N Engl J Med* 345:1719–1726, 2001.

29. Chochinov HM: Dignity-conserving care: a new model for palliative care—helping the patient feel valued, *JAMA* 287:2253–2260, 2002.

30. Frankl V: *The doctor and the soul: an introduction to logotherapy*, New York, 1957, Alfred A. Knopf (Translated by R Winston, C Winston).

31. Greenstein M, Breitbart W: Cancer and the experience of meaning: a group psychotherapy program for people with cancer, *Am J Psychother* 54:486–500, 2000.

32. McClain CS, Rosenfeld B, Breitbart W: Effect of spiritual well-being on end-of-life despair in terminally-ill cancer patients, *Lancet* 361:1603–1607, 2003.

33. Fawzy FI: Psychosocial interventions for patients with cancer: what works and what doesn't, *Eur J Cancer* 35:1559–1564, 1999.

34. Fawzy FI, Fawzy NW, Arndt LA, et al: Critical review of psychosocial interventions in cancer care, *Arch Gen Psychiatry* 52:100–113, 1995.

35. Leubbert K, Dahme B, Hasenbring M: The effectiveness of relaxation training in reducing treatment-related symptoms and improving emotional adjustment in acute non-surgical cancer treatment: a meta-analytic review, *Psycho-oncology* 10:490–502, 2001.

36. Cassem, NH: *The consultation service*. In Hackett TP, Weisman AD, Kucharski A, editors. *Psychiatry in a general hospital: the first fifty years*, Littleton, MA, 1987, PSG Publishing Company, 33–39.

37. Clinical Care Committee of the Massachusetts General Hospital: Optimum care for hopelessly ill patients, *New Engl J Med* 295:362–364, 1976.

38. Cassem EH: Difficult deliberations about care at the end of life. In Dying, decision-making, and appropriate care, *Institute of Medicine Workshop*, Washington DC, 1993.

39. Greenberg DB, Goorin A, Gebhardt MC, et al: Quality of life in osteosarcoma survivors. *Oncology* 8:19–35, 1994.

40. Pirl WF, Siegel GI, Goode MJ, et al: Depression in men receiving androgen deprivation therapy for prostate cancer: a pilot study, *Psycho-oncology* 11:518–523, 2002.

41. Ingram D, Browne G, Reyno L, et al: Prevalence, correlates and cost of anxiety and affective disorder in men with prostate cancer one year after initial assessment, *Psycho-oncology* 12:S1-S277, 2003, (abstract 523).

42. Fernandes PP: Rapid desensitization for needle phobia, *Psychosomatics* 44:253–254, 2003.

43. Seligman MEP: *Helplessness: on depression, development, and death*, San Francisco, 1975, W H Freeman.

44. Fertig DL, Hayes DF: *Psychological responses to tumor markers*. In Holland JC, editor: *Psycho-oncology*, New York, 1998, Oxford University Press.

45. Greenberg DB, Surman OS, Clarke J, et al: Alprazolam for phobic nausea and vomiting related to cancer chemotherapy, *Cancer Treatment Rep* 71:549–550, 1987.

46. Hickok JT, Roscoe JA, Morrow GR, et al: Nausea and emesis remain significant problems of chemotherapy despite prophylaxis with 5-hydroxytryptamine-3 antiemetics, *Cancer* 97:2880–2886, 2003.

47. Andrykowski MA: The role of anxiety in the development of anticipatory nausea in cancer chemotherapy: a review and synthesis, *Psychosom Med* 54:458–475, 1990.

48. Pitman RK, Lanes DM, Williston SK, et al: Psychophysiologic assessment of post-traumatic stress disorder in breast cancer patients, *Psychosomatics* 42:133–140, 2001.

49. Greenberg DB, Kornblith AB, Herndon JE, et al: Quality of life for adult leukemia survivors treated on clinical trials of Cancer and Leukemia Group B during the period 1971–1988; predictors for later psychologic distress, *Cancer* 80:1936–1944, 1997.

50. Kornblith AB, Herndon EJ II, Weiss RB, et al, for the Cancer and Leukemia Group B [CALGB], Chicago, Ill. Long-term adjustment of survivors of early stage breast cancer 20 years after adjuvant chemotherapy, *Cancer* 98:679–689, 2003

51. Stark D, Kiely M, Smith A, et al: Anxiety disorders in cancer patients: their nature, associations, and relation to quality of life, *J Clin Oncol* 20:3137–3148, 2002.

52. Massie MJ: The prevalence of depression in patients with cancer, *J Natl Cancer Inst* (in press).

53. Passik SD, Dugan W, McDonald MV, et al: Oncologists recognition of depression in their patients with cancer, *J Clin Oncol* 16:1594–1600, 1998.

54. Trask PC: Assessment of depression in cancer patients, *J Natl Cancer Inst* (in press).

55. Holland JC: Preliminary guidelines for the treatment of distress, *Oncology (Huntingt)* 11:109–12; 115–117, 1997.

56. Greenberg DB, Sawicka J, Eisenthal S et al: Fatigue syndrome due to localized radiation, *J Pain Symptom Manage* 7:38–45, 1992.

57. Greenberg DB, Gray JL, Mannix CM, et al:. Treatment-related fatigue and serum interleukin-1 levels in patients during external beam irradiation for prostate cancer, *J Pain Symptom Manage* 8:196–199, 1993.

58. Schwartz L: *Les nevroses et la psychologe dynamique de Pierre Janet.* Paris, 1955, Presses Universitaires de France, 248–320.
59. Greenberg D: *Fatigue.* In Holland JC, editor: *Psycho-oncology,* New York, 1998, Oxford University Press, 485–493.
60. Smith IE, Dowsett M: Aromatase inhibitors in breast cancer, *N Engl J Med* 348:2431–2442, 2003.
61. Duffy LS, Greenberg DB, Younger J, et al: Iatrogenic acute estrogen deficiency and psychiatric syndromes in breast cancer patients, *Psychosomatics* 40:304–308, 1999.
62. Stearns V, Beebe KL, Iyengar M, et al: Paroxetine controlled release in the treatment of menopausal hot flashes: a randomized controlled trial, *JAMA* 289:2827–2834, 2003.
63. Loprinzi CL, Kugler JW, Sloan JA, et al: Venlafaxine in management of hot flashes in survivors of breast cancer: a ramdomised controlled trial, *Lancet* 356:2059–2063, 2000.
64. Greenberg DB, Jonasch E, Gadd MA, et al: Adjuvant therapy of melanoma with interferon alpha 2b associated with mania and bipolar syndromes, *Cancer* 89:356–362, 2000.
65. Musselman DL, Lawson DH, Gumnick JF, et al: Paroxetine for the prevention of depression induced by high-dose interferon alfa, *N Engl J Med* 344: 961–966, 2001.
66. Kirkwood JM, Bender C, Agarwala S, et al: Mechanisms and management of toxicities associated with high-dose interferon alfa-2b therapy, *J Clin Oncol* 20:3703–3718, 2002.
67. Carr D, Goudas L, Lawrence D, et al: Management of cancer symptoms: pain, depression, and fatigue. evidence report/technology assessment number 61, *Agency for Healthcare Research and Quality,* Rockville, Md, 2002.
68. Filley CM, Kleinschmidt-DeMasters BK: Toxic leukoencephalopathy, *N Engl J Med* 345: 425–432, 2001.
69. Phillips K-A, Bernhard J: Adjuvant breast cancer treatment and cognitive function: current knowledge and research directions, *J Natl Cancer Inst* 95:190–197, 2003.
70. Crossen JR, Garwood D, Glatstein E, et al: Neurobehavioral sequelae of cranial irradiation in adults: a review of radiation-induced encephalopathy, *J Clin Oncol* 12:627–642, 1994.
71. Auperin A, Arriagada R, Pignon J, et al: Prophylactic cranial irradiation for patients with small-cell lung cancer in complete remission, *N Engl J Med* 341:476–484, 1999.
72. Stern TA, Purcell JJ, Murray GB: Complex partial seizures associated with Waldenstom's macroglobulinemia, *Psychosomatics* 26:890–892, 1985.
73. Crawford J, Cox EB, Cohen HJ: Evaluation of hyperviscosity in monoclonal gammopathies, *Am J Med* 79:13–22, 1985.
74. Dalmau JO, Posner JB: Paraneoplastic syndromes, *Arch Neurol* 56:405–408, 1999.
75. Kung S, Mueller PS, Geda YE, et al: Delirium resulting from paraneoplastic limbic encephalitis caused by Hodgkin's disease, *Psychosomatics* 43:498–501, 2002.
76. Cicerone KD, Dahlberg C, Kalmar K, et al: Evidence-based cognitive rehabilitation: recommendations for clinical practice, *Arch Phys Med Rehabil* 81:1596–1615, 2000.
77. Sawyer M, Antoniou G, Toogood I, et al: Childhood cancer: a two-year prospective study of the psychological adjustment of children and parents, *J Amer Acad Adolesc Psychiatry* 36:1736–1743, 1997.
78. Pirl WF, Baker-Niendorf K, Mahoney-Shannon K, et al: A model of psychosocial care in genetic testing for cancer susceptibility, *Psycho-oncology* 12(suppl):102–103, 2003 (abstract).
79. Horowitz M, Sundin E, Zanko A, et al: Coping with grim news from genetic tests, *Psychosomatics* 42: 100–105, 2001.
80. National Health Interview Survey 1992, National Cancer Institute, Division of Cancer Control and Population Sciences, Office of Cancer Survivorship.
81. Bloom JR, Kessler L: Risk and timing of counseling and support interventions for younger women with breast cancer, *J Natl Cancer Inst Monographs,* 16:199–206, 1994.
82. Siegel K, Mesagno FP, Karus D, et al: Psychosocial adjustment of children with a terminally ill parent, *J Am Acad Child Adolesc Psychiatry* 31(2):327–333, 1992.
83. Silverman PR: *Never too young to know: death in children's lives,* New York, 2000, Oxford University Press.
84. Rauch PK, Muriel AC, Cassem NH: Parents with cancer: who's looking after the children? *J Clin Oncol* 20: 4399–4440, 2002.
85. Rauch PK, Muriel AC: The importance of parenting concerns among patients with cancer. *Crit Rev Oncol/Hematol,* (in press) 2003.
86. Lamont EB, Christakis NA: Complexities in prognostication in advanced cancer, *JAMA* 290:98–104, 2003.
87. Cascino TL: Neurologic complications of systemic cancer, *Med Clin North Am* 77:265–278, 1993.

Chapter 34
The Pregnant Patient

Lee S. Cohen, M.D.
Ruta Nonacs, M.D., Ph.D.
Adele C. Viguera, M.D.

Psychiatric consultation to obstetric patients typically involves the evaluation and treatment of an array of psychopathology. Once thought to be a time of emotional well-being for women,[1] studies now suggest that pregnancy is not protective with respect to the emergence or persistence of psychiatric disorders.[2–7] Given the prevalence of mood and anxiety disorders in women during childbearing years[8,9] and the number of women who receive treatment for these disorders, it is apparent that many women become pregnant either after the recent discontinuation of psychotropic medications or following a decision to maintain treatment during efforts to conceive. With increasing evidence of high rates of relapse following discontinuation of psychotropic medications (e.g., antidepressants,[10] mood stabilizers,[11] antipsychotics,[12] and benzodiazepines[13]) and other data describing new-onset psychiatric illness during pregnancy,[2,6,14] the value of psychiatric consultation during pregnancy and after delivery is evident.

Psychiatric evaluation of pregnant women requires careful assessment of symptoms such as anxiety or depression and decisions about the nature of those symptoms such as (1) normative or pathologic, (2) manifestations of a new-onset psychiatric disorder, or (3) an exacerbation of a previously diagnosed or undiagnosed psychiatric disorder. Unfortunately, screening for a psychiatric disorder during pregnancy or the puerperium is uncommon. Screenings for depression can facilitate thoughtful

treatment planning during pregnancy and the postpartum period.

Pregnancy is an emotionally laden experience that evokes a spectrum of normal reactions, including heightened anxiety and increased reactivity of mood. Normative experience needs to be distinguished from the manifestations of psychiatric disorders. Treatment of psychiatric disorders during pregnancy involves a thoughtful weighing of the risks and benefits of proposed interventions, such as pharmacologic treatment and the documented[15,16] and theoretic risks associated with untreated psychiatric disorders. In contrast to many other clinical conditions, treatment of psychiatric disorders during pregnancy is typically reserved for situations in which the disorder interferes significantly with maternal and fetal well-being; the threshold for the treatment of psychiatric disorders during pregnancy tends to be higher than with other conditions. Moreover, women with similar illness histories often make very different decisions about their care (in collaboration with their physicians) during pregnancy.

Diagnosis and Treatment of Mood Disorder During Pregnancy

Although some reports describe pregnancy as a time of affective well-being[1,17–19] that confers "protection" against psychiatric disorders, at least one prospective study describes equal rates of major and minor depression (approximating 10%) in gravid and nongravid women. Several other recent studies also note clinically significant depressive symptoms during pregnancy (antenatal depression).[2,6,20,21] Furthermore, women with histories of major depression appear to be at high risk for recurrent depression during pregnancy, particularly in the setting of antidepressant discontinuation.[22,23]

Diagnosis of depression during pregnancy can be difficult because disturbance in sleep and appetite, symptoms of fatigue, and change in libido, do not necessarily suggest an evolving affective disorder. Clinical features that may support the diagnosis of major depression include anhedonia, feelings of guilt and hopelessness, and thoughts of suicide. Suicidal ideation is not uncommon[24-26]; however, risk of self-injurious or suicidal behaviors appears to be relatively low in women who develop depression during pregnancy.[25,26]

Treatment for depression during pregnancy is determined by the severity of the underlying disorder. Nonetheless, neurovegetative symptoms that interfere with maternal well-being require treatment. Women with mild to moderate depressive symptoms frequently benefit from nonpharmacologic treatments that include supportive psychotherapy, cognitive therapy,[27] or interpersonal therapy (IPT),[28] all of which may ameliorate depressive symptoms. Given the importance of interpersonal relationships in couples who are expecting a child and the significant role transitions that take place during pregnancy and after delivery, IPT is ideally suited for the treatment of depressed pregnant women; preliminary but encouraging data support the efficacy of this intervention.[29]

Antidepressant Use During Pregnancy

Many reviews have been published[22,23,30-32] that describe available data (from anecdotal case reports and larger, prospectively derived samples) regarding risks associated with fetal exposure to antidepressants. Although accumulated data over the last 30 years suggest that some antidepressants may be used safely during pregnancy,[33-35] information regarding the spectrum of attendant risks of prenatal exposure to psychotropic medications is still incomplete.

As is the case with other medications, four types of risk are typically cited with respect to potential use of antidepressants during pregnancy: (1) risk of pregnancy loss or miscarriage, (2) risk of organ malformation or teratogenesis, (3) risk of neonatal toxicity or withdrawal syndromes during the acute neonatal period, and (4) risk of long-term neurobehavioral sequelae.[34] To provide guidance to physicians seeking information on the reproductive safety of various prescription medications, the Food and Drug Administration (FDA) has established a system that classifies medications into five risk categories (A, B, C, D, and X) based on data derived from human and animal studies. Medications in category A are designated as safe for use during pregnancy, whereas category X drugs are contraindicated and are known to have risks to the fetus that outweigh any benefit to the patient. Most psychotropic medications are classified as category C agents, for which human studies are lacking and for which "risk cannot be ruled out." No psychotropic drugs are classified as safe for use during pregnancy (category A).

Unfortunately, this system of classification is often ambiguous and may lead some to make conclusions that are not warranted. For example, certain tricyclic antidepressants (TCAs) have been labeled as category D agents, indicating "positive evidence of risk," although the pooled available data do not support this assertion and, in fact, suggest that these drugs are safe for use during pregnancy.[36,37] Therefore, the physician must rely on other sources of information when counseling patients about the potential use of psychotropic medications during pregnancy. Randomized, placebo-controlled studies examining the effects of medication use on pregnant populations is unethical for obvious reasons. Therefore, much of the data related to the profile of reproductive safety for a medication is derived from retrospective studies and case reports. More recently, studies that have evaluated the reproductive safety of antidepressants have used a more rigorous prospective design.[36-41]

To date, studies have not demonstrated a statistically increased risk of spontaneous miscarriage or congenital malformations associated with prenatal exposure to antidepressants.

Data supporting reproductive safety of fluoxetine[38,40,42-50] and citalopram[48] are particularly robust. Four prospective studies have evaluated rates of congenital malformations in approximately 1100 fluoxetine-exposed infants.[36,38,43,45,47,51] These data, collected from more than 2500 cases, indicate no increase in the risk of major congenital malformations in fluoxetine-exposed infants.

Information regarding the reproductive safety of other selective serotonin-reuptake inhibitors (SSRIs) including sertraline, paroxetine, fluvoxamine, and the serotonin-norepinephrine reuptake inhibitor (SNRI) venlafaxine[41] is accumulating gradually; however, it is still limited in terms of its sample size.[40,43,48,52,53] Nonetheless, given the frequency of use of these medicines and the frequency of unplanned pregnancy[54] the data supporting safety of SSRIs (as a class) and venlafaxine is increasingly reassuring. To date, prospective data on the use of mirtazapine, nefazodone, and trazodone are not available. Scant information is available regarding the reproductive safety of monoamine oxidase inhibitors (MAOIs). One study in humans described an increase in congenital malformations after prenatal exposure to tranylcypromine and phenelzine, although the sample size was extremely small.[55] Moreover, during labor and delivery, MAOIs may produce a hypertensive crisis if tocolytic medications, such as terbutaline, are used to forestall delivery. Given this lack of data and the cumbersome restrictions associated with their use, MAOIs are typically avoided during pregnancy.

Neonatal toxicity and perinatal syndromes refer to a spectrum of physical and behavioral symptoms observed in the acute neonatal period that are attributed to drug exposure at or near the time of delivery. Over the last 2 decades, a wide range of transient neonatal distress syndromes associated with exposure to (or withdrawal from) antidepressants in utero have been described; however, studies of larger samples suggest that the incidence of these adverse events is low. Anecdotal reports that attribute these syndromes to drug exposure must be interpreted cautiously, and larger samples must be studied to establish a causal link between exposure to a particular medication and a perinatal syndrome.

Various case reports have described perinatal syndromes in infants exposed to TCAs in utero. A TCA withdrawal syndrome, with characteristic symptoms of jitteriness, irritability, and, less commonly, seizure[56–60] has been observed. Withdrawal

seizures from TCAs have been reported only with clomipramine.[56,60] In addition, neonatal toxicity attributed to the anticholinergic effect of TCAs, including symptoms of functional bowel obstruction and urinary retention, also have been reported.[61,62] In all cases, these symptoms have been transient.

The extent to which prenatal exposure to fluoxetine or other SSRIs is associated with neonatal toxicity is still unclear. Case reports and one prospective study have described perinatal complications in fluoxetine-exposed infants, including poor neonatal adaptation, respiratory distress, feeding problems, and jitteriness.[38,63] Although several prospective studies have not observed perinatal distress in infants exposed to fluoxetine,[40,47,49,64] at least one study has described compromised perinatal outcome associated with exposure to SSRIs when compared with nonexposed newborns.[53] The significant limitation of this report, like other reports that describe compromised perinatal outcome associated with fetal exposure to antidepressants, is that the study design does not allow adequate control of the effects of antenatal mood disorder on neonatal outcome. Given data that describe the adverse effects of antenatal mood disorder on neonatal well-being, the absence of adequate measurement of maternal mood across pregnancy in studies that evaluate the effects of antidepressant on fetal and neonatal well-being and longer-term neurobehavioral function[65] must be viewed with caution.

Recently, concern has also been raised regarding the potential for withdrawal syndromes in newborns exposed to shorter-acting SSRIs (i.e., paroxetine) proximate to delivery. Case reports of neonatal withdrawal in neonates exposed to paroxetine refer to transient symptoms of irritability, excessive crying, increased muscle tone, feeding problems, sleep disruption, and respiratory distress.[66–70] In a prospective sample of 55 neonates exposed to paroxetine proximate to delivery (dose range 10 to 60 mg, median 20 mg), 22% (N = 12) had complications that necessitated intensive treatment.[66] The most common symptoms included respiratory distress (N = 9), hypoglycemia (N = 2), and jaundice (N = 1), all of which resolved over 1 to 2 weeks without a specific intervention. The extent to which other SSRIs (with longer half-lives) carry similar risk for neonatal toxicity remains to be explored; however, most prospective studies have not demonstrated significant adverse events in exposed infants.[40,47–49,64] Furthermore, it is crucial to investigate other factors that modulate vulnerability to neonatal toxicity (e.g., prematurity and low birth weight).

Pharmacologic Treatment of Depression During Pregnancy: Clinical Guidelines

The last decade has brought increased attention to the question of how to best manage women who suffer from depression during pregnancy. Although clinical lore previously suggested that women enjoyed positive mood during pregnancy, more recent preliminary data suggest that subpopulations of patients may be at risk for recurrence or new onset of depression during pregnancy. There is also a greater appreciation that depression may exert an effect on fetal and neonatal well-being that needs to be taken into account in the risk-benefit decision-making process.[23,33,35,71] Despite the growing number of reviews on the subject, management of antenatal depression is still largely guided by practical experience, with few definitive data and no controlled treatment studies to inform treatment. The most appropriate treatment algorithm depends on the severity of the disorder and, ultimately, the patient's wishes. Clinicians must work collaboratively with the patient to arrive at the safest decision based on available information. A patient's psychiatric history, her current symptoms, and her attitude toward the use of psychiatric medications during pregnancy must be carefully assessed.

In patients with less severe depression, it is appropriate to consider discontinuation of pharmacologic therapy during pregnancy. IPT or cognitive-behavioral therapy (CBT) may be used prior to conception to facilitate the gradual tapering and discontinuation of an antidepressant medication in a woman planning to become pregnant. These modalities of treatment may reduce the risk of recurrent depressive symptoms during pregnancy, although this has not been studied systematically. Close monitoring during pregnancy is essential, even if all medications are discontinued and there is no need for medication management. Psychiatri-

cally ill women are at high risk for relapse during pregnancy, and early detection and treatment of recurrent illness may significantly reduce the morbidity associated with having an antenatal affective disorder.

Many women who discontinue antidepressant treatment during pregnancy experience recurrent depressive symptoms.[2] Thus, women with recurrent or refractory depressive illness, may decide in collaboration with their clinician that the safest option is to continue pharmacologic treatment during pregnancy. In this setting, the clinician should attempt to select medications during pregnancy that have a well-characterized reproductive safety profile, which may necessitate switching from one psychotropic to another with a better reproductive safety profile. An example would be switching from nefazodone, a medication for which there are sparse data on reproductive safety, to an agent such as fluoxetine. In other situations, one may decide to use a medication for which information regarding reproductive safety is sparse. A scenario that highlights this decision is a woman with refractory depressive illness who has responded only to one antidepressant for which data on reproductive safety are limited (e.g., venlafaxine). She may choose to continue this medication during pregnancy rather than risk relapse if she discontinued this agent or switched to another antidepressant.

Women may also experience the new onset of depressive symptoms during pregnancy. For women who present with minor depressive symptoms, nonpharmacologic treatment strategies should be explored first. IPT or CBT may be beneficial for reducing the severity of depressive symptoms and may either limit or obviate the need for medications.[27–29] In general, pharmacologic treatment is pursued when nonpharmacologic strategies have failed or when it is felt that the risks associated with psychiatric illness during pregnancy outweigh the risks of fetal exposure to a particular medication.

In situations in which pharmacologic treatment is indicated, the clinician should attempt to select the safest medication regimen, using, if possible, medications with the safest reproductive profile. Fluoxetine, with the most extensive literature supporting its reproductive safety, is a first-line choice. The TCAs have been relatively well-characterized in this setting and should also be considered as first-line agents. Among the TCAs, desipramine and nortriptyline are preferred because they are less anticholinergic and the least likely to exacerbate orthostatic hypotension during pregnancy. The amount of literature on the reproductive safety of the newer SSRIs, including citalopram, is growing, and these agents may be useful in certain settings.[40,48] In patients with depression who have not responded to either fluoxetine or a TCA, these newer agents may be considered, acknowledging that information on their reproductive safety is limited. When prescribing medications during pregnancy, every attempt should be made to simplify the medication regimen. For instance, one may select a more sedating TCA for a woman who presents with depression and a sleep disturbance, instead of using an SSRI in combination with trazodone or a benzodiazepine.

In addition, the clinician must use an adequate dosage of medication. Frequently the dosage of a medication is reduced during pregnancy in an attempt to limit risk to the fetus; however, this type of modification in treatment may instead place the woman at greater risk for recurrent illness. During pregnancy, changes in plasma volume and increases in hepatic metabolism and renal clearance may significantly affect drug levels.[72,73] Several investigators have described a significant reduction (up to 65%) in serum levels of TCAs during pregnancy.[37,74] Subtherapeutic levels were associated with depressive relapse[37]; therefore, daily TCA dosage was increased during pregnancy to induce remission. Similarly, many women taking SSRIs during pregnancy require an increase in SSRI dosage to sustain euthymia.[75]

Based on a number of anecdotal reports of toxicity in infants born to mothers treated with antidepressants, some authors have recommended discontinuation of antidepressants several days or weeks prior to delivery to minimize the risk of neonatal toxicity. Given the low incidence of neonatal toxicity with most antidepressants, this practice carries significant risk because it withdraws treatment from patients precisely as they are about to enter the postpartum period, a time of heightened risk for affective illness.

Severely depressed patients who are acutely suicidal or psychotic require hospitalization, and electroconvulsive therapy (ECT) is frequently selected as the treatment of choice. Two recent reviews of ECT during pregnancy note the efficacy and safety of this procedure.[76,77] In a review of the 300 case reports of ECT during pregnancy published over the past 50 years, four premature labors have been reported and no premature ruptures of membranes have been reported. Given its relative safety, ECT may also be considered an alternative to conventional pharmacotherapy for women who wish to avoid extended exposure to psychotropic medications during pregnancy or for women who fail to respond to standard antidepressants.

Some publications have advised antidepressant discontinuation within a week before the estimated date of delivery.[78] These suggestions derive from reports of rare self-limited perinatal sequelae, such as jitteriness, irritability, and neonatal bowel and bladder dysfunction.[56,58,59,61,62,79,80] Given the low incidence of these problems and the extremely high risk of postpartum illness in women with histories of depression or depression during pregnancy,[20] it is unwise to withdraw antidepressants at a time when patients enter this period of risk for recurrent or worsening mood disorder.

Bipolar Disorder During Pregnancy

Women with bipolar disorder (BPD) have at times been counseled to defer pregnancy (given an apparent need for pharmacologic therapy with mood stabilizers) or to terminate pregnancies following prenatal exposure to drugs such as lithium or valproic acid. Concerns regarding fetal exposure to lithium, for example, have typically been based on early reports of higher rates of cardiovascular malformations (e.g., Ebstein's anomaly) following prenatal exposure to this drug.[81,82] More recent data suggest the risk of cardiovascular malformations following prenatal exposure to lithium is smaller than previous estimates (1/2000 versus 1/1000).[83] Prenatal screening with a high-resolution ultrasound and fetal echocardiography is recommended at or about 16 to 18 weeks of gestation to screen for cardiac anomalies. Nonetheless, for the bipolar woman faced with a decision regarding use of lithium during pregnancy, it is appropriate to counsel such a patient about the very small risk of organ dysgenesis associated with prenatal exposure to this medicine.

Compared with lithium, prenatal exposure to some anticonvulsants is associated with a far greater risk for organ malformation. An association between prenatal exposure to mood stabilizers, including valproic acid and carbamazepine, and neural tube defects (3% to 8%) and spina bifida (1%) also has been observed.[84–87] Fetal exposure to anticonvulsants has been associated not only with relatively high rates of neural tube defects (NTD), such as spina bifida, but also with multiple anomalies (including midface hypoplasia [also known as the "anticonvulsant face"], congenital heart disease, cleft lip and/or palate, growth retardation, and microcephaly). Factors that may increase the risk for teratogenesis include high maternal serum anticonvulsant levels and exposure to more than one anticonvulsant. This finding of dose-dependent risk for teratogenesis is at variance with that of other psychotropic medications (e.g., antidepressants). Thus, when using anticonvulsants during pregnancy, the lowest effective dose should be used, and anticonvulsant levels should be monitored closely and the dosage adjusted appropriately.

Information about the reproductive safety of newer anticonvulsants sometimes used to treat BPD including lamotrigine, gabapentin, oxcarbazepine, and topiramate remains sparse.[88] Recent preliminary data on prenatal exposure to lamotrigine monotherapy during the first trimester suggest that the risk of a major malformation is comparable to what is seen in the general nonexposed population.[89] Other efforts are underway to accumulate data from prospective registries regarding teratogenic risks across a broad range of anticonvulsants. The North American Antiepileptic Drug Pregnancy Registry recently was established as a way of collecting such information rapidly and efficiently (http://www.aedpregnancyregistry.org).

Prenatal screening following anticonvulsant exposure for congenital malformations (including cardiac anomalies) with fetal ultrasound at 18 to 22 weeks of gestation is recommended. The possibility of fetal neural tube defects should be evaluated with maternal serum alpha-feto protein (MSAFP) and ultrasonography. In addition, 4 mg a day of folic acid before conception and in the first trimester for women receiving anticonvulsants is recommended. Supplemental folic acid's ability to attenuate the risk of neural tube defects

in the setting of anticonvulsant exposure has not been examined.

Whereas use of mood stabilizers (including lithium and some anticonvulsants) has become the mainstay of treatment for the management of both acute mania and the maintenance phase of BPD, the majority of patients with BPD are not treated with monotherapy. Rather, use of adjunctive conventional and newer antipsychotics has become common clinical practice for many bipolar patients. Moreover, with growing data supporting the use of atypical antipsychotics as monotherapy in the treatment of BPD, patients and clinicians will seek information regarding the reproductive safety of these newer agents. To date, abundant data exist that supports the reproductive safety of typical antipsychotics; these data have been reviewed extensively elsewhere.[33,71] However, despite their growing use in psychiatry, available reproductive safety data regarding the atypical antipsychotics are sparse and thus, they are best avoided if possible; although they are not absolutely contraindicated during pregnancy, atypical antipsychotics should be reserved for use in more refractory clinical situations where treatment with agents for which more conclusive data supporting safety are available, has proven to be less than efficacious.

Although the impact of pregnancy on the natural course of BPD is not well described, studies suggest that any "protective" effects of pregnancy on risk for recurrence of mania or depression in women with BPD are limited[90] and the risk for relapse and chronicity following discontinuation of mood stabilizers is high.[91–93] Given these data, clinicians and bipolar women who are either pregnant or who wish to conceive find themselves between a "teratologic rock and a clinical hard place."[78] The most appropriate treatment algorithm depends on the severity of the individual patient's illness. Patients with histories of a single episode of mania and prompt, full recovery followed by sustained well-being may tolerate discontinuation of mood stabilizer before an attempt to conceive.[83,90] For women with BPD and a history of multiple and frequent recurrences of mania or bipolar depression, several options can be considered. Some patients may choose to discontinue a mood stabilizer prior to conception as outlined above. An alternative strategy for this high-risk group is to continue treatment until pregnancy is verified and then taper off of the mood stabilizer. Because the utero-placental circulation is not established until approximately 2 weeks following conception, the risk of fetal exposure is minimal. Home pregnancy tests are reliable and can document pregnancy as early as 10 days following conception, and with a home ovulation predictor kit, a patient may be able to time her treatment discontinuation accurately. This strategy minimizes fetal exposure to drugs and extends the protective treatment up to the time of conception, which may be particularly prudent for older patients because the time required for them to conceive may be longer than for younger patients. However, a potential problem with this strategy is that it may lead to relatively abrupt discontinuation of treatment, thereby potentially placing the patient at increased risk for relapse. With close clinical follow-up, however, patients can be monitored for early signs of relapse, and medications may be reintroduced as needed.

For women who tolerate discontinuation of maintenance treatment, the decision of when to resume treatment is a matter for clinical judgment. Some patients and clinicians may prefer to await the initial appearance of symptoms before restarting medication; others may prefer to limit their risk of a major recurrence by restarting treatment after the first trimester of pregnancy. Preliminary data suggest that pregnant women with BPD who remain well throughout pregnancy may have a lower risk for postpartum relapse than those who become ill during pregnancy.[90,94]

For women with particularly severe forms of BPD, such as with multiple severe episodes, and especially with psychosis and prominent thoughts of suicide, maintenance treatment with a mood stabilizer before and during pregnancy may be the safest option. If the patient decides to attempt conception, accepting the relatively small absolute increase in teratogenic risk with first—trimester exposure to lithium, for example, may be justified because such patients are at highest risk for clinical deterioration if pharmacologic treatment is withdrawn. For severely depressed or manic patients, hospitalization is required and ECT is frequently the treatment of choice.

Even if all psychotropic medications have been safely discontinued, pregnancy in women with BPD should be considered as a high-risk pregnancy, because the risk of major psychiatric illness during pregnancy is increased without mood-stabilizing medication and is even higher postpartum. Unusually high vigilance is required for early detection of an impending relapse of illness, and rapid intervention can significantly reduce morbidity and improve overall prognosis.

Psychosis During Pregnancy

Although anecdotal reports describe improvement of symptoms in some chronically mentally ill women during pregnancy, as a group these patients are at increased risk for poor fetal outcome.[95,96] Acute psychosis during pregnancy is both an obstetric and psychiatric emergency. Similar to other psychiatric symptoms of new onset, first onset of psychosis during pregnancy cannot be presumed to be reactive; it requires a systematic diagnostic evaluation. Psychosis during pregnancy may inhibit a woman's ability to obtain appropriate and necessary prenatal care or to cooperate with caregivers during delivery.[95–97]

Treatment of psychosis during pregnancy typically requires the use of high-potency neuroleptic medications, such as haloperidol or thiothixene, which have not been associated with an increased risk of congenital malformations when used in the first trimester of pregnancy.[98,99] Historically, lower potency antipsychotics have typically been avoided because of data supporting an increased risk of congenital malformations associated with prenatal exposure to these compounds.[100,101] However, their use is not absolutely contraindicated.

Psychiatric consultation may be requested regarding treatment options for mild or intermittent symptoms of psychosis or for pregnant women with chronic mental illness, such as schizophrenia, who have discontinued therapy with neuroleptic medications. Although as-needed high-potency neuroleptic medications are appropriate for treatment of more mild symptoms of psychosis, consideration should be given to introduction or reintroduction of maintenance high-potency antipsychotics in schizophrenic women who have new-onset illness or a recurrent disorder. This approach can potentially limit overall exposure to these drugs by reducing the need for treatment with higher doses of drug during relapse allowed by drug discontinuation.

Patients with florid psychosis during labor and delivery may benefit from intravenous haloperidol, which may permit cooperation between the patient and the obstetrician, thereby enhancing the overall safety of the delivery.[102,103]

Treatment of Anxiety Disorders During Pregnancy

Although modest to moderate levels of anxiety during pregnancy are common, pathologic anxiety including panic attacks has been associated with a variety of poor obstetric outcomes, including increased rates of premature labor, low Apgar scores, and placental abruption.[104–106] Unfortunately, the course of panic disorder in pregnancy is variable. Pregnancy may ameliorate symptoms of panic in some patients and may provide an opportunity to discontinue medication.[107–110] Other studies have noted the persistence or worsening of panic-related symptoms during pregnancy.[4,5,111,112]

Consultation requests regarding appropriate management of anxiety symptoms during pregnancy are common. The use of nonpharmacologic treatment, such as cognitive-behavioral strategies and supportive psychotherapy, may be of great value in attenuating symptoms of anxiety in some cases.[113,114] For other patients, especially those who experience panic attacks associated with new-onset or recurrent panic disorder or those with severe generalized anxiety, pharmacologic intervention may be necessary. Concerns regarding the potential association between first-trimester exposure to benzodiazepines, such as diazepam, and increased risk for oral clefts have been noted in some studies,[115–117] although other studies do not support this association.[118,119] One meta-analysis that pooled data from multiple samples of patients exposed to different types and doses of benzodiazepines for variable durations of time supported an increased risk of oral clefts following first-trimester exposure to these drugs[33]; a more recent meta-analysis evaluating this potential association did not support the increased risk.[120]

For patients with panic disorder who wish to conceive, slow tapering of antipanic medications is recommended. Adjunctive CBT may benefit in helping patients discontinue antipanic agents and

may increase the time to a relapse.[114] Some patients may conceive inadvertently on antipanic medications and may present for emergent consultation. Abrupt discontinuation of antipanic maintenance medication is not recommended given the risk for rebound panic symptoms or a potentially serious withdrawal syndrome. However, gradual taper of benzodiazepine (>2 weeks) with adjunctive CBT may be pursued in an effort to minimize fetal exposure to medication.

If tapering medication is unsuccessful or if symptoms recur during pregnancy, reinstitution of pharmacotherapy may be considered. For patients with severe panic disorder, maintenance medication may be a clinical necessity. Use of TCAs or fluoxetine are reasonable options for the management of panic disorder during pregnancy.[33] If patients do not respond to these antidepressants, benzodiazepines may be considered.[121] Although some patients may choose to avoid first-trimester exposure to benzodiazepines given the data on the risk for cleft lip and palate, benzodiazepines may be used without significant risk during the second and third trimesters and may offer some advantage over antidepressant treatment because they may be used as needed.

Pharmacotherapy of severe anxiety during pregnancy may include treatment with benzodiazepines, TCAs, SSRIs, or SNRIs. These classes of drugs have all demonstrated efficacy in the management of either GAD[122,123] or panic disorder.[124–126] Pharmacologic treatment of severe anxiety during pregnancy may include the use of TCAs as a nonbenzodiazepine alternative for panic attacks. Nonetheless, patients treated with TCAs alone for management of anxiety symptoms may not respond optimally. For these patients, benzodiazepines represent a reasonable alternative. Lastly, given accumulated data that support the safety of fluoxetine during the first trimester of pregnancy, this SSRI also may be a viable option for management of severe anxiety during pregnancy.

With respect to the use of benzodiazepines during pregnancy at or about the time of labor and delivery, reports of hypotonia, neonatal apnea, neonatal withdrawal syndromes, and temperature dysregulation[127–133] have prompted recommendations to taper and discontinue benzodiazepines at the time of parturition. The rationale for this course is suspect for several reasons. First, given data suggesting a risk for puerperal worsening of anxiety disorders in women with histories of panic disorder and obsessive-compulsive disorder (OCD),[111,134,135] discontinuation of a drug at or about the time of delivery places women at risk for postpartum worsening of these disorders. Second, data describe the use of clonazepam during labor and delivery at doses of 0.5 to 3.5 mg per day in a group of women with panic disorder without evidence of perinatal sequelae.[121]

Electroconvulsive Therapy During Pregnancy

The use of ECT during pregnancy typically raises considerable anxiety among clinicians and patients. Its safety record has been well documented over the last 50 years.[136–138] Requests for psychiatric consultation on pregnant patients requiring ECT tend to be emergent and dramatic. For example, expeditious treatment is imperative in instances of mania during pregnancy or psychotic depression with suicidal thoughts and disorganized thinking. Such clinical situations are associated with a danger from impulsivity or self-harm. The safety and efficacy of ECT in such settings are well described, particularly when instituted in collaboration with a multidisciplinary treatment team, including anesthesiologist, psychiatrist, and obstetrician.[77,138–140] A limited course of treatment may be sufficient followed by institution of treatment with one or a combination of agents, such as antidepressants, neuroleptics, benzodiazepines, or mood stabilizers.

ECT during pregnancy tends to be underused because of concerns that treatment will harm the fetus. Despite one report of placental abruption associated with the use of ECT during pregnancy,[141] considerable experience supports its safe use in severely ill gravid women. Thus, it becomes the task of the psychiatric consultant to facilitate the most clinically appropriate intervention in the face of partially informed concerns or objections.

Breastfeeding and Psychotropic Drug Use

The emotional and medical benefits of breastfeeding to mother and infant are clear. Given the prevalence of psychiatric illness during the postpartum period, a significant number of women may require pharmacologic treatment while nursing. Appropriate concern is raised, however, regarding the safety of psychotropic drug use in women who choose to breastfeed while using these medications. Efforts to quantify psychotropic medications and their metabolites in the breast milk of mothers have been reported. Serum of infants can also be assayed to assess more accurately actual neonatal exposure to medications. The data indicate that all psychotropic medications, including antidepressants, antipsychotic agents, lithium carbonate, and benzodiazepines, are secreted into breast milk. However, concentrations of these agents in breast milk vary considerably. The amount of medication to which an infant is exposed depends on several factors[142]: the maternal dosage of medication, frequency of dosing, and rate of maternal drug metabolism. Typically, peak concentrations in the breast milk are attained approximately 6 to 8 hours after the medication is ingested. Thus, the frequency of feedings *and* the timing of the feedings can influence the amount of drug to which the nursing infant is exposed. By restricting breastfeeding to times during which breast milk drug concentrations would be at their lowest (either shortly before or immediately after dosing medication) exposure may be reduced; however, this approach may not be practical for newborns who typically feed every 2 to 3 hours.

The nursing infant's chances of experiencing toxicity is dependent not only on the amount of medication ingested but also on how well the ingested medication is metabolized. Most psychotropic medications are metabolized by the liver. During the first few weeks of a full-term infant's life, there is a lower capacity for hepatic drug metabolism, which is about one third to one fifth of the adult capacity. Over the next few months, the capacity for hepatic metabolism increases significantly and, by about 2 to 3 months of age, it surpasses that of adults. In premature infants or in infants with signs of compromised hepatic metabolism (e.g., hyperbilirubinemia), breastfeeding typically is deferred because these infants are less able to metabolize drugs and are thus more likely to experience toxicity.

Over the past 5 years, data have accumulated regarding the use of various psychotropic medications during breastfeeding.[143,144] Much data has accumulated on the use of antidepressants in nursing women. The available data on the TCAs, fluoxetine, paroxetine, and sertraline during breast-feeding have been encouraging and suggest that the amounts of drug to which the nursing infant is exposed is low and that significant complications related to neonatal exposure to psychotropic medications in breast milk appear to be rare.[145–151,152] Typically very low or nondetectable levels of drug have been detected in the infant serum, and one recent report indicates that exposure during nursing does not result in clinically significant blockade of serotonin (5-HT) reuptake in infants.[152] Although less information is available on other antidepressants, serious adverse events related to exposure to these medications have not been reported.[143,144]

Given the prevalence of anxiety symptoms during the postpartum period, anxiolytic agents often are used in this setting. Data regarding the use of benzodiazepines have been limited; however, the available data suggest that amounts of medication to which the nursing infant is exposed are low.[145] Case reports of sedation, poor feeding, and respiratory distress in nursing infants have been published[129,153]; however, the data, when pooled, suggest a relatively low incidence of adverse events.[143,145]

Information regarding the use of antipsychotic medications is limited and particularly lacking for the newer atypical agents. Although the use of chlorpromazine has been associated with adverse events, including sedation and developmental delay,[154,155] adverse events appear to be rare when medium- or high-potency agents are used. Data suggest that clozapine may be concentrated in the breast milk[156]; however, no data are available on infant serum levels, making it difficult to interpret the relevance of this finding. Given the severity of adverse events associated with clozapine exposure (i.e., leukopenia), the use of this medication should be reserved for those with treatment-refractory illness, and monitoring of white blood cell (WBC) counts in the nursing infant is mandatory. A recent report demonstrated no adverse events in three infants exposed to olanzapine in breast milk.[157]

For women with BPD, breastfeeding may pose more significant challenges. First, on-demand breastfeeding may significantly disrupt the mother's sleep and thus may increase her vulnerability to relapse during the acute postpartum period. Second, there have been reports of toxicity in nursing infants related to exposure to various mood stabilizers, including lithium and carbamazepine, in breast milk. Lithium is excreted at high levels in the mother's milk, and infant serum levels are relatively high, about one third to one half of the mother's serum levels,[158,159] thereby increasing the risk of neonatal toxicity. Reported signs of toxicity include cyanosis, hypotonia, and hypothermia.[160] Although breastfeeding typically is avoided in women taking lithium, the lowest possible effective dosage should be used and both maternal and infant serum lithium levels should be followed in mothers who breastfeed. In collaboration with the pediatrician, the child should be monitored closely for signs of lithium toxicity.

Similarly, concerns have arisen regarding the use of carbamazepine and valproic acid. Both of these mood stabilizers have been associated in adults with abnormalities in liver function and fatal hepatotoxicity. Hepatic dysfunction associated with carbamazepine exposure in breast milk has been reported several times.[161,162] Most concerning is that the risk for hepatotoxicity appears to be greatest in children younger than 2 years old; thus, nursing infants exposed to these agents may be particularly vulnerable to serious adverse events. Although the American Academy of Pediatrics has deemed both carbamazepine and valproic acid to be appropriate for use in breastfeeding mothers, few studies have assessed the impact of these agents on fetal well-being, particularly in nonepileptic mothers. In those women who choose to use valproic acid or carbamazepine while nursing, routine monitoring of drug levels and liver function tests is recommended. In this setting, ongoing collaboration with the child's pediatrician is crucial.

Consultation about the safety of breastfeeding among women treated with psychotropic medications should include a discussion of the known benefits of breastfeeding to mother and infant and the possibility that exposure to significant levels of medications in the breast milk may occur. Although routine assay of infant serum drug levels was recommended in earlier treatment guidelines, this procedure is probably not warranted; in most instances low infant serum drug levels and, infrequently, serious adverse side effects were reported. This testing is indicated, however, if neonatal toxicity related to drug exposure is suspected. Infant serum monitoring is also indicated when the mother is nursing while taking lithium, valproic acid, or carbamazepine.

Psychiatric Consultation and Postpartum Psychiatric Illness

The postpartum period has typically been considered a time of risk for the development of affective disorder.[18] Although several studies suggest rates of depression during the postpartum period equal to those in nonpuerperal controls, other research has identified subgroups of women at particular risk for postpartum worsening of mood.[20,163–165] At highest risk are women with a history of postpartum psychosis; up to 70% of women who have had one episode of puerperal psychosis will experience another episode following a subsequent pregnancy.[18,165] Similarly, women with histories of postpartum depression are at significant risk, with rates of postpartum recurrence as high as 50%.[166] Women with BPD also appear to be particularly vulnerable during the postpartum period, with rates of postpartum relapse ranging from 30% to 50%[164,167,168] The extent to which a history of major depression influences risk for postpartum illness is less clear. However, in all women (with or without histories of major depression) the emergence of depressive symptoms during pregnancy significantly increases the likelihood of postpartum depression.[20]

Postpartum Mood and Anxiety Disorders: Diagnosis and Treatment

During the postpartum period, about 85% of women experience some degree of mood disturbance. For most women the symptoms are mild; however, 10% to 15% of women experience clinically significant symptoms. Postpartum depressive disorders typically are divided into three categories: (1) postpartum blues, (2) nonpsychotic major depression, and (3) puerperal psychosis. Because these three diagnostic subtypes overlap significantly, it is not clear if they actually represent three distinct disorders. It may be more useful to conceptualize these subtypes as existing along a continuum, where postpartum blues is the mildest and postpartum psychosis the most severe form of puerperal psychiatric illness.

Postpartum blues does not indicate psychopathology, but it is common and occurs in approximately 50% to 85% of women following delivery.[169,170] Symptoms of reactivity of mood, tearfulness, and irritability are, by definition, time limited and typically remit by the tenth postpartum day. As postpartum blues is associated with no significant impairment of functioning and is time-limited, no specific treatment is indicated. Symptoms that persist beyond 2 weeks require further evaluation and may suggest an evolving depressive disorder. In women with histories of recurrent mood disorder, the blues may herald the onset of postpartum major depression.[20,171]

Several studies describe a prevalence of postpartum major depression of between 10% and 15%.[21,169] The signs and symptoms of postpartum depression usually appear over the first 2 to 3 months following delivery and generally are indistinguishable from characteristics of major depression that occur at other times in a woman's life. The presenting symptoms of postpartum depression include depressed mood, irritability, and loss of interest in usual activities. Insomnia, fatigue, and loss of appetite are frequently described. Postpartum depressive symptoms also commingle with anxiety and obsessional symptoms, and women may present with generalized anxiety, panic disorder, or hypochondriasis.[172,173] Although it may sometimes be difficult to diagnose depression in the acute puerperium given the normal occurrence of symptoms suggestive of depression (e.g., sleep and appetite disturbance, low libido), it is an error to dismiss neurovegetative symptoms, such as severe decreased energy, profound anhedonia, and guilty ruminations, as normal features of the puerperium. In its most severe form, postpartum depression may result in profound dysfunction.

A wealth of literature on this topic indicates that postpartum depression, especially when left untreated, may have a significant impact on the child's well-being and development.[174,175] In addition, the syndrome demands aggressive treatment to avoid the sequelae of an untreated mood disorder, such as chronic depression and recurrent disease. Treatment should be guided by the type and severity of the symptoms and by the degree of functional impairment. However, before initiating psychiatric treatment, medical causes for mood disturbance (e.g., thyroid dysfunction, anemia) must be excluded. Initial evaluation should include a thorough history, physical examination, and routine laboratory tests.

Although postpartum depression is relatively common, few studies have systematically assessed the efficacy of nonpharmacologic and pharmacologic therapies in the treatment of this disorder. Nonpharmacologic therapies are useful in the treatment of postpartum depression, and several preliminary studies have yielded encouraging results. Appleby et al.[177] have demonstrated in a randomized study that short-term CBT was as effective as treatment with fluoxetine in women with postpartum depression.[176] IPT has also been shown to be effective for the treatment of women with mild to moderate postpartum depression.

These nonpharmacologic interventions may be particularly attractive to those patients who are reluctant to use psychotropic medications (e.g., women who are breastfeeding) or for patients with milder forms of depressive illness. Further investigation is required to determine the efficacy of these treatments in women who suffer from more severe forms of postpartum mood disturbances. Women with more severe postpartum depression may choose to receive pharmacologic treatment, either in addition to or instead of nonpharmacologic therapies.

To date, only a few studies have systematically assessed the pharmacologic treatment of postpartum depression. Conventional antidepressant medications (e.g., fluoxetine, sertraline, and venlafaxine) have shown efficacy in the treatment of postpartum depression.[176,178,179] In all of these studies, standard antidepressant doses were effective and well tolerated. The choice of an antidepressant should be guided by the patient's prior response to antidepressant medication and a given medication's side-effect profile. SSRIs are ideal first-line agents because they are anxiolytic, nonsedating, and well tolerated. TCAs are used frequently and, because they tend to be more sedating, may be more appropriate for women who have prominent sleep disturbances. Given the prevalence of anxiety in women with postpartum depression,

adjunctive use of a benzodiazepine (e.g., clonazepam or lorazepam) may be very helpful.

Some investigators have also explored the role of hormonal manipulation in women who suffer from postpartum depression. The postpartum period is associated with rapid shifts in the reproductive hormonal environment, most notably a dramatic fall in estrogen and progesterone levels, and postpartum mood disturbance has been attributed to a deficiency (or change in the levels) in these gonadal steroids. Although early reports suggested that progesterone may be helpful,[180] no systematically derived data exist to support its use in this setting. Two studies have described the benefit of exogenous estrogen therapy, either alone or in conjunction with an antidepressant in women with postpartum depression[181-183] Although these studies suggest a role for estrogen in the treatment of women with postpartum depression, these treatments remain experimental. Estrogen delivered during the acute postpartum period is not without risk and has been associated with changes in breast-milk production and more significant thromboembolic events. Antidepressants are safe, well tolerated, and highly effective; they remain the first choice for women with postpartum depression.

In cases of severe postpartum depression, inpatient hospitalization may be required, particularly for patients who are at risk for suicide. In Great Britain, innovative treatment programs involving joint hospitalization of the mother and the baby have been successful; however, mother-infant units are much less common in the United States. Women with severe postpartum illness should be considered candidates for ECT. The option should be considered early in treatment because it is safe and highly effective. In choosing any treatment strategy, it is important to consider the impact of prolonged hospitalization or treatment of the mother on infant development and attachment.

Although symptoms of postpartum panic attacks and OCD symptoms are frequently included in the description of postpartum mood disturbance, a growing literature supports the likelihood that postpartum anxiety disorders are discrete diagnostic entities.[111,173] Several investigators have described postpartum worsening of panic disorder in women with pregravid histories of this anxiety disorder but with an absence of comorbid depressive illness.[4] Postpartum OCD has also been described in the absence of comorbid postpartum major depression. Symptoms often include intrusive obsessional thoughts to harm the newborn in the absence of psychosis. Treatment with antiobsessional agents, such as fluoxetine or clomipramine, has been effective.[135]

Postpartum psychosis is a psychiatric emergency. The clinical picture is most frequently consistent with mania or a mixed state[18] and may include symptoms of restlessness, agitation, sleep disturbance, paranoia, delusions, disorganized thinking, impulsivity, and behaviors that place mother and infant at risk. The typical onset is within the first 2 weeks after delivery, and symptoms may appear as early as the first 48 to 72 hours postpartum. Although investigators have debated whether postpartum psychosis is a discrete diagnostic entity or a manifestation of BPD, treatment should follow the same algorithm to treat acute manic psychosis, including hospitalization and potential use of mood stabilizers, antipsychotic medications, benzodiazepines, or ECT.

Although it is difficult to reliably predict which women will experience a postpartum mood disturbance, it is possible to identify certain subgroups of women (i.e., women with a history of mood disorder) who are more vulnerable to postpartum affective illness. Several investigators have explored the potential efficacy of prophylactic interventions in these women at risk.[184–187]

Several studies demonstrate that women with histories of BPD or puerperal psychosis benefit from prophylactic treatment with lithium instituted either prior to delivery (at 36 weeks gestation) or no later than the first 48 hours following delivery.[184–187] Prophylactic lithium appears to significantly reduce relapse rates and diminish the severity and duration of puerperal illness.

For women with histories of postpartum depression, Wisner et al.[188] have described a beneficial effect of prophylactic antidepressant (either a TCA or a SSRI) administered after delivery. However, a subsequent randomized, placebo-controlled study from the same group did not demonstrate a positive effect in women treatment prophylactically with nortriptyline.[189] The authors have suggested that nortriptyline may be less effective than SSRIs for the treatment of postpartum depression. The efficacy of prophylactic treatment with SSRIs in this population is under investigation.

In summary, postpartum depressive illness may be conceptualized along a continuum, where some women are at lower risk for puerperal illness and others are at higher risk. Although a less aggressive, "wait-and-see" approach is appropriate for women with no history of postpartum psychiatric illness, women with BPD or histories of postpartum psychiatric illness deserve not only close monitoring but specific prophylactic measures.

Psychiatric Consultation to Obstetrics: From Prevention to Treatment

The psychiatric consultant to an obstetric service may evaluate patients experiencing a range of difficulties. Symptoms may be mild, although the consultant is typically requested when symptoms become severe. Psychiatric disorders may emerge anew during pregnancy, although more often clinical presentations represent persistence or exacerbation of already existing illness. Physicians, therefore, should screen more aggressively for psychiatric disorders either prior to conception or during pregnancy, integrating questions about psychiatric symptoms and treatment into the obstetric history. Identification of at-risk women allows the most thoughtful, acute treatment before, during, and after pregnancy and signals the opportunity to institute prophylactic strategies that prevent psychiatric disturbances in women during the childbearing years.

References

1. Zajicek E: *Psychiatric problems during pregnancy.* In Wolkind S, Zajicek E, editors: *Pregnancy: a psychological and social study*, London, 1981, Academic, pp 57–73.
2. Evans J, Heron J, Francomb H, et al: Cohort study of depressed mood during pregnancy and after childbirth, *BMJ* 323:257–260, 2001.
3. Cohen LS, Sichel DA, Dimmock JA, Rosenbaum JF: Impact of pregnancy on panic disorder: a case series, *J Clin Psychiatry* 55:284–288, 1994.
4. Cohen LS, Sichel DA, Faraone SV, et al: Course of panic disorder during pregnancy and the puerperium: a preliminary study, *Biol Psychiatry* 39:950–954, 1996.
5. Northcott CJ, Stein MB: Panic disorder in pregnancy, *J Clin Psychiatry* 55:539–542, 1994.

6. O'Hara MW: Social support, life events, and depression during pregnancy and the puerperium, *Arch Gen Psychiatry* 43:569–573, 1986.

7. Frank E, Kupfer DJ, Jacob M, et al: Pregnancy related affective episodes among women with recurrent depression, *Am J Psychiatry* 144:288–293, 1987.

8. Kessler RC, McGonagle KA, Swartz M, et al: Sex and depression in the National Comorbidity Survey I: lifetime prevalence, chronicity and recurrence, *J Affect Disord* 29:85–96, 1993.

9. Eaton WW, Kessler RC, Wittchen HU, et al: Panic and panic disorder in the United States, *Am J Psychiatry* 151:413–420, 1994.

10. Kupfer D, Frank E, Perel J, et al: Five-year outcome for maintenance therapies in recurrent depression, *Arch of Gen Psych* 49(10):769–773, 1992.

11. Suppes T, Baldessarini RJ, Faedda GL, et al: Risk of recurrence following discontinuation of lithium treatment in bipolar disorder, *Arch Gen Psychiatry* 48:1082–1088, 1991.

12. Dencker SJ, Malm U, Lepp M: Schizophrenic relapse after drug withdrawal is predictable, *Acta Psychiatric Scan* 73:181–185, 1986.

13. Roy-Byrne PP, Dager SR, Cowley DS, et al: Relapse and rebound following discontinuation of benzodiazepine treatment of panic attacks: alprazolam versus diazepam, *Am J Psychiatry* 146:860–865, 1989.

14. Neziroglu F, Anemone R, Yaryura-Tobias JA: Onset of obsessive-compulsive disorder in pregnancy, *Am J Psychiatry* 149:947–950, 1992.

15. Orr S, Miller C: Maternal depressive symptoms and the risk of poor pregnancy outcome: review of the literature and preliminary findings, *Epidemiol Rev* 17:165–171, 1995.

16. Steer RA, Scholl TO, Hediger ML, et al: Self-reported depression and negative pregnancy outcomes, *J Clin Epidemiol* 45:1093–1099, 1992.

17. Kendell RE, Wainwright S, Hailey A: The influence of childbirth on psychiatric morbidity, *Psychol Med* 6:297–302, 1976.

18. Kendell RE, Chalmers JC, Platz C: Epidemiology of puerperal psychoses, *Br J Psychiatry* 150:662–673, 1987.

19. Kumar R, Robson KM: A prospective study of emotional disorders in childbearing women, *Br J Psychiatry* 144:35–47, 1984.

20. O'Hara MW: *Postpartum depression: causes and consequences.* New York, 1995, Springer-Verlag.

21. Gotlib IH, Whiffen VE, Mount JH: Prevalence rates and demographic characteristics associated with depression in pregnancy and the postpartum period, *J Consulting and Clinical Psychol* 57:269–274, 1989.

22. Moline M, Altshuler L, Cohen L, et al: Expert consensus guideline series: treatment of depression in women, *J Psychiatr Practice*, 2001.

23. Altshuler L, Cohen L, Moline M, et al: Expert consensus guideline series: treatment of depression in women, *Postgrad Med Special Rep* 1–116, 2001.

24. Frautschi S, Cervlli A, Maine D: Suicide during pregnancy and its neglect as a component of maternal mortality, *Int. J Gynaecol Obstetrics* 47:275–284, 1994.

25. Appleby L: Suicide during pregnancy and in the first postnatal year. *BMJ* 302:137–140, 1991.

26. Marzuk M, Tardiff K, Leon AC, et al: Lower risk of suicide during pregnancy, *Am J Psychiatry* 154:122–123, 1997.

27. Beck AT, Rush AJ, Shaw BF, et al: *Cognitive therapy of depression,* New York, 1979, Guilford.

28. Klerman GL, Weissman MM, Rounsaville BJ, et al: *Interpersonal psychotherapy of depression,* New York, 1984, Basic Books Inc, 1984.

29. Spinelli M: Interpersonal psychotherapy for depressed antepartum women: a pilot study, *Am J Psychiatry* 154:1028–1030, 1997.

30. Cohen L, Rosenbaum J: Psychotropic drug use during pregnancy: weighing the risks, *J Clin Psychiatry* 59(suppl 2):18–28, 1998.

31. Cohen L, Altshuler L, Heller V, Rosenbaum J: *Psychotropic drug use in pregnancy.* In Bassuk Ga, editor: *The practitioner's guide to psychoactive drugs,* 4 ed, New York, 1998, Plenum Publishing Corporation, pp 417–440.

32. Cott, Wisner: Psychiatric disorders during pregnancy, *Int Rev Psychiatry* 15:217–230, 2003.

33. Altshuler LL, Cohen LS, Szuba MP, et al: Pharmacologic management of psychiatric illness in pregnancy: dilemmas and guidelines, *Am J Psychiatry* 153:592–606, 1996.

34. Cohen L, Altshuler L: *Pharmacologic management of psychiatric illness during pregnancy and the postpartum period.* In Dunner D, Rosenbaum J, editors: *The psychiatric clinics of North America annual of drug therapy,* Philadelphia, 1997, WB Saunders, pp 21–60.

35. Wisner KL, Gelenberg AJ, Leonard H, et al: Pharmacologic treatment of depression during pregnancy, *JAMA* 282:1264–1269, 1999.

36. Pastuszak A, Schick-Boschetto B, Zuber C, et al: Pregnancy outcome following first-trimester exposure to fluoxetine (Prozac), *JAMA* 269:2246–2248, 1993.

37. Altshuler LL, Hendrick VC: Pregnancy and psychotropic medication: changes in blood levels, *J Clin Psychopharmacol* 16:78–80, 1996.

38. Chambers C, Johnson K, Dick L, et al: Birth outcomes in pregnant women taking fluoxetine, *N Engl J Med* 335:1010–1015, 1996.

39. Nulman I, Rovet J, Stewart D, et al: Neurodevelopment of children exposed in utero to antidepressant drugs, *N Engl J Med* 336:258–262, 1997.

40. Kulin N, Pastuszak A, Sage S, et al: Pregnancy outcome following maternal use of the new selective serotonin reuptake inhibitors: a prospective controlled multicenter study, *JAMA* 279:609–610, 1998.

41. Einarson A, Fatoye B, Sarkar M, Lavigne SV, et al: Pregnancy outcome following gestational exposure to venlafaxine: a multicenter prospective controlled study, *Am J Psychiatry* 158:1728–1730, 2001.

42. Dicke JM: Teratology: principles and practice, *Med Clin North Am* 73:567–581, 1989.

43. McElhatton P, Garbis H, Elefant E, et al: The outcome of pregnancy in 689 women exposed to therapeutic doses of antidepressants: a collaborative study of the European network of teratology information services (ENTIS), *Reprod Toxicol* 10:285–294, 1996.

44. Loebstein R KG: Pregnancy outcome and neurodevelopment of children exposed in utero to psychoactive drugs: the Motherisk experience, *J Psychiatry Neurosci* 22:192–196, 1997.

45. Nulman I, Koren G: The safety of fluoxetine during pregnancy and lactation, *Teratology* 53:304–308, 1996.

46. Goldstein DJ, Williams ML, Pearson DK: Fluoxetine-exposed pregnancies, *Clin Res* 39:768A, 1991.

47. Goldstein DJ: Effects of third trimester fluoxetine exposure on the newborn, *Clin Psychopharmacol* 15:417–420, 1995.

48. Ericson A KB, Wilhom B: Delivery outcome after the use of antidepressants in early pregnancy, *Eur J Clin Psychopharm* 55:503–508, 1999.

49. Cohen LS, Heller VL, Bailey JW, et al: Birth outcomes following prenatal exposure to fluoxetine, *Biol Psychiatry* 48:996–1000, 2000.

50. Goldstein DJ, Sundell KL, Corbin LA: Birth outcomes in pregnant women taking fluoxetine, *N Engl J Med* 336:872–873; author reply 873, 1997.

51. Simon G, Korff MV, Heiligenstein J, et al: Initial antidepressant choice in primary care: effectiveness and cost of fluoxetine vs tricyclic antidepressants, *JAMA* 275:1897–1902, 1996.

52. Inman W, Kobotu K, Pearce G, et al: Prescription event monitoring of paroxetine, *PEM Rep* PXL 1206:1–44, 1993.

53. Simon GE, Cunningham ML, Davis RL: Outcomes of prenatal antidepressant exposure, *Am J Psychiatry* 159:2055–2061, 2002.

54. Henshaw S: Unintended pregnancy in the United States, *Fam Plann Perspect* 30:24–29, 1998.

55. Heinonen O, Sloan D, Shapiro S: *Birth defects and drugs in pregnancy*, Littleton, Mass, 1977, Publishing Services Group.

56. Cowe L, Lloyd D, Dawling S: Neonatal convulsions caused by withdrawal from maternal clomipramine, *Brit Med J* 284:1837–1838, 1982.

57. Eggermont E: Withdrawal symptoms in neonates associated with maternal imipramine therapy, *Lancet* 2:680, 1973.

58. Schimmel M, Katz E, Shaag Y, et al: Toxic neonatal effects following maternal clomipramine therapy, *Clin Toxicol* 29:479–484, 1991.

59. Webster PAC: Withdrawal symptoms in neonates associated with maternal antidepressant therapy, *Lancet* 2:318–319, 1973.

60. Bromiker R, Kaplan M: Apparent intrauterine fetal withdrawal from clomipramine hydrochloride, *JAMA* 272:1722–1723, 1994.

61. Falterman LG, Richardson DJ: Small left colon syndrome associated with maternal ingestion of psychotropics, *J Pediatr* 97:300–310, 1980.

62. Shearer WT, Schreiner RL, Marshall RE: Urinary retention in a neonate secondary to maternal ingestion of nortriptyline, *J Pediatr* 81:570–572, 1972.

63. Spencer M: Fluoxetine hydrochloride (Prozac) toxicity in the neonate, *Pediatrics* 92:721–722, 1993.

64. Nulman I RJ, Stewart DE, Wolpin J, et al: Child development following exposure to tricyclic antidepressants or fluoxetine throughout fetal life: a prospective, controlled study, *Am J Psychiatry* 159:1889–1895, 2002.

65. Casper RC, Fleisher BE, Lee-Aneajas JC, et al: Follow-up of children of depressed mothers exposed or not exposed to antidepressant drugs during pregnancy, *J Pediatrics* 142:402–408, 2003.

66. Costei AM, Kozer E, Ho T: Perinatal outcome following third trimester exposure to paroxetine, *Arch Pediatr Adolesc Med* 156:1129–1132, 2002.

67. Dahl M, Olhager E, Ahlner J: Paroxetine withdrawal syndrome in a neonate (letter), *British J Psych* 171:391–392, 1997.

68. Stiskal JA, Kulin N, Koren G, Ho T, et al: Neonatal paroxetine withdrawal syndrome, *Arch Dis Child Fetal Neonatal Educ* 84:F134–F135, 2001.

69. Nordeng H, Lindemann R, Perminov KV, Reikvam A: Neonatal withdrawal syndrome after in utero exposure to selective serotonin reuptake inhibitors, *Acta Paediatr* 90:288–291, 2001.

70. Laine K, Heikkinen T, Ekblad U, Kero P: Effects of exposure to selective serotonin reuptake inhibitors during pregnancy on serotonergic symptoms in newborns and cord blood monoamine and prolactin concentrations, *Arch Gen Psychiatry* 60:720–726, 2003.

71. Cohen LS, Rosenbaum JF: Psychotropic drug use during pregnancy: weighing the risks, *J Clin Psychiatry* 59:18–28, 1998.

72. Krauer: *Pharmacotherapy during pregnancy: emphasis on pharmacokinetics in drug therapy during pregnancy*, 1985, Butterworths, pp 9–31.

73. Jeffries WS, Bochner F: The effect of pregnancy on drug pharmacokinetics, *Med J Aust* 149:675–677, 1988.

74. Wisner K, Perel J, Wheeler S: Tricyclic dose requirements across pregnancy, *Am J Psychiatr* 150:1541–1542, 1993.

75. Hostetter A, Stowe ZN, Strader JR, Jr., et al: Dose of selective serotonin uptake inhibitors across pregnancy: clinical implications, *Depress Anxiety* 11:51–57, 2000.

76. Ferrill MJ, Kehoe WA, Jacisin JJ: ECT during pregnancy: physiologic and pharmacologic considerations, *Convul Ther* 8:186–200, 1992.

77. Miller LJ: Use of electroconvulsive therapy during pregnancy, *Hosp Comm Psychiatry* 45:444–450, 1994.

78. Cohen LS, Heller VL, Rosenbaum JF: Treatment guidelines for psychotropic drug use in pregnancy, *Psychosomatics* 30:25–33, 1989.

79. Eggermont E, Raveschat J, Deneve V: The adverse influence of imipramine on the adaptation of the newborn infant to extrauterine life, *Acta Paediatr Belg* 26:197–204, 1972.

80. Cooper GL: The safety of fluoxetine: an update, *Br J Psychiatry* 153:77–86, 1989.

81. Weinstein MR, Goldfield MD: Cardiovascular malformations with lithium use during pregnancy, *Am J Psychiatry* 132:529–531, 1975.

82. Schou M, Goldfield MD, Weinstein MR, et al: Lithium and pregnancy, I: Report from the register of lithium babies, *Br Med J* 2:135–136, 1973.

83. Cohen LS, Friedman JM, Jefferson JW, et al: A reevaluation of risk of in utero exposure to lithium, *JAMA* 271:146–150, 1994.

84. Rosa FW: Spina bifida in infants of women treated with carbamazepine during pregnancy, *N Engl J Med* 324:674–677, 1991.

85. Lindhout D, Meinardi H: Spina bifida and in-utero exposure to valproate, *Lancet* 2:396, 1984.

86. Lammer EJ, Sever LE, Oakley GP: Teratogen update: valproic acid, *Teratology* 35:465–473, 1987.

87. Omtzigt JGC, Los FJ, Grobbee DE, et al: The risk of spina bifida aperta after first-trimester exposure to valproate in a prenatal cohort, *Neurology* 42:119–125, 1992.

88. Ernst CL, Goldberg JF: The reproductive safety profile of mood stabilizers, atypical antipsychotics, and broad-spectrum psychotropics, *J Clin Psychiatry* 63:42–55, 2002.

89. Corporation GK: Lamotrigine pregnancy registry—interim report, September 1992 through March 2003: Research Triangle (NC), 2003.

90. Viguera AC, Cohen LS, Baldessarini RJ, Nonacs R: Managing bipolar disorder during pregnancy: weighing the risks and benefits, *Can J Psychiatry* 47:426–436, 2002.

91. Faedda GL, Tondo L, Baldessarini RJ, et al: Outcome after rapid vs gradual discontinuation of lithium treatment in bipolar disorders, *Arch Gen Psychiatry* 50:448–455, 1993.

92. Tohen M, Waternaux CM, Tsuang MT: Outcome in mania: a 4-year prospective follow-up of 75 patients utilizing survival analysis, *Arch Gen Psychiatry* 47:1106–1111, 1990.

93. Suppes T, Baldessarini R, Faedda G, et al: Discontinuation of maintenance treatment in bipolar disorder: risks and implications, *Harv Rev Psychiatry* 1:131–144, 1993.

94. Nonacs R VA, Cohen L: Risks of postpartum relapse in pregnant women with bipolar disorder: syllabus and proceedings summary of the 151st Annual Meeting of the American Psychiatric Association 1997, 1998.

95. Spielvogel A, Wile J: Treatment and outcomes of psychotic patients during pregnancy and childbirth, *Birth* 19, 1992.

96. Wrede G, Mednick S, Huttenen M: Pregnancy and delivery complications in the births of unselected series of Finnish children with schizophrenic mothers, *Acta Psychiatr Scand* 62:369–381, 1980.

97. Miller LJ: Psychotic denial of pregnancy: phenomenology and clinical management, *Hosp Comm Psychiatry* 41:1233–1237, 1990.

98. Hanson G, Oakley G: Haloperidol and limb deformity, *JAMA* 231:26, 1975.

99. van Waes A, van de Velde E: Safety evaluation of haloperidol in the treatment of hyperemesis gravidum, *J Clin Psychopharmacol* 224–237, 1969.

100. Rumeau-Rouguette C, Goujard J, Huel G: Possible teratogenic effect of phenothiazines in human beings, *Teratology* 15:57–64, 1977.

101. Edlund MJ, Craig TJ: Antipsychotic drug use and birth defects: an epidemiologic reassessment, *Compr Psychiatry* 25:32–37, 1984.

102. Sos J, Cassem NH: Managing postoperative agitation, *Drug Ther* 10:103–106, 1980.

103. Tesar GE, Stern TA: Evaluation and treatment of agitation in the intensive care unit, *J Intensive Care Med* 1:137–148, 1986.

104. Cohen LS, Rosenbaum JF, Heller VL: Panic attack-associated placental abruption: a case report, *J Clin Psychiatry* 50:266–267, 1989.

105. Crandon AJ: Maternal anxiety and neonatal well-being, *J Psychosom Res* 23:113–115, 1979.

106. Istvan J: Stress, anxiety, and birth outcome: a critical review of the evidence, *Psychol Bull* 100:331–348, 1986.

107. Cowley DS, Roy-Byrne PP: Panic disorder during pregnancy, *J Psychosom Obstet Gynaecol* 10:193–210, 1989.

108. George DT, Ladenheim JA, Nutt DJ: Effect of pregnancy on panic attacks, *Am J Psychiatry* 144:1078–1079, 1987.

109. Klein DF, Skrobala AM, Garfinkel DS: Preliminary look at the effects of pregnancy on the course of panic disorder (technical note), *Anxiety* 1:227–232, 1994.

110. Villeponteaux VA, Lydiard RB, Laraia MT, et al: The effects of pregnancy on pre-existing panic disorder, *J Clin Psychiatry* 53:201–203, 1992.

111. Cohen LS, Sichel DA, Dimmock JA, et al: Postpartum course in women with preexisting panic disorder, *J Clin Psychiatry* 55:289–292, 1994.

112. Cohen LS, Sichel DA, Farone SV, et al: Prospective study of panic disorder during pregnancy, presented at the annual meeting of the American Psychiatric Association, New York, May 4, 1996.

113. Otto M, Pollack M, Sachs G, et al: Discontinuation of benzodiazepine treatment: efficacy of cognitive-behavioral therapy for patients with panic disorder, *Am J Psych* 150:1485–1490, 1993.

114. Robinson L, Walker JR, Anderson D: Cognitive-behavioural treatment of panic disorder during pregnancy and lactation, *Can J Psychiatry* 37:623–626, 1992.

115. Safra MJ, Oakley GP: Association between cleft lip with or without cleft palate and prenatal exposure to diazepam, *Lancet* 2:478–480, 1975.

116. Saxen I: Association between oral clefts and drugs taken during pregnancy, *Int J Epidemiol* 4:37–44, 1975.

117. Aarskog D: Association between maternal intake of diazepam and oral clefts, *Lancet* 2, 1975.

118. Rosenberg L, Mitchell AA, Parsells JL, et al: Lack of relation of oral clefts to diazepam use during pregnancy, *N Engl J Med* 309:1282–1285, 1983.

119. Shiono PH, Mills IL: Oral clefts and diazepam use during pregnancy (letter), *N Engl J Med* 311:919–920, 1984.

120. Dolovich L, Antonio A, Vaillancourt JR, et al: Benzodiazepine use in pregnancy and major malformations or oral cleft: meta-analysis of cohort and case-control studies, *BMJ* 317:839–843, 1998.

121. Weinstock L: Clonazepam use during pregnancy, presented at the annual meeting of the American Psychiatric Society, New York, May 4, 1996.

122. Sheehan DV, Ballenger J, Jacobsen G: Treatment of endogenous anxiety with phobic, hysterical and hypochondriacal symptoms, *Arch Gen Psychiatry* 37:51–59, 1980.

123. Chouinard G, Annable L, Fontaine R, et al: Alprazolam in the treatment of generalized anxiety and panic disorders: a double-blind placebo controlled study, *Psychopharmacology* 77:229–233, 1982.

124. Dunner DL, Ishiki D, Avery DH, et al: Effect of alprazolam and diazepam on anxiety and panic attacks in panic disorder: a controlled study, *J Clin Psychiatry* 47:458–460, 1986.

125. Gorman JM, Liebowitz MR, Fyer AJ, et al: An open trial of fluoxetine in the treatment of panic attacks, *J Clin Psychopharmacol* 7:329–332, 1987.

126. Charney DS, Woods SW, Goodman WK, et al: Drug treatment of panic disorder: the comparative efficacy of imipramine, alprazolam, and trazodone, *J Clin Psychiatry* 47:580–586, 1986.

127. Gillberg C: "Floppy infant death syndrome" and maternal diazepam, *Lancet* 2:244, 1977.

128. Speight A: Floppy infant syndrome and maternal diazepam and/or nitrazepam, *Lancet* 2:878, 1977.

129. Fisher J, Edgren B, Mammel M: Neonatal apnea associated with maternal clonazepam therapy, *Obstet Gynacol* 66:34s–35s, 1985.

130. Mazzi E: Possible neonatal diazepam withdrawal: a case report, *Am J Obstet Gynecol* 129:586–587, 1977.

131. Rementaria JL, Blatt K: Withdrawal symptoms in neonates from intrauterine exposure to diazepam, *J Pediatr* 90:123–126, 1977.

132. Whitelaw A, Cummings A, McFadyen I: Effect of maternal lorazepam on the neonate, *Br Med J* 282:1106–1108, 1981.

133. Rowlatt R: Effect of maternal diazepam on the newborn, *Br J Anaethesiol* 1:985, 1987.

134. Sichel DA, Cohen LS, Dimmock JA, et al: Postpartum obsessive compulsive disorder: a case series, *J Clin Psychiatry* 54, 1993.

135. Sichel DA, Cohen LS, Rosenbaum JF, et al: Postpartum onset of obsessive-compulsive disorder, *Psychosomatics* 34:277–279, 1993.

136. Goldstein H, Weinberg J, Sankstone M: Shock therapy in psychosis complicating pregnancy: a case report, *Am J Psychiatr* 98:201–202, 1941.

137. Impasato DJ, Gabriel AR, Lardara M: Electric and insulin shock therapy during pregnancy, *Dis Nerv Syst* 25:542–546, 1964.

138. Remick RA, Maurice WL: ECT in pregnancy (letter), *Am J Psychiatry* 135:761–762, 1978.

139. Wise MG, Ward SC, Townsend-Parchman W, et al: Case report of ECT during high-risk pregnancy, *Am J Psychiatry* 141:99–101, 1984.

140. Repke JT, Berger NG: Electroconvulsive therapy in pregnancy, *Obstet Gynecol* 63:39s–40s, 1984.

141. Sherer DM, D'Amico LD, Warshal DP, et al: Recurrent mild abruptio placentae occurring immediately after repeated electroconvulsive therapy in pregnancy, *Am J Obstet Gynecol* 165:652–653, 1991.

142. Llewellyn A, Stowe Z: Psychotropic medications in lactation, *J Clin Psychiatry* 59(suppl 2):41–52, 1998.

143. Burt VK, Suri R, Altshuler L, et al: The use of psychotropic medications during breast-feeding, *Am J Psychiatry* 158:1001–1009, 2001.

144. Newport DJ, Hostetter A, Arnold A, et al: The treatment of postpartum depression: minimizing infant exposures, *J Clin Psychiatry* 63:31–44, 2002.

145. Birnbaum CS, Cohen LS, Bailey JW, et al: Serum concentrations of antidepressants and benzodiazepines in nursing infants: a case series, *Pediatrics* 104:e11, 1999.

146. Misri S, Kim J, Riggs KW, et al: Paroxetine levels in postpartum depressed women, breast milk, and infant serum, *J Clin Psychiatry* 61:828–832, 2000.

147. Stowe ZN, Cohen LS, Hostetter A, et al: Paroxetine in human breast milk and nursing infants, *Am J Psychiatry* 157:185–189, 2000.

148. Hendrick V, Fukuchi A, Altshuler L, et al: Use of sertraline, paroxetine and fluvoxamine by nursing women, *Br J Psychiatry* 179:163–166, 2001.

149. Hendrick V, Stowe ZN, Altshuler LL, et al: Fluoxetine and norfluoxetine concentrations in nursing infants and breast milk, *Biol Psychiatry* 50:775–782, 2001.

150. Stowe Z: The pharmokinetics of sertraline excretion into human breast milk: determinants of infant serum concentrations, *J Clin Psychiatry* 64:73–80, 2003.

151. Suri R, Stowe Z, Hendrick V, et al: Estimates of nursing infant daily dose of fluoxetine through breast milk, *Biol Psych* Accepted, 2002.

152. Epperson N, Czarkowsk KA, Ward-O'Brien D, et al: Maternal sertraline treatment and serotonin transport in breast-feeding mother-infant pairs, *Am J Psychiatry* 158:1631–7, 2001.

153. Wesson DR CS, Harkey M, Smith DE: Diazepam and desmethyldiazepam in breast milk, *J Psychoactive Drugs* 17:55–56, 1985.

154. Yoshida K SB, Craggs M, Kumar R: Neuroleptic drugs in breast-milk: a study of pharmacokinetics and of possible adverse effects in breast-fed infants, *Psychol Med* 28:81–91, 1998.

155. Wiles DH OM, Kolakowska T: Chlorpromazine levels in plasma and milk of nursing mothers, *Br J Clin Pharmacol* 5:272–273, 1978.

156. Barnas C, Bergant A, Hummer M, et al: Clozapine concentrations in maternal and fetal plasma, amniotic fluid, and breast milk (letter), *Am J Psychiatry* 151:945, 1994.

157. Goldstein DJ CL, Fung MC: Olanzapine-exposed pregnancies and lactation: early experience, *J Clin Psychopharmacol* 20:399–403, 2000.

158. Schou M, Amdisen A: Lithium and pregnancy: III. lithium ingestion by children breastfed by women on lithium treatment, *Br Med J* 2:138, 1973.

159. Schou M: Lithium treatment during pregnancy, delivery, and lactation: an update, *J Clin Psychiatry* 51:410–413, 1990.

160. Tunnessen WW, Hertz CG: Toxic effects of lithium in newborn infants: a commentary, *J Pediatr* 81:804–807, 1972.

161. Frey BS: Transient cholestatic hepatitis in a neonate associated with carbamazepine exposure during pregnancy and breast-feeding, *Eur J Pediatr* 150:136–138, 1990.

162. Merlob P, Mor N, Litwin A: Transient hepatic dysfunction in an infant of an epileptic mother treated with carbamazepine during pregnancy and breastfeeding, *Ann Pharmacother* 12:1563–1565, 1992.

163. Bratfos O, Haug JO: Puerperal mental disorders in manic depressive females, *Acta Psychiatr Scand* 42:285–294, 1966.

164. Reich T, Winokur G: Postpartum psychosis in patients with manic depressive disease, *J Nerv Ment Dis* 151:60–68, 1970.

165. Davidson J, Robertson E: A follow-up study of postpartum illness, *Acta Psychiatr Scand* 71:451–457, 1985.

166. Kupfer DJ, Frank E: Relapse in recurrent unipolar depression, *Am J Psychiatry* 144:86–88, 1987.

167. Dean C, Williams RJ, Brockington IF: Is puerperal psychosis the same as bipolar manic-depressive disorder? A family study, *Psychol Med* 19:637–647, 1989.

168. Viguera AC, Nonacs R, Cohen LS, et al: Risk of recurrence of bipolar disorder in pregnant and nonpregnant women after discontinuing lithium maintenance, *Am J Psychiatry* 157:179–184, 2000.

169. O'Hara MW, Zekoski EM, Phillips LH, et al: A controlled prospective study of postpartum mood disorders: comparison of childbearing and nonchildbearing women, *J Abnorm Psychol* 99:3–15, 1990.

170. Handley SL, Dunn TL, Waldron G, et al: Tryptophan, cortisol and puerperal mood, *Br J Psychiatry* 136:498–508, 1980.

171. Parekh R: A prospective study of blues, American Psychiatric Association annual meeting, New York, accepted for presentation, 1996.

172. Hendrick V, Altshuler L, Strouse T, et al: Postpartum and nonpostpartum depression: differences in presentation and response to pharmacologic treatment, *Depress Anxiety* 11:66–72, 2000.

173. Buttolph ML, Holland A: *Obsessive compulsive disorders in pregnancy and childbirth*. In Jenike M, Baer L, Minichiello WE, editors: *Obsessive compulsive disorders, theory and management*, Chicago, 1990, Yearbook Medical Publishers.

174. Murray L: Postpartum depression and child development, *Psychol Med* 27:253–260, 1997.

175. Hayworth J, Little BC, Carter SB, et al: A predictive study of post-partum depression: some predisposing characteristics, *Br J Med Psychol* 53:161–167, 1980.

176. Appleby L, Warner R, Whitton A, et al: A controlled study of fluoxetine and cognitive-behavioral counselling in the treatment of postnatal depression, *BMJ* 314:932–936, 1997.

177. O'Hara MW, Stuart S, Gorman LL, et al: Efficacy of interpersonal psychotherapy for postpartum depression, *Arch Gen Psychiatry* 57:1039–1045, 2000.

178. Stowe ZN, Casarella J, Landrey J, et al: Sertraline in the treatment of women with postpartum major depression, *Depression* 3:49–55, 1995.

179. Cohen LS, Viguera AC, Bouffard SM, et al: Venlafaxine in the treatment of postpartum depression, *J Clin Psychiatry* 62:592–596, 2001.

180. Dalton K: Progesterone prophylaxis used successfully in postnatal depression, *Practitioner* 229:507–508, 1985.

181. Gregoire AJ, Kumar R, Everitt B, et al: Transdermal estrogen for treatment of severe postnatal depression, *Lancet* 347:930–933, 1996.

182. Gregoire A: Estrogen supplementation in postpartum depression, Marcé Society Meeting, Cambridge, England, 1994.

183. Ahokas A: Kaukoranta J, Wahlbeck K, Aito M: Estrogen deficiency in severe postpartum depression: successful treatment with sublingual physiologic 17beta-estradiol: a preliminary study, *J Clin Psychiatry* 62:332–336, 2001.

184. Austin M-PV: Puerperal affective psychosis: is there a case for lithium prophylaxis? *Br J Psychiatry* 161:692–694, 1992.

185. Stewart DE, Klompenhouwer JL, Kendall RE, et al: Prophylactic lithium in puerperal psychosis: the experience of three centers, *Br J Psychiatry* 158:393–397, 1991.

186. Sichel DA, Cohen LS, Rosenbaum JF: High dose estrogen prophylaxis in 11 women at risk for recurrent

postpartum psychosis and severe non-psychotic depression, Annual Meeting of the Marcé Society, Einthoven, the Netherlands, November 5, 1993.

187. Cohen LS, Sichel DA, Robertson LM, et al: Postpartum prophylaxis for women with bipolar disorder, *Am J Psychiatry* 152:1641–1645, 1995.

188. Wisner KL, Wheeler SB: Prevention of recurrent postpartum major depression, *Hosp Comm Psychiatry* 45:1191–1196, 1994.

189. Wisner P. Prevention of recurrent postpartum depression: a randomized clinical trial, *J Clin Psychiatry* 62:82–86, 2001.

Chapter 35

Patients with Eating Disorders

Anne E. Becker, M.D., Ph.D.
Esther Jacobowitz Israel, M.D.

Eating disorders are common among adolescent and young adult women and are associated with serious morbidity and mortality. Patients with eating disorders often present a multidimensional clinical challenge in the general hospital setting; they frequently have medical complications, go undetected in clinical settings, and are typically reluctant to accept treatment. Patients with anorexia nervosa (AN), bulimia nervosa (BN), binge-eating disorder (BED), and atypical eating disorders will almost always benefit from integrated multidisciplinary care, with a team that includes primary care and mental health clinicians as well as a nutritionist. Medical and nutri- tional stabilization are clinical priorities but are treatment-specific to managing the psychological and psychiatric dimensions of the illness and can be set into motion as early as they are identified.

Epidemiology

Eating disorders affect over 5 million Americans.[1] Although their prevalence is highest in westernized and postindustrial societies, eating disorders appear to have global distribution.[2] Moreover, recent data have dispelled a previous clinical stereotype that associated eating disorders with affluent white girls and women. Indeed, eating disorders are prevalent among ethnic minority women. Rates among Latinos may be comparable to non-Latino whites, and

rates among Native American women may exceed those among whites.[3] Moreover, rates of binge eating and BED may be elevated in Black and Latino women compared with white women in both community and clinic-based samples.[4–10] Whereas eating disorders and clinically significant disordered eating most commonly occur in the young adult female population, they also occur in males, albeit at lower rates (5% to 15% of cases of AN and BN occur in males).[11] However, the most prevalent eating disorder, BED, is relatively common among men, with 40% of cases occurring in males.[12] Full-syndrome AN occurs at a prevalence of 0.28% in young adult females; BN has a prevalence of approximately 1% in young adult females,[13] The point prevalence of BED in community samples in the United States is 1% to 2%, but the prevalence of BED in weight-treatment–seeking populations ranges up to 30%.[14,15]

Although various guidelines have been proposed to assess subthreshold eating disorders and disordered eating,[16–18] the consensus is that they are prevalent among U.S. females and pose a risk for significant impairment and distress.[19] For example, for U.S. women, lifetime prevalence of anorexia-like syndromes has been reported as over 3%[16] and the lifetime risk for bulimia-like syndromes as 8%.[17] Even higher prevalence rates are reported for specific individual symptoms (e.g., in 2001, 7.8% of adolescent women in the United States reported purging and 19.1% reported fasting in the last month to lose weight).[20] Although the clinical significance of isolated symptoms is debatable, substantial evidence supports the notion that disordered eating is commonly a precursor of a full-syndrome eating disorder[21] and thus likely part of a spectrum of eating disturbances.[16,17]

Etiology, Onset, and Course

The etiology of eating disorders is believed to have genetic, psychodevelopmental, and sociocultural underpinnings, but understanding of their specific contributions is limited. With respect to genetic contributions, whereas twin studies strongly support heritability of eating disorders, attempts to identify candidate genes have yielded mostly inconsistent or negative data thus far. Heritability estimates for AN and BN are impressive, with genetic contributions ranging from 58% to 76% for AN[22] and 30% to 83% for BN.[23,24] Although there are no family or twin studies that have investigated the heritability of BED, a recent study has identified a strong association of binge eating in obese subjects with mutations in the melanocortin receptor gene.[25] On the other hand, variability in the prevalence of disordered eating among culturally distinct populations strongly suggests contributions of sociocultural factors. Whereas social pressures to be thin, exposure to media imagery, westernization, urbanization, and transnational migration have been associated with elevated risk, the mechanisms by which social forces influence pathogenesis remain incompletely understood.[2] An incomplete understanding of etiology to date has thwarted efforts to develop effective primary prevention programs for eating disorders.

AN and BN most commonly have their onset in adolescence; eating disorders are relatively rare in young children compared with postpubertal adolescents and young adults. Although AN can be seen in young children,[26] it is far less common (i.e., only 5%) in prepubertal girls.[27–30] Moreover, the onset of BN is usually late adolescence[28] and prepubertal bulimic behavior is reported to be uncommon.[31] Finally, the onset of BED is typically in the early twenties.[5,32] Despite rapidly evolving pharmacologic and psychosocial treatment strategies for the eating disorders, approximately half of cases of AN and BN follow a chronic course,[33,34] and 43% of individuals with BED continued to be symptomatic in a 6-year longitudinal study of BED.[35] It is not uncommon for individuals with AN, BN, and BED to transition from one diagnostic category to another during the course of their illness.

In addition to their considerable prevalence, eating disorders are associated with serious medical comorbidity and mortality. Eating disorders and substance abuse are associated with the highest risk of premature death compared with all psychiatric illnesses.[36] The mortality rate from AN alone is 0.56% annually.[37] Moreover, AN is associated with an all-cause death risk five times what is expected and BN a risk nine times that expected. It is also important to note that whereas some of the deaths associated with AN were directly attributable to self-starvation, the mortality risk for suicide was 33 times the amount expected.[36] Because of the serious medical complications associated with eating disorders, patients often present to primary care, emergency departments, or hospital inpatient settings—not infrequently with an undisclosed or unrecognized eating disorder. Given that up to half of cases of eating disorders may be undetected in primary care settings,[38–43] inpatient and outpatient medical and pediatric services present significant opportunities to make a new diagnosis of an eating disorder and to initiate treatment. Furthermore, it appears that initiating treatment relatively earlier in the course of the illness may improve outcome.[44]

Differential Diagnosis and Initial Assessment of Eating Disorders

Given that optimal treatment strategies for eating disorders rely on accurate diagnosis, attention must be paid to creation of a careful differential diagnosis during the initial evaluation. This is often less than straightforward, given that there is substantial symptom overlap (Table 35-1) and crossover among diagnostic categories. Moreover, some medical complaints—particularly those associated with gastrointestinal symptoms and weight loss—can obscure an underlying or associated eating disorder. For example, some individuals successfully disguise their restrictive diet as a means to minimize severe bloating, nausea, or constipation. Since a restrictive diet can,

Table 35-1. Differential Diagnosis of Eating Disorders[12]

	Physiologic Symptoms	Cognitive or Emotional Symptoms	Behavioral Symptoms	Associated Distress or Impairment
Anorexia Nervosa (AN)	BMI ≤17.5 or <85% expected body weight Amenorrhea	Fear of weight gain or fatness Body image disturbance: e.g., excessive concern with body weight and shape and undue influence on self-regard; denial of seriousness of medical complications of symptoms, or feeling fat when actually thin	No specific symptoms required to meet DSM diagnostic criteria Almost always associated with restrictive pattern of eating Associated with bingeing or purging behavior in 50% of cases	None required to meet DSM diagnostic criteria; in fact, individuals with anorexia nervosa often are in denial of the serious nature of their illness
Bulimia Nervosa (BN)	BMI can be any range; but a BMI ≤17.5 would likely shift the diagnosis to AN; frequently normal to overweight	Excessive impact of body shape or weight on self-regard Frequently excessively preoccupied with body shape and weight	Frequent and regular binge eating (at least twice weekly for at least 3 months) Frequent and regular inappropriate compensatory behaviors to prevent weight gain (e.g., purging, fasting, excessive exercise; at least twice weekly for at least 3 months)	None required, although many individuals are distressed by their symptoms
Binge-eating Disorder (BED)	BMI can be any range, but a BMI ≤17.5 would likely shift the diagnosis to AN; frequently overweight	Eating symptoms often associated with embarrassment or disgust	Frequent and regular binge eating (on at least 2 days weekly) Binge eating often associated with: Eating rapidly Eating alone Eating while not hungry Eating well past satiety to the point of discomfort No regular inappropriate compensatory behaviors to prevent weight gain	Marked distress about the binge eating is present
Eating Disorder, Not Otherwise Specific (ED NOS)	BMI can be any range, but a BMI ≤17.5 would likely shift the diagnosis to AN	All of the above are possible	All of the above are possible but full-syndrome criteria not met for AN or BN Can be associated with chewing and spitting out food and inappropriate compensatory behaviors following small or normal quantities of food as well	Distress can be present or absent

in fact, *cause* these symptoms, clinicians often find themselves in a clinical catch-22 with such patients.[45] Unfortunately, unless an eating disorder is suspected based on history, patients sometimes only come to psychiatric attention after an extensive medical evaluation has excluded a medical etiology. In other cases, the etiology of symptoms remains unclear and psychiatric consultation is sought to clarify contributions from an eating disorder or other mental illness. Using the same example, in the vast majority of such cases, gastrointestinal symptoms due to disordered eating will remit with nutritional rehabilitation, psychiatric care, and conservative management.[45] Having said this, it is always appropriate to consider the panoply of medical and psychiatric differential diagnoses that could contribute to symptoms. This is particularly true for unexplained weight loss in a demographic group not generally associated with AN or for patients who do not clearly exhibit the excessive concern with weight associated with AN. But it is also true for patients with what appear to be classic symptoms of an eating disorder, given the frequent association between acute weight loss of medical etiology and the onset of a bona fide eating disorder.

Patients with AN are notoriously reluctant to seek or accept treatment for their symptoms; some even go to great lengths to avoid a clinician's detection of their symptoms. If they cannot avoid a visit to the doctor, they will likely avoid being weighed there. They may layer their clothing to give the appearance of normal weight, or, if they anticipate being weighed, they may "water load" (i.e., drink excessive quantities of water) or even tape weights to themselves to make their weight appear closer to normal.

Individuals with BN also commonly avoid treatment, although many eventually become distressed enough by their symptoms to accept it. For these reasons, individuals may only come to medical attention for their eating disorder when they arouse suspicion on a medical or pediatric service, either by unexplained weight changes or by other medical symptoms, or when family members report concerns. For instance, family members might notice restrictive food intake (e.g., a girl becomes a vegetarian or vegan and progressively narrows food selections), secretive

behavior concerning food (e.g., parents notice large quantities of food are consumed after the rest of the family has gone to bed, or cafeteria charges are very high on a term bill), or bathroom use after meals (e.g., a girl is noted to frequently leave the family table to use the bathroom during or just after meals).

Given the prevalence and associated mortality and morbidity of the eating disorders, clinicians should maintain appropriate vigilance for eating disorders in general hospital settings. Obtaining a weight on a patient is frequently a useful probe for concerns about eating disorders (in addition to clarifying the diagnosis and suggesting the most effective therapies). If a patient balks, this can be explored further; however, a weight should be obtained nonetheless if there is a concern about a patient being too underweight. Weighing underweight patients is an inexpensive, convenient, and sensitive procedure; it is an optimal means of establishing nutritional compromise. While the clinician should be sensitive to the patient's discomfort (e.g., by ensuring privacy and offering patients the option of turning their back to the scale if they prefer not to know their weight), he or she should insist on measuring weight and height in the initial evaluation of the patient.

Additional useful probes in exploring the possibility of an eating disorder include taking a relatively straightforward inventory of dietary patterns and any inappropriate compensatory behaviors (Figure 35-1). Patients frequently experience embarrassment when volunteering information about such symptoms and often recall that having a clinician inquire about the symptom was an enormous relief when they felt isolated or unable to disclose their symptoms. Patients are generally heartened to learn that a clinician is savvy about eating disorders, and this expertise is conveyed by a comprehensive inventory of these disordered attitudes and behaviors.

Another useful set of probes focuses on weight and dieting history. Frequent fluctuations in dieting and weight sometimes suggest restrictive and/or binge patterns of eating. When asked about dieting, a patient may disclose that he or she experienced intense family or social pressures to maintain a certain appearance (e.g., mothers who dieted jointly with their young daughters, fathers who were extremely critical of appearance, coaches

Symptom	History	Current	Frequency/Severity	Duration
Restrictive eating (e.g., restricting type or amount of food; skipping meals, fasting)				
Binge eating				
Compulsive overeating				
Vomiting				
Syrup of ipecac use				
Laxative use				
Enema use				
Diuretic use				
Diet pill use (including natural supplements)				
Stimulant use (including caffeine, methylphenidate, and cocaine)				
Inappropriate behaviors related to medical conditions (e.g., withholding of insulin if diabetic, consumption of foods that promote diarrhea in the setting of bowel disease)				
Excessive exercise				

Figure 35-1. Behavioral Symptom Inventory for Assessment of Disordered Eating.

who pressured for a lower weight to enhance athletic performance). This may lead them to disclose extreme dieting or other compensatory behaviors used to manage weight, some of which can be clinically worrisome. It is quite useful to ask patients their current and desired weights as well as what and when their minimum and maximum weights have been. This information will provide a range that will allow assessment of past capacity for nutritional compromise, a gauge of where the patient is now in relation to his or her healthiest and most compromised weights, as well as a realistic assessment of reasonable clinical goals for the weight. Finally, the reported desired weight suggests whether there is a distorted view of the body present, whether the patient desires to be unreasonably thin, and whether the patient and clinician are likely to negotiate common treatment goals with respect to weight. For younger patients whose parents are involved in their care, a question about desired weight is useful to establish that the parent has reasonable expectations for the patient's weight. Psychoeducational information about appropriate weights for height can be reviewed with the patient and others involved in supporting participation in treatment.

Differential Diagnosis

For patients who are more forthcoming about their symptoms, differential diagnosis is relatively straightforward. AN is characterized in the *DSM-IV*[12] by a body weight less than 85% of expected body weight (or body mass index [BMI] ≤17.5), a fear of fatness, some type of body image disturbance (i.e., excessive impact of body shape or weight on self-image, feeling fat when actually thin, denial of seriousness of low weight), and amenorrhea (in women who have passed menarche) (Table 35-1).[12] There have been reports, however, from Asia that fear of fatness is absent in a substantial proportion of cases of AN there,[46,47] so some cultural specificity of the characteristic symptoms appears likely. Moreover, the utility of amenorrhea as a diagnostic criterion for AN has also been questioned.[48] AN occurs as two types, restricting and binge eating/purging. In the latter type, individuals binge and purge in addition to maintaining their low weight; bingeing and purging occurs in about half of anorexics.

Assessment for appropriateness of body weight for height is absolutely essential to evaluation of patients with eating disorders. This is necessary to establish a diagnostic criterion for AN, to assess risk for medical complications due to underweight or obesity, to assess need for active weight management, and to assess need for inpatient-level care. Appropriateness of weight for height and age for children and adolescents can be assessed with standardized weight nomograms. Appropriateness of weight for height for adults can be made with one of two formulae:

BMI = Height (in meters)/ Weight (in kg)^2
Percent expected body weight (%EBW) =
   Actual weight/expected body weight × 100%
Expected body weight =
Women: 100 lb for the first 5 feet + 5 lb/ inch
   above 5 feet ± 10%
Men: 106 lb for the first 5 feet + 6 lb/ inch above
   5 feet ± 10%[49]

BN is characterized by regular binge eating and by inappropriate compensatory behaviors (both at least twice weekly for 3 months) to control weight. In addition, BN is characterized by excessive concern with body shape or weight, which has a major impact on self-regard (Table 35-1). BN can occur as one of two types: purging (i.e., regularly inducing vomiting or using laxatives, diuretics, or enemas) or nonpurging (i.e., not using the aforementioned methods, but controlling weight by restrictive eating or by excessive exercise).[12] Although AN and BN can have substantial phenomenological overlap in symptoms (i.e., excessive concern with weight, binge or restrictive pattern eating, and purging), they are best differentiated by the weight criterion, such that a low-weight individual with bingeing and purging and excessive concern with weight is likely to best fit diagnostic criteria for AN.

BED is primarily characterized by recurrent binge eating (binges on at least 2 days weekly for at least 6 months). A diagnosis of BED is made if the binges occur at least 2 days weekly for the past 6 months, if three of five characteristics associated with binge eating are present— rapid eating; eating past satiety to the point of discomfort; eating a large amount without being hungry; eating alone to avoid embarrassment by the amount one plans to eat; feeling disgust, guilt, or dysphoria after a binge—and if there is marked distress associated with the eating. Patients are not given a diagnosis of BED if there is regular purging or inappropriate compensatory behaviors to control weight nor if diagnostic criteria for AN are met (Table 35-1).[12] BED is, indeed, frequently complicated by obesity. Hospital psychiatric consultation may often not initially identify a patient's BED unless there is a known history or there is a concern about obesity. For these reasons, clinicians should remember to ask about associated symptoms and should be especially vigilant for BED in certain populations of adult patients—for example, those with current obesity, a history of weight fluctuation and dieting, and/or a history of an eating disorder.

Since concern with diet and fitness are virtually normative and often appropriate in American society, it can sometimes be difficult to differentiate appropriate concern with diet, weight, and exercise from excessive concern. For instance, the prevalence of obesity in children is 12% and has more than doubled over the course of the last generation.[50] Moreover, the prevalence of obesity among U.S. adults has steadily increased over the last decades,[51,52] with an estimated 64.5% of adults currently overweight and 30.5% obese.[53] Finally, obesity is associated with substantial medical and psychological complications in both children and adults, and it is the second highest cause of preventable death in the United States.[54] For these reasons, some attention to diet, fitness, and weight is quite appropriate. In addition, the changing American Heart Association guidelines for a desirable amount of daily exercise has been revised upward to a greater frequency and duration of aerobic activity. On the other hand, when an individual's thoughts are dominated by food and weight, when he or she restricts social activity so as to retain control over food intake, when he or she exercises compulsively through sickness, injury, or in addition to team expectations set by the coach, these are causes for concern.

Because many patients with disordered attitudes about eating feel even normal food intake is excessive, it is helpful to establish that binge episodes are consistent with the established definition in the *DSM-IV*[12]. That is, for the purposes of meeting criteria for BN or BED, a binge includes both the consumption of an unusually large amount of food in a discrete time period (2 hours or less) and is associated with a lack of control over the eating.[12] Assessment of the severity and patterning of the binge-eating is essential and is most easily accomplished by requesting that the patient keep a log of food intake (Figure 35-2). Although this log will be generally less useful in the hospital setting given the limited dietary choices and rather structured setting, it can still yield useful diagnostic information and is often therapeutic. Patients are instructed to record foods and beverages consumed, along with the time and place they were consumed. They are directed to also record feelings they experienced prior to, during, and after consuming the food. Patients are encouraged to specify emotional feelings, although physiologic states (e.g., hunger or fullness) can be included. Review of the food log with a patient is often helpful in solidifying the diagnosis and suggesting therapeutic strategies.

Clinicians should maintain vigilance for a broad spectrum of purging and other inappropriate compensatory behaviors in their assessment as well. Although induced vomiting is the most common means of purging associated with eating disorders, laxative abuse is also quite frequently seen. In addition, enema, diuretic, and stimulant use often occur in this population. Clinicians should inquire about prescription stimulants (e.g., methylphenidate), over-the-counter natural supplements (e.g., ephedra or chromium picolinate), and drugs of abuse associated with weight loss. Although its over-the-counter availability often conveys the impression that it is safe, ephedra use has been associated with serious neurologic and cardiovascular complications and even death in young women.[55] Patients with comorbid diabetes should also be assessed for inappropriate withholding of insulin dosing. These patients are at risk for diabetic ketoacidosis or long-term complications of poorly controlled blood sugars. Finally, some individuals with an eating disorder induce vomiting with syrup of ipecac. Again, the ready over-the-counter availability of this medication is often misleading for individuals who wish to use it to purge. Because its chronic use can be associated with cardiomyopathy, myopathy, and death,[56–59] patients should be educated about its associated risk and instructed to discontinue it immediately. Patients who have used it should be evaluated for need for further medical investigation. Patients who cannot reliably agree to discontinue its use should be admitted or remain hospitalized until they are able to abstain from this behavior. Clinicians should also inquire about fasting or dietary restrictions and exercise behavior as modes of preventing weight gain (see Figure 35-1).

Although there is substantial phenomenologic overlap and some crossover among AN, BN, and BED, by definition, they are mutually exclusive diagnoses. As can be seen from the diagnostic criteria, binge eating can be present in all three disorders, and purging and fasting can be present in AN and BN. In addition, excessive concern with weight occurs in both BN and AN. Individuals with BN commonly have amenorrhea as well, but by definition, if they are at or below 85% of their expected body weight, they meet criteria instead for a diagnosis of AN.

Time	Place	Food	Feelings: Before Eating	Feelings: During Eating	Feelings: After Eating	Trigger(s)
7:30 a.m.	Riding on T (subway)	Dunkin Donuts coffee Low fat muffin	Tired; planning to have a good day with food	OK since it is a low fat muffin	OK	Breakfast time; passed by Dunkin Donuts
10:30 a.m.	Desk at work	Coffee	Still tired	OK	OK	Needed a break from work
1:00 p.m.	Desk at work	1 small salad with dressing on the side $\frac{1}{2}$ piece of pita bread diet Coke	Starving	OK	OK; planning to work out later	Hunger/ lunch time
2:30 p.m.	Desk at work	$\frac{1}{2}$ piece of birthday cake	Hungry; thinking about food	?	Wish I hadn't eaten it	Hunger; it was there
3:30 p.m.	Desk at work	2nd $\frac{1}{2}$ piece of birthday cake	Hungry; thinking about food; feeling stressed by work	Zoned out	Have ruined the day; will plan to purge later	Ravenous; $\frac{1}{2}$ piece was there and no one else had taken it
5:30 p.m.	Walking to train	2 large chocolate chip cookies	Upset about eating cake; feeling anxious about family situation	Zoned out	Really disgusted about not resisting the cookies	Already "ruined" day for food; passed by the bakery
7:00 p.m.	Home, in living room in front of TV; roommate gone	Weight Watchers frozen dinner (pasta)	Upset that boyfriend hasn't called	Distracted, watching TV	Fine, was hungry	Dinner time; hungry
8:00 p.m.	Home, still in living room	Vanilla ice cream— finished $\frac{1}{2}$ pint Baked nachos ($\frac{1}{2}$ package) 2 bowls cereal with milk	Got off the phone after calling boyfriend— upset	Numb	Disgusted; purged, needed to get rid of food	Upsetting phone conversation; knowing ice cream was in the fridge

Figure 35-2. Sample Self-Observational Food and Associated Mood Journal.

The majority of patients who present with an eating disorder do not meet full criteria for AN, BN, or BED. Individuals with an eating disorder, not otherwise specified (ED NOS) experience clinically significant disordered eating attitudes or behaviors. Often they meet many criteria of other eating disorders, but they do not meet the frequency the criteria for bingeing or purging in BN or the weight criteria for AN. In some cases, their symptoms are slightly different (e.g., some chew and spit out food, whereas others regularly purge without bingeing).

Medical and other psychiatric causes of poor appetite and weight loss (i.e., the anorexia of depression) should be excluded with appropriate history, examination, and diagnostic tests. The common medical illnesses from which the practitioner needs to differentiate eating disorders include endocrinologic disorders (such as diabetes mellitus and hyperthyroidism), brain tumors, cancer, occult infections, and gastrointestinal disorders. Moreover, because all of the eating disorders are frequently comorbid with mood and anxiety disorders, personality disorders, and substance abuse, a complete assessment of mental status and psychiatric history should be included in the evaluation. Finally, a careful assessment of suicide risk is essential given the frequent association of suicidal ideation and attempts with eating disorders.

Interventions

Although some acute treatment of medical complications, nutritional compromise, and associated acute psychiatric symptoms can commence in the general hospital setting, the majority of the treatment will take place on a longer-term basis either in a psychiatric facility or outpatient setting. It is critical, however, for the consulting psychiatrist to establish a diagnosis and the level of severity that will guide not only inpatient management, but also the development of a disposition and comprehensive treatment plan.

After establishing the diagnosis and symptom severity, psychiatric consultation for eating disorders can be helpful in optimizing an ongoing treatment or developing a treatment plan for a newly diagnosed patient. Interventions in a general hospital setting include (1) education of the clinical staff caring for the patient; (2) patient engagement in treatment and psychoeducation; (3) identification of referral resources for either specialized inpatient eating disorder care or psychotherapy for outpatients; (4) institution of behavioral strategies to control symptoms, when appropriate; (5) initiation of pharmacotherapy, when appropriate; and (6) the elaboration and institution of a plan for nutritional rehabilitation. Also, on occasion, a formal behavioral treatment protocol will be implemented on a general medical or pediatric floor.

Education of the clinical staff on the general medical or pediatric service is essential for two main reasons. It ensures that a thorough targeted workup is complete, and that nutritional and medical complications of restrictive eating, binge eating, and inappropriate compensatory behaviors are addressed. For example, potassium repletion for a patient with chronic vomiting or diuretic or laxative abuse and ensuing hypokalemia, or a suitable bowel regimen for a patient tapering off of laxatives, can be prescribed.

Psychiatric consultation can also assist staff in the management of countertransferential feelings toward patients. These can range from rescue fantasies to anger. Patients with eating disorders are often quite articulate and accomplished. Staff may underestimate their pathology or spend excessive time "talking the patient out of his or her choices." On the other hand, the helplessness that can be engendered in staff and the appearance that the patient is "choosing" the symptoms (e.g., not to eat or to purge, whereas the patient in the next bed may be wasting away from cancer or nauseated by chemotherapy) can lead to anger. Consultation can assist the clinical staff in appropriate (nonpunitive) limit-setting, with empathy, and with realistic expectations.

Engaging the Patient with an Eating Disorder Who Is Reluctant to Accept Treatment

Psychoeducation of the patient, and possibly the family, will be also be an essential step to ensure that all are aware of the serious consequences of the eating disorder and that treatment is available and beneficial. Many individuals with either AN or BN believe their symptoms have an important primary gain—controlling their weight. By definition, individuals with AN and BN unduly base their self-worth on their body shape, weight, and appearance. Sometimes, an initial experience of positive social feedback and self-efficacy is so reinforcing that it will induce them to continue to lose weight. Not infrequently, the restrictive eating gives way to bouts of binge eating, which in turn can segue to purging and other inappropriate compensatory behaviors. Not surprisingly, this cycle is generally ineffective in achieving the desired weight loss. When patients rededicate their efforts to restricting their diet—often in a pattern in which they bank their calories for the end of the day—this frequently results in a pattern of evening binge eating after they become so ravenous that they lose control over their intake and binge. This binge eating is further complicated by a preoccupation with food—undoubtedly somewhat physiologically driven—so extreme that many patients report a constant distraction concerning the tally of calories they have consumed or that they plan to consume during the day. Thus, a viciously self-reinforcing cycle ensues.

Individuals with eating disorders are not always aware of the substantial secondary gains of their symptoms. Many patients experience distraction and emotional numbing as a result of their restrictive and binge-pattern eating and purging behaviors. Commonly they report a general mental dulling with extreme restrictive-pattern eating (consistent with clinically apparent cognitive changes and social withdrawal), a numbing during binge eating, and often a relief after purging. The latter two are almost immediately followed by some dysphoria as well. The net effect of these symptoms is to provide a self-soothing mechanism to individuals who perhaps cannot readily access higher level defenses. Thus, the behavioral symptoms eventually become a core coping strategy for many individuals with eating disorders. Whereas some patients are completely unaware of this function of their symptoms, others have a clear sense that they could not tolerate relinquishing them. Moreover, most patients are convinced that they will gain weight if they establish normal dietary patterns. For these reasons, patients are understandably reticent in disclosing their symptoms and reluctant to impart on any treatment plan that they perceive will result in weight gain and deprive them of sometimes life-saving coping strategies. In addition, extremely low-weight anorexic patients often have a nutritionally related cognitive deficit that impairs their capacity to develop insights about their behavior or consider alternatives to their symptoms.

Thus, engaging a patient in treatment for eating disorders is often challenging since the patient may perceive this as a threat to all the gains he or she experiences from the symptoms. Others—usually those with BED and BED—may quite willingly enter treatment when the symptoms lose their efficacy or purpose in self-soothing, have unwanted weight gain effects, or are too time-consuming or expensive. In addition, some patients finally seek treatment when their living situation (i.e., a roommate and shared bathroom) puts their secrecy in jeopardy or when they are confronted about their symptoms by someone who has adequate leverage to steer them to treatment for their problem.

For reluctant patients, and indeed all others, developing a treatment alliance that will help the therapy survive the patient's reluctance and ambivalence is paramount. It is usually quite helpful to acknowledge empathetically up front how important the symptoms must be to the patient and how frightening it will be to consider giving them up. If the patient is not yet medically or nutritionally compromised but is also utterly dependent on the symptoms, there is considerable latitude for how aggressively symptoms need to be addressed. It is helpful to suggest that the therapy begin by embarking on an understanding of how the patient came to rely on these symptoms. If the symptoms are ego-dystonic, it is helpful to frame the work as an exercise in curiosity while suspending judgment. In the beginning of such a treatment, rather than to feel defeated or to react to symptoms in a self-disparaging way, patients are encouraged to use the opportunity to observe and understand how they could have behaved in a way that seems superficially irrational to them, but that they must have some underlying rationality.

If patients have a history of more harmful behaviors, such as cutting, suicide attempts, or substance abuse, it is sometimes useful to "congratulate" them on finding and using a symptom that is relatively less self-destructive. Indeed, it may be clinically wise to work with the patient to develop more effective and constructive coping strategies prior to eradicating behavioral symptoms of disordered eating that have displaced more self-destructive behaviors. Particularly if patients are in early recovery from substance abuse, are working through sensitive material in psychotherapy, or encountering significant stressors, they might increase their risk for relapse to substance abuse if they are deprived of the self-soothing associated with their disordered eating behaviors.

An important and frequent potential red flag is a call for evaluation of a patient in whom disordered eating has abruptly come to light or who insists on shifting gears in treatment because she wants to address the eating disorder symptoms. Further exploration of the clinical situation often reveals a patient who is having difficulty tolerating the intensity or emotional charge in other areas. Eating behaviors are sometimes appealing to address because they are experienced as more tangible and concrete and the patient hopes the treatment will provide a distraction. In such a situation, the consultant can provide psychoeducation to both the clinician and the treatment team about the risk of controlling the eating disorder symptoms too tightly.

The dilemma between wishing to capitalize on the patient's motivation and to avoid medical and psychosocial complications of the eating disorder (while wishing to prevent a relapse or decompensation to more self-destructive behavior) can be made explicit. The treatment team might decide to reconsider the pace or direction of the therapy. Although appearing somewhat paradoxical, in some cases, patients should actually be encouraged *not* to suppress their disordered eating behaviors if there is a high risk of relapse to substance abuse or of decompensation to other serious self-destructive behaviors. This is not always possible or medically safe, especially if there is any serious medical complication or risk that should result from the behaviors (e.g., an adolescent who refuses to eat and is at risk of growth arrest or a young adult who is seriously hypokalemic and at risk for cardiac dysrhythmias). If eradication of the behaviors is too risky, yet serious medical complications seem possible if they continue, the treatment team should probably consider continuing the treatment in a psychiatric inpatient setting.

Even in such a scenario, it is sometimes appropriate and possible to assist the patient in gaining behavioral control over some of the episodes of bingeing and purging, for example, those that appear to be precipitated by physiologic or environmental cues that could easily be eliminated and those that do not appear to serve a necessary defense for the patient. Extremely useful information about the patterning and stimuli for these episodes can be gleaned from a food journal (Figure 35-2); recommendations can be made to assist the patient to reduce the frequency of episodes without compromising the patient's ability to maintain his or her safety and/ or abstinence.

For individuals who are resistant to treatment of their symptoms, several approaches can be effective. In many cases, the patient can be asked why he or she has agreed to meet or speak with the consultant and what he or she hopes to get out of it. Unfortunately, the reply may be that the patient is hoping to get her parents "off her back" about the situation. In such a scenario, it is helpful to find a specific goal or goals with which to ally with the patient. For example, you might both agree that a goal is health or fitness; in some cases you might only be able to mutually agree that a goal is preventing death. Of note, if no therapeutic alliance can be reached on preserving health and life, an alternative treatment situation—in some cases, possibly involuntary hospitalization,[60] if there is risk of self-harm, passive or otherwise—should be sought.

For the patient who is unable to admit the extent of the symptoms or to acknowledge that symptoms are problematic, gentle confrontation is necessary. This can be accomplished with psychoeducation about clinical signs that are worrisome and with simple-to-understand clinical information about the availability and efficacy of treatment and the substantial risks for not pursuing treatment. Often it will be essential to include the family in the psychoeducational session. This is virtually always true for children, but also often true for young adults who are still living with, or are substantially influenced by, their family.

If laboratory test results are already available, contextualizing abnormal findings that have resulted from the eating disorder is sometimes motivating to the patient, or if not, at least to the family. For example, the results of a dual-energy x-ray absorptiometry (DXA) scan of the lumbar spine showing osteopenia, the results of a brain MRI showing cortical atrophy, or laboratory results indicating hypokalemia as a result of chronic vomiting can all be concrete data that may get the patient's attention. If the threat of compromised health is inadequate, cosmetic considerations (e.g., the dental decay associated with chronic purging, the dry and baggy skin associated with the malnutrition of AN) can be tried to engage the patient's motivation for treatment. For severely nutritionally or medically compromised patients, participation in work or athletic activities may be contraindicated because of impairment or physical risk to the patient. For such patients who are not sufficiently motivated to begin treatment to address health or cosmetic concerns, their desire to continue to work, to perform in a high school ballet production, or to run intercollegiate cross-country may be leveraged into motivation to participate and make concrete improvements in treatment. In such a scenario, parents, coaches, teachers, and overseers of professional standards might be mobilized to clarify and enforce contingencies for continued work or participation in extracurricular activities.

For patients with BN, motivation enhancement therapy has been shown to have some efficacy in addressing symptoms[61]; this therapeutic method is worth consideration for patients who appear unready to commit to treatment. Especially in cases in which motivation is in question and when adherence to treatment or risk of decompensation is high, a treatment contract specifying goals and interim goals and the patient's responsibilities (e.g., the patient may be asked to agree to show up to all appointments, to allow weighing and laboratory work at intervals specified by the team, to agree to communication among all members of the treatment team) should be developed. In addition, parameters to be used in the consideration of intensification of care should be specified so that if a patient's weight is unstable, all team members and the patient are in agreement in advance at what point an increased intensity of care (e.g., adding a group a medications or being admitted to an inpatient unit for eating disorders) are necessary.

Considerations in Initiating Treatment

Goals of the inpatient hospitalization are based on the seriousness of the disease and its complications. These goals include the prevention of death due to starvation, the introduction of a plan for the correction of the malnourished state in a slow and steady manner, the initiation of successful weight gain, stabilization of acute psychiatric illness, and/or prevention of suicide. Thus, initial goals of treatment are medical, nutritional, and psychiatric stabilization, some of which may continue either in a psychiatric hospital, day treatment program, or in multidisciplinary outpatient care.

Depending on clinical staffing, a behavioral protocol can be implemented on a general medical or pediatric service to promote refeeding or control inappropriate compensatory behaviors. Some services have standardized protocols, and in other cases the consulting psychiatrist and staff can develop a plan to meet the needs of individual patients. A description of such protocols are beyond the scope of this chapter, but might include routine weighing, supervised regularly scheduled meals, expectations for participation in meal selection with a nutritionist, expectations for duration of meals, restrictions of bathroom trips within an hour of meals, privileges (i.e., leaving the floor) contingent on meeting a dietary plan and weight goals, and restriction of physical activity. This is also a good opportunity to introduce patients to simple behavioral strategies, such as self-monitoring with a food journal (see Figure 35-2), or controlling stimuli to binge eating, such as hunger, by eating three meals daily with two snacks.

Some patients who have been hospitalized on a medical service because of complications of their eating disorder will benefit from, or require transfer to, psychiatric inpatient care. Others who are well stabilized, or for whom the eating disorder was an incidental finding, will be discharged home for outpatient care. Figure 35-3 shows a partial list of indications for inpatient-level care of patients with an eating disorder. Although psychotherapeutic care (with the exception of supportive or psychoeducational treatment) is unlikely in the general hospital setting, behavioral treatment to support adequate dietary intake can be initiated, pharmacologic therapy—when appropriate—can be started, and an outpatient team can be assembled to ensure smooth transition in care.

Given that the majority of patients present with ED NOS and/or with comorbid psychiatric illness, a flexible, eclectic approach to treatment is often the most appropriate to meet the multifaceted treatment goals of the patient and treatment team. Likewise, treatment strategies suggested by randomized, controlled trials are extremely useful, but clinicians should bear in mind that the frequently broad exclusion criteria and narrowly defined outcomes may limit the generalizability of study findings. The utility and necessity of a multidisciplinary team approach to treatment for eating disorders is well established. Generally, treatment benefits from the inclusion of the primary care

- Body weight   75% expected body weight
- Imminent risk of medical danger (e.g., due to nutritional compromise, dehydration, electrolyte abnormalities, syrup of ipecac use, or organ failure)
- Severe or escalating symptoms (e.g., bingeing and purging so many times in a day that it seriously interferes with work, school, or social function)
- Associated psychiatric emergency, such as suicidal risk or psychosis
- For children and adolescents, serious risk of developmental or growth arrest
- Chronic or intractable symptoms that compromise health or social or occupational function that are not responding to reasonable trial(s) of outpatient psychosocial and/or pharmacologic therapies

Figure 35-3. Indications for inpatient management of an eating disorder.

clinician, a nutritionist, and a mental health clinician or clinicians. It is certainly not essential that the clinicians comprising this team be within one program or institution. However, a clear demarcation of responsibilities and roles (i.e., who will monitor weight if necessary or who will monitor frequency of purging behaviors that may require medical monitoring) and frequent and open communication about the treatment plan, progress, and concerns is optimal. Indeed, clinicians should insist upon permission to communicate all clinical information relevant to treatment planning among members of the team. Because splitting and miscommunication are both strong possibilities in such treatment situations, the team should make every effort to reach a consensus about the treatment plan and contingencies for changes depending on patient progress or difficulties and present a unified front to the patient.

When evaluating an ongoing treatment or the development of a new treatment plan, clinicians should bear in mind that medical, nutritional, and psychological goals are integral to treatment; sometimes progress with psychological symptoms is predicated upon medical and nutritional stabilization. Likewise, if psychological symptoms are not addressed, it is likely that medical complications and nutritional compromise will recur. With respect to the mental health component of treatment, psychosocial therapies and pharmacotherapies both have a role, but the former appear to be more effective. Thus, pharmacotherapy is most appropriately used as an adjunctive treatment to psychotherapy or when access to psychotherapy is otherwise limited. Moreover, there are no randomized controlled trials assessing efficacy and safety of pharmacotherapy for eating disorders in children and adolescents, so the ensuing discussion of

psychopharmacologic agents pertains only to adult patients.

Treatment of Anorexia Nervosa

Poor nutrition associated with restricted diet and low body weight in AN can result in a number of serious medical complications (Table 35-2). A search for these possible sequelae, and their subsequent correction, is a necessary prerequisite to the management of the patient with an eating disorder. The more common problems and the approach to their management are specified here.

Fluid and electrolyte disturbances require immediate attention. The correction of dehydration, hypokalemia, and metabolic alkalosis is a priority. Intravenous (IV) fluids and electrolytes sometimes need to be used to support these patients to improve these parameters.

The electrocardiogram (EKG) must be monitored, looking for signs of hypokalemia and bradycardia. Prolongation of the QT interval—which can be idiopathic in AN[62] or a consequence of hypokalemia—requires immediate medical intervention, since it may increase the risk of ventricular tachycardia and sudden death.

Dental problems in patients with self-induced vomiting may occur due to the effects of gastric acid on teeth enamel and need to be addressed.

Constipation brought on by dehydration, or by long-term laxative abuse often responds to stool softeners and to bulk-forming agents.

Poor gastric emptying may be seen in anorexia presenting with bloating and nausea. Gastric motility agents, such as metoclopramide, and erythromycin, can be used to alleviate the symptoms. Occasionally, marked dilatation of the stomach can be seen in anorexia. The placement of a nasogastric tube

Table 35-2. Selected Medical Complications
of Anorexia Nervosa

Metabolic
Hypokalemia
Hyponatremia
Hyperphosphatemia
Dehydration
Inability to concentrate urine
Decreased glomerular filtration rate
Ketonuria

Endocrine
Euthyroid sick syndrome
Growth retardation and short stature
Delayed puberty
Amenorrhea, oligomenorrhea
Hypercortisolism
Hypothermia
Infertility

Skeletal
Osteopenia/osteoporosis
Fractures

Dermatologic
Acrocyanosis
Yellow skin, secondary to hypercarotenemia
Brittle hair and nails
Lanugo
Hair loss

Cardiovascular
Bradycardia
Orthostatic and non-orthostatic hypotension
Dysrhythmias
EKG abnormalities
    Low voltage
    Prolonged QT interval
Mitral valve prolapse
Congestive heart failure
Pericardial effusion

Gastrointestinal
Parotid hypertrophy
Hematemesis (Mallory-Weiss syndrome)
Delayed gastric emptying
Constipation
Gastric dilatation and rupture
Superior mesenteric artery syndrome
Abnormal liver enzymes with fatty infiltration
Pancreatitis

Neurologic
Seizures
Myopathy
Peripheral neuropathy
Cortical atrophy

Hematologic
Bone marrow suppression

provides symptomatic relief with decompression and avoids the dire consequence of gastric rupture.

Osteopenia is one of the more severe complications of AN. Osteoporosis is one of the most serious clinical concerns accompanying amenorrhea and weight loss. The peak bone mass achieved as a young adult is the major determinant of bone density and fracture risk. AN is associated with markedly reduced bone density, especially at the lumbar spine, but also at the proximal femur and the distal radius.

The importance of nutritional factors, lean body mass, and BMI in determining bone mass cannot be overstated. The duration of estrogen deficiency does not determine the severity of the osteopenia, and hormone replacement has not significantly increased the bone mineral density in anorexic patients.[63–65] The primary therapy is weight gain. The most appropriate recommendations include a plan for nutritional rehabilitation, supplementation with 1000 to 1500 mg/day of calcium if dietary sources are inadequate and 800 IU/day of vitamin D. Individual assessment regarding hormone replacement is made. DXA scanning at the initial medical assessment of a patient with an eating disorder and at varying intervals every 12 to 24 months can assist in counseling those at high risk for fractures and bone loss.

The primary therapy for the amenorrhea associated with anorexia is, as well, the restoration of the nutritional status. Most patients with eating disorders will recover menses within 6 months of reaching 90% of their ideal body weight.[66] The decision to pursue hormone treatment is individualized for each patient.

The most appropriate initial treatment strategy for AN is often weight restoration. This is not only due to the previously mentioned serious medical consequence of low weight and poor nutrition. Low BMI at referral predicts a poor prognosis[67,68] and is associated with significantly higher chronicity and mortality for anorexic patients.[69]

Undernutrition is also suspected to underlie some of the neurocognitive features of AN that may contribute to treatment resistance. Certainly, clinical experience suggests that cognitive inflexibility (e.g., relating to overvalued ideas about body weight) may impede treatment efforts for AN. Indeed, subtle abnormalities in abstraction and cognitive flexibility have been substantiated in studies of anorexic individuals.[70,71] It is noteworthy that some of the cognitive abnormalities in anorexic subjects manifested in attentional domain tasks have been shown to at least partially improve with weight gain (whereas others do not).[72] Interestingly, dilated ventricles and sulcal widening on CT scans as well as global hypometabolism seen in resting PET studies in anorexic subjects improve at least somewhat with weight gain.[72,73]

Therefore, the initial focus of treatment for AN is active weight management with the elaboration and implementation of a nutritional plan. Controlled weight gain of 1 to 1.5 kg per week is the goal for hospitalized patients, and 0.45 kg per week for outpatients. The prescribed intake level needs to be determined with that goal in mind. This is by far the most challenging phase in the treatment of AN since patients usually feel most incapable of tolerating a weight gain when they are underweight. If the patient is not severely underweight, an attempt can be made to manage this phase with nutritional counseling to make adequate dietary selections, restriction of physical activity, and behavioral reinforcement for meeting weight goals. For example, the reinforcement might be to keep the privilege of working as an outpatient or to participate in an extracurricular performance. The treatment team and the patient should identify a weight goal and a timetable for interim goals at the outset of treatment. Generally, a goal weight should be chosen that is consistent with expected weight for height and at which medical complications, such as osteopenia and amenorrhea, are reversed.

Patients with eating disorders are often loathe to meet with a nutritionist, with the excuse that they "know all there is to know" about nutrition themselves. Notwithstanding this attitude, nutritional counseling can be framed as an activity to assist judgment and motivation rather than to educate them about the caloric value of foods. Especially with underweight patients, establishing a caloric requirement and developing a dietary plan to meet the weight goals that are set are highly useful. This plan will include three meals daily to establish expectations of normalized eating and will generally include snacks and/or caloric supplements as well. When such a plan is in place, if a patient is unable to gain weight (i.e., the patient requires more calories or more help to adhere to the plan) can be assessed.

The measurement of the metabolic rate by indirect calorimetry can be helpful in determining the metabolic needs of the patient and thus the caloric goals. However, measurement of resting energy expenditure (REE) is not widely available, so an estimate of energy needs is usually required. Generally, most hospitalized patients with an eating disorder require at least 1500 kcal/day to maintain weight. Their reduced REE may be as low as 800 to 1000 kcal/day and maintenance requirements are 130% to 150% of the REE. Approximately 1 gram of weight is gained for every 5 calories in excess of output, so 5000 extra calories beyond maintenance are necessary for a weight gain of 1 kg. Weight gain may occur rapidly at first because of fluid retention and the baseline low metabolic rate.[74] Intake levels usually begin at 30 to 40 kcal/kg (1000 to 1600 kcal/day). As the patient with an eating disorder begins to gain weight, metabolic demands increase, and the intake needs to be increased considerably to continue to achieve ongoing weight gain.

If patients are severely underweight (e.g., less than or equal to 75% of expected body weight), underweight with rapid weight loss, or remain chronically underweight with medical complications and are unable to gain a reasonable amount of weight as an outpatient, they will require inpatient or partial hospitalization care. In a hospital setting, dietary intake can be more carefully monitored, purging and exercise can be controlled, and behavioral reinforcement can be more easily enforced. In addition, if the patient withstands all feeding efforts, nasogastric feedings or parenteral feedings can be considered in cases of extreme malnutrition and recalcitrance to treatment. Patients who require inpatient level care to gain weight, but who recurrently relapse after discharge, may be best served in a residential care setting for 3 months or more to achieve and stabilize an adequate weight gain.

Great care needs to be taken in the nutritional rehabilitation to avoid the refeeding syndrome, a potentially catastrophic treatment complication in undernourished patients who are being renourished. In this syndrome, the demands that a refilled circulatory system places on a nutritionally depleted cardiac mass result in cardiovascular collapse. This can be seen whether the nutrition is provided orally, enterally, or parenterally.[75] The classic definition of the syndrome refers to the potentiation of refeeding-induced hypophosphatemia, but it can also involve other electrolytes. Phosphate depletion, in turn, produces widespread abnormalities, including cardiac arrest and delirium.[76] Much of the pathophysiology of the refeeding syndrome has been related to the rapid increase of insulin upon refeeding.[77] Carbohydrates stimulate insulin release, which, in turn, increases the cellular uptake of phosphate, glucose, and water, as well as stimulating protein synthesis. Insulin also increases sodium and water reabsorption in the renal tubules. Prolonged starvation results in a reduced cardiac mass and output. During the refeeding, ventricular volume returns to normal while left ventricular mass remains reduced, potentially leading to fluid retention and congestive heart failure (CHF). Sodium and fluid retention compound this problem. Serum phosphate levels may drop precipitously, leading to depletion of phosphorylated compounds with impaired energy stores due to a decrease in intracellular adenosine triphosphate, and tissue hypoxia secondary to reduced levels of erythrocyte 2,3 diphosphoglycerate. Further cardiac compromise may follow. Potassium and magnesium also become depleted during starvation. Upon refeeding, these are deposited intracellularly and serum levels may fall if no supplementation is provided. Therefore, nutritional rehabilitation of the severely malnourished patient needs to be done with extreme care. Vital signs need to be monitored; electrolytes, including sodium, potassium, phosphorus, and magnesium, should be followed every few days; and the patient needs to be regularly examined for signs of edema or CHF. The greatest caution is required during the first weeks after commencing the nutritional support.

Due to concerns regarding refeeding syndrome, patients are cautiously refed with incremental increases of 200 to 300 kcal per day every 3 to 4 days as tolerated and as determined by individual weight gain. As patients near their target weight, they frequently require large amount of calories, upward of 3000 calories/day. Supplements need to be provided. Sodium at 1 mmol/kg/day, potassium at 4 mmol/kg/day, and magnesium at 0.6 mmol/kg/day should be given. Phosphate, up to 1 mmol/kg/day intravenously, and oral supplements up to 100 mmol/day can be given to try to avoid the hypophosphatemia associated with refeeding. Extra calcium may need to be given because hypocalcemia may occur during phosphate

supplementation. Thiamine, folic acid, riboflavin, ascorbic acid, pyridoxine, as well as the fat-soluble vitamins A, D, E, and K, should be supplemented.[78] Trace elements, including selenium, may also be deficient. A good rule of thumb is to provide a multivitamin with minerals on a daily basis.

Because of the desirability of weight gain in the early treatment of AN, there has been interest in identifying pharmacologic agents that promote weight gain in anorexic patients. Efforts to identify pharmacologic agents to treat the primary symptoms of AN have been mostly disappointing. To date, no randomized, controlled, clinical trials have identified an agent that improves clinical outcomes in outpatients with AN. Studies investigating efficacy of chlorpromazine, pimozide, sulpiride, clomipramine, clonidine, and tetrahydrocannabinol[79] in addressing the primary symptoms of AN have all yielded negative results. However, there is a limited role for pharmacologic management of AN (Table 35-3).

Whereas fluoxetine may have a role in stabilizing weight-recovered patients,[80] it does not appear effective addressing anorexic symptoms in patients who are underweight (i.e., those who meet weight criteria for diagnosis). Similarly, despite effecting some theoretically beneficial cognitive changes (with respect to perfectionistic attitudes, sense of ineffectiveness, and lack of interoceptive awareness) sertraline also did not promote significant weight gain in anorexic patients compared with placebo in a controlled study.[81] On the other hand, zinc gluconate (100 mg/day) was found to accelerate weight gain over placebo in anorexic inpatients.[82] While this is encouraging, application to outpatient settings is unclear, as is efficacy or safety of prolonged supplementation.[83,84] Additionally, cyproheptadine (32 mg/day)[85] accelerated weight gain in restricting-type anorexic inpatients in one study. However, cyproheptadine actually worsened the condition of binge/purge type anorexics in this study and was not found superior to placebo in promoting weight gain in another controlled study.[86] Again, utility in outpatient settings or prolonged use has not been established for AN.

Although there are as yet no published controlled studies on the efficacy of atypical antipsychotic agents in treating AN, a number of

Table 35-3. Pharmacologic Strategies for Management of Eating Disorders

	General Considerations	Psychopharmacologic Therapies with Best Support
Anorexia Nervosa	Treat comorbid psychiatric illness as appropriate Avoid agents with side effects that would diminish appetite, cause weight loss, or prolong the QT interval Do not use agents that stimulate weight gain or appetite without negotiating this with the patient and monitoring for onset of binge and purge behavior Pharmacotherapy should augment, not replace, psychotherapy for anorexia nervosa Give multivitamins with 800 IU daily of vitamin D Give calcium supplements (1000 to 1500 mg/day) if dietary sources are inadequate Oral contraceptive pills (OCPs) are sometimes used for alleviation of hypoestrogenemic symptoms but do not provide protection against osteopenia Consider gastric motility agents if there is delayed gastric emptying or transit	Consider fluoxetine 60 mg daily for weight recovered patients (i.e., patients at >85% EBW) Consider olanzapine 2.5 to 15 mg day for underweight patients Consider short-term use of zinc gluconate (100 mg/day)
Bulimia Nervosa	Treat comorbid psychiatric illness as appropriate Avoid agents with side effects that would stimulate appetite, cause weight gain, or prolong the QT interval Pharmacotherapy should augment, not replace, psychotherapy for bulimia nervosa Agents should not be used for a primary effect of weight loss as dieting and active weight loss treatment is contraindicated in bulimia nervosa Agents that cause appetite loss as a side effect are sometimes desirable but should be used with caution as they could exacerbate anorexic or bulimic symptoms or be abused Potassium and magnesium supplementation are sometimes necessary Stool softeners and bulk-forming laxatives (but not cathartic laxatives) can be used to alleviate constipation	Consider one of the following (and consider sequential trials if agents are ineffective or not tolerated): Fluoxetine (60 mg/day) Desipramine (up to 300 mg/day as tolerated) Imipramine (up to 300 mg/day as tolerated) Ondansetron (24 mg/day in 6 divided doses) Trazodone (up to 400 mg/day) Consider a trial of naltrexone 200–300 mg/day with close monitoring for hepatotoxicity for *severe*, treatment-resistant bingeing Avoid bupropion and MAOIs because of specific risks in bulimia nervosa
Binge-eating Disorder	Treat comorbid psychiatric illness as appropriate Avoid agents with side effects that would stimulate appetite or cause weight gain Pharmacotherapy should augment, not replace, psychotherapy for binge-eating disorder	Consider one of the following (and consider sequential trials if agents are ineffective or not tolerated): Fluvoxamine 50–300 mg/day Sertraline (50–200 mg/day) Fluoxetine (20–80 mg/day; mixed data) Topiramate (50–600 mg/day) Sibutramine (15 mg/day)

case reports suggest that risperidone (up to a total of 1.5 mg/day)[87] and olanzapine (2.5 to 15 mg/day total)[88–92] may have a role in promoting weight gain in AN. In addition to promoting clinically significant weight gain, the cases describe additional clinical improvements in compliance and insight, as well as reduced body image disturbance, agitation, and premeal anxiety. A retrospective study of olanzapine in anorexic patients corroborates significant reductions in preoccupation with body image and weight and a more flexible attitude toward eating and weight gain.[93] Finally, an open trial of olanzapine (10 mg/day) also demonstrated clinically significant weight gain over a 10-week period in an outpatient setting.[94]

Whereas controlled data are required to establish whether these medications (and possibly other atypical antipsychotic agents) are effective in treating the primary symptoms of AN, the evidence to date do suggest a trial of olanzapine may be warranted for low-weight anorexic patients. Clinicians should use appropriate caution about potential adverse effects of these medications. For example, AN can present with a prolonged electrocardiographic QT interval (either secondary to hypokalemia or idiopathic); caution should therefore be used with pharmacologic agents that can promote the QT interval, including some of the atypical antipsychotic medications.

While initiating a trial of olanzapine early in the treatment process may be beneficial, the consulting psychiatrist should also make it clear that medication use in anorexia is not only off-label and inconclusively effective, but that it is also an augmentation of—not a replacement for—formal psychotherapeutic treatment. If the patient is to be transferred to a psychiatric unit, psychotherapeutic and milieu care can be initiated there. If the patient is to be discharged to outpatient treatment, identification of a multidisciplinary team with immediate availability is optimal. Psychotherapy generally has limited efficacy with very underweight patients, with the exception of supportive psychotherapy—probably due to the neurocognitive changes described previously. On the other hand, even a few pounds weight gain can have a tremendously positive impact on the insight and behavioral changes necessary for recovery.

A number of psychotherapeutic modalities have support for treatment of AN, including cognitive-behavioral therapy (CBT),[95] psychodynamic psychotherapy,[96] and potentially, interpersonal psychotherapy.[97] Family therapy has a clearly supported role in individuals with nonchronic AN with an onset before age 19,[98] and family involvement for either psychotherapy and/or psychoeducation[99] as well as group therapy[100,101] are often useful as an adjunct to individual psychotherapy. Given that AN frequently occurs with comorbid psychiatric illness and is often associated with some impairment in social function, therapeutic goals will likely be broader than just those addressing AN. In addition, the patient's capacity to do psychotherapeutic work may evolve considerably with improved nutritional status and with developmental maturation. For some, psychotherapy can only be supportive and achieve limited goals until there is initial weight gain. For these reasons, flexibility and some eclecticism are often useful in the treatment of AN.

Psychiatric symptoms (e.g., major depression and obsessive-compulsive disorder) comorbid with AN should be treated, although clinical experience suggests reduced efficacy in the setting of low weight. In all cases, caution should be exercised to avoid agents that promote weight loss or diminish appetite. In addition, agents that prolong the QT interval or that cause orthostatic hypotension should be used with extra caution. Although many clinicians are tempted to use medications that promote appetite or weight gain in anorexic patients, with the exception of risperidone and olanzapine, this has not been shown to be an effective strategy. Indeed, such agents pose a risk of making patients feel out of control with their eating and may intensify restrictive symptoms or precipitate bingeing and purging behaviors. Any potential effects on weight or appetite should be forthrightly communicated to the patient for this reason.

Treatment of Bulimia Nervosa

Individuals with BN are often eventually sufficiently distressed by their symptoms to accept treatment, even if ambivalent about giving them up. As with AN, multidisciplinary team treatment to ensure adequate attention to nutritional and medical issues should be negotiated with the patient at the outset of treatment.

A number of psychosocial treatment modalities have empirical support for the treatment of BN. CBT is the best established treatment. CBT for BN is available in a manual for standardized care and is designed for completion in approximately 20 weeks. The treatment is predicated on the education of the patient on a cognitive model of how symptoms of BN are perpetuated. That is, patients are introduced to a model in which low self-esteem, weight and shape concerns, dieting, binge eating, and purging operate in a self-perpetuating cycle.[102] A recent meta-analysis demonstrated that recovery rates (based on intention to treat) for subjects undergoing CBT for BN were 38%.[103] The major limitation of this approach is that those who did not recover often remained substantially symptomatic[103] and impaired in other domains.[104] Interpersonal psychotherapy (IPT) is as effective, if somewhat slower in effecting progress, as CBT.[105,106] Other therapies that have some empirical support for efficacy for the symptoms of BN include motivational enhancement therapy (MET),[61] dialectic behavioral therapy,[107] psychodynamic psychotherapies,[108] guided imagery,[109] and guided self-change (incorporating a self-care manual).[110]

Psychoeducation about treatment options and the expected course will be helpful in guiding selection of the most effective and acceptable therapeutic modality to the patient. Chronicity, severity of symptoms, comorbid illness, and psychosocial functioning will guide clinician selection as well. Although depending on the clinical situation, psychotherapeutic treatment may not focus on disordered eating symptoms, it is essential that least one member of the treatment team keep tabs on the frequency and severity of purging and on other inappropriate compensatory behaviors to ensure that there is adequate medical monitoring and treatment. Useful behavioral strategies include self-monitoring with a food journal (see Figure 35-2) and stimulus control (keeping "trigger" foods out of sight/reach, eating three meals daily with two snacks to avoid hunger) can be incorporated in the treatment plan relatively easily with supervision from the psychotherapist, the primary care clinician, or the nutritionist.

Although psychotherapy is well established as the core treatment for BN, numerous pharmacologic therapies have proven efficacy in the treatment of BN based on at least one randomized controlled trial. In the limited number of trials conducted, CBT has been more effective than medication in the treatment of BN.[79] Antidepressants as a class have been generally effective in decreasing binge frequency by an average of 56% (vs. 11% with placebo); similar rates of decrease for self-induced vomiting have also been reported.[111] There are few studies to shed light on whether use of pharmacotherapy is effective as an adjunctive treatment to the various psychosocial therapies for BN, but it appears that allowing consecutive trials of adjunctive medication may have some benefit. In addition, patients who have not responded to CBT or IPT have responded to fluoxetine (60 mg/ day).[112]

Of the medications found effective in the short-term treatment of BN in randomized controlled trials (see Table 35-3), only fluoxetine is FDA-approved for the treatment of BN at this time. Fluoxetine (60 mg/day) has been found effective in reducing symptoms of BN and is generally well tolerated in this patient population.[113,114] It is also the only agent to have been shown effective for a year following acute response.[115] Of note, other selective serotonin-reuptake inhibitors (SSRIs) are routinely clinically used for the treatment of BN but have not been studied in published controlled trials to date. Other antidepressant agents found effective, but with less desirable side effect profiles,[116,117] include imipramine (at standard antidepressant doses up to 300 mg/day as tolerated),[118] desipramine (also at standard antidepressant doses up to 300 mg/day as tolerated),[119,120] and trazodone (up to 400 mg/day).[121] Three other antidepressant agents—bupropion,[122] phenelzine,[123] and isocarboxazid[124]—have been found effective in the reduction of bulimic symptoms. However, because of the association with risk for serious adverse events (bupropion was found associated with a 5.8% prevalence of seizures in a study of subjects with BN,[122] and monoamine oxidase inhibitors [MAOIs] have been associated with spontaneous hypertensive crises in bulimic patients),[125,126] these agents are relatively contraindicated for the treatment of BN.

Two other agents have been found effective in controlled studies of subjects with BN. Naltrexone (200 to 300 mg/day) was found effective in reducing symptoms in treatment-resistant patients[127]; its risk of associated hepatotoxicity suggests only a limited role for this therapy. Moreover, a low-dose naltrexone treatment protocol was not found effective in reducing symptoms in another controlled trial.[128] Ondansetron (24 mg/day in six divided doses) was effective in reducing symptoms in bulimic subjects with severe symptoms. Expense is a major limitation in recommending this therapy for use in controlling bulimic symptoms.

The decision to augment a psychosocial therapy with medication in the treatment of BN hinges on comorbid illness, severity, past response to medication, patient preference, and patient commitment to adhering to a medication regimen. Sometimes, the therapeutic alliance is strengthened by the reduction in symptoms in association with a medication. Choice of medication is guided by side effect profile, history of response, and expense, since there are insufficient data to support greater efficacy for any particular agent. However, data do support consecutive trials if a patient does not respond to the first agent. If an agent is prescribed, it is essential to ensure that the dosing schedule is arranged such that the drug is sufficiently absorbed prior to purging behavior.

Medical therapeutic considerations for the comprehensive care of patients with BN include a plan to monitor for and address the most common and serious medical complications, including hypokalemia and cardiac dysrhythmias. Potassium losses occur in the setting of chronic purging behaviors associated with either BN or AN (e.g., induced vomiting, laxative abuse, and diuretic abuse).

The most common side effect of laxative abuse is diarrhea.[129] The diarrhea is often associated with cramping abdominal pain, and rectal pain may accompany defecation. Fecal electrolyte losses can be very high as the daily output increases considerably. Large amounts of sodium may be lost, but hyponatremia is rare because of the concomitant loss of water. The resulting picture of dehydration with hypotension, tachycardia, postural dizziness, and syncope needs to be addressed acutely, usually with IV fluids and electrolytes. Chronic deficiency of sodium and water may lead to increased renin secretion and secondary hyperaldosteronism that may then become autonomous persisting after the laxatives are removed, a pseudo-Bartter's syndrome. Hypo-

kalemia as a result of laxative-related losses may present as generalized muscle weakness and lassitude. More profound levels of hypokalemia may be life-threatening with cardiac arrhythmias. Of particular note, hypokalemia can, and often does, present asymptomatically, so patients with chronic losses through vomiting, laxative abuse, or diuretic abuse must be routinely monitored with serum electrolytes, even in the absence of symptoms. Hyperphosphatemia, hypermagnesemia, and hypocalcemia can also be seen as a result of excessive purging with laxatives, and this behavior needs to be discouraged. If motility is stimulated enough with the cathartic laxatives, absorption of nutrients may be impaired because of decreased transit time. Although laxatives may cause changes in the intestine itself, such as melanosis coli from pigment-laden macrophages within the submucosa of the colon secondary to anthraquinones, there does not appear to be any functional consequence to this. The "cathartic colon" has not truly been observed during the last few decades, presumably because the laxatives causing this are no longer in use.[130] That being said, the preference is to manage frequent complaints of constipation with stool softeners as opposed to cathartic agents (so as not to iatrogenically reproduce the purging behavior, to promote caloric loss, or to waste potassium). Polyethylene glycol solutions, as well as other osmotic agents, such as lactulose, are used to ease evacuation.

Dental hygiene in the bulimic patient (and anorexic patients with vomiting) should also be addressed. Preventive techniques to protect from further dental erosion include fluoride application, the use of brushing techniques, and even the use of mouth guards.[131]

Treatment of Binge-Eating Disorder

BED is the most common eating disorder; it is extremely prevalent in weight treatment–seeking populations. Because bingeing is often associated with shame, individuals are sometimes reluctant to disclose information about bingeing to their clinician. On the other hand, because of its association with distress and obesity, individuals are often quite willing to accept treatment. Although BED is a recently described nosologic category in the *DSM-IV* (currently defined with research criteria), there has been rapid progress in identifying effective psychosocial and pharmacologic treatment.

As with BN, the best-established treatment for BED is CBT. Having said that, few controlled treatment studies have been published[132] and studies are often restricted to obese subjects with BED, making it difficult to generalize to treatment for nonobese subjects. The manual of Fairburn et al.[102] for individual CBT for BN is relatively straightforwardly adapted for the treatment of BED.[102] Individual CBT appears effective in treatment of BED.[133] However, group therapy for BED in several psychotherapeutic modalities also achieves excellent results. Studies have demonstrated 79%, 73%, and 89% remission rates immediately posttreatment for cognitive behavioral group therapy, interpersonal group therapy, and dialectic behavioral therapy, respectively. Follow-up studies have shown some relapse, but remission rates were maintained reasonably well.[134,135]

Pharmacologic therapies for the treatment of BED are being rapidly identified (Table 35-3). Thus far, drugs in several classes (including several SSRIs, centrally acting appetite suppressants, and an anticonvulsant, topiramate) have been found effective. Although these studies show promise for the reduction of binge frequency among individuals with BED, it must be emphasized that more randomized controlled trials are necessary before optimal therapeutic recommendations can be determined. To date, placebo-controlled, randomized studies have found that fluvoxamine (50 to 300 mg/day)[136] and sertraline (50 to 200 mg/day)[137] significantly reduce the frequency of binge eating when compared to placebo. An additional randomized controlled study found fluoxetine (20 to 80 mg/day) effective in reducing binge frequency in BED.[138] However, another controlled randomized study did *not* find fluoxetine (60 mg/day) effective in the treatment of BED[139]; clearly, more trials are required to understand whether and when fluoxetine may be useful in the treatment of BED. In addition, an open-trial of venlafaxine (75 to 300 mg/day) demonstrated a significant reduction of binge frequency in BED.[140] More controlled trials to evaluate the efficacy of pharmacologic therapy in the treatment of BED are warranted and will likely be forthcoming soon in the scientific literature.

Before dexfenfluramine was withdrawn from the U.S. market in 1997, one controlled study had demonstrated its short-term efficacy against placebo in the treatment of BED.[141] Another centrally acting appetite suppressant, sibutramine (15 mg/day), has been shown effective in reducing the number of days with a binge as compared to placebo in a randomized controlled study of obese subjects with BED over a period of 12 weeks.[142] Finally, one randomized placebo-controlled trial of topiramate (mean dosage 212 mg/day; dosage range 50 to 600 mg/day) was found effective in reducing the frequency of binge eating in BED over a 14-week trial.[143] Whereas the SSRIs were generally well tolerated, the adverse event profile of topiramate makes the use of this agent somewhat more problematic in clinical settings.

Although additional agents have not yet been evaluated in the treatment of BED, treatment of symptoms that appear to trigger binges is good clinical practice. For example, in a patient whose binges are a response to anxiety, an anxiolytic agent should be tried. As with the other eating disorders, comorbid psychiatric illness should be treated. Whereas mood, anxiety, psychotic and other disorders should be addressed pharmacologically, clinicians, when possible, should avoid pharmacologic agents associated with weight gain and appetite stimulation if there are more weight-neutral alternatives available. For example, conventional and atypical antipsychotics are frequently associated with clinically significant weight gain, but some are reportedly more weight-neutral than others. By the same token, weight-neutral agents, or even agents that promote weight loss, such as topiramate, if effective in treating the patient's bipolar symptoms, may be an optimal choice for comorbid illness in the setting of BED. When possible, it is advantageous to select an agent that will address both the BED and the comorbid disorders.

Because BED is frequently comorbid with obesity, and because obesity is believed to contribute to risk for BED, weight reduction is often a primary goal of treatment and it can, in contrast to BN, be pursued concurrently or sequentially depending on the clinical situation.[144] For some patients, dieting is likely to exacerbate binge eating; it must be deferred until the binge pattern eating has been controlled. On the other hand, the addition of exercise to CBT appears to improve the outcome of BED.[145]

Notwithstanding the promise of the emerging evidence of efficacy for pharmacotherapy for BED, long-term outcome data are not yet available on which to base recommendations for maintenance therapy strategies for this disorder. Although there are only a few studies that compare efficacy of medication with CBT, one study showed that CBT was superior to either fluvoxamine or fluoxetine in reducing Eating Disorder Examination scores and BMI in subjects with BED. This study further found that augmentation of CBT with fluvoxamine, but not fluoxetine, improved outcome.[146] It must be emphasized that the field is quite rapidly evolving, and it is not yet known which patients might respond favorably to pharmacotherapy. For outpatients, a conservative approach would include starting with one of the proven effective group therapeutic modalities and adding a pharmacologic agent with proven efficacy if symptoms persist. There is no evidence that directly compares any of the agents for treatment of BED, so agents should be chosen based on the patient's history of prior response, comorbid illness, and side effect profile. On the other hand, when a more aggressive approach is desirable, it makes sense to begin with a combination of psychotherapy and pharmacotherapy. In some cases, appropriate psychotherapy may not be available, or the patient may not be amenable to this option; in such cases, it is appropriate to begin treatment with pharmacotherapy.

The most frequent medical complication of BED is obesity, although in many cases obesity occurs first and is complicated by the emergence of BED. Although rare, gastric rupture has also been reported as a sequelae of binge eating. Other medical comorbidities are those associated with overweight and obesity and include an elevated risk of type II diabetes, hypertension, cardiovascular disease, hypercholesterolemia, osteoarthritis, sleep apnea, gall bladder disease, and certain malignancies.

Because of the prevalence of BED in the weight-treatment–seeking population, a high percentage of patients seeking gastric bypass surgery for weight control have comorbid binge eating. For example, studies in different centers found 33.3% of 125 subjects being evaluated for bariatric surgery showing severe binge eating symptoms,[147] 39% of 64 morbidly obese subjects seeking gastric bypass,[148] and 47% of 92 massively obese patients undergoing bariatric surgery meet full criteria for BED.[149] The long-term impact of bariatric surgery on binge eating is still unclear. One short-term follow-up study found that all binge eating ceased in the four months following gastric bypass.[150] However, another study found that 46% of a sample of patients who had undergone gastric bypass within the past 2 to 7 years reported recurrent loss of control over eating; moreover, this group regained more weight than those who did not report such episodes.[151] Obviously, patients who continue to binge eat and thus regain weight after initial weight losses need further study to investigate risk-benefit ratios for proceeding to bariatric surgery and to identify interventions that can assist in suppression of the binge behavior in postoperative patients.

Summary

At Massachusetts General Hospital, and in many general hospital settings, patients with eating disorders frequently present with a serious, chronic, medically complicated, or comorbid illness. In such cases, a more flexible and eclectic treatment approach than is generally studied in clinical trials is frequently warranted. In addition, because of the medical comorbidity frequently associated with BED, a multidisciplinary approach with, at the very least, primary care, mental health care, and nutritional counseling is strongly preferred. Additional medical specialty care and psychopharmacologic specialty care is often optimal as well. Patients should be educated about their medical risk, and appropriate preventive therapy or interventions should be arranged.

An inpatient admission is an excellent time to develop and coordinate a multidisciplinary team and a prime opportunity for discussions about nutrition and psychoeducation. This should by all means be initiated when the patient may be especially motivated to take care or his or her health and have the time to absorb new information.

Inpatient assessment should include determination of nutritional status and medical comorbidities. Interventions typically include assisting the medical team to complete an appropriate diagnostic work-up and address potential medical and nutritional complications as well as develop a plan for any behavioral interventions to be implemented during the admission. Psychoeducation and engagement of the patient and determination of appropriate disposition and available resources are two further goals of psychiatric consultation. Finally, in some cases, behavioral strategies to stabilize weight, eating, or inappropriate compensatory behaviors and pharmacotherapy can be instituted.

References

1. National Institute of Mental Health: *Eating disorders*, Rockville, Md., 1994, NIH Publication No. 94–3477.
2. Anderson-Fye E, Becker AE: *Cultural dimensions of eating disorders: TEN— trends in evidence-based neuropsychiatry 2003*, (in press).
3. Crago M, Shisslak CM, Estes LS: Eating disturbances among American minority groups: a review, *Int J Eating Disord* 19:239–248, 1996.
4. Streigel-Moore RH, Wilfley DE, Pike KM, et al: Recurrent binge eating in black American women, *Arch Fam Med*, 9:83–87, 2000.
5. Spitzer RL, Yanovski S, Wadden T, et al: Binge eating disorder: its further validation in a multisite study, *Int J Eating Disord* 13:137–153, 1993.
6. Yanovski SC, Gormally JF, Leser MS, et al: Binge eating disorder affects outcome of comprehensive very low-calorie diet treatment, *Obes Res* 2:205–212, 1994.
7. Yanovski SC, Nelson JE, Dubbert BK, et al: Associations of binge eating disorder and psychiatric comorbidity in obese subjects, *Am J Psychiatry* 150:1472–1479, 1993.
8. Fitzgibbon ML, Spring B, Avellone ME, et al: Correlates of binge eating in Hispanic, Black, and White women, *Int J Eating Disord* 24:43–52, 1998.
9. Smith JE, Krejci J: Minorities join the majority: eating disturbances among Hispanic and Native American youth, *Int J Eating Disord* 10:179–186, 1991.
10. Bruce B, Agras WS: Binge eating in females: a population-based investigation, *Int J Eating Disord* 12:365–373, 1992.
11. Andersen AE: *Eating disorders in males*. In Brownell KD, Fairburn CG, editors: *Eating disorders and obesity: a comprehensive handbook*. New York, 1995, Guilford Press, 177–187.
12. American Psychiatric Association: *Diagnostic and Statistical Manual of Mental Disorders, ed 4*. Washington, DC, 1994, American Psychiatric Press.
13. Hoek HW: *The distribution of eating disorders*. In Brownell KD, Fairburn CG, editors: *Eating disorders and obesity: a comprehensive handbook*, New York, 1995, Guilford Press, 177–187.
14. Spitzer RL, Devlin M, Walsh BT, et al: Binge eating disorder: a multisite field trial of the diagnostic criteria, *Int J Eating Disord* 11:191–203, 1992.
15. Smith DE, Marcus MD, Lewis C, et al: Prevalence of binge eating disorder, obesity, and depression in a biracial cohort of young adults, *Ann Behav Med* 20:227–232, 1998.
16. Walters E, Kendler K: Anorexia nervosa and anorexic-like syndromes in a population-based female twin sample, *Am J Psychiatry* 152:64–71, 1995.
17. Kendler KS, MacLean C, Neale M, et al: The genetic epidemiology of bulimia nervosa, *Am J Psychiatry* 148:1627–1637, 1991.
18. Stein D, Meged S, Bar-Hanin T, et al: Partial eating disorders in a community sample of female adolescents, *J Am Acad Child Adolesc Psychiatry* 36:1116–1123, 1997.
19. Herzog DB, Delinsky SS: *Classification of eating disorders*. In Striegel-Moore RH, Smolak L, editors: *Eating disorders: innovative directions for research and practice*, Washington, DC, 2001, American Psychological Association, pp 31–50.
20. Center for Disease Control and Prevention: Youth risk behavior surveillance system: adolescent and school health, Available from: http://apps.nccd.cdc.gov/ YRBSS/index.asp. Accessed September 2002.
21. Shisslak CM, Crago M, Estes LS: The spectrum of eating disturbances, *Int J Eating Disord* 18:209–219, 1995.
22. Klump KL, Miller KB, Keel PK, et al: Genetic and environmental influence on anorexia nervosa syndromes in a population-based twin sample, *Psychol Med* 31:737–740, 2001.
23. Kendler KS, Walters EE, Neale MC, et al: The structure of the genetic and environmental risk factors for six major psychiatric disorders in women: phobia, generalized anxiety disorder, panic disorder, bulimia, major depression, and alcoholism, *Arch Gen Psychiatry* 52:374–383, 1995.
24. Bulik CM, Sullivan PF, Kendler KS: Heritability of binge-eating and broadly defined bulimia nervosa, *Biol Psychiatry* 44:1210–1218, 1998.
25. Branson R, Potoczna N, Kral JG, et al: Binge eating as a major phenotype of melanocortin 4 receptor gene mutations, *N Engl J Med* 348:1096–1103, 2003.
26. Bostic JQ, Muriel AC, Hack S, et al: Anorexia nervosa in a 7-year-old girl, *Dev Behav Pediatr* 18:331–333, 1997.
27. Blitzer JR, Rollins N, Blackwell A: Children who starve themselves: anorexia nervosa, *Psychosom Med* 5:369–383, 1961.
28. Halmi KA, Casper RC, Eckert ED, et al: *Unique features associated with the age of onset of anorexia nervosa*. In Nicholi AM, editor: *Harvard guide to psychiatry*. Cambridge, Mass., Belknap Press of Harvard University Press, 1999.
29. Lesser LI, Ashenden BJ, Debuskey M: Anorexia nervosa in children, *Am J Orthopsychiatry* 30:572–580, 1960.
30. Gowers SG, Crisp AH, Joughin N, et al: Premenarcheal anorexia nervosa, *J Child Psychol Psychiatry Allied Disciplines* 32:515–524, 1991.
31. Kent A, Lacey JH, McCluskey SE: Pre-menarchal bulimia nervosa, *J Psychosom Res* 36:205–210, 1992.

32. Mussell MP, Mitchell JE, Weller CL, et al: Onset of binge eating, dieting, obesity, and mood disorders among subjects seeking treatment for binge eating disorder, *Int J Eating Disord* 17:395–401, 1995.

33. Keel PK, Mitchell JE: Outcome in bulimia nervosa, *Am J Psychiatry* 154:313–321, 1997.

34. Steinhausen H: The outcome of anorexia nervosa in the 20th century, *Am J Psychiatry* 159:1284–1293, 2002.

35. Fichter MM, Quadflieg N, Gnutzmann A, et al: Binge eating disorder: treatment outcome over a 6-year course, *J Psychosom Res* 44:385–405, 1998.

36. Harris EC, Barraclough B: Excess mortality of mental disorder, *Br J Psychiatry* 173:11–53, 1998.

37. Sullivan PF: Mortality in anorexia nervosa, *Am J Psychiatry* 152:1073–1074, 1995.

38. King MB: Eating disorders in a general practice population: prevalence, characteristics and follow-up at 12–18 months, *Psychol Med Monographs* 14(suppl):1–34, 1989.

39. Stewart DE, Robinson E, Goldbloom DS, et al: Infertility and eating disorders, *Am J Obstet Gynecol* 163:1196–1199, 1990.

40. Whitehouse AM, Cooper PJ, Vize CV, et al: Prevalence of eating disorders in three Cambridge general practices: hidden and conspicuous morbidity, *Br J Gen Pract* 42:57–60, 1992.

41. Bryant-Waugh RJ, Lask BD, Shafran RL, et al: Do doctors recognise eating disorders in children? *Arch Dis Child* 67:103–105, 1992.

42. Gillberg C, Rastam M, Gillberg IC: Anorexia nervosa: who sees the patients and who do the patients see? *Acta Paediatrica* 83:967–971, 1994.

43. Ogg EC, Millar HR, Pusztai EE, et al: General practice consultation patterns preceding diagnosis of eating disorders, *Int J Eating Disord* 22:89–93, 1997.

44. Schoemaker C: Does early intervention improve the prognosis in anorexia nervosa? A systematic review of the treatment-outcome literature, *Int J Eating Disord* 21:1–15, 1997.

45. Waldholtz BD, Andersen AE: Gastrointestinal symptoms in anorexia nervosa: a prospective study, *Gastroenterology* 98(6):1415–1419, 1990.

46. Lee S: The Diagnostic Interview Schedule and anorexia nervosa in Hong Kong, *Arch Gen Psychiatry* 51:251–252, 1994.

47. Lee S, Ho TP, Hsu LKG: Fat phobic and non-fat phobic anorexia nervosa: a comparative study of 70 Chinese patients in Hong Kong, *Psychol Med* 23:999–1017, 1989.

48. Cachelin FM, Maher BA: Is amenorrhea a critical criterion for anorexia nervosa? *J Psychosom Res* 44:435–440, 1998.

49. Paige DM, editor: *Manual of clinical nutrition.* Pleasantville, NJ, 1983, Nutrition Publications.

50. Crespo CJ, Smit E, Troiano RP, et al: Television watching, energy intake, and obesity in US children: results from the third national health and nutrition examination survey, 1988–1944, *Arch Ped Adolesc Med* 155:360–365, 2001.

51. Mokdad A, Serdula MK, Dietz WH, et al: The spread of the obesity epidemic in the United States, 1991–1998, *JAMA* 282:1519–1522, 1999.

52. Flegal KM, Carroll MD, Kuczmarski RJ, et al: Overweight and obesity in the United States: prevalence and trends, 1960–1994, *Int J Obes* 22:39–47, 1998.

53. Flegal KM, Carroll MD, Ogden CL, et al: Prevalence and trends in obesity among US adults, 1999–2000, *JAMA* 288:1723–1727, 2002.

54. McGinnis M, Foege WH: Actual causes of death in the United States, *JAMA* 270:2207–2212, 1993.

55. Haller CA. Benowitz NL: Adverse cardiovascular and central nervous system events associated with dietary supplements containing ephedra alkaloids, *N Engl J Med* 343:1833–1838, 2000.

56. Dresser LP, Massey EW, Johnson EE, et al: Ipecac myopathy and cardiomyopathy, *J Neurol Neurosurg Psychiatry* 56:560–562, 1993.

57. Schiff RJ, Wurzel CL, Brunson SC, et al: Death due to chronic syrup of ipecac use in a patient with bulimia, *Pediatrics* 78(3):412–416, 1986.

58. Romig RA: Anorexia nervosa, ipecac, and sudden death, *Ann Int Med* 103(4):641, 1985.

59. Friedman EJ: Death from ipecac intoxication in a patient with anorexia nervosa, *Am J Psychiatry* 141:702–703, 1984.

60. Russell GF: Involuntary treatment in anorexia nervosa, *Psychiatric Clin North Am* 24:337–349, 2001.

61. Treasure JL, Katzman M, Schmidt U, et al: Engagement and outcome in the treatment of bulimia nervosa: first phase of a sequential design comparing motivation enhancement therapy and cognitive behavioural therapy, *Behav Res Ther* 37:405–418, 1999.

62. Cooke RA, Chambers JB: Anorexia nervosa and the heart, *Br J Hosp Med* 54:313–317, 1995.

63. Golden NH, Lanzkowsky L, Schebendach J, et al: The effect of estrogen-progestin treatment on bone mineral density in anorexia nervosa, *J Pediatr Adoles Gynecol* 15:135–143, 2002.

64. Grinspoon S, Thomas E, Pitts S, et al: Prevalence and predictive factors for regional osteopenia in women with anorexia nervosa, *Ann Intern Med* 133:790–794, 2000.

65. Jacoangeli F, Zoli A, Taranto A, et al: Osteoporosis and anorexia nervosa: relative role of endocrine alterations and malnutrition, *Eat Weight Disord* 7:190–195, 2002.

66. Golden NH, Jacobson MS, Schebendach J, et al: Resumption of menses in anorexia nervosa, *Arch Pediatr Adolesc Med* 151:16–21, 1997.

67. Hebebrand J, Himmelmann GW, Heseker H, et al: Use of percentiles for the body mass index in anorexia nervosa: diagnostic, epidemiological, and therapeutic considerations, *Int J Eating Disord* 19:359–369, 1996.

68. Howard WT, Evans K, Quintero-Howard C, et al: Predictors of success or failure of transition to day hospital treatment for inpatients with anorexia nervosa, *Am J Psychiatry* 156:1697–1702, 1999.
69. Herzog W, Deter H-C, Fiehn W, et al: Medical findings and predictors of long-term physical outcome in anorexia nervosa: a prospective, 12-year follow-up study, *Psychol Med* 27:269–279, 1997.
70. Koba T, Horie S, Nabeta Y: Impaired performance on Wisconsin Card Sorting Test in patient with eating disorders: a preliminary study, *Clin Psychiatry* 44:681–683, 2002.
71. Fassino S, Piero A, Abbate Daga G, et al: Attentional biases and frontal functioning in anorexia nervosa, *Int J Eating Disord* 31:274–283, 2002.
72. Kingston K, Szmukler G, Andrewes D, et al: Neuropsychological and structural brain changes in anorexia nervosa before and after refeeding, *Psychol Med* 26:15–28, 1996.
73. Delvenne V, Goldman S, DeMaertelaer V, et al: Brain hypometabolism of glucose in anorexia nervosa: normalization after weight gain, *Biol Psychiatry* 40:761–768, 1996.
74. Platte P, Pirke KM, Trimborn P, et al: Resting metabolic rate and total energy expenditure in acute and weight recovered patients with anorexia nervosa and in healthy young women, *Int J Eat Disord* 16:45–52, 1994.
75. Fisher M, Simpser E, Schneider M: Hypophosphatemia secondary to oral refeeding in anorexia nervosa, *Int J Eat Disord* 28:181–187, 2000.
76. Kohn MR, Golden NH, Shenker IR: Cardiac arrest and delirium: presentations of the refeeding syndrome in severely malnourished adolescents with anorexia nervosa, *J Adolesc Health* 22:239–243, 1998.
77. Goulet O: Nutritional support in malnourished pediatric patients, *Bailleres Clin Gastroenterol* 12:843–876, 1998.
78. Afzal NA, Addi S, Fagbemi A, et al: Refeeding syndrome with enteral nutrition in children: a case report, literature review and clinical guidelines, *Clin Nutr* 21:515–520, 2002.
79. Becker AE, Hamburg P, Herzog DB: *The role of psychopharmacologic management in the treatment of eating disorders.* In Dunner DL, Rosenbaum JF, editors: *Psychiatric clinics of North America: annual of drug therapy*, Philadelphia, 1998, WB Saunders, 17–51.
80. Kaye WH, Toshihiko N, Weltzin TE, et al: Double-blind placebo-controlled administration of fluoxetine in restricting- and restricting-purging-type anorexia nervosa, *Biol Psychiatry* 49:644–652, 2001.
81. Santonastaso P, Friederici S, Favaro A: Sertaline in the treatment of restricting anorexia nervosa: an open controlled trial, *J Child Adolesc Psychopharmacol* 11:143–150, 2001.
82. Birmingham CL, Goldner EM, Bakan R: Controlled trial of zinc supplementation in anorexia nervosa, *Int J Eating Disord* 15:251–255, 1994.
83. Fischer PW, Giroux A, L'Abbe MR: Effect of zinc supplementation on copper status in adult man, *Am J Clin Nutr* 40:743–746, 1984.
84. Houston S, Haggard J, Williford J Jr., et al: Adverse effects of large-dose zinc supplementation in an institutionalized older population with pressure ulcers, *J Am Geriatr Soc* 49:1130–1132, 2001.
85. Halmi KA, Eckert E, LaDu TJ, et al: Anorexia nervosa: treatment efficacy of cyprohetadine and amitriptyline, *Arch Gen Psychiatry* 43:177–181, 1986.
86. Vigersky RA, Loriaux DL: *The effect of cyproheptadine in anorexia nervosa: a double-blind trial.* In Vigersky RA, editor: *Anorexia nervosa*, New York, 1977, Raven Press, pp 349–356.
87. Newman-Toker J: Risperidone in anorexia nervosa, *Child Adolesc Psychiatry* 39:941–942, 2000.
88. Hansen L: Olanzapine in the treatment of anorexia nervosa, *Br J Psychiatry* 175:592, 1999.
89. La Via MC, Gray N, Kaye WH: Case reports of olanzapine treatment of anorexia nervosa, *Int J Eating Disord* 27:363–366, 2000.
90. Jensen VS, Mejlhede A: Anorexia nervosa: treatment with olanzapine, *Br J Psychiatry* 177:87, 2000.
91. Mehler C, Wewetzer C, Schulze U, et al: Olanzapine in children and adolescents with chronic anorexia nervosa: a study of five cases, *Eur Child Adolesc Psychiatry* 10:151–157, 2001.
92. Boachie A, Goldfield GS, Spettigue S: Olanzapine use as an adjunctive treatment for hospitalized children with anorexia nervosa: case reports, *Int J Eating Disord* 33:98–103, 2003.
93. Malina A, Gaskill J, McConaha C, et al: Olanzapine treatment of anorexia nervosa: a retrospective study, *Int J Eating Disord* 33:234–237, 2003.
94. Powers PS, Santana CA, Bannon YS: Olanzapine in the treatment of anorexia nervosa: an open label trial, *Int J Eating Disord* 32:146–154, 2002.
95. Bowers WA: Basic principles for applying cognitive-behavioral therapy to anorexia nervosa, *Psychiatr Clin North Am* 24:293–303, 2001.
96. Dare C, Eisler I, Russell G, et al: Psychological therapies for adults with anorexia nervosa: randomised controlled trial of out-patient treatments, *Br J Psychiatry* 178:216–221, 2001.
97. McIntosh VV, Bulik CM, McKenzie JM, et al: Interpersonal psychotherapy for anorexia nervosa, *Int J Eating Disord* 27:125–139, 2000.
98. Russell GF, Szmukler GI, Dare C, et al: An evaluation of family therapy in anorexia nervosa and bulimia nervosa, *Arch Gen Psychiatry* 44:1047–1056, 1987.
99. Geist R, Heinmaa M, Stephens D, et al: Comparison of family therapy and family group psychoeducation

in adolescents with anorexia nervosa, *Can J Psychiatry — Revue Canadienne de Psychiatrie* 45:173–178, 2000.

100. Waisberg JL, Woods MT: A nutrition and behaviour change group for patients with anorexia nervosa, *Can J Diet Pract Res* 63:202–205, 2002.

101. Fernandez-Aranda F, Bel M, Jimenez S, et al: Outpatient group therapy for anorexia nervosa: a preliminary study, *Eating Weight Disord* 3:1–6, 1998.

102. Fairburn CG, Marcus MD, Wilson GT: *Cognitive-behavioral therapy for binge eating and bulimia nervosa: a comprehensive treatment manual.* In Fairburn CG, Wilson GT, editors: *Binge eating: nature, assessment, and treatment,* New York, 1993, 361–404.

103. Thompson-Brenner H, Glass S, Westen D: A multidimensional meta-analysis of psychotherapy for bulimia nervosa, *Clin Psychol* (in press).

104. Zerbe KJ: Feminist psychodynamic psychotherapy of eating disorders: theoretic integration informing clinical practice, *Psychiatr Clin North Am* 19:811–827, 1996.

105. Fairburn DB, Jone R, Peveler RC, et al: Psychotherapy and bulimia nervosa: longer-term effects of interpersonal psychotherapy, behavior therapy, and cognitive behavior therapy, *Year Book Psychiatry Appl Ment Health* 4:110–112, 1995.

106. Agras WS, Walsh BT, Fairburn CB, et al: A multicenter comparison of cognitive-behavior therapy and interpersonal therapy for bulimia nervosa, *Arch Gen Psychiatry* 57:459–466, 2000.

107. Safer DL, Telch CF, Agras WS: Dialectical behavior therapy for bulimia nervosa, *Am J Psychiatry* 158:632–634, 2001.

108. Jager B, Liedtke R, Kunsebeck HW, et al: Psychotherapy and bulimia nervosa: evaluation and long-term follow up of two conflict orientated treatment conditions, *Acta Psychiatrica Scandinavica* 93:268–278, 1996.

109. Esplen MJ, Garfinkel PE, Olmsted M, et al: A randomized controlled trial of guided imagery in bulimia nervosa, *Psychol Med* 28:1347–1357, 1998.

110. Thiels C, Schmidt U, Treasure J, et al: Guided self-change for bulimia nervosa incorporating use of a self-care manual, *Am J Psychiatry* 155:947–953, 1998.

111. Jimerson DC, Herzog DB, Brotman AW: Pharmacologic Approaches in the treatment of eating disorders, *Harvard Rev Psychiatry* 1:82–93, 1993.

112. Walsh BT, Agras WS, Devlin MJ, et al: Fluoxetine for bulimia nervosa following poor response to psychotherapy, *Am J Psychiatry* 157:1332–1334, 2000.

113. Fluoxetine Bulimia Nervosa Collaborative Study Group: Fluoxetine in the treatment of bulimia nervosa: a multicenter, placebo-controlled, double-blind trial, *Arch Gen Psychiatry* 49:139–147, 1992.

114. Goldstein DJ, Wilson MG, Thompson VL, et al: Long-term fluoxetine treatment of bulimia nervosa, *Br J Psychiatry* 166:660–666, 1995.

115. Romano SJ, Halmi KA, Sarkar NP, et al: A placebo-controlled study of fluoxetine in continued treatment of bulimia nervosa after successful acute fluoxetine treatment, *Am J Psychiatry* 159:96–102, 2002.

116. Walsh BT, Hadigan CM, Wong LM: Increased pulse and blood pressure associated with desipramine treatment of bulimia nervosa, *J Clin Psychopharmacol* 12:163–168, 1992.

117. Damlouji NF, Ferguson JM: Trazodone-induced delirium in bulimic patients, *Am J Psychiatry* 141:434–435, 1984.

118. Pope HG, Hudson JI, Jonas JM, et al: Bulimia treated with imipramine: a placebo-controlled, double-blind study, *Am J Psychiatry* 140:554–558, 1983.

119. Hughes PL, Wells LA, Cunningham CJ, et al: Treating bulimia with desipramine: a double-blind, placebo-controlled study, *Arch Gen Psychiatry* 43:182–186, 1986.

120. Barlow J, Blouin J, Blouin A, et al: Treatment of bulimia with desipramine: a double-blind crossover study, *Can J Psychiatry* 33:129–133, 1988.

121. Pope HG, Keck PE, McElroy SL, et al: A placebo-controlled study of trazodone in bulimia nervosa, *J Clin Psychiatry* 9:254–259, 1989.

122. Horne RL, Ferguson JM, Pope HG, et al: Treatment of bulimia with bupropion: a multicenter controlled trial, *J Clin Psychiatry* 49:262–266, 1988.

123. Walsh BT, Gladis M, Roose SP, et al: Phenelzine vs placebo in 50 patients with bulimia, *Arch Gen Psychiatry* 45:471–475, 1988.

124. Kennedy SH, Piran N, Warsh JJ, et al: A trial of isocarboxazid in the treatment of bulimia nervosa, *J Clin Psychopharmacol* 8:391–397, 1988.

125. Keck PE, Pope HG, Nierenberg AA: Autoinduction of hypertensive reactions by tranylcypromine, *J Clin Psychopharmacol* 9:48 51, 1989.

126. Fallon BA, Walsh BT, Sadik C, et al: Outcome and clinical course in inpatient bulimic women: a 2- to 9-year follow-up study, *J Clin Psychiatry* 52:272–278, 1991.

127. Jonas JM, Gold MS: The use of opiate antagonists in treating bulimia: a study of low-dose versus high-dose naltrexone, *Psychiatry Res* 24:195–199, 1988.

128. Mitchell JE, Christenson G, Jennings J, et al: A placebo-controlled, double-blind crossover study of naltrexone hydrochloride in outpatients with normal weight bulimia, *J Clin Psychopharmacol* 9:94–97, 1988.

129. Bake EH, Sandle GI: Complications of laxative abuse. *Annu Rev Med* 47:127–134, 1996.

130. Muller-Lissner SA: Adverse effects of laxatives: fact and fiction, *Pharmacol* 47(suppl 1):138–145, 1993.

131. Sundaram G, Bartlett D: Preventive measures for bulimic patients with dental erosion, *Eur J Prosthodont Restor Dent* 9:25–29, 2001.

132. Ricca V, Mannucci E, Zucchi T, et al: Cognitive-behavioural therapy for bulimia nervosa and binge eating disorder: a review, *Psychother Psychosom* 69:287–295, 2000.

133. Ricca V, Mannucci E, Mezzani B, et al: Fluoxetine and fluvoxamine combined with individual cognitive-behaviour therapy in binge eating disorder: a one-year follow-up study, *Psychother Psychosom* 70:298–306, 2001.

134. Wilfley DE, Welch RR, Stein RI, et al: A randomized comparison of group cognitive-behavioral therapy and group interpersonal psychotherapy for the treatment of overweight individuals with binge-eating disorder, *Arch Gen Psychiatry* 59:713–721, 2002.

135. Telch CF, Agras WS, Linehan MM: Dialectical behavior therapy for binge eating disorder, *J Consult Clin Psychol* 69:1061–1065, 2001.

136. Hudson JI, McElroy SL, Raymond NC, et al: Fluvoxamine treatment of binge eating disorder: a multicenter, placebo-controlled double-blind trial, *Am J Psychiatry* 155:1756–1762, 1998.

137. McElroy SL, Casuto LS, Nelson EB, et al: Placebo-controlled trial of sertraline in the treatment of binge-eating disorder, *Am J Psychiatry* 157:1004–1006, 2000.

138. Arnold LM, McElroy SL, Hudson JI, et al: A placebo-controlled, randomized trial of fluoxetine in the treatment of binge-eating disorder, *J Clin Psychiatry* 63:1028–1033, 2002.

139. Grilo C: A controlled study of cognitive behavioral therapy and fluoxetine for binge eating disorder (abstract), *Eating disorders research society annual meeting scientific program and abstracts* Charleston, SC, November 23, 2002.

140. Malhotra S, King KH, Welge JA: Venlafaxine treatment of binge-eating disorder associated with obesity: a series of 35 patients, *J Clin Psychiatry* 63:1028–1033, 2002.

141. Stunkard A, Berkowitz R, Tanrikut C, et al: d-Fenfluramine treatment of binge eating disorder, *Am J Psychiatry* 153:1455–1459, 1996.

142. Appolinario JC, Bacaltchuk J, Sichieri R, et al: A randomized, double-blind, placebo-controlled study of sibutramine in the treatment of binge eating disorder, *Arch Gen Psychiatry* (in press).

143. McElroy SL, Arnold LM, Shapira NA, et al: Topiramate in the treatment of binge eating disorder associated with obesity: a randomized, placebo-controlled trial, *Am J Psychiatry* 160:255–261, 2003.

144. Devlin MJ: Binge-eating disorder and obesity: a combined treatment approach, *Psychiatr Clin North Am* 24:325–335, 2001.

145. Pendleton VR, Goodrick GK, Poston WSC, et al: Exercise augments the effects of cognitive-behavioral therapy in the treatment of binge eating, *Int J Eating Disord* 31:172–184, 2002.

146. Ricca V, Mannucci E, Messani B, et al: Fluoxetine and fluvoxamine combined with individual cognitive-behaviour therapy in binge eating disorder: a one year follow-up study, *Psychother Psychosom* 70:298–306, 2001.

147. Saunders R: Binge eating in gastric bypass patients before surgery, *Obes Surg* 9:72–76, 1999.

148. Kalarchian MA, Wilson GT, Brolin RE, et al: Binge eating in bariatric surgery patients, *Int J Eating Disord* 23:89–92, 1998.

149. Adami GF, Gandolfo P, Bauer B, et al: Binge eating in massively obese patients undergoing bariatric surgery, *Int J Eating Disord* 17:45–50, 1995.

150. Kalarchian MA, Wilson GT, Brolin RE, et al: Effects of bariatric surgery on binge eating and related psychopathology, *Eating Weight Disord* 4:1–5, 1999.

151. Kalarchian MA, Marcus MD, Wilson GT, et al: Binge eating among gastric bypass patients at long-term follow-up, *Obes Surg* 12:270–275, 2002.

Chapter 36
Organ Failure and Transplantation

Owen S. Surman, M.D.
Laura M. Prager, M.D.

Advances in Transplantation Biology

The past 3 decades have seen dramatic growth in organ transplantation. Kidney transplantation, an uncommon event in the mid-1960s, is now a routine operation. With the advent of cyclosporine, tacrolimus, and other advances in immunosuppressive treatment of graft rejection, transplantation (of livers, hearts, and lungs) became practical in the 1980s; now excellent survival statistics accompany such procedures. These solid organ transplantations (performed as a result of end-organ failure) are the focus of this chapter. Bone marrow transplantation (which has given hope to cancer patients) is beyond the scope of this chapter.[1]

Procedural Limitations

A variety of factors limit organ transplantation; several of these factors will be mentioned here. Rejection and the complications of antirejection therapy remain key biologic factors that limit successful transplantation. Steroid-sparing approaches, such as with sirolimus, have produced progress in pancreatic islet cell transplantation research. Since human organ transplantation has its limitations, work also proceeds on animal models of xenotransplantation. Tissue engineering is at an early, but promising, stage of basic scientific discovery. Immunologic tolerance is essential to transplantation, and one new strategy is to irradiate the bone

marrow of transplant recipients and to perform transplantation of donor marrow as a means of producing temporary immunologic chimerism. This protocol has had initial success in clinical trials with combined bone marrow and renal transplantation for patients with myeloma kidney.[2]

Societal limits are imposed by the shortage of cadaveric organs and in some nations, such as Japan, by the absence of criteria for brain death essential to cadaveric transplantation.[3] While asystolic cadaveric donors are an alternative for renal allografts,[4] other organs are less able to withstand ischemic injury. Fortunately, kidney donation from living donors is common in many countries and participation of unrelated, living donors is now a common and accepted practice in the United States. In addition, parent-to-child liver transplantation is frequently performed using the left lateral lobe, and living-related lung transplantation is an option (with a lung lobe donated by each of two living donors).

Transplantation of the right hepatic lobe from a living adult donor to a recipient has proven life-saving for liver transplant candidates (who face a 10% risk of dying before obtaining a liver from a cadaveric source). The relatively greater morbidity of this type of donor surgery has become a source of ethical deliberation.[5,6] As of March 2003, two donors have died in the United States. In addition, according to a UCLA liver transplant surgeon, Ronald Bussutil, two donors (one in Europe and one in the United States) have required liver transplantation, three donors developed portal vein thrombosis, and several others required *roux y* procedures because of strictures. Other major complications have included bile leaks, secondary biliary cirrhosis, pulmonary embolisms, and bleeding after a liver biopsy. According to Bussutil, two centers in the United States have no cadaveric donor programs.[7] Regulations for partial liver transplantation currently are being developed under the auspices of the New York State Department of Public Health, and there is a transplantation advisory committee for the Department of Health and Human Services. The National Organ Transplant Act upholds ethical practices related to organ donation and prohibits the sale of organs.

The Need for Psychiatric Intervention

Patient and organ donor selection are two areas that require psychiatric input. In some centers a psychiatrist is assigned specifically for this task. However, many transplant centers rely on general hospital psychiatric consultation services for this purpose, and in some centers psychologists and social workers are involved in the psychosocial screening of recipients and donors.

Perioperative psychiatric support of transplant candidates requires an appreciation of the special needs of surgical patients and those with end-stage organ failure.[8] Psychiatrists are typically asked to predict the likelihood of patient compliance after transplantation and to treat preoperative and postoperative psychiatric syndromes. Postoperative sequelae unique to transplantation are a consequence of allograft rejection and use of immunosuppressive agents. Many clinicians refer to the roller coaster-like experience of transplantation, replete with promise and uncertainty.[9]

Organ Failure

Common Features

Functional decline and role loss are inevitable sequelae of end-organ failure; these conditions predispose to adjustment disorders, anxiety syndromes, and depression. Loss of mental acuity, which may progress to frank encephalopathy, also accompanies organ failure.

Renal Failure

Diagnostic Considerations: Renal failure may have either a systemic or local cause. Systemic diseases such as diabetes mellitus (DM), hypertension (HTN), and collagen vascular diseases are associated with greater morbidity than disorders isolated to the kidneys.

Hereditary diseases such as polycystic kidney disease (PCKD) have reduced family donor availability. Afflicted individuals share concern about and emergence of the disorder among younger family members. Acceptance of treatment for renal failure may be affected by adverse experiences of other afflicted family members. This parallels circumstances in cancer care, in which prior treatment experiences of family and friends are important factors in psychological outcome.[10] Patients with diabetes often bear the added burden of retinopathy, sensory deficits, neuropathy, and gastrointestinal dysmotility. Another uncommon cause of nephropathy is chronic lithium therapy; as a consequence, renal function must be monitored when prescribing lithium. Mood stabilizers such as valproate and carbamazepine are therapeutic alternatives.

The availability of dialysis treatment is the feature that most clearly distinguishes renal failure from other types of end-organ disease. Hemodialysis is performed at most acute care centers. Patients are subsequently maintained in chronic-care centers, which provide varying degrees of self-care, or home-based hemodialysis. Hemodialysis is typically performed 3 times weekly for approximately 4-hour sessions. Scheduling of sessions has a significant impact on work and family life. Continuous ambulatory peritoneal dialysis (CAPD) can be performed intermittently, typically 4 times daily or continuously throughout the night. A patient must be capable of meticulous self-care if peritonitis is to be avoided. Lapses may be affected by mood disorders, cognitive impairment, environmental stress, and noncompliance and are indications for psychiatric and social service referral.

Depression has long been considered an important complication of dialysis treatment; moreover, it is more frequent among those with higher levels of morbidity. Some researchers have attempted to standardize measures for medical impairment in this population. An example of this is the end-stage renal disease (ESRD) severity index.[11] Some studies suggest that depression increases mortality among dialysands.[12] Contributing to the depression associated with renal failure are alterations of endocrine function (especially from hyperparathyroidism) and neurotransmission.[13] Anemia, another contributor to depression with renal failure, often responds to erythropoietin.

Encephalopathy is a consequence of uremia. Altered mental status secondary to uremia may be an indication for dialysis. It is especially important to call attention to this abnormality, which may be mistakenly attributed to depression by the nonpsychiatric physician. Neuropsychiatric syndromes specific to renal failure include dialysis dysequilibrium and, rarely, dialysis dementia, which is most commonly ascribed to aluminum encephalopathy.[13] Seizures are common in uremia; complex partial seizures often result in behavioral changes (commonly including agitation and uncommonly catatonia) that respond to anticonvulsant therapy.[14,15] Encephalopathy may also occur in response to activation of cytokines as part of the immunologic activation by synthetic dialysis membranes.[16]

Psychiatric Intervention: Psychopharmacologic care of the patient with renal failure requires dosage adjustments of standard anxiolytics, antidepressants, and neuroleptics as described by Bennett, Singer, and Coggins[17] (Table 36-1). Use of selective serotonin-reuptake inhibitors (SSRIs), bupropion, and psychostimulants for the treatment of depression is preferred.[13,18] Short-acting anxiolytics are generally preferable to longer-acting ones because their use minimizes the build-up of metabolites. Monitoring the blood levels of anticonvulsants can be complicated by low values that may result from changes in protein-binding. More meaningful are unbound or free levels of phenytoin and carbamazepine. Lithium carbonate is readily dialyzed; therefore, it should be administered after dialysis treatments. Some patients require continued administration on the days they do not receive dialysis. Frequent monitoring (especially at the outset of treatment) is essential to detect and to avoid toxicity. Monthly levels, drawn before hemodialysis, are advisable once a satisfactory dosing schedule has been established. When aluminum encephalopathy is suspected,

deferoxamine, an iron-binding and aluminum-binding agent, should be administered.[13]

Psychotherapy (due to medical stressors, decreased autonomy, and in some instances, impaired cognition) is challenging with patients in renal failure. Hypnotherapy may prove beneficial for patients with needle phobias and anxiety. Insight-oriented psychotherapeutic strategies may be unacceptable or destabilizing for those who rely on denial and who lack a sense of control.[19] Cognitive therapy and other active ego-supportive approaches are indicated.

Treatment termination is an option that dialysis patients sometimes choose in the face of an unacceptable reduction in their quality of life.[20,21] The psychiatrist may be called on in such instances to assess the capacity to refuse treatment. When the patient is depressed, one can typically temporize and initiate treatment for depression. The following case examples are illustrative.

Case 1

Mr. A, 40-year-old diabetic man was referred for psychiatric evaluation of depression because he wanted to discontinue hemodialysis. There was no personal or family history of depression. He reported a depressed mood in association with chronic pain from diabetic neuropathy and severe headaches that often followed hemodialysis sessions. Mr. A agreed to a trial of an antidepressant but he did not improve. Fifty milligrams of meperidine, an opiate, was administered by mouth once to twice daily after hemodialysis, and his pain was relieved. Mr. A subsequently underwent successful renal transplantation.

Case 2

Dr. B, a professionally productive, middle-aged physician, developed an infectious complication of CAPD that required acute operative intervention. Psychiatric consultation was requested when he refused surgery. His wife reported that he had never expressed a wish to curtail his medical therapy. On examination, he was alert but looked depressed and felt "overwhelmed." The psychiatrist suggested that he needed to rely on his health care proxy, and he referred to his own history of bereavement regarding the impact of choices. Despite his distress, Dr. B made meaningful eye contact and nodded in apparent acceptance. The psychiatrist recommended that Dr. B undergo laparotomy with the understanding that he could subsequently withdraw from dialysis if operative intervention proved unsuccessful. He acquiesced, and his depression abated following surgery.

Table 36-1. Drug Therapy in Renal Disease *†

Drug	Pharmacokinetic Parameters					Adjustment for Renal Failure GFR (mL/min)				Removed by Dialysis	Toxic Effects and Remarks
	Elimination and Metabolism	Half-life Normal (hr)	Half-life ESRD (hr)	Plasma Protein Binding (%)	Volume of Distribution (L/kg)	Method	>50	10–50	<10		
Antidepressants											
Amoxapine	Hepatic	8–30	?	90	?	D	Unch	Unch	Unch	?	—
Bupropion	Hepatic	9.6–20.9	?	75–85	27–63	D	Unch	Unch	Unch	?	—
Fluoxetine	Hepatic	1–10	Unch	94.5	Large	D	Unch	Unch	Unch	No (H)	—
Maprotiline	Hepatic	48	?	?	?	D	Unch	Unch	Unch	?	—
Barbiturates*											*Group remarks: May increase osteomalacia in hemodialysis patients; half-life decreases with chronic therapy because of hepatic microsomal enzyme induction; hemodialysis more effective than peritoneal dialysis in overdoses; charcoal hemoperfusion best for massive overdoses; all agents in this group may cause excessive sedation.
Hexobarbital	Hepatic	3.5–4.0	?	40–50	1.1	D	Unch	Unch	Unch	No (H)	Group remarks
Pentobarbital*	Hepatic	18–48	Unch	60–70	1	D	Unch	Unch	Unch	No (H)	*Pharmacokinetics of amobarbital are similar ‡Decreased in ESRD
Phenobarbital	Hepatic (renal 30%)	60–150	117–160	40–60	0.7–1.0	1	Unch	Unch	12–16	Yes (H,P)	Group remarks; up to 50% of drug excreted unchanged in alkaline diuresis
Secobarbital	Hepatic	20–35	?	44	1.1–1.25	D	Unch	Unch	Unch	No (H,P)	Group remarks
Thiopental	Hepatic	3.8	?	72–86	1.0–1.5	D	Unch	Unch	75	?	Group remarks

Drug	Metabolism										Comments
Alprazolam	Hepatic	10–19	?	70–80	0.9–1.5	D	Unch	Unch	Unch	?	Group toxicity
Chlordiazep-oxide	Hepatic (renal)*	5–30†	?	94–97	0.3–0.5‡	D	Unch	Unch	Unch	No (H)	Group toxicity
Clonazepam	Hepatic	5–30	?	47	1.5–4.5	D	Unch	Unch	Unch	?	Group toxicity
Clorazepate	Hepatic (renal)	36–200	?	?	?	D	Unch	Unch	Unch	?	Group toxicity
Diazepam	Hepatic (renal,* GI‡)	20–90‡	?	94–98δ	0.7–2.6ll	D	Unch	Unch	Unch	No (H)	Group toxicity
Flurazepam	Hepatic (renal)*	47–100	?	?‡	3.4‡	D	Unch	Unch	Unch	No (H)	Group toxicity

*Group toxicity: All agents in this group may cause excessive sedation or encephalopathy, or both, in chronic hemodialysis patients.

*Active metabolite excreted by kidney.
†Large variability; chronic therapy prolongs half-life.
‡Excessive protein binding leads to underestimation of volume of distribution.

*Active metabolite desmethyl-diazepam excreted by kidney. Enterohepatic circulation exists
‡Increased metabolism with prolonged therapy; extreme variability.
§Variably decreased to about 92% in ESRD; binding higher in males than in females.
llIncreased in ESRD.

*First-pass hepatic metabolism; excretion routes and half-life pertain to active metabolites.
†Protein binding weaker than that of other benzodiazepines.
‡Animal data

continued

Table 36-1. Drug Therapy in Renal Disease *†—cont'd

Pharmacokinetic Parameters

Drug	Elimination and Metabolism	Half-life Normal (hr)	Half-life ESRD (hr)	Plasma Protein Binding (%)	Volume of Distribution (L/kg)	Method	>50	10–50	<10	Removed by Dialysis	Toxic Effects and Remarks
						Adjustment for Renal Failure GFR (mL/min)					
Lorazepam	Hepatic	9–16	32–70	90	1.3	D	Unch	Unch	50	No (H)	Group toxicity
Midazolam	Hepatic	2–3	10–20	90*	1.3	D	Unch	Unch	Unch	No (H)	Group toxicity; *Protein binding decreased in ESRD.
Oxazepam	Hepatic	6–25	25–90	90	1.6*	D	Unch	Unch	75	No (H)	Group toxicity, glucuronide metabolite increases in ESRD. *Increased in ESRD, which accounts for increased half-life.
Triazolam	Hepatic	1.4–3.3	—	85–95	—	D	Unch	Unch	Unch	?	Group toxicity
Nonbenzodiazepine sedative hypnotics											
Buspirone	Hepatic	2–5	5–6	?	?	D	Unch	Unch	50–75*	Yes (H)	*Active metabolite accumulates.
Chloral hydrate	Hepatic	7–14	Unch	35–40	1.6	D	Unch	Avoid	Avoid	Yes (H)	May cause excessive sedation or encephalopathy, or both, in chronic hemodialysis patients.
Ethchlorvynol	Hepatic (renal)*	19–32	Unch	35–50	3–4	D	Unch	Avoid	Avoid	No (H,P)	May cause excessive sedation: nephrotoxic, may be effectively removed by hemoperfusion. *Proportion of hepatic and renal excretion uncertain.
Glutethimide	Hepatic (renal)*	5–22†	Unch	54	2.7	D	Unch	Avoid	Avoid	No (H,P)	May cause excessive sedation. *Enterohepatic circulation exists; active metabolite excreted by kidney. †Half-life increases with dose and hypotension.

Other agents

Drug	Route									Comments
Haloperidol	Hepatic (renal, GI)	10–36	?	90–92	14–21	D	Unch	Unch	Unch	No (H,P)	‡Active metabolite 4 hydroxyglutethimide has long half-life in renal failure. May cause hypotension, excessive sedation.
Lithium carbonate	Renal	14–28*	Prolonged	0	0.5–0.9	D	Unch	50–75	25–50	Yes (H,P)†	Nephrogenic diabetes, insipidus; nephrotic syndrome; renal tubular acidosis; chronic interstitial fibrosis; toxicity when serum levels are >1.2 mEq/L; serum levels 12 hr after a dose should be measured periodically; toxicity enhanced and drug clearance reduced by volume depletion, nonsteroidal anti-inflammatory drugs, and diuretics; excretion enhanced by $NaHCO_3$, acetazolamide, aminophylline, and osmotic diuretics. *Plasma half-life does not reflect extensive tissue accumulation †Plasma levels rise after dialysis as re-equilibration with tissue stores occurs.
Meprobamate	Hepatic (renal 10%)	6–17	Unch	0–20	0.75	1	6	9–12	12–18	Yes (N,P)†	May cause excessive sedation. *Renal excretion may be increased by forced diuresis. †Hemodialysis twice as efficient as peritoneal dialysis.

continued

Table 36-1. Drug Therapy in Renal Disease *† —cont'd

| | Pharmacokinetic Parameters | | | | | Adjustment for Renal Failure GFR (mL/min) | | | | | |
| | | Half-life | | | | | | | | | |
Drug	Elimination and Metabolism	Normal (hr)	ESRD (hr)	Plasma Protein Binding (%)	Volume of Distribution (L/kg)	Method	>50	10-50	<10	Removed by Dialysis	Toxic Effects and Remarks
Methaqualone	Hepatic (0.9 and 16–42)	Biphasic	Unch	80	5–8	D	Unch	Avoid	Avoid	No (H)	May cause excessive sedation; contaminant (O-toluidine) may cause hemorrhagic cystitis. *Biexponential pharmacokinetics; longer half-life more important clinically.
Monoamine oxidase inhibitors											*Group remarks: Hypertensive crisis can be caused by interaction with tyramine in food and beverages or by interaction with sympathomimetics or levodopa. Group remarks
Phenelzine	Hepatic	?	?	?	?	D	Unch	Unch	Unch	?	
Phenothiazines*											*Group toxicity: all agents in this group are anticholinergic; may cause urinary retention, orthostatic hypotension, confusion, and extrapyramidal symptoms; characteristic acute toxic psychosis; >800 mg/day thioridazine causes retinitis; prototype chlorpromazine. Group toxicity *Large volume of distribution after oral dose. †May need to decrease dose and increase interval if excessive sedation occurs.
Chlorpromazine	Hepatic	11–42	?	91–99	8–160*	D	Unch	Unch	Unch	?	
Tricyclic antidepressants*											Group remarks: All agents in this group are anticholinergic and

Drug	Route (renal)									Dialysis	Toxic Effects and Remarks
Amitriptyline	Hepatic* (renal <5%)	32–40	?	96	6–36	D	Unch	Unch	Unch†	No (H,P)	may cause urinary retention; may decrease hypotensive effects of guanethidine, clonidine, and methyldopa; enterohepatic circulation and genetic variation in metabolism exist; increased excretion in acid urine (total remains small); smoking, alcohol, and sedatives induce metabolism; neuroleptics and advanced age inhibit metabolism; may cause excessive sedation; physostigmine. Indicated for life-threatening overdose. Group remarks *Metabolized to nortriptyline. †Reported to stimulate weight gain and appetite in dialysis patients.
Desipramine	Hepatic (renal <5%)	12–54	?	90	28–60	D	Unch	Unch	Unch	No (H,P)	Group remarks
Doxepin	Hepatic	8–25	?	93–95	9–33	D	Unch	Unch	Unch	No (H,P)	Group Remarks
Imipramine	Hepatic* (renal <5%)	6–20	?	96	9–15	D	Unch	Unch	Unch	No (H,P)	Group remarks *Metabolized to desipramine
Nortriptyline	Hepatic (renal <5%)	18–93	15–66	95	15–23	D	Unch	Unch	Unch	No (H,P)	Group remarks
Protriptyline	Hepatic	54–98	?	92	15–31	D	Unch	Unch	Unch	No (H,P)	Group remarks

Adapted from Bennett WM, Singer I, Coggins CJ. *JAMA* 230:1544–1553, 1974.

*Note that footnote symbols within each drug group refer to footnotes in "Toxic Effects and Remarks" column at extreme right.

†ESRD = end-stage renal disease; GFR, glomerular filtration rate: /, interval extension method of dosage adjustment (data units are hours between maintenance doses); D = dose reduction method of dosage adjustment (data units are percent of usual maintenance dose); H = hemodialysis; P = peritoneal dialysis; Unch = unchanged.

Often the patient who wishes to withdraw from therapy has the capacity to refuse treatment. In such instances, it may be necessary for the psychiatrist to support the team and the patient's family while dialysis is discontinued. At Massachusetts General Hospital (MGH) an Optimum Care Committee, comprised of physicians, medical ethicists, clergy, and others, is available for added consultation.

Quality of Life and Choice of Renal Failure Therapy

The benefits of one or another form of ESRD therapy vary with medical circumstances. For a patient with advanced atherosclerosis, a successful vascular anastomosis and transplantation may not be possible. Transplantation will not improve quality of life if a patient is unable to secure funding for the expensive immunosuppressants that are required for the rest of his or her life. Diabetic patients are less tolerant of hemodialysis and are at risk for acceleration of retinopathy. Combined pancreas and kidney transplantation, although associated with an increased risk of postoperative morbidity, offers an advantage because the need for insulin therapy is eliminated. Access to an established transplant center and postoperative follow-up is another consideration, as is the level of individual immunologic sensitization. Historically, there has been some center bias toward either dialytic or transplantation-based treatment of ESRD.[22]

In 1985, Evans et al.[23] reported that 80% of 144 kidney transplant recipients and 48% to 60% of 715 dialysis patients were functioning at a near-normal level. Overall, transplant patients do better than patients receiving dialysis. Improvements in dialysis technique and the availability of erythropoietin to combat the anemia of renal failure have done much to improve the circumstances of those who have high levels of preformed antibody or who are otherwise unsuited to transplantation.

Organ Donation

Further discussion of organ donation and its psychiatric implications is provided later in this chapter. Criteria for unrelated organ donation at MGH have traditionally included documentation of a close bond between the donor and the recipi-

ent, altruistic intent on the part of the donor, and lack of coercion (as evidenced during medical evaluation and a standard psychiatric interview). Participants have included wives, distant relatives, friends, co-workers, and, in one instance, a home health aid. Liberalization of organ donor criteria now allow for selective participation of "Good Samaritan" donors.

Organ donation depends on the willing participation of the donor, the recipient, and the surgical team. Transplant surgeons must decide on their level of acceptance before operating on a healthy individual for purposes of organ donation. Accordingly, there is variability among centers regarding the inclusion of living-donor surgery of any type. In addition, regulations of the United Network for Organ Sharing (UNOS) in the United States require that there be no financial remuneration by a donor for a recipient.[24] Many have recommended that out of pocket costs be available to future donors. Medical ethicists realize that this is an evolving process and subject to change.

Case 3

> Ms. C worked in MGH's medical library in the 1980s. She asked for an opportunity to discuss her own interest in organ donation. In the course of an hour-long office visit, she stated her wish to be an organ donor for anyone in need. There was no discernible psychopathology. The team acknowledged this altruistic request but declined the offer because she did not meet established criteria for a preexisting emotional bond. In 2003, her offer would receive more active consideration.

Case 4

> Ms. D, a 32-year-old woman wanted to be a kidney donor for her divorced boyfriend's ex-wife, whose renal failure had been caused by systemic lupus erythematosus. Psychiatric evaluation revealed that the intended donor was guilt-ridden about the recipient's circumstances. No established bond existed between the two women. The potential donor was, in a manner or speaking, "the other woman," a role in which she had also been cast. She gave a history of physical abuse by her mother and sexual abuse by her mother's three marital partners. Ms. D was tall, edentulous, and modestly attired. She acknowledged a feeling of universal love and a wish to please others. She seemed accepting and possibly relieved when the psychiatrist rejected her

candidacy as a donor. She also pointed out the parallels between her current situation and her past trauma.

At MGH, all potential donors are included in a pretransplant family meeting attended by a nephrologist, the surgical chief of the renal transplant program, the nurse coordinator, the social worker, the consulting psychiatrist, and a representative from the tissue-typing laboratory. The meetings are preceded by an educational and information-gathering session with the social worker and a nurse coordinator. Additional psychiatric evaluation is done for all potential unrelated donors and for any related donors who present with current emotional difficulties, conflicting feelings about the procedure, or a significant psychiatric history. In complicated cases, the pretransplant team requests an independent medical assessment by a team nephrologist who is not the primary caretaker for the recipient.

Allograft survival statistics have improved substantially; participation of a living donor kidney transplant has a half-life of 16 years. Access to cadaver donor renal transplantation now requires an extensive waiting period, averaging 4 to 5 years at MGH. Therefore, the availability of living organ donation is a treasured resource. To deal with the critical shortage of kidneys a donor swap program was started recently. In this program, two donors, each of whom is blood type-incompatible with their intended recipient, can exchange roles, thereby allowing the two recipients to obtain a kidney. In all instances of living donor participation it must be understood that the donor is a patient with rights to medical care independent of the recipient's need or institutional priorities.[25] It is also important to appreciate the tendency of patients and research participants to rely on the physician to decide whether to participate in a protocol or undergo a medical procedure.[26]

Heart Failure

Diagnostic Considerations

Among those who undergo heart transplantation the leading preoperative diagnoses are coronary artery disease (CAD) and cardiomyopathy (CM). On one, occasion a patient presented with alcoholic CM. Need for transplantation was obviated by her response to intense treatment for alcoholism.

Waiting Period

Before transplantation, prolonged intensive care unit (ICU) stays are the rule because medical selection criteria are based on urgency. Many relatively high-functioning younger patients, who risk death from arrhythmia, have lengthier waiting times as outpatients.

Pretransplantation stress is similar to the stress associated with increased cardiac vulnerability in the general population. Major factors include the adverse impact of role loss and of separation from family.[27-30] Fear that transplantation may not be forthcoming or effective also causes anticipatory bereavement. For example, one woman became preoccupied with the thought that her automatic implanted cardiac defibrillator (AICD) would be activated and feared that she would die from arrhythmia and miss out on the experience of grandparenthood.

In other types of organ failure for which there is no sustaining maintenance therapy, a patient who is considered for heart transplantation may express a willingness to proceed and a sense that there is "no other choice." Anger and anxiety may occur as one senses that time is running out. These emotions are also associated with cardiovascular morbidity.[31]

Encephalopathy may develop; Reither et al. have discussed this in detail.[32] Contributing factors include decreased cerebral blood flow, metabolic disorders, and medication effects. Among the latter, lidocaine and β-blocking agents are known to produce cognitive impairment.[33] Also, one must be aware of the potential central nervous system (CNS)-depressing effects of anxiolytics.

Tobacco Abuse

Smoking is an etiologic agent among some patients with heart failure, and it is an exclusion criterion for transplantation at many centers. Historically, tobacco abuse has been more socially acceptable in Europe than it has in the United States. Referral to a hospital-based smoking cessation program is advisable. Some centers follow levels of urinary cotinine to detect and monitor tobacco abuse.

Building a Psychological Bridge

Prolonged ICU stays and their attendant stress call for creative management strategies. Psychopharmacologic support may include use of low-dose anxiolytics and antidepressants (with low risks of cardiotoxicity). Tricyclic antidepressants (TCAs) are disadvantageous in this population prior to transplant surgery because of their potential for causing arrhythmias and orthostatic hypotension. Constipation, a frequent side effect of TCAs, may increase cardiovascular risk by creating the need for Valsalva maneuvers.[34] The use of bupropion and the SSRIs is preferred, with appropriate regard for their potential drug interactions related to their cytochrome P450 isoenzyme effects.

Case 5

> Mr. E, a middle-aged man with a highly counter-dependent style, became depressed after learning that his status on the transplant list had fallen because other patients were more acutely ill. Although he confided that he planned to forego transplantation and leave the ICU, he agreed to a trial of bupropion. Within 3 days, his mood improved and he again elected to undergo transplantation. When pruritus developed, Mr. E chose to add diphenhydramine to his regimen rather than discontinue bupropion. His transplant proceeded uneventfully, and he required no postoperative antidepressant therapy.

Delirium is a common and demanding complication for those patients who require placement of an intra-aortic balloon pump (IABP). Hypotension and microembolic events may be responsible, although cytokine activation might play a role. Use of intravenous (IV) haloperidol is a first-line approach to the management of such agitated delirious states. Adequate analgesia also is essential for patients with severe angina; additional support from a hospital-based pain management team may be required.

Psychotherapy is demanding for clinicians who serve these patients. The consultant visits the ICU each time with the realization that the patient's room may be empty and bed neatly remade (or occupied by a new patient). The effort to diminish one's sense of loss may deter even a seasoned consultant from making an emotional commitment.

Such countertransference features, when acknowledged, add to the psychiatric consultant's appreciation of the level of stress encountered by a patient's relatives and friends and by other members of the heart transplant team.

Hypnotherapy and other cognitively based strategies can enhance the patient's adaptive response. For example, one young mother in her thirties used self-hypnosis to master lonely nights in the ICU; she imagined that the beeping of her monitor represented the sound of a spaceship on which she journeyed each night with her children. Another patient, a middle-aged policeman with intractable chest pain, found relief in frequent images of fishing with a brother who resided out of state. Another man, who proved especially intolerant of medical dependency, was able to use a hypnotic suggestion that he had a double. While engaged in a more active fantasy of managing his horse farm, he could imagine that it was his double that lay in the hospital as a passive recipient of life-saving care.

Case 6

> Mr. F, a middle-aged man, who had enjoyed playing competitive basketball in his youth, experienced an arduous 100-day stay with IABP support. He engaged in spirited banter that centered on the consultant's own athletic incompetence and on the outcome of competition that they might enjoy after his transplant. During the early postoperative period, the consultant gave him a basketball. At a visit following his discharge from the hospital, he reciprocated with a cartoon of two basketball players (with his name and the name of the consultant added in ink).

Liver Failure

Diagnostic Considerations

The most frequent causes of liver failure in the United States are alcoholic cirrhosis and alcoholic hepatitis. Other frequently seen causes of liver failure are infectious and autoimmune hepatitis, primary biliary cirrhosis, and sclerosing cholangitis. Hepatocellular carcinoma is also an indication for transplantation when disease is confined to the liver. Urgency is the deciding factor in allocation of livers. The current MELD system gives priority to ICU-based patients and to medically stable outpatients with good-prognosis hepatocellular carcinoma.[35] The shortage of organs has virtually eliminated liver transplantation as a palliative approach.

At the time of evaluation and listing for transplantation, patients with liver failure have less than a year to live. Recurrent esophageal bleeding, tense ascites, recurrent encephalopathy, nutritional impairment, coagulopathy, and jaundice are common findings. The precarious circumstances of these patients led one hepatologist to comment at rounds, "It's later than you think."[36]

Hepatic Encephalopathy

The principal cause of hepatic encephalopathy is absorption of toxic metabolites from the intestine. The presence of false neurotransmitters may also result in CNS depression. Grading of hepatic encephalopathy has traditionally been accomplished by use of the Parsons-Smith criteria.[37] Some critically ill patients present in frank stupor and may not recall their preoperative course. More subtle cognitive dysfunction may be evident on a standard mental status examination or in behavioral oddities. It is especially important for the consultant to learn about premorbid functioning because patients with so-called subclinical hepatic encephalopathy are likely to improve following transplantation. Neurologic improvement following transplantation may be slow for some patients; in general, transplantation is associated with a significant improvement in the recipient's quality of life.[38,39]

Medical management is the primary approach to these patients. Control of bleeding and infection, reduction of protein intake, and administration of lactulose constitutes the standard approach. Use of anxiolytics and sedatives must be used carefully because most are hepatically metabolized and may precipitate obtundation even when used in relatively modest doses.[36]

Patient Selection and End-Stage Alcoholic Liver Disease (ESALD)

Transplant centers vary considerably in their selection of recipients, as documented by Levenson and Olbrisch.[40] Factors include the experience of the team, the volume of transplant procedures at a given center, the availability of comprehensive psychiatric support, and societal factors.

As in the case of heart transplantation, many of those awaiting liver transplant die before an organ becomes available. Evans[41] reported that 14,400 livers are needed annually. The large number of patients with ESALD has generated considerable controversy. Moss and Siegler[42] argued that patients should be accountable for their histories of substance abuse, even if assignment of fault to such patients leads to second-class status. A risk of such logic is the possibility that patients will become hostages to their past and be excluded by third-party payers from reimbursement of transplantation.[43] Unequal access within a specific category, independent of prognosis, is a form of discrimination incompatible with federal guidelines for the disabled.[44] Confounding the rational selection of patients with ESALD is the challenge inherent in predicting future drinking, the presumed but unproven association between substance abuse and graft loss from noncompliance, the absence of reliable biologic markers, the absence of exclusive pathognomonic biopsy findings for ESALD, the lack of consistently applied criteria for substance abuse, and the difficulty in obtaining reliable historical data from patients and families intent on obtaining advanced medical care.[45]

Case 7

Ms. G, a middle-aged woman presented for liver transplantation; the psychiatric evaluation was noteworthy only for generalized anxiety. Postoperatively, she was tremulous and encephalopathic. Alcohol withdrawal was considered, but her husband steadfastly averred that his wife did not drink. Her condition continued to deteriorate, and she developed hyperbilirubinemia. In a visit to the transplant unit, her husband confided that at home he had unexpectedly discovered a medicine bottle filled with hard liquor. An extensive history of surreptitious drinking was thus implied. She went on to retransplantation and again developed malignant hyperbilirubinemia of unknown cause, which proved fatal.

Experiences with challenging patients have led many liver transplant centers to involve the participation of addiction specialists. The Massachusetts Ethics Committee for Organ Transplantation concurred that active substance abuse or incapacity to benefit from transplantation are appropriate exclusion criteria. MGH's center requires that there be a confirmed history of medical compliance, presence of adequate social support for continued sobriety, absence of dementia or co-morbid alcoholic cardiomyopathy, and active participation in substance abuse counseling and treatment for those perceived to be at risk for relapse or who presented with less than a year of established sobriety. MGH excludes individuals who are actively drinking or who are involved in illicit drug abuse.[35] Participation in a methadone maintenance program has not been a reason for exclusion in our practice.

Beresford et al.[46] advocated a system of inclusion based on Valliant's prognostic criteria. They assessed the extent to which patients and their families recognized alcohol dependence, the current degree of social stability, and the prospect and degree of lifestyle change conducive to long-term sobriety. Yates et al.[47] assessed prognosis with attention to the amount of alcohol consumed and the frequency and success of prior rehabilitation efforts. Knechtle et al.[48] proceeded with liver transplantation in those whose families advocated for transplantation despite failure of the patient to meet criteria for abstinence. This cohort of patients did as well as those with established sobriety. Reported rates of recidivism have varied following transplantation for ESALD. Increasingly, however, it is evident that patient and graft survival for appropriately selected members of this patient population are comparable to those of other groups with liver failure.[49–52]

Whatever the selection process, there should be a clear set of addictions treatment guidelines for patients and their primary support person. MGH requires that patients at risk of relapse sign a formal treatment plan. Centers with stringent exclusion criteria should present information about other programs that can provide a second opinion.

Organ Donorship

The demand for cadaveric livers has led to a number of innovative procedures, including split-liver transplantation and reduced-sized grafts for pediatric recipients.[53] The ethics of partial hepatectomy from parent donors to critically ill offspring was initially explored by Singer et al. in 1989.[54] The authors indicated that there would be a 6-month moratorium on the procedure for review and comment by the medical community,[54] an approach that is now widely accepted. Nonetheless, postoperative risks are greater than in the setting of nephrectomy for living renal transplantation.[55] Right hepatic lobe adult-to-adult transplantation places the live donor at still greater risk but has proceeded without the level of thoughtful deliberation that had marked introduction of parent-to-child partial liver transplantation.[5,56] The approach to live donor organ transplantation has thus become an ethical slippery slope. Confounding the problem is the determination of donors who have made up their mind to proceed and press the surgical team to acquiesce. In an effort to achieve acceptance, the donor candidates sometimes engage in "impression management." Outright deception has been known to occur.[57]

Psychiatric Intervention: Psychopharmacologic limitations are imposed by the metabolism of psychoactive medications and by the role of hepatic enzymes. Preoperative anxiety and agitation can be treated with low doses of short-acting benzodiazepines. In the presence of hepatic encephalopathy, oxazepam is preferred because it does not require oxidative metabolism. A daily dose of 10 mg should not routinely be exceeded. Diphenhydramine is a safe agent in low dosage for nocturnal sedation. Although insomnia is frequent in this patient population, one must treat it gently.

Antidepressants can be used in conjunction with liver transplantation and in those with hepatitis C who develop depression as a side effect of interferon therapy.[58] In some instances it may be advisable to monitor blood levels.[59] We prefer bupropion because of its stimulating effect. SSRIs are also effective. All antidepressants carry a small risk of hepatotoxicity. A "black box" warning to that effect has been included in the package insert for Serzone (nefazodone HCL). Serzone use also risks competitive inhibition of cyclosporine and tacrolimus metabolism through P 450 3A4 isoenzyme system.

The psychotherapeutic approach in this patient population is principally supportive in nature. Lengthy preoperative medical stays may be encountered.

Pulmonary Failure

Lung transplantation is a therapeutic option for many patients with end-stage pulmonary failure. Afflicted patients may suffer from obstructive lung disease (e.g., chronic obstructive pulmonary disease [COPD] or alpha-1-antitrypsin deficiency), restrictive lung disease (e.g., idiopathic pulmonary fibrosis), septic lung disease (e.g., cystic fibrosis or bronchiectasis), or pulmonary vascular disease (that results in pulmonary hypertension). As lung transplantation is a therapy "of last resort," all potential candidates must accept the fact that they have a limited life expectancy without surgery, and they must feel that their current quality of life is unacceptable. At MGH, actuarial 1-year survival after lung transplantation is approximately 85%.[60]

Unfortunately, the number of candidates for lung transplantation exceeds the number of available cadaveric donor organs. Therefore, the waiting list for lung transplantation can be several years long. Ideally, candidates should be referred for evaluation before their pulmonary disease becomes too advanced; otherwise they may be too ill to withstand the long waiting period. When pulmonary failure develops, unlike failure of other solid organs, there is no machine that can provide satisfactory support for patients while awaiting transplantation. In fact, ventilator dependence is usually a contraindication to transplantation. Most candidates, therefore, wait at home for their transplant, often at some distance from the transplant center.

A joint statement by the International Society of Heart and Lung Transplantation, the American Society of Transplant Physicians, the American Thoracic Society, the European Respiratory Society, and the Thoracic Society of Australia and New Zealand offers general guidelines for consideration of lung transplant candidates.[61] Shared guidelines for contraindications to transplantation also exist and include, in addition to active medical problems such as malignancy and HIV infection, many psychosocial parameters. Current, active cigarette smoking and alcohol or recreational drug use/abuse are absolute contraindications to lung transplantation. Other disabling psychological symptoms include ongoing suicidal or homicidal ideation, a history of suicide attempts or chronic self-injurious behaviors, poor compliance with medication regimens, acute psychosis, an eating disorder, and dementia care relative contraindications to transplantation.

At MGH, a psychiatrist is a designated member of the lung transplant team. This physician evaluates all potential lung transplant candidates, follows them both before and after transplantation on an outpatient basis (as needed), and sees them as inpatients during the peri- and postoperative periods.

Because of the scarcity of cadaveric organs, many centers now offer the option of living donor lobar lung transplantation to suitable recipients. Such recipients at MGH are typically young people with cystic fibrosis who are unlikely to survive the long waiting period. These patients are usually small in stature, and therefore, a single lobe from two individuals of average size will provide sufficient pulmonary capacity. Donors must have the same blood type as the recipient but they do not have to be biologically related. Potential donors must undergo a comprehensive psychological evaluation as well as a medical workup to determine motivation and to ensure autonomy, informed consent, and the absence of coercion.

Many psychiatric disorders occur in patients with pulmonary failure. Almost all candidates referred to MGH for lung transplantation have some degree of generalized anxiety and/or panic attacks. Many of them were not anxious premorbidly but instead became anxious in the setting of increasing shortness of breath. They often describe both anticipatory anxiety (particularly in the setting of planned exertion) and panic attacks, despite oxygen supplementation. This behavior is consistent with a study by Pollack, Kradin, and Otto,[60] in which they reported a 17% incidence of panic disorder among 115 patients referred for pulmonary function testing. Adjustment disorder with depressive features is also common in this population, as patients struggle to cope with their progressive inability to perform even simple activities of daily living. In the setting of chronic, debilitating illness, pulmonary patients may develop major depression that requires aggressive psychopharmacologic intervention as well as supportive therapy. Those who are extremely ill may become delirious from hypoxia or hypercapnia. In addition, the medications used to treat the complications of pulmonary disease may precipitate psychiatric problems.

Case 8

Ms. H, a 29-year-old married woman with pulmonary fibrosis, was referred by her pulmonologist so that she could be evaluated for lung transplantation. She had no other medical problems and had no formal psychiatric history. A college graduate, she had worked full-time for several years. During the year prior to her evaluation she had to work fewer hours because of worsening pulmonary function. Although she described herself as "even-keeled," she had noticed becoming increasingly anxious as her pulmonary function worsened. Her pulmonologist started her on continuous oxygen treatment; she remained anxious nevertheless. At the time of her evaluation she was feeling "overwhelmed" and was having intermittent panic attacks, particularly when she anticipated leaving her apartment to go to work. She was also having trouble socializing with her husband and her friends. Her discomfort was such that she considered leaving her job. Panic disorder secondary to pulmonary decline was diagnosed and a selective serotonin re-uptake inhibitor (SSRI) and a benzodiazepine (in a low dose) was prescribed. She did extremely well on this regimen, began a pulmonary rehabilitation program, kept her job, and resumed her social life with her friends.

Case 9

Mr. I, a 27-year-old single man with cystic fibrosis, had been waiting for a transplant for 18 months when he was admitted for a "cleanout." Initially, he did well, but he then developed pneumonia and required additional antibiotics and vigorous chest physical therapy to help him clear his secretions. He had no history of psychiatric illness. Prior to his admission he stayed at home; he was unable to work, but he was able to care for himself and to enjoy being with his friends and family. He was optimistic about his situation and he eagerly anticipated a transplant. During his admission, he developed unremitting chest pain and was started a course of narcotics on an as-needed basis. One morning he complained of vivid, frightening visual hallucinations, which prompted psychiatric consultation. During the exam, his level of consciousness waxed and waned although his oxygen saturation remained above 90%. The psychiatric consultant felt that the narcotics alone could have caused his change in mental status, and asked the medical team to re-check an arterial blood gas (ABG). The ABG showed an acute respiratory acidosis with a pCO_2 of 75. Mr. I's use of narcotics had suppressed his respiratory drive and hypercapnia and delirium developed.

As with other solid organ transplant patients, lung transplant patients are maintained on immunosuppressive drugs for the remainder of their lives. These medications, including, among others, cyclosporine, FK-506 (tacrolimus), and prednisone; each can produce a variety of neuropsychiatric disorders such as mood disorders, psychosis, and leukoencephalopathy.[62] In addition, because of their immunosuppression, these patients are vulnerable to infections such as cytomegalovirus, aspergillus, nocardia, listeria, cryptococcus, and nontubercular mycobacterium that can also cause neuropsychiatric signs and symptoms.

Case 10

Mr. J, a 60-year-old married man with no psychiatric history became quite depressed and developed suicidal thoughts several months after single lung transplantation for COPD. He suffered from anhedonia and felt sleepy all the time (despite receiving adequate rest at night). His medications included cyclosporine and antihypertensives. His prednisone had been tapered slowly to 15 mg per day. He took no pain medications or sedative-hypnotics. He denied any acute psychosocial stressors. Cyclosporine was discontinued and tacrolimus was begun. His mood improved within several weeks and he felt more alert and awake; he began to participate once again in the activities of his household.

Preoperative Psychiatric Considerations

Hope Versus Loss

Typically the first psychiatric encounter with the transplant patient is at the initial medical evaluation for transplantation candidacy. For many, transplantation represents a prospect for autonomy and prolongation of life. A transplant evaluation also implies there will be no spontaneous remission from organ failure. While the patient tries to accept his or her need for transplantation, grief (which varies in intensity with the severity of organ failure and with styles of adaptive function) is manifest.

Preparation for Living Versus Dying

Christopherson[63] described the challenge to families who simultaneously prepared for the alternative outcomes of survival and death for loved ones facing heart transplantation. Our group reported the case of a successful liver transplant candidate whose family was making funeral arrangements when he was placed on the list.[64]

False Starts

Patients awaiting transplantation experience considerable stress. For the cardiac patient waiting in the ICU, the wait for a heart is like the watched pot that never boils. For outpatients waiting in excess of 2 years for lung transplantation, there is the feeling of having been forgotten. For some, the long preparation for transplantation is followed by a call to the hospital for an organ that never materializes. These false starts are expectedly unsettling. In one instance, a patient underwent anesthesia, but the heart transplantation was aborted because the donor organ was inadequate. This patient died before he got a second chance.

Survivor Guilt and Other Variations

Transplantation candidates commonly express guilt about their need for an organ—a need that can only be filled by another person's death. Patients with familial disorders may also be sensitive to a loved one's inability to obtain a successful allograft. Patients who have experienced organ failure often have an opportunity to bond with other candidates undergoing similar evaluations and therapy. As transplantation becomes available, some patients feel sadness for those who continue to wait for a graft, guilt because they received the organ first, or unhappiness because their suffering continues as a result of postoperative complications. At the time of the transplant evaluation, patients often feel guilty about the stress that their illness imposes on family members.

Depression

Depression has long been thought to predispose to postoperative morbidity.[65] Moreover, mood may dramatically improve following operative intervention.[8,66] When a history of affective disorder exists, it is important to ascertain to what extent mood disturbances have affected compliance with prescribed medications and procedures.

Anxiety

Johnston[67] found that preoperative anxiety levels were high and tended to persist for several days following the operation. This pattern is common in living organ donors. Transplant recipients are anxious preoperatively but they feel significantly improved with the return of postoperative end-organ function. Among cadaveric transplant recipients, the hope for an organ is typically followed by anxiety when a graft finally becomes available. On rare occasions such anxiety may lead a patient to turn down an organ. Emergency psychiatric consultation may prove helpful.

Some patients approach surgery with minimal apprehension. Frank denial is problematic for the individual who mistakenly expects that transplantation will be immediately beneficial and uneventful. Psychiatric intervention is recommended for the patient with debilitating anxiety, with unrealistic expectations, and with premorbid anxiety disorders or phobias specific to the planned procedure.[8,9]

Personality Impairment

Trust is essential to successful organ transplantation because of its attendant uncertainties. Patients with personality disorders present a pattern of strained relationships, and they are at higher risk for transplantation complications. Fortunately, most transplant procedures occur in a time frame that allows the team to establish a therapeutic alliance. Overall the best predictor of postoperative compliance is preoperative compliance.[68]

Informed Consent

Teaching and informed consent are the cornerstones of preoperative care. In addition to a declaration of clinical goals and methods for their accomplishment, preoperative discussions between the patient and the transplant team form the basis of a bond that will ultimately allow for the difficult times that occur during the course of solid organ transplantation. The opportunity to shape expectation is especially important. Transplant patients need to understand that hospital care may be prolonged and that recurrent admissions may be necessitated by rejection, infection, and other post-transplant complications. The need for indwelling catheters, drains, and special diets must be addressed and an approach to postoperative pain established. Transplant recipients need to comply strictly with medications, frequent postoperative clinic visits, and the financial demands of transplantation. The process of selection, the contemplated waiting time for transplant, and the rules governing status on the list should be carefully explained. Young people especially must be made aware of the cosmetic impact associated with the use of high doses of steroids following transplantation. The likelihood of weight gain and the potential for diabetes mellitus, cataract formation, mood swings, irritability, impaired concentration, and tremor must be addressed. Potential complications must be presented with sensitivity. It may seem kind to withhold information, but patients who are uninformed and who suffer adverse postoperative effects often feel that they were "led down the garden path." Observation by the team in the course of teaching and informed consent provides important information about mental status and coping styles.[8]

Teaching Venues

Our institution uses a family meeting format for interviewing kidney transplant patients before placing their name on the cadaveric organ list or proceeding with living-donor evaluation. For other types of solid organ transplantation, the patient is admitted when feasible, and a standard series of visits is arranged with surgery, nursing, psychiatry, social service, anesthesiology, and other medical and paramedical subspecialists as indicated. Some insurance plans require that this process occur on an outpatient basis.

Transplant teams typically have a transplant psychiatrist or rely on general hospital psychiatric consultation services. Some teams rely on a psychologist or social worker. The psychiatric interview complements the process of informed consent and provides an excellent opportunity to instruct patients in relaxation techniques, to counsel them about mobilizing an effective support network, and to inform them about the potential for postoperative mental status change

and how it is best addressed. The psychiatrist, consulting psychologist, and social worker are in an optimal position to reinforce adaptive skills and to assist in cognitive refraining and behavioral techniques for the enhancement of perceived control and well-being.[8,69-72] Several studies have demonstrated the favorable postoperative impact of preoperative psychological intervention.[73-75]

Patient-patient interactions provide a valuable adjunct to preoperative teaching. Many successful transplant recipients enjoy the opportunity to "give something back" by sharing their experience with new transplant candidates. Patient groups are similarly effective. They may rely on lay leadership or a skilled group therapist. The format may include didactic teaching sessions to which members of the surgical team are invited. Some groups include patients and family members.

Printed materials are a useful educational supplement. *Organ Transplants: A Patient's Guide*, co-authored by Hank Pizer and the MGH transplant team, is recommended.[76]

Psychotherapy

Indications

Patients with Axis I or Axis II psychiatric disorders should be encouraged to receive essential psychiatric care in preparation for transplantation. When compliance is a concern and when debilitating emotional symptoms exist, MGH requires active treatment before the patient is listed.

Patients who are psychologically asymptomatic or who have mild adjustment disorders are best advised to mobilize whatever resources they find most beneficial. This may include supportive counseling for the patient and family, religious involvement, or community-based support. Patients should also be encouraged to give specific assignments to friends and family who wish to help.

The pretransplant psychiatric evaluation provides a format for brief therapy. It often is useful to tell patients that the purpose of the psychiatric interview is to teach, to form a basis for subsequent *ad hoc* psychiatric referrals, and to ascertain whether any special needs must be addressed for transplantation to be successful.

Goals

Even a one-time psychiatric interview may provide a unique opportunity for listening and debriefing. While underscoring the hope of transplantation, the therapeutic psychological encounter allows for a recognition of loss and grief. Guilt reduction may follow by honoring the sick role. Patients who express feelings of guilt about the need for a cadaveric organ are best reminded of the inevitability of death and of the relief many bereaved families experience when informed of the opportunity for organ donation. Some patients openly express concern about receiving a cadaveric organ. They may require reassurance about body image following transplantation.

The psychiatric interview can be very supportive for patients undergoing a pretransplant evaluation. Patients are best advised that the object is to see whether they can realistically benefit from a transplant and whether there are specific circumstances that need to be addressed before transplantation proceeds. Above all, the pretransplant interview is an excellent opportunity to strengthen the therapeutic alliance.

The psychiatrist can play an important role in shaping expectations. The patient can benefit from learning that adverse events can be managed successfully. For example, liver transplant candidates can be told of a report that pain following liver transplantation required less narcotics than gallbladder surgery.[77] This finding may be the result of denervation that occurs in the process of removing the native liver. Alternatively, one colleague has argued that the teaching process itself may lead to improved pain tolerance.[2]

Put in other terms, the preoperative patient is a "cryptographer" in search of cues that will aid in mastery of events. In an early study, Schacter and Singer[78] found that experimental participants responded differentially to injected adrenaline depending on their exposure to waiting room "stooges" who were either irritable or elated. This is not to say that one should deny pain or tell patients how to feel, but that patients can be taught how to cope within the range of experience that are typically encountered. Egbert et al.[79] demonstrated that patients undergoing abdominal surgery had greater postoperative comfort and required less narcotics when they were taught before their operation about the normalcy of postoperative pain and were encouraged to ask for pain medication as needed. Similarly, one can instruct patients about the risk of postoperative delirium, while emphasizing that some degree of confusion is frequent, that this is temporary, and that it will respond to appropriate adjustments in medication. For example, a liver transplant recipient can imagined that one of his or her surgeons is having a party outside the window of the hospital room.

Phobic disorders relevant to the surgical setting should be identified and plans made to effect desensitization. A technique, postnoxious desensitization, in which individuals are encouraged to fantasize acquisition of a desired goal and then to work backwards imaginally to gain mastery of the steps required for goal attainment, has been described.[80]

Case 11

At the time of transplant evaluation, Ms. K described a dread of endotracheal intubation. At outpatient follow-up, accompanied by her husband, she proved to be an excellent hypnotic subject. Having been asked to imagine under hypnosis that she had completed heart transplantation, she pictured herself sitting in an enclosed porch that her husband had constructed. In subsequent scenes, she was guided in working backward imaginally through an expected sequence of perioperative events and to use her feelings of hope and renewal to interpret the experience favorably.

Following a single outpatient psychiatric visit, she was readmitted for cardiac catheterization. During the procedure, she inquired about the nationality of the attending cardiologist. On learning that her physician was initially from Egypt, she induced self-hypnosis and embarked on a trip by camel to the rug bazaars.[26]

Psychopharmacologic Treatment

Psychopharmacologic care of the transplant patient has been reviewed in depth by Trzepacz et al.[57,81,82] The judicious use of antidepressants, anxiolytics, and antipsychotics can be life-saving. The pretransplant evaluation provides an excellent chance to learn what agents patients have responded best to and to hear of idiosyncratic drug reactions. Some patients give histories of intolerance to benzodiazepines or neuroleptics; this information may prove invaluable on subsequent admissions if the patient's ability to communicate effectively is compromised.

In general, it is essential to tailor psychopharmacologic management to the demands of organ failure and to maintain a close liaison with other medical subspecialists involved in the patient's care. Cassem's[83] dictum, "start low and go slow," is valuable and helps avoid the pitfalls of oversedation and iatrogenesis.

Special Services

Social Service Intervention

It is most helpful to work with a medical social worker who is familiar with the demands of transplantation and who is available to attend work rounds on a weekly basis. The social worker is an invaluable source of patient and family support and plays a pivotal role in ensuring that the patient will be able to access needed health care perioperatively.

Recreation Therapy and Audiovisual Material

Patients who wait for weeks in the hospital require support and distraction. Activities such as card games, board games, and crafts may prove useful. One heart transplant patient who enjoyed oil painting was able to overcome his depression by producing canvases that he offered for sale to the staff.

Relaxation videotapes may be made available through a closed-circuit teaching channel. MGH also uses teaching films for patients and their potential donors when they come to family meetings before transplantation selection. Movies, music, and books on tape may reduce tension during prolonged hospital stays. Complimentary medicine procedures, such as therapeutic touch, may also often prove effective.

Patient Selection

Tragic Choices

Tragic Choices, Calabrese and Bobbit's[84] landmark work in medical ethics, is an apt phrase for the challenge posed by the limitation in resources for solid organ transplantation. Ethical models applied to this task are inevitably in conflict if each is taken to its logical endpoint.[85] Assignment may be made on a basis that is relatively egalitarian or utilitarian in nature. If the decision to transplant is primarily driven by patient demand, unacceptably high-risk candidates are included, and the pool of recipients is larger than if the decision is made on the basis of potential outcome and societal benefit.[86] If wait time is the predominant consideration in listing for transplant, patients in most acute need will not survive long enough to receive an organ, and patients who are relatively healthy will decline in health status before they reach the top of the list.

A rational approach to solid organ transplantation is necessarily multicameral in nature.[87] Current selection procedures are based on urgency and on time waiting. Special consideration among renal transplant recipients is given to patients who are sensitized with high levels of preformed antibody. Availability of a 6-antigen match is considered a priority, independent of other factors. Transplantation is prioritized for patients willing to accept a kidney from older donors whose kidneys would be customarily discarded because of age.

Outcome data are important in patient selection, but some high-risk candidates are accepted. For example, the 1-year survival rate for retransplantation of heart and liver recipients is approximately 38%, yet many centers perform second transplants. Multiple organ recipients are another subgroup at high risk. Some centers offer transplantation to Jehovah's Witnesses who decline use of blood products. Recipients who belong to this religious group may elect to accept blood or plasma. Religious elders can sometimes participate to the advantage of the patient and the surgical team.

Other differences among types of solid organ transplantation are the priority given to patients who require mechanical support. Among lung transplant recipients, ventilator support is a contraindication to transplant, whereas heart and liver candidates are given priority listing when on a ventilator unless the likelihood of a successful outcome is poor because of additional complications, such as active infection or renal failure.

Prioritization in solid organ transplantation has varied over time, beginning with the more selective or parajudicial lifeboat ethics philosophy of the 1960s to our current more egalitarian approach. It is principally, however, a societal consideration. Individual transplant centers may vary in their assessment of a given candidate, but the decision to transplant is driven by a medical model.[88] The team must determine who will benefit within the context of currently accepted norms for selection.

Psychiatrist's Role

The psychiatrist is charged with the task of determining whether the patient is sufficiently able, motivated, and socially supported to follow through with the demands of transplantation. Unfortunately, we lack valid and reliable predictive data. Freeman et al.[89] used the determination "reservation about suitability for transplantation" for 19 of 70 patients who were psychiatrically screened for heart transplantation. Fourteen of the patients who met *Diagnostic and Statistical Manual of Mental Disorders*, third edition (*DSM-III*) criteria for a psychiatric disorder had postoperative surgical or psychiatric complications. Levenson and Olbrisch[40] showed that transplant centers differ in their acceptance of patients with specific psychiatric impairments. Some groups do not accept patients with active schizophrenia. Most centers deny patients with active substance abuse, dementia, current suicidality, past multiple suicide attempts, or severe mental retardation. Mild mental retardation, affective disorder, and commission of a felony are other considerations that may be exclusionary, especially in cardiac and lung transplant programs, which tend to be more selective.[90] In an attempt to standardize patient evaluation and selection, Olbrisch developed the psychosocial assessment of candidates for transplantation (PACT), which rates each of four categories along a five-point semantic difference: social support, psychological health, lifestyle factors, and understanding of transplant and follow-up.[91]

Centers differ in their approach to selection depending on a variety of factors, including volume of cases, outcome statistics, and availability of psychiatric consultation. Larger centers with good results may tolerate higher-risk patients. Experience dictates that solid organ transplantation has been successful in selected patients with schizophrenia, major depression, personality disorder, substance abuse, and moderate mental retardation.[86]

MGH developed a working committee that met weekly to develop selection criteria. Independent of psychiatric diagnostic criteria and items on the PACT, this group ascertained that the ultimate distinction was a perception by the team that a given patient could be medically managed following the transplantation. Operationally, the group strives to delineate the problem areas in a given case and to see what factors might diminish the risk. If the group finds that a workable therapeutic relationship and sufficient availability of social supports exists, the group proceeds with transplantation.

Through active participation with the transplant unit, the psychiatrist gains knowledge about specific concerns that team members bring to the selection process. Patient compliance is an obvious concern. The social worth of the candidate is another.[92] Some who come to transplant evaluation pose a measure of social risk, as in the case of an antisocial patient or the patient whose care will require extensive resources. Team members may also perceive greater tragedy when they have participated in the long-term care of a patient who has experienced multiple setbacks or rejection of a previous allograft. The psychiatrist plays an important role in continuing medical education of the surgical team by sharing current practice standards in psychiatric care and prognostication and by participating in ethical review of complex clinical events.

Noncompliance

Noncompliance is an important source of secondary graft failure, with a reported incidence of up to 5% among renal transplant recipients.[93] Noncompliance may present in various forms, including missed appointments, failure to report important clinical changes in a timely fashion, dietary abuse, and missed medications. Unexpectedly low blood levels of cyclosporine or of other required medications might signal noncompliance. Some patients with recurrent rejection may also stabilize with surprising rapidity following hospital admission and routine monitoring of medications.

Factors in noncompliance include depression, substance abuse, cognitive impairment, and personality disorder. Patients are at increased risk when they live at a distance from the transplant center and when there is insufficient social and financial support. Youth is another risk factor. Young people may be more prone to denial and more reactive to the cosmetic complications of immunosuppressant medications.[94]

Although it is difficult to prognosticate with certainty in individual cases, the patient's history of compliance is a valuable clue to future performance.[68,95] When possible, patients who are at risk by virtue of psychiatric history or social turmoil should have an extended period of follow-up with the understanding that documentation of compliance must precede transplantation. All reasonable efforts should be undertaken to treat ongoing psychiatric impairment and to improve social support. Frequent posttransplant clinic visits may reduce risk of noncompliance among high-risk patients.

Organ Donorship

Types of Donation

In the United States, the principle source of organs available for transplantation is from cadaveric, brain-dead donors with a heartbeat. Hospitals have site-specific criteria for determination of brain death that usually include both diagnostic tests, such as apnea test, EEG, transcranial Doppler, and cerebral blood flow scan, and clinical signs, such as fixed and dilated pupils, absent reflexes, unresponsiveness to external stimuli, and apnea.

The UNOS is the nonprofit agency endowed by the U.S. Congress that regulates the distribution of organs for transplantation. One of its branches, the Organ Procurement and Transplant Networks (OPTN) divides the country into 11 geographic regions in which the allocation of organs proceeds according to local need and priority. Each region has its own organ procurement organization (OPO). The radius of distribution for each type of organ is dependent on how vulnerable each type is to ischemic injury. Donor hearts are limited to a 500-mile radius. Kidneys can be transported across the continent because they can tolerate up to 48 hours of hypothermic perfusion. Lungs can tolerate only 6 hours outside of the body.

The length of time candidates spend on the waiting list for transplantation differs among geographic regions. Furthermore, the waiting list for each organ type is arranged according to different models. For kidney transplantation, the time the candidate has spent waiting is the primary determining factor. However, full HLA compatibility between donor and candidate confers priority for

potential candidates for kidney transplantation. For lung transplantation, the time the candidate has spent waiting is the *only* determining factor. For heart and liver candidates, acuity of illness confers priority on the list. Pediatric candidates have priority on the waiting list for both kidneys and livers.

Many transplant centers support a coordinator for organ donation who usually is a registered nurse. That person serves as a liaison between the transplant team and the local organ procurement organization and also educates the hospital staff and the patients about organ donation and transplantation.

Mechanisms for Increased Organ Donation

The mismatch between the number of persons requiring organ transplantation and the number of available cadaveric organs has prompted investigation into other opportunities for organs, such as extending the age limit on donors, donors without a heartbeat, and living donors. Efforts have also been made to educate the public about the need for organs and to ask patients and relatives to consider the issue and to state their wishes prior to death. In the United States, the "required consent" law protects individuals; all potential organ donors must have provided clear consent for organ donation. In Spain, Belgium, and Singapore, the rule of "presumed consent" applies; all persons are presumed to be organ donors unless they have specifically refused to donate.

The issue of non–heart-beating donors remains controversial at best. Brain dead donors are identified by neurologic criteria. In contrast, the non-heart-beating donor has suffered irreversible cardiac or respiratory failure. Opponents of the use of non–heart-beating donors have emphasized the inevitable period of hypotension in the donor, with potential for hypoperfusion of the organs prior to harvest, leading to the risk for ischemic injury. For this reason, the use of non–heart-beating donors has largely been restricted to kidney transplantation because candidates for kidney transplant can be supported by dialysis should the allograft fail. A recent study by Weber et al.[96] demonstrated no difference in outcome for 122 kidney transplants regardless of whether the transplanted organ was from a heart-beating or non–heart-beating donor.

However, there are not enough data at present to contradict prevailing opinion. In addition, other obstacles to transplantation from non–heart-beating donors remain, including ethical concerns about the actual diagnosis of death and technical difficulties in obtaining consent for donation and arranging for organ procurement.

Living donors represent another source of potential organs. Living donor transplantation is more common in other countries, such as Japan, where religious and cultural norms inhibit the use of cadaveric organs. For many years, living donors were almost always closely related to the recipient. Recently, more transplant centers are willing to accept organ donation from living unrelated donors. However, the use of living donor organs remains controversial because, although the benefit to the recipient is clear, the benefit to the donor is less apparent. Donors who are closely related to the recipient presumably derive psychological benefit because they are potentially extending the life of a loved one.[97] Unrelated donors expose themselves to risk with no clear, direct benefit. The mortality rate for nephrectomy is 0.03% and the risk for morbidity ranges from 1% to 10%.[98] The mortality rate for partial hepatectomy is approximately 0.2% and the morbidity rate is 10%.[99] To date, no deaths have been associated with living lobar lung donation, although the morbidity rate is estimated to be as high as 61% at some centers.[100]

The recent death in New York of a 57-year-old man who donated a lobe of his liver to his brother has led many physicians and ethicists to question once again the cost of such altruism and to examine donor outcome more closely.[101] Small studies of kidney donors have reported improved self-esteem among the donors following donation.[102,103] Gouge, Moore, and Bremer[104] did a retrospective analysis of kidney donors using standing quality of life measurement scales and failed to find enhance quality of life post donation. However, almost all donors reported being glad to have given a kidney. As yet unpublished data from MGH suggests that living lobar lung donors score higher on several subscales of quality of life measures, including emotional well-being, after donation as compared with national norms.

Potential living donors undergo comprehensive medical workups prior to donation. They also undergo psychiatric evaluation to determine motivation and to ensure autonomy, informed consent, and the absence of coercion. As with potential recipients, significant psychiatric illness or substance abuse in the donor is problematic and may preclude donation. Agreeing to organ donation implies acceptance of surgical risk, significant postoperative pain, temporary disability, temporary inability to work, and permanent physical scars. The psychiatric interview can serve as an arena in which potential donors can share their ideas and explore their concerns about donation. Families and patients can put a tremendous amount of pressure on individual family members or friends to donate. There are instances in which patients or other family members have offered a financial incentive to donation or have threatened to withdraw financial support if the potential donor backs out. Sometimes the spouse or significant other of the potential donor objects to donation and withdraws emotional support or even leaves the relationship altogether. The potential donor should always be informed that, should he choose not to donate, the transplant team will not reveal the reason for refusing him as a candidate.

Postoperative Psychiatric Considerations

Improvement in Psychological Function

Improved neuropsychiatric function following transplant surgery accompanies the reversal of end-organ failure; at times it is associated with a sense of rebirth. Improvement in anxiety, depression, and cognition typically occurs most rapidly after renal transplantation, and it is often evident within the first 2 days following transplantation because blood urea nitrogen and creatinine levels decrease. Riether et al.[32] found marked improvement in depression and anxiety within the first 3 months following heart transplantation. Liver recipients improve more slowly; however, some patients have manifest marked progress in well-being as early as 2 to 3 weeks following transplantation. Increased psychological adjustment and quality-of-life following liver transplantation have been well documented and are attributable in part to change in neuropsychiatric function.[39,105]

Organic Brain Syndromes

Intraoperative cerebral ischemia may occur among heart transplant patients as a result of decreased perfusion from hemorrhagic or embolic phenomena. Psychotic reactions are most likely to follow within the first 48 hours after surgery. Hotson and Enzmann[106] pointed out that when psychotic manifestations are delayed by 2 to 5 days with rapid response to neuroleptic treatment and environmental support, the cause is more likely to be multifactorial.

Factors contributing to postoperative delirium include metabolic impairment, infection, and effects of medications. Among the latter, anesthetic agents, analgesics (as in the case of normeperidine toxicity), and antirejection medications should be considered. Prednisone may cause sleep disturbance, emotional lability, and perceptual abnormalities. Affective psychosis was a more frequent finding in the earlier years of transplantation when rapid dose reduction was not yet standard. Both cyclosporine and tacrolimus may be associated with neurologic complications, including seizures, delirium, headache, coma, and, rarely, cortical blindness.[107–111] Hypertension, renal dysfunction, and tremor may serve as clues to cyclosporine or tacrolimus toxicity. Toxic levels may follow from use of cytochrome P450 enzyme inhibitors such as erythromycin, ketoconazole, and diltiazem.[112] In rare instances, liver transplant recipients also develop central pontine myelinolysis, an idiopathic demyelinating disorder that produces a locked-in syndrome.[113,114]

Anxiety

Anxiety in the early postoperative period results from failed expectations or rejection during recovery from major complications that the patient has not yet integrated. Less predictable is anxiety that follows from decreased amounts of medical supervision.

Patients who undergo IV pulses of cortiosteroids may experience mood swings or anxiety that typically subside within in a day or two of completion of rescue therapy. Increasing tremor signals cyclosporine toxicity. OKT3, a monoclonal antibody used for acute rejection, may be associated with severe headache, joint pains, and other anxiety-generating systemic effects.

Posttransplant biopsy procedures are another source of stress. Renal and hepatic biopsies are performed on an *ad hoc* basis. Routine endocardial biopsy and bronchoscopy however, are ordered for heart and lung transplant recipients.

Delays in hospital discharge frequently cause frustration and anxiety. Psychiatric consultation may be required, however, for the patient who avers that discharge is premature. This behavior may result from fear associated with unresolved symptoms or from transition from the close in-hospital monitoring by the surgical team.

Body Image Distortions

Cushingoid changes from prednisone are especially troublesome for young patients undergoing transplantation. One young liver transplant patient chose to undergo a series of cosmetic surgeries to rid herself of areas of adiposity when she reached young adulthood. She did not appear obese, but her newly changed body image was unacceptable.

Cyclosporine may also be associated with hirsutism. Common warts may also prove disfiguring and sometimes improve when immunosuppression is changed from azathioprine to cyclophosphamide.

Castelnuovo-Tedesco[115] and others have been especially interested in the psychological impact of the transplant recipient's incorporation of a body part from the donor. Perhaps the most dramatic account was that of a Ku Klux Klan grand dragon who joined the National Association for the Advancement of Colored People (NAACP) on learning that his donor was an African-American.[116] Some patients comment on changes in their food choices and wonder whether the donor's lifestyle may have been contributory. A middle-aged heart-lung recipient who determined the identity of her cadaveric donor told a national television audience, during an appearance on the Phil Donahue Show, that her subsequent vigor led to an affair with a post-adolescent man whose age was similar to her donor's.

One of the most unusual cases we have encountered was of a 43-year-old heart transplant recipient who reported a recurrent dream in which he was driven by starvation to strip and chew the flesh of his own arm. Preoperatively, he had expressed anxiety about the prospect of receiving a cadaveric organ. When, several months following his operation, a discussion of the dream led to a statement that it sounded like cannibalism. "Yes," he responded, "when I was in the Army working in the motor pool, there was a sign that said, 'Do not cannibalize!'" He explained that it had been an unsanctioned practice to take working parts from other vehicles to service ones in need of repair.

Depression

Postoperative depression may arise as a recurrence of affective illness. Steroid-induced depression is common and tends to be accompanied by irritability that is less evident to the patient than to the family and to the attending surgical staff. Rejection is another common cause of depression, and it may be related to the fear of graft loss, to cytokine production, and to end-organ dysfunction.

Also important for the transplant psychiatrist is awareness of the link between depression and infection. Psychiatric consultation may sometimes precede a request for infectious disease consultation because mood changes may foreshadow a fever spike or evidence of systemic illness. Cytomegalovirus infection is especially common following transplantation, and it is associated with a significant increase in first-time psychiatric consultation.[117] Typically, these patients do not express hopelessness or suicidal ideation. Appetite reduction, lethargy, and psychological withdrawal are common.

Psychological Rejection

Viederman[118] and others have raised the possibility of psychologically induced allograft rejection. This concept is interesting but speculative. More likely, psychologically based rejection results from noncompliance caused by depression, memory impairment, substance abuse, or adjustment reaction related to psychosocial stress or by altered body image. Medication costs thousands of dollars annually, and noncompliance may follow loss of third-party funding or other adverse economic developments.

Postoperative Psychiatric Intervention

Long-term Care

Transplant patients are often told that they will end up with a new set of medical problems once end-organ replacement has occurred. Morbidity may occur as a function of rejection, medication side effects, and progression of systemic disease. The care of transplant patients is thus a long-term prospect, and the consulting psychiatrist may be re-consulted at intervals, especially for those who are most ill or least adaptive.

Patients who are at highest risk psychologically should have follow-up plans created before the operative intervention. Patients with affective disorders, schizophrenia, substance abuse, or moderate mental retardation can be managed with supportive counseling, psychopharmacologic care, and social engineering.

Psychotherapeutic Interventions

Psychotherapy may include the reframing of expectations. For example, a patient who is recovering from a prolonged ICU stay will need help with assessment of his or her progress, which may be measured by absence of a monitor, reduction of IV lines, and signs of early mobilization. Guilt and shame may follow an encounter with delirium or result from the preoperative wish for a donor organ. Patients can be helped to understand that these experiences are common. Daily visits to delirious or acutely depressed patients are advisable and may be a source of relief to the patient, the family, and the surgical staff.

Behavioral interventions may be designed with the nursing staff to assist in the management of excessive dependency, hostility, or resistance. Group therapy is of value for many patients and family members and may be conducted by the psychiatrist, social worker, psychologist, or psychiatric nurse clinician.

Psychopharmacologic Intervention

Treatment with antipsychotics requires modification of immunosuppressant protocols (where feasible), correction of metabolic abnormalities, and treatment of bleeding, infection, and rejection. Complex partial seizures should be considered as a cause of psychosis, but care must be taken in the choice of anticonvulsants. Phenytoin and phenobarbital may decrease levels of immunosuppressants and precipitate rejection. Gabapentin and carbamazepine have been preferred in the management of seizures following transplantation. Haloperidol and morphine sulfate are each of potential benefit in the management of agitated delirious states.

Haloperidol is typically effective at lower dosage levels. Acute psychotic disturbances may respond rapidly IV administration of 0.5 to 1 mg of haloperidol as needed. Steroid-related irritability and hypomania often improve with 0.5 to 2.0 mg of haloperidol at bedtime.

Atypical antipsychotics such as olanzapine and risperidone have also been used in this setting. Olanzapine can be associated with considerable weight gain and elevated triglycerides. Lithium carbonate may be used, but care must be paid to toxicity from its combination with cyclosporine. Neuroleptics increase prolactin levels, but they have no known adverse impact on allograft function.[119]

Use of antidepressants and anxiolytics should proceed with the precautions addressed earlier. A full range of agents, as well as electroconvulsive therapy (ECT) can be used following surgery. TCAs are often preferred for diabetics with peripheral neuropathy, or they may be used in those with migraine or insomnia who are not at cardiovascular risk from these agents. In the setting of hepatic dysfunction, serum levels should be followed. For the most part, bupropion and SSRIs are better tolerated. Strouse and associates[120] have found that fluoxetine does not interfere with cyclosporine levels. Monoamine oxidase inhibitors (MAOIs) are best avoided, but we have encountered one heart transplant patient whose resistant depression responded only to tranylcypromine.

Posttraumatic Stress Disorder

Occasionally one encounters a patient with recurrent nightmares and the spontaneous recollection of medically traumatic events associated with transplantation. The prevalence in transplant recipients is not known. Fukunishi et al.[121] documented post-

traumatic stress disorder (PTSD) in 4 of 40 donors who underwent right lobe hepatectomy. There is no other report of this, but transplantation psychiatrists should be mindful of its potential.[121]

Conclusion

Psychiatric consultation on the transplant unit is highly rewarding and places the psychiatrist in a pivotal role as a member of a multidisciplinary team. The transplant unit is a challenging setting in which a full range of psychiatric skills and sensitivity are employed. The dearth of available organs necessitates a thoughtful and constructive approach to candidate selection. The participation of living donors is a unique circumstance that is worthy of both celebration and support. Transplant patients approach operative intervention with the travail of progressive organ failure and its attendant neuropsychiatric complications. The postoperative course of transplant patients is associated with improved quality of life and a requirement for long-term care.

References

1. Andrykowski MA: Psychiatric and psychosocial aspects of bone marrow transplantation, *Psychosomatics* 35:13–24, 1994.
2. Cosimi AB: Personal communication, 2003.
3. Nudeshima J: Obstacles to brain death and organ transplantation in Japan, *Lancet* 338:1063–1066, 1991.
4. Arnold RM, Youngner SJ: Back to the future: obtaining organs from non-heart-beating cadavers, *Kennedy Inst Ethics J* 3:103–111, 1993.
5. Surman OS: The ethics of partial liver donation (editorial), *N Engl J Med* 346:1038, 2002;
6. Surman OS, Cosimi A B, Fukunishi I, et al: Some ethical and psychiatric aspects of right-lobe liver transplantation in the United States and Japan, *Psychosomatics* 43: 347–353, 2002.
7. Bussutil, RW: Changing faces of liver transplantation: partial grafts for adults. The Paul S. Russell Lecture in Transplantation, Massachusetts General Hospital, Boston March 24, 2003.
8. Surman OS: *The surgical patient.* In Cassem NH, editor: *Massachusetts General Hospital handbook of general hospital psychiatry, ed 3,* St Louis, 1991, Mosby.
9. Surman OS: Psychiatric aspects of organ transplantation, *Am J Psychiatry* 146:972–982, 1989.
10. Abrams HS, Gill BF: Prediction of postoperative psychiatric complications, *N Engl J Med* 265:1163, 1961.

11. Craven J, Littlefields C, Rodin G, et al: The endstage renal disease severity index (ESRD-SI), *Psychol Med* 21:237–243, 1991.

12. Kimmel PL, Weihs K, Peterson RA: Survival in hemodialysis patients: the role of depression, *J Am Soc Nephrol* 4:12–27, 1993.

13. Brown TM, Brown RLS: Neuropsychiatric consequences of renal failure, *Psychosomatics* 20:244–253, 1995.

14. Tyler RH: Neurologic disorders in renal failure, *Am J Med* 44:734–748, 1968.

15. Surman OS, Parker SW: Complex partial seizures and psychiatric disturbance in end-stage renal disease, *Psychosomatics* 22:1077–1080, 1981.

16. Rubin NT: Personal communication.

17. Benett W, Singer I, Coggins CJ: A guide to drug therapy in renal failure, *JAMA* 230:1544–1553, 1974.

18. Stiebel VG: Methylphenidate plasma levels in depressed patients with renal failure, *Psychosomatics* 35:498–500, 1994.

19. Surman OS, Tolkoff-Rubin N: Use of hypnosis in patients receiving hemodialysis for end-stage renal disease, *Gen Hosp Psychiatry* 6:31–35, 1984.

20. Neu S, Kjellstrand CM: Stopping long-term dialysis, *N Engl J Med* 314:14–20, 1986.

21. Hirsch DJ: Death from dialysis termination, *Nephrol Dial Transplant* 4:41–44, 1989.

22. Levy NB: Psychological aspects of renal transplantation, *Psychosomatics* 35:427–433, 1994.

23. Evans RW, Manninen DL, Garrison LP, et al: The quality of life of patients with end-stage renal disease, *N Engl J Med* 312:553–559, 1985.

24. Levey AS, Hou S, Bush HL: Kidney transplantation from unrelated donors: time to reclaim a discarded opportunity, *N Engl J Med* 314:914–918, 1986.

25. Delmonico F, Surman OS, *Transplantation* 2003, in press.

26. Faden RR, Disclosure and informed consent: does it matter how we tell it? *Health Educ Monogr* 3:198–214, 1977.

27. Blumenthal J, Burg MM, Barefoot J, et al: Social support, type A behavior and coronary artery disease, *Psychosom Med* 49:331–340, 1987.

28. Hackett TP, Cassem NH: The psychological adaptation to convalescence of myocardial infarction, *N Engl J Med* 311:552–559, 1984.

29. Ahern DK, Gorkin L, Anderson JL, et al: Biobehavioral variables and mortality for cardiac arrest in the Cardiac Arrhythmia Pilot Study (CAPS*), Am J Cardiology* 66:59–62, 1990.

30. Ruberman W, Weinblatt E, Goldberg JD, et al: Psychosocial influences on mortality after myocardial infarction, *N Engl J Med* 311:552–559, 1984.

31. Vlay SC, Olson LC, Fricchione GL, et al: Anxiety and anger in patients with ventricular tachyarrhythmias: responses after automatic internal cardiovascular defibrillator implantation, *PACE* 12:366–373, 1989.

32. Riether AM, Smith SL, Lewison BJ: Quality of life changes and psychiatric and neurocognitive outcome after heart and liver transplantation, *Transplantation* 54:444–450, 1992.

33. Dimsdale JE: Research links between psychiatry and cardiology: hypertension, type A behavior, sudden death and the physiology of emotional arousal, *Gen Hosp Psychiatry* 10:328–338, 1988.

34. Evans D: Antidepressant adverse effects and antidepressants in the medically ill, *Am Soc Clin Psychopharmacol Progress Notes* 6:22–23, 1995–1996.

35. Onaca NN, Levy MF, Sanchez EQ, et al: A correlation between the pretransplantation MELD score and mortality in the first two years after transplantation, *Liver Transplant* 9:117–123, 2003.

36. Surman OS: Psychiatric aspects of liver transplantation, *Psychosomatics* 35:297–307, 1994.

37. Parsons-Smith BG, Summerskill WHJ, Dawson AAM, et al: The electroencephalogram in liver disease, *Lancet* 2:867–871, 1957.

38. Tarter RE, Switala J, Arria A, et al: Subclinical hepatic encephalopathy: comparison before and after orthotopic liver transplantation, *Transplantation* 50:632–637, 1990.

39. Tarter RE, Switala J, Plail J, et al: Severity of hepatic encephalopathy before liver transplantation is associated with quality of life after transplantation, *Arch Intern Med* 152:2097–2101, 1992.

40. Levenson JL, Olbrisch ME: Psychosocial evaluation of organ transplant candidates: a comparative survey of process, criteria, and outcomes in heart, liver, and kidney transplantation, *Psychosomatics* 34:314–323, 1993.

41. Evans R: Value of the life extended. Paper presented at Massachusetts General Hospital Series in Clinical Ethics, Boston, 1991.

42. Moss AH, Siegler M: Should alcoholics compete equally for liver transplantation? *JAMA* 265:1295–1298, 1991.

43. Surman OS: The morality of transplantation (letter), *JAMA* 266:213, 1991.

44. Merrican KJ, Overcast TD: Patient selection for heart transplantation: when is a discriminating choice discrimination? *J Health Polit Policy Law* 10:7–3, 1985.

45. Field H, Gastfriend DR, Surman OS, et al: Personal communication, 1996.

46. Beresford TP, Turcotte JG, Merion R, et al: A rational approach to liver transplantation for the alcoholic patient, *Psychosomatics* 31:241–254, 1990.

47. Yates B, Reed D, Booth B, et al: A rational approach to liver transplantation for the alcoholic patient, *Psychosomatics* 31:241–254, 1990.

48. Knechtle SJ, Fleming F, Barry KL, et al: Liver transplantation for alcoholic liver disease, *Surgery* 112:694–701, 1992.

49. Kumar S, Stauber RE, Gavaler JS, et al: Orthotopic liver transplantation for alcoholic liver disease, *Hepatology* 11:159–164, 1990.

50. Gastfriend DR, Surman OS, Gaffey GK, et al: Preliminary outcome of liver transplantation in a matched

sample of alcoholics and nonalcoholics. Paper presented at a symposium on selected topics in organ transplantation, American Psychiatric Association Annual Meeting, New Orleans, 1991.

51. Berlakovich G, Rudolf S, Herbst F, et al: Efficacy of liver transplantation for alcoholic cirrhosis with respect to recidivism and compliance, *Transplantation* 58:560–565, 1994.

52. Osorio RW, Ascher NL, Avery M, et al: Predicting recidivism after orthotopic transplantation for alcoholic liver disease, *Hepatology* 20:105–110, 1994.

53. Cosimi AB: Update on liver transplantation, *Transplant Proc* 23:2083–2090, 1991.

54. Singer PA, Seigler M, Whitington PF, et al: Ethics of liver transplantation with living donors, *N Engl J Med* 321:620–622, 1989.

55. Busuttil RW: Living-related liver donation, *Transplant Proc* 23:43–45, 1991.

56. Surman OS, Transplantation of the right hepatic lobe (letter), *N Engl J Med* 347:818, 2002.

57. Olbrisch ME, Bnedict SM, Hatler DL, et al: Psychosocial assessment of living organ donors: clinical and ethical considerations, *Prog Transplant* 11:1–49, 2001.

58. Ondria CG, Yates WR, The use of antidepressants in the treatment of patients with hepatitis C, *Medi Psychiatry* 23–28, 2001.

59. Trzepacz PT, Levenson JL, Tringali RA: Psychopharmacology and neuropsychiatric syndromes in organ transplantation, *Gen Hosp Psychiatry* 13:233–245, 1991.

60. Pollack MH, Kradin R, Otto MW: Prevalence of panic in patients referred for pulmonary function testing at a major medical center, *Am J Psychiatry* 153:110–113, 1996.

61. Joint Statement of ASTP, ATS, ERS, ISHLT: International guidelines for the selection of lung transplant candidates. *Am J Respir Crit Care Med* 158.335–339, 1998.

62. Trzepacz PT, Gupta B, DiMartini AF: *Pharmacologic issues in organ transplantation: psychopharmacology and neuropsychiatric medication side-effects.* In Trzepacz PT, Di Martini AF, editors: *The transplant patient*, 2000, Cambridge University Press, pp 21–41.

63. Christopherson LK: Cardiac transplantation: a psychological perspective, *Circulation* 75:57–62, 1987.

64. Surman OS, Dienstag JL, Cosimi AB, et al: Liver transplantation: psychiatric considerations, *Psychosomatics* 28:615–621, 1987.

65. Kimball CP: Predictive study of adjustment to cardiac surgery, *J Thorac Cardiovasc Surg* 58:891, 1969.

66. Gath D, Cooper P, Day A: Hysterectomy and psychiatric disorder: I. Levels of psychiatric morbidity before and after hysterectomy, *Br J Psychiatry* 140:335–342, 1982.

67. Johnston M: Anxiety in surgical patients, *Psychol Med* 10:145–152, 1980.

68. Wilson P: Psychological risk factors. Paper presented at first working conference on psychological and ethi-

cal aspects of organ transplantation, Toronto, June 1990.

69. Ray C: *The surgical patient: psychological stress and coping resources.* In Eiser JR, editor: *Social psychology and behavioral*, New York, 1982, Wiley & Sons.

70. Andrew JM: Recovery from surgery with and without preparatory instruction for three coping styles, *J Pers Soc Psychol* 15:223–226, 1970.

71. Wilson JF: Behavioral preparation for surgery: benefit or harm? *J Behav Med* 4:79–102, 1981.

72. Johnston M: Preoperative existential status and postoperative recovery, *Adv Psychosom* Med 15:1–20, 1986.

73. Levitan SJ, Kornfeld DK: Clinical and cost benefits of liaison psychiatry, *Am J Psychiatry* 138:790–793, 1981.

74. Mumford E, Schlesinger HJ, Glass GV: The effects of psychological intervention on recovery from surgery and heart attacks: an analysis of the literature, *Am J Public Health* 72:144–151, 1982.

75. Rogers M, Reich P: Psychological intervention with surgical patients: evaluation of outcome, *Adv Psychosom Med* 15:23–50, 1986.

76. Pizer H, Massachusetts General Hospital Transplant Unit: *Organ transplants: a patient's guide*, Boston, 1992, Harvard University Press.

77. Eisenach JC, Plevak DJ, Van Dyke RA, et al: Comparison of analgesic requirements after liver transplantation and cholecystectomy, *Mayo Clin Proc* 64:356–359, 1989.

78. Schacter S, Singer JE: Cognitive, social and physiological determinants of emotional state, *Psychol Rev* 69:379, 1962.

79. Egbert LD, Battit GE, Welch GE, et al: Reduction of postoperative pain by encouragement and instruction of the patient, *N Engl J Med* 270:825, 1964.

80. Surman OS: Psychiatric aspects of organ transplantation, *Am J Psychiatry* 146:972–982, 1989.

81. Trzepacz PT, DiMartini A, Tringali RA: Psychopharmacologic issues in organ transplantation: I. Pharmacokinetics in organ failure and psychiatric aspects of immunosuppressants and anti-infectious agents, *Psychosomatics* 34:199–207, 1993.

82. Trzepacz PT, DiMartini A, Tringali RA: Psychopharmacologic issues in organ transplantation: II. Psychopharmacologic medications, *Psychosomatics* 34: 290–298, 1993.

83. Cassem NH: *Depression.* In Hackett TP, Cassem NH, editors: *Massachusetts General Hospital handbook of general hospital psychiatry, ed 2*, Littleton, Mass, 1986, PSG Publishing Company.

84. Calabrese G, Bobbit P: *Tragic choices*, New York, 1978, Norton.

85. Taylor C: *Sources of the self: the making of the modern identity*, Cambridge, 1992, Harvard University Press.

86. Surman OS, Purtilo R: Reevaluation of organ transplantation criteria: allocation of scarce resources to borderline candidates, *Psychosomatics* 33:202–212, 1992.

87. Surman OS, Cosimi AB: Ethical dichotomies in organ transplantation: a time for bridge building, *Gen Hosp Psychiatry* 18:135–195, 1996.

88. Loewy EH: Drunks, livers, and values: should social value judgments enter into liver transplant decisions, *J Clin Gastroenterol* 9:436–441, 1987.

89. Freeman AM III, Folks DO, Sokol RS, et al: Cardiac transplantation: clinical correlates of psychiatric outcome, *Psychosomatics* 29:47–54, 1988.

90. Olbrisch ME, Levenson JL: Psychosocial assessment of organ transplant candidates: current status of methodological and philosophical issues, *Psychosomatics* 36:236–243, 1995.

91. Olbrisch ME, Levenson JL, Hafner R: The PACT: A rating scale for the study of clinical decision making in psychosocial screening of organ candidates, *Clin Transplant* 3:164–169, 1989.

92. Robertson JA: Patient selection for organ transplantation: age, incarceration, family support, and other social factors, *Transplant Proc* 21:3397–3402, 1989.

93. Didlake RH, Dreyfus K, Kerman RH, et al: Patient noncompliance: a major cause of late graft failure in cyclosporine-treated renal failure, *Transplant Proc* 20(suppl 3):63–69, 1988.

94. Colon EA, Popkin MK, Matas AJ, et al: Overview of noncompliance in renal transplantation, *Transplant Rev* 5:175–180, 1991.

95. Rodriguez A, Diaz M, Colon A, et al: Psychosocial profile of noncompliant transplant patients, *Transplant Proc* 23:1807–1809, 1991.

96. Weber M, Dindo D, DeMartines N, et al: Kidney transplantation from donors without a heartbeat, *N Engl J Med* 347(4) 248–255, 2002.

97. Fabro AJ: Legal aspects of organ transplantation: Strunk vs. Strunk, *Conn Med* 34:583, 1970.

98. Levinsky N: Organ donation by unrelated donors, *N Engl J Med* 434(6): 430–432, 2000.

99. Gridelli B, Remuzzi G: Strategies for making more organs available for transplantation, *N Engl J Med* 343 (6), 404–410, 2000.

100. Battafarano RJ, Anderson RC, Meyers BF, et al: Perioperative complications after living donor lobectomy, *J Thoracic Cardiovasc Surg* 120(5):909–915, 2000.

101. Surman O.S: The ethics of partial-liver donation, *N Engl J Med* 346 (14), 1038.

102. Fellner CH, Marshall JR: Twelve kidney donors, *JAMA* 206:2703–2707, 1968.

103. Simmons RG, Klein SD, Simmons RC: *Gift of life: the social and psychological impact of organ transplantation,* New York, 1977, John Wiley & Sons.

104. Gouge F, Moore J, Bremer CR: The quality of life of donors, potential donors, and recipients of living-related donor renal transplantation, *Transplant Proc* 22:2409–2413, 1990.

105. Moore KA, Jones R, Hardy AK, et al: Psychosocial adjustment to illness: quality of life following liver transplantation, *Transplant Proc* 24:2257–2258, 1992.

106. Hotson JR, Enzmann DR: Neurologic complications of cardiac transplantation, *Neurol Clin* 6:349–365, 1988.

107. de Groen PC, Aksamit AJ, Rakela J, et al: Central nervous system toxicity after liver transplantation: the role of cyclosporine, *N Engl J Med* 317: 861–866, 1987.

108. Vogt DP, Lederman RJ, Carey WD, et al: Neurologic complications of liver transplantation, *Transplantation* 45:1057–1061, 1988.

109. Craven JL: Cyclosporine-associated organic mental disorders in liver transplant recipients, *Psychosomatics* 32:94–102, 1991.

110. Shutteve LA, Green JP, Newman NJ, et al: Cortical blindness and white matter lesions in a patient receiving FK506 after liver transplantation, *Neurology* 43:2417–2418, 1993.

111. Moreno E, Gomez SR, Gonzalez I, et al: Neurologic complications in liver transplantation, *Acta Neural Scanda* 87:25–31, 1993.

112. Castelao AM, Sabate JM, Grino S, et al: Cyclosporine-drug interactions, *Transplant Proc* 20(suppl 6):66–69, 1988.

113. Estol CJ, Fans AA, Martinez AJ, et al: Central pontine myelinolysis after liver transplantation, *Neurology* 39:493–498, 1989.

114. Winnock S, Janvier G, Parmentier F, et al: Pontine myelinolysis following liver transplantation: a report of two cases, *Transpl Int* 6:26–28, 1993.

115. Castelnuovo-Tedesco P: *Transplantation: psychological implications of changes in body image.* In Levy NB, editor: *Psychonephrology: psychological factors in hemodialysis and transplantation,* New York, 1981, Plenum Medical Book Company.

116. Abrams HS: *Repetitive dialysis.* In Hackett TP, Cassem NH, editors: *Massachusetts General Hospital handbook of general hospital psychiatry, ed 2,* St Louis, 1978, Mosby.

117. Hibberd PL, Surman OS, Bass M, et al: Psychiatric disease and cytomegalovirus viremia in renal transplant recipients, *Psychosomatics* 36:561–563, 1995.

118. Viederman M: Psychogenic factors in kidney transplant rejection: a case study, *Am J Psychiatry* 132:957–959, 1975.

119. Surman OS: Possible immunologic effects of psychotropic medication, *Transplantation* 34:139–143, 1993.

120. Strouse TB, Fairbanks LA, Skotzko CE, et al: Fluoxetine and cyclosporine in organ transplantation: failure to detect significant drug interactions or adverse clinical events in depressed organ recipients, *Psychosomatics* 37:23–30, 1996.

121. Fukunishi, I, Sugawara Y, Takayama T, et al: Psychiatric disorders before and after living-related transplantation, *Psychosomatics* 42: 337–343, 2001.

Chapter 37

Patients with HIV Infection and AIDS

B. J. Beck, M.S.N., M.D.
Jonathan L. Worth, M.D.

Human immunodeficiency virus (HIV) infection and acquired immune deficiency syndrome (AIDS) are prevalent in disenfranchised populations, including addicts, the seriously and persistently mentally ill (SPMI), gay men, sex workers, and ethnic minorities. HIV infection is a multisystem disease associated with stigma at the interface of psychiatry and medicine; moreover, it is more prevalent among the mentally ill,[1-3] and mental illness is more prevalent in those who are HIV-positive.[4-6] Even Axis II psychiatric pathology is overrepresented in the HIV-positive population,[7-9] possibly because traits such as impulsivity, reckless disregard for safety, affective instability, or chronic feelings of emptiness may predispose individuals to risky behaviors and to HIV infection. More than a decade ago, HIV infection was a terminal illness; however, as a result of widespread use of complex medication regimens—regimens with unpleasant physical and psychiatric side effects, inconvenient dosing and dietary requirements, and interactions with other medications (including psychotropics) and drugs of abuse—it has become a chronic illness. Complacency, stigma, secrecy, and shame have interfered with detection of HIV infection. Culture, lifestyle, and socioeconomic barriers to appropriate care and to HIV prevention persist.

HIV is a blood-borne, sexually-transmitted retrovirus that contains RNA as its genetic material and the enzyme reverse transcriptase, which facilitates the translation of RNA to DNA in infected human cells. After replication to human DNA, the now-functional virus can go on to infect other cells, preferentially the CD4, T-helper, and lymphocytes, thereby causing severe (primarily cell-mediated) immune dysfunction for which the virus and the resulting syndrome were named. Immune deficiency, a predilection for certain opportunistic infections (OIs), and AIDS-defining conditions correlate with a decline in CD4 lymphocyte count[10] (Table 37-1). This infection-translation-replication-infection cycle repeats billions of times, the host mounts an immune response, and a set point (or dynamic equilibrium) is eventually reached. This set point varies from person to person, and it has been found to be of prognostic significance.[11] The virus also invades the central nervous system (CNS) early, possibly within hours to days of the initial infection.[12]

While the science behind HIV infection and its treatment is changing at a rapid pace, the general tenants of this chapter should provide a consistent framework for the safe and comprehensive psychiatric evaluation and care of adults at risk for, or infected with, HIV. Four general questions help set the context for such an evaluation: (1) At what stage of HIV infection is the patient in terms of symptomatic disease and CD4+ lymphocyte count? (2) Is there evidence of HIV-associated CNS infection? (3) Does the patient have a premorbid psychiatric history? (4) How did the patient become HIV-infected? The important implications of the first

Table 37-1. AIDS-Defining Conditions That Emerge with Advancing Immunosuppression

CD4 Cell Count (cells/mm³)	Condition
200–500	Thrush
	Kaposi's sarcoma
	Tuberculosis reactivation
	Herpes zoster
	Herpes simplex
	Bacterial sinusitis/pneumonia
100–200	*Pneumocystis carinii* pneumonia
50–100	Systemic fungal infections
	Primary tuberculosis
	Cerebral toxoplasmosis
	Progressive multifocal leukoencephalopathy
	Peripheral neuropathy
	Cervical carcinoma
0–50	Cytomegalovirus disease
	Disseminated *Mycobacterium avium-intracellulare complex*
	Non-Hodgkin's lymphoma
	Central nervous system lymphoma
	HIV-associated dementia

Modified from: *APA practice guideline for the treatment of patients with HIV/AIDS*, p 8.

three questions may seem more obvious and should be clear by the completion of the chapter. The fourth question (How did the patient become HIV-infected?) is often a highly personal story, one that reveals the patient as a person. The answer to this question foreshadows how the patient will relate to illness and to medical care. This knowledge informs not only the psychiatrist's evaluation but the patient's individualized treatment and management plans, as well.

Epidemiology

HIV infection and AIDS remains a terminal illness in much of the world; it cuts across all ages and socioeconomic groups, each with specific characteristics and considerations. The United States is the most heavily infected industrialized nation; as of 2001, just shy of a million people were living in this country with the virus (i.e., 0.03% of the population, or 1 in 300 Americans are infected[13,14,]). By contrast, 95% of the estimated 40 million infected people live in the developing world, with more than 25 million of them living in sub-Saharan Africa.[15] The advent of highly active antiretroviral therapy (HAART) in 1996 has decreased the incidence of AIDS and AIDS-related deaths so more people in the United States are living with HIV infection than ever before. Nonetheless, the incidence of HIV infection has not declined over the past decade. A disproportionate number of those 40,000 new infections per year in the United States occur in the ethnic groups, racial minority populations (African-American, Hispanic, Asian, and Pacific Islanders), and heterosexual women.[16] However, recent outbreaks of other sexually-transmitted diseases (STDs) in gay males raise the specter of a possible HIV resurgence in this population and suggest that the success of HAART may have led to complacency and the resumption of unsafe sexual practices in men who have sex with men (MSM).[17,18]

HIV Infection and the Central Nervous System

Within days of the initial infection, the virus is transported to the brain by monocytes that then differentiate into macrophages. These infected but not dead macrophages may be activated randomly, leading over time to excessive secretion of normal inflammatory substances and cell death without neuronal infection. That is, HIV infection causes neuronal destruction without infecting neurons.[19] The CNS appears to be an independent reservoir of HIV replication; CSF viral load does not consistently correlate with plasma levels.[20] HIV in the CNS may also have different characteristics, such as mutations with increased viral resistance or neurotoxicity, than those of the peripherally observed virus. Antiretrovirals have variable blood-brain barrier (BBB) penetrance and may be less potent inhibitors of viral replication within the CNS. There is also evidence that viral particles or proteins, independent of complete, replicating virions, may be responsible for cell damage and death through a variety of mechanisms such as the release of neurotoxic cytokines, attraction or activation of lymphocytes, or activation of receptors that increase central cortisol.[19,21]

Although early studies concentrated on sampling and volume of the frontal cortex, it is now apparent that HIV infection does not uniformly affect the brain; instead, it has a predilection for subcortical structures, such as the hippocampus and basal ganglia, with lower concentrations in the cerebellum and midfrontal cortices.[22,23] This distribution, further differentiation of viral burden within particular basal ganglia regions, and concomitant structural changes in the brain, including ventricular enlargement, hippocampal atrophy, decreased basal ganglia volume, and white matter lesions, may explain the more characteristic cognitive and behavioral impairments associated with HIV infection of the CNS.[19,24,25] These types of lesions in the base of the skull are better visualized by brain magnetic resonance imaging (MRI) than by computed tomography (CT) scanning.

When evaluating neurocognitive impairment in the HIV-positive patient, HIV infection of the CNS should always be a diagnosis of exclusion, made only after a thorough investigation of other possible etiologies for neurocognitive impairment, especially if symptoms are of new or acute onset.[26] OI, neoplasm, other systemic illness, medication side effects, drug-drug interactions, use of recreational drugs, withdrawal syndromes, and metabolic and nutritional derangements should be considered. Primary psychiatric disease should be at the bottom of the list, especially if there is not a significant, preinfection history.[10,27–29]

Although neuropsychological testing may not be specific,[23] it helps to localize and quantify impairments. Recommended neuropsychological tests are an HIV-specific test battery, based on measures found by the AIDS Clinical Trials Group (ACTG) and the Multicenter AIDS Cohort Study to be sensitive to HIV-related cognitive deficits. These measures include Trail Making A & B, WAIS-R Digit Span and Digit Symbol, Grooved Pegboard, Finger Tapping, Stroop Color Word, FAS, Odd Man Out, and computer-based measures of complex reaction time.[30–33] Other measures are added as clinically indicated. Test battery times less than 60 minutes are less likely to produce patient fatigue, which confounds test interpretation and creates significant patient frustration or humiliation.

Medications for HIV Infection[34]

The three classes of antiretroviral medications are nucleoside reverse transcriptase inhibitors (nRTIs), non-nucleoside reverse transcriptase inhibitors (nnRTIs), and protease inhibitors (PIs) (Table 37-2[35]). These medications are generally used in combinations of one or more drugs from more than one class. Single-drug therapy is discouraged because of the rapid development of resistance that may spread to an entire class of medications, thus limiting the prospects for further, effective treatment. The different classes of medications differ in their therapeutic mechanisms and side-effect profiles (Table 37-3[35]).

Nucleoside Reverse Transcriptase Inhibitors

nRTIs are nucleoside analogs that inhibit the action of the enzyme reverse transcriptase. This enzyme inhibition slows or prevents viral replication. Most of the nRTIs require multiple daily doses, do not interact with other drugs, and can be taken with or without food. Didanosine (DDI), however, can decrease the absorption of other antiretrovirals if taken together and must be taken on an empty stomach. All nRTIs have been associated, albeit rarely, with a fatal syndrome of lactic acidosis and hepatic steatosis.

Non-Nucleoside Reverse Transcriptase Inhibitors

Like the nRTIs, the nnRTIs also interfere with reverse transcriptase, but by a different means. They are used in combination with other antiretrovirals. The nnRTIs have been shown to be active against viral strains of HIV that are resistant to nRTIs and PIs. However, if nnRTIs are used alone or with a single nRTI, resistance develops quickly, and usually generalizes to the whole class (i.e., to all the nnRTIs). The nnRTIs can also cause a rash early on; it is thought to be more common and severe (including onset of Stevens-Johnson syndrome) with nevirapine. Drug interactions with PIs and other drugs can occur because of their metabolism by the cytochrome P450 hepatic isoenzyme system.

Table 37-2. Approved Drugs for Antiretroviral Therapy*

Agent	Daily Dose	Frequency	Comment
Nucleoside Reverse Transcriptase Inhibitors (nRTIs)			
Zidovudine (Retrovir, AZT, ZDV)	one 300 mg tab	bid	
	or two 200 mg caps	tid	
Didanosine (Videx, ddI)	two 100 mg tabs	bid	Take on an empty stomach
Zalcitabine (Hivid, ddc)	one 0.75 mg tab	tid	
Stavudine (Zerit, d4T)	one 40 mg cap	bid	
Lamivudine (Epivir, 3TC)	one 150 mg tab	bid	
Combivir (3TC/ZDV)	150/300 mg tabs	bid	
Abacavir (Ziagen)	one 300 mg tabs	bid	
Zidovudine + Lamivudine (Combivir)	one tab	bid	
Non-Nucleoside RT Inhibitors (nnRTIs)			
Nevirapine (Viramune®)	one 200 mg tab	bid	200 mg daily then 200 mg bid
Delavirdine (Rescriptor)	four 100 mg tabs	tid	
Efavirenz (Sustiva)	three 200 mg caps	qd	Avoid high-fat foods
Protease Inhibitors (PIs)			
Saquinavir (Invirase)	six 200 mg caps	tid	High-fat meals/bid are not helpful
Saquinavir soft gel (Fortovase™)	six 200 mg caps	tid	With meals to increase bioavailability
Ritonavir (Norvir®)	six 100 mg caps	bid	Escalating dose required; refrigerate
Indinavir (Crixivan)	two 400 mg caps	Q8h	Empty stomach or light meals
Nelfinavir (Viracept)	three 250 mg tabs	tid	Take with meals
Amprenavir (Agenerase®)	eight 150 mg caps	bid	
Lopinavir + Ritonavir (Kaletra)	400 mg/100 mg caps	bid	Take with meals

*Modified from: *APA HIV-related neuropsychiatric complications and treatment*, HIV-Psychotropic Drug Interactions and Toxicity, slide 21.

Protease Inhibitors

PIs interfere with viral replication, maturation, and new cell infection by inhibiting the enzymatic cleavage of necessary viral protein precursors. Like the nnRTIs, PIs are metabolized by P450 enzymes, leading to drug interactions. PIs can cause gastrointestinal (GI) side effects and liver transaminase elevations. In addition, PIs may worsen or cause new-onset diabetes, insulin resistance, lipodystrophy, and hyperlipidemia. They have also been associated with increased bleeding in hemophiliacs.

Other Medications

HAART regimens are frequently complicated by the addition of antibiotics, antivirals, and/or antifungal medications to prophylaxis against, or to treat, OIs. Lipid-lowering drugs or oral hypoglycemic agents may be necessary to treat the antiretroviral-induced abnormalities in lipid metabolism and glucose control. Antiretroviral GI side effects may require the addition of antidiarrheals, proton pump inhibitors, or H_2 blockers. Pain syndromes may require antiinflammatory or narcotic medications, as well as antiseizure medications or tricyclic antidepressants (TCAs).

Cognitive/Neuropsychiatric Syndromes of HIV-Associated Central Nervous System Infection

HIV-Associated Dementia[36]

Previously known as AIDS dementia complex, HIV-associated dementia (HAD) is a subcortical dementia, similar to that seen in Huntington's disease.[23] HAD is severe enough to cause functional impairment, and it has no other definable cause. HAD is an AIDS-defining condition with a prevalence in the

Table 37-3. Side Effects Profile of Antiretrovirals**

Agent	Side Effects
Nucleoside Reverse Transcriptase Inhibitors (nRTIs)	
Zidovudine (Retrovir, AZT, ZDV)	Depressed bone marrow/anemia, neutropenia, GI symptoms, HA, insomnia
Didanosine (Videx, ddI)	Pancreatitis, peripheral neuropathy, GI symptoms
Zalcitabine (Hivid, ddc)	Peripheral neuropathy, stomatitis
Stavudine (Zerit, d4T)	Peripheral neuropathy, pancreatitis, lactic acidosis
Lamivudine (Epivir, 3TC)	Minimal
Lamivudine + Zidovudine (Combivir™)	As component drugs
Abacavir (Ziagen®)	Hypersensitivity (occasionally fatal), fever, rash, GI symptoms, malaise, anorexia
Non-Nucleoside RT Inhibitors (nnRTIs)	
Nevirapine (Viramune®)	Rash (Steven-Johnson), increased transaminases, hepatitis
Delavirdine (Rescriptor®)	Same, HA
Efavirenz (Sustiva®)	Same, CNS symptoms, teratogenic (monkeys/breast milk), false + marijuana
Protease Inhibitors (PI)	
Saquinavir (Invirase®)	GI symptoms, paresthesias, hepatitis, asthma, lipodystrophy, increased TGC/chol/glucose
Saquinavir soft gel (Fortovase™)	GI symptoms, paresthesias, hepatitis, HA, lipodystrophy, increased TGC/chol/glucose/TSM
Ritonavir (Norvir)	GI symptoms, paresthesias, hepatitis, asthma, lipodystrophy, increased TGC/chol/glucose
Indinavir (Crixivan)	HA, asthma, blurred vision, dizzy, metal taste, thrombocytopenia, increased Glucose, nephrolithiasis, GI symptoms, lipodystrophy, increased TGC/chol, rash
Nelfinavir (Viracept)	GI symptoms, lipodystrophy, increased TGC/chol
Amprenavir (Agenerase)	GI symptoms, asthma, rash, HA
Lopinavir/Ritonavir (Kaletra)	GI symptoms, fatigue, HA, asthenia, increased chol/glucose/transaminases, lipodystrophy, pancreatitis

** From *APA HIV-Related Neuropsychiatric Complications and Treatment*, HIV-Psychotropic Drug Interactions and Toxicity, slide 22. GI = gastrointestinal; HA = headache; chol = cholesterol; TGC = triglyceride.

United States of 21% to 25% prior to the advent of HAART; since then it has decreased to 7% to 10%. Associated with reduced white-matter volume, atrophy of the basal ganglia (reduced gray matter volume) and cell death, HAD is characterized by slowed informational processing, deficits in attention and memory, and impairments in abstraction and fine motor skills.[19,23,37]

Minor Cognitive/Motor Disorder

More common than HAD, minor cognitive/motor disorder (MCMD) had a prevalence prior to HAART of 25% in those with early symptomatic disease and 50% in those with AIDS.[38] Those figures have now declined to 14% and 24.4%, respectively.[19] MCMD is associated with neuronal dysfunction rather than with cell death.

This is important because it suggests that the pathology of MCMD may be treatable and that the syndrome is potentially reversible. Although by definition, the deficits are minor and do not cause obvious functional impairment, such subtle deficits may contribute to poor medication adherence and thus worse overall prognosis. Because of the prevalence, prognostic implications, and possible reversibility, research and improved measurement efforts should focus on MCMD.[19,24,37]

Impairment Without a Definable Syndrome

HAD and MCMD are inadequate descriptors for the wide array of reported and observed neuropsychological symptoms that may occur in 22% to 30% of "asymptomatic" seropositive individuals.[37,39] Given the diagnostic ambiguity of this group, it is not clear whether the prevalence of subsyndromal symptoms has decreased with the advent of HAART.

Differential Diagnosis of Psychiatric Distress

Psychiatric symptoms are common in the HIV-infected population and may meet criteria for *Diagnostic and Statistical Manual for Mental Disorders*, ed 4 (*DSM-IV*) disorders. Or, as with neurocognitive impairments, psychiatric symptoms may be subsyndromal; underlying causes should be identified and reversed when possible, although it may still be necessary to treat the psychiatric symptoms (Table 37-4[40]).

Mental Disorder Due to a General Medical Condition

Differential diagnosis should always begin with Mental Disorder due to a General Medical Condition.[26,27,41] HIV CNS infection, HAD, and MCMD should be considered, along with OIs[42] and neoplasms. Other considerations include side effects of medications (e.g., neurotoxic HIV medications, steroids, antibiotics, antifungals, over-the-counter [OTC] preparations, and herbal supplements, drug-drug interactions (e.g., herbal and OTC preparations), alcohol, and recreational drugs, substance intoxication or withdrawal,[28] nutritional deficits (e.g., thiamine, folate, zinc, cobalamin [vitamin B_{12}], pyridoxine [vitamin B_6]), poor intake (e.g.,

Table 37-4. Differential Diagnosis of Neuropsychiatric Symptoms in Patients with HIV-Infection and AIDS

1. Psychiatric disorders
2. Psychoactive substance intoxication/withdrawal
3. Primary HIV-associated syndromes
   a. Seroconversion illness
   b. HIV CNS infection
   c. HIV-associated dementia
4. CNS opportunistic infections
   a. Fungi: *Cryptococcus neoformans, Coccidioides immitis, Candida albicans, Histoplasma capsulatum, Aspergillus fumigatus,* and mucormycosis
   b. Protozoa/parasites: *Toxoplasma gondii* and amebas
   c. Viruses: CJ virus (progressive multifocal leukoencephalopathy), CMV, adenovirus type 2, herpes simplex virus, and varicella zoster virus
   d. Bacteria: *Mycobacterium avium-intracellulare, M. tuberculosis, Listeria monocytogenes,* gram-negative organisms, *Treponema pallidum,* and *Nocardia asteroides*
5. Neoplasms
   a. Primary CNS non-Hodgkin's lymphoma
   b. Metastatic Kaposi's sarcoma (rare)
   c. Burkitt's lymphoma
6. Medication side effects
7. Endocrinopathies and nutrient deficiencies
   a. Addison's disease (CMV, *Cryptococcus*, HIV-1, and ketoconazole)
   b. Hypothyroidism
   c. Vitamins A, B_6, B_{12}, and E deficiencies
   d. Hypogonadism
8. Anemia
9. Metabolic abnormalities: hypoxia; hepatic, renal, pulmonary, adrenal, and pancreatic insufficiency; hypomagnesemia; hypocalcemia; water intoxication, dehydration; hypernatremia; hyponatremia; alkalosis; and acidosis
10. Hypotension
11. Complex partial seizures
12. Head trauma
13. Non–HIV-related conditions

From: Querques J, Worth JL: *HIV infection and AIDS.* In Stern TA, Herman JB, editors: *Psychiatry update and board preparation,* New York, 2000, McGraw-Hill, p 208.
CJ = Creutzfeldt-Jakob; CMV = cytomegalovirus; HIV = human immunodeficiency virus.

medication or disease-induced nausea, mood disorder, painful oral lesions, or addiction), poor absorption, abnormal losses (e.g., gastritis, diarrhea, vomiting, or nephropathy), or increased demand (e.g., hypermetabolic state due to infection, stress, or neoplasm).[29] Metabolic derangements (e.g., electrolyte abnormalities), renal or hepatic dysfunction, and endocrinopathies (e.g., glucose intolerance, hyperadrenalism, hypocalcemia, or thyroid dysfunction)[21] may also cause psychiatric symptoms.

Delirium

Delirium is a frequent neuropsychiatric complication in hospitalized patients with AIDS.[43] In patients with asymptomatic HIV infection or CD$_4$ lymphocyte counts greater than 500/μL, it is rare to have an HIV-related condition cause delirium; substance intoxication or withdrawal is a more likely cause. This includes drugs used as alternative HIV therapies, such as testosterone and other steroids.

Among patients with symptomatic HIV infection or a CD$_4$ lymphocyte count less than 500/μL, HIV-related conditions and iatrogenic causes (Table 37-5) should be high on the differential diagnosis for delirium and should be at the top of the list for patients at advanced stages of AIDS or when the CD$_4$ lymphocyte count falls below 100/μL. There should be a continued high index of suspicion for substance intoxication and withdrawal. Seizure disorder should also be in the differential diagnosis because HIV-infected patients are at increased risk for new-onset seizures, especially partial complex seizures.[44]

A sudden change in mental status is not characteristic of HAD alone; more frequently, it is because of underlying causes. Patients with advanced HAD experience symptomatic worsening with mild states of delirium during the late afternoon when they are increasingly fatigued or during the night (i.e., sundowning).

The primary goal in the management of delirium is the identification and treatment of causative factors. The need for laboratory tests, including anatomic brain imaging, electroencephalogram (EEG), cerebrospinal fluid (CSF) examination, and blood tests, must be guided by history and clinical examination. If delirium is a treatment-emergent adverse effect, the suspected medication should be discontinued or an alternative agent substituted.

Depression

The most common psychiatric complication of HIV infection or AIDS, depression, should never be considered "appropriate." When a person has sufficient symptoms to meet criteria for depression, the patient deserves to be treated.[45,46] As is the case with certain other medical illnesses, it may be hard to interpret the more somatic neurovegetative symptoms such as fatigue, loss of appetite, altered sleep patterns, or difficulty with concentration.

Fatigue

Fatigue is not pathognomonic for depression. Fatigue may be part of advanced disease or be out of proportion to apparent disease. Reported mood, interest, and guilt may be more significant. Feelings of hopelessness, helplessness, and worthlessness also help make the diagnosis of depression.[5]

Bereavement

The patient with HIV infection or AIDS often suffers multiple losses, including friends, health, physical ability, career, income, housing, child custody, independence, or a sense of freedom or autonomy. Mood and related symptoms require careful evaluation in the setting of loss or bereavement. If the patient meets criteria for major depression, and is not responding to supportive interventions, pharmacologic treatment is warranted.

Suicide

Suicidal thoughts should always be assessed; they are more prevalent in patients with asymptomatic HIV infection than in those with AIDS.[47] The incidence of suicide in patients with HIV infection or AIDS has decreased since the advent of HAART; it is now similar to that seen with other medical illnesses. The incidence of suicide in this population of HIV-infected individuals and those with other medical illnesses, however, is still higher than in the general population. Risk factors include symptomatic depression, persistent pain, drug or alcohol use, altered cognition (i.e., delirium or HAD),

Table 37-5. Neuropsychiatric Side Effects of Medications Commonly Used in Patients with HIV Infection and AIDS

Nucleoside Reverse Transcriptase Inhibitors	Comments
Zidovudine (AZT)	Headache, restlessness, agitation, insomnia, mania, depression, irritability, delirium, somnolence, and peripheral neuropathy
Didanosine (ddI)	Insomnia, mania, and peripheral neuropathy
Zalcitabine (ddC)	Peripheral neuropathy
Stavudine (d4T)	Mania and peripheral neuropathy
Lamivudine (3TC)	Similar to AZT
Abacavir (ABC)	Headache
Non-nucleoside reverse transcriptase inhibitors	
Nevirapine	Headache
Delavirdine	Headache
Efavirenz	False-positive cannabinoid test, agitation, insomnia, euphoria, depression, somnolence, abnormal dreams, confusion, abnormal thinking, impaired concentration, amnesia, depersonalization, and hallucinations
Protease inhibitors	
Indinavir	Headache, asthenia, blurred vision, dizziness, and insomnia
Ritonavir	Circumoral and peripheral paresthesias, asthenia, and altered taste
Saquinavir	Headache
Nelfinavir	Headache and asthenia
Amprenavir	Headache
Lopinavir/ritonavir combination	Asthenia, headache, and insomnia
Other antivirals	
Acyclovir	Headache, agitation, insomnia, tearfulness, confusion, hyperesthesia, hyperacusis, depersonalization, and hallucinations
Ganciclovir	Agitation, mania, psychosis, irritability, and delirium
Antibacterials	
Cotrimoxazole	Headache, insomnia, depression, anorexia, and apathy
Trimethoprim-sulfamethoxazole	Headache, insomnia, depression, anorexia, apathy, delirium, mutism, and neuritis
Isoniazid	Agitation, depression, hallucinations, paranoia, and impaired memory
Dapsone	Agitation, insomnia, mania, and hallucinations
Antiparasitics	
Thiabendazole	Hallucinations and olfactory disturbance
Metronidazole	Agitation, depression, delirium, and seizures (with IV administration)
Pentamidine	Hypoglycemia, hypotension, confusion, delirium, and hallucinations
Antifungals	
Amphotericin B	Headache, agitation, anorexia, delirium, diplopia, lethargy, and peripheral neuropathy
Ketoconazole	Headache, dizziness, and photosensitivity
Flucytosine	Headache, delirium, and cognitive impairment
Others	
Steroids	Euphoria, mania, depression, psychosis, and confusion
Cytosine arabinoside	Delirium with cerebellar signs

From: Querques J, Worth JL: *HIV infection and AIDS.* In Stern TA, Herman JB, editors: *Psychiatry update and board preparation,* New York, 2000, McGraw-Hill, p 210.

social isolation, multiple losses, hopelessness, and Axis II pathology.[10,48] Serious thoughts of self-harm usually indicate the need for inpatient care. Electroconvulsive therapy (ECT) may be a life-saving procedure for individuals who are severely depressed and suicidal, especially when they are medically compromised and unable to tolerate medications or the delay in their effectiveness.

Anxiety

Prevalent in HIV infection, anxiety runs the gamut from an acute response to a devastating diagnosis, to a full-blown anxiety disorder. Patients with a history of an anxiety disorder are at increased risk, as are those with few social supports and poor coping skills. In susceptible patients, onset or recrudescence of anxiety symptoms may be predictably related to disease milestones or to signs of disease progression (e.g., initial diagnosis, declining CD_4 count, increased viral load, onset of OIs, chronic pain or paresthesias, wasting, or physical changes that make the disease more public).[10,49] The somatic symptoms frequently associated with anxiety (e.g., tremor, muscle tension or spasm, shortness of breath, dizziness, headache, sweating, flushing, palpitations, nausea, vomiting, or diarrhea) need to be carefully investigated for possible medical causes, medication side effects, drug interactions, use of activating recreational drugs, and/or withdrawal from opiates or sedative/hypnotics.

Mania

Mania in the setting of a history of recurrent depressive episodes is considered the defining feature of bipolar disorder and is referred to as primary (idiopathic) mania. Without this history or a strong family history of a mood disorder, a first episode of mania in the setting of HIV infection should be considered secondary (organic) mania as a result of the physiologic effects of HIV CNS infection, OIs, neoplasm, medications, or use of substances of abuse.[50] Current or previous treatment with Zidovudine (AZT), which penetrates the BBB, seems to be protective, while less penetrating medications (e.g., ddI and ddC) have not shown such benefit. A positive correlation exists between the manifestation of HIV-associated mania and the eventual development of HAD or MCMD, although mean survival is not adversely affected. HIV-associated structural brain lesions may not be more common in those patients who develop mania.[51]

Psychosis

A preexisting psychotic disorder may be a risk factor for HIV infection, and it is positively associated with psychosis in HIV-positive patients. The literature somewhat suggests that a history of substance abuse, depressive episode, or certain personality disorders may also correlate with the onset of psychotic symptoms in HIV-associated disease, and that antiretroviral therapy may be protective against the development of psychosis.[3,52,53] Secondary causes include more immediate psychoactive substance use, CNS HIV infection (usually a late stage manifestation) or OIs, neoplasms, nutritional deficits, metabolic derangements, or delirium.

Sleep

Sleep, like pain, is a subjective experience. Although HIV-infected patients may underestimate the amount of sleep they get, their experience is that they do not get enough, or good enough, sleep. Patients with HIV infection often report not feeling rested or refreshed after a night's sleep. They feel as though they have "been awake all night." In fact, sleep problems are prevalent (30% to 40%) in HIV infection for a variety of reasons[54,55] and may be related to the stage of HIV disease, persistent pain, other medical conditions (e.g., sleep apnea, congestive heart failure, paroxysmal nocturnal dyspnea, gastroesophageal reflux, polyuria, or delirium), or movement disorders associated with sleep (e.g., restless leg syndrome [RLS] or periodic limb movement disorder [PLMD]).

Medications such as antivirals, interferon, psychostimulants, antidepressants, and bronchodilators and substances such as alcohol, caffeine, nicotine, cannabis, and opiates may interfere with restorative sleep. Psychiatric disorders such as depression, anxiety, adjustment disorders, acute stress, and coping with life events can also disrupt normal sleep. In addition, disordered sleep hygiene may lead to sleep/wake cycle reversal.

Few things in life seem better when one is sleep-deprived. Insufficient or inefficient sleep negatively affects energy, mood, memory, cognition and cognitive speed, work performance and quality, enjoyment, and safety. Insomnia and fatigue also appear to be associated with increased morbidity and disability. One fourth of patients will try OTC sleep aids (e.g., Benadryl, valerian root, or melatonin), 27% will use alcohol, and less than 15% will take prescribed sedative-hypnotics.[56]

Substance Use

Although injection drug use is the second most common HIV infection risk factor,[57] other modes of drug use and alcohol abuse also increase the risk of infection through unsafe sexual practices, drug-induced hypersexuality, disinhibition, impulsiveness, altered cognition, impaired judgment, or prostitution to obtain drugs or money for drugs.[10] In the substance-abusing population, HIV infection is associated with youth, homelessness, being from an ethnic minority, and having a history of sexual victimization. Prior psychiatric illness is also common, with bipolar disorder, major depression, schizophrenia, and schizoaffective disorder being the most prevalent Axis I disorders. Antisocial and borderline personality disorders are the most common Axis II disorders.[58] Injection drug users tend to be diagnosed at a more advanced stage of their disease and may have a more rapid downhill course; they are also seen as a bridge of infection through heterosexual and maternal-child transmission. Continued drug use may speed the patient's decline in several ways: suppressed immune function, increased risk for infections (e.g., STDs, hepatitis C, pneumonia, abscesses, endocarditis, and tuberculosis [TB]), drug interactions with antiretroviral agents, poor ability to adhere to complicated medical regimens, and chaotic lifestyles that make scheduled medical follow-up difficult.[59] This population has a high tolerance to medications and possibly a low tolerance to pain, discomfort, or inconvenience. It is also a population at risk for impaired cognitive function from neurotoxic substances, poor nutrition, metabolic encephalopathies, ischemia, stroke, seizures, and head trauma.

Pain

The evaluation of pain and its adequate treatment and management are essential in the care of patients with HIV infection or AIDS. Pain is a frequent reason for psychiatric consultation and, rather than death, is often what patients fear most.[60] Pain control is one of the cornerstones in the care of patients with end-stage AIDS. Pain syndromes (including neuropathy, myopathies, and headache) are frequent among patients with HIV infection. The psychiatrist may need to intervene when hospital staff who care for a patient with a history of substance disorder fail to distinguish between the management of the patient's addiction and the adequate treatment of pain or fail to provide adequate pain relief to patients from a racial or ethnic minority.[61]

Peripheral neuropathy, the most common pain syndrome in patients with HIV-associated disease, affects up to 35% of patients with AIDS.[62,63] Most commonly the neuropathy presents as a distal, symmetric polyneuropathy that can be caused by HIV infection or by a nucleoside antiretroviral agent, such as zidovudine, didanosine, zalcitabine, and d4T; ddI can cause an irreversible, neuropathy more often than the other agents. The diagnosis is confirmed on the basis of the neurologic examination and laboratory tests, including an electromyelogram and nerve conduction studies. Although the cause of the neuropathy may be unclear in patients with advanced HIV disease, the treatment is nonspecific except for the alteration of the antiretroviral regimen for a secondary neuropathy.

Approach to Psychiatric Care

Prevention

Psychiatrists care for an at-risk population.[64] The first step in prevention is the assessment of the patient for risk factors and behaviors. Knowledge about HIV transmission is essential, but not sufficient. Patients must be able to perceive themselves as "at risk" for counseling to be effective.[65] Prevention models with individuals and groups of chronically mentally ill and substance-abusing patients exist. The program must be specific to the population being addressed, and counselors of similar cultural background to the patient population have proven most effective. Programs geared toward the injection drug use community have enlisted community members as prevention leaders.

Collaboration

Although a number of demonstration projects have shown the efficacy of wrap-around services for HIV-infected patients,[66,67] it is the exception rather than the rule to have medical, mental health, and addiction services, including methadone maintenance, in one coordinated site. More commonly, these multiply-diagnosed individuals on complicated treatment regimens have multiple providers at diverse sites of care, a situation that may parallel the chaos in the rest of their lives. In the absence of single-site treatment, intensive care management can keep all treaters informed, provide outreach to improve attendance at appointments, assist with concrete services (e.g., housing, transportation, and child care), and help devise and implement an individualized medication adherence plan. The consultation psychiatrist has a unique opportunity to facilitate communication and to coordinate care among members of the patient's care team.

Adherence

Adherence is the cornerstone of successful therapy for HIV infection. Missed doses lead to treatment resistance, sometimes to whole classes of medication. This, in turn, is correlated with increased morbidity and mortality. Active substance abuse, homelessness, a lack of social supports, domestic violence, personality disorders, and psychiatric illness, especially major depression,[68,69] are associated with poor adherence.[70] They are not, however, absolute contraindications to nor justifications for exclusion from antiretroviral therapy. The initiation of HAART may be postponed for several months, however, while instituting active addictions and/or psychiatric treatment, along with concurrent medication readiness and adherence education.[71] The patient hospitalized with HIV

infection is a captive audience for the initiation or reinforcement of this preparation for HAART.[41]

Effective adherence programs are tailored to the patient in terms of language, education, culture, lifestyle, and personality. Individualized adherence programs capitalize on or enhance the patient's social supports (e.g., family, friends, and groups), cognitive abilities, and personality style. They require accessibility, flexibility, and positively framed incentives (i.e., rewards, not punishments).[41,72] Adherence is further promoted when the patient understands the importance of taking every dose, believes that missed doses lead to resistance, knows and recognizes each specific medication, and is informed of possible side effects. Simplifying the regimen (e.g., reducing the number of doses and food restrictions) and minimizing the pill burden helps fit the regimen into the patient's lifestyle. Clearly written instructions are helpful, if the patient is literate. Tying pill-taking to daily routines, along with pillboxes, alarms, pagers, directly observed therapy, or other reminder systems, may also increase adherence. Patients who are comfortable taking medications in front of other people also have an easier time incorporating HAART into their lives.[72] Adherence to scheduled medical appointments is associated with optimal viral suppression and may warrant appropriate outreach efforts.[73]

Adherence is not static; it needs to be inquired about, and promoted by, each provider at every visit. Pill fatigue, complacency, transient or prolonged relapse of substance abuse or depression, onset of morphologic or metabolic side effects, onset or exacerbation of other medical conditions, hospitalization, or psychosocial stressors (e.g., financial, housing, insurance and changes, family or relationship issues, and travel) may interrupt or decrease the patient's previous level of adherence.

Treatment

Nonpharmacologic Treatments

Case Management

Case management is often necessary to help with basic needs such as food, shelter, transportation, child care, medical coverage, and other entitlements, which may be of need in this population and are powerful barriers to adequate treatment.

Groups

Groups of various types, often provided in the community or by AIDS activist organizations, offer a supportive, social network and positive affiliations for members of an often disenfranchised and stigmatized population. Self-help, 12-step, and peer counseling are examples of such community-based programs. Therapy groups and other more formalized groups may focus on aspects of living with HIV infection (e.g., disclosure, adherence, and parenting), participant characteristics (e.g., women, particular ethnic minorities, gay men, and substance abusers), or mission (e.g., risk reduction or prevention).[10]

Individual Psychotherapy

Individual psychotherapy may help patients cope with HIV infection or AIDS-related issues and distress, such as coping strategies, problem solving, disclosure of HIV status, discrimination, relationships, sexuality, and bereavement. For patients diagnosed more than a decade ago, issues of facing a foreshortened life span may be replaced by issues of living with a chronic illness.[74] There may be themes of remorse and longing for missed opportunities referent to this erroneous life view. The focus and goals of therapy may be specific to the stage of HIV-associated disease; late in the course of AIDS, therapy may focus on end-of-life issues such as concerns about ongoing childcare and guardianship, coping with loss, progressive disability, and unremitting pain.

For specific diagnoses, including depression or anxiety disorders, proven therapies such as interpersonal psychotherapy or cognitive-behavioral therapy (CBT), respectively, should also be effective in this population.[75–77] Self-hypnosis, guided imagery, meditation, muscle relaxation, yoga, aerobic exercise, or acupuncture may be therapeutic for selected patients.

Adherence to medications for HIV infection and psychotropic medications should be reinforced or explored. It should be stressed that the therapist is a member of the patient's treatment team, and appropriate releases should be obtained to allow all team members to communicate and to coordinate care. The therapist, for instance, may spend more time with the patient and be the first clinician to suspect cognitive dysfunction that requires medical workup and intervention.

Pharmacologic Treatment

Drug-Drug Interactions[78]

Patients with HIV infection or AIDS may be taking HIV-related medications, psychotropics, OTC and herbal preparations, and alcohol or drugs of abuse. Such drug combinations are prone to interactions (Table 37-6),[78] overlapping side effects, and toxicities. Drug side effects such as diarrhea (common to many antiretroviral agents) may decrease the absorption of other drugs. One drug may inhibit or promote the enzymatic degradation of another drug and cause toxicity or a subtherapeutic level, respectively. Some drugs may also switch from being potentiators to inhibitors or vice versa. A drug may induce or inhibit its own metabolism over time. Certain drugs may displace other drugs from plasma protein-binding sites, effectively increasing the concentration of the displaced drug. Potential drug interactions do not necessarily preclude the concomitant use of such medications but require a careful risk/benefit assessment, possible dose adjustment, periodic drug level monitoring, and monitoring for or treatment of side effects. Some general principles and frequently updated resources (Table 37-7) can aid in the safe psychopharmacologic treatment of these patients.

Effects on the cytochrome P 450 enzyme system in the liver account for many of the drug-drug interactions (Table 37-8).[79] Of the five or six P 450 isoenzymes involved in the metabolism of psychotropics and antiretrovirals (1A2, 2C9, 2C10, 2C19, 2D6, and 3A4), 3A4 and 2D6 account for the majority of the metabolism of psychiatric medications. Substances metabolized by a given isoenzyme are referred to as substrates of that enzyme. Allelic differences cause 10% of whites and 1% of Asians to slowly metabolize 2D6 substrates,[80] while 20% of African-Americans and Asians and 5% of whites slowly metabolize 2C19 substrates.[81,82] A drug may be a substrate for more than one enzyme or metabolic pathway. Substances that induce the production of certain

Table 37-6. Drug-Drug Interactions: HIV-Related and Psychotropic Medications Interactions Between HIV-Related Medications and Psychotropic Medications: Indications and Contraindications

Medication	Contraindicated	Use With Caution	Possible Dose Adjustment
Amprenavir	Alprazolam, diazepam, midazolam, triazolam, and zolpidem	Fluoxetine and fluvoxamine may increase Pl concentration and toxicity. Carbamazepine, phenobarbital, phenytoin, primidone, and St. John's wort reduce the level of Pl, and concurrent use should be avoided. Avoid pimozide if possible.	Carbamazepine, phenobarbital, and phenytoin levels rise; monitor levels and adjust as needed.
Clarithromycin	None identified	St. John's wort may decrease the level of clarithromycin.	Carbamazepine level rises; monitor level and adjust as needed. Initial dose of benzodiazepines (e.g., alprazolam or midazolam) should be reduced because clarithromycin may increase their levels.
Delavirdine	Alprazolam, midazolam, and triazolam	Fluoxetine, fluvoxamine, and nefazodone may increase NNRTI levels and increase toxicity. Carbamazepine, phenobarbital, phenytoin, and St. John's wort can lower delavirdine levels; avoid concurrent use, if possible. Avoid pimozide, if possible.	Carbamazepine levels may rise: monitor and adjust as needed.
Didanosine (ddl)	None identified	Gabapentin levels decreased by antacid: ddl should be given 2 hours before or after.	Methadone decreases ddl; consider an increased dose.
Fluconazole	None identified	None identified	Carbamazepine and phenytoin levels rise: monitor level and decrease dose as needed. Due to CNS effects, may need to decrease the dose of benzodiazepines(e.g., alprazolam, and triazolam), methadone, or zolpidem. Levels of amitriptyline and nortriptyline may rise; monitor and adjust as needed.
Indinavir	Diazepam, midazolam, St. John's wort, triazolam, and zolpidem	Fluoxetine, fluvoxamine, and nefazodone increase toxicity. Carbamazepine, phenobarbital, phenytoin, and primidone reduce indinavir levels. Avoid pimozide, if possible.	Carbamazepine level rises; monitor and lower dose as needed.
Ketoconazole	Alprazolam, clonazepam, diazepam, midazolam, and triazolam	None identified	Carbamazepine and ethosuximide levels rise; monitor toxicity and lower dose, if necessary.
Lopinavir/Ritonavir*	Alprazolam, bupropion, clorazepate, clozapine, diazepam, estazolam, flurazepam, midazolam, pimozide, St. John's	Fluoxetine, fluvoxamine, and Pl levels may increase. Mexiletine levels rise and may cause greater cardiac/neurologic toxicity: use with caution. Phenobarbital and	Desipramine levels may rise significantly: consider using a 50% lower dose. Meperidine and methadone levels decrease; may need increased doses.

Continued

Table 37-6. Drug-Drug Interactions: HIV-Related and Psychotropic Medications Interactions Between HIV-Related Medications and Psychotropic Medications: Indications and Contraindications — *Cont'd*

Medication	Contraindicated	Use With Caution	Possible Dose Adjustment
	wort, triazolam, and zolpidem	primidone levels may rise and Pl levels fall; avoid concurrent use, if possible.	Carbamazepine, clonazepam, nefazodone, and sertraline: initial dose should be reduced 70%. Trazodone levels may increase: start low. Phenothiazines, SSRIs, and TCAs should have initial doses reduced by 50% and be monitored closely for toxicity. Valproic acid and phenytoin doses may need to be higher. Ethosuximide level rises; may need to lower the dose.
Nelfinavir	Diazepam, midazolam, St. John's wort, triazolam, and zolpidem	Fluoxetine and fluvoxamine may increase Pl levels. Carbamazepine, phenobarbital, phenytoin, and primidone may decrease Pl; avoid concurrent use, if possible. Avoid pimozide, if possible.	None identified
Nevirapine	St. John's wort	Fluoxetine and fluvoxamine may increase NNRTI levels.	Methadone levels lowered; may need a higher dose. Carbamazepine level rises. Pl levels may drop; avoid concurrent use, if possible.
Pyrimethamine	Lorazepam increases risk of hepatic toxicity (monitor LFTs).	None identified	None identified
Rifabutin and rifampin	None identified	None identified	Methadone levels decrease, and higher doses may be needed. Carbamazepine, phenytoin, and valproic acid levels may decrease: may need to increase dose based upon levels.
Ritonavir*	Alprazolam, bupropion, clorazepate, clozapine, diazepam, estazolam, flurazepam, midazolam, pimozide, St. John's wort, triazolam, and zolpidem	Fluoxetine, fluvoxamine, and Pl levels may increase. Mexiletine levels rise and may cause greater cardiac/neurologic toxicity: use with caution. Phenobarbital and primidone levels may rise and Pl level fall; avoid concurrent use if possible.	Desipramine levels may rise significantly: consider lowering dose by 50%. Meperidine and methadone levels decrease: may need to increase the dose. Carbamazepine, clonazepam, nefazodone, and sertraline: initial dose should be reduced by 70%. Trazodone levels may increase: start low. Phenothiazines, SSRIs and the initial dose of TCAs should be reduced by 50% and be monitored closely for toxicity. Valproic acid and phenytoin doses may need to be higher. Ethosuximide levels rise: may need to lower the dose.
Saquinavir	Diazepam, midazolam, St. John's wort, triazolam, and zolpidem	Fluoxetine and fluvoxamine may increase Pl levels and toxicity. Phenobarbital and primidone	Carbamazepine levels rise (may need to lower the dose as needed) and Pl fall when co-administered.

Continued

Table 37-6. Drug-Drug Interactions: HIV-Related and Psychotropic Medications Interactions Between HIV-Related Medications and Psychotropic Medications: Indications and Contraindications — *Cont'd*

Medication	Contraindicated	Use With Caution	Possible Dose Adjustment
		can lower Pl: avoid pimozide, if possible.	
Stavudine	None identified	None identified	None identified
Zalcitabine (ddC)	None identified	Disulfiram and phenytoin may increase the risk for peripheral neuropathy.	None identified
Zidovudine	None identified	Methadone and valproic acid increase zidovudine levels: monitor for toxicity.	None identified

*Dose of ritonavir is lower than when used as a single Pl, and the drug-drug impact of ritonavir may be less significant. However, as pharmacologic data are limited, at this time the same cautions and contraindications as with full-dose ritonavir are repeated. From 1) APA Neuropsychiatric Curriculum, *HIV-related neuropsychiatric complications and treatments,* 2002. 2) Klein R. Struble K. *The protease inhibitors: backgrounder,* Food and Drug Administration, September 1996. 3)Preston SL, Stein DS: Drug Interactions and adverse drug reactions with protease inhibitors, *Primary Psychiatry* 64–69, 1997. 4) *Physicians' desk reference,* Oradell, NJ, 1997, Medical Economics Company Inc.

Table 37-7. HIV/AIDS Resources on the Internet Recommended by American Psychiatric Association Office of HIV Psychiatry (May 2002)

AIDS Clinical Trials Information Service (ACTIS)
www.actis.org
Provides quick and easy access to information on federally and privately funded clinical trials for adults and children.

American Psychiatric Association AIDS Resource Center
www.psych.prg/aids
Includes a searchable database of mental health resources, policy statements, training, and education information.

Bastyr University AIDS Research Center
www.bastyr.edu/research/buarc
Provides PWA resources links; general research links; and reports on patterns of use of alternative medicine, evaluation of naturopathic therapies, and consultation to the medical and research community.

Center for AIDS Prevention Studies (CAPS)
www.caps.ucsf.edu
This site links to prevention fact sheets, which are one-page, science-based summaries of what works in prevention programs, and list research projects taking place at CAPS.

HIV/AIDS Treatment Information Service
www.hivatis.org
This web site allows you to view and download HIV treatment guidelines, general HIV treatment information, and more.

Printable HIV/AIDS Glossary of Terms
HIV Insight/Medical
hivinsite.ucsf.edu/medical
Includes full text of *The AIDS Knowledge Base*, listing of clinical trials, science and treatment of HIV-related infections and malignancies, drug database, treatment guidelines, conference updates, medication programs, journals, and fact sheets.

Indiana University Department of Medicine
http://medicine.iupui.edu/flockhart
Cytochrome P450 Drug Interaction Table.

John Hopkins AIDS Service
www.hopkins-aids.edu
Prepared by faculty from The John Hopkins University Division of Infectious Disease. Site features clinical news, conference calendar, prevention and treatment information, case studies, expert questions and answers, and a full-text version of the reference book, *Medical Management of HIV Disease.*

Continued

Table 37-7. HIV/AIDS Resources on the Internet Recommended by American Psychiatric Association Office of HIV Psychiatry (May 2002) — *Cont'd*

Journal of the American Medical Association HIV/AIDS Information Center

www.ama-assn.org/aids

Organized into sections containing news, literature reports, treatment, prevention, education and policy information areas. The literature section offers a list of abstracts of recently published articles on HIV/AIDS.

Medscape HIV/AIDS

Hiv.medscape.com/Home/Topics/AIDS/AIDs.html

News, treatment updates, clinical management, practice guidelines, conference summaries, library, links, and online CME.

National Institute of Allergy and Infections Disease (NIAID)

www.niaid.nih.gov

Program announcements, news, and links to a searchable database of federally funded biomedical research projects and the National Neuro AIDS Tissue Consortium—established to standardize protocols to obtain CNS tissues from HIV-infected individuals.

New Mexico AID Infonet

www.aidsinfonet.org

This excellent site provides regularly updated information for patients, clients, consumers, including easy-to-read FACT SHEETS in English and Spanish on "conventional" and "complementary" HIV treatment that can be downloaded and printed for distribution. This site provides an extensive listing of categorized web sites in all major professional and non-professional fields and interests. Very highly recommended.

Toronto General Hospital University Health Network

www.tthhivclinic.com

Provides medication fact sheets and drug interaction tables.

Patient Information

The Body

www.thebody.com

Critical Path AIDS Project

www.critpath.org

Gay Men's Health Crisis

www.gmhc.org

National Association of People with AIDS

www.napwa.org

Project Inform

www.projinf.org

San Francisco AIDS Foundation

www.sfaf.org

New Mexico AIDS Infonet

See above

Other Useful Sites

Aegis

www.aegis.com

American Red Cross

www.redcross.org/hss/HIV/AIDS

International Association of Physicians in AIDS Care

www.iapac.org

Knowledge Exchange Network

www.mentalhealth.org/cmhs/HIVAIDS/index.htm

National Minority AIDS Council

www.nmac.org

UNAIDS

www.unaids.org/index

Table 37-8. Important Substrates, Inhibitors, and Inducers of Cytochrome P450 Isoenzymes* CYP

Isoform	Substrates		Inhibitors	Inducers
1A2	Caffeine	Imipramine	Fluvoxamine (+++)	*Ritonavir**
	Clomipramine	Methadone		
	Clozapine	Mirtazapine		
	Fluvoxamine	Zolpidem		
2C9			*Ritonavir** (++)	
	Fluoxetine		Fluoxetine (+)	Phenobarbital
			Paroxetine (+)	Rifampin
2D6				
	*Ritonavir**	Ecstasy	*Ritonavir** (++)	
	*Nelfinavir**	Olanzapine	*Indinavir** (+)	
	*Indinavir**	Paroxetine	Cocaine (+++)	
	Amphetamines	Perphenazine	Fluoxetine (+++)	
	Clozapine	Risperidone	Methadone	
	Codeine	Sertindole	Paroxetine (+++)	
	Fluvoxamine	TCAs	Perphenazine	
	Mirtazapine	Thioridazine	Sertindole	
	Venlafaxine		Sertraline (++)	
			Venlafaxine (+)	
3A family				
	*Amprenavir**	Clomipramine	*Amprenavir**	*Efavirenz†*
	*Ritonavir**	Clonazepam	*Indinavir** (+++)	*Nevirapine†*
	*Nelfinavir**	Diazepam	*Nelfinavir** (++)	*Ritonavir**
	*Saquinavir**	Imipramine	*Ritonavir** (+++)	Barbiturates
	*Indinavir**	Midazolam	*Saquinavir** (+)	Carbamazepine
	Nevirapine†	Nefazodone	*Efavirenz†*	Dexamethasone
	Alprazolam	Pimozide	Fluvoxamine (+)	Rifabutin
	Buspirone	Sildenafil	Nefazodone (+++)	Rifampin
	Carbamazepine	Trazodone	Sertindole	
	Citalopram	Triazolam	Thioridazine	

*Protease inhibitor.
†Non-nucleoside-analogue reverse transcriptase inhibitor.
Note: Antiretroviral drugs are in italics; +, ++, and +++ represent relative inhibitory potencies.
TCAs = tricyclic antidepressants.
From: Gillenwater DR, McDaniel JS: Rational Psychopharmacology for patients with HIV infection and AIDS, *Psychiatric Ann* 31:30; 2001.

P 450 isoenzymes, increase the metabolism (i.e., decrease the effective level) of metabolic substrates of that enzyme. Enzyme inhibitors cause an increase in the effective level of substrates. Inhibitors may cause direct inhibition of enzyme action, or may inhibit by means of substrate displacement from the enzyme. Substances may be weak, moderate, or strong inhibitors of one or more isoenzymes, and certain drugs may rely more or less on different metabolic pathways. In vitro studies of drug metabolism do not adequately portray the human experience that is complicated by individual genetic and nutritional differences and multidrug/substance regimens.[79,80] The protease inhibitors, followed by the nnRTIs, have the broadadest effects on the P 450

system. The PI ritonavir also induces glucuronyl transferase, a non–P 450, metabolic enzyme.[79]

Antidepressants. Antidepressants are largely metabolized, though not exclusively, by 2D6. Citalopram and nefazodone, for instance, are primarily metabolized by 3A4. The selective serotonin-reuptake inhibitors (SSRIs) (paroxetine, fluoxetine, sertraline, citalopram [minimal], but not fluvoxamine) also are inhibitors of 2D6 isoenzymes. Ritonavir, and to a lesser extent indinavir, inhibit metabolism of 2D6 substrates; all of the PIs inhibit 3A4 metabolism to varying degrees.[83] Inhibition of the metabolism of the SSRIs, venlafaxine, and mirtazapine by ritonavir and indinavir increases the levels of the antidepressants, which may allow for a therapeutic response at a low or moderate dose. Although high doses of the antidepressants could lead to serotonin syndrome (SS)[84] or other toxicities, a wide range of concentrations are generally well tolerated. TCAs, however, have a narrower therapeutic window; metabolic inhibition at 2D6, from PIs or SSRIs, can lead to serious toxicity. Concurrent use of these medicines requires low doses of TCAs and close monitoring of levels, electrocardiograms (ECGs), and side effects.[79]

Bupropion continues to be in a class by itself. Initially thought to be a substrate of 2D6, bupropion was considered to be contraindicated in patients taking PIs because of the potential for seizures. It turns out, however, that a little studied isoenzyme, 2B6, is responsible for bupropion metabolism. Low doses and conservative titration are still recommended, but the actual risk seems much less than previously thought.[10,79] There has been one report of in vitro 2B6 inhibition by ritonavir, nelfinavir (PIs), and efavirenz (nnRTI) causing significant interference with bupropion metabolism.[85] Whether this interference is significant in vivo is unclear. A recent prospective study that included the administration of bupropion to patients on PIs reported no serious adverse events, and, specifically, no seizures.[86]

Nefazodone is a 3A4 substrate and inhibitor. When teamed with the PIs, a potentially dangerous synergistic inhibition diminishes the metabolism of other 3A4 substrates.[81,87] Use of this combination with astemizole, cisapride, or pimozide can cause cardiac arrhythmias, with benzodiazepines respiratory depression, with clozapine seizures, with ergot alkaloids systemic vasoconstriction, and with sildenafil, priapism.[79]

Mirtazapine and venlafaxine may prove to have the least clinically significant drug interactions.[82]

Psychostimulants, such as methylphenidate[88] and dextroamphetamine,[89] may be used to treat depression, to augment antidepressant therapy, or to treat the symptoms of fatigue and cognitive decline associated with HIV infection.[90] Methylphenidate may inhibit 2C9 and 2C19 metabolism, leading to increased levels of certain TCAs (i.e., desipramine, clomipramine, and imipramine), barbiturates, and warfarin. Dextroamphetamine, however, is a 2D6 substrate that neither inhibits nor induces the P 450 isoenzymes, but may compete at active sites.[10,79] Modafinil is a new psychostimulant that appears to inhibit 2D6 metabolism.

Benzodiazepines. Benzodiazepines are primarily 3A4 substrates, with the exception of lorazepam, oxazepam, and temazepam, which are metabolized by glucuronyl transferase. For this reason, these three exceptions are the drugs of choice when patients on (3A4 inhibiting) PIs require treatment with a benzodiazepine. Other benzodiazepines would be expected to have increased levels when co-administered with PIs, leading to possibly dangerous sedation or respiratory depression. However, use of these glucuronyl transferase substrates (e.g., lorazepam, oxazepam, and temazepam) with that enzyme's inducer, ritonavir, may require higher doses of benzodiazepines.[10,79] The nnRTIs efavirenz and nevirapine, along with the PI ritonavir, also induce the 3A isoenzymes. This 3A induction may be delayed and cause a drop in previously elevated benzodiazepine levels, resulting in decreased efficacy or withdrawal. This unpredictability precludes the regular use of such short-acting agents (e.g., alprazolam) because of the risk of withdrawal precipitating seizures.[91]

Mood Stabilizers. Mood stabilizers include the anticonvulsants carbamazepine, valproic acid, and others, as well as lithium carbonate. Although lithium does not interface with the P 450 system, it should be avoided in HIV-positive patients because of its potential for toxicity with fluid and electrolyte shifts. Carbamazepine induces 3A4, lowering levels of the PIs and other antiretrovirals, a situation that could foster resistance, possibly to a whole class of medications.[79] It might be possible in certain instances to avert this resistance by using higher doses of the antiretroviral. However, carbamazepine is also relatively contraindicated in immune-suppressed patients because of its potential to cause leukopenia.[10] Valproic acid inhibits glucuronyl transferase, the major metabolic pathway of zidovudine.[92] Gabapjentin, useful for mood stabilization as well as chronic pain and possibly anxiety, does not interact with the P 450 system. Lamotrigine also bypasses the P 450 system, but is a glucuronyl transferase substrate.[79]

Neuroleptics. Levels of clozapine, a 2D6 substrate, may increase with concomitant use of the PIs, ritonavir, and indinavir. Because of the risk of seizures and hypotension, co-administration of ritonavir and clozapine is contraindicated.[93] (The non–dose-dependent clozapine-induced agranulocytosis would also seem an unacceptable risk in this population). Pimozide, a 3A4 substrate, can cause fatal arrhythmias at high levels; therefore, it is contraindicated with the use of any 3A4 inhibitor and thus all PIs.[94]

Substance-Drug Interactions

Opiates also interface with hepatic metabolism, affecting and being affected by interactions with antiretroviral medications. Meperidine may be cleared more quickly, leaving a higher concentration of its neurotoxic metabolite that causes delirium and possibly seizures. Clearance of fentanyl, a 3A4 substrate, is decreased by ritonavir, which can cause nausea, dizziness, and possibly respiratory depression. Codeine and its derivatives are prodrugs that need conversion to analgesic agents. PIs can block this conversion and make pain control more difficult. PIs may also induce withdrawal in heroin-addicted individuals or patients on methadone maintenance. Conversely, ritonavir inhibits metabolism of ecstasy, ketamine, cocaine and other stimulants, and gamma-hydroxybutyrate (GHB). Fatal interactions between ecstasy and ritonavir have been reported.[79,95]

Pharmacologic Treatment Considerations

Depression

For a variety of reasons, patients with HIV infection are very sensitive to small doses of medications, similar to what is seen in geriatric patients. Helping the patient tolerate medications is ultimately more important than raising the dose quickly. So, the general principle is "start low and go slow." Because of the pill burden and complicated schedules patients with HIV infection must often endure, once-a-day antidepressant therapy is generally preferable. Anticholinergic medications should be avoided or minimized because of their deleterious effects on cognition, the possibility of delirium, or even seizures. Decreased saliva can also predispose to the development of thrush.[27]

SSRIs. The SSRIs remain the drugs of choice for depressive disorders because they offer once-a-day dosing and tolerable side effects that may dissipate over time. Fluoxetine, with the longest half-life ($t_{1/2}$), is a good option for patients who have tumultuous lives and who may miss doses. Use of fluoxetine weekly is also an option. On the other hand, if there is a side effect or an unpleasant interaction, it will take 2 weeks or more for it to clear. Citalopram and its L-enantiomer escitalopram are the SSRIs that may have the fewest interactions and possibly side effects. All SSRIs are associated with sexual side effects, SS when toxic levels are present, as well as GI symptoms, akathisia, and apathy.

TCAs. The TCAs are often used in small doses for neuropathic pain, insomnia, or headaches. The side effect of constipation may be helpful in some HIV-infected patients with diarrhea. They can be lethal with ingestion of a 2-week supply. The least anticholinergic ones, nortriptyline and desipramine, should be used with an awareness that anticholinergia may worsen cognition.

Venlafaxine. The extended release form of venlafaxine is a reasonable first-line medication because of its once-a-day dosing. Initially stimulating, some patients will have difficulty tolerating it. It may raise blood pressure unacceptably in hypertensive patients. It also has GI side effects.

Bupropion. The antidepressant least likely to have sexual side effects, bupropion, does not treat anxiety. Bupropion's continued stimulant effect, if tolerable, may benefit patients with fatigue or apathy, although, unlike psychostimulants, bupropion tends not to improve HIV-related cognitive slowing.[27] Even the slow-release form is not considered a once-a-day medication. There may be GI side effects. Bupropion lowers the seizure threshold, which is a concern in patients who have a history of seizures, poorly controlled seizure disorders, head trauma, or other threshold-lowering pathology (e.g., space-occupying lesions, infections, or alcohol or psychoactive substance abuse). Patients with eating disorders or metabolic derangements from drug side effects such as vomiting or diarrhea may be at increased risk of seizures. The slow-release form may have less of an effect on the seizure threshold.

Trazodone. Primarily used for its major side effect, trazodone makes people very sleepy within 20 to 30 minutes of ingestion. In low doses, it is minimally anticholinergic. Men of all ages must always be informed of its rare but serious side effect, priapism (prevalence ~1/7000).

Mirtazapine. At low doses, mirtazapine is useful for patients who have difficulty eating and sleeping, even in the absence of clear depression. At higher doses, it is also an effective antidepressant with the advantage of minimal metabolic interaction with antiretrovirals. However, it is fairly anticholinergic.

Monoamine Oxidase Inhibitors (MAOIs). Because of the myriad drugs patients with HIV infection may need over time, MAOIs are relatively contraindicated in these patients. They should specifically not be co-administered with zidovudine.

Psychostimulants. In low doses, psychostimulants may improve appetite, energy, and mood. They work quickly, often within hours, and have few side effects or interactions. Especially useful in patients who are unresponsive to or intolerant of other antidepressants, stimulants also effectively improve the early symptoms of cognitive decline; they help patients attend and stay more focused and organized. In late HAD, however, they can become toxic. Stimulants should also be avoided in the presence of psychotic symptoms or in those with a history of seizures. Abuse is rare in patients who have no history of a substance disorder. A history of a substance disorder is not a contraindication to the use of stimulants but it does require that the prescriber be more cautious.

Anxiety

Anxiolytic Antidepressants. For prolonged use in anxiety disorders, the SSRIs are beneficial, and will decrease the effective dose of benzodiazepines, when these medications are co-administered. TCAs and venlafaxine also have anti anxiety effects.

Benzodiazepines. For more time-limited episodes of intolerable anxiety, short- to medium-acting benzodiazepines without active metabolites and the least drug-drug interactions such as lorazepam or oxazepam should be used. Alprazolam may be helpful for procedures in which a very quick onset and short duration are required. For more continuous use, however, the rapid offset of alprazolam predisposes to mild withdrawal or rebound anxiety. This rapid offset leads to extreme discomfort several times a day or to a gradually increased frequency of dosing. Lorazepam, oxazepam, or temazepam are the preferred choices if the patient is taking a PI. However, if co-administered with ritonavir, higher doses of these benzodiazepines may be required to maintain their therapeutic effects (and avoid withdrawal in benzodiazepine—dependent patients).[79]

Buspirone. An option for patients on PIs, buspirone unfortunately takes several weeks to become effective. Concomitant use of benzodiazepines may be necessary to help the patient through this initiation/titration period. In advanced systemic illness, but not less symptomatic disease, buspirone has worsened cognition and triggered mania.[27]

Gabapentin. An antiseizure medication that seems to have antianxiety properties, gabapentin has the added benefit of minimal drug-drug interactions. Unlike older medications in this class, it requires no serum levels or blood monitoring. A wide dose range is tolerable, but it generally requires dosing 3 times daily.

Neuroleptics. Although generally not recommended for anxiety, low doses of atypical neuroleptics may be effective if fear or pain is a major precipitant.

Mania

Although lithium bypasses hepatic metabolism, it carries the risk of serious neurotoxicity and nephrotoxicity in patients prone to fluid loss from diarrhea, vomiting, inadequate intake, or HIV nephropathy. Valproic acid may be more effective for patients with secondary mania and brain abnormalities on MRI.[96] Carbamazepine is less useful because of its potent induction of the 3A4 isoenzyme (increased clearance of PIs) and possible blood dyscrasia. Gabapentin has been used successfully and is a safe alternative. Clonazepam also has antimanic properties, but it carries a risk of disinhibition, anterograde amnesia, and confusion.

Psychosis

Neuroleptics are the treatment of choice for psychotic symptoms of any cause. Patients with HIV infection, however, are extremely sensitive to side effects of neuroleptics and are at risk for extrapyramidal symptoms and neuroleptic malignant syndrome with high-potency agents and confusion or seizures with low-potency agents.[10,53,97] The newer, atypical antipsychotics appear to be effective and better tolerated, though little is known about their interactions with antiretroviral medications. Very low starting doses and cautious titration are recommended. Risperidone and olanzapine have each been used effectively for HIV-related psychosis without causing undue sedation or cognitive impairment.[10,98] The deleterious effect of olanzapine on glucose metabolism, however, may limit its usefulness, especially in patients already at risk for diabetes, such as those taking PIs. Quetiapine is the least apt to induce parkinsonian symptoms of these newer agents, making it a reasonable first-line medication for advanced neuropsychiatric disease. Clozapine and pimozide are contraindicated with the PI ritonavir. (As mentioned previously, clozapine is generally contraindicated in patients with HIV infection or AIDS).

Substance Abuse

The treatment and management of hospitalized patients with HIV infection and substance abuse disorders has five main features, depending on the patient's level of addiction or recovery: (1) prophylaxis against or treatment of withdrawal, (2) encouragement to enter a recovery program, including referral to a comprehensive addictions program, (3) maintenance of recovery during the stress of hospitalization, (4) adequate pain control, including the use of narcotic medications, if appropriate, and (5) careful monitoring for drug-drug interactions, especially for patients on methadone maintenance.

If the patient is on methadone maintenance and opiate analgesia is required, an agent other than methadone should be used to maintain clear boundaries for the patient and the methadone maintenance program. For patients with active addictions problems, HIV infection and AIDS community-based organizations may have addictions outreach programs that send a worker to the patient's bedside. Prescribed medications that are being abused may need to be discontinued, an intervention that does not appear to precipitate dropping out of HIV-associated medical care.[99] There are limitations to the model of "harm reduction" used in many addiction treatment programs, and the psychiatrist should know that prescribing oral forms of abused injection drugs does not promote recovery from substance disorder. This practice may only introduce the problems of dependence on high doses of oral substances.[100] For patients on methadone maintenance with symptomatic HIV infection or with CD4 lymphocyte counts below $500/\mu L$, the initiation of some antimicrobial agents can have pharmacologic consequences.[101] For example, methadone increases zidovudine serum levels, which can lead to increased toxicity. Treatment with rifampin can increase methadone metabolism and potentially precipitate acute opiate withdrawal. In this instance, the daily methadone dose needs to be increased. The discharge plan would need to include notification of the patient's methadone clinic of this dose change.

Pain

The treatment of HIV-related neuropathy is similar to the approach used with a chronic pain syndrome. Low doses of TCAs can be effective, either alone or in combination with other analgesic therapies. No systematic studies have been conducted to compare the effectiveness of different TCAs, and no evidence exists for the superiority of amitriptyline for HIV-related neuropathy. Desipramine and nortriptyline are better tolerated and appear to be as effective.

Anticonvulsants in low doses can be effective for neuropathic pain, either alone or in combination with other analgesic therapies. Both carbamazepine and valproic acid have been effective, but hematopoietic and hepatic side effects and drug interactions must be monitored. Gabapentin may be effective for neuropathic pain; its use avoids hematopoietic and hepatic side effects. Low-dose clonazepam can be particularly effective for hyperpathic pain.

Some antiarrhythmics also have local anesthetic properties and can be useful for some types of pain syndromes. Postherpetic neuralgia can be highly disabling in HIV-infected patients, particularly those who have had multidermatomal Herpes zoster. IV lidocaine can offer relief, often with once- or twice-weekly infusions, and a significant dose reduction in narcotic analgesics. The oral antiarrhythmic mexiletine may be neither effective nor well tolerated.[102]

Opiates are beneficial for short-term use or for periods of pain exacerbation, but they may induce tolerance and abuse or dependence. A history of a substance disorder does not preclude the use of opiates required for adequate analgesia, but it requires careful monitoring to prevent unauthorized dosage escalation. In discharge planning for patients with advanced HIV disease, the psychiatrist should remember that cognitive impairment can make compliance with as-needed dosing schedules difficult, and patients may accidentally overuse analgesics. The use of a pill alarm or box can help. If long-term therapy with opiates is needed, the psychiatrist should consider long-acting oral or transdermal formulations. The latter are particularly helpful in the care of terminally ill patients, many of whom have odynophagia or dysphagia.

Conclusion

Neuropsychiatric symptoms are part of the HIV infection and AIDS and have multiple etiologies. HIV CNS infection and primary psychiatric disorders should always be considered. CNS other infections or lesions, medications, drugs of abuse, drug-drug interactions, and metabolic derangements need to be explored. Whenever identified, underlying causes should be treated, but the psychiatric symptoms may require more immediate treatment. Nonpharmacologic treatments should be tried whenever feasible, but many patients will require medications, as well. For a number of reasons, patients with HIV infection are sensitive to small amounts of medication, and they should generally be given geriatric doses with careful monitoring and slow dosage titration. The PIs, and to a lesser extent the nnRTIs, are responsible for the majority of the drug-drug interactions with psychotropic medications. These interactions are largely because of interference with the hepatic P 450 enzyme system. Having access to frequently updated and reliable resources assists with the choice of safe pharmacologic alternatives in this population.

References

1. Cournos F, McKinnon K: HIV seroprevalence among people with severe mental illness in the United States: a critical review, *Clin Psychol Rev* 17:259–269, 1997.
2. Cournos F, McKinnon K, Rosner J: HIV among individuals with severe mental illness, *Psychiatr Ann* 31:50–56, 2001.
3. Susser E, Colson P, Jandorf L, et al: HIV infection among young adults with psychotic disorders, *Am J Psychiatry* 154:864–866, 1997.
4. Cohen MA, Hoffman RG, Cromwell C, et al: The prevalence of distress in persons with human immunodeficiency virus infection, *Psychosomatics* 43:10–15, 2002.
5. Lyketsos CG, Treisman GJ: Mood disorders in HIV infection, *Psychiatr Ann* 31:45–49, 2001.
6. Rabkin JG: Prevalence of psychiatric disorders in HIV illness, *Int Rev Psychiatry* 8:157–166, 1996.
7. Brooner RK, Greenfield L, Schmidt CW, Bigelow GE: Antisocial personality disorder and HIV infection among intravenous drug abusers, *Am J Psychiatry* 150:53–58, 1993.
8. Golding M, Perkins DO: Personality disorder in HIV infection, *Int Rev Psychiatry* 8:253, 1996.
9. Perkins DO, Davidson EJ, Leserman J, et al: Personality disorder in patients infected with HIV: a controlled study with implications for clinical care, *Am J Psychiatry* 150:309–315, 1993.
10. APA: Practice guideline for the treatment of patients with HIV/AIDS, *Am J Psychiatry* 157S:1–62, 2000.
11. Ho DD: Viral counts count in HIV infection, *Science* 272:1124–1125, 1996.
12. Palmer DL, Hjelle BL, Wiley CA, et al: HIV-1 infection despite immediate combination antiviral therapy after infusion of contaminated white cells, *Am J Med* 97:289–295, 1994.
13. Centers for Disease Control and Prevention: HIV/AIDS surveillance report, 1999. Cited in APA: Practice guideline for the treatment of patients with HIV/AIDS, *Am J Psychiatry* 157S:4, 2000.
14. De Cock KM, Janssen RS: An unequal epidemic in an unequal world, *JAMA* 288:236–238, 2002.
15. Satcher D: The global HIV/AIDS epidemic, *JAMA* 281:1479, 1999.
16. Centers for Disease Control and Prevention: HIV and AIDS—United States, 1981–2000, *JAMA* 285:3083–3084, 2001.

17. Centers for Disease Control and Prevention: The global HIV and AIDS epidemic, *JAMA* 285:3081–3083, 2001.
18. Katz MH, Schwarcz SK, Kellog TA, et al: Impact of highly active antiretroviral treatment on HIV seroincidence among men who have sex with men: San Francisco, *Am J Public Health* 92:388–394, 2002.
19. Goodkin K, Baldewicz TT, Wilkie FL, et al: HIV-1 Infection of the brain: a region-specific approach to its neuropathophysiology and therapeutic prospects, *Psychiatr Ann* 31:182–192, 2001.
20. Schrager LK, D'Souza MP: Cellular and anatomical reservoirs of HIV-1 in patients receiving potent antiretroviral combination therapy, *JAMA* 280:67–71, 1998.
21. Kumar M, Goodkin K, Kumar AM, et al: HIV-1 infection, neuroendocrine abnormalities, and clinical outcomes, *CNS Spectrums* 5:55–65, 2000.
22. Harrison MJG, Newman SP, Hall-Craggs MA, et al: Evidence of CNS impairment in HIV infection: clinical, neuropsychological, EEG, and MRI/MRS study, *J Neurol Neurosurg Psychiatry* 65:301–307, 1998.
23. Wilkie FL, Goodkin K, van Zuilen MH, et al: Cognitive effects of HIV-1 infection, *CNS Spectrums* 5:33–51, 2000.
24. Paul RH, Cohen RC, Stern RA: Neurocognitive manifestations of human immunodeficiency virus, *CNS Spectrums* 7:860–866, 2002.
25. Shapshak P, Fujimura R, Srivastava A, Goodkin K: Dementia and the neurovirulence of HIV-1, *CNS Spectrums* 5:31–42, 2000.
26. APA Commission on AIDS: Policy guideline on the recognition and management of HIV-related neuropsychiatric findings and associated impairments, *Am J Psychiatry* 155:1647, 1998.
27. Martin L, Tummala R, Fernandez F: Psychiatric management of HIV infection and AIDS, *Psychiatr Ann* 32:133–140, 2002.
28. Ferrando S: Substance abuse and HIV infection, *Psychiatr Ann* 31:57–62, 2001.
29. Baldewicz TT, Brouwers P, Goodkin K, et al: Nutritional contributions to the CNS pathophysiology of HIV-1 infection and implications for treatment, *CNS Spectrums* 5:61–72, 2000.
30. Stern Y, Marder K, Bell K, et al: Multidisciplinary assessment of homosexual men with and without immunodeficiency virus infection: III. Neurologic neuropsychological findings, *Arch Gen Psychiatry* 48:131–138, 1991.
31. Portegies P, Enting RH, de Gans J, et al: Presentation and course of AIDS dementia complex, *AIDS* 7:669–675, 1993.
32. Miller EN, Satz P, Visscher B: Computerized and conventional neuropsychological assessment of HIV-1 infected homosexual men, *Neurology* 41:1608–1616, 1991.
33. Worth JL, Savage C, Baer L, et al: Computer-based screening for AIDS dementia complex, *AIDS* 7:677–681, 1993.
34. *The Medical Letter, Inc*: Drugs for HIV infection. 42:1–6, 2000.
35. APA Commission on AIDS: *HIV-related neuropsychiatric complications and treatment* (Neuropsychiatric training curriculum published by APA), 2002.
36. American Academy of Neurology AIDS Task Force: Nomenclature and research case definitions for neurologic manifestations of human immunodeficiency virus-type 1 (HIV-1) infection, *Neurology* 41:778–785, 1991.
37. Goodkin K, Baldewicz TT, Wilkie FL, Tyll MD: Cognitive-motor impairment and disorder in HIV-1 infection, *Psychiatr Ann* 31:37–44, 2001.
38. The Dana Consortium on Therapy for HIV Dementia and Related Cognitive Disorders: Clinical confirmation of the American Academy of Neurology algorithm for HIV-1-associated cognitive/motor disorder, *Neurology* 47:1247–1253, 1996.
39. Albert SM, Marder K, Dooneief G, et al: Neuropsychologic impairment in early HIV infection, *Arch Neurol* 52:525–530, 1995.
40. Querques J, Worth JL: *HIV infection and AIDS*. In Stern TA, Herman JB, editors: *Psychiatry update and board preparation*, New York, 2000, McGraw-Hill.
41. Treisman GJ, Angelino AF, Hutton HE: Psychiatric issues in the management of patients with HIV infection, *JAMA* 286:2857–2864, 2001.
42. Concha M, Rabinstein A: Central nervous system opportunistic infections in HIV-1 infection, *CNS Spectrums* 4:43–60, 2000.
43. Buhrich N, Cooper DA: Requests for psychiatric consultation concerning 22 patients with AIDS and ARC, *Aust NZ J Psychiatry* 21:346–353, 1987.
44. Wong MC, Suite NDA, Labar DR: Seizures in human immunodeficiency virus infection, *Arch Neurol* 47:640–642, 1990.
45. Sherbourne CD, Hays RD, Fleishman JA, et al: Impact of psychiatric conditions on health-related quality of life in persons with HIV infection, *Am J Psychiatry* 157:248–254, 2000.
46. Morrison MF, Petitto JM, Have TT, et al: Depressive and anxiety disorders in women with HIV infection, *Am J Psychiatry* 159:789–796, 2002.
47. O'Dowd MA, Biderman DJ, McKegney FP: Incidence of suicidality in AIDS and HIV-positive patients attending a psychiatry outpatient program, *Psychosomatics* 34:33–40, 1993.
48. Johnson JG, Williams JBW, Rabkin JG, et al: Axis I psychiatric symptoms associated with HIV infection and personality disorder, *Am J Psychiatry* 152:551–554, 1995.
49. Roy KF (in collaboration with the APA Commission on AIDS): *HIV fact sheet: HIV and anxiety*, American Psychiatric Association, 2002.
50. Lyketsos CG, Schwartz J, Fishman M, Treisman G: AIDS mania, *J Neuropsychiatry Clin Neurosci* 9:277–279, 1997.

51. Mijch AM, Judd FK, Lyketsos CG, et al: Secondary mania in patients with HIV infection: Are antiretrovirals protective? *J Neuropsychiatry Clin Neurosci* 11:475–480, 1999.

52. De Ronchi D, Faranca I, Forti P, et al: Development of acute psychotic disorders and HIV-1 infection, *Intl J Psychiatry Med* 30:173–183, 2000.

53. Sewell DD, Jeste DV, Atkinson JH, et al: HIV-associated psychosis: a study of 20 cases. San Diego HIV Neurobehavioral Research Center Group, *Am J Psychiatry* 151:237–242, 1994.

54. Rubinstein ML, Selwyn PA: High Prevalence of insomnia in an outpatient population with HIV infection, *J Acquir Immune Defic Syndr Hum Retrovirol* 19:260–265, 1998.

55. Darko DF, McCutchan JA, Kripke DF, et al: Fatigue, sleep disturbance, disability, and indices of progression of HIV infection, *Am J Psychiatry* 149:514–520, 1992.

56. APA Office of HIV Psychiatry: *HIV-related sleep disorders.* Fast Facts, 2002.

57. Centers for Disease Control and Prevention: U.S. HIV and AIDS cases reported through December 1998. *HIV/AIDS Surveillance Report*, www.cdc.gov/ hiv/stats/ hasr/002.htm.

58. APA Office of HIV Psychiatry: *HIV-related substance use disorder.* Fast Facts, 2002.

59. Solomon L, Frank R, Vlahov D, Astemborski J: Utilization of health services in a cohort of intravenous drug users with known HIV-1 serostatus. *Am J Public Health* 81:1285–1290, 1991.

60. Lenderking WR, Cleary PD, Drey EA, et al: Communication about quality of life and treatment preferences between HIV-infected psychiatric outpatients and their primary care physicians. Scientific program and abstracts, Quality of Life and HIV Infection Conference, Amsterdam, 1992.

61. Todd KH, Samaroo N, Hoffman JR: Ethnicity as a risk factor for inadequate emergency department analgesia, *JAMA* 269:1537–1539, 1993.

62. So YT, Holtzman DM, Abrams DI, et al: Peripheral neuropathy associated with acquired immunodeficiency syndrome, *Arch Neurol* 45:945–948, 1988.

63. Verma A, Bradley WG:HIV-1-associated Neuropathies, *CNS Spectrums* 5:66–72, 2000.

64. Chung JY, Suarez AP, Zarin DA, Pincus HA: Psychiatric patients and HIV, *Psychiatr Serv* 50:487, 1999.

65. Chung JY: Prevention of HIV infection in psychiatric patients, *Psychiatr Ann* 31:21–25, 2001.

66. Friedmann PD, Alexander JA, Jin L, D'Aunno TA: On-site primary care and mental health services in outpatient drug abuse treatment units, *J Behav Health Serv Res* 26:80–94, 1999.

67. Gomez MF, Klein DA, Sand S, et al: Delivering mental health care to HIV-positive individuals: a comparison of two models, *Psychosomatics* 40:321–324, 1999.

68. Singh N, Squier C, Sivek C, et al: Determinants of compliance with antiretroviral therapy in patients with human immunodeficiency virus: prospective assessment with implications for enhancing compliance, *AIDS Care* 8:261–269, 1994.

69. Paterson DL, Swindells S, Mohr J, et al: Adherence to protease inhibitor therapy and outcomes in patients with HIV infection, *Ann Intern Med* 133:21–30, 2000.

70. Chesney MA: Factors affecting adherence to antiretroviral therapy, *Clin Infect Dis* 30 (suppl 2):177–176, 2000.

71. Sherer R: Adherence and antiretroviral therapy in injection drug users, *JAMA* 280:567–568, 1998.

72. Panel on Clinical Practices for Treatment of HIV Infection, Deptartment of Health and Human Services and H J Kaiser Family Foundation: *Guidelines for the use of antiretroviral agents in HIV-infected adults and adolescents.* http://www.hivatis.org, 2001.

73. Lucas GM, Chaisson RER, Moore RD: Highly active antiretroviral therapy in a large urban clinic: risk factors for virologic failure and adverse drug reactions, *Ann Intern Med* 131:81–87, 1999.

74. Liang WM, Goodkin K, Stasko RS: Psychological issues of people living longer with HIV. Component workshop 52, 155th American Psychiatric Association Annual Meeting, Philadelphia, 2002.

75. Eller LS: Effectts of two cognitive-behavioral interventions on immunity and symptoms in persons with HIV, *Ann Behav Med* 17:339–347, 1995.

76. Kelly JA, Murphy DA, Bahr GR, et al: Outcome of cognitive-behavioral and support group brief therapies for depressed, HIV-infected persons, *Am J Psychiatry* 150:1679–1686, 1993.

77. Markowitz JC, Kocsis JH, Fishman B, et al: Treatment of depressive symptoms in human immunodeficiency virus-positive patients, *Arch Gen Psychiatry* 55:452–457, 1998.

78. APA Neuropsychiatric Curriculum: Drug-drug interactions: HIV-related and psychotropic medications. *HIV-related neuropsychiatric complications and treatments*, American Psychiatric Association, 2002.

79. Gillenwater DR, McDaniel JS: Rational psychopharmacology for patients with HIV infection and AIDS, *Psychiatric Annals* 31:28–34, 2001.

80. Nemeroff CB, DeVane CL, Pollock BG: Newer antidepressants and the cytochrome P450 system, *Am J Psychiatry* 153:311–320, 1996.

81. Greenblatt DJ, von Moltke LL, Harmatz JS, Shader RI: Drug interactions with newer antidepressants: role of human cytochromes P450, *J Clin Psychiatry* 59(suppl):19–27, 1998.

82. Richelson E: Pharmacokinetic drug interactions of new antidepressants: a review of the effects on the metabolism of other drugs, *Mayo Clin Proc* 72:835–847, 1997.

83. Deeks SG, Smith M, Holodniy M, Kahn JO: HIV-1 protease inhibitors: a review for clinicians, *JAMA* 277:145–153, 1997.

84. DeSilva KE, Le Flore DB, Marston BJ, Rimland D: Serotonin syndrome in HIV-infected individuals receiving antiretroviral therapy and fluoxetine, *AIDS* 15:1281–1285, 2001.

85. Hesse LM, von Moltke LL, Shader RI, Greenblatt DJ: Ritonavir, efavirenz, and nelfinavir inhibit CYP2B6 activity in vitro: potential drug interactions with bupropion, *Drug Metab Dispos* 29:100–102, 2001.

86. Currier MB, Molina G, Kato M: A prospective trial of sustained-release bupropion for depression in HIV-seropositive and AIDS patients, *Psychosomatics* 44:120–125, 2003.

87. von Moltke, Greenblatt DJ, Grassi JM, et al: Protease inhibitors as inhibitors of human cytochromes P450: high risk associated with ritonavir, *J Clin Pharmacol* 38:106–111, 1998.

88. Fernandez F, Levy JK, Samley HR, et al: Effects of methylphenidate in HIV-related depression: a comparative trial with desipramine, *Int J Psychiatry Med* 25:53–67, 1995.

89. Wagner GJ, Rabkin R: Effects of dextroamphetamine on depression and fatigue in men with HIV: a double-blind, placebo-controlled trial, *J Clin Psychiatry* 61:436–440, 2000.

90. Hinkin CH, Castellon SA, Hardy DJ, et al: Methylphenidate improves HIV-1–associated cognitive slowing, *J Neuropsychiatry Clin Neurosci* 13:248–254, 2001.

91. Greenblatt DJ, von Moltke LL, Daily JP, et al: Extensive impairment of triazolam and alprazolam clearance by short-term low-dose ritonavir: the clinical dilemma of concurrent inhibition and induction, *J Clin Psychopharmacol* 19:293–296, 1999.

92. Akula SK, Rege AB, Dreisbach AW, et al: Valproic acid increases cerebrospinal fluid zidovudine levels in a patient with AIDS, *Am J Med Sci* 313:244–246, 1997.

93. Preston SL, Stein DS: Drug interactions and adverse drug reactions with protease inhibitors, *Prim Psychiatry* July:64–69, 1997.

94. Mechcatie E: Orap manufacturer warns of sudden deaths, *Clin Psychiatry News*, November 4, 1999.

95. Henry JA, Hill IR: Fatal interaction between ritonavir and MDMA, *Lancet* 352:1751–1752, 1998.

96. Halman MH, Worth JL, Sanders KM, et al: Anticonvulsant use in the treatment of manic syndromes in patients with HIV-1 infection, *J Neuropsychiatry Clin Neurosci* 5:430–434, 1993.

97. Hriso E, Kuhn T, Masdeu JC, Grundham M: Extrapyramidal symptoms due to dopamine blocking agents in patients with AIDS encephalopathy, *Am J Psychiatry* 148:1558–1561, 1991.

98. Repetto MJ, Evans DL, Cruess DG, et al: Neuropsychopharmacologic treatment of depression and other neuropsychiatric disorders in HIV-infected individuals, *CNS Spectrums* 8:59–63, 2003.

99. Freedman JB, O'Dowd, McKegney FP, et al: Managing diazepam abuse in an AIDS-related psychiatric clinic with a high percentage of substance abusers. Scientific program and abstracts, 40th Annual Meeting of Academy of Psychosomatic Medicine, New Orleans, 1993.

100. Ronald PJM, Robertson JR, Elton RA: Continued drug use and other cofactors for progression to AIDS among injecting drug users, *AIDS* 8:339–343, 1994.

101. Kosten T: *Treatment of substance abusing AIDS patients: psychopharmacology and HIV-1 infection: clinical challenges and research directions.* NIMH, Washington, DC, 1993.

102. Kemper CA, Ganer A, Kent G, et al: Double-blind placebo-controlled cross-over study fails to show benefit of mexiletine in painful HIV neuropathy, program and abstracts. 2nd National Conference on Human Retroviruses, Washington, DC, 1995.

Chapter 38
Burn Patients

Frederick J. Stoddard, Jr., M.D.
Gregory L. Fricchione, M.D.

Burns are as ancient as fire. To cope, all patients need help and many require psychiatric consultation. The patient with severe burns is as challenging to treat psychiatrically as surgically.[1] In the burn unit, new physicians and nurses may deeply fear seeing burned patients, but this feeling moderates as they relieve pain, help patients survive, and see the repair of disfiguring scars. Nevertheless, the stress of the burn unit is trying to all—viewing an acutely burned infant, child, or adult can meet the stressor criteria for posttraumatic stress disorder (PTSD) and evoke nightmares in some staff and patients. Some individuals need reminding at times that the child or adult with the scarred face is not a monster and that his or her feelings are hurt by avoidance or by ridicule from peers.

Burn units bring together specialists from several disciplines to provide specialized care to those with critical injuries. The Massachusetts General Hospital (MGH) Level 1 Trauma Center treats burned adults at the MGH and children at the affiliated Shriners Burns Hospital, staffed by many of the same MGH physicians. The MGH Burn Unit admits about 200 adult burn patients annually, and the Shriners Burns Hospital, located across the street from the MGH, is the pediatric burn center has about 200 acute pediatric burn and 700 plastic surgical admissions each year. Together staff follow thousands of outpatients recovering from burns.

History

The current era of burn treatment and research began more than 60 years ago at MGH after the Coconut Grove Fire on November 28, 1942. Cobb and Lindemann,[2] eminent early MGH psychiatrists, collaborated with other physicians and surgeons and chronicled the deliria and posttraumatic reactions of the survivors of that terrible fire in which 491 people died. Lindemann, in a classic paper,[3] reported for the first time the symptoms and psychotherapeutic management of acute grief, based in part on his work with 13 bereaved disaster victims (Coconut Grove Fire) and their close relatives and with relatives of members of the armed forces. Their studies involved psychiatric treatment and subsequent research on grief that would be applied to soldiers, civilians, and the bereaved.

In 2003, as in the Coconut Grove fire, The Station nightclub fire in Rhode Island wreaked havoc. It resulted in 100 deaths and tested emergency and burn trauma disaster plans at the MGH, the Shriners Burns Hospital, and the entire region; the triage system worked superbly. Unlike the September 11, 2001 terrorist attacks when staff readied for transfers to their burn units but were disappointed with how few survived to be treated, scores survived (despite severe burns to the lungs, face, hands and upper body) The Station nightclub fire due to the advances in modern burn care. Use of

697

Table 38-1. Ten-Point Plan for Consulting to Burned Patients

1. Speak with the patient at the bedside, and ensure the patient's safety.
2. Consult directly to the burn or trauma team, the surgeons and other physicians, nurses, social worker, and others, about the patient, clarifying your time availability and role. Within psychiatry, arrange for supervision, peer consultation, and departmental support.
3. Obtain the history of the burn circumstances, psychopathology, or substance abuse, and social and family functioning.
4. Diagnose the patient: Assess the developmental stage, burn severity, other stressors, mental status (including pain, stress, memory), psychiatric risk (delirium, suicide, child abuse), prognosis, medical and surgical issues including medications and their interactions, alcohol or drug withdrawal, current risk factors, language/cultural factors, legal status, and staff or family concerns. Recommend special studies or consultations as indicated.
5. Monitor, explain, and treat pain, delirium, stress, insomnia, and depression. Provide staff support and, for complex cases, plan a team conference.
6. Assess, treat, and support the dying child or adult and the family, and assist the clarification and the resolution of ethical dilemmas.
7. When the patient has survived the acute phase, progress to treating residual mental disorders, substance abuse, and other problems.
8. Facilitate grieving and adaptation of the patient and family to cosmetic or functional losses.
9. Collaborate in planning plastic and reconstructive surgical follow-up if possible and communicate psychiatric findings and recommendations to the primary care physician. Support reentry to school or work, including special education and rehabilitation services.
10. Remain available for follow-up consultation to patient and caregivers, clarifying the psychiatric issues, and assist the patient and family in obtaining psychiatric services if needed.

dental records and genetic testing enabled identification of some severely burned patients. As described earlier by Erich Lindemann and Stanley Cobb, these survivors, their children, and other relatives experienced and were treated for survivor guilt, traumatic grief, and what is now recognized as PTSD.

In the last 35 years, strong leadership and new research have led to improved methods of resuscitation and transport, excision and grafting,[4] anesthesia,[5] pain control,[6,7] anxiety management,[8] pulmonary care,[9] cardiovascular and infection control, artificial skin and skin substitutes,[10] psychiatric assessment and treatment (see Table 38-1), plastic surgical techniques,[11] and rehabilitative efforts that include interventions that benefit those with disfiguring facial and body burns. Taken together, these innovations have dramatically improved both mortality rates and the morbidity associated with burn injuries in the United States.

Just as Cobb and Lindemann did for adults, Bernstein,[12] Galdston,[13] and others pioneered the psychiatric care of burned children and their families; moreover, they conceptualized consultations to the burn team. Childhood injuries, including burns, now, after years of neglect are a priority for medical research and treatment.[14] The principal

resource regarding education about and research for burn care is the American Burn Association, which is linked to federal agencies, a variety of foundations, and the International Society for Burn Injuries.[15] Many patients also benefit from a self-help group called the Phoenix Society, which is an international organization for children and adults with burns (and their families).[16] Its mission is to better understand burned individuals and to support their care.

Epidemiology

Because of improved fire and burn prevention, and the expansion of burn centers in the United States, acute hospitalizations for burn injuries were cut in half between 1971 and 1991.[17] Roughly 1.25 to 2.5 million burns occur annually in the United States, accounting for about 5500 deaths,[14] of which about 35% occur in children. Each year about 51,000 people (many of whom are children) are hospitalized for burns. Burns are the leading cause of accidental deaths in children ages 1 to 4, and are the sixth leading cause of injury and death for children ages 5 to 9.[18] Similarly the elderly are at risk for severe burns because of mental impairment, isolation, substance abuse, and depression. Most burns are preventable; many are cigarette-related. Many infants and young children are burned as a result of scalds. Other burns are secondary to flames, electrical equipment, ingestions, and chemicals.[18]

Risk Factors

A combination of developmental and familial factors contribute to the risk of burns in children. Increased exploration by young child, access to scalding or flammable liquids or flame, childhood depression, behavioral disturbances, and parental psychopathology each predispose children to burns. Children's burns should not be indiscriminately labeled as due to neglect or abuse because, on careful assessment, they may be the result of a combination of developmental, environmental, and family variables. However, child neglect or abuse accounts for between 6% and 20% of pediatric burns; the age of maximum risk of abuse is 13 to 24 months, and scalds are the most common type of inflicted burn.[19] Factors suggestive of abuse include a caretaker who changes the story of what occurred from one interview to the next, prior injuries or accidents, a parent who neither visits nor is inattentive, a consistently awake but withdrawn child who appears immune to pain, a burn distribution inconsistent with the history, and other signs of abuse (e.g., fractures).[20] Suspected abuse must be reported to the appropriate state agency in most states.

The risk factors for burns are shown in Tables 38-2 and 38-3.[21–27]

Table 38-2. Risk Factors for Burns in Adults

Alcoholism
Drug abuse
Depression
Suicide attempts
Antisocial personality disorder
Schizophrenia
Bipolar disorders
Chronic medical illness
Dementia
Abuse/homicide
Occupational hazards

Table 38-3. Risk Factors for Burns in Child and Adolescents

Neglect
Abuse
Poverty
Unsafe housing
Family discord
Risk-taking behaviors
Learning disabilities
Depression
Fire setting

Severe Preexisting Psychopathology

Individuals with self-inflicted burns are, in general, the most severely mentally ill. Patients with bipolar disorder, especially when manic, are at risk for burning themselves and others; patients with schizophrenia may also burn themselves, as can depressed or conduct-disordered children. Addicts who free-base cocaine and alcoholics who smoke in a drunken stupor may also suffer severe burns, possibly because their intent remains uncertain as a form of parasuicide. Self-inflicted burns are common; small ones may serve as a warning for some as to how painful burns can be. Attempts at suicide via self-immolation occur worldwide and often result in massive, disfiguring burns.[28] Such suicide attempts often are kept secret by families and even by referring physicians. Because individuals with burns as a result of suicide attempts tend to have long lengths of stay, many adult burn units have at least one such patient at any given time.

A study of adolescent self-immolators revealed serious untreated or partially treated psychopathology, including drug abuse, guilt, psychosis, intense conflict with parents, and histories of physical or sexual abuse. They induced intense staff hostility and conflict, and some remained suicidal after discharge. Studies of adults similarly have found elevated rates of alcoholism, depression, psychosis, and personality disorder as preexisting factors.[29–31] These patients arouse intense feelings in caregivers and are among the most difficult surgical and psychiatric patients; typically, they are managed by both the surgical and psychiatric services. Despite their burns and severe psychopathology, most patients cope well with sound long-term psychiatric treatment that is initiated on the burn unit. Among young children, intentional self-inflicted burns are rare, although accidental self-injury is common.

Treating the Patient with Acute Burns: Essential Elements

Diagnosis and Developmental Assessment

Thorough diagnostic assessment is necessary to plan treatment. Initial assessment may be difficult; history must often be obtained from others,[32] as the patient's condition may be critical.[33] Special studies (e.g., toxicologic drug screening, brain imaging, electroencephalography [EEG], and neuropsychological testing) are often indicated. The assessment usually proceeds with multiple, relatively brief visits to the patient beginning at or near admission; it incorporates changes in clinical status into the formulation. The developmental model described below for assessing burned children,[32] has been supplemented by a developmental model that is useful throughout the life cycle.[34]

Developmental Stage and Burns: Case Examples

Infant

A 4-month-old girl was admitted with a 20% total body surface area (TBSA) scald to the face, neck, and chest. The parents responded with intense self-reproach and fears of future scars; they had intermittent difficulty soothing her because of their own distress. Psychiatric consultation was requested to deal with her refusal to eat, her crying in anticipation of painful dressing changes, and her anxiety that was aroused by her mother's departure for home to be with her older children. With support of nursing, social work, and child psychiatric staff, the mother roomed with the infant, pain was reduced with opiates, and the infant healed (over a 2-week period that involved skin grafting) and appeared to resume her normal developmental course. This case illustrated typical signs of distress and regression in a burned infant, manifestations of parental stress, and a dyadic (parent-child) approach to intervention.

Child

A 3-year-old boy with smoke inhalation and 30% TBSA, mostly partial thickness, burns became increasingly withdrawn following the burn, except when in his brother's company; when with his brother he would play with toys and be more outgoing. He was interpersonally inhibited and afraid of dressing changes. His pain was only partially relieved by oral morphine and lorazepam, he clung to nursing staff, and he appeared to regress. His speech was indistinct; what he did say was repeated over and over. Consistently somber, he stared silently at staff and did not speak or interact in a meaningful way. A psychiatric assessment suggested that he suffered from a combination of acute stress disorder and a mild anoxic brain injury. Regression, a slow recovery associated with anoxic brain injuries, an acute stress disorder,[35,36] and possible depression were the consequences of his burn.

Adolescent

A 15-year-old boy sustained 85% TBSA flame and inhalation injuries in a grease fire from a cookstove; a friend perished in the fire. Trouble sleeping, bad dreams, and flashbacks of the fire plagued him. Nightmares persisted for 6 weeks. He tried to think about "positive things during the day" so that when he slept his dreams would be positive. He continued to dream about activities he had done and took pleasure from before his injuries. One month later, he described a different type of dream. He described romantic fantasies about a female staff member caring for him. He was relieved to hear from the psychiatrist that such thoughts were not unusual when a close relationship develops between a patient and a caregiver. He became able to acknowledge age-appropriate emotions. Near discharge, his nightmares recurred, as did positive dreams related to returning home and resuming his life. This case illustrates how dreams of many burned patients can evolve and how they can be used to adapt to severe injury. Posttraumatic nightmares may follow sleep deprivation, delirium, and painful procedures. As patients enter the rehabilitative phase, their outlook often becomes more positive and the content of their dreams may become more developmentally normal and less anxiety provoking.

Young Adult

A 23-year-old father of two was admitted with 40% TBSA burns to his face, neck, upper torso, and arms following a house fire. He received morphine for pain and diazepam for anxiety. He became acutely delirious (with agitation, disorientation, and combativeness), which required physical restraints and 10 to 20 mg of intravenous (IV) haloperidol per day for the first few days of the admission. The delirium seemed to be due to smoke inhalation and cerebral anoxia. He healed well over a 2-week period, and all medications (except for morphine that was used for dressing changes) were tapered. He was observed to be "strange," to be "more like a kid," and to have inappropriate behavior, apparently because of ongoing delirium. Psychiatric reassessment, however, indicated terror with severe sleep deprivation and posttraumatic nightmares (both sleeping and waking) of the fire. He faced several stressors (e.g., severe burns suffered by his wife, two young sons, and younger brother); his grief was intense once his medications were reduced. He recalled, but was unable to cope with, images of the fire and the injuries to himself and his loved ones; they were all nearby, in various stages of recovery from their burns. He responded well to emotional support, to clarification, and to reassurance, as well as to tranquilizers that restored adequate sleep and reduced the intensity of his terror. This case illustrates the combined effects of anoxic brain injury, delirium, acute stress, and acute grief in a young adult.

Elderly

A 77-year-old woman caught her housecoat on a gas stove, which resulted in a cooking-related clothing ignition. She was admitted with 15% TBSA first-degree and second-degree burns to her left side. According to observers she was "lovely" and "intact." She had a history of valvular disease with congestive heart failure (CHF), metastatic breast carcinoma (status postbilateral mastectomies), and deep venous thrombosis (DVT). Psychiatric consultation was obtained because of confusion, which lessened when doses of diazepam and morphine were reduced. No neurologic basis for her confusion was found. This case involved an ill, elderly, and cognitively impaired woman who responded slowly but well to acute care.

Managing Acute Pain

Pain is often underestimated and undertreated (because staff fear that respiratory depression or death will result from treatment).[37] Organizational approaches to monitor and reduce this problem include the creation of pain management guidelines, the implementation of educational programs for pain management, and attendance at pain service rounds. In responding to this, Szyfelbein, et al.[38] and others used self-rated scales and measured serum endorphin levels; they proved that high-dose IV opiates were needed to provide relief from pain for those who were severely burned. Improving pain relief[39,40] and sharpening the focus on psychological as well as pharmacologic interventions is important to improve outcomes; nonetheless, pain in burn patients remains undertreated in many hospitals.[41]

The pain experienced by burn patients is mainly acute, although the itching that occurs during healing can be chronic. The addition of short-acting IV and oral agents (especially opiates, midazolam, and propofol) to target acute pain and anxiety has dramatically lessened the suffering from acute burns. Initially the location(s), source, quality, intensity, course, and duration of pain are identified; then, with nursing staff, self-reported ratings of pain (from 0 to 10 with 10 equaling the most pain) are monitored in response to treatment. Burn pain correlates with endorphin levels and with the extent and depth of the burn.[42] Because infants cannot provide self-reported ratings, behavioral measures (e.g., facial expressions, body movements, and crying) and physiologic parameters (e.g., heart rate, blood pressure, respiratory rate, oxygen saturation, and if available, levels of epinephrine, norepinephrine, growth hormone, and cortisol) are useful in monitoring pain responses.[43] For children who are able to communicate, self-reported measures, such as the Faces Scale, the Visual Analogue Scale, and the Oucher Scale are useful; among staff-observed scales the Children's Hospital of Eastern Ontario Pain Scale (CHEOPS) has utility.[44] The most easily used self-rating scales for verbal burn patients are 0 to 10 visual analogue scales, which rate pain from 0 to 10, with 0 as no pain and 10 being the most severe pain experienced. Management of pain in burned adults also involves pain ratings (e.g., a visual analogue scale) and multimodal treatment with opiates, anxiolytics, and nonsteroidal anti-inflammatory drugs (NSAIDs) together with psychological methods (see Chapter 21). For patients unable to communicate (e.g., owing to use of paralytic agents or to intubation), estimates of maximum analgesic requirement for body weight are recommended.

Psychological Treatment

Psychological techniques to ease burn pain include education, hypnosis, relaxation, patient participation in dressing changes, and biofeedback; these techniques do not predispose to side effects or toxic effects as do medications. Patients can be trained to use these methods,[41] and they can discover that they are capable of dissociating and using hypnosis. Developmentally targeted psychological approaches to pain management are effective for both children and adults. Hypnosis for burn pain is effective and practical,[45–47] but it requires more staff time than when relying solely on the use of analgesics. Hypnosis and simple and complex relaxation techniques such as focused imagery are in wide use and are practical for children (who are the most hypnotizable subjects) and for adults. Spiegel and Spiegel[48] described a method that is generally applicable for burn patients. Intriguingly, Ewin[49] has reported that hypnosis can acutely prevent the postburn inflammatory response, thereby lessening burn severity. Patient-mediated methods involve the patient's active participation and are designed to shift the locus of control in burned children to themselves.[39,50] This involves preparation for painful procedures and increases the patient's ability to choose when, for how long, and who will perform invasive procedures by encouraging their participation at each step. This structured method can lead to fewer maladaptive behaviors, to improved outcomes, and to lower dosages of narcotics.

Pharmacologic Treatment

Psychopharmacologic treatment of mental disorders in both adults and children with burn patients is increasing, primarily with use of anxiolytics, neuroleptics, antidepressants, stimulants, and mood stabilizers. Because of efforts to improve pain management, opiate use has also increased in burn centers. Pharmacologic treatment of patients with burns is often complicated by prior substance use and abuse, the possibility that use of pharmacologically active agents will adversely alter mental state, the critical condition of the patient (especially respiratory failure or renal insufficiency), drug interactions, altered pharmacodynamics, and the need to balance the benefits of the medication against the risks of unwanted side effects or toxicity.[51] In some cases, reducing the dosage of medications will result in less confusion, anorexia, somnolence, insomnia, lethargy, depression, and irritability and more alertness and cooperation with procedures and physical therapy. Psychotherapeutic interventions may also be more feasible at this point.

Despite wide use of psychotropics for patients with burns, few studies demonstrate symptom relief (except for pain). Patients often require psychotropics for alcohol or drug withdrawal, agitation, psychosis, or mood disorders. The IV sedative-hypnotic propofol (Diprivan) is now being used as a bolus with good effect during painful procedures and for adults, as an IV infusion. It is excreted within approximately 30 minutes.

Opiates

The most common agent for relief of acute burn pain is morphine, but benzodiazepines also relieve pain and anxiety.[52] For the acutely burned child, morphine sulfate is often started as a continuous infusion (starting at 0.05 mg/kg/hour with intermittent IV boluses of 0.05 to 0.1 mg/kg every 2 hours); the guideline for midazolam (if anxiety is otherwise unrelieved) is to start at 0.04 mg/kg/hour and then administer an intermittent IV slow push every 4 to 6 hours (0.04 mg/kg/hour). Respiratory depression may require use of opiate or benzodiazepine antagonists. Reversible neurologic abnormalities have been reported in children following long-term midazolam use.[52] With acutely burned adults, morphine sulfate is often begun at 5 to 10 mg intramuscularly or intravenously every 1 to 4 hours and diazepam 5 mg IM or IV every 1 to 4 hours. Continuous IV drip morphine sulfate or midazolam is often needed with selected patients (e.g., those with large burns).

Pain reduction is effective whether the cause is biologic or psychological because pain "disrupts metabolic, autonomic, and thermoregulatory" as well as immune functions.[53] Studies have clarified the efficacy of high-dose morphine for relief of burn pain, using either IV or oral administration. Patient-controlled analgesia (PCA) with burned adults has been universally useful, but PCA is still useful in selected patients, usually after the first few days of treatment. Adjuvants, such as methylphenidate, tricyclic antidepressants, and even haloperidol, among others, can enhance the effectiveness of opiates.

Benzodiazepines

A host of benzodiazepines are available for use; each has a different side effect profile. There are short-acting agents (e.g., midazolam, which has rapidly assumed a significant place for brief procedures,[54] lorazepam,[55,56] oxazepam, and triazolam) and long-acting agents (e.g., chlordiazepoxide, diazepam, clonazepam, and flurazepam). There are few indications for use of psychotropics in recently burned children other than for the management of pain, anxiety, or delirium. As is true for pain, anxiety is often undertreated.

Neuroleptics

Major tranquilizers are, at times, necessary to control delirium, agitation, or severe insomnia in older adolescents and adults. Initially, IV haloperidol, used in low doses (0.5 to 2.0 mg IV) (although not approved by the Food and Drug Administration [FDA] for IV use may be used) while the cause for the target symptoms is being identified and specifically treated; phenothiazines are less often used because of their propensity to induce hypotension. Much higher doses have been used safely and with good results.[57] Extrapyramidal side effects (e.g., dystonia) may occur, but their incidence is exceedingly low,[58] and dystonia can be largely prevented by use of antiparkinsonian agents. Occasionally, when severe agitation occurs, a propofol drip and/or IV haloperidol, lorazepam, and a narcotic may be necessary when the goal is to enhance deep sedation. This state reduces the metabolic demand imposed by agitation, minimizes pain, and produces amnesia that may decrease the vulnerability to PTSD. Haloperidol is not indicated for use in young children with burns due to risk of hypotension that is common. Such children usually respond to benzodiazepines.

Newer oral, atypical antipsychotics are increasingly used in use with adult burn patients, adolescents, and (primarily risperidone) with some children. These drugs include risperidone, ziprasidone, olanzapine, and clozapine. Long-term use may cause severe weight gain with all of the above except ziprasidone.

Drug Side Effects, Toxicity, and Adverse Interactions

Side effects, toxicity, and adverse interactions can occur with just about any agent used in burn care. Opiates, benzodiazepines, various sedatives, antidepressants, and antipsychotics (especially haloperidol or droperidol) are among the more noteworthy psychotropics. These and many other agents are managed in collaboration with surgeons, anesthesiologists, and other physicians and nurses. Rarely, neuroleptic malignant syndrome (NMS) may develop following neuroleptic use; its symptoms are similar to those of malignant hyperthermia induced by anesthetics. An uncommon cardiac complication, torsades de pointes, has been associated with haloperidol use (among other antipsychotics and antidepressants), especially in alcoholic and metabolically compromised patients.[59] Opiate or benzodiazepine tolerance, dependence, and withdrawal also occur. Opiate withdrawal may be reversed by opiate agonists and a clonidine patch can be used for symptoms of minor withdrawal. Benzodiazepine withdrawal may cause anxiety, dysphoria, insomnia, and a full-scale syndrome with abdominal cramps, vomiting, sweating, tremors, and convulsions. Some of these symptoms continue even days after the drug is stopped, especially in those individuals with hepatic or renal impairment. Resuming the prewithdrawal dose and initiating a slower taper of the benzodiazepine usually minimizes or eliminates the withdrawal symptoms. Although patients with burns may develop physical dependence on analgesics and anxiolytics, addiction is almost never caused by use of these agents in the context of burns, despite concerns of staff about those with a history of substance abuse; moreover, substance abusers may at first require higher doses of opiates than do others without similar histories. The interaction of opiates and benzodiazepines may cause delirium, excess sedation, and respiratory depression.[60] Opiate toxicity can be reversed by naloxone while benzodiazepine toxicity can be reversed by use of flumazenil; however, seizures may be induced with this medication in benzodiazepine-dependent individuals. Recognizing these risks and carefully monitoring use of medications typically results in reductions in, and relief of, pain, delirium, and anxiety.

Postburn Phases: Acute, Intermediate, and Long-Term Adaptation

To review the clinical models of postburn adaptation is to review most of the major clinical models of psychiatry and psychology in the last 50 years.

The models have included ego psychological,[61] sociologic/adaptational,[12] crisis,[62] psychopathologic,[63,64] existential,[12,34] developmental, empiric/evaluative, and behavioral/rehabilitative/ therapeutic. Some of these models have essential neurobiologic and pharmacotherapeutic components. As the field progresses, few models are wholly discarded, but the trend is toward less theory and more empiric measurement of symptoms and well-defined interventions.

Acute Phase

Diagnostic Assessment

From admission, assessment and treatment proceed hand in hand. Orientation to and explanation about the burn and its treatment are followed by assessment of the effectiveness of these interventions. Communication should involve a vocabulary that the patient can understand and should be appropriate to the patient's cognitive and emotional ability. Because a burned patient may be confused, afraid of death or dismemberment, and anxious about pain, the initial history may need to be obtained from other individuals. Explanation, reassurance, and relief of pain help to reduce fear and confusion. A formal mental status evaluation is necessary to diagnose subtle changes in mental functioning. The patient's initial emotional reactions (e.g., denial, fear, guilt, grief, anger, or withdrawal) should be noted. A history of developmental, mental or substance abuse disorders, medical illness, and psychiatric treatment, should be obtained; the social context should also be established. When family members understand, feel supported, and are reassured, they are better able to calm their loved one; however, when this support is absent the opposite is often true. As an alliance with the patient and family develops, additional history typically clarifies the circumstances of the injury.

Burn-Induced Delirium

Burn-induced delirium or encephalopathy usually occurs soon after injury and signals an increased risk of death. The confused, agitated, or aggressive patients can hit staff, attempt to leave the hospital, fall, self-extubate, and dislodge intravascular lines and skin grafts. Early studies confirmed that delirium was associated with EEG and other neurologic abnormalities in both children and adults.[65,66] Delirium may occur in 10% to 30% of burn patients and signal the patient's unstable condition; the more severe the burn the more likely will be a delirious state. Current burn treatment renders it less common. With severe burns, patients are often kept anesthetized and intubated until grafting is completed; thus, acute delirium is often masked. Delirium can be caused by opiates or by other medications, infection, metabolic disturbance, hypoxia, central nervous system (CNS) injury, or other factors. Prompt evaluation and the maintenance of safety (which may necessitate the use of restraints), diagnosis and treatment of the causative factors, environmental change, and increased supportive personal contact with staff and family are indicated.[67,68]

Acute Stress Disorder

The *Diagnostic and Statistical Manual of Mental Disorders (DSM-IV)*[69] criteria for acute stress disorder include symptoms of dissociation, reexperience of the trauma, avoidance, and anxiety or arousal. The symptoms must last for at least 2 days and occurs within 4 weeks of the trauma; the condition is not due to drugs or medications or to the patient's medical condition. Acute stress disorder in burned children and adults predicts the later occurrence of PTSD.[26,89] At some point following the burn, most patients become increasingly aware of their burn and recall the acute burn experience. These symptoms usually coincide with the hypermetabolic and hypercatecholaminergic postburn state. Awareness and recall may be delayed until opiates and benzodiazepines are tapered, at which time the intrusive recollections, nightmares or night terrors, and associated arousal states may begin abruptly. When the hypermetabolic response later subsides, a state of depression may develop, with depressive mood, interpersonal withdrawal, and decreased appetite. Some of the postburn phenomena affecting and being affected by neurobiologic systems include the effects of neurotoxins (e.g., carbon monoxide, smoke, and anoxia), catecholamine depletion, anesthetics, opiates, and benzodiazepines. Brief supportive psychotherapy usually focuses on developing an alliance with the patient, assessing pain and anxiety, determining orientation, and providing appropriate reassurance. These interventions assist the patient in making sense of the burn, and of treatments for a burn of the type and location that the patient has sustained.

Intermediate Phase

The intermediate phase, during which the patient is healing, is less stressful. Hospitalization, however, is the period for which the term *continuous traumatic stress* may be most fitting.[70] Stress occurs throughout burn treatment. Vulnerable patients with prior comorbid conditions have special difficulty adapting to the frequent stresses of burn care and they benefit from individualized psychological and psychopharmacologic treatment.

Psychological Interventions

There is a shift from the acute to the intermediate phase when survival is assured, when most burn wounds are grafted, and when the patient approaches ambulatory status. At this time, it is possible to assess more fully the mental status and to begin differentiating issues of mourning the prior body image, grieving the loss of loved ones, depression, and PTSD. In addition, assessment and diagnosis of neurologic or pre-existing psychiatric impairment becomes feasible. The patient's awareness of functional losses and disfigurement is eased by responsive staff and by supportive, informed family members. Psychotherapeutic interventions also focus on phase-related issues (e.g., forthcoming surgery, return to home and school, and rehabilitation).

Adaptation of the family usually follows the course of the patient's recovery. Remarkably similar feelings and defensive responses are observed in the patient and his or her family. Psychotherapeutic support (often several sessions per week) during this phase, especially regarding guilt feelings and grief, assists the family and enables them to support the patient's coping through this phase.

Some hospitals provide groups that offer brief psychotherapy, education, and rehabilitation. Several types of group interventions have been used: a children's group structured to encourage expressive drawing and puppet play, an adolescent or adult group for hospitalized patients, and family groups for parents or families of acutely ill patients. These group interventions focus on education about treatment, grief, and one's response to hospitalization, surgery, stigmatization, discharge, and reentry into society. In England, Rivlin et al.[71] conducted parent groups using a multidisciplinary approach, which the parents rated as helpful.

Rehabilitative Phase

Body Image and Plastic and Reconstructive Surgery

After the burn heals, ongoing care may be transferred to the plastic and reconstructive surgeon. Certain problems or mental disorders should prompt psychiatric consultation in those returning for postburn plastic and reconstructive surgery. For children, lack of age-appropriate preparation, preoperative panic, PTSD, parent-child disturbances, attention deficit hyperactivity disorder (ADHD), depression, and enuresis or encopresis are not unusual. For adults, PTSD, psychosis, substance abuse, malingering, or factitious disorder may occur. Certain burns that require cosmetic surgery (e.g., of the face and head, breasts, or genitalia) and are associated with functional deficits (e.g., burns to the mouth, hands, arms, and lower extremities), including amputations and revisions, require special consideration and, at times, special expertise in preoperative psychological assessment and postoperative management.

Plastic surgeons develop psychological skills for the evaluation of burned patients and may seek psychiatric consultation for their patients.[72] Because much of acute treatment, even with recent improvements in care, is outside the control of the patient and the family, a central psychological goal at this point is to increase the patient's and the family's role in the treatment, its timing, and the long-term plans. Although staff assist the patient to see himself or herself anew,[73] the consultant, in turn, becomes aware of the experience of being burned through the eyes of the patient. By age 2 to 3, body image is a relatively stable part of the self-concept, although it is modified by growth, puberty, trauma, and aging.

Interviewing a burned patient provides a window to the development of body image and, usually, on the adaptation and recovery that follows. Attitudes of family and staff toward the patient's physical defects helps to shape body image. Burns in children and adults may profoundly alter the subsequent body image, level of self-esteem, interpersonal relations, and ego function,[74,75] but body image disturbances are not inevitable. Body image revision occurs through plastic surgery, allowing another stage of reintegration of body image and healing of the damage to appearance and to self-image. Focused, short-term supportive and educational psychotherapy is helpful, and protocols for these treatments are being developed.[76]

The capacity to tolerate fear and anxiety associated with rehospitalization should be assessed before embarking upon plastic and reconstructive surgery. Anxiety often blocks one's understanding, and multiple explanations may be necessary. If there is significant psychopathology, review of records and a preoperative assessment are indicated to reduce postoperative complications. Preoperative problems include phobic reactions to surgery, unrealistic expectations of "perfect" surgical results, embarrassment or shame related to severe disfigurement, and resurgence of PTSD symptoms (e.g., flashbacks or nightmares). Reality-oriented preoperative psychotherapeutic interventions support the patient's coping and facilitate a positive attitude following surgery.

Massively Burned Persons

Prior to the advances in burn care over the past 30 years, most patients with massive burns died. Today, children and adults usually survive once they reach an acute burn unit, even with massive burns. Despite suffering severe burns to the bronchial tree, face, torso, or extremities, which may require deep, disfiguring excisions of fat and muscle, or amputations, people survive. Many of these survivors draw on personal strengths and family supports and are incredibly resilient. Psychiatric treatment of those with massive burns initially focuses on the management of pain, stress, or delirium, then deals with grief and injury to body image. Next, treatment focuses on support, restoration of mobility, self-esteem, and hope. Finally, treatment helps the burn survivor resume educational, occupational, and social function. Encouragement, education, and advocacy for the massively burned patient is crucial to mobilize resources so that life, school, and work outside the hospital can be resumed and that the social stigma of disfigurement can be endured.

Less Severely Burned Persons

Those with less severe burns do not necessarily have fewer or less severe psychiatric problems. Some studies of children and adults have found as many or more psychiatric problems with small burns than with large burns,[77] but other studies have found the opposite. In either case, children or adults with small burns may have severe psychiatric or substance abuse problems and may be at risk of neglect or abuse; especially in this era of managed care, the opportunity for psychiatric intervention may be fleetingly.

Outcome after a Burn

Many small studies of varying quality and a few larger ones relate to outcome after a burn.[78–80] Clearly, the quality of burn and reconstructive treatment has improved; this makes conclusions based on earlier studies unreliable when attempting to predict current outcomes. Tarnowski and Rasnake,[78] in a review of child outcome studies, believed that "collectively, findings indicate that little empirical data exists to support the contention that the majority of pediatric burn victims exhibit severe poor post-burn adjustment." Patterson et al.[79] essentially agreed with these conclusions for adults from a rehabilitation psychology perspective. They suggested that poor outcomes were mainly a result of severe preburn psychopathology, which is significant. Although there is much preburn psychopathology in adults and some in children, this theory underemphasizes the severity and chronicity of posttraumatic reactions. Issues of vulnerability, resilience, and the effects of traumatic stress on emerging personality development[81] have been thoroughly summarized. Although pessimistic conclusions about outcomes are unwarranted, serious psychiatric and psychological morbidity after severe, disfiguring burns merit attention, especially for adolescents who are more vulnerable to depression.

For instance, Stoddard et al.,[82] in a cross-sectional follow-up study of children age 7 to 19 with severe burns (mean injury, 38% TBSA) readmitted for plastic surgery, found that a majority had mental disorders (including PTSD, depression, and enuresis) at some time following the burn, whereas 20% developed no disorders. Blakeney et al.,[80] while following 47 of 72 children with over 80% TBSA burns, found that the 47 achieved "positive psychosocial adaptation" with moderate to severe difficulties in 24% to 30%, a comparable level to those seen with lesser burn injuries. Outcome studies in burned adults have not met the criterion of controlled psychiatric research (using structured diagnostic interviews that evaluate all disorders).

In child and adult studies, the prevalence of PTSD after burns ranges from 20% to 40%, but partial PTSD is more frequent. As the patient improves medically, an acute stress disorder may emerge as full-syndrome PTSD. For children, *DSM-IV* PTSD criteria include "disorganized or agitated behavior" in response to trauma and posttraumatic play, "frightening dreams without recognizable content," and "trauma-specific reenactment" as symptoms of re-experiencing. In a study of PTSD, 60 burned children readmitted for plastic surgery, Stoddard et al.[82] found that about one third had full-syndrome *DSM III-R*-defined PTSD, and more than half had post-traumatic symptoms. Similarly, Kravitz et al.[83] found both a high incidence of sleep disorders in 82 children and, like Stoddard et al.,[82] enuresis in 24%. In adult burn survivors, PTSD occurred among 20% to 40% of subjects, often with associated sleep disorders. Roca, Spence, and Munster[84] followed 43 patients (from discharge to follow-up with 314 months later): 7% initially fulfilled criteria for PTSD; this increased to 22% at 4 months. Perry et al.[85] also found an increase from 35% at 2 months to 45% at 12 months. Powers et al.[86] found similar findings a year following discharge from the burn unit, with 38% fulfilling *DSM-III-R* criteria and 43% using the *DSM-IV* criteria. Most studies and clinical observation indicated a gradual attenuation of PTSD symptoms, but these studies suggested that it might not be so. Behavioral, cognitive, and pharmacologic therapies all have a place in treatment of PTSD; new short-term treatments are being tested.[87]

Surgical reconstruction improves appearance and strikingly enhances social and emotional adjustment. Outcome studies in adults suggest that a majority have adjusted well to their burns over the long term but that those with facial burns are more likely to experience social rejection, impaired self-esteem, and withdrawal. These results do not resolve the likelihood of severe burn-related emotional disability in burned adults. As with children, improved treatment methods appear to improve outcomes, but definitive studies are lacking.

End-of-life Care

The mortality rate on adult units is much higher than on pediatric burn units because of more extensive burns, severe medical and psychiatric risk factors, an increased mortality risk associated with being older, and the limits of what medical care can achieve. Most deaths as a result of burns occur during the initial phases, but some patients survive for months before death arrives. The psychiatrist is often consulted to assist in the care of dying patients and their families to minimize pain and suffering and to assist in the process of decision-making at the end of life.[88–90] Although it is often traumatic when an adult dies, it is always emotionally traumatic when a child dies from burns.[88–91] It is essential to provide accurate explanations about the risk of death to families and to patients when possible, as well as emotional preparation for this possibility. Support in their grieving is helpful to relatives of burn patients who die; many are very grateful for the care their loved ones have received.

Staff Support, Staff Stress, and Burnout Prevention

Psychiatric skills are especially valuable and valued by burn patients; stressed staff also know their benefits. It is useful to understand organizations in which one works, the rapid changes that affect hospitals and health care, and the virtues of developing a relationship with a multidisciplinary team to care for severely traumatized patients. One's introduction to the unit may be followed by shock, dismay, fear, frustration, and sadness as the full meaning of burn care takes hold.[12,88] Respect for the coping styles of the staff is crucial, since it may at times appear that individuals are harsh, regressed, or overinvolved.

The psychiatrist on the team, simply by her or his presence, encourages communication; a reflective attitude about staff members' own feelings as well as those of their patients is helpful. Encouraging staff to ask questions, the psychiatrist can enable them to think diagnostically and therapeutically about their patients' and their future and provide them with a sense of satisfaction and hope. Gratitude for sharing the burden of tragic or irreversible situations and for lending an ear may be forthcoming. The psychiatrist is often able to place trauma in a positive perspective and to broaden and deepen the psychiatric knowledge of the entire burn team.

Ethical Considerations

Ethical issues stimulated by burn care may be a source of difficulty for staff and the family; these issues may be magnified by costs, which may exceed $1 million for a single patient. Ethical issues[33] include consent to treatment, quality of life, prevention of intolerable pain, organ donation, decisions about resuscitation or withdrawal of life support, cost of care versus potential benefit, responsibility for long-term care of most severely burned, right to treatment, and determination of disability. Consultation by the ethics committee to the burn team in difficult cases is often helpful to provide optimal care to the patient and family.

References

Internet information sources are available online regarding burns (American Burn Association), pain (American Pain Society), psychopharmacology, traumatic stress (International Society for Traumatic Stress Studies; Dartmouth traumatic stress library), American Psychiatric Association, and American Academy of Child and Adolescent Psychiatry.

1. Stoddard FJ: *Care of infants, children, and adolescents with burn injuries.* In Lewis M, editors: *Child and adolescent psychiatry: a comprehensive textbook,* ed 3, Baltimore, 2002, Williams and Wilkins, pp 1188–1208.
2. Cobb S, Lindemann E: Neuropsychiatric observations after the Cocoanut Grove fire, *Ann Surg* 117:814–824, 1943.
3. Lindemann E: Symptomatology and management of acute grief, *Am J Psychiatry* 101:141–148, 1994.
4. Sheridan RL, Tompkins RG, Burke JF: Management of burn wounds with prompt excision and immediate closure, *J Intens Care Med* 9:6–19, 1994.
5. Martyn JAJ, Szyfelbein SK: *Anesthetic management of the burned patient.* In Martyn JAJ, editor: *Acute management of the burned patient,* Philadelphia, 1990, WB Saunders.
6. Stoddard FJ, Martyn J, Sheridan R: Psychiatric issues in pain of burn injury, *Curr Rev Pain* 1(2):130–136, 1996.
7. Stoddard FJ, Sheridan RL, Saxe G, et al: Treatment of pain in acutely burned children, *J Burn Care Rehabil* 23: 135–156, 2002.
8. Sheridan R, Stoddard F, Querzoli E: Management of background pain and anxiety in critically burned children requiring protracted mechanical ventilation, *J Burn Care Rehabil* 22:150–153, 2001.
9. Demling RH: Pulmonary function in the burn patient, *Semin Nephrol* 13(4):371–381, 1993.
10. Sheridan RL, Hegarty M, Tompkins RG, et al: Artificial skin in massive burns: results to ten years, *Eur J Plast Surg* 17:91–93, 1994.
11. Salisbury RE, guest editor: Burn rehabilitation and reconstruction, *Clin Plast Surg* 19:551–756, 1992.
12. Bernstein N: *Emotional care of the facially burned and disfigured,* Boston, 1976, Little, Brown.
13. Galdston R: The burning and healing of children, *Psychiatry* 35:57, 1957.
14. Stoddard FJ, Saxe G: Ten year research review of physical injuries, *J Am Acad Child Adolesc Psychiatry* 40 (10):1128–1145, 2001.
15. American Burn Association. Available at www.ameriburn.org.
16. The Phoenix Society. Available at info@phoenixsociety.org.
17. Brigham PA, McLoughlin E: Burn incidence and medical care use in the United States: estimates, trends and data sources, *J Burn Care Rehabil* 17:95–107, 1996.
18. Scheidt PC, Harel Y, Trumble AC, et al. The epidemiology of nonfatal injuries among US children and youth, *Am J Public Health* 85(7):932–938, 1995.
19. McLaughlin E, Crawford JD: Types of burn injury, *Pediatr Clin North Am* 23:41, 1985.
20. Renz BM, Sherman R: Abusive scald burns in infants and children: a prospective study, *Am Surg* 59:329–334, 1993.
21. Rockwell E, Dimsdale JE, Carroll W, et al: Preexisting psychiatric disorders in burn patients, *J Burn Care Rehabil* 9:83–86, 1988.
22. Haum A, Perbix W, Hack AJ, et al: Alcohol and drug abuse in burn injuries, *Burns* 21:194–199, 1995.
23. Kolman PBR: Incidence of psychopathology in burned adult patients, *J Burn Care Rehabil* 4:430–36, 1984.
24. Stoddard FJ, Frumin M, Ryan CM, et al: Psychiatric and medical conditions associated with severe burns in adults: abstracts of Academy of Psychosomatic Medicine, Annual Meeting, 1995, Palm Springs.

25. Kelley D, Lynch JB: Burns in alcohol and drug users result in longer treatment times with more complications, *J Burn Care Rehabil* 13:218, 1992.

26. Difede J, Ptacek JT, Roberts J, et al: Acute stress disorder after burn injury: a predictor of posttraumatic stress disorder? *Psychosomatic Medicine* 64(5):826–834, 2002.

27. Fauerbach JA, Lawrence JW, Schmidt CW, et al: Personality predictors of injury-related posttraumatic stress disorder, *J Nerv Ment Dis* 188(8):510–517, 2000.

28. Stoddard FJ: A psychiatric perspective on self-inflicted burns, *J Burn Care Rehabil* 14:340, 1993.

29. Andreason NC, Noyes R: Suicide attempted by self-immolation, *Am J Psychiatry* 132:554–556, 1975.

30. Daniels SM, Fenley JD, Powers PS, et al: Self-inflicted burns: a ten year retrospective study, *J Bum Care Rehabil* 12:144–147, 1991.

31. Tuohig GM, Saffle JR, Sullivan JJ, et al: Self-inflicted patient burns: suicide versus mutilation, *J Burn Care Rehabil* 16:429–436, 1995.

32. Stoddard FJ: Coping with pain: a developmental approach to treatment of burned children, *Am J Psychiatry* 139: 6:736, 1982.

33. Stoddard FJ, Sheridan R, Selter L: General surgery: basic principles. In Stoudemire, editor: *Psychiatric Care of the Medical Patient, ed 2*, New York: Oxford University Press.

34. Watkins PN, Cook EL, May SR, et al: Psychological stages in adaptation following burn injury: a method for facilitating psychological recovery of burn victims, *J Burn Care Rehabil* 9:376, 1988.

35. Scheeringa M, Zeanah C, Drell MJ, et al: New finding on alternative criteria for PTSD in preschool children, *J Am Acad Child Adolesc Psychiatry* 42:5:561–570, 2003.

36. Stoddard FJ, Ronfeldt H, Saxe G, et al: Identification of symptoms of stress in 12–48 month old burn patients, *J Burn Care Rehabil* 24:2:S 160.

37. Perry SW: Undermedication for pain on a burn unit, *Gen Hosp Psychiatry* 6:308–316, 1984.

38. Szyfelbein SK, Osgood PF, Carr DB: The assessment of pain and plasma β-endorphin immunoactivity in burned children, *Pain* 22:173, 1985.

39. Kavanaugh CK, Lasoff E, Eide Y, et al: Learned helplessness and the pediatric burn patient: dressing change behavior and serum cortisol and beta endorphin, *J Pain Symp Manage* 6:106–177, 1991.

40. Ptacek JT, Patterson DR, Montgomery BM, et al: The relationship between pain during hospitalization and disability at one month post-burn, Proceedings of the American Burn Association, 1994, Orlando, Fla.

41. Marvin JA, Carrougher G, Bayley B, et al: Burn nursing delphi study: setting research priorities, *J Burn Care Rehabil* 12:190–197, 1991.

42. Atchison NE, Osgood PF, Carr DB, et al: Pain during burn dressing changes in children: relationship to burn area, depth, and analgesia regimen, *Pain* 47:41–45, 1991.

43. Porter F: *Pain assessment in children: infants.* In Schechter NL, Berde CB, Yaster M, editors: *Pain in infants, children, and adolescents*, Baltimore, 1993, Williams & Wilkins.

44. Mathews JR, McGrath PJ, Pigeon H: Assessment and measurement of pain in children. In Schechter NL, Berde CB, Yaster M, editors: *Pain in infants, children, and adolescents*, Baltimore, 1993, Williams & Wilkins.

45. Patterson DR, Burns GL, Everett JJ, et al: Hypnosis for the treatment of burn pain, *J Consult Clin Psychol* 60:5:713–717, 1992.

46. Kuttner L: Hypnotic interventions for children in pain. In Schechter N, Berde CB, Yaster M, editors: *Pain in infants, children, and adolescents.* Baltimore, 1993, Williams & Wilkins.

47. Foertsch CE, O'Hara MW, Stoddard FJ, et al: Treatment-resistant pain and distress during pediatric burn-dressing changes, *J Burn Care Rehabil* 19:219–224, 1998.

48. Spiegel H, Spiegel D: *Trance and treatment: clinics uses of hypnosis*, New York, 1978, Basic Books.

49. Ewin DM: Emergency room hypnosis for the burned patient, *Am J Clin Hypn* 26:5–8, 1983.

50. Tarnowski KJ, McGrath ML, Calhoun MB, et al: Pediatric burn injury: self-versus therapist-mediated debridement, *J Pediatr Psychol* 12:567–579, 1987.

51. Cassem EH, Lake CR, Boyer WF: Psychopharmacology in the ICU. In Chernow B: *The pharmacologic approach to the critically ill patient*, Baltimore, 1994, Williams & Wilkins.

52. Daly W, Sheridan R, Stoddard F, et al: Taking the conflict out of pain management: an institutional approach, Proceedings of the 26th Annual Meeting of the American Burn Association, 1994, Orlando, Fla.

53. Carr DB, Osgood PF, Szyfelbein SK: Treatment of pain in acutely burned children. In Schechter N, Berde CB, Yaster M, editors: *Pain in infants, children, and adolescents*, Baltimore, 1993, Williams & Wilkins.

54. Sheridan RL, McEttrick M, Bacha G, et al: Midazolam infusion in pediatric patients with burns who are undergoing mechanical ventilation, *J Bum Care Rehabil* 15:515–518, 1994.

55. Martyn JAJ, Greenblatt DJ, Quinby WC: Diazepam kinetics in patients with severe burns, *Aneth Analg* 62: 293–297, 1983.

56. Martyn JAJ, Greenblatt DJ: Lorazepam conjugation unimpaired in burned patients, *Clin Pharmacol Ther* 43:250–255, 1988.

57. Brown RL, Henke A, Greenhalgh DG, et al: The use of haloperidol in the agitated, critically ill pediatric patient with burns, *J Bum Care Rehabil* 17:34–38, 1996.

58. Sanders KM, Minnema AM, Murray GB: Low incidence of extrapyramidal symptoms in treatment of delirium with intravenous haloperidol and lorazepam in intensive care units, *J Intens Care* 4:201–204, 1989.

59. Aeifman CW, Breidman B: Torsades de pointes: potential consequence of intravenous haloperidol in the intensive care unit, *Intensive Careworld* 63:109–112, 1994.

60. American Psychiatric Association: Benzodiazepine dependence, toxicity, and abuse: a task force report of the American Psychiatric Association, Washington, DC, 1990, American Psychiatric Association.

61. Hamburg DA, Hamburg B, deGoza S: Adaptive problems and mechanisms in severely burned patients, *Psychiatry* 16:1–20, 1953.

62. Steiner H, Clark WB: Psychiatric complications of burned adults: a classification, *J Trauma* 17:134–143, 1977.

63. Andreasen NJC, Norris AS, Hartford CE: Incidence of long-term psychiatric complications in severely burned adults, *Ann Surg* 174:725–733, 1971.

64. Stoddard FJ, Norman DK, Murphy JM, et al: Psychiatric outcome of burned children, *J Am Acad Child Adolesc Psychiatry* 28:589–595, 1989.

65. Andreasen NJ, Hartford CE, Knott JR, et al: EEG changes associated with burn delirium, *Dis Nerv Sys* 38:27–31, 1977.

66. Antoon AY, Volpe JJ, Crawford JD: Burn encephalopathy in children, *Pediatrics* 50:609–616, 1972.

67. Blank K, Perry S: Relationship of psychological processes during delirium to outcome, *Am J Psychiatry* 141:843–847, 1984.

68. Stoddard FJ, Wilens TE: *Delirium*. In Jellinek MS, Herzog DB, editors: *Psychiatric aspects of general hospital pediatrics*, Chicago, 1990, Yearbook Medical Publishers.

69. American Psychiatric Association: *Diagnostic and statistical manual of mental disorders, ed 4*, Washington, DC, 1994, American Psychiatric Association.

70. Gilboa G, Friedman M, Tsur H: The burn as a continuous traumatic stress: implications for emotional treatment during hospitalization, *J Burn Care Rehabil* 15:86, 1994.

71. Rivlin E, Forshaw A, Polowyi G, et al: A multidisciplinary group approach to counseling the parents of burned children, *Burns* 12:479, 1986.

72. Goin JM, Goin MK: *Changing the body: psychological effects of plastic surgery*, Baltimore, 1981, Williams and Wilkins.

73. Solnit AJ, Priel B: Psychological reactions to facial and hand burns in young men, *Psychoanal Study Child* 30:549–566, 1975.

74. Stoddard FJ: Body image development in the burned child, *J Am Acad Child Psychiatry* 21:502–507, 1982.

75. Fauerbach JA, Heinberg LJ, Lawrence JW, et al: Effect of early body image dissatisfaction on subsequent psychological and physical adjustment after disfiguring injury, *Psychosom Med* 62(4):576–582, 2000.

76. Pruzinsky T, Doctor M: *Body images and pediatric burn injury*. In Tarnowski KJ, editor: *Behavioral aspects of pediatric burn injuries*, New York, 1994, Plenum Press.

77. Blumenfield M, Reddish PM: Identification of psychologic impairment in patients with mild-moderate thermal injury: small burn, big problem, *Gen Hosp Psychiatry* 9:142–146, 1987.

78. Tarnowski KJ, Rasnake LK: *Long-term psychosocial sequelae*. In Tarnowski KJ, editor: *Behavioral aspects of pediatric burns*, New York, 1994, Plenum Press.

79. Patterson DR, Everett JJ, Bombardier CH, et al: Psychological effects of severe burn injuries, *Psychol Bull* 113:362–378, 1993.

80. Blakeney P, Meyer W, Robert R, et al: Long-term psychosocial adaptation of children who survive burns involving 80% or greater total body surface area, *J Trauma Injury Infec Crit Care* 44(4):625–634, 1998.

81. Pynoos RS: Traumatic stress and developmental psychopathology in children and adolescents, *Rev Psychiatry* 12:205–238, 1993.

82. Stoddard FJ, Norman DK, Murphy JM, et al: Psychiatric outcome of burned children, *J Am Acad Child Adolesc Psychiatry* 28:589–595, 1989.

83. Kravitz M, McCoy BJ, Tompkins DM, et al: Sleep disorders in children after burn injury, *J Burn Care Rehabil* 14:83–90, 1993.

84. Roca RP, Spence RJ, Munster AM: Posttraumatic adaptation and distress among adult burn survivors, *Am J Psychiatry* 149:1234–1238, 1992.

85. Perry SJ, Difede J, Musngi G, et al: Predictors of posttraumatic stress disorder after burn injury, *Am J Psychiatry* 149:931–935, 1992.

86. Powers PS, Cruse W, Daniels S, et al: Posttraumatic stress disorder in patients with burns, *J Burn Care Rehabil* 15:147–153, 1994.

87. Solomon SD, Gerity ET, Muff AM: Efficacy of treatments for posttraumatic stress disorder, *JAMA* 268:633–638,1992.

88. Jellinek MS, Todres ID, Catlin EA, et al: Pediatric intensive care training: confronting the dark side, *Crit Care Med* 21:775–779, 1993.

89. Saxe G, Chawla N, Stoddard F, et al: The child stress disorders checklist: a measure of ASD and PTSD in children, *J Am Acad Child Adolesc Psychiatry* 42(8):972–978, 2003.

90. Field MJ and Cassel CK, Eds. *Approaching death: improving care at the end of life*, Washington, DC, Institute of Medicine, National Academy Press, 1997.

91. Schnitzer J, Nankin M, Stoddard FJ: Death and grief counseling in children and adolescents. In Stoudemire, editor: *Psychiatric care of the medical patient, ed 2*, NewYork, 2000, Oxford University Press, pp 1127–1131.

Chapter 39
Chronic Medical Illness and Rehabilitation

Terry Rabinowitz, M.D., D.D.S.
Thomas D. Stewart, M.D.
Gregory L. Fricchione, M.D.

For most of us, optimal physical functioning is part of the normal fabric of our everyday lives. Routine tasks, such as opening a tube of toothpaste, answering the telephone, tying our shoelaces, using the toilet, or combing our hair, take place without much conscious thought or effort. We grow accustomed to these behaviors, forgetting that each one of them took considerable time and effort to master.

Likewise, most of us take good physical health for granted. When we wake each day, we expect that our legs will carry us to the shower, then to work or school, and so forth. We do not expect (or accept) that the slightest exertion will lead to breathlessness or that we might need to check various physiologic parameters throughout the day lest we become hypoglycemic, dehydrated, or more seizure-prone. When we are still quite young, the large majority of us depend on the "autopilot" capabilities of our bodies to get us from place to place, to keep us out of danger, and to adjust to changing environmental demands seamlessly and without much mindful input.

Imagine if you were not born with perfect health. Life is dramatically changed when the ravages of rheumatic fever scar one's heart, or when one's legs are weakened by polio, or mucous plugs caused by cystic fibrosis constantly encumber one's lungs. Life also changes when one suffers a traumatic amputation, hemiparesis, or the complete loss of speech.

These are some of the challenges that face those with chronic medical illnesses or those who need rehabilitation. The behaviors, functions, and outcomes that most of us expect in response to our brain's "request" that our body perform, may never again be available to some of these individuals. Indeed, many of them have never experienced a "normal" response to such demands. Many others may take considerable time before they return to anything that approaches normal or baseline functioning. This chapter addresses the unique problems and challenges faced by patients with chronic medical illnesses and by the psychiatrists who treat them.

Psychiatric Complications Seen in the Context of Chronic Medical Illness and Rehabilitation

Rapid discharge of patients from acute care facilities as quickly as possible is the rule rather than the exception in the United States. Moreover, there is an increasing tendency to divert patients from acute care hospitals to other (lower cost) facilities in order to keep costs in check.[1] Thus, there is a growing need for appropriate aftercare following acute treatment. Many larger hospitals have rehabilitation hospitals attached to them or close by; smaller hospitals often rely on distant rehabilitation centers to provide the specialized, long-term care that they cannot offer.

Unfortunately, many who require rehabilitation and who have a chronic illness are at substantial risk for developing one or more psychiatric complications. Rates of depression, for example, among amputees range from 35% to 58%, while for those with multiple sclerosis it ranges from 6% to 27%, and for those with cancer 6% to 25%.[2] Suicide intent[3] and suicide prevalence rates are also substantially higher among those with chronic illnesses compared to those without such problems. Compared with those with chronic illness, people with cancer have suicide rates that are 15 to 20 times greater, those with spinal cord injuries, 15 times greater, and those with multiple sclerosis, 14 times greater.[2,4]

The consulting psychiatrist will often be asked to help care for patients from among many different diagnostic groups while they are receiving rehabilitative care. Among those patients, the most challenging will be those who have sustained traumatic brain injuries, injuries to their spinal cord, and prolonged and catastrophic medical illnesses. Adding to this, there are patients with preexisting psychiatric conditions, most notably personality disorders, who may decompensate under the stress of prolonged hospitalization, sometimes leading to a sense of powerlessness among their caregivers.[5–7]

Problems that may be Experienced During Rehabilitation

Patients receiving rehabilitative treatments tend to spend a large portion of their time worrying about the future. They anticipate, correctly or incorrectly, difficulties that they will face while adjusting to their new (more medically compromised) lives. Among the domains a patient may worry about are problems with returning home, obtaining financial independence, driving, returning to work, adjusting to changes in appearance, socializing, dealing with stigmatization, engaging in sexual activities, and managing decreased functional capacity.[8–11]

Rehabilitative services may be obtained in a rehabilitation hospital or as an outpatient. This component of their treatment may continue for months or years, much longer than their acute treatment, and it may cause serious disturbances in their usual schedules. During this phase of treatment, patients are usually exposed to a variety of new caregivers,

including physiatrists, nurses, occupational therapists, physical therapists, social workers, vocational therapists, recreational therapists, psychologists, clergy, and psychiatrists. Interactions with so many personnel may be difficult for the patient in ways that are bound to affect the quality of the relationships. Likewise, patients receiving rehabilitative treatments may be exposed to many new, uncomfortable, or painful procedures.

Not uncommonly, we have experienced situations during which significant differences between us and those on whom we are consulting impede empathic connectedness. These obvious differences are often been brought more fully to light when noncaregiver personnel of similar or identical ethnic or cultural backgrounds easily make a connection with someone who has not yet learned to trust the new (and foreign) consultant. Table 39-1 lists some characteristics that may be different between a patient and his or her caregivers that should be considered when a clinician, especially a consulting psychiatrist, tries to make an empathic connection with a patient undergoing rehabilitation.

The Rehabilitation Environment

In addition to the large number of rehabilitation personnel that might be involved in any patient's care, the rehabilitation setting is often different,

Table 39-1. Some Differences Between Psychiatrist and Patient That May Affect the Quality of the Interaction

Gender
Race
Sexual orientation
Age
Religion
Education
Appearance
Financial status
Health
Personality
Profession
Partner/Marital status
Living situation

Adapted from Rabinowitz T, Stern TA: *The patient requiring rehabilitation*. In Stern TA, Herman JB, Slavin PL, editors. *The MGH guide to primary care psychiatry, ed 2*, New York, McGraw-Hill, 2004.

from a patient's perspective, from the acute hospital setting in several important ways. Perhaps most important for the rehabilitation patient is the possibility of physical displacement. With separation from loved ones as well as familiar objects and surroundings, receiving treatment far from home for an extended period may be particularly troublesome and lead to depressed mood, apathy, or hopelessness.

Other problems that may surface during rehabilitation may hinder timely and successful recovery and produce long-term negative effects for a recovering patient. These include disruptions in school or work attendance as well as stresses on a marriage/partnership and parent-child relationships as a direct result of prolonged hospitalization or incapacity. A patient may also believe that they and their illnesses have caused a financial and/or emotional burden for loved ones, and they feel guilty about the large blocks of time spent on them and the care they require.

Common Psychiatric Problems in Patients Undergoing Rehabilitation and in Those with Chronic Medical Illnesses

The consulting psychiatrist should expect to encounter the full spectrum of psychiatric conditions among their patients with chronic illness who require rehabilitation. However, certain psychiatric diagnoses and conditions are more common in this population. These include depression, cognitive impairment, adjustment disorders, and behavioral difficulties.[1,2]

Although diagnostic criteria for these conditions do not change in the setting of chronic illness or among patients receiving rehabilitative services, it often is more difficult to obtain sufficient data to satisfy the *Diagnostic and Statistical Manual of Mental Disorders Fourth Edition (DSM-IV)* criteria in this setting. Our clinical experience leads us to conclude that, in these circumstances, it is most appropriate to treat symptoms rather than diagnoses. Although a large proportion of patients who are receiving rehabilitative care and coping with chronic medical illnesses appear depressed, confused, or anxious, when certain clinical assessment instruments are employed a sizable proportion of these patients do not meet diagnostic criteria for

the condition. However, clinicians know that symptoms should be treated.

This inability to reach a diagnostic threshold may be due in part to shared communication deficits between the clinician and the patient. Many of the conditions that afflict rehabilitating patients wreak havoc on their ability to communicate their most basic feelings and emotions. Likewise, clinicians may be fooled because the usual affective "music" associated with various mood states in the healthy population may not be present in the chronically ill. In these circumstances, we believe that it is far better to err on the side of too much treatment than too little treatment, so that this population has the greatest chance of improving.

Delirium is of particular importance in rehabilitation patients. An acute confusional state is at times present during an acute hospitalization, and it may "follow" the patient to the rehabilitation center without ever having been detected. Its presence may adversely affect prognosis and lead to an increased length of stay or the need for a nursing home placement.[13] However, it is also possible for delirium to develop during rehabilitation when, for example, a new medication is administered or an infection develops.[14]

Several important predisposing and precipitating risk factors for the development of delirium are often present among patients undergoing rehabilitation and management of chronic illness. Risk factors include visual or hearing impairment, cognitive impairment, history of stroke, presence of an intracranial lesion, ongoing infection, and regular use of psychotropic drugs.[12]

Chronic or Disabling Conditions and Their Impact on Psychiatric Diagnosis and Treatment

Disabling conditions can confound both psychiatric diagnosis and treatment. For example, the pathophysiology of strokes can interfere with the expression of cognition or affect, functions often required by psychiatrists to make a diagnosis.[15] Treatment can be influenced as well, for example, when acute cervical spinal cord injury is accompanied by psychosis and delirium. Oculogyric crisis related to use of neuroleptics for treatment of psychosis can generate further spinal cord injury. This section will explore these disabilities and others that complicate psychiatric diagnoses and treatment.

Strokes can generate disorders of communication that can mislead treating physicians. Aprosodia is an underappreciated example of dysfunctional post-stroke communication. It involves an impaired ability to convey affect through inflection, gesture, and facial expression.[16] The damage is in the nondominant frontotemporal region and is an analogue of aphasia, which is associated with the frontotemporal region of the dominant hemisphere. Expressive aprosodia disrupts the music of communication that supports the lyrics that are affected by aphasia.

Aprosodic patients sometimes have depressive cognitions, but they cannot convey their depressive mood; this leads to underdiagnosis of depression. On the other hand, a patient with an expressive aprosodia is sometimes misdiagnosed as having depression when his or her unemotional speech is taken as a sign of a mood disorder. Several approaches can detect defects in prosody. First one wants to know if the nondominant hemisphere is damaged; this can be gleaned from detection of hemi-plegia and by associated head magnetic resonance imaging (MRI) findings. Then the examiner can ask the patient to repeat a neutral sentence, such as, "I am going to the store," in an emotional way that signifies happiness, sadness, and anger in succession. Failure to do these well suggests expressive aprosodia. If the patient cannot detect changes in tonality of the examiner when reciting the phrase (when the patient cannot see the examiner's face) then a receptive aprosodia is suggested. In aprosodic patients, careful observation of vegetative signs, such as decreased appetite, take on a greater significance, as does a personal and family history of depression.

Strokes in the nondominant parietal lobe can produce anosognosia, as originally described by Babinski. This condition involves denial of deficits on the left side of the body; however, it can also involve irritability, crying, and denial of depression that are all too evident to family and staff. The patient's failure to report depressive experience in anosognosia can also lead to underdiagnosis.

Dominant hemisphere lesions generate confounds for psychiatric diagnosis as well. The most prominent are the aphasias. Fluent aphasia, such as Wernicke's, presents with well-articulated incoherence and failure to comprehend without a motor/sensory deficit. This disordered, fluent speech can be confused with the loose thinking found in schizophrenia. History is the key for differentiating fluent aphasia with sudden onset in a previously well-functioning patient from schizophrenia, where an insidious onset along with emotional and social impoverishment is evident. It is the rare consulting psychiatrist who has not been called to see a patient with a fluent aphasia (who has recently had a stroke) in order to rule out schizophrenia.

Nonfluent aphasia, such as seen with a Broca's aphasia, features slow, telegraphic, but coherent speech with impaired word-finding ability. Through yes-no questions, such patients can be helped to express their feelings. Facial expressions associated with depression remain intact.

Strokes and multiple sclerosis can lead to the overdiagnosis of major depressive disorder (MDD). For example, lesions of the frontal lobe can produce abulia, a syndrome featuring apathy, a loss of motivation, and a loss of goal-directed behavior. Stroke- and multiple sclerosis–related abulia can lead to the misdiagnosis of depression as the cause for the observed amotivational state.

A few observations can reduce the likelihood of diagnostic error in abulia. Sudden onset is characteristic of cerebrovascular accident (CVA)-related abulia, but not of MDD. Abulic, but not depressed, patients may display a wide affective range despite lacking motivation. They are also less apt to be preoccupied with suicide. As is true of the aprosodias, careful observation of vegetative symptoms along with knowledge of the patient's history can help one differentiate neurologic conditions from psychiatric ones.

Pathologic crying and pseudobulbar affect can mislead clinicians and patients regarding the presence of MDD. This type of crying, or sometimes laughing, is spontaneous and incongruent with the thought content. Neurovegetative symptoms of depression are minimal or absent between affective displays. For unclear reasons, pathologic crying is often ameliorated with use of low-dose tricyclics, even in the absence of an associated change in mood.

Other brain-related disabilities (e.g., Parkinson's disease [PD], Alzheimer's dementia [AD], and temporal lobe epilepsy [TLE]) also create perplexing problems for the diagnosis and treatment of depression. Apathy, masked facies, cognitive slowing, sleep disturbance, and fatigue are features of PD and depression that complicate diagnosis. It is not surprising that several studies have shown that, in general, neurovegetative symptoms do not help separate depression from underlying PD. However, two symptoms—appetite disturbance and early morning awakening—do have discriminative power to help diagnose depression. The symptoms that correlate most significantly with depression in PD patients, as measured by the Hamilton Depression Scale, are suicidal thoughts and feelings of guilt.[17] The highest correlations using the Montgomery-Asberg Depression Rating Scale were observed for depression (0.75) and anhedonia (0.74).[18]

The pathophysiology of PD overlaps with that of MDD. Reduced catecholamine neurotransmitter release in the midbrain is implicated in both, thus raising interesting possibilities for treating both conditions with the same medication. Unfortunately, convincing evidence is lacking regarding the notion that improvement in dyskinetic movements with dopaminergic treatment lessens depression. Selective serotonin-reuptake inhibitors (SSRIs), on the other hand, can lessen depression in this population; unfortunately, they may worsen dyskinesia through reductions in dopamine release that accompany increased serotonin receptor activity. Conclusive evidence that dyskinesia worsens in PD with the use of SSRIs is lacking. Electroconvulsive therapy (ECT) is effective in both MDD and PD, relieving depression and reducing parkinsonian symptoms for up to several weeks.

Alzheimer's disease shares several features with both PD and MDD.[19] All three have depleted brainstem aminergic nerve cell functioning. This common pathology contributes to apathy, impaired concentration, and reduced short-term memory seen in all three. The high comorbidity of MDD in AD and PD is understandable. MDD may be the initial presentation in late-life AD and is prominent in the differential diagnosis for reversible dementias.[20] In addition depression at anytime in life appears to increase risk for AD.

What distinguishes the presentation of depression of MDD in late life in those with and without AD? Those with AD and MDD are less apt to experience excessive guilt, disturbed sleep, and feelings of worthlessness; however, they are more apt to

describe indecisiveness and an inability to concentrate, which is consistent with cognitive decline. It is noteworthy that there is no change in the frequency of the features of MDD with the severity of AD, except for psychosis, which increases with the severity of AD.

Successful treatment of MDD in AD can reduce agitation, improve quality of life, and reduce caretaker stress. Antidepressants with significant anticholinergic properties, such as tricyclic antidepressants, should not be used because they undermine the already depleted cholinergic reserves seen in those with AD. In apathetic AD patients, it is reasonable to use antidepressants that increase synaptic catecholamines, such as bupropion and venlafaxine (with a dose greater than 200 mg/day). For those who are anxious and agitated, SSRIs or mirtazapine are appropriate, although definitive studies to support these choices are lacking.

Of the epilepsies, TLE, including complex partial seizures, is the most commonly (roughly 20%) associated with psychiatric findings; 14% of these patients exhibit psychosis during postictal and interictal states.[21,22] Care is needed to make psychiatric diagnoses associated with TLE while patients have a clear sensorium, not when they are ictal or in a postictal state.

According to Geschwind,[23] psychopathology exists during interictal periods in those with TLE. The interictal syndrome (named after Geschwind) also features hypergraphia, seriousness, humorlessness, and an intense interest in philosophic, moral, or religious issues. In addition, afflicted patients tend to be viscous, that is, having a tendency to talk on and on and circumstantially about a restricted range of topics. One famous person with these traits, Dostoyevsky, is thought to have had TLE.

Two clues can raise suspicion that TLE, and not primary psychiatric illness, is the driving force behind persistent psychiatric symptoms. The first is treatment-resistant psychosis. Neuroleptics can reduce seizure threshold and can make the psychosis related to TLE worse.

Another clue is the incongruity between severe psychosis and the patient's ability to function socially when psychotic symptoms are quiescent. In essence, the gut feeling that the patient is not schizophrenic is critical to assessing a recurrently psychotic individual. Making the correct diagnosis of TLE leads to treatment of the underlying seizure disorder and to the amelioration of psychosis. Nevertheless there is a risk of interictal psychosis in these patients, which increases with the frequency of the seizure episodes.

TLE is difficult to diagnose because the seizure activity may be deeply imbedded in the limbic system; deep electric signals are not easily accessible to surface electrodes or even to sphenoidal electrodes used during sleep. The failure to find those signals can lead to an incorrect diagnosis of conversion disorder or of malingering. However, the diagnosis of seizures and epilepsy is based largely on the clinical state and not solely on the electroencephalogram (EEG).

Spinal cord injury can also confound psychiatric diagnosis and treatment. Acute high cervical injury can lead to sensory deprivation due to the sudden loss of sensory input from the neck down coupled with head restraint by tongs. The apathy and withdrawal under these conditions can be misread as MDD. Treatment of depression should not start before the first month postquadriplegia to allow for increased sensory input as more stimulation becomes possible and depression-inducing steroids are no longer being used to quell spinal cord edema. Should symptoms of major depression persist 1 month after the injury, then it is reasonable to begin treatment. Another potential psychiatric issue following spinal cord injury is the persistence of body perception; that is, of being in the same position as one was in at the time of the injury, for example, on a motorcycle. The patient knows this compelling perception is untrue and may secretly feel insane. The question, "Do you have any strange sensations?" can unearth this problem and allow for a reassuring explanation.

Treatment considerations exist as well. Oculogyric crisis following neuroleptic use in acute cervical injury, mentioned earlier, can be minimized by the use of atypical neuroleptics. Should an injectable neuroleptic be required for severe agitation in the setting of acute cervical injury, intramuscular ziprasidone would be preferable to intramuscular haloperidol due to a lower incidence of extrapyramidal effects, or one can use intravenous haloperidol.

Orthostasis is a problem in quadriplegia due to disruption of central nervous system (CNS) controls, both excitation and inhibition, over the paraspinal sympathetic ganglia. This autonomic vulnerability requires that psychotropic medication with potent α-blocking properties be avoided as much as possible in the immediate postinjury period.

Sexual dysfunction is a major concern in the spinal cord injury patient. Male patients with upper motor neuron lesions above S4 have fairly good outcomes in terms of ability to achieve stimulated or manipulated erections, whereas those with lower motor neuron damage to the sacral plexus have poorer outcomes. Sildenafil-treated patients have improved erection response rates and a substantial number of individuals with complete lesions, regardless of level or lower motor neuron lesions, also benefit from it.[24]

Being depressed is sometimes viewed as a natural sequelae of cardiovascular disease (CVD), and thus depression may not be recognized as an independent clinical entity. Morbidity and mortality due to CVD transcends that of any other disability in the Western world. Detection and treatment of depression in this population is critical, because an expanding literature demonstrates that depression and CVD are highly comorbid and that depression, independent of CVD severity, increases CVD-related morbidity and mortality.

Depression is an independent risk factor for coronary artery disease. MDD at the time of myocardial infarction (MI) increases mortality 3.5-fold over a 2-year period, and this depression does not correlate with MI severity. Major depression, as well as ejection fraction, also predicts MI survival.

The potential mechanisms for this impact are unfolding. Depression activates platelets in those with CVD, and fibrinogen and factor VII levels increase. Depression also reduces heart rate variability (HRV), which is a risk factor for cardiac events. Atherosclerosis is an inflammatory disease as indicated by the fact that the presence of C-reactive protein increases cardiac risk. Depression is associated with increases in macrophage activity and the presence of proinflammatory cytokines like interleukin-6 (IL-6). In light of the foregoing, it is becoming more understandable that cardiac mortality increases with depressed mood and increases even more so with major depression.

Selection of antidepressants may be critical in the management of CVD. There is evidence from a large retrospective study of depressed patients after an MI showing a confound-adjusted 35% reduction in second MI occurrence over a 28-month period with sertraline treatment, compared to those lacking treatment for depression.[25]

Putative mechanisms for this risk reduction are unfolding. SSRIs reduce platelet activation in those with CVD. They also reduce IL-6 levels. SSRIs increase HRV in the immediate post-MI period, thus correcting the cardiac rhythm overregularization found in depression. Recent literature suggests, but does not prove, that SSRI treatment post-MI reduces cardiovascular sudden death over a 1-year period.[25] One such study established that sertraline has no inotropic or chronotropic effects 1 month post-MI, and thus it appears to be safe in this population. This finding may represent a class effect.

Depression is commonly comorbid with CVD. As such, it increases morbidity and mortality, as much as hypertension does with comorbid diabetes. Aggressive treatment of hypertension in diabetics lengthens the quality and quantity of life. Similarly, treatment of depression in CVD may not only improve mood and related self-care, but may possibly address the pathologic processes of CVD, such as platelet activation and reduced HRV.

Consulting psychiatrists face a perplexing problem when asked to assess physically disabled patients for whom there is no established pathophysiologic basis. The framed question is: "Does this patient have conversion disorder?" The importance of this question is underlined by the finding that as many as 50% of those diagnosed as having conversion disorder subsequently develop medical diagnoses consistent with a disability at a later date. Usually multiple sclerosis is involved. More recent literature, possibly reflecting improved diagnostic techniques, finds only 4.3% of those with conversion disorder developed subsequent medical illness that could have explained the prior presenting findings in conversion disorder.[26] This same study, however, revealed substantial psychiatric comorbidity (with 50% meeting the *International Statistical Classification of Diseases and Related Health Problems, revision 10* [*ICD-10*] criteria for mental illness, especially personality disorder) in this population.

Although undetected medical illnesses in conversion disorder now appear common, paraneoplastic disorders are an infrequent but important exception. Paresthesias or memory loss are two findings that can appear without a supporting medical diagnosis until is it discovered as a *forme fruste* of cancer. These symptoms appear to be mediated by the immunologic response to the tumor that attacks neural tissue. Thus, an oncologic evaluation and work-up for otherwise unexplained memory loss or paresthesia is warranted.

Conversion disorders can produce medical complications. For example, conversion-based lower extremity paralysis can lead to Achilles tendon contracture, decubiti, and pulmonary emboli. Psychiatric consultation in these patients should thus draw attention to their prevention. In addition aggressive treatment of comorbid psychiatric conditions, such as depression and psychosis, can reduce emotional suffering. However, addressing psychiatric comorbidity does not usually ameliorate the conversion-based physical findings.

Medical disabilities influence psychiatric diagnosis and treatment in ways that are specific for each condition. Lack of standardized and validated depression screening instruments for chronic medically ill patients compounds the problem of detecting depression in chronically ill people with malaise. Proper psychiatric diagnosis and treatment can enhance quality of life in those with disability.

Diagnosis and Treatment

Psychiatric treatment in the context of rehabilitative medicine or chronic illness may bear little resemblance to routine psychiatric care. Patients from these groups may be engaged in so many activities during the day that it is often impossible to sit with them for long periods at a time. They may require intensive physical and occupational therapy, time-consuming diagnostic studies, and longer and more frequent rest periods. In addition, many of these persons will be far from home and loved ones. Visits from these important people will likely take precedence over prescribed and/or necessary treatments and interviews. These and other activities will compete for (and usually win) the time necessary to accurately assess, diagnose, and treat psychiatric conditions in this population.

Psychiatrists unfamiliar with this milieu may quickly become frustrated by their lack of success in capturing enough "quality time" with a patient. However, rather than becoming frustrated, we suggest they think of this as an opportunity to practice and fine-tune their skills with this challenging group. Over this period for the patient in rehabilitation, assessment and treatment can effectively take place. The rehabilitation hospital setting provides the consulting psychiatrist with an opportunity to get to know his or her patient; to do so requires that he or she accurately identify the oftentimes unclear question or questions embedded in the request for consultation. It is also of key importance for the psychiatrist to assess the personality and coping styles the patient facing the protracted challenges of rehabilitation in chronic medical illness. Oftentimes it is maladaptive coping that delays or even prevents improvement in the patient's condition. Supporting adaptive strategies and helping to build social support are important in the psychiatric care of these patients. Table 39-2 presents some key domains that should be explored *before* a consultation is begun. Table 39-3 provides important core questions to be

Table 39-2. Questions To Be Addressed Prior to Consultation

Who is requesting the consultation?
What is the problem(s)?
　This is best determined from personal contact with the consultees or their designee, not from information obtained by secretaries or others.
Who will implement the recommendations?
　This may seem obvious, but many recommendations are never implemented because of miscommunication between the consultant and consultee.
　We recommend that orders be written by the consultee except when waiting would significantly compromise patient care.
Does the patient know that a consultation has been requested?
　If not, why?
　Is there a concern about capacity/competence?
　If there is no concern about competence or capacity, the patient should be informed of the request for consultation and consent to its performance.
When is the best time to see the patient?
Can time be reserved for an interview?
　If not, what are potentially available times?
Can family/friends and important others (e.g., RN, LPN, MD) be available if necessary?

Table 39-3. Core Questions for All Patients Receiving Rehabilitation or with Chronic Illnesses

Have they ever been under the care of the psychiatrist or received psychiatric treatment?
Do they take any medications for a psychiatric condition?
Have they ever been suicidal or made a suicidal gesture or attempt?
Is there any history of violence?
Have they ever received inpatient or outpatient treatment for substance abuse or dependence?
Have they ever been in trouble with the law?
　Now or in the past?
　Any jail or prison time?
Have they ever received rehabilitative treatment before?
　How did it go?
　Where they cooperative, disruptive, threatening, or violent?
Is there any history of delirium?
Is there any history of brain injury?
What is the level of intellectual/cognitive functioning?
　Is this a change from baseline?
What are their social supports?
　Are they reliable?
　How have they performed in the past?
Do they know someone who has an illness like them or
　Who has received rehabilitative care?
　How did that person do?
How did they do:
　In school?
　At work?
　With their partner or spouse and family?
　In the military?

Adapted from Rabinowitz T, Stern TA: *The patient requiring rehabilitation.* In Stern TA, Herman JB, Slavin PL, editors. *The MGH guide to primary care psychiatry, ed 2,* New York, McGraw-Hill, 2004.

answered for all rehabilitation and chronic illness patients, and Table 39-4 offers more specific questions for this population.

We can divide possible treatments into two broad categories: psychotherapeutic and pharmacologic/somatic. However, although these categories may kindle specific ideas in the minds of most psychiatrists, the way these treatments are delivered to this patient population will often be very different from what may have been learned or practiced elsewhere. Specific pharmacologic indications and recommendations as well as the use of and indications for ECT are covered elsewhere in this text.

Considering psychotherapy, any modality may be appropriate for some patients in this group,[2] but some may be more suitable than others. Many

Table 39-4. Focused Questions for All Patients in Rehabilitation or Chronic Illness Settings

What is the meaning of the illness or injury to the patient?
Is their condition hereditary?
  Are there affected relatives?
  If yes, how are they doing?
  If the condition is hereditary, are there markers that can be searched for in others?
  How do they feel about such searches?
How has the condition or situation affected their self-esteem?
  Do not ask *if* self-esteem has been affected—this will give the patient the unfortunate opportunity to say "No" and shut down the interview.
How do they feel their condition has affected family and friends?
How are they adjusting to change or loss of function in the following areas:
  Academic
  Athletic
  Creative
  Intellectual
  Occupational
  Sex
  Other
Are they taking medication(s)?
  Is it helping?
  Are there side effects?
  What are they?

Adapted from Rabinowitz T, Stern TA: *The patient requiring rehabilitation.* In Stern TA, Herman JB, Slavin PL, editors. *The MGH guide to primary care psychiatry, ed 2*, New York, McGraw-Hill, 2004.

patients may have never received psychotherapy before and may be suspicious or doubtful of its efficacy. It has been our experience that this is not the time for deep explorations into the unconscious or for a passive psychotherapeutic approach that may be fitting in other settings. These patients often struggle with some very basic problems: learning to walk with a prosthesis following a traumatic amputation, adjusting to the new need for continuous oxygen, and adapting to significant loss of cognitive functioning. When conducting psychotherapy with these patients, we recommend focusing on the chief complaint; we pay much less attention to other areas that might be of interest but that must take a "backseat" in these patients who have so little free time and energy. The psychiatrist should expect to take a more active role in the psychotherapy of these individuals. That is, he or she should expect to give advice and guidance where appropriate, and not necessarily wait for a patient to experience an epiphany that may take too long (or forever) to arrive.

Facilitating questions and applying limbic probes may prove useful in the psychotherapeutic arsenal. For instance, commenting on a patient's affect by saying something like: "You seem so down today. Are you feeling blue?" may give a patient who is emotionally defended the opportunity to connect with their internal world and to release stored-up emotional pressure. Likewise, a nonoffensive joke or silly gesture may slide past cortical "sentinels" directly into the limbic system and evoke an expansive smile or a hearty laugh in someone who is despondent but who wants to feel better.

Conclusion

Patients with chronic illnesses or those who are receiving rehabilitation may evoke strong emotions in their caregivers. Psychiatrists who perform consultations on these patients are not immune to these emotions. We may find ourselves thanking our stars that we have escaped such unfortunate circumstances or, at the other extreme, we may find that we are imagining ourselves in such desperate straits. In either case, we have a mandate to bind our anxiety and perhaps our horror at what has occurred to a fellow human being and to make an empathic connection so that someone can benefit from our expertise. There are few rewards as great as seeing the smile on the face or the twinkle in the eye of someone who just a short while ago considered throwing in the towel.

References

1. Rabinowitz T, Stern TA: *The patient requiring rehabilitation.* In Stern TA, Herman JB, Slavin PL, editors: *The MGH guide to primary care psychiatry, ed 2*, New York, McGraw-Hill, 2004.
2. Bishop DS, Pet LR: *Physical medicine and rehabilitation.* In Wise MG, Rundell JR, editors: *Textbook of consultation-liaison psychiatry: psychiatry in the medically ill, ed 2*, Washington, DC, 2002, American Psychiatric Publishing, pp 729–751.
3. Feinstein A: An examination of suicidal intent in patients with multiple sclerosis. [comment], *Neurology* 59:674–678, 2002.

4. Stewart TD: *Spinal cord-injured patients: the Massachusetts General Hospital handbook of general hospital psychiatry, ed 4*, St. Louis, 1997, Mosby.

5. Groves JE: Taking care of the hateful patient, *N Engl J Med* 298:883–887, 1978.

6. Groves JE: *Personality disorders I: general approaches to difficult patients*. In Stern TA, Herman JB, Slavin PL, editors: *The MGH guide to psychiatry in primary care*, New York, 1998, McGraw-Hill, pp 591–598.

7. Groves JE: *Personality disorders II: approaches to specific behavioral presentations*. In Stern TA, Herman JB, Slavin PL, editors: *The MGH guide to psychiatry in primary care*, New York, 1998, McGraw-Hill, pp 599–604.

8. Mazaux JM, Richer E: Rehabilitation after traumatic brain injury in adults, *Disability Rehabil* 20:435–447, 1998.

9. Grosbois JM, Douay B, Fortin F, et al: Effects of ambulatory respiratory rehabilitation on exercise tolerance and quality of life in chronic obstructive lung disease patients [comment], *Rev Malad Respir* 13:61–67, 1996.

10. Coyle CP, Santiago MC, Shank JW, et al: Secondary conditions and women with physical disabilities: a descriptive study, *Arch Phys Med Rehabil* 81:1380–1387, 2000.

11. O'Neill ES: Illness representations and coping of women with chronic obstructive pulmonary disease: a pilot study, *Heart Lung* 31:295–302, 2002.

12. American Psychiatric Association: *Diagnostic and statistical manual of mental disorders, ed 4*, Washington, DC, 1994, American Psychiatric Press.

13. Rabinowitz T: Delirium: an important (but often unrecognized) clinical syndrome, *Curr Psychiatry Rep* 4:202–208, 2002.

14. Rabinowitz T, Murphy KM, Nagle KJ, et al: Delirium: pathophysiology, recognition, prevention, and treatment, *Expert Rev Neurotherapeu* 3:89–101, 2003.

15. Black KJ: Diagnosing depression after stroke, *South Med J* 88:699–709, 1995.

16. Ross ED: The aprosodias: functional-anatomic organization of the affective components of language in the right hemisphere, *Arch Neurol* 38:561–569, 1981.

17. Leentjens AFG, Marinus J, Van Hilten JJ, et al: The contribution of somatic symptoms to the diagnosis of depressive disorder in Parkinson's disease: a discriminant analytic approach, *J Neuropsychiatry Clin Neurosci* 15:74–77, 2003.

18. Burn DJ: Depression in Parkinson's disease, *Eur J Neurology* 9(suppl 3):44–54, 2002.

19. Zubenko GS, Zubenko WN, McPherson S, et al: A collaborative study of the emergence and clinical features of the major depressive syndrome of Alzheimer's disease, *Am J Psychiatry* 160:857–866, 2003.

20. Green RC, Cupples A, Kurz A: Depression as a risk factor for Alzheimer disease, *Arch Neurol* 60:753–759, 2003.

21. Tisher PW, Holzer JC, Greenberg M, et al: Psychiatric presentations of epilepsy, *Harvard Rev Psychiatry* 1:219–227, 1993.

22. Onuma T: Classification of psychiatric symptoms in patients with epilepsy, *Epilepsia* 4:1(suppl 9):43–48, 2000.

23. Geshwind, N: Behavioral change in temporal lobe epilepsy, *Arch Neurol,* 34:453, 1977.

24. Derry F, Hultling C, Seftel AD et al. Efficacy and safety of sildenafil citrate (Viagra) in men with erectile dysfunction and spinal cord injury: a review, *Urology* 60(suppl 2):49–57, 2002.

25. Glassman AH, O'Connor, Califf RM, et al: Sertraline treatment of major depression in patients with acute MI or unstable angina, *JAMA* 288:701–709, 2002.

26. Crimlisk HL, Bhatia K, Cope H, et al: Slater revisited: 6 year follow up study of patients with medically unexplained motor symptoms, *Br Med J* 316:582–586, 1998.

Chapter 40
Genetics and Genetic Disorders

Christine T. Finn, M.D.
Joan M. Stoler, M.D.
Jordan W. Smoller, M.D., Sc.D.

Many genetic syndromes and metabolic diseases have psychiatric symptoms as part of their observed presentation. In fact, behavioral manifestations may be as important as other clinical features for identification of underlying genetic illness. While some patients may meet full *DSM-IV* criteria for psychiatric disorders, others may have more general symptoms, like hyperactivity, anxiety, aggression, or cognitive deficits.

This chapter provides a brief overview of a subset of genetic syndromes and inborn errors of metabolism that the general psychiatrist may encounter in the hospital or clinic setting. Although the disorders presented in this chapter are relatively rare, knowing when to suspect that a genetic or metabolic issue may be contributing to the presenting condition of a patient is important in formulating a differential diagnosis. Proper identification of genetic and metabolic illness may allow for new opportunities for treatment or intervention directed at the primary process (e.g., correction of hyperammonemia in urea cycle disorders) rather than management of its downstream effects (e.g., delirium).

For the most part, the disorders reviewed here may present in late childhood to adulthood; the chapter specifically excludes those disorders that are lethal in infancy or early childhood. While it is not considered the role of the psychiatrist to diagnosis specific genetic and metabolic illnesses, knowledge of these disorders aids clinical decision-making for all specialties. When an underlying genetic syndrome or metabolic disease is suspected, a consultation by a geneticist may greatly benefit the patient and help to direct clinical management.

Genetic Syndromes

The normal number of human chromosomes is 46, organized into 23 pairs. Chromosomes numbered 1 to 22 are autosomes; sex chromosomes make up the remaining pair. The sex chromosomes are made up of two X chromosomes in females (46, XX), and one X and one Y chromosome in males (46, XY). Abnormalities of chromosomes may include whole chromosomes (aneuploidy), chromosomal rearrangements (translocations or inversions), small deletions or duplications, or mutations in single genes. Visualization of chromosome number and gross structure is accomplished by karyotype analysis. More recently, other cytogenetic and molecular techniques have allowed for focused study of smaller regions of chromosomes or individual genes. Fluorescent in-situ hybridization (FISH) is a cytogenetic technique that uses florescent probes to investigate the presence of small, submicroscopic chromosomal changes that are beyond the resolution of karyotype analysis.

Genetic syndromes are disorders with a characteristic set of features that are due to an underlying common mechanism. Features can include congenital anomalies, specific physical features, associated medical disorders, cognitive deficits, and psychiatric or behavioral symptoms. When considering a diagnosis of a genetic syndrome, clinicians may be guided by several web-based resources (OMIM, Geneclinics) and software packages (POSSUM) that allow the option of searching for disorders based on observed findings and historical information.

Currently, there are no available treatments that can "cure" genetic syndromes or replace missing genetic material. For this reason, treatment is directed at symptomatic management of physical malformations, surveillance for associated medical conditions, and early developmental interventions. Special education or additional academic supports may be needed. Management of psychiatric and behavioral symptoms is accomplished by a combination of pharmacologic treatment and other therapies, including behavioral techniques.

Assessment of the Patient for Genetic Syndromes

Certain features of the medical history, family history, and physical examination may indicate the possibility of a genetic syndrome that underlies observed psychiatric and behavioral symptoms. In addition to the comprehensive review of systems and medical history completed during the initial assessment of patients, inclusion of questions about pregnancy and the perinatal period, birth defects, and surgeries in infancy or early childhood that may have been performed to correct congenital anomalies may provide valuable clues to an underlying genetic syndrome. In addition, careful review of the developmental history (with special attention paid to early developmental milestones) may reveal the presence of specific developmental delays, mental retardation, or learning disabilities. When inquiring about family history, specific questions about recurrent miscarriages, stillborn children, early infant deaths, a family history of mental retardation, seizures, or congenital illness may help in uncovering an underlying genetic disease, especially when the pattern of illness appears to be Mendelian (e.g., dominant, recessive, or X-linked inheritance). Physical examination may reveal abnormalities of growth, dysmorphic features, or involvement of various organ systems. Results of imaging studies may aid in the assessment of underlying malformations suggested by physical examination (e.g., echocardiogram to rule out structural heart defects when a murmur is appreciated).

Selected Genetic Disorders

Ms. A, an 18-year-old girl, presented to the psychiatric emergency room with auditory hallucinations and paranoid ideation. She had a history of attention deficit hyperactivity disorder (ADHD) and oppositional behavior. Her full-scale IQ was 78, and her verbal IQ was 15 points greater than her performance IQ, characteristic of a nonverbal learning disorder. Review of systems revealed surgery in infancy for correction of a congenital heart defect, and frequent episodes of sinusitis, otitis media, and pneumonia. On physical examination, she was short with a flat facial expression. Facial features included a high-arched palate, a small chin, and a nose with a broad, square nasal root. Ms. A was admitted to the inpatient psychiatric service and treated with atypical neuroleptics with a good result. Consultation with the Genetics service for her dysmorphic facial features and congenital heart defect, along with her cognitive and psychiatric symptoms, resulted in a diagnosis of velocardiofacial syndrome (VCFS).

Disorders Due to Chromosomal Abnormalities and Microdeletions

Velocardiofacial Syndrome/DiGeorge Syndrome. The cohort of patients diagnosed with VCFS, which also includes most patients previously diagnosed with DiGeorge syndrome, is due to a microdeletion on chromosome 22q11.2, which results in the loss of up to 60 known and predicted contiguous genes. VCFS has been called a "genetic subtype of schizophrenia," and it is estimated that as many as 2% of schizophrenics may have this disorder undiagnosed.[1] This rate may be even higher among patients with childhood-onset schizophrenia.[2] Psychiatric symptoms in VCFS patients with schizophrenia do not appear to differ from those in other schizophrenics based on factors such as description of psychosis or comorbid illnesses. Overall, between 60% and 75% of patients with VCFS have significant psychiatric morbidity, including mood disorders, ADHD, autism, substance abuse, anxiety disorders, and oppositional defiant disorder, among others.[3-9] The physical features of those with VCFS include a characteristic facial appearance (broad and squared nasal root, midface hypoplasia, short palpebral fissures, retruded chin), cleft palate, and velopharyngeal insufficiency (which may manifest as hypernasal speech, nasal regurgitation in infancy, or frequent ear infections), congenital heart defects, aplasia of the thymus (leading to immune problems), problems with calcium homeostasis, low muscle tone, and scoliosis. Facial hypotonia may result in a somewhat flat, expressionless appearance. Learning disabilities, especially nonverbal learning disorder, are common. However, patients can exhibit only some of these features and the spectrum of findings may vary even within families. Diagnostic testing is available on a clinical basis and involves testing for the microdeletion with FISH techniques.

Smith-Magenis Syndrome.   Smith-Magenis syndrome is due to a microdeletion of chromosome 17p11.2, resulting in the loss of several contiguous genes at that location. In infancy, these patients may exhibit failure to thrive and hypotonia. Physical findings, which may change over time, include short stature, scoliosis, eye abnormalities, renal problems, heart defects, peripheral neuropathy, and hearing loss (both conductive and sensorineural). Characteristic facial features include a square face with prominent forehead, deep set and upslanting eyes, a broad nasal bridge with a short nose and fleshy nasal tip, full cheeks, and a "cupid's bow" tented upper lip. The jaw becomes more prominent with age. Although they may have hypersomnolence in infancy, a striking feature of this syndrome is marked sleep disturbance, with absence of REM sleep in some patients. In addition, abnormalities of circadian rhythms and melatonin secretion have been documented.[10–12] Most patients have developmental delay, and their IQs may range from borderline intelligence to moderate mental retardation. Patients are described with symptoms of ADHD, tantrums, impulsivity, and a variety of self-injurious behaviors, including onychotillomania (pulling out finger and toe nails) and polyembolokoilamania (insertion of foreign bodies), head banging, face slapping, and skin picking.[13–15] In addition, they may show stereotypies, most commonly a "self hug" when happy.[16] Abnormalities of lipid profiles have been seen in these patients, with elevations of cholesterol, triglycerides, and LDL.[17] Diagnostic testing involves testing for the microdeletion with FISH techniques.

Williams Syndrome.   A microdeletion on chromosome 7q11.23 results in Williams syndrome. Loss of the gene for elastin *(ELN)* is hypothesized to contribute to at least some of the observed phenotypic features, including short stature and microcephaly, cardiac defects (most often supravalvular aortic or supravalvular pulmonic stenosis), and connective tissue disease (joint laxity, hernias, soft skin). Patients with Williams syndrome are described as having an "elfin" facial appearance with a broad forehead that narrows at the temples, a short nose with a fleshy nasal tip, large prominent ear lobes, a wide mouth with full lips, and a small jaw. The iris of the eye has a stellate or lacey appearance. Other characteristics include a hoarse voice and hyperacusis (hypersensitivity to sounds). Mental retardation in the mild-severe range is usually present, with an average IQ of 56. Specific learning deficits in visual-spatial skills are in marked contrast to strengths in verbal and language domains and are important for the identification and care of these patients. Psychiatric symptoms and conditions include autism, ADHD, depression, and anxiety. Patients with this syndrome may show circumscribed interests or obsessions and may be somatically focused. Despite being socially disinhibited and overly friendly, they tend to have difficulty with peer relationships and may become socially isolated.[18,19] Affected individuals are described as overly talkative, a feature that may be, in part, reflective of generalized anxiety.[20] Diagnostic testing involves the detection of the microdeletion with FISH techniques.

Prader-Willi Syndrome.   Although several genetic mechanisms may result in Prader-Willi syndrome, the absence of a critical region of the paternally inherited chromosome 15q11-q13 is central to the disorder. This region of chromosome 15 undergoes the process of imprinting, by which genes are switched on or off depending on whether they are of maternal or paternal origin. In contrast to Prader-Willi syndrome, the absence of the maternally derived region results in Angelman's syndrome (manifest by severe mental retardation, seizures, ataxia, and characteristic behaviors). Prader-Willi patients may be hypotonic and show failure to thrive in infancy. Most have short stature, and have small hands, feet, and external genitalia; some have fair skin and hair coloring. A characteristic facial appearance with upslanting almond-shaped eyes and a thin upper lip is seen. The hallmark behavior of this disorder is hyperphagia, with resultant morbid obesity, which develops early in childhood. Behavioral interventions have been effective in controlling this behavior if started at an early age. Psychiatric symptoms and conditions include obsessional thoughts, compulsions, repetitive behaviors, mood disorders, anxiety, psychosis, ADHD, autism, skin picking, and temper tantrums.[21–25] Afflicted individuals may have a high pain threshold, and they rarely vomit. These patients may show decreased IQ and learning problems, although they also show areas of relative strength in visual-spatial skills (e.g., as with jigsaw puzzles). Diagnostic testing for Prader-Willi syndrome involves analysis of the critical region for methylation status (the process that determines if genes are turned on or off) or the detection of the deletion by FISH techniques.

Down Syndrome. The majority of individuals with Down syndrome are diagnosed soon after birth. This disorder is included in this chapter because of its known association with Alzheimer's dementia, where cognitive decline or changes in behavior in adults with Down syndrome may prompt psychiatric consultation. In 95% of cases, Down syndrome is due to an extra free copy of chromosome 21; the remainder of cases are due to unbalanced translocations or duplications involving the Down syndrome critical region on chromosome 21. Down syndrome is the most common genetic cause of mental retardation; an increased incidence is observed with older maternal age. Most clinicians recognize the characteristic Down's face, which consists of eyes with upslanting palpebral fissures, epicanthal folds, and Brushfield's spots (white spots in the iris), a flat nasal bridge, low-set ears, and a protruding tongue. In addition, they have a short neck, short stature, and single transverse palmar crease. These patients may also have a variety of congenital malformations, including heart defects and duodenal atresia, and they have high rates of hypothyroidism. Mental retardation is seen in the majority of patients, with an average IQ of 24. Social skills are usually more advanced than would be expected based on their level of mental retardation. Decline in cognition or changes in behavior in middle-aged adults with Down syndrome should raise one's suspicion for Alzheimer's disease. The presence of an extra copy of the amyloid precursor protein (*APP*) gene (one of

the causative genes in early onset Alzheimer's disease) on chromosome 21 is thought to contribute to increased rates of dementia in these patients. Nonspecific behavioral symptoms, depression, and anxiety may also be seen.[26–28] Diagnostic testing for Down syndrome involves karyotype analysis of chromosomes.

Turner's Syndrome. The majority of cases of Turner's syndrome are due to the loss of an entire X chromosome, which is designated as 45, X. These patients are females, with physical characteristics of short stature, a webbed neck, and a flat, broad chest. Diagnosis may be delayed until adolescence, when these girls fail to develop secondary sexual characteristics (due to gonadal dysgenesis). Use of hormonal therapy can help to achieve pubertal changes but will not result in fertility. These patients may also have involvement of other organ systems, including congenital heart or kidney disease. Psychiatric symptoms and conditions include ADHD, depression, anxiety, and problems with social skills. Specific learning disabilities (especially visual-spatial deficits) have been reported.[29–31] Diagnostic testing for Turner's syndrome involves karyotype analysis of chromosomes.

Klinefelter's Syndrome. Klinefelter's syndrome is due to the addition of an extra X chromosome, resulting in 47, XXY. These patients are males and usually are described as tall, and they may be somewhat hypotonic and clumsy. They typically have a small penis and testes. Contrary to earlier descriptions, they have a male distribution of body fat and hair, although gynecomastia may be seen. Again, these patients may first be diagnosed in adolescence, due to failure to go through puberty, or as part of an infertility work-up. Use of testosterone can help with the development of secondary sexual characteristics. There have been reports of an increased incidence of ADHD, immaturity, and depression in these patients.[32–34] Cognitively, specific learning disabilities are seen. Diagnostic testing for Klinefelter's syndrome involves karyotype analysis of chromosomes.

47, XYY. Males with an extra copy of the Y chromosome have been of interest to the psychiatric profession for many years, due to reports of increased criminality and antisocial behaviors in these patients. While early studies conducted on criminal populations were limited by ascertainment bias, more recent studies have continued to show small increases in these behaviors in 47, XYY males compared to controls. However, increased rates of antisocial or criminal behavior appear to be related to the cognitive deficits seen in some of these patients.[35] Physical findings may include accelerated linear growth in childhood and tall stature as adults. They may have a lower than average IQ or specific learning disabilities, especially in reading and language domains. Psychiatric conditions include ADHD and conduct disorders.[36] Overall, the majority of these patients may never come to medical attention, as they can be without any identifying features. Diagnostic testing for 47, XYY involves karyotype analysis of chromosomes.

Autosomal Dominant Single-Gene Disorders

Huntington's Disease. Huntington's disease is due to an increased number of CAG triplet repeats in the *HD* gene on chromosome 4p16. The normal number of CAG repeats ranges from 10 to 26 in unaffected individuals, where patients with Huntington's disease have between 36 and 121 repeats. The number of repeats may expand from one generation to the next, and increased severity and earlier onset of illness (known as anticipation) may be seen in subsequent generations. Psychiatric symptoms are prominent in the early presentation of this disorder and may include changes in personality, depression, or apathy. Later, progressive cognitive decline and dementia occur. Mood lability and psychosis may also be seen. A high suicide rate is reported in these patients.[37,38] Early physical findings include dysarthria and clumsiness with deterioration in both voluntary and involuntary movements and the development of chorea. The abnormal movements are often treated with high-potency neuroleptics, but there is no treatment that stops the progressive neurologic decline in this disease. Characteristic atrophy of the caudate and putamen may be apparent on MRI or CT of the brain. Diagnostic testing involves molecular detection of increased number of CAG repeats in the *HD* gene.

Tuberous Sclerosis. Tuberous sclerosis is due to mutations in the *TSC1* (on chromosome 9q23) or *TSC2* (on chromosome 16p13.3) genes. Patients with tuberous sclerosis exhibit characteristic skin findings of flat hypopigmented macules (ash leaf spots), shagreen patches (raised area with dimpled texture), and angiofibromas (red papular lesions). They may have small pits in their tooth enamel. Tumors occurring in different organ systems are seen, including central nervous system (CNS) tubers, retinal hamartomas, cardiac rhabdomyomas, and renal angiomyolipomas. Seizures are a common feature of this disorder. Patients with tuberous sclerosis have been reported to have symptoms of pervasive developmental disorder (PDD) and of ADHD.[39,40] Mental retardation may occur, depending on the extent of CNS involvement. The diagnosis is most often made on a clinical basis, but mutation analysis of the *TSC1* and *TSC2* genes is now available.

Neurofibromatosis Type I. Neurofibromatosis type I (NF1), previously known as von Recklinghausen's disease, is due to a mutation in the *NF1* gene on chromosome 17q11.2, which is believed to result in loss of tumor suppressor function. Abnormalities of skin pigmentation (*café au lait* spots, freckling in axilla or groin), Lisch nodules (small brown spots) on the iris, bony abnormalities, neurofibromas (cutaneous, subcutaneous, or plexiform), and macrocephaly are some of the physical findings in NF1. Complications may arise depending on the size or location of neurofibromas or due to development of malignant tumors. Psychiatric symptoms may include learning disabilities and ADHD.[41,42] Diagnosis is usually made on a clinical basis; mutation analysis of the *NF1* gene is available on a limited basis.

X-Linked Dominant Disorders

Fragile X Syndrome. In contrast to Down syndrome, which is the most common *genetic* cause of mental retardation, Fragile X syndrome is the most common *inherited* (i.e., transmitted from a parent who carries the abnormal gene) cause of mental retardation. Fragile X is the result of dysfunction of the *FMR1* gene at Xq27.3 due to increased numbers of trinucleotide repeats. Normal alleles have approximately 5 to 44 repeats, and borderline alleles have approximately 45 to 58 repeats. Having greater than approximately 200 CGG repeats results in the full syndrome; a "premutation" allele with approximately 59 to 200 repeats may expand to the full syndrome when passed on from a mother to her children. The full syndrome is most often found in males, but females who carry a full-length mutation on one of their X chromosomes may have features of the disorder of variable severity. Approximately one third of females with a full-length mutation are thought to be normal, one third are mildly affected, and the remaining one third have findings similar to the full syndrome in males. In addition to mental retardation in the moderate to severe range, physical features, such as large testes, connective tissue disease (loose joints), low muscle tone, and characteristic facial appearance (large head with prominent forehead and jaw, long face with large ears) may help identify males with this disorder. Of note, the facial features and testicular size may be more apparent after puberty. Psychiatric symptoms include autistic features, ADHD, oppositional defiant disorder, mood disorders, and avoidant personality disorder and traits.[43–45] Although carrying a premutation-length allele has not traditionally been associated with cognitive or behavioral findings, a variety of studies have shown increased rates of psychiatric symptoms, including social phobia and mood disorders, in these women.[46–48] Diagnostic testing to determine the number of trinucleotide repeats in the *FMR1* gene is widely available.

Rett Syndrome.   Rett syndrome is due to a mutation in the *MECP2* gene on chromosome Xq28. This syndrome is described in girls who appear normal at birth and during the first several months or years of life. They then experience a progressive loss of developmental skills associated with acquired microcephaly. Additional features include impaired language, loss of purposeful hand movements (replaced by stereotyped hand movements), gait abnormalities, seizures, and bruxism. It is classified as a pervasive developmental disorder in *DSM-IV*. Mutations in the *MECP2* gene, once thought to be fatal in males, have been recognized as a cause of developmental disorders in boys.[49] Diagnostic testing for analysis of the *MECP2* gene is available.

Metabolic Disease

Inborn errors of metabolism are a class of genetic disorders that result in dysfunction of production, regulation, or function of enzymes or enzyme cofactors. The disruption of normal metabolic processes may lead to a build up of pathway by-products or production of alternate substances that cause toxicity. In addition, the absence of essential pathway end-products may lead to disease states. Classically, disorders of metabolism have been described in children. However, presentation or recognition of disease may be delayed in patients with relative preservation of enzyme activity that is seen in milder forms of disease, and many disorders have later-onset forms. Metabolic disorders are most often classified based on the abnormal substances involved or by the cell location where the enzyme dysfunction occurs.

Testing for metabolic illness begins at birth, by population screening for a variety of illnesses by state-mandated newborn screening programs. However, the number of diseases tested for varies widely by state, and even the most comprehensive testing has been available only for the past several years. Thus, it is unlikely that older children and adults would have benefited from these screening programs. Furthermore, even the most comprehensive state panels do not rule out all, or even most, genetic and metabolic diseases. For this reason, suspicion of a metabolic disease should be pursued vigorously. Early identification of metabolic illness is crucial to maximize good outcome.

Assessment of the Patient for Metabolic Illness

Essential to the evaluation for possible metabolic illness is careful history-taking. Questions about dietary history (e.g., food intolerances, unusual food preferences, and colic/reflux), a history of decompensation associated with minor illness, or history of transient neurologic symptoms (e.g., lethargy, encephalopathy, ataxia, and confusion) may lead to detection of an underlying metabolic illness. In addition, careful review of developmental history, especially a history of a developmental regression, loss of skills, or decline in cognition, is important to elicit. As many metabolic illnesses are inherited in an autosomal recessive fashion, a review of family history should include questions about consanguinity and ethnicity. In addition, a history of stillbirths or early infant deaths may prove informative. For example, it is thought that many children who died of Reye's syndrome (manifest by vomiting, liver dysfunction with fatty infiltration, and hypoglycemia) may have had underlying problems with disorders of fatty acid oxidation.

Abnormal results of routine and specialized laboratory studies may indicate a primary metabolic illness. Of note, laboratory findings may be abnormal only during the period of acute illness or metabolic decompensation. For this reason, following up on a suspicion of metabolic illness with prompt collection of indicated specimens is crucial for diagnosis. Some general laboratory tests to consider when evaluating a patient for metabolic illness are listed in Table 40-1. Abnormal results on preliminary testing may direct more specific assessment of certain metabolic pathways.

Many patients with metabolic illness have completely normal physical features, although characteristic findings, when applicable, are indicated below. Thorough ophthalmologic examination may prove particularly helpful when evaluating metabolic illnesses, as the retina provides a window through which to observe the metabolic processes in the brain.

Many metabolic illnesses may affect the brain, either directly (e.g., via destruction of white matter in metachromatic leukodystrophy) or indirectly (e.g., as encephalopathy in urea cycle disorders). For this reason, neuropsychiatric symptoms associated with metabolic disease may vary widely. Conversely, many metabolic illnesses may have similar acute presentations (e.g., delirium). As is the case with genetic syndromes, some patients may meet full criteria for psychiatric disorders, while others may exhibit nonspecific behavioral findings.

Selected Metabolic Disorders

Mr. B, a 57-year-old man, was admitted to the medical service for a change in mental status. He was reported to have prominent mood lability, disorientation, and disorganized and racing thoughts. His medical history was significant for hypertension, dental surgery, and a history of hepatitis 6 months previously (attributed to alcohol intake and medication side effects). Mr. B had been consuming six beers at a time several times a week. His family history was unremarkable. On evaluation, he appeared anxious and restless, and a tremor was noted. He had difficulty with speech and had abnormal facial movements. He exhibited mood lability and had difficulty completing cognitive tasks. Laboratory studies showed a mild elevation of liver transaminases, a low serum ceruloplasmin, and a greatly increased urine copper excretion, which led to a diagnosis of Wilson disease.

Autosomal Dominant Disorders

Porphyrias/Acute Intermittent Porphyria. The porphyrias are a group of disorders with dysfunction of heme biosynthesis. One of the more common porphyrias is acute intermittent porphyria (AIP), which results from mutations in the *hydroxymethylbilane synthase (HMBS)* gene on chromosome 11q23.3 that causes decreased activity of porphobilinogen (PBG) deaminase. AIP is inherited in an autosomal dominant manner. Episodic "neurovisceral" attacks are the predominant manifestations of AIP; they consist of recurrent abdominal pain, vomiting, generalized body pain, and weakness. Photosensitivity is not a feature of AIP as it is with some types of porphyria. Psychiatric symptoms and

Table 40-1. Laboratory Studies to Evaluate Metabolic Illness

Laboratory Test	Metabolic State/Disorders Tested For
Electrolyte panel	Acidosis, calculation of anion gap
Liver function tests	Storage of abnormal substances in liver
Blood gas	Determination of pH (acidosis vs. alkalosis)
Ammonia (NH_3)	Urea cycle disorders-primary elevation organic acidemias, disorders of fatty acid oxidation-secondary elevation
Lactate, pyruvate	Disorders of energy metabolism
Plasma amino acids	Amino acid disorders (e.g., urea cycle defects, homocystinuria)
Urine organic acids	Organic acidemias
Acylcarnitine profile	Disorders of fatty acid oxidation, organic acidemias
Very long chain fatty acids	Peroxisomal disorders
Urine mucopolysaccharides	Lysosomal storage disorders
Urine oligosaccharides	Lysosomal storage disorders

conditions, such as delirium, psychosis, depression, and anxiety, may accompany the acute attacks. In between attacks, constitutional and psychiatric symptoms resolve, although anecdotally these patients are often described as having a distinct personality with longstanding histrionic traits. Over time, indications of demyelination may develop. Of importance to the psychiatric consultant is that medications that upregulate heme biosynthesis may worsen attacks. For this reason, patients treated with medications that up-regulate the cytochrome P450 system may make symptoms worse, as heme is an essential part of the cytochrome ring; these patients may be incorrectly labeled as treatment-refractory. Offending agents include benzodiazepines, some tricyclic antidepressants, barbiturates, some anticonvulsants (valproate and carbamazepine), oral contraceptives, cocaine, and alcohol, among others.[50-53] Diagnostic testing focuses on identification of by-products of heme synthesis in the urine, or measurement of PBG deaminase levels in the blood. Urine that is left standing may discolor, turning dark red or brown due to the presence of porphobilinogen and aminolevulinic acid. Treatment for AIP includes supportive care during attacks and the avoidance of offending agents. In addition, a high-carbohydrate diet, folic acid (a PBG diamine cofactor), and the use of medications that suppress heme synthesis may be helpful.

Autosomal Recessive Disorders

Homocystinuria. Classic homocystinuria is due to mutations of the *cystathionine β-synthase (CBS)* gene on chromosome 21q22.3 that results in decreased enzymatic activity of cystathionine β-synthase and problems with conversion of homocystine to cystine and remethylation of homocystine to methionine. Patients with preservation of some enzyme activity may respond to high dosages of pyridoxine (vitamin B_6), which acts as a cofactor for cystathionine β-synthase. Deficiencies of other enzyme cofactors (e.g., B_{12} and folate) may also lead to symptoms. Patients with homocystinuria usually have unremarkable early histories, with development of symptoms in childhood. The patients tend to be tall and thin and are sometimes described as "marfanoid." They may have features of connective tissue disease, such as a pectus excavatum, lens dislocation, scoliosis, and a high-arched palate. Unlike patients with Marfan's syndrome, they may have restricted mobility of their joints. It is thought that high levels of homocystine may interfere with collagen cross-linking, which results in connective tissue symptoms. In addition, abnormalities in collagen can lead to disruptions of the vascular endothelium and thrombotic events with disabling or fatal consequences. High levels of homocystine, or other factors, are also thought to be neurotoxic and, when left untreated, lead to mental retardation and learning disabilities. During the 1960s and 1970s, these patients were reported to have increased rates of schizophrenia, which was attributed to the hypothesized central role of methionine in both disorders.[54] More recent studies have not supported an increased risk of schizophrenia or psychosis but have shown depression, OCD, personality disorders, and other behavioral disturbances.[55] Urinary nitroprusside testing for disulfides and measurement of high levels of homocystine and methionine (the precursor of homocystine) in the blood help to make the diagnosis. Newborn screening for homocystinuria has been available in some states for more than 30 years. Molecular testing is also available. Treatment focuses on providing a diet low in methionine and supplementation with vitamin cofactors and cystine (which becomes an essential amino acid in these patients). Use of the supplement betaine also aids in lowering homocystine levels.

Wilson's Disease. Wilson's disease is due to mutations in the *ATP7B* gene, located on chromosome 13q14.21, which lead to copper deposition in the CNS as a result of decreased levels of copper-transporting adenosine triphosphatase (ATPase). Signs and symptoms of liver dysfunction, such as jaundice, hepatomegaly, cirrhosis, and hepatitis, may be present, along with abnormal liver function tests. Of particular importance to psychiatrists are changes in personality, mood lability (including pseudobulbar palsy), cognitive decline, and other behavioral changes that may be among the earliest symptoms of Wilson's disease.[50,56,57] Neurologic symptoms are most often extrapyramidal in nature and can include tremor, dysarthria, muscular rigidity, parkinsonism, dyskinesia, dystonia, and chorea. Seizures may also occur. The hallmark of this disorder is the Kayser-Fleischer ring, a yellow-brown ring (a consequence of copper deposition in the cornea) that is visible on slit lamp ophthalmologic examination. Accumulations of copper in other organ systems may result in a variety of complications, including arthritis, renal tubular dysfunction, and cardiomyopathy. Confirmatory diagnostic testing includes measurement of reduced bound copper and ceruloplasmin in the serum and increased copper excretion in the urine. Copper deposits may be seen on head MRI, or in the liver via a liver biopsy. Treatment, in the form of chelation of copper (with medications such as d-penicillamine) and supplementation with antioxidants, is available. Avoidance of copper-rich foods, like shellfish, liver, chocolate, and nuts, is recommended. Unfortunately, liver damage may progress to liver failure and necessitate liver transplantation in some patients.

Metachromatic Leukodystrophy. Metachromatic leukodystrophy (MLD) is a lysosomal storage disorder with deficiency of the enzyme aryl-sulfatase A and mutations in the *ARSA* gene located on chromosome 22q13.31. As a result, abnormal storage of galactosyl sulfatide (cerebroside sulfate) occurs in the white matter of the central and peripheral nervous systems. The disorder may present in infancy, childhood, or adulthood. For the later-onset forms, psychiatric symptoms may be an earlier manifestation of the disease, with a decline in cognition, personality changes, and psychotic features (including hallucinations and delusions). In some cases, psychosis may predate the onset of other symptoms by several years.[50,58,59] Neurologic symptoms may include ataxia and walking difficulties, dysarthria and dysphagia, and pyramidal signs. Vision loss may also occur. Brain MRI may show periventricular changes; eventually white matter atrophy due to loss of myelin may be noted. Diagnostic testing involves measurement of elevated urine sulfatides and decreased levels of aryl sulfatase-A in blood. No treatment is currently available, although bone marrow transplantation may delay the progression of symptoms.

Niemann-Pick Disease, Type C. Niemann-Pick disease, type C, (NPC) is a condition that results in abnormal cholesterol esterification and lipid storage in lysosomes due to mutations in the *NPC1* gene on chromosome 18q11-q12. The disorder may present in childhood or adolescence (and rarely in adulthood) with early findings of

ataxia, coordination problems, and dysarthria. Vertical supranuclear palsy is the hallmark of the disorder. Seizures and hepatosplenomegaly may be present. Psychiatric symptoms include progressive cognitive decline and dementia. In addition, several reports have documented the initial presentation of this disorder as psychosis or schizophrenia.[60,61] Diagnosis is based on demonstration of characteristic pathologic findings in the skin or in the bone marrow, abnormal cholesterol esterification in fibroblasts, and molecular analysis of the *NPC1* gene, which is positive in 95% of cases. Of note is that panels that test blood and urine specimens for lysosomal storage diseases will be normal in NPC, so diagnostic suspicion must direct a more comprehensive work-up.

Tay-Sachs Disease, Late-Onset Type. Tay-Sachs disease is another lysosomal storage disease, with accumulation of GM2 gangliosides in neurons. Mutations in the *HEXA* gene on chromosome 15q23-q24, which encodes the alpha subunit of hexosaminidase A, lead to an enzyme deficiency. Most clinicians are familiar with the infantile-onset form of the disorder but may not be aware of the later-onset forms that can occur with preservation of some enzymatic activity. Patients may present with psychiatric symptoms of psychosis, mood lability, catatonia, and cognitive decline.[62,63] Physical findings are those of progressive neurologic dysfunction and include early ataxia, coordination problems, dysarthria, and progressive neurologic dysfunction (e.g., with dystonia, spasticity, and seizures). Macular cherry-red spots, the hallmark of the early-onset form, are not present in the later-onset form. Diagnosis is based on analysis of enzyme levels in the blood, or mutation analysis. Tay-Sachs may occur in people of various ethnic and racial backgrounds, and prenatal screening is offered, especially to those of Ashkenazi Jewish descent, where the carrier rate is estimated to be 1:30, and to French Canadians, who have a carrier rate of 1:50. There is no treatment available for Tay-Sachs disease.

X-Linked Disorders

X-Linked Adrenoleukodystrophy. X-linked adrenoleukodystrophy (XLD) is also a disorder of abnormal storage but in the peroxisome instead of the lysosome. In this disorder, deficiency of lignoceroyl-CoA ligase results from mutations in the *ABCD1* gene on Xq28 and leads to accumulation of very long chain fatty acids (VLCFA) in the cerebral white matter and adrenal cortex. Due to its X-linked manner of inheritance, males are described with the full syndrome. Female carriers, however, can also exhibit a spectrum of associated symptoms with varying degrees of severity, and they may be misdiagnosed with other disorders, including multiple sclerosis. Often, the first signs and symptoms of the disorder result in a diagnosis of ADHD for affected males. In the adult-onset form, high rates of mania and psychosis are reported.[64,65] Other early signs may include difficulty with gait, handwriting, or speech. Progressive loss of motor skills, vision, and hearing, accompa-

nied by continued decline in cognition, occurs over a period of months to years. Accumulation of VLCFA in the adrenal cortex may cause elevation of adrenocorticotropic hormone (ACTH) and other findings associated with adrenal dysfunction. These adrenal abnormalities, brain MRI findings, and elevated levels of VLCFA in the blood can lead to the diagnosis. Confirmatory molecular testing for mutations in the *ABCD1* gene is available. Treatment for adrenal dysfunction is recommended, but there is no treatment available for the neurologic sequelae of this disease, as the use of "Lorenzo's Oil" has not proven to be effective. Bone marrow transplantation has been proposed as a possible treatment for this disorder, but concerns about the high morbidity and mortality rate associated with the procedure have limited its use.

Table 40-2. Additional History and Physical Examination Assessment for Genetic and Metabolic Illness

Prenatal History
Any complications with pregnancy?
Timing of complication(s)?
Maternal diabetes, systemic illness?
Maternal hypertension, eclampsia, or toxemia?
HELLP (*H*emolysis, *E*levated *L*iver enzymes,
   *L*ow *P*latelets)?
Maternal infection or high fevers?
Toxic exposures (medications, illicit substances,
   alcohol, radiation, chemicals)?
Any abnormalities on ultrasound?
Any indications for amniocentesis/chorionic villus
   sampling (CVS)? Amniocentesis/CVS results?

Birth/Perinatal History
Mode of delivery (vaginal vs. cesarean
   section, natural vs. induced vs. emergent)?
Complications with delivery?
NICU or prolonged hospital stay in infancy?
Issues with feeding or growth?

Developmental History
Timing of major verbal and motor milestones?
History of developmental regression?
History of speech, occupational or physical therapy?
Decline in school performance?
History of special education services, academic supports?

Family History
Ethnicity/race of parents?
History of consanguinity?
Patterns of illness in family members?
History of infertility, miscarriages?
History of infant/child deaths?
Family members with surgeries in childhood?

Multiorgan Review of Systems
History of decompensation with illness?
Dietary history of food intolerances, or unusual food preferences?
Episodic neurologic symptoms?
Problems with linear growth or weight gain?

Physical Examination
Asymmetry of features?
Presence of dysmorphic features?
Signs of neurologic dysfunction?

Psychiatric Review of Systems
Nonspecific behavioral problems (e.g., tantrums, violent
   outbursts, hyperactivity)?
Self-injurious behaviors?
Difficulties with sleep?

Table 40-3. Selected Disorders with Associated Cognitive Decline/Dementia

Genetic Syndromes	Inborn Errors of Metabolism
Rett syndrome	Wilson's disease
Huntington's disease	Homocystinuria
Down syndrome (with associated Alzheimer's disease)	X-linked adrenoleukodystrophy
	Niemann-Pick disease, type C
	Metachromatic leukodystrophy
	Tay-Sachs disease
	Mitochondrial disease

Table 40-5. Selected Disorders with Associated Psychosis

Genetic Syndromes	Inborn Errors of Metabolism
Velocardiofacial syndrome/DiGeorge syndrome	Acute intermittent porphyria
	X-linked adrenoleukodystrophy
	Niemann-Pick disease, type C
Prader-Willi syndrome	Metachromatic leukodystrophy
Huntington's disease	Tay-Sachs disease
	Wilson's disease
	Mitochondrial disease

Urea Cycle Defects—Ornithine Transcarbamylase Deficiency. Disorders of the urea cycle interfere with the normal urinary excretion of excess nitrogen via conversion to urea. Several enzymes comprise the urea cycle, and deficiencies of these enzymes lead to variable failure to manage nitrogenous waste from protein. Ornithine transcarbamylase (OTC) deficiency is one of the more common urea cycle disorders, and it is inherited in an X-linked manner due to mutations in the *OTC* gene on Xp21.1. Although males with this disorder most often present in the neonatal period with marked hyperammonemia and resultant sequelae, female carriers of the *OTC* gene may have a more variable course, owing to lyonization of X chromosomes. Their presentations may occur at any age and range from being asymptomatic to being as severely affected as are males. Psychiatric symptoms in affected carrier females may include intermittent episodes of delirium, ataxia, lethargy, and confusion.[66–68] Patients may report a history of self-restriction of protein in the diet, or severe decompensations with vomiting illnesses or fasting (which may result in an endogenous protein load via catabolism of muscle). During symptomatic episodes, elevations of ammonia, urine orotic acid, and liver function, accompanied by a characteristic pattern of plasma amino acids, aid in

Table 40-4. Selected Disorders with Associated Delirium

Acute intermittent porphyria
Wilson's disease
Ornithine transcarbamylase deficiency (including female carriers)
Mitochondrial disease

diagnosis. Confirmatory molecular diagnostic testing by mutation analysis, or enzymatic assay of liver tissue, is available. Treatment is focused on maintaining a low intake of dietary protein and providing supplemental essential amino acids and urea cycle intermediates. Acutely, medications that allow alternate excretion of nitrogen compounds may be used for high ammonia levels; in some cases hemodialysis is required for rapid control of hyperammonemic episodes. Of note, the use of valproate has been reported to cause acute liver failure in patients with OTC and also to precipitate a hyperammonemic crisis in carrier females. It is thought that valproate inhibits urea synthesis and can lead to hyperammonemia.[69–72]

Lesch-Nyhan Syndrome. Lesch-Nyhan syndrome is a disorder of purine metabolism owing to deficiency of hypoxanthine-guanine phosphoribosyltransferase (HPRT), caused by mutations in the *HPRT1* gene at Xq26-27.2. Hyperuricemia and hyperuricuria occur and can result in deposition of urate crystals in the joints, kidneys, and bladder. Affected males exhibit hallmark behaviors of self-injury and self-mutilation (including head banging and biting of lips and fingers). Mutilation may be severe enough to warrant removal of teeth or the use of restraints.[73] Mental retardation may occur, although progressive loss of cognition does not. Diagnostic testing reveals increased uric acid production and excretion, decreased HPRT activity, and confirmatory molecular analysis of the *HPRT1* gene. Although allopurinol may control sequelae of high uric acid, it does not ameliorate the neurologic or psychiatric symptoms. There is some suggestion that dysfunction of dopamine metabolism may be related to the CNS pathology in this disorder.[74]

Mitochondrial Disorders

Disorders that involve dysfunction of the mitochondria are diverse and include disorders of fatty acid beta-oxidation or pyruvate metabolism and dysfunction of the Krebs cycle or oxidative phosphorylation by the electron transport chain. Commonly, they may be thought of as disorders of energy metabolism. Mitochondrial disorders are inherited from the mother, in the case of those coded for by genes located in the mitochondrial genome, or from either or both parents in those coded for by genes located in the nuclear genome. Mitochondrial syndromes may be characterized as specific disorders (e.g., mitochondrial encephalopathy with lactic acidosis and stroke-like episodes [MELAS]) or may involve dysfunction of multiple organ systems (e.g., cardiomyopathy, diabetes, and hearing loss). Body tissues with high energy demands, including the brain, may be preferentially affected. Psychiatric symptoms and conditions in mitochondrial disorders are largely uncharacterized but may include depression, delirium, dementia, and psychosis.[75] Mitochondrial dysfunction may be suggested by elevations of lactate or pyruvate or by presence of by-products of fatty acid oxidation or other mitochondrial pathways. Diagnosis by analysis of specific mutations is available for some disorders, while others rely on functional analysis of pathways using skin or muscle tissue. Dietary and vitamin supplementation, prevention of lactic acidosis with acute decompensations, as well as management of associated medical conditions, are the mainstays of treatment for mitochondrial disorders.

Teratogen Exposure

A variety of reproducible syndromes and characteristic features are associated with prenatal exposure to prescribed medications, alcohol and drugs of abuse, maternal illnesses (e.g., diabetes) and infectious agents, chemicals, radiation, and other toxins. Observed physical, cognitive, and psychiatric findings may vary, based on the amount and timing of exposure. When possible, a detailed prenatal history should be obtained as part of a comprehensive evaluation of a patient.

Fetal Alcohol Syndrome. Alcohol is the major teratogen to which fetuses are exposed; it can result in a wide spectrum of cognitive, behavioral, and physical findings known as fetal alcohol syndrome (FAS). The severity of symptoms appears to be dose-related, although a critical threshold of alcohol intake has not been identified. High levels of blood alcohol (achieved by binge drinking) may result in more severe manifestations. Psychiatric symptoms and conditions include ADHD, depression, mood lability, anxiety, aggression, and oppositional-defiant behaviors.[76–78] Physical features include prenatal and postnatal growth deficiency and a characteristic facial appearance manifest by a small head, a flattened mid face, the presence of epicanthal folds, a flat philtrum with a thin upper lip, and small jaw. Learning disabilities and cognitive limitations are common. Diagnosis rests on clinical features with recognition of characteristic findings in the context of a known history of prenatal alcohol exposure. Diagnosis of FAS spectrum, partial FAS, or alcohol-related neurodevelopmental disorder (ARND) may also be made. Exposure to multiple drugs in utero should also be considered in all patients evaluated for FAS. No confirmatory laboratory or imaging tests are available, although recent MRI studies have documented structural abnormalities of the brain with absence or small size of the corpus callosum being reported in FAS patients.[79]

Conclusions

While many psychiatric disorders are thought to have a genetic component, the underlying etiologies of the major psychiatric diseases have not been fully characterized. In contrast, the genetic mechanisms and modes of inheritance for the disorders described in this chapter are well understood.[80–85] Their relatively frequent association with psychiatric symptoms makes an awareness of these disorders important for the general psychiatrist. A comprehensive assessment that includes attention to family history (see Tables 40-2 to 40-5) (highlighting psychiatric and neurologic disease, dementia, or other medical illness in family members), review of systems (including developmental and cognitive status, dietary history, and involvement of other organ systems) and noted abnormalities on physical examination (especially neurologic findings and dysmorphic features) may uncover clues that can help to determine which psychiatric patients may require more extensive organic workups. Consultation by a geneticist can help with diagnostic and management issues in individual patients with known or suspected genetic and metabolic disorders.

Advances flowing from the Human Genome Project are rapidly expanding knowledge in all areas of medicine. Clarification of the molecular and physiologic basis of psychiatric and behavioral symptoms in disorders where the underlying cause is known may add to our understanding of psychiatric disorders as a whole, aid in refinement of diagnostic criteria, and offer novel treatment approaches to common psychiatric disease.

General References and Web-Based Resources

Gene Clinics web site *http://www.Geneclinics.org*
Online Mendelian Inheritance in Man (OMIM) web site *http://www.ncbi.nlm.nih.gov/omim/*
POSSUM web site and software *http://www.possum.net.au/*

References

1. Bassett AS, Chow EW: 22q11 deletion syndrome: a genetic subtype of schizophrenia, *Biol Psychiatry* 46:882–891, 1999.
2. Usiskin SI, Nicolson R, Krasnewich DM, et al: Velocardiofacial syndrome in childhood-onset schizophrenia, *J Am Acad Child Adolesc Psychiatry* 38:1536–1543, 1999.
3. Pulver AE, Nestadt G, Goldberg R, et al: Psychotic illness in patients diagnosed with velo-cardio-facial syndrome and their relatives, *J Nerv Ment Dis* 182:476–478, 1994.
4. Gothelf D, Frisch A, Munitz H, et al: Clinical characteristics of schizophrenia associated with velo-cardio-facial syndrome, *Schizophr Res* 35:105–112, 1999.
5. Bassett AS, Hodgkinson K, Chow EW, et al: 22q11 deletion syndrome in adults with schizophrenia, *Am J Med Genet* 81:328–337, 1998.
6. Arnold PD, Siegel-Bartelt J, Cytrynbaum C, et al: Velo-cardio-facial syndrome: implications of microdeletion 22q11 for schizophrenia and mood disorders, *Am J Med Genet* 105:354–362, 2001.
7. Papolos DF, Faedda GL, Veit S, et al: Bipolar spectrum disorders in patients diagnosed with velo-cardio-facial syndrome: does a hemizygous deletion of chromosome 22q11 result in bipolar affective disorder? *Am J Psychiatry* 153:1541–1547, 1996.
8. Murphy KC: Schizophrenia and velo-cardio-facial syndrome, *Lancet* 359:426–430, 2002.
9. Murphy KC, Owen MJ: Velo-cardio-facial syndrome: a model for understanding the genetics and pathogenesis of schizophrenia, *Br J Psychiatry* 179:397–402, 2001.
10. Greenberg F, Guzzetta V, Montes de Oca-Luna R, et al: Molecular analysis of the Smith-Magenis syndrome: a possible contiguous-gene syndrome associated with del(17)(p11.2), *Am J Hum Genet* 49: 1207–1218, 1991.
11. De Leersnyder H, De Blois MC, Claustrat B, et al: Inversion of the circadian rhythm of melatonin in the Smith-Magenis syndrome, *J Pediatr* 139:111–116, 2001.
12. Smith AC, Dykens E, Greenberg F: Sleep disturbance in Smith-Magenis syndrome (del 17 p11.2), *Am J Med Genet* 81:186–191, 1998.
13. Greenberg F, Lewis RA, Potocki L, et al: Multi-disciplinary clinical study of Smith-Magenis syndrome (deletion 17p11.2), *Am J Med Genet* 62:247–254, 1996.
14. Smith AC, Dykens E, Greenberg F: Behavioral phenotype of Smith-Magenis syndrome (del 17p11.2). *Am J Med Genet* 81, 179–185, 1998.
15. Smith AC, McGavran L, Robinson J, et al: Interstitial deletion of (17)(p11.2p11.2) in nine patients, *Am J Med Genet* 24:393–414, 1986.
16. Finucane BM, Konar D, Haas-Givler B, et al: The spasmodic upper-body squeeze: a characteristic behavior in Smith-Magenis syndrome, *Dev Med Child Neurol* 36:78–83, 1994.
17. Smith AC, Gropman AL, Bailey-Wilson JE, et al: Hypercholesterolemia in children with Smith-Magenis syndrome: del (17) (p11.2p11.2), *Genet Med* 4:118–125, 2002.
18. Gosch A, Pankau R: Personality characteristics and behaviour problems in individuals of different ages with Williams syndrome, *Dev Med Child Neurol* 39:527–533, 1997.
19. Davies M, Udwin O, Howlin P: Adults with Williams syndrome: preliminary study of social, emotional and behavioural difficulties, *Br J Psychiatry* 172:273–276, 1998.
20. Morris CA: *Adults with Williams syndrome: natural history and recommendations for management*, San Diego, 2003, American College of Medical Genetics.
21. Demb HB, Papola P: PDD and Prader-Willi syndrome, *J Am Acad Child Adolesc Psychiatry* 34:539–540, 1995.
22. Descheemaeker MJ, Vogels A, Govers V, et al: Prader-Willi syndrome: new insights in the behavioural and psychiatric spectrum, *J Intellect Disabil Res* 46:41–50, 2002.
23. Dykens EM, Hodapp RM, Walsh K, et al: Adaptive and maladaptive behavior in Prader-Willi syndrome, *J Am Acad Child Adolesc Psychiatry* 31:1131–1136, 1992.
24. Holland AJ, Whittington JE, Butler J, et al: Behavioural phenotypes associated with specific genetic disorders: evidence from a population-based study of people with Prader-Willi syndrome, *Psychol Med* 33:141–153, 2003.
25. Clarke DJ, Boer H, Whittington J, et al: Prader-Willi syndrome, compulsive and ritualistic behaviours: the first population-based survey, *Br J Psychiatry* 180: 358–362, 2002.

26. Collacott RA, Cooper SA, McGrother C: Differential rates of psychiatric disorders in adults with Down's syndrome compared with other mentally handicapped adults, *Br J Psychiatry* 161:671–674, 1992.

27. Cooper SA, Collacott RA: Clinical features and diagnostic criteria of depression in Down's syndrome, *Br J Psychiatry* 165:399–403, 1994.

28. Myers BA, Pueschel SM: Psychiatric disorders in persons with Down syndrome, *J Nerv Ment Dis* 179:609–613, 1991.

29. Delooz J, Van den Berghe H, Swillen A, et al: Turner syndrome patients as adults: a study of their cognitive profile psychosocial functioning and psychopathological findings, *Genet Couns* 4: 169–179, 1993.

30. Kleczkowska A, Kubien E, Dmoch E, et al: Turner syndrome: II. Associated anomalies, mental performance and psychological problems in 218 patients diagnosed in Leuven in the period 1965–1989, *Genet Couns* 1:241–249, 1990.

31. Siegel PT, Clopper R, Stabler B: The psychological consequences of Turner syndrome and review of the National Cooperative Growth Study psychological substudy, *Pediatrics* 102:488–491, 1998.

32. Bender BG, Puck MH, Salbenblatt JA, et al: Dyslexia in 47,XXY boys identified at birth, *Behav Genet* 16:343–354, 1986.

33. Mandoki MW, Sumner GS, Hoffman RP, et al: A review of Klinefelter's syndrome in children and adolescents, *J Am Acad Child Adolesc Psychiatry* 30:167–172, 1991.

34. Ratcliffe SG, Bancroft J, Axworthy D: Klinefelter's syndrome in adolescence, *Arch Dis Child* 57:6–12, 1982.

35. Gotz MJ, Johnstone E, Ratcliffe SG: Criminality and antisocial behavior in unselected men with sex chromosome abnormalities, *Psychol Med* 29(4):953–962, 1999.

36. Ratcliffe S: Long term outcome in children of sex chromosome abnormalites, *Arch Dis Child* 80(2):192–195, 1999.

37. Kirkwood SC, Su JL, Conneally P, et al: Progression of symptoms in the early and middle stages of Huntington disease, *Arch Neurol* 58 273–278, 2001.

38. Paulsen JS, Ready RE, Hamilton JM, et al: Neuropsychiatric aspects of Huntington's disease, *J Neurol Neurosurg Psychiatry* 71:310–314, 2001.

39. Gillberg IC, Gillberg C, Ahlsen G: Autistic behaviour and attention deficits in tuberous sclerosis: a population-based study, *Dev Med Child Neurol* 36:50–56, 1994.

40. Hunt A, Dennis J: Psychiatric disorder among children with tuberous sclerosis, *Dev Med Child Neurol* 29: 190–198, 1987.

41. Koth CW, Cutting LE, Denckla MB: The association of neurofibromatosis type 1 and attention deficit hyperactivity disorder, *Neuropsychol Dev Cogn Sect C Child Neuropsychol* 6:185–194, 2000.

42. Mautner VF, Kluwe L, Thakker SD, et al: Treatment of ADHD in neurofibromatosis type 1, *Dev Med Child Neurol* 44:164–170, 2002.

43. Backes M, Genc B, Schreck J, et al: Cognitive and behavioral profile of fragile X boys: correlations to molecular data, *Am J Med Genet* 95:150–156, 2000.

44. Freund LS, Reiss AL, Abrams MT: Psychiatric disorders associated with fragile X in the young female, *Pediatrics* 91:321–329, 1993.

45. Hatton DD, Hooper SR, Bailey DB, et al: Problem behavior in boys with fragile X syndrome, *Am J Med Genet* 108:105–116, 2002.

46. Franke P, Leboyer M, Gansicke M, et al: Genotype-phenotype relationship in female carriers of the premutation and full mutation of FMR-1, *Psychiatry Res* 80:113–127, 1998.

47. Franke P, Maier W, Hautzinger M, et al: Fragile-X carrier females: evidence for a distinct psychopathological phenotype? *Am J Med Genet* 64:334–339, 1996.

48. Johnston C, Eliez S, Dyer-Friedman J, et al: Neurobehavioral phenotype in carriers of the fragile X premutation, *Am J Med Genet* 103:314–319, 2001.

49. Clayton-Smith J, Watson P, Ramsden S, et al: Somatic mutation in MECP2 as a non-fatal neurodevelopmental disorder in males, *Lancet* 356:830–832, 2000.

50. Estrov Y, Scaglia F, Bodamer OA: Psychiatric symptoms of inherited metabolic disease, *J Inherit Metab Dis* 23:2–6, 2000.

51. Crimlisk HL: The little imitator: porphyria—a neuropsychiatric disorder, *J Neurol Neurosurg Psychiatry* 62:319–328, 1997.

52. Santosh PJ, Malhotra S: Varied psychiatric manifestations of acute intermittent porphyria, *Biol Psychiatry* 36:744–747, 1994.

53. Tishler PV, Woodward B, O'Connor J, et al: High prevalence of intermittent acute porphyria in a psychiatric patient population, *Am J Psychiatry* 142:1430–1436, 1985.

54. Bracken P, Coll P: Homocystinuria and schizophrenia. literature review and case report, *J Nerv Ment Dis* 173:51–55, 1985.

55. Abbott MH, Folstein SE, Abbey H, et al: Psychiatric manifestations of homocystinuria due to cystathionine beta-synthase deficiency: prevalence, natural history, and relationship to neurologic impairment and vitamin B6-responsiveness, *Am J Med Genet* 26:959–969, 1987.

56. Dening TR, Berrios GE: Wilson's disease. psychiatric symptoms in 195 cases, *Arch Gen Psychiatry* 46: 1126–1134, 1989.

57. Dening TR, Berrios GE: Wilson's disease: a longitudinal study of psychiatric symptoms, *Biol Psychiatry* 28:255–265, 1990.

58. Hyde TM, Ziegler JC, Weinberger DR: Psychiatric disturbances in metachromatic leukodystrophy. insights into the neurobiology of psychosis, *Arch Neurol* 49:401–406, 1992.

59. Waltz G, Harik SI, Kaufman B: Adult metachromatic leukodystrophy. value of computed tomographic scanning and magnetic resonance imaging of the brain, *Arch Neurol* 44:225–227, 1987.

60. Fink JK, Filling-Katz MR, Sokol J, et al: Clinical spectrum of Niemann-Pick disease type C: *Neurology* 39:1040–1049, 1989.

61. Turpin JC, Masson M, Baumann N: Clinical aspects of Niemann-Pick type C disease in the adult, *Dev Neurosci* 13:304–306, 1991.

62. Navon R, Argov Z, Frisch A: Hexosaminidase A deficiency in adults, *Am J Med Genet* 24:179–196, 1986.

63. MacQueen GM, Rosebush PI, Mazurek MF: Neuropsychiatric aspects of the adult variant of Tay-Sachs disease, *J Neuropsychiatry Clin Neurosci* 10:10–19, 1998.

64. Kitchin W, Cohen-Cole SA, Mickel SF: Adrenoleukodystrophy: frequency of presentation as a psychiatric disorder, *Biol Psychiatry* 22:1375–1387, 1987.

65. Rosebush PI, Garside S, Levinson AJ, et al: The neuropsychiatry of adult-onset adrenoleukodystrophy, *J Neuropsychiatry Clin Neurosci* 11:315–327, 1999.

66. Gilchrist JM, Coleman RA: Ornithine transcarbamylase deficiency: adult onset of severe symptoms, *Ann Intern Med* 106:556–558, 1987.

67. Rowe PC, Newman SL, Brusilow SW: Natural history of symptomatic partial ornithine transcarbamylase deficiency, *N Engl J Med* 314:541–547, 1986.

68. Legras A, Labarthe F, Maillot F, et al: Late diagnosis of ornithine transcarbamylase defect in three related female patients: polymorphic presentations, *Crit Care Med* 30:241–244, 2002.

69. Hjelm M, Oberholzer V, Seakins J, et al: Valproate-induced inhibition of urea synthesis and hyperammonaemia in healthy subjects, *Lancet* 2:859, 1986.

70. Honeycutt D, Callahan K, Rutledge L, et al: Heterozygote ornithine transcarbamylase deficiency presenting as symptomatic hyperammonemia during initiation of valproate therapy, *Neurology* 42:666–668, 1992.

71. Kay JD, Hilton-Jones D, Hyman N: Valproate toxicity and ornithine carbamoyltransferase deficiency, *Lancet* 2:1283–1284, 1986.

72. Tripp JH, Hargreaves T, Anthony PP, et al: Sodium valproate and ornithine carbamyl transferase deficiency, *Lancet* 1:1165–1166, 1981.

73. Robey KL, Reck JF, Giacomini KD, et al: Modes and patterns of self-mutilation in persons with Lesch-Nyhan disease, *Dev Med Child Neurol* 45:167–171, 2003.

74. Ernst M, Zametkin AJ, Matochik JA, et al: Presynaptic dopaminergic deficits in Lesch-Nyhan disease, *N Engl J Med* 334:1568–1572, 1996.

75. Spellberg BRM, Carroll RM, Robinson E, et al: mtDNA disease in the primary care setting, *Arch Intern Med* 161(20):2497–2500, 2001.

76. Sood B, Delaney-Black V, Covington C, et al: Prenatal alcohol exposure and childhood behavior at age 6 to 7 years: I. dose-response effect, *Pediatrics* 108:E34, 2001.

77. Thackray H, Tifft C: Fetal alcohol syndrome, *Pediatr Rev* 22:47–55, 2001.

78. O'Malley KD, Nanson J: Clinical implications of a link between fetal alcohol spectrum disorder and attention-deficit hyperactivity disorder, *Can J Psychiatry* 47:349–354, 2002.

79. Swayze VW, Johnson VP, Hanson JW: Magnetic resonance imaging of brain anomalies in children prenatally exposed to ehtanol, *Pediatrics* 99:232–240, 1997.

80. Golomb M: Psychiatric symptoms in metabolic and other genetic disorders: is our "organic" workup complete? *Harv Rev Psychiatry* 10(4):242–248, 2002.

81. Jones KL, Smith DW: *Smith's recognizable patterns of human malformation, ed 5*, Philadelphia, 1997, Saunders.

82. Korf BR: *Human genetics: a problem-based approach, ed 2*, Malden, Mass., 2000, Blackwell Science.

83. Lyon G, Adams RD, Kolodny EH: *Neurology of hereditary metabolic diseases of children, ed 2*, New York, 1996, McGraw-Hill Health Professions Division.

84. Moldavsky M, Lev D, Lerman-Sagie T: Behavioral phenotypes of genetic syndromes: a reference guide for psychiatrists, *J Am Acad Child Adolesc Psychiatry* 40:749–761, 2001.

85. Scriver CR: *The metabolic & molecular bases of inherited disease, ed 8*, New York, 2001 McGraw-Hill.

Chapter 41
Culture and Psychiatry

David C. Henderson, M.D.
Dana Diem Nguyen, M.D.
Marketa M. Wills, M.D.
Gregory L. Fricchione, M.D.

Gender, race, ethnicity, and culture may all have a tremendous impact on the diagnosis, treatment, and outcome for many individuals with psychiatric and medical problems. While it is impossible to understand every culture, there are basic principles that should be utilized to minimize clashes of cultures and to lessen the risk of providing compromised medical care. When evaluating and treating a patient from a different culture, care must be taken when making observations or applying stereotypes. A clinician must be aware at all times of his or her own feelings, biases, and stereotypes. Additionally, the consulting psychiatrist must assess the impact of the hospital environment, the attitudes of the medical and ancillary care team, and the patient's experience within the health care system. Mistrust of the health care system is common and may influence a patient's behavior, level of cooperation, and adherence with recommendations. On the other hand, disparities in health care delivery exist and are influenced by factors such as gender, race, ethnicity, and culture.[1] Understanding a patient's culture will aid in the delivery of high-quality medical and psychiatric care. However, a little knowledge may be a dangerous thing. Interindividual variability is common; an individual may not fit into preconceived notions of his or her culture. One must probe for cultural clues while remaining flexible enough to recognize that a patient's patterns and behaviors do not necessarily match the clinician's expectations.

Culture

Culture comprises a pattern of beliefs, customs, and behaviors, which a group (or people) acquire socially and transmit from one generation to another through symbols, shared meanings, teachings, and life experiences. It provides the tools by which people of a given society adapt to their physical environment, their social environment, and one another. It organizes groups with ready-made solutions to the problems and challenges that a people often face. Culture (as exemplified by art, literature, architecture, tools, machines, food, clothing, and means of transportation) can be observed directly through the five senses and/or through items collected in a museum or recorded on film. Other aspects of culture must be observed indirectly, usually through the behavior of people. These include the beliefs and values of the people, the reasons for holding some things sacred and other things ordinary, the things and events of which they are proud or ashamed, and the sentiments that underlie patriotism or chauvinism.

Each society establishes its own criteria regarding which forms of behavior are acceptable or abnormal and which represent a medical problem. Understanding an individual's culture, or working with bicultural and bilingual interpreters, may help clarify normal and abnormal behaviors. The consulting psychiatrist must often employ the skills of a detective to verify whether a patient's statements or beliefs are appropriate to their environment, heritage, and culture.

Cultural Assessment

A cultural assessment related to diagnosis and treatment should be included in one's formulation of a patient and their problems. The *Diagnostic and Statistical Manual, Fourth Edition (DSM-IV)*,[2] Appendix I, provides an outline for cultural formulations. The *DSM-IV* emphasizes that a clinician must take into account an individual's ethnic and cultural context in the evaluation of each of the *DSM-IV* axes. This process, called *cultural formulation*, contains the following components:

1. Determination of cultural identity. Ethnic or cultural references and the degree to which an individuals are involved with their culture of origin and their host culture are important. It is crucial to listen for clues about culture and to ask specific questions concerning a patient's cultural identity. For instance, an Asian-American male who grew up in the Southern United States may exhibit patterns, behaviors, and views of the world more consistent with those of a Caucasian southerner. Attention to language abilities and preferences must also be addressed.
2. Determination of cultural explanations. How an individual understands distress or the need for support is often communicated through symptoms (e.g., nerves, possession by spirits, somatic complaints, and misfortune); therefore, the meaning and severity of an illness in relation to one's culture, family, and community should be determined. This explanatory model may be helpful when developing an interpretation, a diagnosis, and a treatment plan.
3. Determination of psychosocial function. Cultural factors can have a significant impact on the psychosocial environment and on function. Cultural interpretations of social stress, support, and one's level of disability and function must also be addressed. It is the physician's responsibility to determine the level of disability, and to help the patient and his or her family adjust to role changes caused by illness.
4. Determination of the relationship between the clinician and the patient. Cultural aspects of the relationship between the individual and the clinician need to be considered. Moreover, cultural differences and their impact on the treatment must not be ignored. Language difficulties, difficulties eliciting symptoms or understanding their cultural significance, difficulties negotiating the appropriate relationship, and difficulties determining whether a behavior is normal or pathologic are common barriers to care. In the hospital, the consulting psychiatrist must also attend to the environment in which the patient is receiving treatment. An intervention of this nature may improve the comfort of patients and their health care providers and the quality of the care provided.

Impact of Ethnicity on Psychiatric Diagnosis

In the United States, race and ethnicity have a significant impact on psychiatric diagnosis and treatment.[3-5] Moreover, the need to reduce disparities in the mental health care of racial and ethnic minorities was recently underscored by the United States Surgeon General.[6] African-Americans are frequently misdiagnosed as having schizophrenia when instead they have bipolar disorder or a psychotic depression. Moreover, treatment approaches and responses often differ depending on the diagnosis. The reasons for misdiagnosis are complicated. They include the fact that individuals from some ethnic or cultural backgrounds may present to the medical system later in the course of their illness than do Caucasian individuals; this results in the perception of a more severe illness.[5] The late presentation may, in part, be related to mistrust of the health care system. Physician biases also play a major role in misdiagnosis. Psychiatric diagnoses are often established by eliciting symptoms from patients that are then interpreted by the psychiatric expert. Many disorders have overlapping symptoms and can be used to support one diagnosis or to disregard another. In the case, of African-Americans, affective symptoms are frequently ignored and psychotic symptoms are emphasized. This pattern has also been seen in other ethnic populations, including Hispanics, some Asian populations, and the Amish in the United States). African-American patients are also more likely to receive higher doses of antipsychotics, to receive depot preparations, to have higher rates of involuntary psychiatric hospitalizations, and to have significantly higher rates of seclusion and restraints while in psychiatric hospitals.[3,5,7] The tendency is to oversedate such patients to reduce their "risk of violence" despite, in some cases, little evidence that the patient has ever been violent. These biases in psychiatric treatment continue and must be addressed.

Differences in Presentation of Illness

Cultural differences in the presentation of psychiatric illnesses abound. For instance, a Cambodian woman may present with complaints of dizziness, fatigue, and back pain, while she ignores other neurovegetative symptoms and is unable to describe feelings of dysphoria. American mental health care providers are generally unfamiliar with various Indo-Chinese culture-bound syndromes and with the meaning attributed to those symptoms by various cultures.[8,9] For example, common American expressions such as "feeling blue" cannot be readily translated into Indo-Chinese languages. A Cambodian clinician will ask Cambodian patients if they "feel blue" by using Cambodian terms which literally translate into "'heavy, overcast, gloomy." The Laotian way of describing "feeling tense" is feeling like a "balloon blown up until it is about to burst." Westermeyer,[10] in a case-controlled study in Laos, documented the general inability of Western psychiatrists to recognize the Laotian symptoms of depression.

Depression may be missed by psychiatrists and by primary care physicians who search for biologic and structural reasons for complaints such as back pain, headaches, and dizziness. Oftentimes afflicted patients are treated with meclizine for dizziness and analgesics for pain, where an antidepressant would have been most appropriate.

From a cross-cultural perspective, evaluating the meanings of bizarre delusions, hallucinations, and psychotic-like symptoms remains a clinical challenge. A nonpsychotic patient may admit to hearing voices of her ancestors (a feature that is culturally appropriate in certain cultural groups). In many traditional, non-Western societies, spirits of the deceased are regarded as capable of interacting with and possessing those still alive. It is difficult to determine whether symptoms are bizarre enough to yield a diagnosis of schizophrenia without an adequate understanding of a patient's sociocultural and religious background. On the other hand, caution must be taken not to assume that bizarre symptoms are culturally appropriate when in fact they are a manifestation of psychosis. The use of bicultural and bilingual interpreters, along with the search for information from other sources, such as family, community leaders, or religious officials, may help to determine whether an individual's experience is culturally appropriate or acceptable.

Additionally, while a great deal of attention has been paid to the study of panic disorder in Caucasians, little empirical research within the United States has looked at the phenomenology of panic disorder among minority groups. Compared to Caucasians, African-Americans with panic disorder report more intense fears of dying or going crazy, higher levels of numbing and tingling in their extremities, and higher rates of comorbid posttraumatic stress disorder (PTSD) and depression. African-Americans also use somewhat different coping strategies (e.g., religious practice and counting one's blessings) and endorse less self-blame. The incidence of isolated sleep paralysis is also higher in African-Americans.[11]

Acculturation and Immigration

Recent immigrants or refugees arrive in the United States with a host of difficulties and psychosocial problems. A physician must ask about and make an effort to understand the circumstances surrounding immigration. An individual may have been a political prisoner or a victim of trauma and torture, or may have been lost or separated from family members. Under these circumstances, the level of depression and PTSD experienced may be high. Literature on the contribution of acculturative stresses to the emergence of mental disorder is abundant.[12] The impact of acculturation may also lead to symptoms of depression, anxiety, "culture shock," and even to PTSD-like symptoms.

The trauma and torture experienced by many refugees are also unfamiliar to the majority of American practitioners.[8] In spite of the numerous reports of the concentration camp experiences in Cambodia, the sexual abuse of Vietnamese boat-women, and the serious emotional distress associated with escape, refugee camps, and resettlement experiences, limited research exists on refugee trauma and trauma-related psychiatric disorders and social handicaps.

Culture-Bound Syndromes

A culture-bound syndrome is a collection of signs and symptoms that is restricted to a limited number of cultures by reason of certain psychosocial features. Culture-bound syndromes are usually restricted to a specific setting, and they have a special relationship to that setting. Culture-bound syndromes are classified on the basis of common etiology (e.g., magic, evil spells, or angry ancestors), so clinical pictures may vary.

Projection is a common ego defense mechanism in many non-Western cultures. Guilt and shame are often projected into cultural beliefs and ceremonies. Guilt and shame are attributed to other individuals, to groups, or to objects, and may involve acting out, blaming others, and needing to punish others. Projection is also seen in magic and in supernatural perspectives of existence. This leads to projective ceremonies and may lead to illness when the ceremonies are not performed.

Cultural psychoses are difficult to define. In cultural syndromes, hallucinations may be viewed as normal variants. Delusions and thought disorder must be reevaluated within a particular cultural setting. A culture may interpret abnormal behavior as relating to some kind of voodoo or anger and may regard the symptoms as normal even though symptoms are consistent with schizophrenia. Table 41-1 lists a number of culture-bound syndromes and the countries or regions where they have been described.

In the past, it was believed that culture-bound syndromes only occurred in the country or region of origin. However, with significant population movements and the tendency for immigrants to remain within their culture (though they have moved to a new country), culture-bound syndromes have been observed in other parts of the world. One common culture-bound syndrome is *ataque de nervios*, which is commonly known and observed in Hispanic populations. As with many culture bound syndromes, there may be significant overlap with *DSM-IV* psychiatric diagnoses. In one study, 36% of Dominican and Puerto Rican subjects[13] diagnosed with *ataque de nervios* also met the criteria for panic attacks, while the features did not necessarily present together during the *ataque* episode.[13]

Table 41-1. Culture-Bound Syndromes

Syndrome	Culture
Sleep paralysis (*amafufanyane*)	Zulu population of southern Africa
Sudden mass assault (*amok/benz*)	Malaysia, Indonesia, Laos, Philippines, Polynesia (called *cafard* or *cathard*), Papua New Guinea, Puerto Rico (called *mal de pelea*), and the Navajo (*itch'aa*)
Ataque de nervios	Latin-American and Latin-Mediterranean groups
Boufée delirante	West Africa and Haiti
Genital retraction (*koro*)	China and Malaysia
Startle-matching (*Latah*)	Malaysia and Indonesia
Running (*piblokto*)	Eskimos
Falling-out or blacking-out	Southern United States and Caribbean groups
Fright illness (hexing, voodoo, ghost illness)	Africa, Brazil, and native West Indians in Haiti
Ghost sickness	Kiowa Apache Indians
Mal de ojo "evil eye"	Mediterranean cultures and elsewhere
Qi-gong psychotic reaction	Chinese
Taijin kyofusho	Japan
Shenjing shuairo or neurasthenia	China
Susto (meaning fright or soul loss)[17]	Hispanics in the United States, Mexico, Central America, and South America

Working with Interpreters

Communication problems are common even between English-speaking doctors and patients from similar socioeconomic backgrounds. Therefore, it is not difficult to imagine the challenges and obstacles that a physician faces when working with limited-English–speaking patients whose culture may be very different and unfamiliar to the doctor. Misunderstandings or a lack of comprehension about a patient's physical or psychiatric complaints may lead to misdiagnosis and result in unnecessary or inappropriate treatment. Patients, in turn, may feel frustrated, discouraged, or dissatisfied with their health care; this may lead them to refuse treatment or terminate their visits altogether.[14] Fortunately, interpreters can help bridge the communication gap between doctors and non–English-speaking patients.

Many states now have laws that require federally funded medical facilities to provide interpreters for their non–English speaking patients. While many interpreters are trained and certified to work with medical providers, translating for a mental health professional is very different, and it can be challenging. Both interpreters and clinicians need to be aware of issues that may arise when using interpreters in psychiatric settings. Some of the issues that clinicians face when working with interpreters may include[15]:

- Clinicians may feel they have less control in their work because their direct contact with the patient is decreased by the presence of the interpreter.
- Clinicians may feel uncertain about their role when working with interpreters who are more active and involved in the treatment process.
- Clinicians may have transference issues toward the interpreter.
- Conflicts may arise when clinicians and interpreters hold opposing views on a patient's diagnosis and treatment plans.
- Interpreters may find it difficult to work with clinicians of a different gender than their own.
- Clinicians may feel frustrated when they cannot verify what is being said to the patient.
- Clinicians may feel left out if the patient appears to have more of a connection with the interpreter.

- Interpreters may feel uncomfortable when asked to translate certain issues such as sexual history or childhood abuse.

Recommendations When Working with Interpreters

When clinicians work with interpreters, they need to know their qualifications. Do the interpreters have experience working with psychiatrists and psychologists? How much do they know about mental illness and mental health services? What are their personal views about mental illness? Interpreters who come from cultures where mental illness is highly stigmatized may bring biases or beliefs into the therapeutic process. It is well known that patients from certain cultures have been advised by their interpreters not to seek mental health services because only "crazy" people see psychiatrists and psychologists.

Clinicians should avoid using family members, friends, or clerical staff as interpreters.[16] Patients may not be able to disclose certain information in front of their spouse or child. At the same time, it may be too difficult or distressing for a young child to have to hear certain details about his or her parent. In addition, family members have been known to omit or to alter information they feel is too embarrassing or inappropriate to reveal to the clinician. In the past, janitors and clerical staff were used as interpreters. This, of course, is strongly discouraged since cleaning and clerical staff may not have adequate medical or mental health language skills to provide accurate translations for clinicians. Unless there are no other alternatives, clinicians should avoid using family members and clerical employees as interpreters.

Trained interpreters should be treated as professional colleagues by clinicians.[16,17] Most interpreters are now well trained and can offer important cultural knowledge that can help promote the doctor-patient relationship. Clinicians should use the interpreters' language skills as well as their cultural expertise to help increase the clinician's understanding of the patient's culture, religion, and worldview. For some clinicians, interpreters are used only as voices to communicate with his or her patients. They prefer word-for-word translations and do not want the interpreter to filter or alter what they say. While this allows the clinician to maintain his or her role as the primary caregiver, and to a certain extent, control for what is being said to the patient, using direct translations can often lead to misunderstandings and confusions for both the patient and the clinician.

Literal translations from one language to another can be inaccurate and inappropriate. For example, "feeling blue," when translated word for word into Vietnamese, does not make any sense to the patients because it literally translates to "*cam giac xanh*," which means "feeling color blue." Certain words or concepts, such as depression and mental health, may not exist in the country of origin of the patient. Interpreters may have to explain or to describe the concept of depression to the patient, which requires much more time than what the clinician might expect. Clinicians must be patient, keeping in mind that it may take 10 minutes to translate one word. In addition, certain issues may be culturally inappropriate to ask or to say to a patient. Most women from an Asian or Hispanic background feel uncomfortable if asked directly about sensitive topics such as sexual abuse or family discord. Interpreters can be used as cultural consultants to assist clinicians with these more complex cases. Allowing interpreters the freedom and flexibility to rephrase or to summarize what is being said can help prevent misunderstandings and improve the exchange between the clinician and the patient.

Clinicians should meet with the interpreter briefly before each session to discuss expectations and to clarify any issues or points that the clinician would like to address during the session.[15,16] Patients do not get as much time with the clinicians when they have to go through interpreters. Everything has to be translated back and forth; hence, clinicians may find that they do not get as much accomplished in their session as they do with English-speaking patients. Time is a crucial factor when interpreters are involved. Thus, one should protect the patient's time by avoiding any discussions with the interpreters that can wait until after the session.

Be sure to introduce the interpreter to the patient at the start of the session if they have not met. Reaffirm issues of confidentiality.[15,16] Often, a patient may feel uneasy about revealing personal issues or conflicts to individuals from his or her own community. As most ethnic communities are small and close-knit, patients may fear that the interpreter will divulge their private information to those in the community. Patients are more likely to open up if they feel reassured that what they share with the clinician and interpreter will be kept in strict confidence. If possible, try to use the same interpreter to help build trust and continuity of care for the patient.[18]

During sessions, clinicians should face and speak directly to the patients instead of to the interpreters.[15–17] While the patient and the clinician may not be able to communicate through language, they can communicate and connect through eye contact, gestures of acknowledgment, and other nonverbal behaviors. It is helpful for the interpreter if the clinician can speak slowly and avoid using long and complicated sentences. Stay away from technical or psychological terminology that does not translate well. Pause often to allow the interpreter to translate. Ask for clarification if there is any confusion.[17] Avoid two-way conversations. Just as clinicians and interpreters should not engage in lengthy discussions in front of the patient, clinicians should interrupt when a patient and an interpreter are talking too long. Tension may arise when someone in the group feels left out.

After each session, encourage the interpreters to give their impression about the session; he or she can often provide important observations and feedback.[15] Ask the interpreter to clarify any issues or points that were not clear during the session. Clinicians can use this time to learn more from the interpreter about their patient's culture. The clinician and interpreter can also provide feedback about each other's performances. Good communication and trust between clinicians and interpreters are essential to care for patients with little or limited English.

Ethnicity and Psychopharmacology

There is emerging research on transcultural psychopharmacology ("ethnopsychopharmacology")[19,20] that may aid the clinician's effective treatment of diverse populations. An understanding of ethnicity and its psychopharmacology and psychobiology is necessary to ensure quality care for ethnic minorities. Biologic and nonbiologic issues have a significant impact on the use of psychotropic medications.

Culturally shaped beliefs play a major role in determining whether an explanation about an illness and a treatment plan will make sense to a patient ("explanatory models"); e.g., Hispanics or Asians often expect rapid relief with treatment and are cautious about potential side effects induced by Western medicine. Concerns about addictive and toxic effects of medications also arise. Some populations continue to use a mixture of herbal medicines and typically believe that polypharmacy is more effective. The use of herbal medicines is of great concern secondary to the risk of drug interactions and the risk of medical or psychiatric side effects or toxicity. The Food and Drug Administration (FDA) has issued a number of warnings on herbal medicine products, including the most popular weight loss products containing *Ephedra sinica* (*ma huang*), which is the main plant source of ephedrine and which has been reported to cause mania, psychosis, and sudden death.

Patient compliance may be affected by incorrect dosing, medication side effects, and polypharmacy. Other factors include a poor therapeutic alliance and a lack of community support, money, or transportation; in addition, substance abuse or concerns about the addictiveness of a medication may be crucial. Communication difficulties and divergence between a patient's and a clinician's explanatory model play an important role in why a patient from an ethnic minority is significantly more likely to drop out of treatment. Exploring these beliefs will improve communication, adherence, and outcome.

Examining social support systems in each patient is vital. The ways in which a family interacts and functions has a significant impact on psychiatric treatment. For example, some Hispanics have more interactions with relatives and may become increasingly demoralized when the involvement of relatives in their treatment does not occur. Hispanics and Asians typically have a "closed network," which consists of family members, kin, and intimate friends.

Biologic Aspects of Psychopharmacology

Pharmacokinetics deal with metabolism, blood levels, absorption, distribution, and excretion of medications. However, other pharmacokinetic variables, such as conjugation, plasma protein–binding, and oxidation by the cytochrome (CYP) isoenzymes also play a role. Pharmacokinetics may be influenced by genetics, age, gender, total body weight, environment, diet, toxins, drugs, and use of alcohol, as well as disease states. Environmental factors include medications, drugs, herbal medicines, steroids, dietary factors, sex hormones, and use of caffeine or tobacco.

The activity of CYP liver enzymes is controlled genetically, although environmental factors can alter their activity. Understanding how pharmacokinetics and environmental factors relate to different populations will help to predict side effects, blood levels, and potential drug-drug interactions. For example, CYP 2D6 is the isoenzyme that metabolizes many antidepressants, including the tricyclic and heterocyclic antidepressants, and the selective serotonin-reuptake inhibitors (SSRIs); SSRIs can inhibit this enzyme, leading to accumulations of other substrates. CYP 2D6 also plays a role in metabolizing antipsychotics, for example, clozapine, haloperidol, perphenazine, risperidone, thioridazine, and sertindole. While much emphasis has been placed on the CYP 2D6 metabolism of psychotropics, it is a major enzyme for the metabolism of numerous nonpsychotropic medications as well. This, while often ignored clinically, can have a significant effect on the tolerability or toxicity of medications.

The incidence of "poor metabolizers" (i.e., those individuals with little enzyme activity) at the CYP 2D6 is roughly 3% to 10% in Caucasians, 0.5% to 2.4% in Asians, 4.5% in Hispanics, and approximately 1.9% in African-Americans.[19] Individuals from these backgrounds are at great risk for toxicity, even when medications are used at low doses. For instance, a woman who develops hypotension and a change in mental status several days after starting 20 mg of nortriptyline may be found to have toxic blood levels and require cardiac monitoring. Table 41-2 lists drugs that are metabolized through different CYP enzyme systems.

Recently a genetic variation of the extensive metabolizer gene that decreases activity at the CYP 2D6 enzymes by approximately 50% ("slow metabolizer") was discovered. This group appears to have enzyme activity levels that are intermediate between poor and extensive metabolizers.[19] Approximately 18% of Mexican-Americans and 33% of Asians and

Table 41-2. Cytochrome P450 Isoenzymes, Substrates, Inhibitors and, Inducers

CYP	CYP 1A2	CYP 2C9/10	CYP 2C19	CYP 2D6	CYP 2E1	CYP 3A3/4
Inhibitors						
	Fluvoxamine	Fluvoxamine	Fluoxetine	Bupropion	Diethylithio-carbamate (Disulfiram)	Fluoxetine
	Moclobemide	Disulfiram	Fluvoxamine	Fluoxetine		Fluvoxamine
	Cimetidine	Amiodarone	Imipramine	Fluvoxamine		Nefazodone
	Fluoroquinolones	Azapropazone	Moclobemide	Hydroxybupropion		Sertraline
	Ciprofloxacin/ norfloxacin	D-propoxyphene	Tranylcypromine	Paroxetine		Diltiazem
	Naringenin (grapefruit)	Fluconazole	Diazepam	Sertraline		Verapamil
	Ticlopidine	Fluvastatin	Felbamate	Moclobemide		Dexamethasone
		Miconazole	Phenytoin	Fluphenazine		Gestodene
		Phenylbutazone	Topiramate	Haloperidol		Clarithromycin
		Stiripentol	Cimetidine	Perphenazine		Erythromycin
		Sulfaphenazole	Omeprazole	Thioridazine		Troleandomycin
		Zafirlukast		Amiodarone		Fluconazole
				Cimetidine		Itraconazole
				Methadone		Ketoconazole
				Quinidine		Ritonavir
				Ritonavir		Indinavir
						Amiodarone
						Cimetidine
						Mibefradil
						Naringenin (grapefruit)
Inducers						
	Tobacco	Barbiturates	Rifampin		Ethanol	Carbamazepine
	Omeprazole	Phenytoin			Isoniazid	Barbiturates
		Rifampin				Phenobarbital
						Phenytoin
						Dexamethasone
						Rifampin
						Troglitazone

Substrates

Tertiary Amine TCAs	THC	Citalopram	Fluoxetine	Ethanol	Carbamazepine	Amiodarone
Clozapine	NSAIDs	Moclobemide	Mirtazapine	Acetaminophen	Alprazolam	Disopyramide
Olanzapine	Phenytoin	Tertiary Amine TCAs	Paroxetine	Chlorzoxazone	Diazepam	Lidocaine
Caffeine	Tolbutamide	Diazepam	Venlafaxine	Halothane	Midazolam	Propafenone
Methadone	Warfarin	Hexobarbital	Secondary & Tertiary Amine TCAs	Isoflurane	Triazolam	Quinidine
Tacrine	Losartan	Mephobarbital	Trazodone	Methoxyflurane	Buspirone	Erythromycin
Acetaminophen	Irbesartan	Omeprazole	Clozapine	Sevoflurane	Citalopram	Androgens
Phenacetin		Lansoprazole	Haloperidol		Mirtazapine	Dexamethasone
Propranolol		Phenytoin	Fluphenazine		Nefazodone	Estrogens
Theophylline		S-Mephenytoin	Perphenazine		Reboxetine	Astemizole
Warfarin		Nelfinavir	Risperidone		Sertraline	Loratadine
		Warfarin	Sertindole		Tertiary Amine TCAs	Terfenadine
			Thioridazine		Sertindole	Lovastatin
			Codeine		Quetiapine	Simvastatin
			Dextromethorphan		Ziprasidone	Atorvastatin
			Hydrocodone		Diltiazem	Cerivastatin
			Oxycodone		Felodipine	Cyclophosphamide
			Mexiletine		Nimodipine	Tamoxifen
			Propafenone		Nifedipine	Vincristine
			(IC antiarrhythmics)		Nisoldipine	Vinblastine
			β-Blockers		Nitrendipine	Ifosfamide
			Donepezil		Verapamil	Cyclosporine
			D & L fenfluramine		Acetaminophen	Tacrolimus
					Alfentanil	Cisapride
					Codeine	Donepezil
					Fentanyl	Lovastatin
					Sufentanil	Protease inhibitors
					Ethosuximide	Sildenafil
					Tiagabine	Disopyramide
					Warfarin	Losartan

African-Americans have this gene variation. This may explain ethnic differences in the pharmacokinetics of neuroleptics and antidepressants. While these individuals are not as likely to experience toxicity at extremely low doses (e.g., poor metabolizers). They are likely to experience significant side effects at lower doses. These individuals may quickly be classified as the "difficult patients" because they complain of side effects at unexpectedly low doses. The above information is striking considering that numerous studies, for instance, have shown that African-Americans receive higher doses of antipsychotics, are more frequently treated with depot neuroleptics, and have higher rates of involuntary commitments and seclusion and restraints than do Caucasians. While data on pharmacokinetics of neuroleptics have been mixed in African-Americans, Asians have been shown to have a higher "area under the curve" for haloperidol.[20,21] Korean-Americans have also been found to have higher blood levels of clozapine and to respond to lower doses of clozapine when compared to Caucasians. In fact, though sertindole, metabolized by the CYP 2D6, did not make it to the United States market, the phase II clinical trials included enough African-Americans to determine that their sertindole blood levels were 50% higher than Caucasian subjects who took the same dose.

The CYP 2C9 isoenzyme is involved in the metabolism of ibuprofen, naproxen, phenytoin, warfarin, and tolbutamide. Approximately 18% to 22% of Asians and African-Americans are poor metabolizers of these drugs. CYP 2C19 is involved in the metabolism of diazepam, clomipramine, imipramine, and propranolol; it is inhibited by fluoxetine and sertraline. The rates of poor metabolizers of this enzyme are approximately 3% to 6% in Caucasians, 4% to 18% in African-Americans, and 18% to 23% in Asians.[19,20]

Finally, lithium appears to be a drug with significant differences in dosing and tolerability across populations. African-Americans are more likely to experience lithium toxicity and delirium compared to Caucasians (likely related to a slower lithium-sodium pathway and connected to higher rates of hypertension). Some Asian populations respond to lower doses and have lower serum levels of lithium (0.4 to 0.8 mEq/L).[19,22]

Also the choice of medications, particularly atypical antipsychotics, should be tempered by an understanding of individual and population risk factors for medical morbidities, such as obesity, hypertension, diabetes mellitus, and cardiovascular disease. For instance, many of the reports of diabetic ketoacidosis (DKA) secondary to atypical agents have been in African-Americans who are at higher risk for diabetes.[23,24]

The "Medical Ombudsman" Role

In 1988, Pasnau[25] enumerated six fundamental functions of the consultation-liaison psychiatrist including the role of "medical ombudsman" for the patient. While the use of this term has not caught on, it signified the sometimes important need of medical and surgical teams to be reminded of the unique human nature of each patient being cared for by them. Racial, ethnic, and cultural factors are obviously important characteristics of individuals. Psychiatrists in the general hospital can present these factors in their consultations and as a result, enrich patient care.

Techniques to Minimize Cultural Clashes and Misdiagnosis

There are certain techniques that may be utilized to avoid misdiagnosis, mistreatment, and cultural clashes. The first moments of an encounter are often crucial. A clinician must be respectful to all patients and address them formally (e.g., Mr., Ms., or Mrs.). In some cultures, an informal introduction is considered disrespectful and may have a lasting impact on the physician-patient relationship.

The relationship will be more complex and it will take longer to develop trust and an alliance. It will also take time to assure patients about confidentiality and to educate patients about mental illness to reduce stigmas that may be influenced by culture. Also, if the diagnosis is unclear or is affected by ethnicity or culture, consider a structured diagnostic interview (e.g., the SCID), to reduce the possibility of misdiagnosis. Finally, it is important to acknowledge the need to spend more time with a patient from a different culture. A clinician must have patience and should expect longer sessions when using an interpreter.

References

1. Johnson PA, Fulp RS: Racial and ethnic disparities in coronary heart disease in women: prevention, treatment, and needed interventions, *Womens Health Issues* 12(5):252–271, 2002.

2. American Psychiatric Association: *Diagnostic and statistical manual of mental disorders, ed 4*, Washington, DC, 1994, American Psychiatric Association.

3. Harper G: Cultural influences on diagnosis, *Child Adolesc Psychiatr Clin North Am* 10:711–728, 2001.

4. Kales HC, Blow FC, Bingham CR: Race, psychiatric diagnosis, and mental health care utilization in older patients, *Am J Geriatr Psychiatry* 8:301–309, 2000.

5. Rayburn TM, Stonecypher JF: Diagnostic differences related to age and race of involuntarily committed psychiatric patients, *Psychol Rep* 79:881–882, 1996.

6. United States Public Health Service, Office of the Surgeon General: *Mental health: culture, race, and ethnicity: a supplement to mental health: a report of the surgeon general*, Washington, DC, 2001, U.S. Public Health Service.

7. Grekin PM, Jemelka R, Trupin EW: Racial differences in the criminalization of the mentally ill, *Bull Am Acad Psychiatry Law* 22:411–420, 1994.

8. Mollica RF, Wyshak G, Lavelle J: The psychosocial impact of war trauma and torture on Southeast Asian refugees, *Am J Psychiatry* 144:1567–1572, 1987.

9. Mollica RF, Lavelle J: *Southeast Asian refugees*. In Comas-Diaz L GE, editor: *Clinical guidelines in cross-cultural mental health*, New York, 1988, Wiley, pp 262–304.

10. Westermeyer J: Lao folk diagnosis for mental disorders: comparison with psychiatric diagnosis and assessment with psychiatric rating scales, *Med Anthropol* 5:425–443, 1981.

11. Friedman S, Paradis C: Panic disorder in African-Americans: symptomatology and isolated sleep paralysis, *Cult Med Psychiatry* 26(2):179–198, 2002.

12. Bhugra D, Bhui K: Transcultural psychiatry: do problems persist in the second generation? *Hosp Med* 59(2):126–129, 1998.

13. Lewis-Fernandez R, Guarnaccia PJ, Martinez, IE et al: Comparative phenomenology of ataques de nervios, panic attacks, and panic disorder, *Cult Med Psychiatry* 26(2):199–223, 2002.

14. Marcos L: Effects of interpreters on the evaluation of psychopathology in non-English speaking patients, *Am J Psychiatry* 136:171–174, 1979.

15. Tribe RRH, editor: *Working with interpreters in mental health*, New York, 2003, Brunner-Routledge.

16. McPhee SJ: Caring for a 70-year old Vietnamese woman, *JAMA* 287:495–504, 2002.

17. Profession Update: *RN* 11–12, 1996.

18. Peterson DE, Remington PL, Kuykendall MA: Behavioral risk factors of Chippewa Indians living on Wisconsin reservations, *Public Health Rep* 109(6):820–823, 1994.

19. Lin KM: Psychopharmacology in cross-cultural psychiatry, *Mt Sinai J Med* 63(5–6):283–284, 1996.

20. Herrera JM, Lawson W, Sramek JJ: *Cross cultural psychiatry*, New York, 1999, Wiley.

21. Lin KM, Poland RE, Nuccio I et al: A longitudinal assessment of haloperidol doses and serum concentrations in Asian and Caucasian schizophrenic patients, *Am J Psychiatry* 146:1307–1311, 1989.

22. Lin TY: Psychiatry and Chinese culture, *West J Med* 139(6):862–867, 1983.

23. Henderson DC: Clinical experience with insulin resistance, diabetic ketoacidosis, and type 2 diabetes mellitus in patients treated with atypical antipsychotic agents, *J Clin Psychiatry* 62(suppl 27):10–14; discussion 40–41, 2001.

24. Henderson DC: Atypical antipsychotic-induced diabetes mellitus: how strong is the evidence? *CNS Drugs* 16(2):77–89, 2002.

25. Pasnau RO: Consultation-liaison psychiatry: progress, problems, and prospects, *Psychosomatics* 29:4–15, 1988.

Chapter 42
Behavioral Medicine

Bruce J. Masek, Ph.D.
Lisa Scharff, Ph.D.

The field of behavioral medicine, now 25 years old, began when applied behavior analysis, behavior therapy, and psychophysiology emerged as clinical sciences. The field's inception drew inspiration from other sources, notably a vision of the limitations of the biomedical model, the value associated with the recognition that behavioral factors broaden our understanding of health and illness,[1] and dissatisfaction with the long-standing dominance of the psychoanalytic approach in psychosomatic medicine.[2]

Behavioral medicine was initially viewed in broad terms as an interdisciplinary field concerned with the development of knowledge in the behavioral sciences and techniques relevant to prevention, diagnosis, treatment, and rehabilitation of physical illness.[3] It grew rapidly in the 1980s. By the end of that decade, curricula in behavioral medicine were found in most medical schools and graduate programs in clinical psychology, and clinical units and research programs in behavioral medicine were operational in most major universities and medical centers. Even a few academic departments changed their names to incorporate *behavioral medicine* into their titles.[4] Thus, the stage was set in the 1990s for the pursuit of a scientific agenda that was ambitious and broad in scope to identify behavioral factors that influence the development and course of organic disease, to develop psychosocial interventions that reduce the effect of these behavioral factors, and to demonstrate that such psychosocial interventions improve clinical outcomes in organic disease through direct effects on the underlying pathology.[5] This last proposition could well be considered the Holy Grail for the field.

Just how good is the clinical evidence from the past quarter century with respect to these propositions? Many believe that the evidence supports the notion that behavioral factors are involved in the development and course of most major diseases, and that psychosocial interventions effectively reduce the risk of illness, decrease morbidity and mortality, and improve health-related quality of life.[6–10] However, a small but vocal minority views the same evidence as the product of seriously, if not fatally flawed studies.[11–13] Both sides seem to agree that the mind can influence the body to the betterment or the detriment of one's health and that some of the evidence is worthy of further scrutiny in large-scale prospective, rigorously controlled clinical trials with hard biologic endpoints.[14]

Currently, behavioral medicine still draws heavily on the theory and practice of applied behavior analysis, behavioral therapy, and psychophysiology for interventions to modify the risk, course, and effect of organic disease. Stress, negative emotions, lifestyle, and quality of life among other factors are frequent targets for interventions. Clinical topics under the umbrella of behavioral medicine have expanded over the last

2 decades,[9] reflecting advances in biomedical science (e.g., organ transplantation), changing public health priorities (e.g., AIDS prevention), and innovative applications of existing technologies (e.g., aging). For those readers interested in a comprehensive review of the evolution of the field, a special issue of the *Journal of Consulting and Clinical Psychology*[15] is an excellent source.

The goals of this chapter are more modest. We present an overview of clinically important psychosocial factors that mediate health and illness and discuss the most frequently employed interventions used in behavioral medicine to modify their impact. We conclude with an examination of behavioral medicine's role in the management of two very common clinical problems, irritable bowel syndrome and recurrent abdominal pain, to provide perspective on the practice of behavioral medicine in a hospital setting.

Psychosocial Factors Affecting Health and Illness

Stress

Stress has been implicated directly or indirectly in the development and clinical course of a host of physical ailments, from the common cold[16] to coronary heart disease (CHD).[17] Stress is thought to play an important role in the development and maintenance of risk factors for organic disease, such as smoking, obesity, and physical inactivity.[18] The view that stress is ubiquitous and that it has harmful effects on the body's organ systems and defenses has infiltrated the public's consciousness. This view has been succinctly summed up as "a mania for pop psychosomatics, which writes off to stress everything from athlete's foot to cancer" (p. 739).[19]

From a clinical perspective the pathologic effects of stress are of concern. In susceptible individuals, chronic and persistent exposure to stressors, be they real (physical) or perceived (psychological), lead to a dampening of homeostatic mechanisms that restore internal stability and defend against disease.[20] As homeostatic mechanisms become less effective or break down completely under the pressure of chronic stress, susceptible individuals are subject to exacerbations of existing illnesses or are predisposed to new diseases. The outcome of pathologic stress depends on a variety of factors including the type of stressor, the length of exposure, one's genetic predisposition, preexisting coping strategies, and the presence of social and environmental supports.[21] Behavioral medicine's answer to stress is a collection of techniques known as stress management. These techniques teach patients to cultivate low levels of stress arousal, particularly in stressful social environments.

Negative Emotions

Interest in how emotional states affect health and illness is probably as old as medicine itself. Negative emotional states may be precursors of organic disease as suggested by recent studies of CHD[15] and essential hypertension.[22] Moreover, morbidity and a decreased quality of life are often seen in association with chronic pain disorders[23] and with cancer.[24]

Negative emotions such as anger, sadness, and pessimism are part of the human condition and are not necessarily harmful to health. The damaging effects are thought to occur when these emotions are expressed in their chronic forms: hostility, depression, and helplessness, respectively. Interventions used in behavioral medicine for negative emotional states have focused on the development of cognitive coping skills to replace the maladaptive thoughts, feelings, and behavior that are the basis of negative emotional states.

Risk Factors

Nonadherence with Medical Therapy

Nonadherence with medical therapy occurs throughout the life span, and there is little doubt that low rates of adherence to established medical therapies contribute to increased morbidity, increased health care costs, and adverse consequences for public health.[25] Many theories explain why some patients are nonadherent with diagnostic maneuvers and treatment. Belief in the efficacy of treatment, complexity of medical regimens, passive self-care decision-making, and problems with doctor-patient communication are some of the reasons put forth to explain why some patients fail to follow through with prescribed medical therapy.[26] Behavioral medicine interventions are based on the premise that nonadherence is a behavioral problem that is particularly suited to applied behavior analysis methods that aim to modify overt behavior. The patient's beliefs about health and illness and the doctor-patient relationship are not considered relevant targets for intervention. The behavioral procedures of reinforcement and stimulus control have been shown as effective methods for the improvement of adherence from simple to complex medical regimens.[27]

Obesity and Smoking

Despite a long and concerted effort to develop effective interventions to reduce the health risks associated with obesity and smoking, behavioral medicine approaches arguably have had limited success. Obesity has reached epidemic proportions in this country; 61% of adults are either overweight or obese and the prevalence appears to be rising steadily.[28] In contrast, smoking and other forms of tobacco use were declining steadily until 1991, when the prevalence of smoking failed to decrease and the number of individuals who quit smoking failed to increase for the first time in over 35 years.[29] About the same time the effects of smoking-cessation approaches used in behavioral medicine appeared to have stagnated.[30] The situation has changed little since then.[31] Experts agree that the task of reversing these disturbing trends is daunting. It requires the design of new behavioral medicine treatments (based on a better understanding of the causes of obesity and smoking) and public policy initiatives focused on prevention.[32,33]

Behavioral Medicine Interventions

Stress Management

The goal of stress management is to teach patients skills that relieve them from the harmful effects of stress. First, patients must learn to identify thought patterns and social situations that produce stress. Second, patients are taught relaxation techniques that cultivate low states of arousal. A host of relaxation techniques exist in the marketplace; none has been proven to be more therapeutic than any other for stress reduction. Some of the most commonly taught techniques are progressive muscle relaxation, deep breathing, imagery, and meditation. To become skilled in relaxation, patients must practice these techniques daily for 3 to 4 weeks. It is most helpful to provide patients with an audiocassette version of the relaxation instructions that facilitates adherence with practice at home. Children as young as 7 years old can learn relaxation techniques.[34] The final step to prevention involves guiding patients in the use of relaxation techniques in their natural environment, replete with stressful stimuli.

Biofeedback is sometimes used to help patients learn about relaxation techniques. Immediate feedback about muscle tension, heart rate, surface skin temperature, and respiration can facilitate the learning process, particularly for patients who present with high levels of arousal, harbor skepticism about the approach, or doubt their ability to learn relaxation.

Cognitive Coping

Cognitive coping involves teaching a patient to identify negative thoughts and behaviors that increase their stress burden and the situations where stress occurs. Then, positive coping strategies (e.g., positive reappraisal, diverting attention, problem-solving, coping self-statements, disengagement, and relaxation techniques) are taught that replace negative patterns. Rehearsal of coping strategies during therapy sessions is critical for the successful application in the natural environment. Patients are encouraged to start using coping strategies at the first opportunity. Self-monitoring tools such as diaries and checklists are used first to assess maladaptive coping and then to monitor progress and to refine coping strategies as needed.

Behavioral Procedures

One of the most effective techniques to improve adherence is to provide feedback to patients on their adherence early in the course of therapy when they are most at risk to develop patterns of nonadherence.

Objective measures of adherence, such as serum drug levels, urine metabolites, or physiologic markers (e.g., blood glucose level or pulmonary functioning), when feasible, are the feedback methods of choice in this regard.[35] Positive and negative reinforcement are often employed to promote adherence with treatment regimens that extend over long periods. Positive reinforcement is the process by which rewards, such as parking vouchers, gift certificates, negotiated privileges, are provided to the patient contingent on observed or objectively measured adherence at specified intervals. Negative reinforcement is the converse process by which patients lose the opportunity to earn money or privileges if they are nonadherent; they must remain adherent to avoid this possibility. Stimulus-control techniques include teaching patients to self-monitor adherence behaviors, structure their medical therapy to have it occur while performing daily routines, and enlist the social environment to generate external cues for adherence, such as a telephone call, email, or postcard reminder.

Clinical Applications

Irritable Bowel Syndrome and Recurrent Abdominal Pain

A strong, documented relationship exists between stress and abdominal pain. Most people are familiar with the sensation of "butterflies" in the stomach when facing stress, and when bad news is delivered it can be referred to as "a kick in the stomach." Individuals with irritable bowel syndrome (IBS) or its childhood counterpart, recurrent abdominal pain (RAP), almost unanimously endorse stress as a trigger of their symptoms. Abundant and growing research evidence reveals that IBS and RAP may be related to autonomic nervous system function and to an increased sensitivity to physiologic changes in the gut that are also highly responsive to stress.

Behavioral medicine treatments have been highly effective for IBS and RAP[36,37]; they usually involve relaxation training to activate the parasympathetic nervous system and cognitive techniques to decrease the effects of stress on the body. Education is crucial to the process, because a patient needs to understand the rationale for treatment to be invested in it. Biofeedback can also be a useful

training strategy; patients can receive immediate feedback and learn that they can have a significant amount of control over their own bodies. Finally, self-hypnosis has also been successfully used as a pain management strategy that can be integrated into a pain management program.

Education

Patients with IBS or RAP frequently report that they have gotten the message from health care providers that the pain is "in my head." Often the explanation for pain provided by a family physician or gastroenterologist is designed to comfort a patient and to emphasize that no organic cause for the pain can be found, and therefore, there is no disease process to worry about. What the patient hears instead is a dismissal of the pain as not being real or a statement that the doctor cannot be of help with their suffering. One of the significant contributions that behavioral medicine has made in the treatment of stress-related disorders is to focus on the importance of communicating with patients. Simply validating the pain, providing education about the physical affect of stress, and explaining that there are skills that can be learned to manage stress and pain can be extremely beneficial. A shift in perception from being a victim to having options (i.e., to take more control) can be an important first step in the management of chronic pain.

Of course, patients must believe in the efficacy of treatment and in their ability to do what it takes to be successful in the treatment (self-efficacy); one must be motivated to participate. Moreover, the extent to which individuals believe that what they do influences their health (internal locus of control) versus the extent to which they believe health care professionals or others influence their health (external locus of control) varies greatly. For a behavioral medicine intervention to work well, the individual needs to be invested in the work and involved in the treatment program.

Relaxation Training

Stress triggers of IBS or RAP initiate activity in the sympathetic nervous system and affect multiple physiologic activities, including digestion, breathing, and heart rate. The cultivation of a state of low arousal by activating the parasympathetic nervous system is antithetical to this aroused state: one simply cannot be stressed and relaxed at the same time. Relaxation training is designed to teach parasympathetic arousal during times of stress, so symptoms of pain and resultant bowel functioning can be reduced or even eliminated. As reviewed earlier in this chapter, many types of relaxation training are available.

Cognitive Coping Skills

Cognitive treatments for IBS and RAP tend to focus on the identification of stressful situations that may lead to symptoms, examining the thoughts or "internal dialogue" that takes place in these situations, and learning how to change the stressful situation itself, the reaction to the situation, or both. Usually the focus is specifically aimed at stressful situations that can lead to episodes of pain. The symptoms themselves or worries about them can also be significant stressors. Individuals with diarrhea-predominant IBS, for example, often state that concerns about being far from a bathroom and worries about being able to access a bathroom when needed can trigger an episode of pain and diarrhea.

Biofeedback

Biofeedback can aid relaxation training and allow patients to gain insight into their own ability to control different aspects of their bodies. Many individuals who suffer from pain can become distanced from their bodies and lack insight as to what relaxation feels like. They can be taught, however, what relaxation looks like on a monitor, and learn through this method what they need to do in order to achieve that state.

Several types of biofeedback have been used with IBS patients. Thermal biofeedback is often used because it assesses a generalized relaxation response. A thermal sensor is applied to the finger and relaxation techniques are employed to relax the muscles and activate the parasympathetic nervous system, thereby allowing an increase in blood flow to the hand with a resultant increase in temperature. Electromyographic biofeedback can also be used to teach relaxation of specific muscle groups. Another type of biofeedback that has been used specifically with IBS patients is bowel-sound feedback, during which a stethoscope is used to teach patients to change their bowel sounds. No studies have investigated the efficacy of thermal or EMG biofeedback alone for IBS or RAP, and most treatments incorporate elements of other behavioral medicine strategies. Evidence in support of bowel-sound feedback as a treatment for IBS has been mixed.

Hypnosis

Hypnosis can be a very powerful and useful technique when put to use by a trained and experienced clinician. Because the use of hypnotic trance and suggestion tends to focus on changing perceptions and directed attention, it is a particularly useful strategy when working with patients who have chronic or episodic pain.

After the induction is taught, specific images and suggestions can be used to induce a state of relaxation. Often "ego-strengthening" suggestions are used to help deepen the trance and allow the patient to focus. Several different types of images and metaphors can then be used to help the patient gain control of his or her symptoms. Images of flowing water in streams or waterfalls can be used as a metaphor for the GI tract working smoothly, or suggestions of having possession of a switchboard that can be used to manipulate different parts of the body are often used to allow the patient to gain a sense of control over symptoms. As in relaxation training, an audiotape or CD can be made for the patient to practice at home.

References
1. Engel GL: The need for a new medical model: a challenge for biomedicine, *Science* 196:129–136, 1977.
2. Gatchel RJ: *Psychophysiological disorders: past and present perspectives*. In Gatchel RJ, Blanchard EB, editors: *Psychophysiological disorders: research and clinical applications*, Washington, DC, 1993, American Psychological Association, pp 1–21.
3. Schwartz GE, Weiss SM: Yale conference on behavioral medicine: a proposed definition and statement of goals, *J Behav Med* 1:3–13, 1978.

4. Pattishall EG: The development of behavioral medicine: historical models. *Ann Behav Med* 11:43–48.

5. Williams RB, Schneiderman N: Resolved: psychosocial interventions can improve clinical outcomes in organic disease (pro), *Psychosom Med* 64:552–557, 2002.

6. Krantz DS, McCeney MK: Effects of psychological and social factors on organic disease: a critical assessment of research on coronary heart disease, *Annu Rev Psychol* 53:341–369, 2002.

7. Krantz DS, Sheps DS, Carney RM, Natelson BH: Effects of mental stress in patients with coronary artery disease: evidence and clinical implications, *JAMA* 283:1800–1802, 2000.

8. Schneiderman N, Antoni MH, Saab PG, Ironson G: Health psychology: psychosocial and biobehavioral aspects of chronic disease management, *Annu Rev Psychol* 52:555–580, 2001.

9. Keefe FJ, Buffington AL, Studts JL, Rumble ME: Behavioral medicine: 2002 and beyond, *J Consult Clin Psychol* 70:852–856, 2002.

10. Sobel DS: Mind matters, money matters: the cost-effectiveness of mind/body medicine, *JAMA* 284:1705, 2000.

11. Angell M: Disease as a reflection of the psyche, *N Engl J Med* 312:1570–1572, 1985.

12. Relman AS, Angell M: Resolved: psychosocial interventions can improve clinical outcomes in organic disease (con), *Psychosom Med* 64:558–563, 2002.

13. Scheidt S: The current status of heart-mind relationships, *J Psychosom Res* 48:317–320, 2000.

14. Williams R, Schneiderman N, Relman A, Angell M: Resolved: psychosocial interventions can improve clinical outcomes in organic disease—rebuttals and closing arguments, *Psychosom Med* 64:564–567, 2002.

15. Smith TW, Kendall PC, Keefe FJ: Behavioral medicine and clinical health psychology: introduction to the special issue, a view from the decade of behavior, *J Consult Clin Psychol* 70:459–462, 2002.

16. Cohen S, Tyrell DA, Smith AP: Psychological stress and susceptibility to the common cold, *N Engl J Med* 325:606–612, 1991.

17. Smith TW, Ruiz JM: Psychosocial influences on the development and course of coronary heart disease: current status and implications for research and practice, *J Consult Clin Psychol* 70:548–568, 2002.

18. Baum A, Poloszny DM: Health psychology: mapping biobehavioral contributions to health and illness, *Ann Rev Psychol* 50:137–163, 1999.

19. Levenstein S: Psychosocial factors in peptic ulcer and inflammatory bowel disease, *J Consult Clin Psychol* 70:739–750, 2002.

20. Chrousos GP, Gold PW: The concepts of stress and stress system disorders: overview of physical and behavioral homeostasis, *JAMA* 267:1244–1252, 1992.

21. Mayer EA: The neurobiology of stress and gastrointestinal disease, *Gut* 47:861–869, 2000.

22. Blumenthal JA, Sherwood A, Gullette EC, et al: Biobehavioral approaches to the treatment of essential hypertension, *J Consult Clin Psychol* 70:569–589, 2002.

23. Turk DC, Okifuji A: Psychological factors in chronic pain: evolution and revolution, *J Consult Clin Psychol* 70:678–690, 2002.

24. Andersen BL: Biobehavioral outcomes following psychological interventions for cancer patients, *J Consult Clin Psychol* 70:590–610, 2002.

25. McDonald HP, Garg AX, Haynes RB: Interventions to enhance patient adherence to medication prescriptions: scientific review, *JAMA* 288:2868–2879, 2002.

26. Kyngas H, Duffy ME, Kroll T: Conceptual analysis of compliance, *J Clin Nurs* 9:5–12, 2000.

27. Mathews JR, Spieth LE, Christophersen ER: *Behavioral compliance in a pediatric context*. In Roberts, MC editor: *Handbook of pediatric psychology*, ed 2, New York, 1995, Guilford Press, pp 617–632.

28. Prevalence of overweight and obesity among adults: United States, 1999, National Center for Health Statistics, 1999.

29. CDC: Surveillance of smoking-attributable morbidity and years of potential life lost, by state: United States, 1990, *MMWR*, 43:1–8, 1994.

30. Shiffman S: Smoking cessation treatment: any progress? *J Consult Clin Psychol* 61:718–722, 1993.

31. Brandon TH: Behavioral tobacco cessation treatments: yesterday's news or tomorrow's headlines? *J Clin Oncol* 19:64S–68S, 2001.

32. Niaura R, Abrams DB: Smoking cessation: progress, priorities, and prospectus, *J Consult Clin Psychol* 70:494–509, 2002.

33. Wadden TA, Brownell KD, Foster GD: Obesity: responding to the global epidemic, *J Consult Clin Psychol* 70:510–525, 2002.

34. Fentress DW, Masek BJ, Mehegan JE, Benson H: Biofeedback and relaxation-response training in the treatment of pediatric migraine, *Dev Med Child Neurol* 28:139–146, 1986.

35. Dunbar J, Wazak L: *Patient compliance: pediatric and adolescent populations*. In Gross AM, Drabman RS, editors: *Handbook of clinical behavioral pediatrics*, New York, 1990, Plenum, pp 365–382.

36. Blanchard EB: *Long-term follow-up of psychological treatments for irritable bowel syndrome*. In Blanchard, Edward B, editor: *Irritable bowel syndrome: psychosocial assessment and treatment*, Washington, DC, 2001, American Psychological Association, pp 309–314.

37. Blanchard EB, Scharff L: Psychosocial aspects of assessment and treatment of irritable bowel syndrome in adults and recurrent abdominal pain in children, *J Consult Clin Psychol,* 70:725–738, 2002.

Chapter 43

Complementary Medicine and Natural Medications

Felicia A. Smith, M.D.

Complementary and alternative medical (CAM) therapies constitute a diverse spectrum of practices and beliefs in current medical practice. The National Institutes of Health (NIH) defines CAM as "healthcare practices outside the realm of conventional medicine, which are yet to be validated using scientific methods."[1] The term *natural medications* refers to medications derived from natural products which are not approved by the Food and Drug Administration (FDA) for their proposed indication.[2] Natural medications fall under the category of CAM and may include hormones, vitamins, plants, herbs, fatty acids, amino acid derivatives, and homeopathic preparations, among others. Although natural medications have been used for thousands of years, their use in the United States has increased dramatically over the past decade. In fact, a recent study found that in an American ambulatory adult population, 40% of patients routinely used one or more vitamin or mineral supplements.[3] Moreover, between 1990 and 1997 the prevalence of herbal remedy use increased by 380%, while high-dose vitamin use increased by 130%.[4] The consultation psychiatrist must therefore be informed about these medications in order to provide comprehensive patient care. This chapter provides an overview of the use of natural medications in psychiatry. Issues pertaining to general safety and effectiveness are discussed first, followed by a more specific look at some of the remedies used for mood disorders,

anxiety and sleep disorders, menstrual disorders, and dementia. The final section is devoted to a description of two nonmedication alternative therapies: acupuncture and hypnosis.

Efficacy and Safety

Although there has been a recent increase in both governmental and industry sponsorship of clinical research involving natural medications, data regarding effectiveness still lag behind. The true benefits of natural remedies are often unclear given that few systematic studies have addressed the question of effectiveness.[5] Since the FDA does not routinely regulate natural medications, issues of safety remain problematic. One concern flows from the belief that because a remedy is "natural," it is therefore safe. Reports of toxicity may not reach the populations using the remedies because they are often purchased over-the-counter (OTC). Moreover, data are limited regarding the safety and efficacy of combining natural medications and their use with more conventional medications.[5] This situation is very important to the consultation psychiatrist given the prevalence of polypharmacy often seen in inpatient medical settings. It is also noteworthy to mention that patients frequently do not disclose their use of CAM therapies to their physicians. In one study, fewer than 40% of CAM therapies used were disclosed to a physician,[4] thereby making it essential to ask patients specific questions about their use of pre-scribed and OTC medications. Finally, significant variability exists among different preparations of natural medications. Preparations often vary in purity, quality, and potency, and efficacy and side effects may vary accordingly. As mentioned earlier, government- and industry-sponsored studies are increasingly being undertaken to further elucidate the potential uses, safety, and efficacy of these med-ications. The remainder of this chapter outlines what is currently known in this regard for a few such natural medications.

Mood Disorders

Omega-3 fatty acids, St. John's wort (SJW), S-adenosyl methionine (SAMe), folic acid, vitamin B_{12}, and inositol have all been used for mood disorders. The following section describes the efficacy, possible mechanisms of action, dosing, adverse effects, and drug interactions of each of these medications. A particular emphasis is placed on the interface between their psychiatric and other medical uses, as well as on drug interactions, given the nature of consultation psychiatry.

Omega-3 fatty acids are polyunsaturated lipids derived from fish oil that have been shown to have benefits in a variety of health domains including rheumatoid arthritis, Crohn's disease, ulcerative coli-tis, psoriasis, and systemic lupus erythematosus.[6] Cardioprotective effects have also been demon-strated as have several neuropsychiatric benefits. Eicosapentaenoic acid (EPA) and docosahexanoic acid (DHA) are thought to be psychotropically active omega-3 fatty acids.[2] Lower rates of depression and bipolar disorder have been detected in countries where more fish is consumed, suggesting that omega-3 fatty acids may play a protective role in these disorders.[7] Omega-3 fatty acids also may have a role in the treatment of both bipolar disor-der and unipolar depression; positive studies have been reported in each of these domains.[8,9] Further-more, early benefits have been shown in the areas of postpartum depression and schizophrenia.[10–13] Although their mechanism of action is not com-pletely clear, omega-3 fatty acids may function in a similar fashion to mood stabilizers by inhibiting G-protein signal transduction via reduced hydrolysis of phosphatidylinositol and

other membrane phospholipids.[2] Commercially available preparations of omega-3 fatty acids vary in composition, and the suggested ratio of EPA:DHA is controversial. Psychotropically active doses are generally thought to be in the range of 1 to 2 g per day, with the major side effect being dose-related gastrointestinal distress. There is also a theoretical risk of increased bleeding, so concomitant use with high-dose nonsteroidal anti-inflammatory drugs (NSAIDs) or anticoagulants is not recommended. In sum, the use of omega-3 fatty acids is promising, particularly given the range of potential benefits and the relatively low toxicity seen thus far. However, larger studies are still needed.

St. John's wort (SJW) (*Hypericum perforatum L.*) has been shown to be more effective than placebo in the treatment of mild to moderate depression.[14] Studies have suggested that SJW is as effective as low-dose tricyclic antidepressants (TCAs) (e.g., imipramine 75 mg, maprotiline 75 mg, or amitriptyline 75 mg).[2,14] Data comparing SJW and selective serotonin reuptake inhibitors (SSRIs) is more mixed, although in at least two cases SJW was shown to be as effective as sertra-line and fluoxetine in the treatment of mild to moderate depression.[15,16] SJW has not shown an advantage over placebo in other studies[17,18]; how-ever, some believe that a more severely depressed study population may have contributed to these outcomes.[2,5] While *Hypericum* is thought to be the main antidepressant ingredient in SJW, polycy-clic phenols, pseudohypericin, and hyperforin are also thought to be active ingredients. Possible mechanisms of action include: the inhibition of cytokines, a decrease in serotonin (5-HT) receptor density, a decrease in reuptake of neurotransmit-ters, and monoamine oxidase inhibitor (MAOI) activity.[2,5] Of note is that SJW should not be com-bined with SSRIs because of its MAOI activity and the possible development of serotonin syndrome (SS). The metabolism of SJW is not well under-stood, but it is thought to be hepatic. Suggested doses range from 300 to 1800 mg three times per day depending on the preparation, and adverse effects include dry mouth, dizziness, constipation, and phototoxicity. A switch to mania in patients with bipolar disorder may also occur.[19] Finally, there are a number of important drug-drug inter-actions with SJW that are particularly noteworthy for the consultation psychiatrist. Since hyperforin induces CYP-3A4 expression, therapeutic activity of the following medications may be reduced: warfarin, cyclosporine, oral contraceptives, theophylline, digoxin, and indinavir.[2,5] Transplant rejections have been reported as a result of interactions between SJW and cyclosporine; therefore, transplant recipients should not use SJW. Individuals with HIV infection on protease inhibitors also should avoid SJW because of drug interactions. In conclusion, SJW appears to be better than placebo and equivalent to low-dose TCAs for the treatment of mild depression. It may also compare favorably to SSRIs, though more data is needed. It may not be as effective for more severe forms of depression. Care should also be taken given the drug-drug interactions as outlined above.

SAMe in doses of up to 1600 mg per day has been shown to elevate mood in depressed patients. Meta-analyses support antidepressant efficacy of SAMe when compared with placebo and TCAs.[20] However, many studies have used intramuscular (IM) and intravenous (IV) preparations because of the instability of oral SAMe. Oral preparations may require high doses for adequate bioavailability; the medication is relatively expensive. SAMe is the principal methyl donor in the one carbon cycle, and SAMe levels depend on levels of the vitamins, folate and B_{12}. It donates methyl groups to hormones, neurotransmitters, nucleic acids, proteins, and phospholipids. In this light, SAMe may work as an antidepressant by providing methyl groups in the reactions that result in the synthesis of norepinephrine, serotonin, and dopamine.[2,5,21] Potential adverse effects are relatively minor and include anxiety, agitation, a switch to mania, insomnia, dry mouth, bowel changes, and anorexia. Sweating, dizziness, palpitations, and headaches have also been reported. At least one case has been reported of suspected SS when SAMe was combined with clomipramine in an elderly woman.[22] No significant drug-drug interactions have been reported, and there is no apparent hepatotoxicity. SAMe, therefore, is a natural medication that shows promise as an antidepressant. It appears to be relatively safe and is without significant interactions thus far. Further study will help clarify issues of efficacy and safety.

Folate and vitamin B_{12} are vitamins obtained in the diet that play important roles in the synthesis of CNS neurotransmitters (e.g., serotonin, dopamine, and norepinephrine). Sequelae of folate and vitamin B_{12} deficiency include a variety of neuropsychiatric and general medical conditions (e.g., macrocytic anemia, neuropathy, cognitive dysfunction/dementia, and depression). Folate deficiency may result from inadequate dietary intake, malabsorption, inborn errors of metabolism, or an increased demand (e.g., as seen with pregnancy, infancy, bacterial overgrowth, and rapid cellular turnover). Certain drugs may also cause folate deficiency. These include anticonvulsants, oral contraceptives, sulfsalazine, methotrexate, triamterene, trimethoprim, pyrmethamine, and alcohol, among others.[23] Vitamin B_{12} deficiency states also may result from inadequate dietary intake, malabsorption, impaired utilization, and interactions with other drugs. Included in such drugs are colchicine, H_2 blockers, metformin, nicotine, oral contraceptive pills, cholestyramine, K-Dur, and zidovudine.[23] Folate deficiency may also hinder antidepressant response,[24] and folate supplementation may be a beneficial adjunct to SSRI-refractory depression.[25] Vitamin B_{12} deficiency, in turn, may cause an earlier age of onset of depression.[2] The recommended daily dose of vitamin B_{12} is 6 μg, while that of folate is 400 μg. Since both vitamins are involved in the synthesis of CNS neurotransmitters, adequate levels provide for optimal neurotransmitter synthesis that may aid in reversing depression. Finally, folate may "mask" vitamin B_{12} deficiency by correcting macrocytic anemia while neuropathy continues, so vitamin B_{12} levels should be routinely measured when high doses of folate are given. Folate may also reduce effectiveness of phenytoin, methotrexate, and phenobarbital.[26] In summary, correction of folate and B_{12} deficiency may improve depression or augment other antidepressant therapy. Psychiatrists should be mindful of potential deficiency states as outlined here and should check serum levels in patients at risk of deficiencies or who have not responded to antidepressant treatment.

Inositol is a natural isomer of glucose that is present in common foods. It has been found in small studies to be effective in the treatment of depression, panic disorder, obsessive-compulive disorder (OCD), and possibly bipolar depression.[27–30] Effective doses range from 12 to 18 g per day. Negative monotherapy trials with inositol have been seen in schizophrenia, dementia, attention deficit hyperactivity disorder (ADHD), premenstrual dysphoric disorder, autism, and electroconvulsive therapy (ECT)-induced cognitive impairment.[5,30] Inositol is a polyol precursor in brain second messenger systems that may reverse desensitization of serotonin receptors.[2,5] Mild adverse effects include gastrointestinal (GI) upset, headache, dizziness, sedation, and insomnia. There is no apparent toxicity or known drug interactions at this time.[2,5] Treatment with inositol for the above indications currently appears safe and remains promising. The following section will move from the treatment of mood disorders to those of anxiety and insomnia. Three natural agents often used for their anxiolytic and hypnotic properties will be discussed: valerian, melatonin, and kava.

Anxiolytics and Hypnotics

Valerian (*Valeriana officinalis*) is a sedating plant extract that has been used for over 2000 years. It is thought to promote natural sleep after several weeks of use by decreasing sleep latency and by improving overall sleep quality. The effects on slow-wave sleep increase with time. Valerian is thought to work by decreasing gamma amino-butyric acid (GABA) breakdown.[2,5] Sedative effects are dose-related with usual dosages in the range of 450 to 600 mg about 2 hours before bedtime. Dependence has not been an issue, nor has daytime drowsiness. Adverse effects are thought to be uncommon and include blurry vision, GI symptoms, headache, and dystonia. Because of potential hepatotoxicity, valerian should be avoided in patients with liver dysfunction. Major drug interactions have not been reported. In sum, valerian has been used as a hypnotic for many years with relatively few reported adverse effects. More trials are needed to further quantify efficacy and safety issues.

Melatonin is a hormone made in the pineal gland that has gained popularity for its use by travelers to avoid "jet lag." It is derived from serotonin and is thought to play a role in the organization of circadian rhythms via interaction with the suprachiasmatic nucleus.[31] Melatonin generally facilitates falling asleep within 1 hour, no matter what time of day it is taken. Optimal doses are

controversial although they are thought to be in the range of 0.25 to 0.30 mg per day. Some preparations, however, contain as much as 5 mg of melatonin.[2,5] Daytime sleepiness and confusion have been noted with high doses. Other adverse effects include a decreased sex drive, retinal damage, hypothermia, and fertility problems. Moreover, melatonin is contraindicated in pregnancy and in immunocompromised patients.[2,5] There are few reports of drug-drug interactions. In conclusion, melatonin is a promising and relatively safe hypnotic and organizer of circadian rhythms. Caution should be taken in patients at risk as noted above.

Kava (*Piper methysticum*) is derived from a root originating in the Polynesian Islands. Though it is believed to have a mild anxiolytic effect, study results have been mixed. The mechanism of action is attributed to kavapyrones, which are central muscle relaxants involved in GABA receptor binding and norepinephrine uptake inhibition.[2,5] The suggested dose is 60 to 120 mg per day with GI upset, headaches, and dizziness being the major adverse effects. Toxic reactions, however, have been seen at high doses or with prolonged use including: ataxia, hair loss, respiratory problems, yellowing of the skin, and vision problems. Even more worrisome are reports of severe hepatotoxicity, including some requiring liver transplantation.[2,5] For this reason, the FDA is currently investigating the safety of kava and is recommending that the duration of use not exceed 3 months. While kava appears to be somewhat efficacious in the treatment of mild anxiety, current concerns about safety make cautious use essential.

Premenstrual and Menopausal Symptoms

Black cohosh (*Cimicifuga racemosa*) at a dose of 40 mg per day has been shown to reduce physical and psychological menopausal symptoms.[32] Active ingredients are thought to be triterpenoids, isoflavones, and aglycones, which may participate in suppression of luteinizing hormone in the pituitary gland.[2,5] Mild side effects include headache, dizziness, GI upset, and weight gain. Limited data have not revealed specific toxicity or drug interactions. Black cohosh is not recommended for individuals who are pregnant or have heart disease or hypertension. More data are needed to further specify beneficial effects as well as safety profiles.

Cognition and Dementia

Ginkgo biloba comes from the seed of the Ginkgo tree and has been a part of Chinese medicine for thousands of years. It has generally been used for the treatment of impaired cognition and affective symptoms in dementing illnesses; however, a possible new role has emerged in the management of antidepressant-induced sexual dysfunction.[33] Memory and abstract thinking are target symptoms when used for individuals with dementia. At doses of 120 mg per day, studies have shown modest but significant improvements in both cognitive performance and social functioning.[34] Progression of disease may be delayed by 6 to 12 months. Further evidence suggests greater improvement for those with mild dementia and stabilization at most with more severe disease.[35] *Ginkgo biloba* may also enhance learning capacity as evidenced by one study of healthy young volunteers who made significant improvements in speed of information processing, executive processing, and working memory on the medication.[36] The active components of ginkgo, flavonoids, and terpene lactones, stimulate nerve cells that are still functional,[2,5] which seems to provide protection from pathologic effects like hypoxia, ischemia, seizures, and peripheral damage. Since ginkgo has been shown to inhibit platelet activating factor, it should be avoided in those at high risk of bleeding. Other side effects include headache, gastrointestinal distress, headache, seizures in epileptics, and dizziness. The suggested dose of ginkgo biloba is 120 to 240 mg per day with a minimum 8-week course of treatment. However, full benefit may not be seen for a year. In conclusion, gingko biloba appears to be a safe and efficacious cognition-enhancing medication. It may also have a role in reducing antidepressant-induced sexual dysfunction. Further studies are needed to fully understand its complete and long-term effects.

Dehydroepiandrosterone (DHEA) is an androgenic hormone synthesized primarily in the adrenal glands, which is converted to testosterone and estrogen.[20] Although study results have been somewhat mixed, DHEA is thought to play a role in enhancing memory and in improving depressive symptoms.[20,37–39] Mechanisms of action may include modulation of NMDA receptors and GABA (A) receptor antagonism.[20] Synthetic DHEA is available in an oral formulation and an intra-oral spray with doses range from 5 to 100 mg per day. Like many other natural remedies, strength and purity are not regulated. In women there is a risk of weight gain, hirsutism, menstrual irregularity, voice changes, and headache. Men may experience gynecomastia and prostatic hypertrophy, and the effects on hormone-sensitive tumors are not known.[20] While early data is promising for DHEA, larger studies must be undertaken to clarify risks versus benefits before it may be safely recommended.

Nonmedication Therapies

Acupuncture has been employed in Eastern countries for several millennia for the treatment of neuropsychiatric disorders, especially pain. Acupuncture is quite safe with no major adverse events reported in a recent review of over 65,000 treatments.[40] Although there are some data to support its use to treat a wide range of psychiatric disorders including schizophrenia, bipolar disorder, substance abuse, and mood and anxiety disorders, the lack of an ideal placebo has been a major barrier in establishing its efficacy in Western studies. However, recent findings in the arena of functional neuroimaging may provide a deeper understanding of the role of acupuncture in mediating pain perception.[41] Further study will help elucidate potential neuropsychiatric benefits of this ancient Eastern treatment.

Hypnosis may be defined as "an event or ritual between a hypnotist and an hypnotic subject in which both agree to use suggestion to bring about a change in perception or behavior."[42] Hypnosis is thought to depend on the dissociative and imaginative abilities of the subject, motivation of the subject, and on the relationship between the hypnotist and subject.[42] Mechanisms are unclear, though levels to which a patient can be hypnotized tend to fall on a bell-shaped curve. Although hypnosis may be used for a wide variety of medical and psychiatric conditions, the following disorders often respond better than others: anxiety, pain, asthma, phobias, nausea, vomiting, and bulimia.[42] Contraindications include unwillingness to be hypnotized, a history of paranoia, and an inexperienced hypnotist. Since hypnosis may be employed at the bedside, it is particularly attractive to the consultation psychiatrist. Finally, hypnosis is a powerful tool when administered by properly trained individuals, and it may be used alone or as an adjunct in the treatment of a wide array of medical disorders.

Conclusion

The spectrum of CAM therapies is quite diverse in current medical practice and is gaining significant popularity in the United States. Historical lack of scientific research in this area has contributed to deficiencies in knowledge with respect to safety and efficacy of many of the natural remedies on the market today. A recent surge in funding by governmental and industry sources should help in this regard. Current knowledge about a few such therapies has been outlined in this chapter, including proposed treatments for mood disorders, anxiety and sleep disorders, menstrual disorders, and dementia. Many of these therapies may prove to be a valuable addition to the armamentarium of treatments available to psychiatrists in the future. A particular emphasis was placed on potential adverse effects and drug-drug interactions given the nature of consultation psychiatry. A general knowledge of these therapies and routine questioning about their use is an essential part of comprehensive care by the consultation psychiatrist.

References

1. Eisenberg DM: *Epidemiology of complementary and alternative medicine (cam) and integrative medicine*. Division for Research and Education in Complementary and Integrative Medical Therapies, Harvard Medical School, 2003.
2. Mischoulon D, Nierenberg AA: *Natural medications in psychiatry*. In Stern TA, Herman JB, editors: *Psychiatry update and board preparation*, ed 2, New York, 2004, McGraw-Hill.
3. Kaufman DW, Kelly JP, Rosenberg L, et al: Recent patterns of medication use in the ambulatory adult population of the United States: the Slone survey, *JAMA* 287(3):337–344, 2002.
4. Eisenberg DM, Davis RB, Ettner SL, et al: Trends in alternative medicine use in the United States, 1990–1997: results of a follow-up national survey, *JAMA* 280(18):1569–1575, 1998.
5. Mischoulon D, Nierenberg AA: *Natural medications in psychiatry*. In Stern TA, Herman JB, Slavin PL, editors: *The Massachusetts General Hospital guide to primary care psychiatry*, ed 2, New York, 2004, McGraw-Hill.
6. Simopoulos AP: Omega-3 fatty acids in inflammation and autoimmune diseases, *J Am Coll Nutr* 21(6):495–505, 2002.
7. Hibbeln JR, Salem N Jr: Dietary polyunsaturated fatty acids and depression: when cholesterol does not satisfy, *Am J Clin Nutr* 62(1):1–9, 1995.
8. Stoll AL, Severus WE, Freeman MP, et al: Omega 3 fatty acids in bipolar disorder: a preliminary double-blind, placebo-controlled trial, *Arch Gen Psychiatry* 56(5):407–412, 1999.
9. Nemets B, Stahl Z, Belmaker RH: Addition of omega-3 fatty acid to maintenance medication treatment for recurrent unipolar depressive disorder, *Am J Psychiatry* 159(3):477–479, 2002.
10. Hibbeln JR: Seafood consumption, the DHA content of mothers' milk and prevalence rates of postpartum depression: a cross-national, ecological analysis, *J Affect Disord.* 69(1–3):15–29, 2002.
11. Hibbeln JR, Makino KK, Martin CE, et al: Smoking, gender, and dietary influences on erythrocyte essential fatty acid composition among patients with schizophrenia or schizoaffective disorder, *Biol Psychiatry* 53(5):431–441, 2003.
12. Horrobin DF: The membrane phospholipid hypothesis as a biochemical basis for the neurodevelopmental concept of schizophrenia, *Schizophr Res* 30(3):193–208, 1998.
13. Peet M, Brind J, Ramchand CN, et al: Two double-blind placebo-controlled pilot studies of eicosapentaenoic acid in the treatment of schizophrenia, *Schizophr Res* 49(3):243–251, 2001.
14. Linde K, Ramirez G, Mulrow CD, et al: St John's wort for depression: an overview and meta-analysis of randomised clinical trials, *BMJ* 313(7052):253–258, 1996.
15. Brenner R, Azbel V, Madhusoodanan S, Pawlowska M: Comparison of an extract of hypericum (LI 160) and sertraline in the treatment of depression: a double-blind, randomized pilot study, *Clin Ther* 22(4):411–419, 2000.
16. Schrader E: Equivalence of St John's wort extract (Ze 117) and fluoxetine: a randomized, controlled study in mild-moderate depression, *Int Clin Psychopharmacol* 15(2):61–68, 2000.
17. Shelton RC, Keller MB, Gelenberg A, et al: Effectiveness of St John's wort in major depression: a randomized controlled trial, *JAMA* 285(15):1978–1986, 2001.
18. Hypericum Depression Trial Study Group: Effect of *Hypericum perforatum* (St John's wort) in major depressive disorder: a randomized controlled trial, *JAMA* 287(14):1807–1814, 2002.

19. Nierenberg AA, Burt T, Matthews J, Weiss AP: Mania associated with St. John's wort, *Biol Psychiatry* 46(12):1707–1708, 1999.

20. Crone C, Gabriel G, Wise TN: Non-herbal nutritional supplements—the next wave: a comprehensive review of risks and benefits for the C-L psychiatrist, *Psychosomatics* 42(4):285–299, 2001.

21. Mischoulon D, Fava M: Role of *S*-adenosyl-L-methionine in the treatment of depression: a review of the evidence, *Am J Clin Nutr* 76(5):1158S–1161S, 2002.

22. Iruela LM, Minguez L, Merino J, Monedero G: Toxic interaction of *S*-adenosylmethionine and clomipramine, *Am J Psychiatry* 150(3):522, 1993.

23. Snow CF: Laboratory diagnosis of vitamin B12 and folate deficiency: a guide for the primary care physician, *Arch Intern Med* 159(12):1289–1298, 1999.

24. Fava M, Borus JS, Alpert JE, et al: Folate, vitamin B12, and homocysteine in major depressive disorder, *Am J Psychiatry* 154(3):426–428, 1997.

25. Alpert JE, Mischoulon D, Rubenstein GE, et al: Folinic acid (Leucovorin) as an adjunctive treatment for SSRI-refractory depression, *Ann Clin Psychiatry* 14(1):33–38, 2002.

26. Reynolds EH: Benefits and risks of folic acid to the nervous system, *J Neurol Neurosurg Psychiatry* 72(5):567–571, 2002.

27. Levine J, Barak Y, Kofman O, Belmaker RH: Follow-up and relapse analysis of an inositol study of depression, *Isr J Psychiatry Relat Sci* 32(1):14–21, 1995.

28. Benjamin J, Agam G, Levine J, et al: Inositol treatment in psychiatry, *Psychopharmacol Bull* 31(1):167–175, 1995.

29. Palatnik A, Frolov K, Fux M, Benjamin J: Double-blind, controlled, crossover trial of inositol versus fluvoxamine for the treatment of panic disorder, *J Clin Psychopharmacol* 21(3):335–339, 2001.

30. Fux M, Levine J, Aviv A, Belmaker RH: Inositol treatment of obsessive-compulsive disorder, *Am J Psychiatry* 153(9):1219–1221, 1996.

31. Zhdanova IV, Wurtman RJ: Efficacy of melatonin as a sleep-promoting agent, *J Biol Rhythms* 12(6):644–650, 1997.

32. McKenna DJ, Jones K, Humphrey S, Hughes K: Black cohosh: efficacy, safety, and use in clinical and preclinical applications, *Altern Ther Health Med* 7(3):93–100, 2001.

33. Ashton AK, Ahrens K, Gupta S, Masand PS: Antidepressant-induced sexual dysfunction and *Ginkgo biloba*, *Am J Psychiatry* 157(5):836–837, 2000.

34. Le Bars PL, Katz MM, Berman N, et al: A placebo-controlled, double-blind, randomized trial of an extract of Ginkgo biloba for dementia: North American EGb Study Group, *JAMA* 278(16):1327–1332, 1997.

35. Le Bars PL, Velasco FM, Ferguson JM, et al: Influence of the severity of cognitive impairment on the effect of the *Ginkgo biloba* extract EGb 761 in Alzheimer's disease, *Neuropsychobiology* 45(1):19–26, 2002.

36. Stough C, Clarke J, Lloyd J, Nathan PJ: Neuropsychological changes after 30-day *Ginkgo biloba* administration in healthy participants, *Int J Neuropsychopharmacol* 4(2):131–134, 2001.

37. Wolkowitz OM, Reus VI, Roberts E, et al: Dehydroepiandrosterone (DHEA) treatment of depression, *Biol Psychiatry* 41(3):311–318, 1997.

38. Wolkowitz OM, Reus VI, Keebler A, et al: Double-blind treatment of major depression with dehydroepiandrosterone, *Am J Psychiatry* 156(4):646–649, 1999.

39. Bloch M, Schmidt PJ, Danaceau MA, et al: Dehydroepiandrosterone treatment of midlife dysthymia, *Biol Psychiatry* 45(12):1533–1541, 1999.

40. Yamashita H, Tsukayama H, White AR, et al: Systematic review of adverse events following acupuncture: the Japanese literature, *Complement Ther Med* 9(2): 98–104, 2001.

41. Hui KK, Liu J, Makris N, et al: Acupuncture modulates the limbic system and subcortical gray structures of the human brain: evidence from fMRI studies in normal subjects, *Hum Brain Mapp* 9(1): 13–25, 2000.

42. Kulleseid S, Surman OS: *Hypnosis*. In Stern TA, Herman JB, editors: *Psychiatry update and board preparation*, New York, 2000, McGraw-Hill, pp 467–470.

Chapter 44

Collaborative Care: Psychiatry and Primary Care

B. J. Beck, M.S.N., M.D.

The convergence of several historic trends[1] in the health care system has necessitated novel approaches to the psychiatric care of patients in the general medical setting. Such approaches must meet the mandates of cost containment and appropriate allocation of limited resources and are potentiated by advances in psychopharmacology. Previously considered a hospital-based specialist, the psychiatric consultant now must be comfortable in the outpatient medical clinic because shorter medical/surgical hospitalizations and more outpatient procedures, such as same-day surgery, have transitioned the locus of care for medically ill patients from inpatient to outpatient settings.[2] At the same time, primary care providers (PCPs) are seeing more seriously ill psychiatric patients in their outpatient practices as shorter psychiatric hospitalizations have transitioned these patients back to their communities more quickly, without a concomitant increase in community mental health resources.[3] Consultation psychiatrists are well positioned to collaborate with their medical colleagues in the development and implementation of pragmatic and cost-effective outpatient models of care.

Burgeoning medical cost and subsequent need to allocate limited health care resources in the United States have moved the focus from patient to population-based care.[4] In a society that so highly values the individual, this painful transition has, nonetheless, exposed the tremendous fiscal burden of psychiatric morbidity. The psychiatrically disordered population experiences increased *physical* health care utilization, work absenteeism, unemployment, subjective disability,[5–7] and mortality. Though more difficult to demonstrate, there is also evidence of the cost-offset value of appropriate and timely psychiatric treatment.[8,9]

Changes in health care reimbursement have resulted in conflicted PCP incentives to recognize and treat psychiatric problems.[10] On the one hand, prepaid, provider-risk plans, such as health maintenance organizations (HMOs) and other capitated programs, have exposed the expensive use of general medical services by patients with untreated or poorly managed psychiatric illness. This statistic serves as an incentive for the PCP to initiate treatment for the more common psychiatric problems seen in primary care. On the other hand, the PCP gate-keeper system, which evolved to manage the expense of specialty care, can be a disincentive to the recognition of more serious mental illness or any mental condition the PCP is not comfortable treating. Managed care organizations (MCOs) often carve out "behavioral health care" to managed behavioral health organizations (MBHOs)[11] that may have limited referral networks not inclusive of the PCP's psychiatric colleagues. This situation makes the referral process a time-consuming disincentive and complicates future communication and collaboration between mental health and physical health providers.

Many of the MBHOs have spearheaded initiatives to promote treatment of common psychiatric problems in the primary care setting. (Yet, most do not credential or contract with nonpsychiatric physicians, so the PCP's treatment of psychiatric problems essentially cost-shifts to the [medical] MCOs.)

Epidemiology

The large Epidemiologic Catchment Area (ECA) Study found that during a 6-month interval, roughly 7% of community residents seek help for a mental health problem. More than 60% of these individuals never see a mental health professional; they seek care in a general medical setting, often from their PCP.[12] Even those with full-criteria mental disorders are more than three times as likely to see a general medical clinician than a mental health professional.[13] Psychiatric distress, therefore, is exceedingly common among primary care populations. About half of general medical outpatients have some psychiatric symptoms. The use of structured diagnostic interviews has detected a prevalence of 25% to 35% for diagnosable psychiatric conditions in this patient population. However, roughly 10% of primary care patients have significant psychiatric symptomatology that does not meet criteria for a recognizable, *Diagnostic and Statistical Manual for Mental Disorders*, fourth edition (*DSM-IV*) psychiatric disorder.[14] Of the full criteria disorders, the vast majority are mood disorders (80%), with depression being the most prevalent (60%) and anxiety a distant second (20%). The more severe disorders (e.g., psychotic) are more likely to be treated by mental health professionals.[13]

Multiple studies have suggested that PCPs routinely diagnose less than half of the full criteria mental disorders present in their patients.[15,16] However, newer information suggests that PCPs do recognize more seriously depressed[17] or anxious[18] patients. These same studies have demonstrated that higher functioning, less severely symptomatic primary care patients have relatively good outcomes, even with short courses of relatively low-dose medication. This highlights the diagnostic difficulty in the primary care setting. Primary care patients are different than those who seek specialty care, (which is a population in whom most psychiatric research is done). Primary care patients may present earlier in the course of their illness, since they have an established relationship with their PCP that is not dependent on their having a psychiatric disorder. They frequently present with somatic complaints, rather than psychiatric symptoms. Since the *soma* is the rightful domain of the PCP, this further obscures the diagnosis. Primary care patients also may have acute psychiatric symptoms that clear relatively quickly and before medication has had time to become therapeutic, which suggests that such individuals might benefit as much from watchful waiting and from empathic support of their PCP. There is a high noise-to-signal ratio in psychiatrically distressed primary care patients. That is, as many as a one third of these significantly distressed patients have subsyndromal disorders, which are symptoms that do not meet full, *DSM-IV* criteria for a diagnosable mental disorder. This diagnostic ambiguity in the general medical setting is paralleled by the relatively good outcomes that primary care patients experience on what most psychiatrists would consider nontherapeutic doses and duration of pharmacotherapy[15,19] and calls into question the significance of the PCP's failure to diagnose.

Barriers to Treatment

Although symptom recognition is necessary, it is not sufficient to ensure treatment of psychiatric problems in the primary care setting.[20] Even when PCPs are informed of the results of standardized screening tests, they may not initiate treatment. PCP, patient, and systems factors collude to inhibit the discussion necessary to promote treatment ("don't ask/don't tell").[21]

Physician factors, the "don't ask" part of the equation, include the failure to take a social history or to perform a mental status examination (MSE).[22] This behavior has been attributed to deficits in training of medical students and residents,[23] time and productivity pressures, and to personal defenses such as identification, denial,[24] or isolation of affect. PCPs are experienced and more comfortable addressing their patients' physical complaints. Some PCPs fear their patients will leave their practice if asked about mental health issues. The PCP, like many patients, may not believe treatment will help. Not having a ready response or approach to a problem is a major deterrent to identification of a new problem within the context of a 15-minute primary care visit. Denial or avoidance may prevail when the time-pressured PCP feels unsure of how or whether to treat or refer.

Stigma, which is prevalent among patients and providers, is a major patient deterrent to initiating a discussion of psychiatric symptomatology. Often patients "don't tell" because of shame or embarrassment. They may believe psychiatric problems are a personal weakness, and they may perceive that their PCP shares this belief. Patients may not know they have a diagnosable or treatable mental disorder.[25] These are among the reasons that primary care patients more frequently have physical complaints. Somatic complaints also increase the diagnostic complexity[26] since medical disorders may simulate psychiatric disorders, psychiatric disorders may lead to physical symptoms, and psychiatric and medical disorders may coexist.

Systems factors already alluded to include financial imperatives to contain cost and increase efficiency. Mental health carve-outs have either eliminated or greatly complicated, the possibility of reimbursing PCP treatment of mental disorders. Prepaid plans, such as HMOs, significantly decrease incentives to offer anything "extra."[27] The necessity to increase productivity has excessively shortened the "routine visit," now often less than 15 minutes, while the tremendous burden of required documentation further erodes clinically available time. (The implementation in some practices of the electronic medical record [EMR] has standardized and improved documentation, but has brought about its own time-consuming offsets.) At this point, the pressures are so overwhelming that few PCPs can sustain full-time clinical practice.

The Goals of Collaboration

The four major goals of collaboration are to improve access, treatment, outcomes, and communication.

Access

Collaborative care in the primary care setting, addresses both physician and patient factors that limit the patient's access to appropriate assessment and treatment. Most patients are not new to the general medical setting and, therefore, feel relatively comfortable and unstigmatized in that setting. Conversely they may believe the mental health clinic is for "crazy people," and that they do not identify with the (perceived) clientele (it's not that they *believe* they don't identify, it's that they *don't* identify). A specified mental health wing or floor in the primary care setting may hold that same stigma and act as a disincentive for patients to access treatment. Most patients do not know of a psychiatrist or how to access care from one and may not feel certain that they need one. The unaided decision to foray into the mental health arena may be fraught with shame and anxiety, powerful deterrents to making that first call. Calling the PCP's office and making an appointment for fatigue, sleep problems, weight loss, or palpitations is infinitely less threatening.

An established relationship between the PCP and a trusted, accessible psychiatric consultant removes the onus of recognizing, treating, or referring patients with mental disorders. With this availability of expert opinion and back-up, PCPs more readily identify psychiatric distress in their patients and are more likely to initiate treatment.

Treatment

In the past, PCPs often prescribed insufficient doses of medications, such as amitriptyline (25 mg) for major depression.[28] Since the advent of safer, well-tolerated medications, such as selective serotonin-reuptake inhibitors (SSRIs), the selection of medications by PCPs has improved,[29,30] although the dose chosen often remains suboptimal. Benzodiazepines have been prescribed by PCPs more frequently than any other class of psychotropic medication, even for major depression,[31] although they now are appropriately surpassed by antidepressant prescriptions.[30] Collaboration with the consultation psychiatrist can improve the choice, dose, and management of psychotropic medications.

Outcomes

Several studies have demonstrated better outcomes for seriously depressed primary care patients treated collaboratively by their PCP and a psychiatrist.[32–34] Cost offset, however, is difficult to demonstrate because of the hidden costs of psychiatric disability. Nonetheless, there is some evidence for a decrease in total health care spending when mental health problems are adequately addressed. Even if this were not so, the case for cost-effectiveness could be made.[35,36] That is, care for the patient's psychiatric problem is more cost-effective than spending the same amount of money addressing the often nonresponsive, somatic complaints of high-maintenance, high-cost medical patients.

Communication

Collaboration ends the PCP's justifiable complaint of the "black box" of psychiatry because communication is implicit in these models of care. The flow of information is useful for the psychiatrist and the PCP, and hence, must be bidirectional. PCP referrals provide pertinent information and state the clinical question. In addition to the target psychiatric symptoms, the PCP has important information about the medical history, allergies, treatments, and medications. The collaborating psychiatrist shares findings, diagnostic impressions, and treatment recommendations. Information about referrals and consultations should be written, and, whenever possible, provided verbally. This protocol improves documentation and ensures an understanding between collaborating care providers. Secure e-mail environments may also provide a venue for almost immediate feedback and a focus on the pertinent details for the busy PCP.

Patients, of course, must be aware of the collaborative relationship between the PCP and the psychiatrist, as well as their shared communication.

Roles, Relationships, and Expectations

Successful collaboration requires a clear understanding and definition of roles. All parties, including the patient, should recognize the PCP's responsibility for the patient's overall care. The PCP is the broker and overseer of all specialty services. The psychiatrist is a consultant to the PCP and sometimes a cotreater, depending on the model employed. Collaboration does not breach patient confidentiality because the PCP and the psychiatrist are now within the circle of care, and the patient is informed of this relationship.

However, this free flow of communication and documentation has reasonable limitations. If a patient asks that particular details not be placed in their general medical record and these details do not directly affect their medical care (e.g., a history of childhood incest), it is reasonable to respect this wish. The pertinent information (e.g., the experience of childhood trauma) can be expressed in more general terms. However, information that affects medical treatment, such as current or past drug addiction, or safety, such as suicidal or homicidal intent, or previous suicide attempt, cannot be withheld from the PCP, and the patient should be so informed.

When the PCP refers the patient to the psychiatrist, the patient should understand what to expect from the visit. At the start of the visit, the psychiatric consultant also should clearly and consistently state the parameters of the contact (e.g., whether it will be a one-time consultation, with or without the possibility of medication follow-up, or possible referral for therapy). If the psychiatrist sees the patient more than once, the relationship between the PCP and psychiatrist may need to be restated. The clarity of the providers' roles and relationship serves to spare the patient a sense of abandonment, either by the PCP when the patient is referred to the psychiatrist, or by the psychiatrist when the patient is returned to the PCP for ongoing psychiatric management.

In collaborative models of care, it is common for the psychiatric notes to be placed in the general medical record, which may raise issues of confidentiality and privacy. Most states require a specific release for mental health or substance abuse treatment records. Psychiatric or mental health notes in the general medical record should be color-coded or otherwise flagged, so they can be removed when records are copied for general medical release of information. In practices with an EMR, some coding system must also be in place to avoid the inadvertent release of this information.

Models of Collaboration

Collaborative models differ in a number of ways, such as where the patient is seen, whether there is a single medical record, how providers communicate, whether the consultant recommends or initiates treatment, and whether the psychiatrist sees the patient (at all, once, more than once) or is an ongoing treater. Other differences include whether both providers are part of the same medical staff and how physically or telephonically available the psychiatrist is to the PCP.

Outpatient Consultation Models

Consultation implies collaboration in that the PCP refers the patient to the psychiatrist, or the PCP presents the patient to the psychiatrist to obtain expert advice or recommendations. Depending on the setting or the system, one medical record may be shared or providers may maintain separate records and share pertinent information. Patients may be seen in either the psychiatric or the primary care setting.

Some have asked how outpatient consultation differs from the practice of private psychiatrists who may have established referral sources in the primary care sector. Such psychiatrists generally do not develop truly collaborative relationships, with ongoing communication or shared records. They treat in parallel, not in collaboration.

Specialty Psychiatric Clinics

Specialty psychiatric clinics such as an eating disorders clinic generally maintain separate records, require the patient to be seen in the psychiatric clinic, and develop some means of ongoing, clinically relevant communication with the PCP. Patients typically need to have well-defined and recognized problems to get referred, and such clinics usually exist in teaching hospitals or tertiary care centers, as opposed to the PCP's practice setting. Although stigma may interfere with patient adherence to such a referral, one major advantage of such clinics is the expert, multidisciplinary approach they provide for patients with complex psychiatric and medical problems.

Consultation Psychiatrists[37,38]

Consultation psychiatrists may render a one-visit opinion in the primary care clinic. (Sometimes patients are sent to the consultant psychiatrist's office, just as with other specialty consultations). This model is similar to the consultation model used in the inpatient medical setting. The consultation should be written or transcribed into the primary care record. Immediate verbal communication, in person, whenever possible, or by phone or voice mail, greatly enhances the utility of such consultations. The consultant generally does not initiate treatment but makes practical recommendations. The role of the PCP and occurrence in the primary care setting enhances patient participation and decreases stigma. This model also promotes opportunities for ongoing informal education between the PCP and the consultant.

Psychiatric Teleconsultation

Psychiatric teleconsultation is a service with full-time, experienced consultation psychiatrists available for immediate telephone consultation to PCPs. This service, which is not accessible to patients, can provide general psychiatric information, consultation about pharmacologic or behavioral management, or triage and referral functions. Computer technology is used to maintain a database, promote timely referrals, and generate follow-up letters to PCPs. There is currently no direct third-party reimbursement for the full-time teleconsultant's services. At one time, increased capitation was expected to provide a funding source because of the cost-offset of this timely service. That expectation, however, was never realized, which effectively terminated some of these services. (This might be a single, viable option for psychiatric consultation in some remote areas of the country, where it might be tacked onto already established, more general teleconsultation services. This possibility, however, still begs the question of reimbursement).

Psychiatrist on the Primary Care Clinic Medical Staff

When the psychiatrist is a medical staff colleague of the PCP, there are enhanced possibilities for collaboration and shared care. This PCP-consultant proximity facilitates communication, formal and informal education, immediate access to curbside consultation, and heightened PCP awareness of psychiatric problems in their patients. This arrangement can also provide an excellent opportunity for training of both psychiatric and primary care residents. Patients appreciate being seen in the more familiar primary care setting, and they feel less stigmatized.

Several models of care have evolved or been developed to utilize the services of an in-house psychiatrist. The psychiatrist may (1) consult as a member of the medical team, (2) evaluate and treat patients in parallel with the PCP, (3) alternate visits with the PCP while treatment is initiated, or (4) evaluate, stabilize, and return the patient to the PCP with recommendations for continued care, or facilitate referrals to outside mental health providers.

Staff Consultant

Consultations, as above, are written in the regular medical record. The permanency of the psychiatrist allows for a more finely tuned consultant-PCP relationship. For instance, with a previously established agreement, the consultant may initiate the recommended treatment. The consultation psychiatrist may offer clinically relevant suggestions during case conferences or discussions of more complex patients. The psychiatrist may also see the patient with the PCP during the primary care visit, capitalizing on the PCP's extensive knowledge of and long-term relationship with the patient to provide more timely treatment recommendations.

Parallel Care

If the psychiatrist assumes the ongoing psychiatric care of patients in parallel with the PCP, some clinics have separate mental health charts. This option requires some overt means of communication to keep all providers informed. In clinics with an EMR, a single up-to-date medication list will at least keep both providers aware of current medications and medication changes.

Some primary care clinics incorporate a mental health unit or clinic. If this is an identifiable, special area within the clinic, it is fraught with the same stigma that occurs when the clinics are truly separate. Although still within the circle of care, the larger the clinic and more separate the clinical services, the greater the diligence required on the part of each provider to meet the challenge of continued communication.

The psychiatric capacity of primary care clinics that offer these services is often inadequate to meet the needs of the total patient population. This situation can be problematic and delay access because most patients would like to be treated in this setting. Uniform criteria facilitate the triage of patients for in-house treatment or outside referral. These criteria include such justifiable considerations as diagnosis, available community resources, language requirements, or payment source. Certain unstable or less common psychiatric problems may be better served in the mental health sector, either in community clinics with wrap-around services or in specific subspecialty clinics. In most communities, English-speaking patients have more options for treatment. Depending on the location and availability of appropriate, non–English-speaking services, patients may be preferentially kept in house, or referred out. When otherwise appropriate, capitation will favor treating the patient in-house. Patients with insurance will generally have more options outside the primary care setting, and some insurance plans with mental health carve-outs may not cover psychiatric care in the same setting in which they cover medical services.

Collaborative Management[34,39,40]

In collaborative management, the patient alternates visits between the psychiatrist and the PCP in the primary care setting during initiation of treatment (i.e., the first 4 to 6 weeks). The PCP then assumes responsibility for the patient's continued psychopharmacologic treatment. This model was developed as a research protocol for the treatment of depressed, primary care patients. Patients are referred by the PCP, usually after an initial ineffective trial of medication. This intensive program of care has been cost-effective for more severely depressed primary care patients.

Implicit to this model are certain underlying assumptions. Collaborative management assumes that PCPs can initiate appropriate treatment for depression, manage the care of patients stabilized on antidepressant medications, and better care for more seriously depressed patients with the collaboration of in-house psychiatric consultation.[41] This model also assumes that such collaboration begins with PCP education and training. In addition, they participate in regular teaching conferences. A psychoeducational module for patients is also an integral part of the treatment.

Primary Care–Driven Model

The primary care–driven model evolved from the practical necessity to assist PCPs in the provision of quality psychiatric care for their own primary care patients with limited psychiatric resources.[42] This model incorporates elements of consultation, teleconsultation, and collaborative management, with the goal of maximizing the treatment of appropriate primary care patients, in the primary care setting. Established criteria are used for triage, with the appropriateness of PCP management being the first consideration. Photocopies or electronic copies of all psychiatric notes and evaluations are sent to the PCP and placed in the regular medical record. The clinic provides psychiatric training for both psychiatric and primary care residents. Underlying assumptions of this model include those of the Collaborative Management model, but are more extensive, reflective of the broader diagnostic scope. These assumptions are listed in Table 44-1.

Table 44-1. Underlying Assumptions of the Primary Care-Driven Model

---

Collaboration begins with education of primary care physicians (PCPs) *and* psychiatrists.

Patients' psychiatric needs should be met in the primary care setting when consistent with good care.

PCPs can manage the care of patients stabilized on psychiatric medications.

PCPs can initiate appropriate treatment for some psychiatric disorders.

PCPs can better care for the psychiatric needs of more patients with the collaboration of in-house psychiatric consultation.

Some patients and some disorders are unlikely to be stable enough for PCP management.

Responsibility for total care requires communication between the PCP and any other involved care provider or consultant.

In this model, the written request for consultation or referral comes from the PCP. The referral includes the clinical question or problem to be addressed and any PCP-initiated medication trials. PCPs are also encouraged to call or stop by the psychiatrist's office, located within the primary care clinical area, for more general information about diagnoses, medications, or psychiatric and behavioral management.

Psychiatric services include formal evaluation, stabilization over several visits, and return of the patient to the PCP's care (with recommendations on how to take and how long to continue medications and when to re-refer). The psychiatrist also provides informal "curbside" consultation (it is not considered "curbside" because the patient is present; rather, this is another type of brief consultation), brief consultation with the patient and the PCP during the patient's primary care visit, and behavioral treatment planning for the difficult-to-manage patient. Re-evaluation of patients previously seen occurs when there is a change, such as roughening, or the recurrence of symptoms, the development of new psychiatric symptoms, medication side effects, or a change in the medical condition or medications that affect psychiatric symptoms or medications. When a patient does not meet criteria for in-house treatment, the psychiatrist facilitates the referral to an outside psychiatrist and/or therapist. Other mental health services include focused, short-term, and goal-oriented, individual or group therapy (with master's level clinicians located within the primary care clinical areas they serve). Collaborative care management is another service that helps broker and coordinate the care of patients with complicated medical, mental health, and/or addiction problems who utilize services in multiple settings.

A premise of the primary care-driven model is that not all patients are appropriate for PCP management. The psychiatrist should help the PCP recognize which patients need ongoing specialty care and assist with appropriate referral. Patients not recommended for PCP management include those with inherently unstable conditions, or complicated medication regimens, (i.e., those who require close monitoring) or those who require close monitoring. Such patients include those with bipolar disorder, psychotic disorders, suicidal ideation, severe personality disorders, or primary substance abuse or dependence problems.

Collaborative care management is a program that bridges the needs for communication and coordination when patients must access services outside the primary care setting. It improves the care of patients with complex medical, psychiatric, and addiction problems that often require treatment spanning several community agencies. After a comprehensive diagnostic and functional assessment, necessary releases are signed so that the care manager can serve as a liaison between the PCP and all other care providers. The care manager involves the patient and all treaters in the development of a comprehensive treatment plan within a network of services, and tracks the patient from site to site throughout this plan. As a member of the discharge planning team, the care manager ensures that the patient returns to the appropriate network of services after care in a hospital, a detoxification program, or another residential/institutional setting. Like teleconsultation, the existence of this useful program has been severely limited by the lack of sustainable reimbursement sources.

Choosing the Right Model

The choice of model for a given clinical setting depends on a variety of factors, such as patient population, payor mix, range of available community resources, and the location, type and size of the practice. Patients with higher educational or socioeconomic status may feel less stigmatized and be more able and willing to seek and pay for outside psychiatric services.[43] Some patients feel more comfortable in private practice settings that allow the greatest possible privacy. Mental health problems are less acceptable or even shameful in some cultures. These patient populations will favor a more integrated and "invisible" system of care in the primary care setting. Capitation would most clearly demonstrate the cost-offset and cost-effectiveness of in-house, collaborative models (and teleconsultation, if the market penetration is ever high enough). The primary care-driven model requires adequate community resources to refer patients not considered appropriate for primary care management. Suburban or rural areas

that lack these resources are better served by parallel, or shared, care models. Small groups or solo practitioners may favor consultation models, either with a part-time, but regularly scheduled consultant or through access to an outside consultant or teleconsultant as needed. Large practices, and especially training facilities, will benefit most from the full range of in-house consultative and collaborative services that include formal education, case conferences, curbside consultation, and collaborative care management.

Summary

Though mandated by changes in the health care system, collaborative models serve to increase access and improve treatment for patients who would be unable or unlikely to receive psychiatric care outside of the primary care setting. A number of considerations determine the best model for a given practice setting. Such factors include size, patient population, available community resources, payor mix, and other reimbursement sources. To remain viable, high-quality and cost-effective models will need to adapt and evolve with the changing health care system. Psychiatrists and PCPs will need to be flexible and innovative in their approaches to patient care and to be diligent in the documentation of cost-offset to encourage payors to reimburse their services.[44,45] Medical,[46] psychiatric, and patient education will need to reflect these changes in caregiver roles and expectations.

References

1. McKegney FP: After a century of C-L psychiatry, whither goest C-L in the 21st? Abstract. *Psychosomatics* 36:202–203, 1995.
2. Simon GE, Walker EA: *The primary care clinic.* In Wise MG, Rundell JR, editors: *Textbook of consultation-liaison psychiatry: psychiatry in the medically ill,* ed 2, Washington, DC, 2002, American Psychiatric Publishing Inc, pp 917–925.
3. Leslie DL, Rosenheck R: Shifting to outpatient care? Mental health care use and cost under private insurance, *Am J Psychiatry* 156:1250–1257, 1999.
4. Katon W, Von Korff M, Lin E, et al: Population-based care of depression: effective disease management strategies to decrease prevalence, *Gen Hosp Psychiatry* 19:169–178, 1997.

5. Broadhead WE, Blazer DG, George LK, Tse CK: Depression, disability days, and days lost from work in a prospective epidemiological study, *JAMA* 264:2524–2528, 1990.

6. Johnson J, Weissman MM, Klerman GL: Service utilization and social morbidity associated with depressive symptoms in the community, *JAMA* 267:1478–1483, 1992.

7. Wells KB, Stewart A, Hays RD, et al: The functioning and well-being of depressed patients: results from the Medical Outcomes Study, *JAMA* 262:914–919, 1989.

8. Katon WJ, Roy-Byrne P, Russo J, Cowley D: Cost-effectiveness and cost offset of a collaborative care intervention for primary care patients with panic disorder, *Arch Gen Psychiatry* 59:1098–1104, 2002.

9. Zhang M, Rost KM, Fortney JC: Earnings changes for depressed individuals treated by mental health specialists, *Am J Psychiatry* 156:108–114, 1999.

10. Pincus HA: Assessing the effects of physician payment on treatment of mental disorders in primary care, *Gen Hosp Psychiatry* 12:23–29, 1990.

11. Frank RG, Huskamp HA, McGuire TG, Newhouse JP: Some economics of mental health 'carve-outs,' *Arch Gen Psychiatry* 53:933–937, 1996.

12. Regier DA, Narrow WE, Rae DS, et al: The de facto US mental health and addictive disorders service system, *Arch Gen Psychiatry* 50:85–94, 1993.

13. Shapiro S, Skinner EA, Kessler LG, et al: Utilization of health and mental health services: three Epidemiologic Catchment Area sites, *Arch Gen Psychiatry* 41:971–978, 1984.

14. Barrett JE, Barrett JA, Oxman TE, Gerber PD: The prevalence of psychiatric disorders in a primary care practice, *Arch Gen Psychiatry* 45:1100–1106, 1988.

15. Ormel J, Koeter WJ, van den Brink W, van de Willige G: Recognition, management, and course of anxiety and depression in general practice, *Arch Gen Psychiatry* 48:700–706, 1991.

16. Zung WWK, Magill M, Moore JT, George DT: Recognition and treatment of depression in a family medicine practice, *J Clin Psychiatry* 44:3–6, 1983.

17. Coyne JC, Schwenk TL, Fechner-Bates S: Nondetection of depression by primary care physicians reconsidered, *Gen Hosp Psychiatry* 17:3–12, 1995.

18. Roy-Byrne PP, Katon W, Cowley DS, et al: Panic disorder in primary care: biopsychosocial differences between recognized and unrecognized patients, *Gen Hosp Psychiatry* 22:405–411, 2000.

19. Tiemens BG, Ormel J, Simon GE: Occurrence, recognition, and outcome of psychological disorders in primary care, *Am J Psychiatry* 153:636–44, 1996.

20. Shapiro S, German PS, Skinner EA, et al: An experiment to change detection and management of mental morbidity in primary care, *Med Care* 25:327–339, 1987.

21. Eisenberg L: Treating depression and anxiety in primary care: closing the gap between knowledge and practice, *N Engl J Med* 326:1080–1084, 1992.

22. Schwab JJ: Psychiatric illness in medical patients; why it goes undiagnosed, *Psychosomatics* 23:225–229, 1982.

23. Weissberg M: The meagerness of physicians' training in emergency psychiatric intervention, *Acad Med* 65:747–750, 1990.

24. Ness DE, Ende J: Denial in the medical interview: recognition and management, *JAMA* 272:1777–1781, 1994.

25. Karlsson H, Lehtinen Vjoukamaa M: Psychiatric morbidity among frequent attender patients in primary care, *Gen Hosp Psychiatry* 17:19–25, 1995.

26. Bridges KW, Goldberg DP: Somatic presentation of DSM III psychiatric disorders in primary care, *J Psychosom Res* 29:563–569, 1985.

27. Wells KB, Hays RD, Burnam MA, et al: Detection of depressive disorder for patients receiving prepaid or fee-for-service care, *JAMA* 262:3298–3302, 1989.

28. Katon W, Von Korff M, Lin E: Adequacy and duration of antidepressant treatment in primary care, *Med Care* 30:67–76, 1992.

29. Olfson M, Marcus SC, Druss B, et al: National trends in the outpatient treatment of depression, *JAMA* 287:203–209, 2002.

30. Pincus HA, Tanielian TL, Marcus SC, et al: Prescribing trends in psychotropic medications: primary care, psychiatry and other specialties, *JAMA* 279:526–531, 1998.

31. Wells KB, Katon W, Rogers B, Camp P: Use of minor tranquilizers and antidepressant medications by depressed outpatients: results from the Medical Outcomes Study, *Am J Psychiatry* 151:694–700, 1994.

32. Druss BG, Rohrbaugh RM, Levinson CM, Rosenheck RA: Integrated medical care for patients with serious psychiatric illness, *Arch Gen Psychiatry* 58:861–868, 2001.

33. Robinson P: Integrated treatment of depression in primary care, *Strategic Med* 1:22–29, 1997.

34. Katon W, Von Korff M, Lin E, et al: Collaborative management to achieve treatment guidelines: impact on depression in primary care, *JAMA* 273:1026–1031, 1995.

35. Smith GR, Rost K, Kashner M: A trial of the effect of standardized psychiatric consultation on health outcomes and costs in somatizing patients, *Arch Gen Psychiatry* 52:238–243, 1995.

36. Strum R, Wells KB: How can care for depression become more cost-effective? *JAMA* 273:51–58, 1995.

37. Kates N, Craven MA, Crustolo A, et al: Sharing care: the psychiatrist in the family physician's office, *Can J Psychiatry* 42:960–965, 1997.

38. Nickels MW, McIntyre JS: A model for psychiatric services in primary care settings, *Psychiatric Services* 47:522–526, 1996.

39. Katon W, Von Korff M, Lin E, et al: Stepped collaborative care for primary care patients with persistent symptoms of depression, *Arch Gen Psychiatry* 56:1109–1115, 1999.

40. Unutzer J, Katon W, Callahan CM, et al: Collaborative care management of late-life depression in the primary care setting, a randomized controlled trial, *JAMA* 288:2836–2845, 2002.

41. Simon GE: Can depression be managed appropriately in primary care? *J Clin Psychiatry* 59(suppl. 2):3–8, 1998.

42. Pirl WF, Beck BJ, Safren SA, Kim H: A descriptive study of psychiatric consultations in a community primary care center, *Primary Care Companion J Clin Psychiatry* 3:190–194, 2001.

43. Simon GE, Von Korff M, Durham ML: Predictors of outpatient mental health utilization by primary care patients in a health maintenance organization, *Am J Psychiatry* 151:908–913, 1994.

44. Smith GR, Hamilton GE: The importance of outcomes research for the financing of care, *Harvard Rev Psychiatry* 2:288–289,1995.

45. Pincus HA, Zarin DA, West JC: Peering into the 'black box': measuring outcomes of managed care, *Arch Gen Psychiatry* 53:870877, 1996.

46. Cole SA, Sullivan M, Kathol R, Warshaw C: A model curriculum for mental disorders and behavioral problems in primary care, *Gen Hosp Psychiatry* 17:13–18, 1995.

Chapter 45

Billing Documentation and Cost-Effectiveness of Consultation

Robert M. Stern, M.D.
Vincent Alessandrini
Theodore A. Stern, M.D.

The purpose of this chapter is to provide psychiatric providers of Consultation-Liaison (C-L) services with an understanding of the complex business aspects of C-L psychiatry. Understanding and appropriately adhering to the often-confusing guidelines for reimbursement can be stressful to clinicians and expose them to painful audits and to substantial penalties, both personally and for their institutions. In this atmosphere, providing ethical, legal, and appropriate services can be a daunting task.

A fuller understanding of coding and billing will also help psychiatrists, C-L hospital-based programs, and hospital administrators to bill and to collect the appropriate reimbursement for services rendered.

In this chapter, we will address the principle of coding and billing that will improve medical documentation for C-L clinicians as well as address improvements in clinical outcome and economic benefits accrued to the general hospital by operating a C-L service. Adherence to the following principles for coding, billing, and documentation should help keep the work of the C-L clinician more clinically focused and facilitate capture of appropriate revenue for the services delivered. Pitfalls of "routine care" will also be explored.

Documentation Should Reflect the Service Actually Performed

Successful C-L services rely on the establishment of cooperative and collaborative relationships with medical colleagues. Hospital-based physicians are exposed to psychiatric comorbidity on a daily basis. Their need for consultation may range from an opportunity to review their approach to a patient, to a request for a comprehensive assessment. The needs of a physician do not always mirror the severity of the medical condition of the patient. *Billing, however, is always geared to the patient's illness*. The insurance company or other third party payor is paying for a service for an individual patient, rather than purchasing the expertise of the clinician.

Bill Only for Services Documented in the Medical Record

The overriding principle for third party reimbursement is to bill for only those services documented in the medical record. The charge for service and the reimbursement available for the service are guided by definitions established by Current Procedure Terminology (CPT) codes. A brilliant, life-saving consultation that goes undocumented is not billable. The effectiveness and expertise of the consultant is not an issue for the collection of reasonable fee. Moreover, significant pressure may be placed on clinicians to "maximize revenue" for the services they provide. This is especially true during difficult financial times. Efforts to "game" the system, by "up-coding," that is, charging for a more intensive service than delivered, are illegal and unethical.

Utilize the Medicare Guidelines for All Entries in the Medical Record

Medicare is the predominant insurance coverage in the general hospital. This is especially so for a psychiatric consultation service that is called upon to consult on elderly or disabled patients. CPT codes were developed by the American Medical Association (AMA) and adopted by the Health Care Financing Administration (HCFA) in the early 1990s. The guidelines were established as mandatory for Medicare and Medicaid billing but are essentially "universal," that is, they are applicable to most insurance plans. More importantly, Medicare guidelines for reimbursement are the strictest among insurance plans. *Adhering to the Medicare guidelines will ensure that the provider will be in compliance with all the insurance plans for appropriate coding for reimbursement purposes*.

For many psychiatrists, documentation requirements for in-patient psychiatric and consultation services are different in form and content from the documentation that might be employed in outpatient practices. Codes for billing in-patients reflect the need for the consultant to be aware of the physical status of the patient as well as the patient's psychiatric complications. A premium is paid for thoroughness and attention to "process of care." Thus, *documentation for in-patient consultative psychiatric services requires documentation of the comorbid medical problems*. An extensive psychiatric examination, including recommendations for treatment and/or medication without the inclusion of elements of the review of systems, for example, can be billed only for the lowest consultation service code. Billing is otherwise considered "up-coding" and is prohibited by law.

The critical ingredients of an appropriate note congruent with an appropriate billing code will be addressed in the section on documentation and coding.

Obtain Preauthorization for Services Whenever Necessary

Health insurance companies vary in their requirements for precertification (i.e., permission for providing a consultation prior to the delivery of the service to enable payment for that service). Medicare, for example, does not require precertification, whereas most Behavioral Health Organizations (BHOs) require such precertification. Precertification is the rule for carve-out BHOs that are subcontracted to manage the mental health and substance abuse benefit for the larger medical insurance plan. A patient may be authorized by the primary insurance carrier for the medical admission, authorizing payment for all physicians performing medical consultations save the psychiatrist who requires specific and separate authorization from the carve-out company for payment for the psychiatric consultation.

Critical to the financial viability of C-L services is the management and monitoring of the billing and collection of third party claims. Consultation services are often not billed for,[1] and the tracking of payments goes unmonitored. Each phase of the process between the provision of service and the receipt of payment for services presents its own dilemmas.

Identifying the Payor

During the admission process, most hospitals will have identified the primary, secondary, and supplementary insurance coverage.

It is critical for the managers of a C-L service to understand how each type of insurance adjudicates claims for professional services. Health insurance claims for hospital services are separated into two components: the technical or hospital charge and the professional or physician charges. For some insurers these charges are billed together, whereas for others they are billed separately.

Medicare, nonmanaged Medicaid, Blue Cross, and commercial indemnity plans will each pay both the technical (hospital) and professional (physician) components. Payments for each component are based upon a previously agreed upon fee schedule or percentage of charges submitted. Managed care plans will typically negotiate an "all-inclusive fee" for services rendered and will not pay for the professional (physician) charges separately unless they are specifically contracted for, apart from the day rate for the hospital charge.

When a patient is insured by a managed care plan, C-L services must be contracted for separately to be reimbursed beyond the "all-inclusive rate" the hospital receives through the day rate. If the insurer carves out the management of its mental health and substance abuse benefit to a behavioral health subcontractor, separate professional bills will have to be submitted to the carve-out behavioral health subcontractor. A common error for C-L services is the sending of the C-L consultation claim to the primary insurance carrier rather than to the behavioral health subcontractor and receiving rejection for "service not covered" or "bill to carve-out." Too often these rejected claims are written off, which engenders increased irritation with the primary carrier or blaming the C-L service for not obtaining prior authorization. The best method for ensuring that the correct payor is billed is to confirm with the medical insurer, usually by telephone, in advance of the treatment to determine whether the mental health benefit is carved out and, if so, to what organization. Then, one should contact the carve-out company to obtain prior authorization for the service. The critical request should be for both the initial consultation and follow-up visits, if necessary.

Develop a Standard Format for Writing the Consultation Note

Several standards and guidelines collide when writing an efficient and effective consultation note. Standards established by the American Psychiatric Association (APA) Practice Guidelines for Psychiatric Evaluation of Adults[2] address the content of an appropriate psychiatric examination; they then must be adapted to the special conditions of the consultative examination. As noted by the Academy of Psychosomatic Medicine (APM): Practice Guidelines for Psychiatric Consultation in the General Medicine Setting,[3] the psychiatric consultation should also address the consultee-stated versus the consultant-assessed reason for referral, the extent the patient's psychiatric disturbance was caused by the medical/surgical illness, the adequacy of pain management, the extent of the psychiatric disturbance caused by medications or substance abuse, disturbances in cognition, the patient's character style, thoughts of dying, and psychiatric symptomatology.

The consultation note should include the chief complaint, the history of the present illness, the medical and psychiatric history, the social and family history, the review of systems, the mental status examination, and an impression and treatment plan (Table 45-1). It should also include data to support the billing code for reimbursement-submitting that documents the appropriate level of care. Given this level of complexity, even the most competent and organized physicians may find it difficult to keep these guidelines in mind when they are writing a note.

One of the authors (T.A.S.) has developed a working template for documentation that facilitates compliance with HCFA and Medicare guidelines (Figure 45-1). Templates should be considered works in progress, since standards shift with respect to required content; the format presented is intended as a guide to a flexible document that can be amended as needed (see Figure 45-1). An additional excellent consultation form was developed by Worley et al.[4]

We believe that the use of such a template facilitates more complete consultations, serves as a teaching tool for trainees, and improves communication with medical providers. Templates also lend themselves to inclusion in computerized medical records, prevent loss of critical observations and recommendations secondary to illegible notes, and decrease medical errors. Furthermore, from a time-management perspective, such templates make clinicians more efficient with regard to documentation of information relevant to the consultation. With the developing capacity to import computerized (observational and laboratory) results, vital signs, recent laboratory values, medication orders, and drug administration, data can be more easily included in the consultation note. Utilizing the capabilities of the hospital information

Table 45.1. Key Elements of the Initial Consultation Note

1. Document the date and time of the visit; write "psychiatry" at the top of the note.
2. Document the name of the doctor who requested the consultation and the reason for the consultation request.
3. Provide a chief complaint.
4. Provide a summary of the patient's medical history relevant to the current psychiatric situation; do not just duplicate information in the medical record and the problem list (provide at least four of seven categories of information, e.g., timing, severity, duration of symptoms, associated features).
5. Provide a description of current psychiatric symptoms (or events leading up to the psychiatric consultation).
6. Document the psychiatric history; be specific about medication and other treatment effects and adverse reactions.
7. Document the family psychiatric history (include drug/alcohol use), including medication and other treatment responses.
8. Document the social history—work and school history, sexual history, drug and alcohol use history, legal history, social supports, and current living arrangements.
9. Provide the past medical history.
10. Document that a review of systems has been performed.
11. Provide a complete mental status examination, with at least nine fields of the following—appearance, behavior, speech, affect/mood, thought content (suicidal, homicidal, delusions, hallucinations), orientation, memory, attention, and other cognitive tests, language, fund of knowledge, insight, and judgment.
12. List the current medications—review hospital medication records as well as doctor's orders
13. Document recent and pertinent tests and procedures performed—e.g., laboratory studies, roentgenography (computed tomography, magnetic resonance imaging), electrocardiography, and electroencephalography.
14. Document pertinent aspects of the physical examination—e.g., vital signs, neurologic examination findings, and abnormal movements.
15. Provide your impression; use DSM-IV diagnoses and readily understandable terminology (avoiding psychiatric jargon) as well as a formulation.
16. Provide your recommendations; be clear and concise, list medications exactly how you wish them given (including suicide precautions, recommendations for restraints or other consultations, and so on). N.B.: All notes from consultations and follow-up visits should be written with discretion; keep in mind that medical-surgical charts frequently are read by hospital staff and sometimes by patients and their families.
17. Document the date of next follow-up visit and the planned frequency of visits.
18. Sign and print your (i.e., the consultant's) name, along with a telephone and/or pager number.

system also increases opportunities for programmatic and clinical research.

Bill the Appropriate Code

CPT Evaluation and Management (E & M) codes (99251–99255) have become the standard codes for the initial inpatient psychiatric consultation, while others (99261–99263) are typically used for follow-up consultations (Table 45-2). The E & M codes are now used for inpatient services in preference to the psychotherapy codes, although in some cases, the psychotherapy codes (90810–90847) may be employed. *To use consultation codes properly, it must be clear that the consultation is a service requested by another physician or another provider rather than by the patient or the patient's family.*

The content of the history, the comprehensiveness of the examination, the complexity of

medical decision-making, and the average time required to complete the consultation determine the reimbursement that will be provided (Table 45-3). Engaging the assistance of a professional coder to perform periodic audits and training sessions for physicians is essential to remain abreast of changes in federal auditing guidelines. Additionally, providing psychiatrists with simplified pocket billing guidelines and definitions of terms for selecting the appropriate CPT code can be helpful.

Evaluation of the Costs and Benefits of a Consultation Service

C-L services are rarely lucrative cost centers.[5] Moreover, providing fee-for-service psychiatric consultation by independent practitioners rarely leads to a financially viable service or career. By its nature, clinicians must expend significant time away from

MASSACHUSETTS GENERAL HOSPITAL
BOSTON, MASSACHUSETTS

Enter name and unit number on both sides of EVERY sheet.
Name and unit number to be written distinctly when plate is
not available.

Psychiatric Consultation Note

Date:_____/_____/_____Time:_____am/pm

Consult Log #: _____
☐ Inpt   ☐ ED   ☐ OPD
Request Type: Urgent w/in 24hrs. Convenience
                  ☐   ☐   ☐

Asked to see this ___y/old ☐M ☐F for eval of:

☐ ΔMS   ☐ depress.   ☐ capacity to... ☐ agitation   ☐ anxiety
☐ PTSD   ☐ dementia   ☐ suicidality   ☐ Etoh/subs.   ☐ psychosis
☐ coping   ☐ pharm eval. ☐ eating dis.   ☐ grief   ☐ school probs.
☐ obs./comp. ☐ sex disfunct. ☐ relationship probs.   ☐ transpl. eval.
☐ sleep disturb. ☐ homicidal ideation   ☐ inadequate self care
☐ Attention/impulse dis. ☐ psychol. components ☐ aggress. behavior
☐ Other / describe _____

PCP: _____ Tele: _____
Pt's Tele: (h) _____ Pharmacy Tele: _____
          (w) _____ Contact Person: _____

by:
(Dr./Service) _____

Use superscripts to indicate source of information. (1 = MD 2 = RN 3 = Pt 4 = Family 5 = Other)

HPI:
(please check off and
include descriptions
of at least 4 of the
following features)

☐ Timing
☐ Severity
☐ Duration
☐ Quality
☐ Context
☐ Modifying Facts
☐ Assoc. Signs/sx

(check if abnormal and indicate direction)

Depression:		Mania:		Risk factors for stress:		
☐ Sleep ↑ ↓	☐ Concentration ↓	☐ Distractibility	☐ Ideas that race	☐ Chronic disease	☐ Irritability	☐ Learning Disab.
☐ Interest ↓	☐ Appetite ↑ ↓	☐ Talkativeness	☐ Grandiosity	☐ Poor peer relat.	☐ Perceives threat	☐ Insecure attach.
☐ Guilt +	☐ Psychomotor ↑ ↓	☐ Recklessness	☐ Hypersexuality	☐ Poverty	☐ Unstable/safe envir.	☐ Hyperactivity
☐ Energy ↓	☐ Suicidal +	☐ Hyposomnia		☐ Impulsivity	☐ Inattentiveness	☐ School failure

Psychiatric History: *(check if present and inidcate pertinent details)* -or check-   ☐ UNREMARKABLE

☐ Care by physician of same group practice w/in 3 years.

	HP (√)	Admissions (√)(Date)	Details / Medication trials
Depression			
Anxiety			
Psychosis			
Bipolar			
Personality Dis.			
Subs. Abuse			
DTs			
W/D sz			
Other: (specify)			

Abuse:
(check: ☐ = current   ○ = past)   ☐○ Physical Absue   Sexual Abuse

Psychiatric Treaters: Name   tel. #
                         1. _____   _____

USE REVERSE SIDE   PLEASE DO NOT WASTE SPACE

MGH 81560 REV 11/95

Figure 45-1. MGH Psychiatric Consultation Note Template.

MASSACHUSETTS GENERAL HOSPITAL
BOSTON, MASSACHUSETTS

Enter name and unit number on both sides of EVERY sheet.
Name and unit number to be written distinctly when plate is
not available.

*** Review of Systems: (○ = normal   □ = abnormal)

○ Constitutional	○ ENT	○ Resp	○ Lymph	○ Eyes	○ Neuro
□ △ appetite	□ hearing	□ Cough	□ lymph nodes	□ △ vision	□ numbness/tingle □ confusion
□ fever		□ SOB			□ speech diff. □ imp. memory
□ △ weight	○ Cardiac		○ Musculo	□ Psych	□ personality△ □ diff. swallowing
□ △ energy	□ Chest pain	○ GU	□ weakness		□ lethargy □ incontinence
		□ urinary freq.	□ pain	○ Skin	□ H/A □ diff. w/ coord.
○ Immune	○ GI			□ rash	□ dizziness □ gait disturb.
□ freq. infections	□ abdom. pain				□ syncope

Details of above:

Allergies: _____

or: ○ Refer to note/worksheet of _____ (date)____/____/____ □ changes as above □ unchanged
(check)

Medical History (check if present and indicate pertinent details) -or check-   □ *UNREMARKABLE*

Constitutional	Eyes	GI	Endocrine	Skin	Respiratory	Mus./Skel.	Immune	Reproductive:
□ Fatigue	□ Cataracts	□ PUD	□ Diabetes	□ Burns	□ Pneumonia	□ Fractures	□ HIV	□ Ammenoria
□ CFS	□ Glaucoma	□ Hepatitis	□ Hypothyroidism	□ Psoriasis	□ Asthma	□ Fibromyalgia	□ S/P Transplant	□ Pregnancies
□ Sleep dist.	□ Blindness	□ Crohn's	□ Hyperthyroidism	□ Other:	□ COPD	□ Other:	□ Other:	□ Prior births
□ Dizziness	□ Other:	□ Bowel dysf.	□ Other:		□ Other:			□ Currently preg.
		□ Other:						□ LMP

ENT	Hem./Onc.	GU	Cardiac	Neuro:		Immunizations	List others:
	□ XRT	□ Bladder dysf.	□ CHF	□ Dementia	□ H/A	□ Polio	
□ ↓ Hearing	□ Chemotx	□ UTI	□ AFIB	□ CVA	□ Gait dist.	□ DPT	
□ Vertigo	□ Multmyeloma	□ BPH	□ VT	□ MS	□ Syncope	□ Chicken Pox	
□ Other:	□ CA colon	□ CRF	□ MI	□ Parkinsons	□ Neuro/musc. dis.	□ M/M/R	
	□ CA prostate	□ ARF	□ HTN	□ Meningitis	□ Disc disease	□ Hepatitis	
	□ CA breast	□ Other:	□ CAD	□ Head Trauma	□ Neuropathy	□ Influenza	
	□ CA Other:		□ Other:	□ Sz Disord.			
	□ Anemia			□ Other:			
	□ CNS tumor						

□ Prior Hospitalizations

Surgical History: *(provide dates of surgery where relevant)*

Cardio/vasc.	Ortho:			
□ CABG	□ AKA	□ Appendectomy	□ Trach	Neuro:
□ MVR	□ BKA	□ Cholecystectomy	□ G-Tube	□ Craniotomy
□ AVR	□ THR	□ Gastrectomy	□ T&A	
□ Pacemaker	□ Laminectomy	□ Nephrectomy		Others:
□ AICD		□ Portocaval shunt	Transplant:	
□ AAA	General:	□ TAH	□ Heart	_____
□ CEA	□ Colon resection	□ BSO	□ Kidney	_____
□ Peripheral bypass	□ Colostomy	□ Thyroidectomy	□ Liver	_____
	□ Splenectomy	□ Laryngectomy	□ Lung	_____
		□ Skin grafting	□ Bone marrow	

Medical Pharmacology: (Check: □ = current use) □ *NONE*

MGH 81560 REV 11/95

Figure 45-1. *Continued*

**MASSACHUSETTS GENERAL HOSPITAL
BOSTON, MASSACHUSETTS**

Enter name and unit number on both sides of EVERY sheet.
Name and unit number to be written distinctly when plate is
not available.

Date: _____ Psychiatric Consultation Note

Psychiatric Pharmacology: (check: □ = current use ○ = past use) △ = *NONE*

Neuroleptics:	TCAs:	SSRIs:	Mood Stab./Anti-Conv:	
□○ Haloperidol	□○ Amitriptyline	□○ Fluoxetine	□○ Carbamazepine	□○ Tacrine
□○ Olanzapine	□○ Desipramine	□○ Sertraline	□○ Valproic acid	□○ Pemoline
□○ Clozapine	□○ Nortriptyline	□○ Paroxetine	□○ Phenytoin	□○ Clonidine
□○ Resperidol	□○ Other:	□○ Fluvoxamine	□○ Gabapentin	□○ Disulfiram
□○ Perphenazine		□○ Other:	□○ Phenobarbitel	□○ Zolpidem
□○ Other:			□○ Other:	□○ Propofol

MAOIs:	Other Antidepressants:	Bzs:	Others:
□○ Phenelzine	□○ Trazodone	□○ Alprazolam	□○ Buspirone
□○ Tranylcypramine	□○ Bupropion	□○ Clonazepam	□○ Lithium
□○ Other:	□○ Nefazodone	□○ Diazepam	□○ Methylphenidate
	□○ Other:	□○ Lorazepam	□○ Dextroamphetamine
		□○ Other:	

Social & Developmental History:

Employment/Education: (check)   description

current: _____

past: _____

Marital Status:
□S □M □D
□W □Sep.

Education Level: □ < High School   Legal Problems: □ Current ○ Past
□ High School Grad   Details:
□ College   _____

	yes / no
Advanced Directive	□ ○
Power of Attorney	□ ○
Developmentally Disabled □	○

Etoh/Subs. Abuse: (check: □ = current use ○ = past use; give dates of use on line)

□○ Alcohol _____   □○ Benzos _____   □○ Stimulants/Cocaine _____   □○ Other:
□○ Narcotics _____   □○ Hallucinogens _____   □○ IVDA _____   _____

Details:

Family Medical History: (check appropriate box)

	CAD	HTN	DM	Sz Dis.	CVD	Others
Father:						
Mother:						
Sibs:						
Children:						
Grandparents:						
Other:						

Family Psychiatric History: (check appropriate box)

	Deceased	Suicide	Depres.	Anxiety	Bipolar	Psychotic	Personality Dis.	Other
Father								
Mother								
Sibs (#)								
Children (#)								
Other:								

Family of Origin: □ Stable □ Chaotic

Relevant Details:

USE REVERSE SIDE   PLEASE DO NOT WASTE SPACE

MGH 81560 REV 11/95

Figure 45-1. *Continued*

MASSACHUSETTS GENERAL HOSPITAL
BOSTON, MASSACHUSETTS

Enter name and unit number on both sides of EVERY sheet.
Name and unit number to be written distinctly when plate is
not available.

Labs and Records: (Insert values in appropriate areas)

Na	Cl	BUN
K	CO_2	Cr

GLU

WBC — Hb — MCV / Plt

Hct — RDW

	Reviewed	Results Gathered by Review *(summarize)*
Labs:		
U/A		
ABGs		
LFTs		
TFTs		
B12		
Folate		
Other:		
X-Rays: CXR		
Other:		
LP:		
EKG:		
EEG:		
CT: (type)		
MRI: (type)		
Other:		
Old Records:		
Tox Screen: *drugs:*		
levels:		

*** Vital signs:

☐ Temp_____ ☐ HR_____ ☐ BP_____ ☐ Resp. Rate_____ ☐ HT_____ ☐ WT_____

◯ (check)   Refer to note/worksheet of _____ (date)___ /___ /___

Physical exam:
relevant features:

Corotid bruits   Pupils:
Hearing: EOMS:
Cranial nerves: Reflexes:
Coordination/gait:
Motor tone:
Visual acuity: If date of last physical > 6 months, has pt been referred? ☐

MGH 81560 REV 11/95

USE REVERSE SIDE   PLEASE DO NOT WASTE SPACE

Figure 45-1. *Continued*

**MASSACHUSETTS GENERAL HOSPITAL
BOSTON, MASSACHUSETTS**

Enter name and unit number on both sides of EVERY sheet.
Name and unit number to be written distinctly when plate is
not available.

Mini-Mental State Examination

(Add points for each correct response)

			Score	Points
Orientation				
1.	What is the	Year?	_____	1
		Season?	_____	1
		Date?	_____	1
		Day?	_____	1
		Month?	_____	1
2.	Where are we?	State?	_____	1
		Country?	_____	1
		Town or city?	_____	1
		Hospital	_____	1
		Floor	_____	1

Registration
3.   Name three objects, taking one second to say each. Then
        ask the patient all three after you have said them.
        Give one point for each correct answer.
        Repeat the answers until the patient learns all three.   _____   3

Attention and calculation
4.   Serial sevens. Give one point for each correct answer.
        Stop after five answers.
        Alternate: Spell WORLD backwards.   _____   5

Recall
5.   Ask for names of three objects learned in Q.3. Give one point
        for each correct answer.   _____   3

Language
6.   Point to a pencil and a watch. Have the patient name them as
        you point.   _____   2
7.   Have the patient repeat "No ifs, ands or buts."   _____ 1
8.   Have the patient follow a three-stage command: 'Take a paper
        in your right hand. Fold the paper in half. Put the paper on the
        floor.'   _____   3
9.   Have the patient read and obey the following:
        'CLOSE YOUR EYES.' (Write it in large letters.)   _____ 1
10.   Have the patient write a sentence of his or her choice.
        (The sentence should contain a subject and an object, and should
        make sense. Ignore spelling errors when scoring).   _____   1
11.   Enlarge the design printed below to 1.5 cm per side, and have
        the patient copy it. (Give one point if all sides and angles are
        preserved and if the intersecting sides form a quadrangle.)   _____   1

_____ = Total 30

References:
1. Folstein MF, Folstein SE, McHugh PR: "Mini-Mental State" A practical method for grading
   the cognitive state of patients for the clinician. J Psychiat Res. 1975; 12: 89-198.

2. Tombaugh T. McIntyre NJ: The Mini-Mental State examination: A comprehensive review.
   J Am Geriatr Soc. 1992; 40:922–935.

MGH 81560 REV 11/95

USE REVERSE SIDE   PLEASE DO NOT WASTE SPACE

Figure 45-1. *Continued*

CLOSE YOUR EYES

Write a sentence below

MGH 81560 REV 11/95

Copy design below

USE REVERSE SIDE   PLEASE DO NOT WASTE SPACE

Figure 45-1. *Continued*

MASSACHUSETTS GENERAL HOSPITAL
BOSTON, MASSACHUSETTS

Enter name and unit number on both sides of EVERY sheet.
Name and unit number to be written distinctly when plate is
not available.

Psychiatric Consultation Note

Date: _____

Mental Status
(Check ○ if category is normal, otherwise check abnormality ☐)

General Appearance:
○ *Normal* Abnormal
☐ agitated
☐ unkempt
☐ psychomotor ret.
☐ SOB
☐ uncomfortable
☐ bruised
☐ hyperactive
☐ slumped
☐ fidgeting
☐ other:

Speech:
○ *Normal* Impaired
☐ non-verbal
☐ slurring
☐ paraphasic errors
☐ rapid
☐ pressured
☐ monotonous
☐ non-fluent
☐ sparse
☐ non spontaneous
☐ verbose
☐ loud
☐ soft
☐ other:

☐ belligerent/hostile
☐ uncooperative
☐ evasive
☐ guarded
☐ impulsive
☐ passive
☐ withdrawn
☐ laughs
☐ smiles
☐ other:

Suicidal Ideation:
○ No Yes
☐ ideation
☐ plan
☐ attempts

Judgement & Insight:
○ *Normal* Abnormal
☐ poor
☐ confused
☐ other:

Thought process:
○ *Normal* Abnormal

HEENT:
○ *Normal* Abnormal
☐ oral thrush
☐ neck stiffness
☐ staring
☐ averts gaze
☐ other:

Language:
○ *Normal* Impaired Ability
☐ naming objects
☐ repeating phases
☐ writing sentences
☐ other:

Hallucinations:
☐ Vis ☐ Aud ☐ Tact
☐ Gust ☐ Sens ☐ other:

☐ impaired abstraction
☐ assoc. loose
☐ tangential
☐ perseverative
☐ delusional
☐ obsessed
☐ circumstantial

Memory:
○ *Normal* Abnormal
☐ short-term
☐ long-term
☐ other:

Attention Span:
○ *Normal*
☐ Impaired

Musculo./Skel:
○ *Normal* Abnormal
☐ rigid
☐ cogwheeling
☐ flaccid
☐ myoclonus
☐ oral-buccal movements
☐ tremor
☐ tics
☐ other:

Level of Vocabulary:
○ *Normal*
☐ Impaired

Mood/Affect:
○ *Normal* Abnormal
☐ anxious
☐ depressed
☐ angry
☐ flat
☐ labile
☐ sad
☐ fearful
☐ constricted
☐ tearful

Calculation Ability:
○ *Normal*
☐ Impaired

Sensorium / Orientation:
○ *Normal* Disoriented
☐ Time
☐ Place
☐ Person

Thought content:
○ *Normal*
☐ delusions
☐ ideas of ref.
☐ SI
☐ HI
☐ obsessions

Homicidal Ideation:
○ No Yes
☐ ideation
☐ plan
☐ attempts

Gait:
○ *Normal*
☐ Abnormal

MGH 81560 REV 11/95

Diagnostic Impressions: _____

Please detail all abnormal findings:

Axis I:	Vascular:	Etoh:	☐ Schizophrenia paranoid (295.30)	☐ Panic disorder w/o agoraphobia (300.01)	Adjustment disorder:
☐ Delirium (293.0) due to	☐ uncomplicated (.40)	☐ dependence (303.90)	☐ Schizophrenia undiff. (295.90)	☐ Anxiety NOS (300.00)	☐ w/ depressed mood (309.0) ☐ w/ anxiety (309.24)
☐ Delrium (780.09)	☐ w/ delirium (.41)	☐ abuse (305.00)	☐ Scz-affective (295.70)	☐ PTSD acute (309.81)	☐ w/ mixed features (309.28)
☐ Dementia (290.xx)	☐ w/ delusions (.42)	☐ intox (303.00)		☐ PTSD chronic (309.81)	
Early Alzheimer's:	☐ w/ depression (.43)	☐ w/d (291.8)	☐ Major Depression	☐ Somatization disorder (300.81)	☐ Neuroleptic-induced Parkins. (332.1)
☐ uncomplicated (.10)	☐ Dementia NOS (294.80)	Opioid:	☐ single episode (296.2)	☐ Conversion (300.11)	☐ NMS (333.99)
☐ w/ delirium (.11)	☐ Demntia from HIV (294.9)	☐ dependence (304.00)	☐ recurrent (296.3)	☐ Pain disorder (307.xx)	☐ Med-induced movement disorder (333.90)
☐ w/ delusions (.12)	☐ Dementia from head trauma (294.1)	☐ abuse (305.0)	☐ Depres. disor. NOS (311)	☐ Hypochondriasis (300.7)	
☐ w/ depression (.13)	☐ Dementia from Parkinson's (294.1)	Sed-hyp:	☐ Dysthymia (300.4)	☐ Breathing rel. sleep dis. (780.59)	Others:
Late onset Alzheimer's:	☐ Personality change (310.1)	☐ dependence (304.10)	☐ Bipolar I (296.xx)		☐ ADHD (314.01)
☐ uncomplicated (.10)	from _____	☐ w/d (292.0)	☐ Bipolar II (296.89)		☐ Conduct Disorder (312.20)
☐ w/ delirium (.3)	☐ Catatonia (293.89)	☐ Polysubs depend (304.80)	☐ Panic disorder w/ agoraphobia (300.21)	☐ Psych. fators affecting Physical Illness (316.00)	☐ Anorexia Nervosa (307.10)
☐ w/ delusions (.20)		☐ Psychosis NOS (298.9)			☐ Bulimia Nervosa (307.51)
☐ w/ depression (.21)		☐ Psychosis med. condt. _____ (293.xx)			

Other Axis I:
Axis II: ☐ Borderline (301.83)   ☐ Antisocial (301.7)   ☐ Personality disorder NOS (301.9)   Others: _____
Axis III: (see pages 1 & 2)
Axis IV:
☐ Problems w/ primary support group ☐ Problems related to social environment   ☐ Educational problems ☐ Occupational problems ☐ Housing problems
☐ Economic problems   ☐ Problems w/ access to health care services   ☐ Problems related w/ legal system/crime   ☐ Other psych. social & environmental problems
Axis V: GAF Score: [   ]

☐ 100–91 ☐ 90–81 ☐ 80–71 ☐ 70–61 ☐ 60–51 ☐ 50–41 ☐ 40–31 ☐ 30–21 ☐ 20–11 ☐ 10–0 ☐ 0
Superior function   Mild sx   Serious sx/ impaired fx   Seriously impaired Danger to self/others   Inadequate information

USE REVERSE SIDE   PLEASE DO NOT WASTE SPACE

Figure 45-1. *Continued*

**MASSACHUSETTS GENERAL HOSPITAL
BOSTON, MASSACHUSETTS**

Enter name and unit number on both sides of EVERY sheet.
Name and unit number to be written distinctly when plate is
not available.

Psychiatric Consultation Note

Date: _____

Impression: _____

Plan: (Dx'tic w/u; lab tests; pharm Tx; psychological Tx; mgmt. strategies;)

1. _____
2. _____
3. _____
4. _____
5. _____

Currently
lacks capacity to:
☐ Make Tx decisions re: _____
☐ make disposition decisions
☐ leave AMA

suicide precautions: ☐ recommended ☐ ordered
sitter: ☐ recommended ☐ ordered
restraints: ☐ recommended ☐ ordered

Goals & Objectives	Tx Plan (Modality & Freq.)	Risks discussed	Side Effects Experienced
☐ Tx anxiety ☐ Tx Depression ☐ Tx Psychosis ☐ Provide support ☐ Improve function ☐ Improve relatshps. ☐ Return to work ☐ other:	☐ Psychotherapy Psychopharm: ☐ continue w/o ☐ ↑ dose: ☐ ↓ dose: ☐ Add: ☐ D/C: Check labs ☐ BUN/Cr ☐ LFTs ☐ TFTs ☐ CBC ☐ Levels ☐ Lytes ☐ other:	☐ Bleeding tendency ☐ sedation ☐ H/A ☐ wt gain ☐ EPS ☐ hypohtyroidism ☐ ↓ WBC ☐ polyuria ☐ anemia ☐ drug-drug inter. ☐ ↑ LFTs ☐ other: ☐ rash/allergy ☐ ataxia ☐ hypotension/dizziness ☐ sex. dysf. ☐ GI distress ☐ insomnia	☐ sedation ☐ dry mouth ☐ sex. dysf. ☐ palp ☐ GI upset ☐ rash ☐ other:

Consultant Name: _____ Signature: _____

Beeper #:_____ Date: ___/___/___ ☐ Attending ☐ Fellow ☐ Resident ☐ Med. Student

USE REVERSE SIDE   PLEASE DO NOT WASTE SPACE

Figure 45-1. *Continued*

Table 45.2. Inpatient Initial Psychiatric Consultation Codes

Code	Time (minutes)	History	Examination	Decision-making
99251	20	Problem-focused	Problem-focused	Straightforward
99252	40	Expanded	Expanded	Straightforward
99253	55	Detailed	Detailed	Low complexity
99254	80	Comprehensive	Comprehensive	Moderate complexity
99255	110	Comprehensive	Comprehensive	High complexity
Definitions of Terms				
	HPI	**ROS**	**Psych/FHx/SHx**	**MSE**
Problem-focused	1–3 items	None	None	1–5 elements
Expanded problem-focused	1–3 items	1 system	None	6–8 elements
Detailed	4 or more items	2–9 systems	1 field	9–13 elements
Comprehensive	4 or more items	10 + systems	3 fields	14–15 elements

HPI, History of Present Illness; ROS, Review of Systems; Psych/FHx/SHx, Psychiatric/Family History/Social History; MSE, Mental Status Examination.

Table 45.3. Definitions of Medical Decision-Making

Code	Decision-Making	No. of Diagnoses/Options	Complexity of Data Reviewed	Risk of Complications
99251/2	Straight-forward	Minimal	Minimal or none	Minimal
99253	Low complexity	Limited	Limited	Low
99254	Moderate complexity	Multiple	Moderate	Moderate
99255	High complexity	Extensive	Extensive	High

Straightforward: One or more self-limiting minor problem.
Low complexity: Two or more self-limiting or minor problems or one stable problem.
Moderate complexity: One or more chronic illnesses with mild exacerbations or progression of, or side effects, or two or more stable chronic diseases.
High complexity: One or more chronic illness with severe exacerbation or progression, or side effects of treatment, or acute or chronic illness that poses a threat to life or bodily functions.

the bedside to provide meaningful consultation. Necessary tasks include the review of the medical record and case discussion before and after the consultation with the referring physician, nursing staff, and social service. Ancillary meetings with family members are often necessary to collect critical information unobtainable from a medically compromised patient. A cost-benefit analysis that sees cost as the psychiatrists' salary and the benefit as the lowest expenditure of finances to provide the service without severely compromising the service is far too common.

In contrast to the above, we support a "value accounting" methodology that approaches the consultation service in a broader systemic manner.[6] This methodology looks at cost, clinical outcome, and consumer satisfaction as interrelated domains. With a broader view, we can examine the impact

of a C-L service on the financial functioning of the hospital, the care of the patient, and their impact on consumers of care (i.e., patients, families, and the medical staff).

From a fiscal perspective, the availability of C-L services results in decreased length of stays (LOS)[7] and recidivism rates, outcomes especially critical in a capitated, managed care environment. Decreasing the LOS lowers overall hospital costs.[8] Moreover, a proactive C-L service identifies comorbid medical, psychiatric, and substance abuse problems that result in increased payments to the hospital under the Diagnosis-Related Groups (DRG) payment system by including previously overlooked complications and comorbid diagnoses.[8] For example, delirium is significantly underrecognized with a prevalence of approximately 10% of hospitalized patients. Alcoholism in the general hospital has been reported in 20% to 40% of hospitalized patients.[9] Identifying and treating comorbid delirium, substance abuse, and psychiatric problems have a salutary impact on patient outcome as well as on the financial health of the general hospital. There is some evidence that effective consultation reduces the use of other medical services as well.[8] This additional revenue is quite separate from the financial savings in staff time expended while managing aggressive, confused, uncooperative, or "undesirable" patients, the costs of security, the use of restraints, and secondary problems of injuries or infections (e.g., from catheters placed in agitated elderly patients, or pneumonias or aspirations secondary to patients being restrained in bed to control aggression and agitation).

From a public health perspective, the involvement of the C-L psychiatrist may lead to improved "disease management protocols," and "best practices," helping patients understand and cope with their diabetes; chronic pain; or gastrointestinal, respiratory, or cardiac disease. Enrolling patients in smoking cessation or weight control programs may initiate or support patient's general health and wellness. Consider that 25% to 40% of patients in the general hospital are being treated for ailments secondary to alcoholism and that the societal loses secondary to alcoholism may exceed $115 billion per year.[8,9] With effective interventions as part of the medical team, future medical utilization and cost may be reduced.[10,11]

The impact on "consumers of consultation," with a focus on medical providers, results in many of the less tangible or "nonspecific" outcomes of that consultation. These outcomes include dramatically increasing opportunities for training that result in a deeper and more substantial appreciation of the biopsychosocial perspective. The C-L psychiatrist's participation with the house staff in ethic rounds, end-of-life decisions, and collaborative cancer care management (or care of other feared illnesses) provides an understanding of the patient and facilitates patient satisfaction. Addressing the inner experience of the medically compromised psychiatric patient may also serve to reduce the stigma associated with mental illness.

Diligent attention to rules and regulations associated with billing and documentation can help improve patient care and help C-L services become financially viable.

References

1. Kunkel EJS, Worley LL, Monti DA, et al: Follow-up consultation billing and documentation, *Gen Hop Psychiatry* 21:197–208,1999.
2. American Psychiatric Association: *Practice guidelines for psychiatric evaluation of adults*, Arlington, VA., 1995, American Psychiatric Press.
3. Bronheim HE, Fulop G, Kunkel EJ, et al: The Academy of Psychosomatic Medicine practice guidelines for psychosomatic consultation in the general medical setting, *Psychosomatics* 39:S8–S30, 1998.
4. Worley LL, Kunkel EJS, Hilty DM: How C-L services can comply with new HCFA guidelines, *Gen Hosp Psychiatry* 20:160–169, 1998.
5. Anotnowicz J: Medicare revenue enhancement and consultation-liaison psychiatry, *Psychiatr Times*, 15(10): 1998.
6. Butler SF, Docherty JP: A comprehensive system for value accounting in psychiatry, *J Ment Health Adm*, 23(4):479–491, 1996.
7. Saravay SM, Lavin M: Psychiatric comorbidity and length of stay in the general hospital, *Psychosomatics* 35:233–252,1994.
8. Hall RCW, Rundell JR, Hirsch: Developing a financially viable consultation-liaison service, *Psychosomatics* 35: 308–318, 1994.
9. Schneekloth TD, Morse RM, Herrick LM, et al: Point prevalence of alcoholism in hospitalized patients: continuing challenges of detection, assessment, and diagnosis, *Mayo Clin Proc* 76:460–466, 2001.
10. Mumford E, Schlesinger HJ, Glass GV, et al: A new look at evidence about reduced cost of medical utilization following mental health treatment, *Am J Psychiatry* 10:1145–1148, 1984.
11. Saravay SM: Psychiatric interventions in the medically ill: outcome and effectiveness research, *Psychiatric Clin N Am* 19(3):467–480, 1996.

Chapter 46
Medical Psychiatry and Its Future

Paul Summergrad, M.D.
Scott L. Rauch, M.D.
Gregory L. Fricchione, M.D.

The formal introduction of psychiatric services into general hospitals in the 1930s and their subsequent growth have been among the most important institutional developments that have affected modern American psychiatric practice. Psychiatric units in general hospitals have proliferated since 1934, when 96% of psychiatric beds were under government control and generally found in state or veterans hospitals.[1–5] Consultation, outpatient, and emergency psychiatric services in general hospitals have grown dramatically during this period as well.[6–8] Including data on the admission of patients to general medical services for primary psychiatric illness, it has been estimated that general hospitals provide nearly 60% of all inpatient psychiatric care in the United States.[9–12]

Reviews of the growth in general hospital psychiatry have often attempted to define its proper role. Commentators about these issues have generally split into two groups. The social/reformist group has seen the development of general hospital psychiatry as a function of its social position. General hospital psychiatry emerged in this view because it was seen as the setting in which mental illness could be treated in a more open manner, replacing custodial state hospital care. The general hospital's proximity to family and community resources was perceived as a central therapeutic element in this clinical efficacy.[11–15] Psychiatric wards should be therapeutic communities, and psychiatric consultants should be standard-bearers for a biopsychosocial model of illness, who would educate physicians to this new style of medical practice.[16,17]

The medical group, especially Hackett,[6] emphasized the links to medicine as central to the identity and growth of general hospital psychiatry. These authors stressed the development of psychopharmacology and the need for consultation services for patients with serious medical illness.[18–20] Institutional expressions of this perspective include the development of medical/psychiatric units, psychiatric consultation services stressing the medical care of patients rather than the education of caregivers, and the growing use of neurobiologic discoveries in many areas of psychiatric practice.[21,22] The development of a sophisticated psychiatric pharmacopoeia, new insights into the molecular biology of psychiatric illness, and this handbook are a testimony to the correctness of this latter point of view.

This chapter reviews the forces that are currently affecting general hospital psychiatry and its major responses: medical/psychiatry units, consultation-liaison services, psychiatric neuroscience, and psychiatry within integrated medical delivery systems.

Forces Affecting General Hospital Psychiatry

Forces that contribute to change within contemporary general hospital psychiatry include intense economic pressures to reduce costs, restrictions on access to health care by insurers, new theoretical models within psychiatry, larger populations in need of psychiatric care, and privatization of public mental health care.

Controlling Health Care Costs

Attempts to control health care expenditures in the United States abound. Faced with budget deficits at home and fierce international industrial competition abroad, the pressures applied by government and industry to reduce these expenditures have been unrelenting.[23–25]

These pressures have led to significant changes in the way expenditures for health care services have been monitored and controlled. The growth of health maintenance organizations (HMOs) and prepaid health plans, including capitation and other forms of health care financing that shift risk to providers, are among mechanisms that attempt to reduce the duration of hospitalization and the cost of health care. The net effect of these changes has been to shorten hospital stays for all classes of medical and psychiatric patients and to increase the acuity of illness necessary to allow admission to the general hospital.[26,27]

The growth of carve-outs (the removal of contracts for psychiatric services from the rest of medical services so that they are independently bid on and separately managed) has been one of the most difficult developments affecting general hospital psychiatry. These carve-out arrangements are particularly pernicious for medical psychiatry, placing newer and more competitive pressures on services and limiting the quality of care. In this model psychiatry is divorced from primary care. Patients are unable to be cared for by psychiatrists who in the past were well-known colleagues of primary care physicians (PCPs). Additionally, carve-out models falsely assume that the medical and psychiatric needs of patients are distinct (both clinically and fiscally)—often to the detriment of patient care.

New Treatments and New Technologies

The development of new treatments and technologies has some roots in the development of effective psychopharmacologic agents in the mid 1950s.[7] Medica-

tions previously used in other areas of medicine have been used to treat psychiatric illness. Psychopharmacologic evaluation and treatment are often a focus of psychiatric hospitalization, especially for patients not safely treated outside of the hospital.

The efficacy of these new agents has also increased the emphasis on accurate diagnosis in psychiatry. Semistructured diagnostic interviews and rating scales have targeted observable elements in psychiatric illness.[28] Newer neuroimaging techniques, such as magnetic resonance imaging (MRI) or positron emission tomography (PET) scanning, have revealed evidence of previously unsuspected abnormalities, such as enlarged lateral ventricles in patients with schizophrenia or abnormal white matter in elderly patients with affective illness.[29] Studies using these technologies have begun to define fundamental neurobiologic abnormalities underlying major psychiatric disorders. The combined effect of these changes is to make psychiatric care even more focused on neuromedical diagnostic evaluation, on medical care, and on psychopharmacologic management.

New Populations in Psychiatric Treatment

Changing populations have also affected the focus and organization of general hospital psychiatric care. This happened, in part, due to the willingness of general hospital psychiatrists to care for a broader range of patients: elderly patients, demented patients, patients with concomitant medical and psychiatric illness, and patients with other neurobehavioral disorders. Psychiatrists are now established caregivers in intensive care and critical care settings.

New patient populations, including patients with drug-induced illness and those with human immunodeficiency virus (HIV)-related illness, have emerged that have required psychiatric care. Acquired immune deficiency syndrome (AIDS) has now been recognized to have significant psychological, psychiatric, and neuropsychiatric sequelae. The capacities of the medical/psychiatric unit are an important resource for the response to the HIV epidemic.[30–33]

At the same time, new medical technologies, while sometimes life-saving, have in some instances put individuals at risk for psychiatric morbidity. For example, undergoing cardiac electrophysiologic studies, having an automatic implanted cardiac defibrillator (AICD) implanted, and then having it discharge appears to lower the threshold for panic/phobic anxiety and for posttraumatic stress disorder (PTSD).[34]

Changing Relationship with State Hospital Systems

Another factor that has affected the use and demographics of general hospital inpatient services has been the attempt to increase the admission of patients previously cared for in state hospital systems.[35–38]

Medical/Psychiatric Units

The development of medical/psychiatric units has represented the most important conceptual shift in general hospital inpatient psychiatric care during the past decade.[39–50]

The development of the medical/psychiatric concept has been, in some measure, a response to the limitations of the therapeutic milieu model. The medical/psychiatric unit established the appropriate medical role of the attending physician. Where traditional units required attendance at group meetings as a condition for admission, patients on medical/psychiatric units might be so ill (e.g., with catatonia, feeding tubes, central lines, or severely psychotic behavior) that they may not be able to leave their bed, let alone their room. Patients with severe medical/psychiatric illness, excluded from traditional general hospital units, became the *raison d'être* of medical/psychiatric units. Such populations require traditional medical rounds, physical examinations, and the use of active treatments (such as psychopharmacologic agents). The role of the general hospital psychiatric unit, as it transitioned into a medical/psychiatric unit, became more medically traditional. Patients needed to receive an active medical intervention to get well. Community activities were relatively deemphasized, and a normative medical hierarchy was approximated.[39,40,47,48]

Models

Kathol and others[51–54] have described a typology of medical/psychiatric units that has been useful in defining levels of medical/psychiatric acuity and the physical and staff organization to manage such services appropriately. Kathol defined four types of medical psychiatry units; Type I and II units are traditional psychiatric units without medical capacity and standard medical units, while Types III and IV units are medical/psychiatry units proper. They differ predominately in the severity of medical illness that they can care for. Both Types III and IV units can care for patients needing intravenous fluids or medications, blood products, hemodialysis, peritoneal dialysis, or the care of other acute medical conditions. Type IV units are usually staffed by both internists and psychiatrists. These units can care for patients with high medical acuity (up to, but not including, patients who might require intensive care unit admission). Patients on such units may include those with significant congestive heart failure and comorbid depression, delirium while undergoing chemotherapy, or peritransplantation issues.

All medical/psychiatry units require cross-training of nursing and medical staff to allow for the provision of high-quality care for patients with comorbid acute medical and psychiatric illness. Psychiatrists on such units need to be able to provide general medical care and to collaborate with medical consultants. This conjoint care should include in-house internists for medical emergencies and possibly hired internal medicine consultants. Some units have handled this by hiring directors who are double-boarded in psychiatry and either internal medicine or neurology.

In an environment that tends to carve out psychiatric care from medical care, close attention needs to be paid to define how medical/psychiatry units are reimbursed. To the extent that such units can shorten the overall length of stay for patients with combined medical and psychiatric illness, they may be fiscally advantageous, especially in a capitated environment.

As medical/psychiatry services become more oriented to acute symptomatic care, a variety of outpatient, partial hospital, and holding facilities are being created both to decrease the need for hospitalization and to provide for the longer-term psychological, social, and medical rehabilitation of psychiatric patients. It is clear that medical/psychiatric units need to be closely integrated with such outpatient and partial hospital facilities to allow medical/psychiatry units to be used for patients in need of acute care; moreover, this will facilitate shorter admissions and successful operation within integrated delivery systems.

Consultation-Liaison Psychiatry

Kornfeld[55] recently wrote an elegant review on the impact of consultation-liaison (C-L) psychiatry on medical care in general hospitals. He surveyed, among others, the major contributions of Hackett and Cassem, and Frasure-Smith and Reich in psychocardiology; his own team in helping to understand why some patients want to sign out against medical advice; Sutherland, Holland, Oken, and Spiegel in psychooncology; Abrams, Denour, Levy, and Viederman in psychonephrology; Robinson in poststroke syndromes; Perry in HIV care; and Musselman on the relationship between interferon and depression. He then recounted the effects of C-L psychiatry on cost-benefit analyses, medical teaching, clinical ethics, end-of-life care, and clinical genetics. He concluded that psycho- somatic medicine through C-L psychiatry has substantially influenced medical practice for the better, and he predicted that the field will flourish especially, ironically, as medicine becomes increasingly technologic.

Here at MGH, advances in the psychopharmacology of medical psychiatry patients are worth noting. The use of intravenous haloperidol for agitated delirium, the use of methylphenidate for depression in medically ill patients, and the first-line use of intravenous lorazepam for catatonic states were pioneered and then advocated by MGH consulting psychiatrists; these have become part of standard medical practice.[56–58]

Alert and well-trained consulting psychiatrists will continue to make key contributions to our understanding of pathophysiology and therapeutics. More and more will be learned from clinical experience and from research about how the visceral paralimbic and limbic brain influences human disease processes, and vice versa. Take the so-called "functional gastrointestinal disorders," for example. Up to 50% of all patients who present with gastrointestinal (GI) complaints have such a disorder with no known pathophysiologic basis for their complaints or have complaints that are out of proportion to their physiologic abnormalities.[59] In the future, the intricate interrelationship between the intrinsic enteric nervous system of the gut and the extrinsic peripheral and central nervous systems will be better understood, thereby improving our ability to manage these painful and costly disorders. Consulting psychiatrists have the skill set and knowledge of both the brain and the body to make major contributions in this effort.

Outpatient Consultation-Liaison Psychiatry

As general hospitals shorten medical admissions and shift more care to observation, nonacute settings, and ambulatory settings, traditional inpatient C-L activities will need to shift as well. In many cases, this will require the location of these services within PCP groups.

Approximately 6% of all patients receive psychiatric services within the general medical sector. Additionally, other patients who present for medical care have undiagnosed or undertreated psychiatric or substance abuse disorders. In situations in which PCPs are financially at risk for all medical services, the ability of outpatient C-L psychiatrists to offset unneeded medical utilization will be important in reducing the cost of care and improving outcome.

The co-location of psychiatrists who are able to provide immediate consultation to PCPs in a variety of non–in-patient settings, while caring for patients in the specialty care sector, will be important for the further development of medical psychiatry. Medical psychiatrists are also performing teleconsultations and using computer-based systems to provide immediate consultations to a larger network of PCPs and their patients at risk. Such teleconsultation services allow PCPs to consult with psychiatrists in real-time, while their patients are still in their office.

Psychiatric Neuroscience

Looking forward to the future of psychiatry, in the best tradition of the medical model, pathophysiology-based diagnostic entities will be ascertained through history and examination, as well as more direct tests of brain structure and function (e.g., neuroimaging tests) and by probes of genotype. Thus, the diagnostic process and classification system in psychiatry will inevitably evolve in tandem, incorporating contemporary advances in psychiatric neuroscience.[60]

The emergence of contemporary neuroimaging techniques has provided a new class of information, allowing for characterization of regional brain activity or chemistry in time and in three dimensions of space.[61] Investigators have quickly come to realize that psychiatric diseases will not simply be reducible to a three-dimensional map of generic regional brain dysfunction. Rather, neuroimaging will help to characterize pathophysiology in terms of dysfunctional distributed networks and provide for multidimensional assessments of computational deficits at any given locus.

Psychiatric neuroscience in the twenty-first century will continue to rely heavily on neurotransmitter pharmacology, as well as on the newly found power of neuroimaging methods, to establish phenotypes at the level of the brain. However, there will be a progressive focus on molecular biology, which is necessary to understand the genetic bases of selected vulnerabilities as well as the presynaptic and postsynaptic and second messenger processes that mediate neural dysfunction.

Implications for Psychiatric Treatment in the General Hospital

Developing valid and reliable predictors of treatment response will enhance treatment efficacy. If such predictors can be gleaned from easily accessible clinical information (e.g., age, gender, and constellation of symptoms), this would be most cost effective. However, it may be that the most powerful predictors of treatment response will be ascertained via more fine-grained probes of brain function, such as those obtained via neuroimaging. Already, brain imaging studies have produced preliminary findings that suggest that particular brain activity profiles predict antidepressant and antiobsessional responses to medication.[62,63] Such predictors of treatment response will be most important in the context of candidate treatments that are of long duration, high cost, or great risk (e.g., antiobses-

sional medication trials, electroconvulsive therapy [ECT], or neurosurgical treatment).[64] Here it should also be emphasized that reliable predictors of bad outcomes can be just as valuable as reliable predictors of treatment success.

New Concepts in Somatic Therapies

As we discover the core pathophysiology of particular diseases, optimal therapies might include a capacity to direct medications to specific cell types or brain regions. It is difficult to know whether or not transplantation methods will evolve into useful interventions for psychiatric conditions. To date, this strategy has been adopted as a means to compensate for gross degeneration, such as in the neurologic condition Parkinson's disease.[65]

Advances in psychiatric neurosurgical treatments have accelerated over the past decade. Vastly different from the crude freehand lobotomies of the mid twentieth century, much refined stereotactic procedures have emerged in the last 25 years, culminating in noninvasive ablative radiosurgical applications using the gamma knife.[66,67] Most recently, deep brain stimulation (DBS) methods have been adapted for use in psychiatric conditions. Paralleling advances in surgical treatment for Parkinson's disease, DBS promises the potential for adjustable and reversible means of modulating brain function and hence ameliorating psychiatric symptoms.[68]

Over the next decade, the early promise of transcranial magnetic stimulation (TMS) as an alternative to ECT will be rigorously tested.[69] While it is appealing to propose that localized brain stimulation could provide advantages in terms of efficacy and adverse effects, this remains an empirical matter. Certainly, advances in our understanding of pathophysiology will help guide the study of this potential treatment modality.

Building Integrated Delivery Systems

Managed care organizations (MCOs) are able to lower costs in part by controlling where the large number of patients they insure will receive care. In an environment in which the supply of hospital services (e.g., inpatient beds) is high and the demand for services is dropping (as in managed care), prices for care (e.g., hospital per diems) decline. In response to this concentration of buying power by payers, providers have formed integrated delivery systems.

The growth of such integrated delivery systems allows for the creation of a balance between the payers and providers. Also, integrated delivery systems allow the management of care to be returned to providers. Many integrated delivery systems organize around PCP groups or physician hospital organizations. Such integrated delivery systems often place PCPs at financial risk (in a gatekeeper role) and discourage excessive care by specialists and hospitals.

How does medical psychiatry fare within these integrated delivery systems? In large measure, it depends on the available conditions in given localities. In some areas, separate psychiatric or behavioral health integrated delivery systems may be strong. If these are also areas where carve-out models of care are also prominent among payers, the task facing medical psychiatrists may be more complex and difficult. Psychiatrists in these circumstances may need to fight a two-front war— building relationships with primary care, while competing for carve-out contracts and internally reintegrating care. Given that a significant percentage of all primary care visits are psychiatric in nature, psychiatrists need to be actively involved in the creation of integrated delivery systems and in the education of payers, PCPs, and others about the suboptimal nature of disaggregated care.

Medical Psychiatry in a Managed Environment

Medical psychiatrists have to struggle with a variety of tensions regarding how to provide effective care in the context of managed care.

Length of Stay

Medical/psychiatry units are under intense pressure to reduce hospital length of stay. Frequently, clinicians must explain to cost-conscious reviewers why their patients who have recently been suicidal require continued hospitalization or why

their elderly patients cannot safely receive the rest of their ECT on an ambulatory basis. MCOs, operating within a carve-out model (and thus eager to shift costs) may ask why they should pay for the care of a patient with poststroke depression. When conflicts arise with reviewers, physicians should request a formal review by a physician who is board-certified in psychiatry. Such physicians often have greater latitude in allowing extended stays for patients with complex medical/psychiatric illness. In other situations, patients may fall under a catastrophic case definition, which may allow for greater flexibility of care.

National managed care benchmarks for average length of stay or for days of inpatient care per 1000 covered members may reflect distinctly different psychiatric populations. It is important for clinical and administrative leadership in general hospitals to be aware of this population variability before agreeing to contract benchmarks or payments that may compromise patient care.

The efficacy of a medical-psychiatry service that operates in a carve-out environment requires careful education of payers, administrators, clinical leadership, and the general physician community. Because psychiatric illness is common in the primary care setting and because effective care requires the availability of psychiatric services, the lower cost of a mental health carve-out may be both short-lived and illusory— especially in a capitated environment. Unless these groups are aware of the impact of carve-out models, they will not be able to prevent the exclusion of psychiatrists from contracts or the erosion of clinical standards. Many patients cared for on medical/psychiatry units are elderly or disabled; these groups are covered by the Medicare insurance system. The impact of the legislatively mandated shift from a cost-based to a prospective payment system for inpatient psychiatry has yet to be determined.

Summary and Conclusions

As we face the future, we can anticipate continuing pressures on general hospital services that will require local and national responses. It is unlikely that pressures to decrease length of stay, to admit sicker patients, or to respond to the competition inherent in managed care will diminish. In some locations, general hospitals may be asked to assume more responsibilities for state hospital care. It is likely that overall economic pressures will require a coherent system of care that may, with local variations, include private psychiatric hospitals, state hospitals, and outpatient and partial hospital functions as well as integration with the general medical care system. General hospital in-patient services may have to offer involuntary locked care or other specialized psychiatric units and emphasize attending physician involvement and daily walk-rounds. Developments in the neurosciences are likely to enhance the role of medical/psychiatry physician leadership.

The decision about how much general hospital psychiatric services should specialize will be affected by the range of psychiatric and medical services available in a particular area. Affiliation agreements between private and general hospital units, as well as the types of general hospital units in a community, will also affect these decisions. As pressures intensify from large managed care contracts to provide extensive integrated systems of care, general hospital psychiatric services may be forced to provide specialty medical/psychiatric or psychiatric services for more severely ill populations. Such networking arrangements may create fiscal risks for the care of patients with combined medical and psychiatric illness as these individuals may not be easily discharged into available aftercare resources. When constructing integrated systems, we need to attend to the continuity of care and minimize the number of transitions between providers.

The concept of the general hospital developed in the nineteenth and early twentieth centuries in response to advances in medical science, urbanization, and economic forces that surrounded the practice of medicine.[70] It was not until the early 1930s that a similar movement in psychiatry began, bringing psychiatry into the general hospital. Beginning in the 1930s,[71] general hospital psychiatry was poised for the rapid growth of the postwar years that was to make it the dominant institution in American psychiatry.

The entry of psychiatry into the general hospital meant more than a change of locale. It meant a shift from a "moral" to a medical model of psychiatric illness. It was a shift from methods of investigation and treatment that ran counter to the ethos of the general hospital and academic medicine to methods that were consonant with it. Psychiatry's entry into the general hospital brought it closer to the thinking of medicine, which was transforming illness into a treatable and comprehensible phenomenon.

The period that lies ahead will provide great opportunities for general hospital psychiatry in training, models of clinical care, and medical/psychiatric treatment and research. Advances in neurobiology and psychopharmacology, as well as the broadening clinical population of general hospital psychiatry, will make it the setting in which the most sophisticated and comprehensive psychiatric care can and should take place. In this era of growing efficacy and research, attention to these opportunities and to the pressures outlined herein is crucial for the further development and viability of medical/psychiatry, of general hospital psychiatry, and of psychiatry as a whole.

References

1. Summergrad P, Hackett TP: Alan Gregg and the rise of general hospital psychiatry, *Gen Hosp Psychiatry* 9:439–445, 1987.
2. Summergrad P: General hospital inpatient psychiatry in the 1990's: problems and possibilities, *Gen Hosp Psychiatry* 13:79–82, 1991.
3. Summergrad P: Medical/psychiatry units and the roles of the inpatient psychiatric service in the general hospital, *Gen Hosp Psychiatry* 16:20–31, 1994.
4. Bryan WA: Relationship of psychiatry to medicine, *N Engl J Med* 205:195–198, 1931.
5. Taube CA, Barren SA, editors: *Mental health, United States, 1983*, Rockville, Md., 1983, DHSS Publication Number (Adm) 83–1275, National Institute of Mental Health.
6. Hackett TP: The psychiatrist: in the mainstream or on the banks of medicine, *Am J Psychiatry* 134:432–434, 1977.
7. Klerman GL: *The psychiatric revolution of the past twenty-five years*. In Gove WR, editor: *Deviance and mental illness*, Beverly Hills, 1982, Sage.
8. Bassuk EL: The impact of deinstitutionalization on the general hospital psychiatric emergency ward, *Hosp Com Psychiatry* 31:623–627, 1980.
9. Kiesler CA, Sibulkin AE: Episodic rate of mental hospitalization: stable or increasing, *Am J Psychiatry* 141:44–48, 1984.
10. Schulberg HC, Burns BJ: The nature and effectiveness of general hospital psychiatric services, *Gen Hosp Psychiatry* 7:249–257, 1985.

11. Bachrach LL: General hospital psychiatry: overview from a sociological perspective, *Am J Psychiatry* 138:879–887, 1981.

12. Lipsitt DR: Psychiatry and the general hospital: an editorial, *Gen Hosp Psychiatry* 1:1–2, 1979.

13. Greenhill MH: Psychiatric units in general hospitals: 1979, *Hosp Com Psychiatry* 30:169–182, 1979.

14. Flamm GH: The expanding roles of general hospital psychiatry, *Hosp Com Psychiatry* 30:190–192, 1979.

15. Schulberg HC: Psychiatric units in general hospitals: bone or band? *Am J Psychiatry* 120:30–35, 1963.

16. Leeman CP, Autio S: Milieu therapy: the need for individualization, *Psychother Psychosom* 29:84–92, 1978.

17. Vistosky HM, Plaut EA: Psychiatry in the general hospital: visualizing the changes, *Hosp Com Psychiatry* 33:739–741, 1982.

18. Lebensohn ZM: General hospital psychiatry U.S.A.: retrospect and prospect, *Comp Psychiatry* 21:500–509, 1980.

19. Sanders CA: Reflections on psychiatry in the general hospital setting, *Hosp Com Psychiatry* 30:185–189, 1979.

20. Jones RE: Issues facing general hospital psychiatry, *Hosp Com Psychiatry* 30:183–184,1979.

21. Herz MI: Short term hospitalization and the medical model, *Hosp Com Psychiatry* 30:117–121,1979.

22. Cooper AM: Will neurobiology influence psychoanalysis? *Am J Psychiatry* 14:1395–1402, 1985.

23. Sederer LI, St. Clair RL: Managed health care and the Massachusetts experience, *Am J Psychiatry* 146:1142–1148, 1989.

24. Sederer LI: Utilization review and quality assurance: staying in the black and working with the blues, *Gen Hosp Psychiatry* 9:210–219, 1987.

25. Editorial: The states of the Union, *New Republic* 3919:7–9, 1990.

26. Billig N, Leibenluft E: Special considerations in integrating elderly patients into a general hospital unit, *Hosp Commun Psychiatry* 38:277–281, 1987.

27. Schoonover SC, Bassuk EL: Deinstitutionalization and the private general hospital inpatient unit. Implications for clinical care, *Hosp Commun Psychiatry* 34:135–139, 1983.

28. Perry S, Cooper AM, Michels R: The psychodynamic formulation: its purpose, structure and clinical application, *Am J Psychiatry* 144:543–550, 1987.

29. Summergrad P, Peterson B: Binswangers disease: the clinical recognition of subcortical arteriosclerotic encephalopathy in elderly neuropsychiatric patients, *J Ger Psychiatry Neurol* 2:123–133, 1989.

30. Gottlieb MS, Schroff R, Shanker HM, et al: *Pneumocystis carinii* pneumonia and mucosal candidiasis in previously healthy homosexual men: evidence of a new acquired cellular immunodeficiency, *N Engl J Med* 305:1425–1431, 1981.

31. Navia BA, Price RW: The acquired immunodeficiency syndrome dementia complex as the presenting or sole manifestation of human immunodeficiency virus infection, *Arch Neural* 44:65–69, 1987.

32. Beckett A, Summergrad P, Manschreck T, et al: Symptomatic HIV infection of the central nervous system in a patient without evidence of immune deficiency, *Am J Psychiatry* 144:1342–1344, 1987.

33. Summergrad P, Glassman RS: *Human immunodeficiency virus and other infections affecting the central nervous system*. In Stoudemire A, Fogel B, editors: *Medical-psychiatric practice*, Washington, DC, 1991, American Psychiatric Press.

34. Fricchione GL, Vlay SC: *Neuropsychiatric aspects of arrhythmia evaluation and management*. In Vlay SC, editor: *Manual of cardiac arrhythmias: a practical guide to clinical management*, vol 2, Boston, 1996, Little, Brown and Company, 438–450.

35. Klerman GL: National trends in hospitalization, *Hosp Commun Psychiatry* 30:110–113,1979.

36. Bachrach LL: The effects of deinstitutionalization on general hospital psychiatry, *Hosp Commun Psychiatry* 32:786–790, 1981.

37. Goldman HH, Adams NH, Taube CA: Deinstitutionalization: the data demythologized, *Hosp Commun Psychiatry* 34:124–134, 1983.

38. Thompson JW, Burns BJ, Taube CA: The severely mentally ill in general hospital psychiatric units, *Gen Hosp Psychiatry* 10:1–9, 1988.

39. Stoudemire A, Fogel BS: Organization and development of combined medical-psychiatric units: II. *Psychosomatics* 27:341–345, 1986.

40. Fogel BS: A psychiatric unit becomes a psychiatric medical unit: administrative and clinical implications, *Gen Hosp Psychiatry* 7:26–35, 1985.

41. Stoudemire A, Trig Brown J, McLeod M, et al: The combined medical specialties unit: an innovative approach to patient care, *N C Med J* 44:365–367, 1983.

42. Burke GF: Caring for the medically ill psychiatric patient on a psychiatric unit, *Psychiatry Ann* 13:627–634, 1983.

43. Molnar G, Fava GA, Zielezny MA: Medical-psychiatric unit patients compared with patients in two other services, *Psychosomatics* 26:193–209, 1985.

44. Koran LM: Medical-psychiatric units and the future of psychiatric practice, *Psychosomatics* 26:171–175, 1985.

45. Goodman B: Combined psychiatric-medical inpatients: the Mount Sinai model, *Psychosomatics* 26:179–189, 1985.

46. Young LD, Harsch HH: Inpatient unit for combined physical and psychiatric disorders, *Psychosomatics* 27:53–57, 1986.

47. Fogel B, Stoudemire A: Organization and development of combined medical-psychiatric units: II. *Psychosomatics* 27:417–428, 1986.

48. Fogel D, Stoudemire A, Houpt TL: Contrasting models for combined medical and psychiatric inpatient treatment, *Am J Psychiatry* 142:1085–1089, 1985.

49. Fogel BS: Med-psych units financial viability and quality assurance, *Gen Hosp Psychiatry* 11:17–22,1989.

50. Hoffman RS: Operation of a medical-psychiatric unit in a general hospital setting, *Gen Hosp Psychiatry* 6:93–99, 1984.
51. Kathol RG, Harsch HH, Hall RCW, et al: Categorization of types of medical/psychiatry units based on level of acuity, *Psychosomatics* 33:376–386, 1992.
52. Hall RCW, Kathol RG: Developing a level III/IV medical/psychiatry unit: establishing a basis, design of the unit and physician responsibility, *Psychosomatics* 33:368–375, 1992.
53. Kathol RG, Harsch HH, Hall RCW, et al: Quality assurance in a setting designed to care for patients with combined medical and psychiatric disease, *Psychosomatics* 33:387–396, 1992.
54. Fogel BS, Summergrad P: *Evolution of the medical/psychiatric unit in the general hospital.* In Judd FK, Burrows GD, Lipsitt DR, editors: *Handbook of studies on general hospital psychiatry*, Amsterdam, 1991, Elsevier Science.
55. Kornfeld, DS: Consultation-liaison psychiatry: contributions to medical practice, *Am J Psychiatry* 159: 1964–1972, 2002.
56. Sos J, Cassem NH: *The intravenous use of haloperidol for acute delirium in intensive care settings.* In Speidel H, Rodewald G, editors: *Psychic and neurological dysfunctions after open heart surgery*, Stuttgart, 1980, George Thieme Verlag.
57. Kaufmann MW, Cassem N, Murray G, et al: The use of methylphenidate in depressed patients after cardiac surgery, *J Clin Psychiatry* 45:82–84, 1984.
58. Fricchione GL, Cassem NH, Hooberman D, et al: Intravenous lorazepam in neuroleptic induced catatonia, *J Clin Psychopharmacology* 3:338–342, 1983.
59. Ringel Y, Drossman DA: From gut to brain and back: a new perspective into functional gastrointestinal disorders, *J Psychosomatic Res* 47:205–210, 1999.
60. Rauch SL: *Preparing for psychiatry in the 21st century.* In Stern TA, Herman JB, editors: *Massachusetts General Hospital Psychiatry Update & Board preparation, ed 2*, New York, 2004, McGraw-Hill, 581-585.
61. Dougherty DD, Rauch SL, editors. *Psychiatric neuroimaging research: contemporary strategies*, Washington, DC, 2001, American Psychiatric Publishing.
62. Mayberg HS, Brannan SK, Mahurin RK, et al: Cingulate function in depression: a potential predictor of treatment response, *Neuroreport* 8:1057–1061, 1997.
63. Rauch SL, Shin LM, Dougherty DD, et al: Predictors of fluvoxamine response in contamination-related obsessive compulsive disorder: a PET symptom provocation study, *Neuropsychopharmacol* 27:782–791, 2002.
64. Rauch SL, Dougherty DD, Cosgrove GR, et al: Cerebral metabolic correlates as potential predictors of response to anterior cingulotomy for obsessive compulsive disorder, *Biol Psychiatry* 50:659–667, 2001.
65. Redmond DE Jr: Cellular replacement therapy for Parkinson's disease: where we are today?, *Neuroscientist* 8(5):457–88, 2002
66. Greenberg BD, Price LH, Rauch SL, et al: Neurosurgery for intractable obsessive-compulsive disorder and depression: critical issues, *Neurosurg Clin North Am* 14:199–212, 2003.
67. Rauch SL, Greenberg BD, Cosgrove GR: *Neurosurgical treatments and deep brain stimulation.* In Sadock BJ, Sadock V, editors: *Comprehensive textbook of psychiatry, ed 8*, Baltimore, Lippincott, Williams & Wilkins (in press).
68. Nuttin B, Cosyns P, Demeulemeester H, et al: Electrical stimulation in anterior limbs of internal capsules in patients with obsessive-compulsive disorder, *Lancet* 354:1526, 1999.
69. George MS, Belmaker R, editors: *Transcranial magnetic stimulation in neuropsychiatry*, Washington, DC, 2000, American Psychiatric Press.
70. Starr P: *The social transformation of American medicine*, New York, 1982, Basic Books.
71. Goldman HH: Integrating health and mental health services: historical obstacles and opportunities, *Am J Psychiatry* 139:616–620, 1982.

Index